HEALTH FOOD INGREDIENTS AND SCIENTIFIC NAMES

Food and Drug classification in Japan

学名でひく食薬区分リスト

健康食品・医薬品に区分される成分

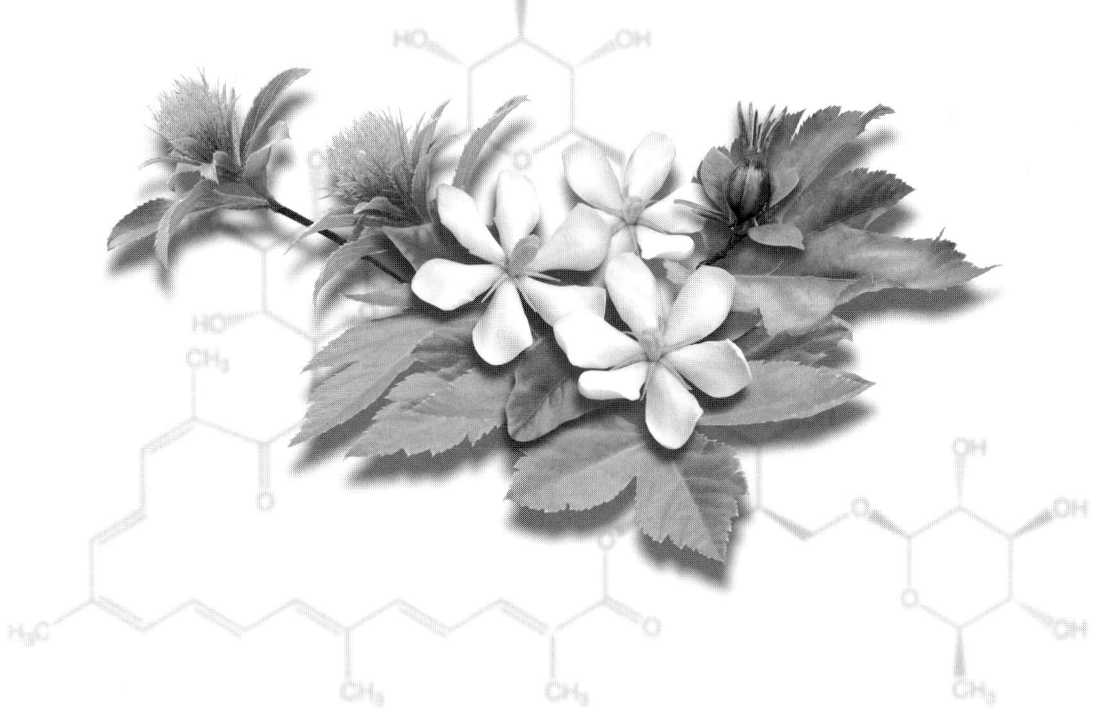

佐竹元吉［監修］

Edited by Motoyoshi Satake

関田節子／大濱宏文／池田秀子［著］

Setsuko Sekita / Hirobumi Ohama / Hideko Ikeda [Authors]

一般財団法人医療経済研究・社会保険福祉協会
「健康食品の安全性および品質管理のための研究会」

Association for Health Economics Research and Social Insurance and Welfare (ASIW)
"Research on Quality and Safety of Health Foods"

薬事日報社 Yakuji Nippo Ltd.

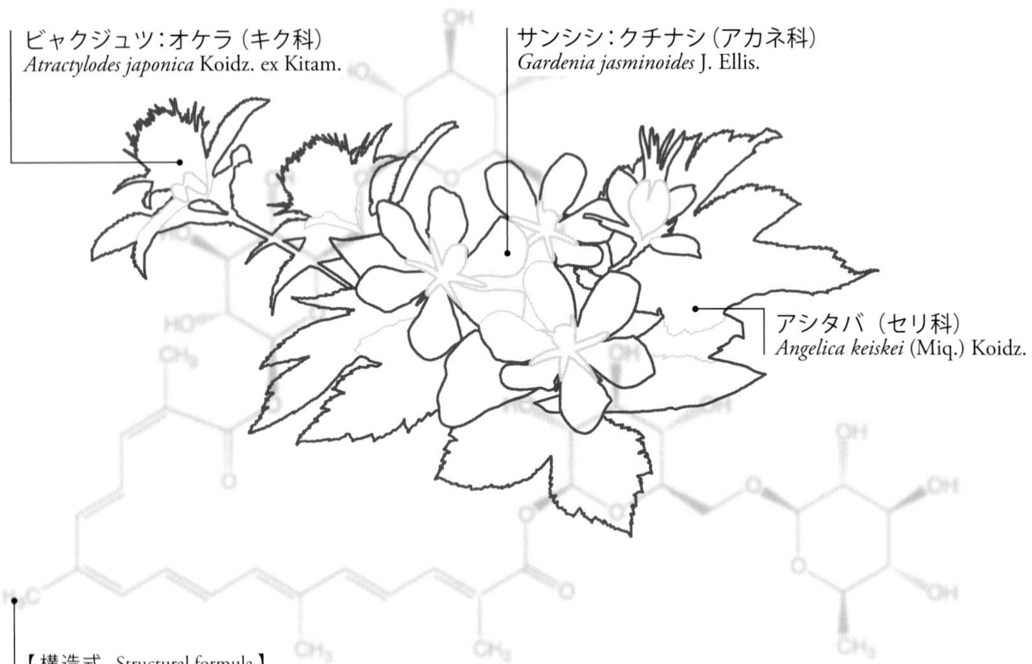

【構造式 Structural formula】
クチナシの色素成分 (Pigment of *Gardenia jasminoides* J. Ellis)，クロシン (crocin)

HEALTH FOOD INGREDIENTS AND SCIENTIFIC NAMES

Food and Drug classification in Japan

Association for Health Economics Research and Social Insurance and Welfare (ASIW)
"Research on Quality and Safety of Health Foods"

序　　文

1971年、薬事法に基づく食薬区分に関する通知「無承認無許可医薬品の指導取締りについて」（昭和46年６月１日、薬発第476号）が出された。これが通称46通知として知られる最初の食薬区分であり、行政の手の届かないところで医薬品と誤認させる効能効果を標榜した品質の保証のない製品が、健康食品と称して流通し出したことに対応するものであった。この通知により、医薬品として認可されていないものに対する効能効果の表示は激減した。

一方、食品の第三次機能が注目されるようになり、健康食品分野の企業は、食薬区分における「専ら医薬品として使用される成分本質（原材料）」に該当しない素材を対象に、食品に新たな機能性を見出す研究を活発化させてきた。また海外では、1994年にアメリカでダイエタリーサプリメント健康教育法が施行され、日本に向けた輸出も検討されるようになった際、日本の食薬区分が貿易障壁であるとされ、規制緩和の名目で開放の要求がなされた。

その結果、ビタミン、ミネラル、ハーブの食品成分への追加及び錠剤、カプセル状等の剤形規制の緩和等が行われた。また、それまでの46通知における食薬区分リストが６分類と煩雑であったため、今日の２分類の形式に改定されて、より判断しやすいものとなった。これらの対応もあり、食薬区分の改正は、2013年７月10日薬食発0710第２号に至るまでに13回行われた。

アメリカのダイエタリーサプリメントを嚆矢として、サプリメントが急速に世界的に流通し出すと共に、健康被害情報も各国から伝えられるようになった。わが国でも、2002年にダイエットを目的とする健康食品による死亡例が発生し、2003年に創設された食品安全委員会においても、健康食品の安全性について一部検討されることとなった。しかし、市場に流通する多くの健康食品の安全性は、未だ十分に担保されていない。

健康食品が国民の健康の維持・増進に資するものとなるためには、使用される素材が明らかにされ、その機能性と安全性が十分に確保されることが、極めて重要である。本書は、学名による素材の特定を容易にするための、46通知が公表されて以来、初めての本格的な取り組みとなるものであり、諸外国の方々の利用にも資するものとなっている。健康食品の科学的な安全性の検討に、本書が多大な貢献をするものであることを確信しており、多くの方の利用を期待している。

なお、生物多様性条約（Convention on Biological Diversity: CBD）が、日本を含む多くの国で締結されている。CBDには「遺伝資源の取得の機会及びその利用から生ずる利益の公正かつ衡平な配分（ABS：Access and Benefit-Sharing）」が含まれている。本書には、原材料として多くの生物資源が記載されている。
これらのものをCBD締結国から輸入する場合は、ABSに十分注意しなければならない。

Preface

The notification on food and drug classification based on the Pharmaceutical Affairs Act (PAA). entitled "Regulatory control of unapproved/unpermitted drugs" (PAB Notification No. 476, 1 June 1971). was issued in 1971. This first food and drug classification, popularly known as Notification 46, dealt with products of no guaranteed quality that could be mistaken for drugs because of efficacy claims but which the authorities could not regulate as they were being distributed as so-called health foods. Notification 46 resulted in a dramatic decrease in labeling that claimed efficacy of substances not permitted as drugs.

At the same time, the tertiary functions of foods began to draw attention, and companies in the health food sector became increasingly involved in research to give foods new functions, targeting ingredients not classified as "ingredients (raw materials) used exclusively for drugs" in the food and drug classification. Overseas, the Dietary Supplement Health and Education Act was enacted in the US in 1994 and exports to Japan came under consideration. The US requested that Japan ease its regulations concerning food and drug classification in the name of deregulation, on the grounds that they acted as a trade barrier.

The MHLW responded by adding vitamins, herbs, and minerals to food ingredients and easing the regulations on tablets, capsules, and other dosage forms. The food and drug classification in Notification 46 was complex, including six different categories, so it has been revised to two categories to make assessments easier. Partly because of these changes, the food and drug classification has been amended 13 times until the latest PFSB Notification 0710 No. 2 issued on 10 July 2013.

The US regulatory changes on dietary supplements resulted in supplements spreading rapidly around the world. Information on their side effects began to be reported from various countries as well. In Japan, the use of weight-loss supplements resulted in deaths in 2002. The Food Safety Commission was founded in 2003 and gave some consideration to the safety of health foods. However, many health foods on the market are still not properly guaranteed as safe.

If health foods are to contribute to maintaining and improving the health of the public, it is of vital importance that the ingredients used are clearly labeled and systems are in place to ensure their functionality and safety. This publication is the first real attempt since the issue of Notification 46 to provide an easy way to access information on specific ingredients using scientific nomenclature. I hope that it will also provide a useful resource for other countries. I am confident that this publication will make an enormous contribution to scientific studies of the safety of health foods and hope that it is widely used.

In addition, the Convention on Biological Diversity (CBD) has been concluded by many courtiers including Japan. "Access to genetic resources and the fair and equitable sharing of benefits arising from their Utilization" which is known as Access and Benefit-Sharing (ABS) is included in the CBD. A number of biological resources as ingredients (raw materials) are listed up in this book. For importing these resources from the CBD parties, very careful approach and treatment must be taken in consideration of the ABS.

最後に、本書は健康食品の安全性及び品質確保のための研究会（Research on Quality and Safety of Health Foods, RQSHF）の研究成果の一環として出版するものである。RQSHFは2011年（平成23年）10月5日に一般財団法人医療経済研究・社会保険福祉協会（社福協）の研究プロジェクトとして発足した。以来、RQSHFは研究活動を続けてきたが、本研究の推進にあたり、当初より多大な支援を頂いている社福協に深甚なる謝意を表したい。

2014年9月

健康食品の安全性及び品質確保のための研究会（RQSHF）
代表　佐竹元吉

Finally, this publication is being published as part of the research output of the Research on Quality and Safety of Health Foods (RQSHF). an ongoing research project initiated on October 5, 2011 by the Association for Health Economics Research and Social Insurance and Welfare (ASIW). I would like to close this preface by expressing my particular gratitude to the ASIW for its tremendous support for this project right from its inception.

September 2014

Motoyoshi Satake
Lead Researcher
Research on Quality and Safety of Health Foods (RQSHF)

刊行にあたり

一般財団法人医療経済研究・社会保険福祉協会では2004年以来、健康食品の正しい知識の普及啓発事業とともに科学的根拠に基づいた調査研究を数々行ってきた。その一つとして既に公開中の「健康食品素材の科学的実証データベース（HFS：Health Food Material Scientific Database）」は、2014年１月に完成した。

健康食品業界では2013年６月、食品の機能性表示の規制緩和などを織り込んだ規制改革会議の答申が閣議決定され、米国のダイエタリーサプリメントの表示制度を参考に、企業責任において健康食品を含む食品の機能性表示が認められるのではないかと期待が高まっている。これはこれなりに画期的なことであり、今後の成り行きを注視していく必要がある。

健康食品の機能性と安全性は、よく車の両輪に例えられるが、まず安全性があっての機能性であり、安全性は何を差し置いても最優先されるべき課題である。日本では、欧米のようなサプリメントに対する法整備が完全でないこともあって、通常、「健康食品」として扱われるもののうち、特定保健用食品を除く栄養機能食品といわゆる健康食品の安全性と品質の確保は、基本的に個々の企業の自主的取り組みに委ねられている。健康食品には、国内外からの数千種類に上るといわれる原材料が使用されているが、その安全性と品質が十分確認されているとは限らず、消費者保護の観点からも実効性のある対応策の確立が喫緊の課題となっている。

厚生労働省は、「錠剤、カプセル状等食品の原材料の安全性に関する自主点検ガイドライン」及び「錠剤、カプセル状等食品の適正な製造に係る基本的考え方について」（GMPガイドライン）を最終製品および原材料を対象として、2005年２月１日付通知で公表している。また、厚生労働省の「健康食品の安全性確保に関する検討会」は、業界の取り組みとして、一定の安全性と品質が確保された原材料及び最終製品に対して第三者認証機関による認証とマークの付与等の対策を提言している。現在安全性認証は１機関が、GMPは２機関がこれにあたっている。

いうまでもなく、健康食品の安全性と品質確保は、一定の科学水準と客観性をもとに企業規模にかかわらず、企業が取り組んで実効性を上げることが必要である。そのために、厚生労働省が示すガイドラインに従って、十分に目的を果たすことが可能なシステムが求められ、最終的に消費者の信頼に足るものでなければならない。

このような観点から当協会では、2011年10月から別記研究者による「健康食品の安全性および品質確保のための研究会（RQSHF：Research on Quality and Safety of Health Foods）」を立ち上げ、厚生労働省の安全性及び品質に係る上記ガイドラインを基本に、栄養機能食品及びいわゆる健康食品の安全性及び品質確保のための方法と基準の策定及び事業者の自主点検に活用可能なデータベース（食薬区分・食経験・文献検索・毒性調査情報）の構築に着手した。研究は、ワーキンググループ（WG）１～５によって構成されている。

On this publication

The Association for Health Economics Research and Social Insurance and Welfare (ASIW) has since 2004 been pursuing numerous scientific studies as well as programs to promote knowledge and awareness of health foods. Forming part of these activities is the development of a database called the "Health Food Material Scientific Database" (HFS), which has been already publicly accessible in January 2014.

Since the Japanese cabinet's approval in June 2013 of the findings of the Council for Regulatory Reform, which cover among other things deregulation of food functionality labeling requirements, there have been growing expectations within the health food industry over the possibility that companies may be allowed, on their own responsibility, to label foods (including health foods) to show their functionality based on a system of labeling similar to that used for dietary supplements in the United States. This would be quite groundbreaking and developments will have to be watched closely.

The functionality and safety of health foods are often likened to the two wheels of a car. However, functionality is entirely dependent on safety, and safety must take precedence above all else. Partly due to the incomplete development of Japanese legislation on supplements compared with Europe and North America, of foods generally considered to be "health foods" (*kenkô shokuhin*), the safety and quality of "foods with nutrient function claims" (*eiyô kinô shokuhin*) is, with the exception of "foods for specified health uses" (*tokutei hokenyô shokuhin*), basically left to the independent initiative of individual enterprises. Thousands of ingredients from Japan and overseas are thought to be used in health foods. They are not always properly confirmed to be safe and of good quality, however, and effective measures are urgently needed to protect consumers.

In a notice dated February 1, 2005, the Japanese Ministry of Health, Labour and Welfare (MHLW) published two sets of guidelines covering end products and ingredients : the "Voluntary Inspection Guideline on Safety of Ingredients of Foods in Tablet, Capsule, and Similar Form" and the "Basic Approaches to Proper Manufacture of Foods in Tablet, Capsule, and Similar Form" ("GMP Guideline"). The MHLW's Investigative Commission on Ensuring the Safety of Health Foods is in addition recommending that the industry too should take certain steps, including the adoption of certification and awarding of "marks" by third-party certifying bodies of ingredients and end products that meet certain safety and quality standards. Safety certification is currently performed by one organization, and good manufacturing practice (GMP) is certified by two organizations.

Ensuring health food safety and quality naturally requires that companies of all sizes act to raise effectiveness based on fixed scientific standards and objectivity. Arrangements are therefore needed to allow this to be properly achieved following the guidelines laid down by the MHLW, and these must ultimately be worthy of the consumer's trust.

To this end, the ASIW launched a project in October 2011 called "Research on Quality and Safety of Health Foods" (RQSHF) involving the researchers stated elsewhere. This has begun formulating methods and standards to ensure the safety and quality of so-called health foods and foods with nutrient function claims based on the above MHLW guidelines on safety and quality, and it is also developing a database (food and drug classification, eating experiences, literature searches, and toxicity studies) that can be used by businesses to assist their own voluntary inspections. Five working groups are carrying out the research.

食薬区分は原材料の安全性点検に際して、最初に確認すべき事項である。今般、食薬区分に関する情報のデータベース化に先立って、「学名でひく食薬区分リスト　－健康食品・医薬品に区分される成分－」を出版することにした。

本書の特徴としては、

1．食薬区分に収載された「医」リスト332成分、「非医」リスト1037成分すべてを網羅した。
2．海外でも参照できるように各成分のローマ字表記や必要事項の英訳を付した。
3．各成分に関する文献検索や関連情報の入手を学名に基づいて行うために、学名には異名（Synonym(s)）も併記した。
4．食薬区分リスト掲載成分のうち、米国で使用実績のある植物成分として Herbs of Commerce（第2版、American Herbal Products Association発行、2000年）に掲載されているものに＊印を付して示した。
5．食薬区分に係る通知及び欧米におけるハーブ関連情報を付した。

本書は、元お茶の水女子大学の佐竹元吉教授を筆頭に、植物等については一般社団法人日本健康食品規格協会の大濱宏文前理事長、池田秀子理事長、化学物質については昭和薬科大学の関田節子特任教授による永年にわたっての研究成果でもある。特に大濱先生、池田先生には、休日を返上し昼夜を惜しんでの、細やかで地道なご尽力をいただいた。頭が下がる思いで一杯である。

勿論、別記研究会の多くの先生方にも支えていただいたが、特に動物並びにきのこ類については富山大学和漢医薬学総合研究所の紺野勝弘教授に、さらに動物については独立行政法人国立科学博物館動物研究部の川田伸一郎研究員に、微生物関連情報については前国立医薬品食品衛生研究所衛生微生物部長で麻布大学の小西良子教授に貴重なアドバイスをいただいた。

また、当協会の蓑田由紀子研究員並びに鬼頭志保研究員の体系的フォローアップ作業が、本書の完成に到った大きな力となったことも忘れることができない。

なお、出版全般については薬事日報社の河邉秀一執行役員に何かとお世話になり心より感謝申し上げる。

本書が国内外において有効に活用され、さらに日本の健康食品の安全性及び品質確保に寄与できれば幸甚である。

一般財団法人医療経済研究・社会保険福祉協会
前常務理事　斎 場　仁

平成25年9月18日、一般社団法人日本健康食品規格協会 前理事長の大濱宏文氏が急逝された。

本書の刊行のため、亡くなられる直前まで、データ編集、校正に当たられた。

改めて、これまでのご貢献に感謝申し上げるとともに、追悼の誠を捧げたい。

Food and drug classification is the first thing that should be verified when checking the safety of ingredients, and it is for this reason that the ASIW decided to publish this *Health food ingredients and Scientific names–Food and Drug classification in Japan* ahead of developing a database of information on food and drug classification.

This publication is distinguished by the following features :

1. It covers all 332 ingredients on the "drug" list and all 1,037 ingredients on the "non-drug" list recorded in the food and drug classification.
2. Each ingredient is also romanized and English translations of necessary matters are provided so that it can also be used overseas.
3. So that literature searches on ingredients can be made and relevant information obtained using their scientific names, synonyms are provided alongside scientific names.
4. Of the ingredients included in the food and drug classification list, those included in the *Herbs of Commerce* (2nd Ed., by American Herbal Products Association, 2000) that details the plant ingredients actually used in the US are marked with an asterisk (*).
5. Notices pertaining to food and drug classification and herb-related information in Europe and North America are provided.

This publication is the product of long years of research by Professor Motoyoshi Satake, formerly of Ochanomizu University, Hirobumi Ohama and Hideko Ikeda, respectively the former Chairman and Chairman of the Japanese Institute for Health Food Standards, who contributed mainly to the sections on plants, and Setsuko Sekita, specially appointed Professor at Showa Pharmaceutical University, whose focus was on chemicals. I am particularly overwhelmed by the meticulous, hard effort put in by Dr. Ohama and Ms. Ikeda, who devoted their time and gave up their holidays to make this publication possible.

Alongside, of course, the assistance of the many researchers involved in RQSHF, particularly valuable advice was received from Professor Katsuhiro Konno of the University of Toyama's Institute of Natural Medicine regarding animals and mushrooms, Shinichiro Kawada, researcher in the Department of Zoology at the National Museum of Nature and Science, regarding animals, and Professor Yoshiko Konishi of Azabu University and formerly director of the Division of Microbiology at the National Institute of Health Sciences regarding information on microorganisms.
The major contribution made to the completion of this publication by the follow-up work of Yukiko Minoda and Shiho Kito, researchers at the ASIW, must also not be forgotten.
Thanks are additionally due to Shuichi Kawabe, executive director of Yakuji Nippo, for his assistance on the publishing side.

I hope that this publication finds effective use both in Japan and abroad, and that it makes a contribution to ensuring the safety and quality of health foods in Japan.

Hitoshi Saiba
Former Executive Managing Director
Association of Health Economics Research and Social Insurance and Welfare

Hirobumi Ohama Ph.D., the former Chairman of the Japanese Institute for Health Food Standards, passed away suddenly on 18 September 2013.
Dr. Ohama was involved in editing data and proofreading for this publication right up to his death. We would like to express our gratitude, once again, for his contributions and pay tribute to his memory.

RQSHF研究会メンバー

（アルファベット順）

秋田　徹	AKITA, Toru 日本新薬株式会社　機能食品カンパニー　食品開発研究所長
早川　堯夫	HAYAKAWA, Takao (Chair of WG1/ RQSHF) 近畿大学　薬学総合研究所 所長，大阪大学大学院医学系研究科招聘教授
本田　清隆	HONDA, Kiyotaka 一般財団法人　医療経済研究・社会保険福祉協会　常務理事
池田　秀子	IKEDA, Hideko (Chair of WG5/ RQSHF) 一般社団法人　日本健康食品規格協会　理事長
金澤　惠子	KANAZAWA, Keiko 一般財団法人　医療経済研究・社会保険福祉協会　健康食品グループ　研究員
川田　伸吉	KAWADA, Shinkichi 株式会社サンメディア　リサーチソリューションズ　執行役員
鬼頭　志保	KITO, Shiho 一般財団法人　医療経済研究・社会保険福祉協会　健康食品グループ　研究員
小林　公子	KOBAYASHI, Kimiko 病院薬剤師
近藤　和雄	KONDO, Kazuo お茶の水女子大学大学院　教授，生活環境教育研究センター長
黒柳　正典	KUROYANAGI, Masanori 静岡県立大学薬学部　客員教授
蓑田　由紀子	MINODA, Yukiko 一般財団法人　医療経済研究・社会保険福祉協会　健康食品グループ　研究員
森本　隆司	MORIMOTO, Takashi 三栄源エフ・エフ・アイ株式会社　検査部 担当次長
大濱　宏文	OHAMA, Hirobumi (Chair of WG4/ RQSHF) 一般社団法人　日本健康食品規格協会　前理事長
大塩　稔	OHSHIO, Minoru 株式会社サンメディア　リサーチソリューションズ
斎場　仁	SAIBA, Hitoshi 一般財団法人　医療経済研究・社会保険福祉協会　前常務理事
佐竹　元吉	SATAKE, Motoyoshi (Chair of RQSHF and WG3) お茶の水女子大学　元教授
関田　節子	SEKITA, Setsuko 昭和薬科大学　薬学部　特任教授
渋谷　淳	SHIBUTANI, Makoto 東京農工大学大学院　教授
清水　浩一	SHIMIZU, Koichi 一般財団法人　医療経済研究・社会保険福祉協会　部長
正山　征洋	SHOYAMA, Yukihiro (Chair of WG2/ RQSHF) 長崎国際大学　薬学部薬学科　教授
多田　澄恵	TADA, Sumie 一般財団法人　医療経済研究・社会保険福祉協会　健康食品グループ　研究員
高橋　功	TAKAHASHI, Isao 一般財団法人　医療経済研究・社会保険福祉協会　次長
内田　智明	UCHIDA, Chiaki 一般財団法人　医療経済研究・社会保険福祉協会　次長
和仁　皓明	WANI, Kohmei 西日本食文化研究会
山田　和彦	YAMADA, Kazuhiko 女子栄養大学　栄養学部　実践栄養学科　教授
義平　邦利	YOSHIHIRA, Kunitoshi 東亜大学　元副学長
吉岡　加奈子	YOSHIOKA, Kanako 一般財団法人　医療経済研究・社会保険福祉協会　健康食品グループ　主任研究員

Members of the RQSHF

(alphabetic order)

AKITA, Toru, Ph.D.
General Manager, Food Development Labs., NIPPON SHINYAKU CO., LTD.

HAYAKAWA, Takao, Ph.D. (Chair of WG1/ RQSHF)
Director, Pharmaceutical Research and Technology Institute, KINKI UNIVERSITY
Visiting Professor, Graduate School of Medicine, OSAKA UNIVERSITY

HONDA, Kiyotaka
Executive Managing Director, Association for Health Economics Research and Social Insurance and Welfare

IKEDA, Hideko (Chair of WG5/ RQSHF)
Chairman of the Board, The Japanese Institute for Health Food Standards

KANAZAWA, Keiko
Researcher, Association for Health Economics Research and Social Insurance and Welfare

KAWADA, Shinkichi
Chief Research Solutions Officer, SUNMEDIA Co., Ltd. Research Solutions

KITO, Shiho
Researcher, Association for Health Economics Research and Social Insurance and Welfare

KOBAYASHI, Kimiko
Hospital Pharmacist

KONDO, Kazuo, M.D., Ph.D.
Professor, Ochanomizu University

KUROYANAGI, Masanori, Ph.D.
Visiting Professor, School of Pharmaceutical Sciences, UNIVERSITY OF SHIZUOKA

MINODA, Yukiko
Researcher, Association for Health Economics Research and Social Insurance and Welfare

MORIMOTO, Takashi, Ph.D.
Deputy General Manager, Quality Assurance Laboratory San-Ei Gen F.F.I., Inc.

OHAMA, Hirobumi, Ph.D. (Chair of WG4/ RQSHF)
Former Chairman of the Board, The Japanese Institute for Health Food Standards

OHSHIO, Minoru
SUNMEDIA Co., Ltd. Research Solutions

SAIBA, Hitoshi
Former Executive Managing Director, Association for Health Economics Research and Social Insurance and Welfare

SATAKE, Motoyoshi, Ph.D. (Chair of RQSHF and WG3)
Former Professor, Ochanomizu University

SEKITA, Setsuko, Ph.D.
Professor, Showa Pharmaceutical University

SHIBUTANI, Makoto, D.V.M., Ph.D.
Professor, Tokyo University of Agriculture and Technology Graduate School, Institute of Agricultural Science, Division of Animal Life Science

SHIMIZU, Koichi
Department Director, Association for Health Economics Research and Social Insurance and Welfare

SHOYAMA, Yukihiro, Ph.D. (Chair of WG2/ RQSHF)
Professor, Faculty of Pharmaceutical Science Nagasaki International University

TADA, Sumie
Researcher, Association for Health Economics Research and Social Insurance and Welfare

TAKAHASHI, Isao
Deputy General Manager, Association for Health Economics Research and Social Insurance and Welfare

UCHIDA, Chiaki
Deputy General Manager, Association for Health Economics Research and Social Insurance and Welfare

WANI, Kohmei, Ph.D.
Research Group of Western Japan Dietary Culture

YAMADA, Kazuhiko, Ph.D.
Professor, Department of Applied Nutrition Undergraduate School of Nutrition Kagawa Nutrition University

YOSHIHIRA, Kunitoshi, Ph.D.
Former Vice President, University of East Asia

YOSHIOKA, Kanako
Senior Researcher, Association for Health Economics Research and Social Insurance and Welfare

目　次
Contents

序文 …… 2
Preface

刊行にあたり …… 6
On this publication

凡例 …… 14
How to use this book

食薬区分における成分本質（原材料）についての考え方 …… 22
Fundamental policies of ingredients (raw materials) in the food and drug classification in Japan

学名について …… 26
About scientific names for botanicals and animals

第１部「非医」リスト［医薬品的効能効果を標ぼうしない限り医薬品と判断しない成分本質（原材料）リスト］ …… 33
Part 1　Non-Drug List
(List of ingredients (raw materials) not deemed drugs unless claiming medicinal efficacy)

1．植物由来物等 …… 35
Substances originated in plants

2．動物由来物等 …… 221
Substances originated in animals

3．その他（化学物質等） …… 239
Other substances (chemicals, vitamins and minerals, etc.)

第２部「医」リスト［専ら医薬品として使用される成分本質（原材料）リスト］ …… 289
Part 2　Drug List
(List of ingredients (raw materials) used exclusively for drugs)

1．植物由来物等 …… 291
Substances originated in plants

2．動物由来物等 …… 345
Substances originated in animals

3．その他（化学物質等） …… 353
Other substances (chemicals, vitamins and minerals, etc.)

第３部　添付資料 …… 379
Part 3　Appendix

1．既存添加物名簿収載品目リスト …… 381
List of existing food additives

2．天然香料基原物質リスト …… 419
List of plant or animal sources of natural flavorings

3．一般に食品として飲食に供されている物であって添加物として使用される品目リスト …… 437
List of substances which are generally provided for eating or drinking as foods and which are also used as food additives

4．無承認無許可医薬品の指導取締りについて（昭和46年６月１日薬発第476号） 445
Regulatory control of unapproved/unpermitted drugs (1 June 1971, PAB Notification No. 476)

5．無承認無許可医薬品の監視指導について（昭和62年９月22日薬監第88号） 463
Inspection and guidance of unapproved/unpermitted drugs (22 September 1987, PAB Notification No. 88)

6．「「医薬品的効能効果を標ぼうしない限り医薬品と判断しない成分本質（原材料）」の食品衛生法上の取り扱いの改正について」の一部改正について（平成26年３月14日食安基発0314第１号） 509
Partial amendments to the 'Amending the handling of "Ingredients (raw materials) not deemed drugs unless claiming medicinal efficacy" under the Food Sanitation Act' (14 March 2014, Department of Food Safety, Standards and Evaluation Division Notification No. 0314-1)

7．欧州医薬品庁(EMA)ハーブ医薬品委員会によるハーブ素材評価リスト（2014年７月８日現在） 519
List of herbal substances designated for assessment by the European Medicines Agency's Committee on Herbal Medicinal Products (HMPC) (as of July 8, 2014)

8．第36改正 米国薬局方及び第31改正 国民医薬品集におけるダイエタリーサプリメント，オフィシャルモノグラフ（2013） 527
Lists of USP 36-NF 31 (2013) Dietary Supplements, Official Monographs

9．日本薬局方（第16改正）収載生薬の学名表記について 535
On the scientific names of crude drugs listed in the Japanese Pharmacopoeia (The 16th Edition)

〈１．～３．〉平成22年10月20日消食表第377号通知「食品衛生法に基づく添加物の表示等について」の別添１、２、３
〈１．～３．〉Labeling of additives based on the Food Sanitation Act (Food Labeling Division, Consumer Affairs Agency Notification No. 377) Attachment table 1, 2 and 3

参考文献 549
References

索引 555
Index

和名索引 555
Japanese name index

学名索引 592
Scientific name index

英名索引 619
English name index

監修者・著者略歴 652
Profiles of editor and authors

凡　例

本書は、厚生労働省による「医薬品的効能効果を標ぼうしない限り医薬品と判断しない成分本質（原材料）リスト（「非医」リスト）」及び「専ら医薬品として使用される成分本質（原材料）リスト（「医」リスト）」（両リストを合わせて、以下食薬区分リストと記す）に示された成分本質（原材料）を学名、化学名などによって確認することを目的とし、さらに異名等についても確認できるようにしたものである。

我が国における食品／健康食品の成分リストは海外においても高い関心を引いている。したがって、リストに示された成分、使用部位、関連事項を海外でも参照できるようにするために、本書に示された事項に対して可能な限り英訳を付すことにした。また、成分の英語名についても可能な限り収載するようにした。植物の一般的事項の英訳は、主に文部省「学術用語集　植物学編（増訂版、丸善株式会社、1990)」を参考に行った。

成分本質の収載は厚生労働省の食薬区分リストに従い、「非医」リスト及び「医」リストのそれぞれについて植物由来物等、動物由来物等、その他（化学物質等）の順に行った。また、これらの区分における各成分本質の掲載順も食薬区分リストの順序に従った。なお、本書に収載した成分数は以下の通りである。

	食薬区分リスト収載成分数（平成25年７月10日現在）	
	「医」リスト	「非医」リスト
1．植物由来物等	236	817
2．動物由来物等	21	65
3．その他（化学物質等）	75	155
小計	332	1,037
合計	1,369	

各成分の表記方法について以下に示す。

1．網掛け部分について

網掛け部分には「名称」、「他名等」、「部位等」、「備考」の４項目が含まれる。これらの項目は食薬区分リストの表記に準拠し、そのまま一切の変更を加えずに記載したものである。

2．その他の記載事項について

2.1　植物由来物等及び動物由来物等成分

植物由来物等及び動物由来物等成分については、以下の項目が含まれる。

▶ **他名（参考）**：食薬区分リストに示されていないものであって、実際に使用されている名称を収載した。

How to use this book

The purpose of this publication is to enable the ingredients (raw materials) listed in the Ministry of Health, Labour and Welfare's (MHLW) "List of ingredients (raw materials) not deemed drugs unless claiming medicinal efficacy" ("non-drug list") and "List of ingredients (raw materials) used exclusively for drugs" ("drug list") (referred to collectively below as the "food and drug classification lists") to be checked by means of their scientific or chemical names, etc. It is also designed to allow the user to check for synonyms and other names.

Lists of ingredients of foods and health foods in Japan are attracting strong interest overseas. To enable overseas users to look up listed ingredients, parts of use, and related information, therefore, English translations of as much of the relevant content of this publication as possible have been provided. The English names of components have also been included where possible. The English translations of general information on plants have been made based mainly on the translations provided in Japanese Scientific Terms "Botany" (Revised and enlarged editing, Compiled by Ministry of Education Science and Culture, Japan, Maruzen, 1990).

Ingredients (raw materials) on the non-drug and drug lists are respectively listed in order of plant origin, etc., animal origin, etc., and others (chemicals, etc.) in accordance with the MHLW's food and drug classification lists. Additionally, each ingredient (raw material) in these categories appears in the same order as in the food and drug classification lists. This publication contains the following numbers of ingredients.

	Ingredients on the food and drug classification lists (as of July 10, 2013)	
	Drug list	Non-drug list
1. Plant origin, etc.	236	817
2. Animal origin, etc.	21	65
3. Others (chemicals, etc.)	75	155
Subtotal	332	1,037
Overall total	1,369	

Each ingredient is described as follows.

1. Shaded section

The shaded section consists of four items : Name, Other name(s), Part of use, and Remarks. These items are shown exactly as recorded in the food and drug classification lists without any changes having been made whatsoever.

2. Other items

2.1 Plant origin and animal origin ingredients

The entries on plant origin and animal origin ingredients include the following items.

▶ **Other name(s) (for reference)** : Names in actual use but not recorded in the food and drug classification lists appear here.

▶ **漢字表記・生薬名等**：名称及び他名等の漢字表記、並びに生薬、漢方等で使用されている名称（漢字）を収載した。

▶ **Name (romaji)**：食薬区分リストの名称のローマ字表記を記載した。

▶ **Other name(s) (romaji)**：食薬区分リストの他名等のローマ字表記を記載した。

▶ **学名**：学名は巻末に掲載した参考文献を用い、また主に米国のNational Center for Biotechnology Information（NCBI）のデータベースを根拠として、食薬区分リストに示されている名称に該当するものを記載した。同様に、各学名のSynonyms（異名）についても併記した。なお、食薬区分リストの名称及び他名等の項目には分類上異なる種が２種類以上収載されている場合があるので、その場合にはそれぞれに該当する学名を記載すると同時に、学名と共に和名を（　）内に記載した。

学名はラテン語の二名法により属名と種小名をイタリック体で示し、そのあとに命名者名を示した。命名者名は、省略形が決まっている場合には省略形を用いた。なお、学名の取り扱いについての詳細は別項の解説「学名について」を参考にされたい。

▶ **科名**：科名として日本語名とラテン語名を併記した。科名の取り扱いについても別項の解説「学名について」を参考にされたい。

▶ **英名**：英名は、上記の学名に対応する英語名を“Herbs of Commerce（第２版、American Herbal Products Association発行、2000年）”、“NCBI Database”、“世界有用植物事典（平凡社、第４版、1996）”、“園芸植物大事典（小学館、第１版、1994）”を主に参考にして、可能な範囲で収載した。

▶ **Part of use**：食薬区分リストに記載されている「使用部位」（網掛け部分）の英訳である。

▶ **Note 1**：食薬区分リストに記載されている「備考」（網掛け部分）の英訳である。

▶ **Note 2**：下記「注」の英訳である。

▶ **注**：食薬区分リストには名称の誤りと考えられる部分、同一成分が別名等によって二か所以上にわたって収載されている場合等、若干の見直しが必要と考えられるものがみられたので、このような場合についてその内容を記載した。

▶ **＊印**：本書に掲載した学名が“Herbs of Commerce（第２版、American Herbal Products Association発行、2000年）”に収載されている場合は、当該学名に＊印を付すとともに、食薬区分リストの名称及びローマ字表記による名称にも＊印を付した。

実例を以下に示す。

▶ **Kanji notation and crude drug name** : The kanji notations of "Names" and "Other names" appear here, along with the names (kanji) used in crude drug and Kampo medicine (traditional Japanese medicine), etc.

▶ **Name (romaji)** : The names recorded in the food and drug classification lists appear here in the Roman alphabet (romaji).

▶ **Other names (romaji)** : Other names recorded in the food and drug classification lists appear here in the Roman alphabet (romaji).

▶ **Scientific name** : This is the scientific name corresponding to that given in the food and drug classification, and was determined using the works cited in the references at the end of this publication and mainly the database of the U.S. National Center for Biotechnology Information (NCBI). Similarly determined synonyms are also given alongside each scientific name. As the "Name" and "Other name(s)" entries of an ingredient in the food and drug classification sometimes include two or more taxonomically different species, in such cases the scientific name is given for each and the Japanese name (*wamei*) is given in parentheses alongside the scientific name.
The scientific name is the Latin binomial. This consists of a generic name and a specific name, both of which are italicized, followed by the name(s) of the author(s). Author names are given in abbreviated form where an accepted abbreviation exists. For further details on the treatment of scientific names, see the section entitled "Scientific Names."

▶ **Family name** : The family name is given in both Japanese and Latin. For further details on family names, see "Scientific Names."

▶ **English name** : The English name corresponding to the above scientific name is given wherever possible based mainly on *Herbs of Commerce* (2nd Ed. by American Herbal Products Association), *NCBI Database*, *Useful Planets of the World* (Heibonsha, 4th Edition, 1996), and *The Grand Dictionary of Horiticulture* (Shogakukan, 1st Edition, 1994).

▶ **Part of use** : An English translation of the "Part of use" entry (shown in the shaded section) given in the food and drug classification lists appears here.

▶ **Note 1** : This is an English translation of the content of "Remarks" (in the shaded section) appearing in the food and drug classification lists.

▶ **Note 2** : This is an English translation of the "Note (注)" in the next item.

▶ **Note** : Where a slight revision seems necessary because, for example, a name in the food and drug classification lists appears to contain an error or the same appears in two or more locations under different names, the relevant details appear here.

▶ **Asterisk (*)** : If a scientific name given in this publication is recorded in *Herbs of Commerce* (2nd Ed. by American Herbal Products Association), it is marked with an asterisk (＊). Names in the food and drug classification lists and Romanized names are similarly asterisked.

A sample entry is shown below.

名　称　**オウギ***

他名等　キバナオウギ／ナイモウオウギ
部位等　茎・葉
備　考　根は「医」

他名(参考)　タイツリオウギ（鯛釣黄耆）
漢字表記・生薬名等　黄耆（オウギ）、黄花黄耆（キバナオウギ）、内蒙黄耆（ナイモウオウギ）
Name (Romaji)　ÔGI*
Other name(s) (Romaji)　KIBANA ÔGI, NAIMÔÔGI
学名　*Astragalus membranaceus* (Fisch. ex Link) Bunge*（キバナオウギ）
Astragalus mongholicus Bunge（ナイモウオウギ）
Astragalus membranaceus (L.) (Fish. ex Link) Bunge var. *mongholicus* (Bunge) P.K.Hsiao*（ナイモウオウギ）
科名　Leguminosae（マメ科）
英名　huang qi / astragarus / membranous milkvetch / Mongholian milkvetch
Part of use　stem, leaf
Note 1　root：drug category
Note 2　ÔGI is identical with TÔHOKUÔGI, but their parts of use are different each other.
TÔHOKUÔGI is also listed in the item of "Name".
KIBANAÔGI and NAIMÔÔGI in the item of "Other names" are different species.
注　オウギは別項のトウホクオウギと同一。ただし、「部位等」の記載が異なっている。
「他名等」のキバナオウギ と ナイモウオウギは別種。

2.2 その他（化学物質等）成分

その他（化学物質等）成分については、多様な物質が含まれるので、記述内容が成分によって若干異なる場合があるが、原則として、以下の項目を含む。

- **Name**：成分の英名を記載した。
- **Other name(s)**：他名等の英名を記載した。
- **IUPAC Name**
- **CAS registry number**
- **Synonyms**
- **分子式**
- **特性・カテゴリー**
- **Note 1**：食薬区分リストの「部位等」及び「備考」の英訳を記載した。
- **Note 2**：下記「注」の英訳である。

名　称　**オウギ***

他名等　キバナオウギ／ナイモウオウギ
部位等　茎・葉
備　考　根は「医」

他名(参考)　タイツリオウギ（鯛釣黄耆）
漢字表記・生薬名等　黄耆（オウギ）、黄花黄耆（キバナオウギ）、内蒙黄耆（ナイモウオウギ）
Name (Romaji)　ÔGI*
Other name (s) (Romaji)　KIBANA ÔGI, NAIMÔÔGI
学名　*Astragalus membranaceus* (Fisch. ex Link) Bunge*（キバナオウギ）
Astragalus mongholicus Bunge（ナイモウオウギ）
Astragalus membranaceus (L.) (Fish. ex Link) Bunge var. *mongholicus* (Bunge) P.K.Hsiao*（ナイモウオウギ）
科名　Leguminosae（マメ科）
英名　huang qi / astragarus / membranous milkvetch / Mongholian milkvetch
Part of use　stem, leaf
Note 1　root：drug category
Note 2　ÔGI is identical with TÔHOKUÔGI, but their parts of use are different each other.
TÔHOKUÔGI is also listed in the item of "Name".
KIBANAÔGI and NAIMÔÔGI in the item of "Other names" are different species.
注　オウギは別項のトウホクオウギと同一。ただし、「部位等」の記載が異なっている。
「他名等」のキバナオウギ と ナイモウオウギは別種。

2.2 Other ingredients (chemicals, etc.)

As other ingredients (chemicals, etc.) comprise a diversity of substances, the content of this item can differ slightly according to the ingredient concerned. As a rule, however, it includes the following information.

- **Name**：English name of the ingredient.
- **Other name (s)**：English translation of "Other names".
- **IUPAC Name**
- **CAS registry number**
- **Synonyms**
- **Molecular formula**
- **Properties and category**
- **Note 1**：This is an English translation of the "Part of use" and "Remarks" information given in the food and drug classification lists.
- **Note 2**：This is an English translation of the "Note (注)" in the next item.

▶ **注**：「非医」リストに収載された化学物質等成分の取り扱いについては、関連通知により既存添加物に準拠すべき旨等の規定があるため、その内容を記載した。「医」リストについては、収載された化学物質等成分に関する説明等を記載した。

必要に応じて成分・組成等を記載した。酵素の場合は、CAS registry numberに加えて国際生化学分子生物学連合（IUBMB）の酵素委員会によるEC番号（酵素番号、Enzyme Commission number）を記載した。項目の最後に構造式を示した。

実例を以下に示す。

名　称　**アスタキサンチン**

他名等　－
部位等　ヘマトコッカス藻の主成分
備　考　ヘマトコッカス藻は「非医」

Name　Astaxanthin
Other name(s)　－
IUPAC Name　(6S)-6-hydroxy-3-[(1E,3E,5E,7E,9E,11E,13E,15E,17E)-18-[(4S)-4-hydroxy-2,6,6-trimethyl-3-oxocyclohexen-1-yl]-3,7,12,16-tetramethyloctadeca-1,3,5,7,9,11,13,15,17-nonaenyl]-2,4,4-trimethylcyclohex-2-en-1-one
CAS No.　472-61-7
Synonims　Astaxanthine / Ovoester / 3,3'-Dihydorxy- beta- carotene-4,4' -dione
分子式　$C_{40}H_{52}O_4$
特性・カテゴリー　カロテノイド／carotenoid
Note 1　Main component of *Haematococcus pulvialis*.
Haematococcus pulvialis is in the “non-drug” list.
Note 2　Fall under the category of existing food additive.
注　既存添加物に該当する

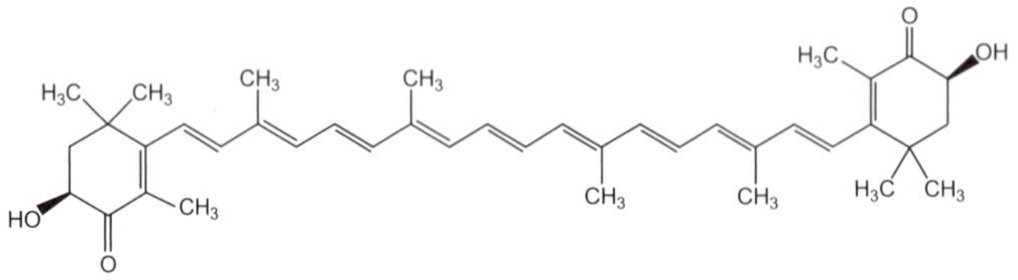

3．参考資料

本書の巻末に参考資料として、厚生労働省による食薬区分関連通知のほか、日本薬局方収載生薬リストを掲載し、さらに、海外情報として欧州医薬品庁ハーブ製品委員会によるハーブ成分評価リスト、及び米国USPによるサプリメント成分モノグラフリストを添付した。また、本書作成に際して使用した参考文献等を掲載した。

▶ **Note**：The handling of ingredients (chemicals etc.) included in the non-drug list is given in detail because the relevant notifications include regulations such as standards to be followed for existing food additives. For ingredients (chemicals etc.) included in the drug list, an explanation of the chemical or other ingredient listed is provided.

Components and composition are included where necessary. In the case of enzymes, the Enzyme Commission (EC) number assigned by the Enzyme Commission of the International Union of Biochemistry and Molecular Biology (IUBMB) is included along with the CAS registry number. The structural formula is shown at the end of the entry.

A sample entry is shown below.

名　称　**アスタキサンチン**

他名等　–
部位等　ヘマトコッカス藻の主成分
備　考　ヘマトコッカス藻は「非医」

Name　Astaxanthin
Other name (s)　–
IUPAC Name　(6S)-6-hydroxy-3-[(1E,3E,5E,7E,9E,11E,13E,15E,17E)-18-[(4S)-4-hydroxy-2,6,6-trimethyl-3-oxocyclohexen-1-yl]-3,7,12,16-tetramethyloctadeca-1,3,5,7,9,11,13,15,17-nonaenyl]-2,4,4-trimethylcyclohex-2-en-1-one
CAS No.　472-61-7
Synonims　Astaxanthine / Ovoester / 3,3'-Dihydorxy- beta- carotene-4,4' -dione
分子式　$C_{40}H_{52}O_4$
特性・カテゴリー　カロテノイド／carotenoid
Note 1　Main component of *Haematococus pulvialis*.
Haematococus pulvialis is in the "non-drug" list.
Note 2　Fall under the category of existing food additive.
注　既存添加物に該当する

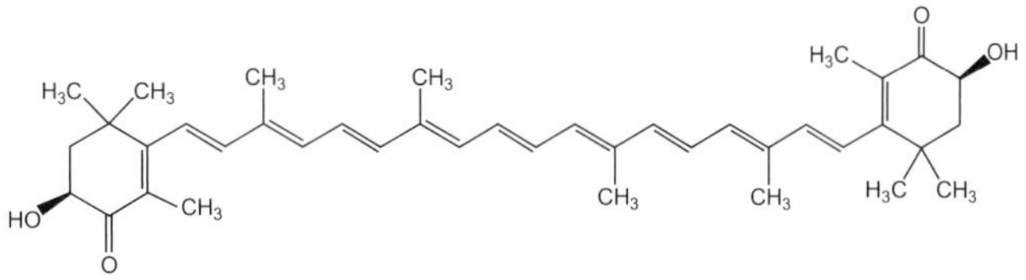

---

3. Reference materials

The following reference materials are to be found at the end of this publication：food and drug classification-related notices issued by the MHLW and a list of crude drugs contained in the Japanese Pharmacopoeia. Regarding overseas sources, a list of assessments of herbal substances made by the Committee on Herbal Medicine Products (HMPC) of the European Medicines Agency (EMA) and a list of monographs for dietary supplements and ingredients produced by the U.S. Pharmacopeial Convention (USP) are included. Sources used in the production of this publication are also listed.

食薬区分における成分本質（原材料）についての考え方

1．収載品目数

厚生労働省は、経口的に服用する製品の原材料となるものについて、医薬品としての使用実態、毒性、麻薬様作用等を考慮し、「医薬品に該当するか否か」の判断を示している。

医薬品区分に該当する成分本質（原材料）については、「専ら医薬品として使用される成分本質（原材料）リスト」（以下「医」リスト）に、医薬品区分に該当しない成分本質（原材料）については、参考として「医薬品的効能効果を標榜しない限り医薬品と判断しない成分本質（原材料）リスト」（以下「非医」リスト）にその例示が掲げられている。

2013年７月10日現在、食薬区分リストの収載品目数は、「医」リスト及び「非医」リストそれぞれ332品目、1,037品目である。

2．食薬区分の判断基準の考え方

(1) 成分本質（原材料）の判断基準については、我が国における医薬品による保健衛生上の危害を防止するため、専ら医薬品としての使用実態のあるもの、毒性及び麻薬覚せい剤様作用をもつもの、医薬品に相当する成分を含むもの等、医薬品として規制すべき成分本質を判断するために必要と考えられている。

(2) 食品との関係については、我が国において一般に食品として飲食に供されている物については、食品として取り扱われるべき旨、判断基準上に明記されている。

(3) 「非医」リストについては、「医薬品の範囲基準の見直しに関する検討会報告書」（2000年３月23日公表）を踏まえ、「医薬品の範囲に関する基準の一部改正について（医薬発第392号、2000年４月５日付厚生省医薬安全局長通知）において、関係者等の利便を考え、参考として作成すべきとされているものであり、あくまで、専ら医薬品として使用される成分本質（原材料）に対する該当性の問い合わせがあったもののうち、その成分本質（原材料）からみて、「医」区分に該当しないと判断したものの例であり、食品の範囲を定めているものではない。

(4) 従来の食薬区分の「１-a」成分（専ら医薬品として使用される物）が改正によって全て自動的に「医」リストに移行するわけではなく、当該判断基準に照らし、改めて「専ら医薬品として使用される成分本質（原材料）」に該当するか否かを判断するものである。

(5) 医薬部外品として経口摂取される物、食品添加物として区分されるもの、諸外国において医薬品として使用されているものについても同様に、全てが自動的にどちらかのリストに移行するものではなく、当該判断基準に照らし、「専ら医薬品として使用される成分本質」に該当するか否かを判断するものである。

3．毒性について

(1) 毒性が強いものにあっては、その作用の強さから医薬品として使用されてきたものもあり、我が国における医薬品に該当するものによる保健衛生上の危害を防止する観点から、毒性の程度を判断基準の一つとしたものである。但し、食品衛生法で規制される食品等に起因して中毒を起こす物など、食品として規制されるべき物は除く旨、判断基準上に明記されている。

(2) 現在までに種々の毒性成分の含有が定性的に知られている原材料であっても、それぞれの毒性成分の含有量が定量的に明らかにされている場合は少なく、また、同じ原材料であっても含有量に差があるとの知見があることなどから、毒性成分の量に基づく基準化については困難であると考えられている。但し、毒性成分

Fundamental policies of ingredients (raw materials) in the food and drug classification in Japan

1. Number of items listed

The Ministry of Health, Labour and Welfare (MHLW) issues rulings on whether or not the raw materials used in products for oral ingestion "correspond to drugs" taking into consideration factors such as their actual usage as drugs, toxicity, and narcotic-like effect.
Examples are provided of ingredients (raw materials) that are classified as falling in the drug category on the "List of ingredients (raw materials) used exclusively for drugs" (referred to below as the "drug list"), and of ingredients (raw materials) that are classed outside the drug category on the "List of ingredients (raw materials) not deemed drugs unless claiming medicinal efficacy" (referred to below as the "non-drug list").
As of July 10, 2013, there were 332 and 1,037 items listed on the drug list and the non-drug list, respectively.

2. Approach to the evaluation criteria for food and drug classification

(1) Classification standards are considered necessary for determining whether ingredients (raw materials) such as those used exclusively for drugs, those with toxic and narcotic/stimulant-like effects, and those containing the entity of ingredients corresponding to drugs should be subject to regulation as drugs in order to prevent harm to public health caused by drugs in Japan.
(2) Regarding foods, the classification standards clearly state that substances generally used to eat or drink as food in Japan should be treated as "foods."
(3) Regarding the non-drug list, based on the "Report of the Investigative Commission on Revision of the Standards on Scope of Drugs" (issued March 23, 2000), "Partial amendments to the Standards on Scope of Drugs" (Notice of the Director General of the Pharmaceutical Safety Bureau, The Ministry of Health and Welfare (MHW), dated April 5, 2000, PMSB Notification No.392) states that it was prepared as a convenient reference for the relevant parties, and that it does not define the scope of foods but instead simply provides examples of ingredients (raw materials) that had been the subject of inquiries concerning their classification as ingredients (raw materials) used exclusively for drugs and that had been deemed not to fall in the "drug" category.
(4) Ingredients classed as "1-a" materials under the old food and drug classification (ingredients used exclusively for drugs) are not all automatically transferred to the "drug" list as a result of the revision. Instead, it is re-determined in each case whether they fall in the category of "ingredients (raw materials) used exclusively for drugs" in light of the classification standards concerned.
(5) Materials taken orally as quasi-drugs, used as food additives, or used as drugs in other countries are similarly not all automatically transferred to either list, but instead it is determined in each case whether they fall in the category of "ingredients (raw materials) used exclusively for drugs" in light of the classification standards concerned.

3. Toxicity

(1) As some highly toxic ingredients have been classified as drugs due to the strength of their action, degree of toxicity has been adopted as a classification standard in order to prevent harm to public health caused by ingredients corresponding to drugs in Japan. However, the classification standards clearly state that ingredients that should be regulated as foods, such as ingredients causing poisoning attributable to foods etc. that are typically regulated under the Food Sanitation Act, are excluded.
(2) The toxic content of raw materials known to contain toxic constituents is often only known qualitatively. Given that the same raw materials have been found in some cases to contain varying quantities

の含有量等について、科学的なデータが十分に得られ、摂取量等からみて安全性が担保できる場合には、「医」リストから「非医」リストに移行させる場合もあり得ると考えられている。

(3) 毒性の判断は経口投与による毒性が基本となると考えられている。なお、経口での毒性に関する資料が整備されておらず、静脈投与のみの毒性が判明している場合などにあっては、毒薬・劇薬指定成分の判断基準を参考に当該成分本質の毒性を判断することとされている。

4．麻薬等の構造類似物

麻薬等との化学構造上の類似物については、同様の作用が合理的に予測されるものについて規制すべきと考えられており、その旨、判断基準上に明記されている。

5．薬理作用等用語の定義

「薬理作用が明確であるもの」、「同一性」及び「劇性」については定義が不明確であるため、「処方箋医薬品に相当する成分を含むもの」及び「毒劇薬指定成分に相当する成分を含むもの」とし、基準の明確化が図られた。

6．抽出物の取扱い

抽出物の取扱いについては、水、エタノール以外による抽出物が全て食品に使用できないとする趣旨ではなく、成分本質（原材料）が「非医」リストに収載されていたとしても、水、エタノール以外で抽出を行った場合には、その抽出物については、毒性等の観点から改めて判断を行うとする趣旨であるため、その旨、判断基準上に明記されている。

佐竹　元吉

of such constituents, it is considered difficult to establish standards based on quantities of toxic constituents. However, where sufficient scientific data on such matters as toxic content has been obtained and safety can be ensured from the point of view of intake, etc., it may be possible for ingredients (raw materials) containing toxic constituents to be transferred from the drug list to the non-drug list.

(3) Toxicity should, as a rule, be determined on the basis of toxicity when administered orally. In cases where, for example, there is insufficient data on oral toxicity and only intravenous toxicity has been determined, the toxicity of the ingredient (raw material) concerned shall be determined based on the criteria for ingredients in drugs designated poisonous or deleterious.

4. Structural analogs of narcotics, etc.

Chemical structural analogs of narcotics, etc. that may reasonably be expected to have a similar effect should be subject to regulation, and the classification standards make provision to that effect.

5. Definition of pharmacological action and other terms

As "ingredients having a clear pharmacological effect," "identity," and "powerful" have not been clearly defined, standards have been clarified by defining them as "ingredients containing constituents equivalent to ethical drugs" and "ingredients containing constituents equivalent to constituents of drugs designated as poisonous or deleterious".

6. Treatment of extracts

Rather than saying that no extracts other than those obtained using water and/or ethanol may be used in food products, the classification standards clearly state that extracts obtained other than with water or ethanol shall be re-evaluated from the point of view of their toxicity, etc. even where ingredients (raw materials) are listed on the non-drug list.

Motoyoshi Satake

学名について

1．学名とは

学名（ラテン語：binomen、英語：scientific name）とは、生物につけられた世界共通の名称である。命名には一定の規則があり、ラテン語で表記される。この規則は、それぞれの生物分野の命名規約により取り決められている。動物には「国際動物命名規約」International code of zoological nomenclatureがあり、藻類・菌類と植物には「国際藻類・菌類・植物命名規約」International code of botanical nomenclatureが、細菌には「国際細菌命名規約」International code of nomenclature of bacteriaがある。学名は属名と種小名（細菌の場合には属名と種形容語）で構成される。この表し方を二名法という。二名法は「分類学の父」と呼ばれるリンネ（Carl von Linné, 1707-1778）によって体系化された。

学名が全世界で通用するものとするために、1つの種に対し有効な学名が1つだけとなるように規則が定められている。各国語で呼ばれる生物名は普通名（通俗名）common nameで、日本語の場合は和名という。

属名とは、分類上近い種をまとめて取り扱う分類単位の名称で、同じ属に分類される全ての種に共通する名前となる。種小名を属名と組み合わせる事により、その種に固有の学名となる。

属名と種小名の後ろに命名者名が記載されるが、種の発見者が命名者になるとは限らない。その種の特徴、近縁種との区別を明確に示した「論文」の発表者が命名したことになり、命名者として扱われる。

学名をさらに細分するのに用いられる表現形として「〜の変種」は「var.」、「〜の型」は「f.」または「forma」、「〜の園芸品種」は「cv.」、「〜属の一種」は「sp.」、「〜属の数種類」は「spp.」、「〜の亜種」は「subsp.」または「ssp.」、「〜と〜の交雑種」は「〜 × 〜」（×はクロスと読む）等がある。
尚、属名と種小名はイタリック体（斜体）で、命名者名は立体で記載される。

2．学名表記の例

2.1 クチナシ

Gardenia	*jasminoides*	J.Ellis
属名	種小名	命名者名

*Gardenia*は、クチナシが分類されるクチナシ属の属名で、属名は必ず大文字から書き始める。次に*jasminoides*は種小名で、属名との組合せによりこの植物（種）をあらわす学名となる。種小名は原則としてその種の特徴をよく表現する形容詞、名詞の所有格または人名や地域名に基づく固有名詞が用いられる。最後のJ.Ellisは、この学名を発表した研究者（命名者）の名前で、学名の正確さを期する意味で命名者の名前を最後に付すことになっている。

About scientific names for botanicals and animals

1. What are scientific names?

Scientific names (binomina in Latin) are the common international names given to organisms. The nomenclature is governed by certain rules and written in Latin. These rules are set by naming conventions in each branch of biology : the scientific names of animals are ruled by the International Code of Zoological Nomenclature, while the names of algae, fungi, and plants and of bacteria are respectively ruled by the International Code of Botanical Nomenclature and the International Code of Nomenclature of Bacteria. Scientific names consist of two parts : the generic name and the specific name (or the generic name and specific epithet in the case of bacteria). This method of representing scientific names is known as the binomial nomenclature and was systematized by Carl von Linné (1707-1778), the "father of taxonomy."

To ensure that scientific names are accepted around the world, rules are provided to ensure each species has only one valid scientific name. The organism name used in each country is the "common name," which in Japanese is the wamei.

The generic name is the name of the taxonomic unit into which taxonomically similar species are grouped, and all species in the same genus share this name. Combining the specific name with the generic name gives each species its own scientific name.

The name of the "author" who named the species can come after the generic name and specific name. This is the name of the author of the paper or other publication in which the species was first clearly distinguished from related species and its characteristics described, and is not necessarily the name of the person who discovered the species.

Several forms of expression are used to subdivide scientific names. These include "var." for variety, "f." or "forma" for forma, "cv." for cultivar, "sp." for one species in a genus, "spp." for plural species in a genus, "subsp." or "ssp." for subspecies, and "x" (pronounced "cross") for crossbreeds between two species.
The generic and specific names are italicized, while the author name is not italicized.

2. Examples of how scientific names are written

2.1 Cape jasmine

Gardenia	*jasminoides*	J. Ellis
Generic name	**Specific name**	**Author's name**

Gardenia is the name of the genus to which Cape jasmine belongs. Note that the generic name is always capitalized. Next comes *jasminoides*, which is the specific name. Combined with the generic name, this gives the scientific name of this plant (species). The specific name is as a rule an adjective or a noun in the genitive case that expresses well the characteristics of the species concerned, or a proper noun based on the name of a person or region. Last comes J. Ellis, which is the name of the author who announced the scientific name. The author's name comes last, and is added to make sure of the accuracy of the scientific name.

2.2 カンゾウ

Glycyrrhiza	*glabra*	L.
属名	種小名	命名者名

*Glycyrrhiza*は、カンゾウが属するカンゾウ属を示す属名である。種小名の*glabra*は「無毛の」を意味する形容詞である。次のL.はこの学名を発表したリンネ（命名者）の名前の省略記載である。

2.3 バショウ

Musa	*basjoo*	Siebold et Zuccarini
属名	種小名	命名者名（２人）

バショウはバショウ属（Musa）に属し、日本名にちなんだ種小名basjooが付けられている。命名者名は２名で、「et」は「および」を意味し、シーボルト氏とツッカリニ氏の共同命名であることを示す。etは＆と記載されることもある。Siebold とZuccariniはそれぞれSieb.とZucc.のように省略形で記載されることもある。

3．科名とは

科（familia）はフランスの植物学者、ピエール・マニョールが1689年の著作で用いた用語である。カール・フォン・リンネは、分類学の方法論について述べた1751年の著作 Philosophia botanica『植物哲学』において、植物には７つのfamiliaがあると述べている（78節）。７つとは、菌、藻、コケ、シダ、草、ヤシ、木であるが、このときは植物の形態を区分しているだけで、分類体系のための用語として用いた訳ではなかった。

分類体系のための科名の使用は、ドイツのエングラーが1900年ごろに提唱し、その後、修正を加えながら発展したものである。単純な構造の花から、複雑な構造の花へと進化した、との考えに基づいている。現在、最も一般的に使われており、日本で目にする植物図鑑や植物ガイドブックのほぼ全てで、新エングラー体系に基づく分類が採用されていると言って過言ではない。

新エングラー体系では、花の咲く被子植物を、まず、双子葉類と単子葉類に大別している。双子葉とは、いわゆる「ふたば」のことで、種から発芽した時に、最初に出てくる２枚の葉のことである。これが出てくるのが双子葉類、２枚ではなく１枚の葉が伸びるのが単子葉類である。単子葉類に比べると双子葉類は種類の多い大きな仲間なので、双子葉類はさらに、花びらが分かれる離弁花類と、花びらが分かれない合弁花類とに分けられる。

1980年代に提唱されたクロンキスト体系では、ストロビロイド説を採用する。ストロビロイド説は単純な構造を出発点とするのではなく、「花被・おしべ・めしべ等が多数、軸の周りを螺旋状に配列している両性花を出発点とし、この原始的被子植物から種々の植物群が進化した」とする仮説である。単純な構造の尾状花序群などは、原始的被子植物の構造の一部が退化して生成したとする。この分類体系では、原始的被子植物の形態的特徴をもっともよく保存しているモクレンの仲間を最初に配列する。逆に双子葉植物の最後に位置するのは、もっとも進化した形態特徴をもつとされるキクの仲間である。

2.2 Licorice

Glycyrrhiza	*glabra*	L.
Generic name	**Specific name**	**Author's name**

Glycyrrhiza is the name of the genus to which licorice belongs. The specific name *glabra* is an adjective meaning "glabrous," i.e., hairless. Last comes L., which is an abbreviation of the name of the author (Linnaeus) who announced the scientific name.

2.3 Japanese banana

Musa	*basjoo*	Siebold et Zuccarini
Generic name	**Specific name**	**Authors' names (2 individuals)**

Japanese banana belongs to the Musa genus. To this is added the specific name, basjoo, which derives from the Japanese name. The two authors' names are joined by "et" which is the Latin for "and" signifying that the scientific name was announced by joint authors, Siebold and Zuccarini. Et is also sometimes written as &. The two authors, Siebold and Zuccarini, are also sometimes written in abbreviated form as Sieb. and Zucc.

3. Family

Family (familia) is a term used by the French botanist Pierre Magnol in a work published 1689. The taxonomic methodology described by Carl von Linné in his Philosophia botanica (Botanical philosophy), published in 1751, divides plants into seven families (principle §78). These are : fungi, algae, mosses, ferns, grasses, palms, and trees. At this time, however, plants were classified only by form, and family was not used as a taxonomic term.

Taxonomic use of families was advocated by the German botanist Adolf Engler in around 1900, and the concept subsequently developed as modifications were made. It was based on the idea that flowers evolved from simple structures to complex structures. This system is now the most commonly used, and it is safe to say that virtually all illustrated encyclopedias of flowers and botanical guidebooks encountered in Japan employ a system of classification based on the modified Engler system.

The modified Engler system begins by broadly dividing flowering plants into dicotyledons and monocotyledons, known for short as dicots and monocots. Cotyledons are the "seed leaves" that appear first when a seed germinates ; hence plants that have two such leaves are called dicotyledons and those that have just one are called monocotyledons. As there are more dicots than monocots, the dicots are further divided into Choripetalae (which have divided petals) and Sympetalae (which have fused petals).

The Cronquist system put forward in the 1980s uses the Strobiloid theory. Rather than taking simple structures as its starting point, the Strobiloid theory hypothesizes that "androgynous flowers whose perianth, stamens, pistils, and so forth are arranged spirally in large numbers around a stem comprise the starting point, and various flora evolved from these primitive angiosperms." Simply structured plants such as Amentiferae are believed to have been formed by the atrophy of part of the structure of a primitive angiosperm. In this taxonomy, the magnolias come first, as they best preserve the morphological characteristics of primitive angiosperms. Conversely, at the far end of the dicots are relatives of the chrysanthemum, which are regarded as being morphologically the most evolved.

クロンキスト以後、1990年代以降は、DNA解析による分子系統学が大きく発展してきた。DNA解析による知見をもとに植物の分類体系も、さらに見直された。特に葉緑体DNAの解析から、被子植物の分岐を調査する研究は近年飛躍的に進み、新しい知見は被子植物系統グループ（Angiosperm Phylogeny Group；APG）に集約されている。

4．本書で用いた科名

本書で用いた科名は、新エングラー分類体系[1]に基づく。現在、遺伝子解析による新しい分類体系APG II (2003)[2]が構築されてきている。しかしこの分類はまだ確定されているとはいえない。本書では広く使われてきた新エングラー分類体系の科名を採用したが、APG II分類体系やクロンキスト分類体系[3]による科名と一部異なるので下記に主なものを示す。

Japanese Family Name	Engler (1964)[1] Family Name	APG II (2003)[2] Cronquist (1981)[3] Family Name
ヤシ科	Palmae	Arecaceae
イネ科	Gramineae	Poaceae
マメ科	Leguminosae	Fabaceae
アブラナ科	Cruciferae	Brassicaceae
シソ科	Labiatae	Lamiaceae
セリ科	Umbelliferae	Apiaceae
キク科	Compositae	Asteraceae

1) H. G. A. Engler, H. Melchior：Engler's Syllabus der Pflanzenfamilien (1964)
2) APG II (An update of the Angiosperm Phylogeny Group Classification for the orders and families of flowering plants. Botanical Journal of the Linnean Society 141：399-436, 2003)
3) Arthur Cronquist：An Integrated System of Classification of Flowering Plant (1981)

佐竹　元吉
関田　節子

Since the 1990s following Cronquist, considerable developments have occurred in molecular phylogenetics using DNA analysis, and the taxonomy of plants has been further revised based on the findings of such analysis. Chloroplast DNA analysis in particular has propelled dramatic advances in research into the divergence of angiosperms in recent years, and the new findings are being aggregated by the Angiosperm Phylogeny Group (APG).

4. Family names used in this publication

The family names used in this publication are given according to the widely used modified Engler system of classification[1). A new taxonomy, APG II (2003)[2), is now being developed using genetic analysis, but is not yet completely finalized. As the family names used by the modified Engler system and the APG II and Cronquist systems[3) differ in part, the main differences are shown below.

Japanese Family Name	Engler (1964)[1) Family Name	APG II (2003)[2) Cronquist (1981)[3) Family Name
ヤシ科 (Yashi-ka)	Palmae	Arecaceae
イネ科 (Ine-ka)	Gramineae	Poaceae
マメ科 (Mame-ka)	Leguminosae	Fabaceae
アブラナ科 (Aburana-ka)	Cruciferae	Brassicaceae
シソ科 (Shiso-ka)	Labiatae	Lamiaceae
セリ科 (Seri-ka)	Umbellliferae	Apiaceae
キク科 (Kiku-ka)	Compositae	Asteraceae

1) H. G. A. Engler, H. Melchior：Engler's Syllabus der Pflanzenfamilien (1964)
2) APG II (An update of the Angiosperm Phylogeny Group Classification for the orders and families of flowering plants. Botanical Journal of the Linnean Society 141：399-436, 2003)
3) Arthur Cronquist：An Integrated System of Classification of Flowering Plant (1981)

Motoyoshi Satake
Setsuko Sekita

第 1 部 「非医」リスト
［医薬品的効能効果を標ぼうしない限り医薬品と判断しない成分本質（原材料）リスト］

Part 1 Non-Drug List
(List of ingredients (raw materials) not deemed drugs unless claiming medicinal efficacy)

1．植物由来物等
Substances originated in plants

2．動物由来物等
Substances originated in animals

3．その他（化学物質等）
Other substances (chemicals, vitamins and minerals, etc.)

1．植物由来物等

1. Substances originated in plants

網掛け部分：網掛け部分には「名称」、「他名等」、「部位等」、「備考」の４項目が含まれる。これらの項目は食薬区分リストの表記に準拠し、そのまま一切の変更を加えずに記載した。

注１）「名称」及び「他名等」の欄については、生薬名、一般名及び起源植物等を記載している。

注２）リストに掲載されている成分本質（原材料）のうち、該当する部位について、「部位等」の欄に記載している。

注３）他の部位が別のリストに掲載されている場合等、その取扱いが紛らわしいものについては、備考欄にその旨記載している。

注４）備考欄の「医」は「専ら医薬品として使用される成分本質（原材料）リスト」に掲載されていることを示す。

Shaded section：The shaded section consists of four items：Name, Other name(s), Part of use, and Remarks. These items are shown exactly as recorded in the food and drug classification lists without any changes having been made whatsoever.

1) The “Name” and “Other name(s)” entries include the crude drug name, common name, source plant, and other names.
2) Of the ingredients (raw materials) included in the list, the relevant part used is included in the “Part of use” entry.
3) Where other parts are included in other lists, notes are entered in the “Remarks” column if there could be any confusion over the handling.
4) Where the “Remarks” column shows “drug (医)”, the substance is included in the “List of ingredients (raw materials) used exclusively for drugs”.

植物由来等の原材料の見方
(Notation of a substance originated in plant(s).)

名　称 **他名等** **部位等** **備　考**	**Name** **Other name(s)** **Part of Use** **Remarks**	食薬区分リストの記載事項とその内容。 The shaded section consists of the following four items which are exactly shown as recorded in the food and drug classification lists without any changes.
他名(参考)		食薬区分リストには載っていないが、実際に使用されている名称。 **Other name(s) (for reference)**：Names in actual use but not recorded in the food and drug classification list.
漢字表記・生薬名等		「名称」「他名等」の漢字表記と読み。それらの生薬、漢方等における名称の漢字表記と読み。 **Kanji notation and crude drug name**：The kanji notations of "Name" and "Other name(s)" along with the names (kanji) used in crude drug and/or Kampo medicine (traditional Japanese medicine), etc.
Name(Romaji)		「名称」のローマ字表記。 Roman alphabet (romaji) of the "Name" in the food and drug classification list.
Other name(s) (Romaji)		「他名等」のローマ字表記。 Roman alphabet (romaji) of the "Other name(s)" in the food and drug classification list.
学名 **科名** **英名**	**Scientific name(s)** **Family name** **English name(s)**	「名称」または「他名等」の学名、科名、英名。 Scientific name(s), Family name and English name(s) of the "Name" or "Other name(s)".
Part of use		「部位等」の英訳。 English translation of the "Part of use" in the food and drug classification list.
Note 1		「備考」の英訳。 English translation of the content of "Remarks" in the food and drug classification list.
Note 2		下記「注」の英訳。 English translation of "Note (注)" in the last item.
注		食薬区分リストの記載事項についての補足情報等。 **Note**：Comments or supplementary information on the content of the food and drug classification records are given.

＊印：本書に掲載した学名が "*Herbs of Commerce* (2nd Ed. by American Herbal Products Association)" に収載されている場合は、当該「学名」と「名称」、「Name(Romaji)」表記に＊印を付した（ただし、植物の「非医」と「医」リストに限る）。

Asterisk (*)：If a scientific name given in this publication is recorded in *Herbs of Commerce* (2nd Ed. by American Herbal Products Association), it is marked with an asterisk (*)."Name"and its Romanized name are also asterisked.

ア行

名　称　アイギョクシ

他名等　―
部位等　寒天様物質
備　考　―

他名(参考)　―
漢字表記・生薬名等　愛玉子（アイギョクシ）
Name(Romaji)　AIGYOKUSHI
Other name(s) (Romaji)　―
学名　*Ficus awkeotsang* Makino
科名　Moraceae（クワ科）
英名　jelly fig
Part of use　agar like substance
Note 1　―
Note 2　―
注　―

名　称　アイスランド苔*

他名等　―
部位等　植物体
備　考　―

他名(参考)　―
漢字表記・生薬名等　依蘭苔（エイランタイ）
Name(Romaji)　AISURANDOGOKE*
Other name(s) (Romaji)　―
学名　*Cetraria islandica* (L.) Ach.*
科名　Parmeliacea（ウメノキゴケ科）
英名　alga perlada / Bejin gwenn / British agar / carrageen / carrageenan / carragheen moss / carraigín / chondrus / gristle moss / curly moss / dorset weed / Ezo-tsunomata / Irish moss / Iceland moss
Part of use　whole plant
Note 1　―
Note 2　―
注　―

名　称　アイブライト*

他名等　―
部位等　全草
備　考　―

他名(参考)　コゴメグサ（小米草）
漢字表記・生薬名等　―
Name(Romaji)　AIBURAITO*
Other name(s) (Romaji)　―
学名　*Euphrasia officinalis* L.*
Euphrasia stricta J.P. Wolff ex J.F. Lehm.*
Euphrasia rostkoviana F. Hayne*
科名　Scrophulariaceae（ゴマノハグサ科）
英名　eyebright / eye bright
Part of use　whole plant
Note 1　―
Note 2　AIBURAITO is identical with KOGOMEGUSA. KOGOMEGUSA is also listed in the item of "Name".
注　アイブライトは別項のコゴメグサと同一。

名　称　アオギリ

他名等　―
部位等　種子
備　考　―

他名(参考)　ゴウシュウアオギリ（豪州アオギリ）
漢字表記・生薬名等　青桐（アオギリ）、梧桐子（ゴトウシ）
Name(Romaji)　AOGIRI
Other name(s) (Romaji)　―
学名　*Firmiana simplex* (L.) W.F. Wight
Firmiana plantanifolia (L. f.) Schott et Endl.
Hibiscus simplex L.
科名　Sterculiaceae（アオギリ科）
英名　bottle tree / Chinese parasol tree
Part of use　seed
Note 1　―
Note 2　―
注　―

名　称　アオダモ

他名等　コバノトネリコ／トネリコ／Fraxinus lanuginosa／Fraxinus japonica
部位等　樹皮
備　考　―

他名(参考)　ケアオダモ（毛青梻）
漢字表記・生薬名等　秦皮（シンピ）

Name (Romaji)　AODAMO
Other name (s) (Romaji)　KOBANOTONERIKO／TONERIKO
学名　*Fraxinus lanuginosa* Koidz.（コバノトネリコ）
Fraxinus japonica Bl.（トネリコ）
科名　Oleaceae（モクセイ科）
英名　—
Part of use　bark
Note 1　—
Note 2　—
注　—

名　称　アガーベ

他名等　テキラリュウゼツ
部位等　球茎
備　考　—

他名(参考)　—
漢字表記･生薬名等　—
Name (Romaji)　AGÂBE
Other name (s) (Romaji)　TEKIRARYÛZETSU
学名　*Agave tequilana* J.H. Weber
科名　Agavacaceae（リュウゼツラン科）
英名　tequila agave / blue agave
Part of use　corn
Note 1　—
Note 2　—
注　—

名　称　アカザ

他名等　—
部位等　葉
備　考　—

他名(参考)　—
漢字表記･生薬名等　藜（アカザ）
Name (Romaji)　AKAZA
Other name (s) (Romaji)　—
学名　*Chenopodium album* L. var. *centrorubrum* Makino
Chenopodium centrorubrum (Makino) Nakai
科名　Chenopodiaceae（アカザ科）
英名　goosefoot / fat hen / lamb's quarters / pigweed
Part of use　leaf
Note 1　—
Note 2　—
注　—

名　称　アカショウマ

他名等　—
部位等　根
備　考　ショウマの根茎は「医」

他名(参考)　—
漢字表記･生薬名等　赤升麻（アカショウマ）
Name (Romaji)　AKASHÔMA
Other name (s) (Romaji)　—
学名　*Astilbe thunbergii* (Sieb. et Zucc.) Miq.
科名　Saxifragaceae（ユキノシタ科）
英名　plume flower / Japanese astilpe
Part of use　root
Note 1　rhizome of *Cimicifuga simplex* (DC.) Wormusk. ex Turcz.：drug category
Note 2　—
注　—

名　称　アカツメクサ*

他名等　コウシャジクソウ／ムラサキツメクサ／レッド・クローバー
部位等　葉・花穂（序）
備　考　—

他名(参考)　—
漢字表記･生薬名等　紅車軸草（コウシャジクソウ）
Name (Romaji)　AKATSUMEKUSA*
Other name (s) (Romaji)　KÔSHAJIKUSÔ／MURASAKITSUMEKUSA／REDDO・KURÔBÂ
学名　*Trifolium pratense* L.*
科名　Leguminosae（マメ科）
英名　red clover / purple clover / peavine clover / cow clover
Part of use　leaf, inflorescence
Note 1　—
Note 2　—
注　—

名　称　アカテツ

他名等　—
部位等　果肉・葉
備　考　—

他名(参考)　—
漢字表記･生薬名等　赤鉄（アカテツ）
Name (Romaji)　AKATETSU
Other name (s) (Romaji)　—

学名 *Pouteria obovata* (R. Br.) Baehni
Planchonella obovata (R. Br.) Pierre
科名 Sapotaceae（アカテツ科）
英名 lucma / Ecuador sapote
Part of use sarcocarp, leaf
Note 1 —
Note 2 —
注 —

名 称 **アカニレ***

他名等 スリッパリーエルム
部位等 全草
備 考 —

他名(参考) —
漢字表記・生薬名等 赤楡（アカニレ）
Name (Romaji) AKANIRE*
Other name (s) (Romaji) SURIPPARÎERUMU
学名 *Ulmus fulva* Michx.*
Ulmus rubla Muhl.*
科名 Ulmaceae（ニレ科）
英名 slippery elm
Part of use whole plant
Note 1 —
Note 2 —
注 —

名 称 **アカバナムシヨケギク**

他名等 —
部位等 葉
備 考 —

他名(参考) ペルシアジョチュウギク（ペルシア除虫菊）
漢字表記・生薬名等 紅花除虫菊（アカバナムシヨケギク）
Name (Romaji) AKABANAMUSHIYOKEGIKU
Other name (s) (Romaji) —
学名 *Chrysanthemum coccineum* Willd.
Pyrethrum coccineum (Willd.) Voroch.
Tanaceum coccineum (Willd) Grieson
Chrysanthemum roseum weberet Moor
Chrysanthemum arneum Bieb.
科名 Compositae（キク科）
英名 pyrethrum / pyrethurum gardens / Persian pellitory / common pyrethurum / Persian insect flower / painted daisy
Part of use leaf
Note 1 —
Note 2 —
注 —

名 称 **アカメガシワ**

他名等 —
部位等 樹皮
備 考 —

他名(参考) ゴサイバ（五菜葉）、サイモリバ（菜盛葉）
漢字表記・生薬名等 赤芽柏（アカメガシワ）、将軍木皮（ショウグンボクヒ）、野梧桐（ヤゴドウ）
Name (Romaji) AKAMEGASHIWA
Other name (s) (Romaji) —
学名 *Mallotus japonicus* (Thunb.) Müll. Arg.
科名 Euphorbiaceae（トウダイグサ科）
英名 red oak / Japanese mallotus
Part of use bark
Note 1 —
Note 2 —
注 —

名 称 **アガリクス**

他名等 アガリクス・ブラゼイ／ヒメマツタケ
部位等 子実体
備 考 —

他名(参考) —
漢字表記・生薬名等 姫松茸（ヒメマツタケ）
Name (Romaji) AGARIKUSU
Other name (s) (Romaji) AGARIKUSU・BURAZEI／HIMEMATSUTAKE
学名 *Agaricus blazei* Murrill
科名 Agaricaceae（ハラタケ科）
英名 agaricus
Part of use fruit body
Note 1 —
Note 2 —
注 —

名 称 **アギタケ**

他名等 阿魏茸
部位等 子実体
備 考 —

他名(参考) —
漢字表記・生薬名等 阿魏茸（アギタケ）
Name (Romaji) AGITAKE

Other name (s) (Romaji)　AGITAKE
学名　*Pleurotus eryngii* var. *ferulae* (Lanzi) Sacc.
科名　Pleurotaceae (ヒラタケ科)
英名　—
Part of use　fruit body
Note 1　—
Note 2　—
注　—

名　称　**アキノキリンソウ***

他名等　—
部位等　全草
備　考　—

他名(参考)　—
漢字表記・生薬名等　秋の麒麟草(アキノキリンソウ)、泡立草(アワダチソウ)
Name (Romaji)　AKINOKIRINSÔ*
Other name (s) (Romaji)　—
学名　*Solidago virgaurea* var. *asiatica* Nakai*
Solidago japonica Kitam.
Solidago virgaurea L. ssp. *asiatica* Kitam. ex H. Hara
科名　Compositae (キク科)
英名　golden rod / woundwort / Aaron's rod / Japanese goldenrod / virgaurea
Part of use　whole plant
Note 1　—
Note 2　—
注　—

名　称　**アケビ***

他名等　モクツウ
部位等　実
備　考　つる性の茎は「医」

他名(参考)　—
漢字表記・生薬名等　木通・通草(アケビ)、木通(モクツウ)、果実：八月札(ハチガツサツ)、預知子(ヨチシ)
Name (Romaji)　AKEBI*
Other name (s) (Romaji)　MOKUTSÛ
学名　*Akebia quinata* (Thunb. ex Houtt.) Decne.*
Rajania quinata Thunb. ex Houtt.
科名　Lardizabalaceae (アケビ科)
英名　chocolate vine / five leaf akebia / akebia
Part of use　fruit
Note 1　vine stem：drug category
Note 2　—
注　—

名　称　**アサ***

他名等　—
部位等　発芽防止処理されている種子
備　考　発芽防止処理されていない種子は「医」

他名(参考)　タイマ(大麻)、オノミ(苧実)、アサノミ(麻実)
漢字表記・生薬名等　麻(アサ)、麻子仁(マシニン)、火麻仁(カマニン)、大麻仁(タイマニン)
Name (Romaji)　ASA*
Other name (s) (Romaji)　—
学名　*Cannabis sativa* L.*
Cannabis sativa L. ssp. *sativa**
科名　Cannabidaceae (アサ科)
英名　chingma / hemp / linen / Indian hemp / marijuana
Part of use　seed treated for prevention of germination
Note 1　seed not treated for prevention of germination：drug category
Note 2　—
注　—

名　称　**アサガオ***

他名等　—
部位等　葉・花
備　考　種子は「医」

他名(参考)　—
漢字表記・生薬名等　朝顔(アサガオ)、牽牛子(ケンゴシ)
Name (Romaji)　ASAGAO*
Other name (s) (Romaji)　—
学名　*Ipomoea nil* (L.) Roth*
Pharbitis nil (L.) Choisy*
Convolvulus nil L.
科名　Convolvulaceae (ヒルガオ科)
英名　morning glory / white-edge morning glory / Japanese morning glory
Part of use　leaf, flower
Note 1　seed：drug category
Note 2　—
注　—

名　称　**アサツキ**

他名等　—
部位等　茎葉・鱗茎
備　考　—

他名(参考)　イトネギ（糸葱）、エゾネギ（蝦夷葱）、センボンワケギ（千本分葱）
漢字表記・生薬名等　浅葱（アサツキ）
Name (Romaji)　ASATSUKI
Other name (s) (Romaji)　—
学名　*Allium ledebourianum* Roem. et Schult.
Allium schoenoprasum L. var. *foliosm* Regel
科名　Liliaceae（ユリ科）
英名　chive / asatsuki
Part of use　stem and leaf, bulb
Note 1　—
Note 2　"茎葉（stem-leaf）in the item of "Part of use" written in Japanese should be replaced by "茎・葉（stem and leaf）".
注　「部位等」の "茎葉" は "茎・葉"。

名　称　**アシ***

他名等　ヨシ
部位等　全草（根茎を除く）
備　考　根茎は「医」

他名(参考)　—
漢字表記・生薬名等　葦・蘆（アシ）、葭（ヨシ）
Name (Romaji)　ASHI*
Other name (s) (Romaji)　YOSHI
学名　*Phragmites australis* (Cav.) Trin. ex Steud.*
Phragmites communis Trin.*
科名　Gramineae（イネ科）
英名　common reed / reed grass / reed / phragmites
Part of use　whole plant (except rhizome)
Note 1　rhizome：drug category
Note 2　—
注　—

名　称　**アジサイ**

他名等　シヨウカ／ハチセンカ
部位等　全草
備　考　—

他名(参考)　シチヘンゲ（七変化）
漢字表記・生薬名等　紫陽花（シヨウカ、アジサイ）、八仙花（ハチセンカ、アジサイ）
Name (Romaji)　AJISAI
Other name (s) (Romaji)　SHIYÔKA／HACHISENKA
学名　*Hydrangea macrophylla* (Thunb. ex J. Murr.) Ser. f. *macrophylla*
Viburnum macrophyllum Thunb.
Hydrangea hortensis Sm.
科名　Saxifragaceae（ユキノシタ科）
英名　hydrangea / common hydrangea / Japanese hydrangea
Part of use　whole plant
Note 1　—
Note 2　—
注　—

名　称　**アシタバ**

他名等　—
部位等　葉
備　考　—

他名(参考)　アシタグサ（明日草）
漢字表記・生薬名等　明日葉（アシタバ）、明日草（アシタグサ）
Name (Romaji)　ASHITABA
Other name (s) (Romaji)　—
学名　*Angelica keiskei* (Miq.) Koidz.
Angelica utilis Makino
科名　Umbelliferae（セリ科）
英名　angelica / Keiske angelica
Part of use　leaf
Note 1　—
Note 2　—
注　—

名　称　**アシドフィルス菌**

他名等　—
部位等　菌体
備　考　—

他名(参考)　ニュウサンキン（乳酸菌）
漢字表記・生薬名等　乳酸桿菌（ニュウサンカンキン）
Name (Romaji)　ASHIDOFIRUSU-KIN
Other name (s) (Romaji)　—
学名　*Lactobacillus acidophilus*
科名　Lactobacillaceae（乳酸桿菌科）
英名　lactobacillus acidophilus
Part of use　mycelium
Note 1　—
Note 2　ASHIDOFIRUSU-KIN is icluded in NYÛSAN-

KIN. NYÛSAN-KIN is also listed in the item of "Name".
注　アシドフィルス菌は別項の乳酸菌に含まれる。

名　称　アズキ*

他名等　セキショウズ
部位等　種子
備　考　—

他名(参考)　—
漢字表記・生薬名等　小豆（アズキ）、赤小豆（セキショウズ）
Name (Romaji)　AZUKI*
Other name (s) (Romaji)　SEKISHÔZU
学名　*Vigna angularis* (Willd.) Ohwi et Ohashi*
Azukia angularis (Willd.) Ohwi
Phaseolus radiatus L. var. *aurea* Prain
Dolichos angularis Willd.
科名　Leguminosae（マメ科）
英名　adzuki bean / aduki bean
Part of use　seed
Note 1　—
Note 2　—
注　—

名　称　アスナロ

他名等　—
部位等　葉
備　考　—

他名(参考)　ヒノキアスナロ（檜翌檜）
漢字表記・生薬名等　翌檜（アスナロ）、檜葉（ヒバ）
Name (Romaji)　ASUNARO
Other name (s) (Romaji)　—
学名　*Thujopsis dolabrata* (L.f.) Sieb. et Zucc.
Thujopsis dolabrata (L.f.) Sieb. et Zucc. var. *hondae* Makino
科名　Cupressaceae（ヒノキ科）
英名　asunaro / false arborvitae / hiba arbovitae / hiba
Part of use　leaf
Note 1　—
Note 2　—
注　—

名　称　アセロラ*

他名等　バルバドスサクラ
部位等　果実
備　考　—

他名(参考)　バルバドスチェリー
漢字表記・生薬名等　—
Name (Romaji)　ASERORA*
Other name (s) (Romaji)　BARUBADOSUSAKURA
学名　*Malpighia punicifolia* L.*
Malpighia glabra L.*
Malpighia emarginata Sésse et Moç. ex DC.*
科名　Malpighiaceae（キントラノオ科）
英名　acerola / Barbados cherry / West Indian cherry / Puertorican cherry
Part of use　fruit
Note 1　—
Note 2　—
注　—

名　称　アセンヤク*

他名等　ガンビール
部位等　葉及び若枝の乾燥水製エキス
備　考　—

他名(参考)　ホウジチャ（方児茶）
漢字表記・生薬名等　阿仙薬（アセンヤク）、孩児茶（ガイジチャ）
Name (Romaji)　ASEN'YAKU*
Other name (s) (Romaji)　GANBÎRU
学名　*Uncaria gambir* (W. Hunt.) Roxb.*
科名　Rubiaceae（アカネ科）
英名　cube gambir / gambir / brown cutch / pale catechu / white cutch
Part of use　dried extract with water of leaf and branch
Note 1　—
Note 2　—
注　—

名　称　アッケシソウ

他名等　—
部位等　全草
備　考　—

他名(参考)　サンゴソウ／ヤチサンゴ／ハママツ
漢字表記・生薬名等　厚岸草（アッケシイソウ）、珊瑚草（サンゴソウ）、谷地珊瑚（ヤチサンゴ）

Name (Romaji)　AKKESHISÔ
Other name (s) (Romaji)　—
学名　*Salicornia europaea* L.
Salicornia herbacea L.
科名　Chenopodiaceae（アカザ科）
英名　samphire / slender glasswort / saltwort / glasswort / crab grass / pickle plant
Part of use　whole plant
Note 1　—
Note 2　—
注　—

名　称　**アップルミント**

他名等　ラウンドリーミント
部位等　葉
備　考　—

他名（参考）　—
漢字表記・生薬名等　円葉薄荷（マルバハッカ）
Name (Romaji)　APPURUMINTO
Other name (s) (Romaji)　RAUNDORÎMINTO
学名　*Mentha suaveolens* Ehrh.
Mentha rotundifolia Hudson (Lamiac.)
Mentha rotundifolia auct. non (L.) Huds.
科名　Labiatae（シソ科）
英名　round-leaved mint / apple mint
Part of use　leaf
Note 1　—
Note 2　—
注　—

名　称　**アニス***

他名等　ピンピネラ
部位等　果実・種子・種子油・根
備　考　—

他名（参考）　—
漢字表記・生薬名等　茴芹（ウイキン）、欧茴香（オウウイキョウ）
Name (Romaji)　ANISU*
Other name (s) (Romaji)　PINPINERA
学名　*Pimpinella anisum* L.*
Anisum vulgare Gaertn.*
Anism officinarum Moench
科名　Umbelliferae（セリ科）
英名　anise / aniseed / anis seed / sweet cumin
Part of use　fruit, seed, seed oil, root
Note 1　—
Note 2　—
注　—

名　称　**アファニゾメノン**

他名等　—
部位等　全藻
備　考　—

他名（参考）　シアノバクテリア
漢字表記・生薬名等　—
Name (Romaji)　AFANIZOMENON
Other name (s) (Romaji)　—
学名　*Aphanizomenon* A. Morren ex Bornet et Flahault
Aphanizomenon flos-aquae Ralfs ex Bornet et Flahault
科名　Nostocaceae（ネンジュモ科）
英名　blue-green algae / cyanobacteria
Part of use　whole algae
Note 1　—
Note 2　AFANIZOMENON is one of blue-green algae.
注　アファニゾメノンは藍藻類の一種。

名　称　**アフリカマンゴノキ**

他名等　オボノ／アポン（種子）／ティカナッツ／ブッシュマンゴー／ワイルドマンゴー
部位等　種子
備　考　—

他名（参考）　—
漢字表記・生薬名等　—
Name (Romaji)　AFURIKAMANGONOKI
Other name (s) (Romaji)　OBONO／APON (SHUSHI)／TIKANATTSU／BUSSHUMANGÔ／WAIRUDOMANGÔ
学名　*Irvingia gabonensis* (Aubry-Lecomt ex O'Rorke) Baill.
Irvingia barteri Hook. f.
科名　Irvingiaceae（ニガキ科）
英名　wild mango / African mango / African wild mango / bush mango / dika / dikanut / dikabread tree / ogbono / rainy season bush-mango / sweet bush-mango
Part of use　seed
Note 1　—
Note 2　—
注　—

名　称　**アボガド***

他名等　—
部位等　果実・葉
備　考　—

他名(参考)　ワニナシ（鰐梨）
漢字表記・生薬名等　油梨（アボカド）
Name(Romaji)　ABOGADO*
Other name(s) (Romaji)　—
学名　*Persea americana* Mill.*
Persea gratissima Gaertn.*
Laurus persea L.*
科名　Lauraceae（クスノキ科）
英名　avocado / alligator pear / butter pear / butter fruit / aguacate
Part of use　fruit, leaf
Note 1　—
Note 2　ABOKADO is the KATAKANA notation based on the English general name.
注　英語名に基づくカタカナ表記は、アボカドとなる。

名　称　**アマ***

他名等　アマシ／アマニン／アマニ油
部位等　種子・種子油
備　考　—

他名(参考)　ゴマシ（胡麻子）
漢字表記・生薬名等　亜麻（アマ）、亜麻仁（アマニン）、亜麻子（アマシ）
Name(Romaji)　AMA*
Other name(s) (Romaji)　AMASHI／AMANIN／AMANI-YU
学名　*Linum usitatissimum* L.*
科名　Linaceae（アマ科）
英名　linum / flax / linseed
Part of use　seed, seed oil
Note 1　—
Note 2　—
注　—

名　称　**アマチャ**

他名等　—
部位等　枝先・葉
備　考　—

他名(参考)　—
漢字表記・生薬名等　甘茶（アマチャ）
Name(Romaji)　AMACHA
Other name(s) (Romaji)　—
学名　*Hydrangea macrophylla* Seringe var. *thunbergii* Makino
Hydrangea serrata Seringe var. *thunbergii* Sugimoto
Hydrangea macrophylla Seringe var. *oamacha* Makino
科名　Saxifragaceae（ユキノシタ科）
英名　sweet tea / sweet hydrangea
Part of use　tip of branch, leaf
Note 1　—
Note 2　—
注　—

名　称　**アマチャヅル***

他名等　コウコラン
部位等　全草
備　考　—

他名(参考)　—
漢字表記・生薬名等　甘茶蔓（アマチャヅル）、七葉胆（シチヨウタン）、紋股藍（コウコラン）
Name(Romaji)　AMACHAZURU*
Other name(s) (Romaji)　KÔKORAN
学名　*Gynostemma pentaphyllum* (Thunb.) Makino*
科名　Cucurbitaceae（ウリ科）
英名　sweet tea vine / gynostemma / blue ginseng / sweet-tea vine
Part of use　whole plant
Note 1　—
Note 2　—
注　—

名　称　**アマナ**

他名等　サンジコ
部位等　鱗茎
備　考　—

他名(参考)　コウジコ（光慈姑）、ムギグワイ（麦慈姑）
漢字表記・生薬名等　甘菜（アマナ）、山慈姑（サンジコ）
Name(Romaji)　AMANA
Other name(s) (Romaji)　SANJIKO
学名　*Amana edulis* (Miq.) Honda
Tulipa edulis (Miq.) Bak.
科名　Liliaceae（ユリ科）
英名　shan tzu ku / amana
Part of use　bulb
Note 1　—

Note 2 —
注 —

名 称 **アメリカサンショウ***

他名等 —
部位等 全草
備 考 —

他名(参考) —
漢字表記・生薬名等 アメリカ山椒(アメリカサンショウ)
Name(Romaji) AMERIKASANSHÔ*
Other name(s) (Romaji) —
学名 *Zanthoxylum americanum* Mill.*
科名 Rutaceae(ミカン科)
英名 prickly ash / northen prickly ash / toothache tree
Part of use whole plant
Note 1 —
Note 2 —
注 —

名 称 **アメリカニンジン***

他名等 カントンニンジン/セイヨウジン/セイヨウニンジン/Panax quinquefolium
部位等 根茎・根・茎・葉
備 考 —

他名(参考) —
漢字表記・生薬名等 広東人参(カントンニンジン)、西洋人参(セイヨウニンジン)、西洋参(セイヨウジン)
Name(Romaji) AMERIKANINJIN*
Other name(s) (Romaji) KANTONNINJIN/SEIYÔJIN/SEIYÔNINJIN
学名 *Panax quinquefolius* L.*
科名 Araliaceae(ウコギ科)
英名 American ginseng
Part of use rhizome, root, stem, leaf
Note 1 —
Note 2 —
注 —

名 称 **アメリカホドイモ**

他名等 —
部位等 塊根
備 考 —

他名(参考) ポテイトウ・ビーン
漢字表記・生薬名等 アメリカ塊芋(アメリカホドイモ)
Name(Romaji) AMERIKAHODOIMO
Other name(s) (Romaji) —
学名 *Apios americana* Medik.
Apios tuberosa Moench
Glycine apios L.
科名 Leguminosae(マメ科)
英名 ground nut / groundnut / potato bean
Part of use root tuber
Note 1 —
Note 2 —
注 —

名 称 **アラガオ**

他名等 —
部位等 葉
備 考 —

他名(参考) —
漢字表記・生薬名等 —
Name(Romaji) ARAGAO
Other name(s) (Romaji) —
学名 *Premna odorata* Blanco
科名 Verbenaceae(クマツヅラ科)
英名 fragrant premna / alagaw / alagau / argaw
Part of use leaf
Note 1 —
Note 2 ARAGAO is the general Tagalog name. Tagalog is the Filipino official language.
注 アラガオはタガログ語(フィリピン公用語)の名前である。

名 称 **アラビアゴム***

他名等 アラビアゴムノキ
部位等 乾燥ゴム質(枝・葉)
備 考 —

他名(参考) —
漢字表記・生薬名等 —
Name(Romaji) ARABIAGOMU*
Other name(s) (Romaji) ARABIAGOMUNOKI
学名 *Acacia senegal* (L.) Willd.*
Acacia verek Guill. et Perr.*
Mimosa senegal L.
科名 Leguminosae(マメ科)
英名 gum arabic / gum arabic tree / thorny acacia / gum Senegal / Sudan gum Arabic
Part of use dried gum (branch, leaf)

Note 1 —
Note 2 —
注 —

名 称 **アラメ**

他名等 —
部位等 全草
備 考 —

他名(参考) —
漢字表記･生薬名等 荒布・骨海藻・阿良米（アラメ）
Name(Romaji) ARAME
Other name(s) (Romaji) —
学名 *Eisenia bicyclis* (Kjellman) Setch.
科名 Lessoniaceae（レッソニア科）
英名 arame / kajimi / sagarame / eisenia / aramu
Part of use whole algae
Note 1 —
Note 2 ARAME is one of algae.
注 アラメは海藻の一種。

名 称 **アリタソウ***

他名等 ドケイガイ
部位等 茎・葉
備 考 —

他名(参考) ケアリタソウ（毛有田草）
漢字表記･生薬名等 有田草（アリタソウ）、土荊芥（ドケイガイ）
Name(Romaji) ARITASÔ*
Other name(s) (Romaji) DOKEIGAI
学名 *Chenopodium ambrosioides* L.*
Chenopodium anthelminticum L.*
Ambrina ambrosioides (L.) Spach
科名 Chenopodiaceae（アカザ科）
英名 wormseed / epazote / American wormseed / Mexican tea / Indian wormseed
Part of use stem, leaf
Note 1 —
Note 2 —
注 —

名 称 **アルテア***

他名等 ビロードアオイ／マーシュマロウ
部位等 根・葉
備 考 —

他名(参考) ウスベニタチアオイ（薄紅立葵）
漢字表記･生薬名等 薄紅立葵（ウスベニタチアオイ）
Name(Romaji) ARUTEA*
Other name(s) (Romaji) BIRÔDOAOI／MÂSHUMARÔ
学名 *Althaea officinalis* L.*
科名 Malvaceae（アオイ科）
英名 althea / marsh mallow / marshmallow / althaea
Part of use root, leaf
Note 1 —
Note 2 —
注 —

名 称 **アルファルファ***

他名等 ウマゴヤシ／ムラサキウマゴヤシ
部位等 全草
備 考 —

他名(参考) —
漢字表記･生薬名等 紫苜蓿（シモクシュク）、紫馬肥（ムラサキウマゴヤシ）
Name(Romaji) ARUFARUFA*
Other name(s) (Romaji) UMAGOYASHI／MURASAKI-UMAGOYASHI
学名 *Medicago sativa* L.*
科名 Leguminosae（マメ科）
英名 alfalfa / blue alfalfa / lucerne
Part of use whole plant
Note 1 —
Note 2 —
注 —

名 称 **アロエ***

他名等 キュラソーアロエ／ケープアロエ
部位等 根・葉肉
備 考 葉の液汁は「医」

他名(参考) —
漢字表記･生薬名等 蘆薈（ロカイ）
Name(Romaji) AROE*
Other name(s) (Romaji) KYURASÔAROE／KÊPU-AROE
学名 *Aloe vera* (L.) Burm. f.*

Aloe africana Mill.
Aloe barbadensis Mill.*
Aloe ferox Mill.*

科名 Liliaceae（ユリ科）

英名 aloe / aloe vera / barbados aloe / Curaçao aloe / true aloe / Cape aloe

Part of use root, leaf inner gel

Note 1 juice of leaf：drug category

Note 2 —

注 —

名　称 **アンゼリカ***

他名等 **ガーデンアンゼリカ**

部位等 全草

備　考 —

他名(参考) —

漢字表記・生薬名等 西洋当帰（セイヨウトウキ）、ヨーロッパ当帰（ヨーロッパトウキ）

Name(Romaji) ANZERIKA*

Other name(s) (Romaji) GÂDEN'ANZERIKA

学名 *Angelica archangelica* L.*
Angelica officinalis Moench*
Archangelica officinalis (Moench) Hoffm.*

科名 Umbelliferae（セリ科）

英名 angelica / arcangel / European angelica / garden angelica

Part of use whole plant

Note 1 —

Note 2 —

注 —

名　称 **アンソクコウノキ***

他名等 —

部位等 樹脂

備　考 —

他名(参考) —

漢字表記・生薬名等 安息香（アンソクコウ）

Name(Romaji) ANSOKUKÔNOKI*

Other name(s) (Romaji) —

学名 *Styrax benzoin* Dryand.*

科名 Styracaceae（エゴノキ科）

英名 styrax / Sumatra benzoin / Benjamin gum / storax / gum benzoin / gum Benjamin / Siam benzoin / Sumatra benzoin / benzoin tree / Benjamin tree

Part of use resin

Note 1 —

Note 2 —

注 —

名　称 **アンティリス・ブルネラリア**

他名等 —

部位等 根・葉・花

備　考 —

他名(参考) アンティリス・ウルネラリア、クマノアシツメクサ、ワタゲツメクサ

漢字表記・生薬名等 —

Name(Romaji) ANTIRISU・BURUNERARIA

Other name(s) (Romaji) —

学名 *Anthyllis vulneraria* L.

科名 Leguminosae（マメ科）

英名 kidney vetch / spring vetch / lady's finger / wounder wort

Part of use root, leaf, flower

Note 1 —

Note 2 —

注 —

名　称 **イグサ***

他名等 **イ／トウシンソウ／Juncus effusus**

部位等 地上部の熱水抽出（100℃ 8分以上又は同等以上の方法）後の残渣

備　考 全草は「医」

他名(参考) —

漢字表記・生薬名等 藺草（イグサ）、藺（イ）、燈芯草（トウシンソウ）

Name(Romaji) IGUSA*

Other name(s) (Romaji) I／TÔSHINSÔ

学名 *Juncus effusus* L.*
Juncus effusus L. var. *decipiens* Buchenau
Juncus decipiens (Buchenau) Nakai

科名 Juncaceae（イグサ科）

英名 mat rush / common rush / soft rush / bul rush / lump rush

Part of use residue of boiled water extraction of aerial part (longer than 8 minutes at 100℃ or equivalent methods)

Note 1 whole plant except the edible part of this plant as non-drug：drug category

Note 2 —

注 —

名 称　イクリニン*

他名等　コニワザクラ／チョウコウイクリ／ニワウメ
部位等　種子・根
備　考　—

他名(参考)　—
漢字表記・生薬名等　郁李仁（イクリニン）、庭梅（ニワウメ）
Name (Romaji)　IKURININ*
Other name(s) (Romaji)　KONIWAZAKURA／CHÔKÔIKURI／NIWAUME
学名　*Prunus japonica* Thunb.*
Cerasus japonica (Thunb.) Loisel.*
Prunus humilis Bunge
科名　Rosaceae（バラ科）
英名　Korean cherry / Japanese bush cherry / dwarf flowering cherry / flowering almond / niwa-ume
Part of use　seed, root
Note 1　—
Note 2　IKURININ is the name of traditional Japanese herbal medicine and its Japanese name is KONIWAZAKURA or NIWAUME. It is also called CHÔKÔIKURI.
注　イクリニンは生薬名である。和名はコニワザクラ、ニワウメ。チョウコウイクリと呼ばれることもある。

名 称　イズイ*

他名等　アマドコロ／ギョクチク
部位等　根茎
備　考　—

他名(参考)　—
漢字表記・生薬名等　萎蕤（イズイ）、玉竹（ギョクチク）、甘野老（アマドコロ）
Name (Romaji)　IZUI*
Other name(s) (Romaji)　AMADOKORO／GYOKUCHIKU
学名　*Polygonatum officinale* All.*
Polygonatum odoratum (Mill.) Druce*
Convallaria odorata Mill.
Polygonatum odoratum (Mill.) Durce var. *pluriflorum* (Miq.) Ohwi
科名　Liliaceae（ユリ科）
英名　dwarf Solomon's seal / aromatic Solomon's seal / fragrant Solomon's seal
Part of use　rhizome
Note 1　—
Note 2　—
注　—

名 称　イソマツ

他名等　ウコンイソマツ
部位等　全木
備　考　—

他名(参考)　キバナイソマツ（黄花磯松）
漢字表記・生薬名等　磯松（イソマツ）、鬱金磯松（ウコンイソマツ）
Name (Romaji)　ISOMATSU
Other name(s) (Romaji)　UKON'ISOMATSU
学名　*Limonium wrightii* (Hance) O. Kuntze
Limonium wrightii (Hance) O. Kuntze f. *arbusculum* (Maxim.) Hatusima
Limonum wrightii (Hance) O. Kuntze var. *wrightii*
科名　Plumbaginaceae（イソマツ科）
英名　Japanese limonium / limonium
Part of use　whole tree
Note 1　—
Note 2　—
注　—

名 称　イタドリ*

他名等　—
部位等　若芽
備　考　根茎は「医」

他名(参考)　—
漢字表記・生薬名等　虎杖（コジョウ、イタドリ）
Name (Romaji)　ITADORI*
Other name(s) (Romaji)　—
学名　*Polygonum cuspidatum* Sieb. et Zucc.*
Reynoutria japonica Houtt.
Pleuropterus cuspidatus (Sieb. et Zucc.) Gross
科名　Polygonaceae（タデ科）
英名　Japanese knotweed / Japanese fleeceflower / giant knotweed / flowering bamboo / Mexican bamboo
Part of use　sprout
Note 1　rhizome：drug category
Note 2　—
注　—

名　称　**イチイ**

他名等　アララギ
部位等　果実
備　考　枝・心材・葉は「医」

他名(参考)　オンコ［アイヌ語起源］
漢字表記・生薬名等　一位（イチイ）、蘭葱（アララギ）、紫杉（シサン：イチイの枝や葉）
Name (Romaji)　ICHII
Other name (s) (Romaji)　ARARAGI
学名　*Taxus cuspidata* Sieb. et Zucc.
Taxus baccata ssp. *cuspida* (Sieb. et Zucc.) Pilg.
Taxus baccata var. *microcarpa* Trautv.
Taxus sieboldii hort.
科名　Taxaceae（イチイ科）
英名　Japanese yew
Part of use　fruit
Note 1　branch, heart wood and leaf : drug category
Note 2　—
注　—

名　称　**イチジク***

他名等　—
部位等　花托・根・葉
備　考　—

他名(参考)　トウガキ（唐柿）、ナンバンガキ（南蛮柿）
漢字表記・生薬名等　無花果（ムカカ、イチジク）、無花果根（ムカカコン）、無花果葉（ムカカヨウ）
Name (Romaji)　ICHIJIKU*
Other name (s) (Romaji)　—
学名　*Ficus carica* L.*
科名　Moraceae（クワ科）
英名　fig / sycamore / common fig / fig tree
Part of use　receptacle, root, leaf
Note 1　—
Note 2　—
注　—

名　称　**イチビ***

他名等　—
部位等　種子・葉
備　考　—

他名(参考)　ボウマ（苘麻）、キリアサ（桐麻）、ホクチガラ（火口ガラ）
漢字表記・生薬名等　冬葵子（トウキシ：種子）、苘麻（ケイマ）
Name (Romaji)　ICHIBI*
Other name (s) (Romaji)　—
学名　*Abutilon avicennae* Gaertn.（イチビ）
Abutilon theophrasti Medik.（イチビ）
Malva verticillata L.*（フユアオイ）
科名　Malvaceae（アオイ科）
英名　China jute / Chinese jute / button weed / velvet weed / butter-print / Indian mallow / pie-marker / velvet-leaf
Part of use　seed, leaf
Note 1　—
Note 2　Nowadays it is said that all of TÔKISHI sold in China is KEIMASHI, seed of ICHIBI. TÔKISHI is also listed in the item of “Name”.
注　今日の中国では、トウキシ（冬葵子）として売られているのは、すべてケイマシ（イチビの種子）であるという。トウキシは別項に記載されている。

名　称　**イチヤクソウ***

他名等　ロクテイソウ／Pyrolaceae japonica
部位等　全草
備　考　—

他名(参考)　ロクジュソウ（鹿寿草：イチヤクソウの全草）
漢字表記・生薬名等　一薬草（イチヤクソウ）、鹿蹄草（ロクテイソウ）
Name (Romaji)　ICHIYAKUSO*
Other name (s) (Romaji)　ROKUTEISÔ
学名　*Pyrola japonica* Klenze
Pyrola rotundifolia L.*
Pyrola asarifolia Michx. ssp. *asarifolia**
Pyrola rotundifolia ssp. *asarifolia* (Michx.) A. et G. Löve*
Pyrola incarnata Fisch. var. *japonica* (Klenze) Koidz.
科名　Pyrolaceae（イチヤクソウ科）
英名　liver-leaf wintergreen / pink wintergreen
Part of use　whole plant
Note 1　—
Note 2　Pyrolaceae japonica written in the item of “Other names” should be replaced by “*Pyrola japonica*”. ROKUTEISÔ also in the item of “Other names” is *Pyrola rotundifolia* native to China.
注　イチヤクソウの「他名等」に記載されたPyrolaceae japonicaは*Pyrola japonica*の誤りである。「他名等」のロクテイソウは中国原産の*Pyrola rotundifolia*である。

名　称　**イチョウ***

他名等　**ギンナン／ハクカ**
部位等　種子・葉
備　考　—

他名(参考)　—
漢字表記･生薬名等　公孫樹・鴨脚樹（イチョウ）、銀杏葉（イチョウヨウ）、白果（ハクカ）
Name (Romaji)　ICHÔ*
Other name (s) (Romaji)　GINNAN／HAKUKA
学名　*Ginkgo biloba* L.*
科名　Ginkgoaceae（イチョウ科）
英名　ginkgo / gingko / maidenhair tree
Part of use　seed, leaf
Note 1　—
Note 2　—
注　—

名　称　**イナゴマメ***

他名等　**アルガロバ／キャロブ**
部位等　果肉・葉・豆
備　考　—

他名(参考)　ヨハンパンノキ
漢字表記･生薬名等　蝗豆（イナゴマメ）
Name (Romaji)　INAGOMAME*
Other name (s) (Romaji)　ARUGAROBA／KYAROBU
学名　*Ceratonia siliqua* L.*
科名　Leguminosae（マメ科）
英名　carob / locust bean / St. John's bread / karoub / algaroba / algarroba bean / caroubier
Part of use　sarcocarp, leaf, bean
Note 1　—
Note 2　—
注　—

名　称　**イヌサンショウ***

他名等　—
部位等　果実・根
備　考　—

他名(参考)　—
漢字表記･生薬名等　犬山椒（イヌザンショウ）
Name (Romaji)　INUSANSHÔ*
Other name (s) (Romaji)　—
学名　*Zanthoxylum schinifolium* Sieb. et Zucc.*
　Fagara schinifolium (Seib. et Zucc.) Engl.
　Fagara mantchurica
科名　Rutaceae（ミカン科）
英名　Sichuan pepper / Sichuan peppercorn
Part of use　fruit, root
Note 1　—
Note 2　INUSANSHÔ is incorrect. The collect name is INUZANSHÔ.
注　イヌサンショウは、通常、イヌザンショウと呼ばれる。

名　称　**イヌナズナ**

他名等　—
部位等　種子
備　考　—

他名(参考)　—
漢字表記･生薬名等　犬薺（イヌナズナ）、葶藶子（テイレキシ）
Name (Romaji)　INUNAZUNA
Other name (s) (Romaji)　—
学名　*Draba nemorosa* L.
　Draba nemorosa L. var. *hebecarpa* Ledeb.
科名　Cruciferae（アブラナ科）
英名　draba / Japanese draba
Part of use　seed
Note 1　—
Note 2　—
注　—

名　称　**イヌノフグリ**

他名等　—
部位等　全草
備　考　—

他名(参考)　ジキン（地錦）
漢字表記･生薬名等　婆婆納（ババノウ）
Name (Romaji)　INUNOFUGURI
Other name (s) (Romaji)　—
学名　*Veronica didyma* Tenore var. *lilacina* (Hara) Yamazaki
科名　Scrophulariaceae（ゴマノハグサ科）
英名　grey field-speedwell / Japanese speedwell
Part of use　whole plant
Note 1　—
Note 2　—
注　—

名　称　イヌハッカ*

他名等　チクマハッカ
部位等　葉・花穂
備　考　—

他名(参考)　—
漢字表記・生薬名等　白花荊芥（ビャッカケイガイ）、犬薄荷（イヌハッカ）、筑摩薄荷（チクマハッカ）
Name (Romaji)　INUHAKKA*
Other name (s) (Romaji)　CHIKUMAHAKKA
学名　*Nepeta cataria* L.*
Cataria vulgaris Moench
科名　Labiatae（シソ科）
英名　catnip / catnep / catmint / common nep
Part of use　leaf, florescence
Note 1　—
Note 2　—
注　—

名　称　イヌホオズキ*

他名等　リュウキ
部位等　全草
備　考　—

他名(参考)　—
漢字表記・生薬名等　竜葵（リュウキ）、竜葵子（リュウキシ）、犬酸漿（イヌホオズキ）
Name (Romaji)　INUHÔZUKI*
Other name (s) (Romaji)　RYÛKI
学名　*Solanum nigrum* L.*
Solanum incertum Dunal.*
Solanum rubrum auct. non L.*
科名　Solanaceae（ナス科）
英名　black nightshade / makoi / wonderberry
Part of use　whole plant
Note 1　—
Note 2　Caution：INUHÔZUKI contains toxic alkaloids such as solanine.
注　ソラニンなどの有毒なアルカロイドを含むので注意を要する。

名　称　イネ*

他名等　—
部位等　刈株の二番芽
備　考　—

他名(参考)　—
漢字表記・生薬名等　稲（イネ）
Name (Romaji)　INE*
Other name (s) (Romaji)　—
学名　*Oryza sativa* L.*
科名　Gramineae（イネ科）
英名　paddy / rice / rice plant / rice leaf
Part of use　second sprout after reaping
Note 1　—
Note 2　—
注　—

名　称　イブキジャコウソウ*

他名等　—
部位等　葉
備　考　—

他名(参考)　セルピウムソウ
漢字表記・生薬名等　伊吹麝香草（イブキジャコウソウ）、百里香（ヒャクリコウ）
Name (Romaji)　IBUKIJAKÔSÔ*
Other name (s) (Romaji)　—
学名　*Thymus serpyllum* L.*
Thymus serpyllum L. ssp. *quinquecostatus* (Celak.) Kitam.
Thymus quinquecostatus Celak.
科名　Labiatae（シソ科）
英名　wild thyme / creeping thyme / mother-of-thyme / lemon thyme
Part of use　leaf
Note 1　—
Note 2　IBUKIJAKÔSÔ is identical with SERUPIUMUSÔ, but their parts of use are different each other. SERUPIUMSÔ is also listed in the item of "Name".
注　イブキジャコウソウは別項のセルピウムソウと同一。但し、「部位等」の記載が異なっている。

名　称　イボツヅラフジ

他名等　Tinospora crispa
部位等　全草
備　考　—

他名(参考)　—
漢字表記・生薬名等　疣葛藤（イボツヅラフジ）
Name (Romaji)　IBOTSUZURAFUJI
Other name (s) (Romaji)　—
学名　*Tinospora crispa* (L.) Hook. f. et Thoms.
Tinospora tuberculata (Lam.) Hayne

Tinospora rumphii Boerl.
科名 Menispermaceae（ツヅラフジ科）
英名 tinospora
Part of use whole plant
Note 1 —
Note 2 —
注 —

名 称 イラクサ属

他名等 ウルチカソウ／ネットル
部位等 茎・種子・根・葉
備 考 —

他名(参考) —
漢字表記・生薬名等 刺草・蕁麻（イラクサ）
Name (Romaji) IRAKUSA-ZOKU
Other name (s) (Romaji) URUCHIKASÔ／NETTORU
学名 *Urtica* L.（イラクサ属）
Urtica thunbergiana Sieb. et Zucc.
科名 Urticaceae（イラクサ科）
英名 nettle / stinging nettle
Part of use stem, seed, root, leaf
Note 1 —
Note 2 —
注 —

名 称 イレイセン*

他名等 シナボタンヅル
部位等 葉
備 考 根・根茎は「医」

他名(参考) シナセンニンソウ（支那仙人草）、サキシマボタンヅル（先島牡丹蔓）
漢字表記・生薬名等 威霊仙（イレイセン）
Name (Romaji) IREISEN*
Other name (s) (Romaji) SHINABOTANZURU
学名 *Clematis chinensis* Osbeck*
科名 Ranunculaceae（キンポウゲ科）
英名 wei ling xian / Chinese clematis
Part of use leaf
Note 1 root and rhizome：drug category
Note 2 IREISEN is the name of traditional Japanese herbal medicine and several different herbs are used as IREISEN. The scientific name of SHINABOTANZURU written in the "Other names" is described here.
注 イレイセンは生薬名であり、数種の植物がイレイセンとして使用される。本項では「他名等」に記載されたシナボタンヅルの学名を記載した。

名 称 イワタバコ

他名等 —
部位等 全草
備 考 —

他名(参考) イワジシャ（岩萵苣）
漢字表記・生薬名等 岩煙草（イワタバコ）、岩萵苣（イワジシャ）、岩千佐（イワチサ）、苦苣苔（クキョタイ）
Name (Romaji) IWATABAKO
Other name (s) (Romaji) —
学名 *Conandron ramondioides* Sieb. et Zucc.
科名 Gesneriaceae（イワタバコ科）
英名 Japanese gesneria
Part of use whole plant
Note 1 —
Note 2 —
注 —

名 称 イワニガナ

他名等 ジシバリ
部位等 全草
備 考 —

他名(参考) —
漢字表記・生薬名等 岩苦菜（イワニガナ）、菊葉地縛（キクバジシバリ）、地縛（ジシバリ）
Name (Romaji) IWANIGANA
Other name (s) (Romaji) JISHIBARI
学名 *Ixeris stolonifera* A. Gray
科名 Compositae（キク科）
英名 creeping lettuce / creeping ixeris
Part of use whole plant
Note 1 —
Note 2 —
注 —

名 称 イワベンケイ*

他名等 コウケイテン
部位等 全草
備 考 —

他名(参考) —
漢字表記・生薬名等 岩弁慶（イワベンケイ）、紅景天（コウケイテン）

Name (Romaji)　IWABENKEI*
Other name (s) (Romaji)　KÔKEITEN
学名　*Rhodiola rosea* L.*
　　Sedum roseum (L.) Scop.*
科名　Crassulaceae（ベンケイソウ科）
英名　rose root / rose wort / snowdown rose / rhodiola / arctic rose / golden root / rose root / king's crown
Part of use　whole plant
Note 1　—
Note 2　—
注　—

名　称　**インゲンマメ***

他名等　フジマメ
部位等　種子
備　考　—

他名(参考)　サイトウ（菜豆）、サンドマメ（三度豆）、トウササゲ（唐豇）、ゴガツササゲ（五月豇）
漢字表記・生薬名等　隠元豆（インゲンマメ）、藤豆（フジマメ）、白扁豆（ビャクヘンズ）
Name (Romaji)　INGENMAME*
Other name (s) (Romaji)　FUJIMAME
学名　*Phaseolus vulgaris* L.*（インゲンマメ）
　　Lablab purpureus (L.) Sweet*（フジマメ）
　　Dolichos lablab L.*（フジマメ）
科名　Leguminosae（マメ科）
英名　bayo / butter bean / fagiolo / frijol / frijole / haricot / haricot bean / marrow bean / pinto bean / common bean / kidney bean / French bean / green bean / hyacinth bean / bonavit bean / lablab bean
Part of use　seed
Note 1　—
Note 2　INGENMAME and FUJIMAME are different species. FUJIMAME is also written in the item of "Other names" of HENZU.
注　インゲンマメとフジマメは別種。フジマメはヘンズの「他名等」にも記載されている。

名　称　**インスリーナ***

他名等　アニール・トレバドール
部位等　葉
備　考　—

他名(参考)　—
漢字表記・生薬名等　—
Name (Romaji)　INSURÎNA*
Other name (s) (Romaji)　ANÎRU・TOREBADÔRU
学名　*Cissus verticillata* (L.) Nicolson et C.E. Jarvis*
　　Cissus sicyoides L.*
科名　Vitaceae（ブドウ科）
英名　princess vine
Part of use　leaf
Note 1　—
Note 2　—
注　—

名　称　**インドアマチャ**

他名等　—
部位等　葉
備　考　—

他名(参考)　—
漢字表記・生薬名等　印度常山（インドアマチャ）、根：常山（ジョウザン）、葉：蜀漆（ショクシツ）
Name (Romaji)　INDOAMACHA
Other name (s) (Romaji)　—
学名　*Dichroa febrifuga* Lour.
科名　Hydrangeaceae（アジサイ科）
英名　Chinese quinine / fever flower
Part of use　leaf
Note 1　—
Note 2　AMACHA is written in Chines character as "常山（JÔZAN）". INDOAMACHA could be derived from the "印度常山（INDOJÔZAN）".
注　アマチャは常山とも書かれる。インドアマチャは印度常山に由来すると思われる。

名　称　**インドカラタチ***

他名等　ベールフルーツ／ベンガルカラタチ
部位等　果実・樹皮
備　考　—

他名(参考)　—
漢字表記・生薬名等　印度枳（インドカラタチ）
Name (Romaji)　INDOKARATACHI*
Other name (s) (Romaji)　BÊRUFURÛTSU／BENGARU-KARATACHI
学名　*Aegle marmelos* (L.) Correa ex Roxb.*
科名　Rutaceae（ミカン科）
英名　Indian bael / bael tree / bel / Bengal quince / Bengal fruit
Part of use　fruit, bark
Note 1　—
Note 2　INDOKARATACHI is identical with BERUNOKI.
注　インカドカラタチは別項のベルノキと同一。

名　称　**インドナガコショウ***

他名等　ヒハツ
部位等　果穂
備　考　—

他名(参考)　—
漢字表記・生薬名等　印度長胡椒（インドナガコショウ）、蓽茇・蓽撥（ヒハツ）
Name (Romaji)　INDONAGAKOSHÔ*
Other name (s) (Romaji)　HIHATSU
学名　*Piper longum* L.*
科名　Piperaceae（コショウ科）
英名　long pepper / jaborandi pepper / Indian long pepper
Part of use　matured spike
Note 1　—
Note 2　—
注　—

名　称　**インドボダイジュ***

他名等　Ficus religiosa
部位等　樹皮
備　考　—

他名(参考)　—
漢字表記・生薬名等　印度菩提樹（インドボダイジュ）
Name (Romaji)　INDOBODAIJU*
Other name (s) (Romaji)　—
学名　*Ficus religiosa* L.*
科名　Moraceae（クワ科）
英名　sacred fig / Bodhi tree / peepal / peepul / Bo-tree
Part of use　bark
Note 1　—
Note 2　—
注　—

名　称　**インドヤコウボク**

他名等　—
部位等　葉・花
備　考　—

他名(参考)　ヨルソケイ（夜素馨）
漢字表記・生薬名等　印度夜香木（インドヤコウボク）
Name (Romaji)　INDOYAKÔBOKU
Other name (s) (Romaji)　—
学名　*Nyctanthes arbor-tristis* L.
科名　Verbenaceae（クマツヅラ科）
英名　night jasmine / tree of sadness / coral jasmine
Part of use　leaf, flower
Note 1　—
Note 2　—
注　—

名　称　**インペティギノサ***

他名等　—
部位等　全草
備　考　—

他名(参考)　—
漢字表記・生薬名等　—
Name (Romaji)　INPETIGINOSA*
Other name (s) (Romaji)　—
学名　*Tabebuia impetiginosa* (Mart. ex DC.) Standl.*
Tabebuia avellanedae Lorentz ex Griseb.*
Tabebuia heptaphylla (Vell.) Toledo*
Tecoma impetiginosa Mart. ex DC.*
科名　Bignoniaceae（ノウゼンカズラ科）
英名　pau d'arco / ipe roxo / lapacho / taheebo / trumpet tree
Part of use　whole plant
Note 1　—
Note 2　INPETIGINOSA is identical with both of PAUDARUKO and TABEBUIA. But parts of use of INPETIGINOSA is different form those of other two species. The former is whole plant and the latter is bark and leaf, but bark and/or leaf of these trees are commonly used.
注　インペティギノサはパウダルコ及びタベブイアと同一。インペティギノサの「部位等」は全草であるが、タベブイアとパウダルコは“樹皮・葉”とされている。通常は樹皮と葉が使用される。

名　称　**インペラトリア***

他名等　—
部位等　根
備　考　—

他名(参考)　—
漢字表記・生薬名等　—
Name (Romaji)　INPERATORIA*
Other name (s) (Romaji)　—
学名　*Imperatoria ostruthia* L.*
Peucedanum ostruthium (L.) W.D.J. Koch*
科名　Umbelliferae（セリ科）
英名　masterwort

Part of use　root
Note 1　—
Note 2　—
注　—

名　称　**ウイキョウ***

他名等　フェンネル
部位等　果実・種子・根・葉
備　考　—

他名(参考)　—
漢字表記・生薬名等　茴香（ウイキョウ）
Name(Romaji)　UIKYÔ*
Other name(s)(Romaji)　FENNERU*
学名　*Foeniculum vulgare* Mill.*
　Anethum foeniculum L.
　Foeniculum officinale All.
科名　Umbelliferae（セリ科）
英名　fennel
Part of use　fruit, seed, root, leaf
Note 1　—
Note 2　—
注　—

名　称　**ウキヤガラ**

他名等　—
部位等　塊茎
備　考　—

他名(参考)　—
漢字表記・生薬名等　浮矢柄（ウキヤガラ）、三稜（サンリョウ）、荊三稜（ケイサンリョウ）
Name(Romaji)　UKIYAGARA
Other name(s)(Romaji)　—
学名　*Bolboschoenus fluviatilis*（Torr.）T. Koyama ssp. *yagara*（Ohwi）T. Koyama
　Scirpus fluviatilis auct. non（Torr.）A. Gray
　Scirpus yagara Ohwi
　Scirpus maritimus auct. non L.
科名　Cyperaceae（カヤツリグサ科）
英名　river bulrush / Japanese scirpus
Part of use　tuber
Note 1　—
Note 2　—
注　—

名　称　**ウコギ***

他名等　—
部位等　葉
備　考　—

他名(参考)　ゴカ（五加：中国名）
漢字表記・生薬名等　五加（ゴカ）、根皮：五加皮（ゴカヒ）
Name(Romaji)　UKOGI*
Other name(s)(Romaji)　—
学名　*Acanthopanax sieboldianus* Makino
　Acanthopanax pentaphyllus（Sieb. et Zucc.）Marchal
　Acanthopanax gracilistylus W.W. Sm.*
　Eleutherococcus gracilistylus（W.W. Sm.）S.Y. Hu*
科名　Araliaceae（ウコギ科）
英名　eleutherococcus gracilistylus
Part of use　leaf
Note 1　—
Note 2　—
注　—

名　称　**ウコン***

他名等　—
部位等　根茎
備　考　—

他名(参考)　—
漢字表記・生薬名等　鬱金＝宇金（ウコン）（注：日本のウコン（根茎）は、中国の姜黄（キョウオウ））
Name(Romaji)　UKON*
Other name(s)(Romaji)　—
学名　*Curcuma longa* L.*
　Curcuma domestica Valet.*
科名　Zingiberaceae（ショウガ科）
英名　curcuma / turmeric / common turmeric / Indian saffron / yellow ginger
Part of use　rhizome
Note 1　—
Note 2　—
注　—

名 称 ウショウ

他名等 クロモジ／チョウショウ
部位等 幹皮・根皮
備 考 —

他名(参考) —
漢字表記・生薬名等 烏樟（ウショウ）、釣樟（チョウショウ）、黒文字（クロモジ）
Name(Romaji) USHÔ
Other name(s) (Romaji) KUROMOJI／CHÔSHÔ
学名 *Lindera umbellata* Thunb.
Lindera hypoglauca Maxim.
Lindera obtusa Franch. et Sav.
Benzoin thunbergii Sieb. et Zucc.
Benzoin umbellatum (Thunb.) O. Kuntze
科名 Lauraceae（クスノキ科）
英名 lindera / kuromoji
Part of use bark, root bark
Note 1 —
Note 2 —
注 —

名 称 ウスベニアオイ*

他名等 ゼニアオイ
部位等 葉・花
備 考 —

他名(参考) マロー、ゼニバアオイ（銭葉葵）
漢字表記・生薬名等 薄紅葵（ウスベニアオイ）、銭葵（ゼニアオイ）、錦葵葉（キンキヨウ）、錦葵花（キンキカ）
Name(Romaji) USUBENIAOI*
Other name(s) (Romaji) ZENIAOI
学名 *Malva sylvestris* L.*
Malva sylvestris L. var. *mauritiana* (L.) Boiss.
Malva mauritiana L.
Malva neglecta Wallr.*
科名 Malvaceae（アオイ科）
英名 common mallow / blue mallow / high mallow / tall mallow / cheeses / tree mallow / dwarf mallow / malva
Part of use leaf, flower
Note 1 —
Note 2 USUBENIAOI is identical with ZENIAOI. ZENIAOI is also listed in the item of “Name”.
注 ウスベニアオイは別項のゼニアオイと同一。

名 称 ウチワサボテン属*

他名等 ウチワサボテン／フィクスインディカ
部位等 全草
備 考 —

他名(参考) —
漢字表記・生薬名等 団扇仙人掌（ウチワサボテン）
Name(Romaji) UCHIWASABOTEN-ZOKU*
Other name(s) (Romaji) UCHIWASABOTEN／FIKUSUINDIKA
学名 *Opuntia ficus-indica* (L.) Mill.*
Opuntia ficus-indica (L.) Mill. var. *saboten* Makino
科名 Cactaceae（サボテン科）
英名 opuntia / Indian fig / cactus pear / cardon pear (fruit) / prickly pear / nopal (leaf) / tuna (fruit)
Part of use whole plant
Note 1 —
Note 2 —
注 —

名 称 ウチワヤシ*

他名等 パルミラヤシ
部位等 全草
備 考 —

他名(参考) オウギヤシ（扇椰子）
漢字表記・生薬名等 団扇椰子（ウチワヤシ）
Name(Romaji) UCHIWAYASHI*
Other name(s) (Romaji) PARUMIRAYASHI
学名 *Borassus flabellifer* L.*
科名 Palmae（ヤシ科）
英名 palmyra palm
Part of use whole plant
Note 1 —
Note 2 —
注 —

名 称 ウド

他名等 Aralia cordata
部位等 軟化茎
備 考 根茎は「医」、シシウド（Angelica pubescens／Angelica bisserata）の根茎・軟化茎は「非医」

他名(参考) ドクカツ（独活）、キョウカツ（羌活）、ワキョウカツ（和羌活）
漢字表記・生薬名等 独活（ウド）
Name(Romaji) UDO

Other name(s) (Romaji)　—
学名　*Aralia cordata* Thunb.
　　Aralia edulis Sieb. et Zucc.
科名　Araliaceae（ウコギ科）
英名　udo
Part of use　soft stem
Note 1　rhizome of *Aralia edulis* Sieb. et Zucc.：drug category
　　rhizome and softened stem of *Angerica pubescens* Maxim. and *Angerica bisserata*（R.H. Shan et C.Q. Yuan）C.Q. Yuan et R.H. Shan：non-drug category
Note 2　—
注　—

名　称　**ウベ***
他名等　**ダイショ**
部位等　根茎
備　考　—

他名(参考)　ダイジョ（大薯）、オキナワヤマイモ（沖縄山芋）、タイワンヤマイモ（台湾山芋）
漢字表記・生薬名等　大薯（ダイショ）、参薯（サンショ）、田薯（デンショ）（ウベはフィリピン語）
Name(Romaji)　UBE*
Other name(s) (Romaji)　DAISHO
学名　*Dioscorea alata* L.*
科名　Dioscoreaceae（ヤマノイモ科）
英名　yam / greater yam / water yam / winged yam / white yam / Guyana arrowroot / ten-months yam / ube
Part of use　rhizome
Note 1　—
Note 2　UBE derives from Filipino and its Japanese name is DAISHO or DAIJO.
注　ウベはフィリピン語であり、和名はダイショ又はダイジョ。

名　称　**ウマノアシガタ**
他名等　**キンポウゲ**
部位等　全草
備　考　—

他名(参考)　アンデスポテト
漢字表記・生薬名等　金鳳花（キンポウゲ）、馬の足形（ウマノアシガタ）
Name(Romaji)　UMANOASHIGATA
Other name(s) (Romaji)　KINPÔGE
学名　*Ranunculus japonicus* Thunb.
科名　Ranunculaceae（キンポウゲ科）
英名　buttercup / Japanese buttercup
Part of use　whole plant
Note 1　—
Note 2　—
注　—

名　称　**ウメ***
他名等　**ウバイ**
部位等　果肉・未成熟の実
備　考　—

他名(参考)　—
漢字表記・生薬名等　梅（ウメ）、烏梅（ウバイ：未熟果実をくん製）
Name(Romaji)　UME*
Other name(s) (Romaji)　UBAI
学名　*Prunus mume* Sieb. et Zucc*
　　Armeniaca mume Sieb.*
科名　Rosaceae（バラ科）
英名　Japanese apricot / mume / ume
Part of use　sarcocarp, unriped fruit
Note 1　—
Note 2　—
注　—

名　称　**ウメガサソウ***
他名等　**オオウメガサソウ**
部位等　全草
備　考　—

他名(参考)　—
漢字表記・生薬名等　梅笠草（ウメガサソウ）、大梅笠草（オオウメガサソウ）
Name(Romaji)　UMEGASASÔ*
Other name(s) (Romaji)　ÔUMEGASASÔ
学名　*Chimaphila japonica* Miq.（ウメガサソウ）
　　Chimaphila umbellata（L.）W.C. Barton*（オオウメガサソウ）
　　Chimaphila umbellata（L.）W.C. Barton ssp. *cisatlantica*（Blake）Hultén*（オオウメガサソウ）
科名　Pyrolaceae（イチヤクソウ科）
英名　pipsissewa / prince's pine / wintergreen / wax-flower / small spotted wintergreen / spotted wintergreen
Part of use　whole plant
Note 1　—
Note 2　UMEGASASÔ and ÔUMEGASASÔ written in

the item of "Other names" are different species.
注　ウメガサソウと「他名等」に記載されているオオウメガサソウは別種。

名　称　**ウヤク***

他名等　テンダイウヤク
部位等　葉・実
備　考　根は「医」

他名(参考)　—
漢字表記・生薬名等　烏薬（ウヤク）、天台烏薬（テンダイウヤク）
Name(Romaji)　UYAKU*
Other name(s)(Romaji)　TENDAIUYAKU
学名　*Lindera strychnifolia* (Sieb. et Zucc.) F. Vill.*
Lindera aggregata (Sims) Kosterm.*
Benzoin strychnifolium (Sieb. et Zucc.) O. Kuntze
Daphnidium strychnifolium Seib. et Zucc.
科名　Lauraceae（クスノキ科）
英名　lindera / black medicine / Chinese allspice
Part of use　leaf, fruit
Note 1　root：drug category
Note 2　—
注　—

名　称　**ウラジロガシ**

他名等　—
部位等　葉
備　考　—

他名(参考)　—
漢字表記・生薬名等　裏白柏（ウラジロガシ）
Name(Romaji)　URAJIROGASHI
Other name(s)(Romaji)　—
学名　*Quercus salicina* Bl.
Cyclobalanopsis salicina (Bl.) Oerst.
Quercus stenophylla Makino
科名　Fagaceae（ブナ科）
英名　Japanese willow oak
Part of use　leaf
Note 1　—
Note 2　—
注　—

名　称　**ウワミズザクラ**

他名等　—
部位等　花穂
備　考　—

他名(参考)　クソザクラ、コンゴウザクラ、ハハカ、メズラ、ヨグソザクラ
漢字表記・生薬名等　上溝桜（ウワミゾザクラ）、杏仁香（アンニンゴ）、波波迦（ハハカ）
Name(Romaji)　UWAMIZUZAKURA
Other name(s)(Romaji)　—
学名　*Prunus grayana* Maxim.
Padus grayana (Maxim.) C.K. Schneid.
科名　Rosaceae（バラ科）
英名　Japanese bird cherry / Gray's bird cherry
Part of use　florescence
Note 1　—
Note 2　—
注　—

名　称　**エーデルワイス**

他名等　Leontopodium alpinum
部位等　地上部
備　考　—

他名(参考)　セイヨウウスユキソウ（西洋薄雪草）
漢字表記・生薬名等　西洋薄雪草（セイヨウウスユキソウ）
Name(Romaji)　ÊDERUWAISU
Other name(s)(Romaji)　—
学名　*Leontopodium alpinum* Cass.
Leontopodium nivale (Ten.) Huet ex Hand.-Mazz. ssp. *alpinum* (Cass.) Greuter
科名　Compositae（キク科）
英名　edelweisse / Alpine edelweisse / common edelweisse
Part of use　aerial part
Note 1　—
Note 2　—
注　—

名　称　**エキナケア***

他名等　パープルコーンフラワー／プルプレア／ムラサキバレンギク
部位等　全草
備　考　—

他名(参考)　—
漢字表記・生薬名等　紫馬簾菊（ムラサキバレンギク）

Name (Romaji)　EKINAKEA*
Other name (s) (Romaji)　PÂPURUKÔNFURAWÂ／PURUPUREA／MURASAKIBARENGIKU
学名　*Echinacea angustifolia* DC.*
Echinacea pallida (Nutt.) Nutt.*
Echinacea purpurea (L.) Moench*
科名　Compositae（キク科）
英名　Echinacea / Echinacea angustifolia / Echinacea pallida / Echinacea purpurea / purple cone flower / cone flower
Part of use　whole plant
Note 1　—
Note 2　—
注　—

名　称　**エストラゴン***
他名等　タラゴン
部位等　葉
備　考　—

他名(参考)　—
漢字表記・生薬名等　—
Name (Romaji)　ESUTORAGON*
Other name (s) (Romaji)　TARAGON
学名　*Artemisia dracunculus* L.*
科名　Compositae（キク科）
英名　estragon / French tarragon / tarragon
Part of use　leaf
Note 1　—
Note 2　—
注　—

名　称　**エゾウコギ***
他名等　シゴカ／シベリアニンジン
部位等　幹皮・根・根皮・葉・花・果実
備　考　—

他名(参考)　—
漢字表記・生薬名等　五加参（ゴカジン）、蝦夷五加（エゾウコギ）、刺五加（シゴカ）
Name (Romaji)　EZOUKOGI*
Other name (s) (Romaji)　SHIGOKA／SHIBERIANINJIN
学名　*Acanthopanax senticosus* (Rupr. et Maxim.) Harms*
Eleutherococcus senticosus (Rupr. et Maxim.) Maxim.*
科名　Araliaceae（ウコギ科）
英名　eleutherococcus / eleuthero / Siberian ginseng / Ussurian thorny pepper bush
Part of use　dried bark, root, root bark, leaf, flower, fruit
Note 1　—
Note 2　—
注　—

名　称　**エゾチチコグサ**
他名等　—
部位等　花
備　考　—

他名(参考)　エゾノチチコグサ（蝦夷父子草）
漢字表記・生薬名等　蝦夷父子草（エゾノチチコグサ）
Name (Romaji)　EZOCHICHIKOGUSA
Other name (s) (Romaji)　—
学名　*Antennaria dioica* (L.) Gaertn.
科名　Compositae（キク科）
英名　cat's foot / pied-de-chat
Part of use　flower
Note 1　—
Note 2　The correct "Name" of this herb is EZONOCHICHIKOGUSA.
注　正しい「名称」はエゾノチチコグサ。

名　称　**エゾヘビイチゴ***
他名等　—
部位等　全草
備　考　—

他名(参考)　ベスカイチゴ
漢字表記・生薬名等　蝦夷蛇苺（エゾヘビイチゴ）
Name (Romaji)　EZOHEBIICHIGO*
Other name (s) (Romaji)　—
学名　*Fragaria vesca* L.*
科名　Rosaceae（バラ科）
英名　Alpine strawberry / strawberry / wild strawberry
Part of use　whole plant
Note 1　—
Note 2　—
注　—

名 称 エニシダ*

他名等 —
部位等 花
備 考 枝・葉は「医」

他名(参考) —
漢字表記・生薬名等 金雀枝（エニシダ）
Name(Romaji) ENISHIDA*
Other name(s) (Romaji) —
学名 *Cytisus scoparius* (L.) Link*
Sarothamnus scoparius (L.) Wimm. ex W.D.J. Koch*
Spartium scoparium L.*
科名 Leguminosae（マメ科）
英名 broom / common broom / yellow broom / Scotch broom / scoparium
Part of use flower
Note 1 branch and leaf : drug category
Note 2 —
注 —

名 称 エノキタケ

他名等 —
部位等 子実体
備 考 —

他名(参考) ナメタケ（滑茸）、カキノキバナ、ユキノシタ（雪下）、ユキモタセ
漢字表記・生薬名等 榎茸（エノキダケ）
Name(Romaji) ENOKITAKE
Other name(s) (Romaji) —
学名 *Flammulina velutipes* (Curtis : Fr.) Singer
科名 Tricholomataceae（キシメジ科）
英名 Flammulina velutipes / velvet foot / winter mushroom
Part of use fruit body
Note 1 —
Note 2 —
注 —

名 称 エビスグサ*

他名等 ケツメイシ／ケツメイヨウ
部位等 種子・葉
備 考 —

他名(参考) ロッカクソウ（六角草）、ソウケツメイ（草決明）
漢字表記・生薬名等 決明子（ケツメイシ）、決明葉（ケツメイヨウ）、夷草（エビスグサ）
Name(Romaji) EBISUGUSA*
Other name(s) (Romaji) KETSUMEISHI／KETSUMEIYÔ
学名 *Cassia obtusifolia* L.*
Senna obtusifolia (L.) H.S. Irwin et Barnedy
Cassia tora auct. non. L.*
科名 Leguminosae（マメ科）
英名 cassia seed and leaf / sickle-pod senna / oriental senna / sickle sennna
Part of use seed, leaf
Note 1 —
Note 2 —
注 —

名 称 エルカンプーレ

他名等 Hercampure
部位等 全草
備 考 —

他名(参考) —
漢字表記・生薬名等 チャビン茶
Name(Romaji) ERUKANPÛRE
Other name(s) (Romaji) —
学名 *Gentianella alborosea* (Gilg) Fabris
科名 Gentianaceae（リンドウ科）
英名 hercampuri / hercampure
Part of use whole plant
Note 1 —
Note 2 —
注 —

名 称 エンショウ

他名等 —
部位等 全草
備 考 —

他名(参考) セキレンカ（石連花）、カゲツ（花月）、オウゴンカゲツ（黄金花月）、フチベニベンケイ（縁紅弁慶）
漢字表記・生薬名等 燕子掌（エンシショウ）
Name(Romaji) ENSHISHÔ
Other name(s) (Romaji) —
学名 *Crassula ovata* (Mill.) Druce
Crassula argentea L. f.
Crassula argentea Thunb.
Crassula obliqua Haw.

Crassula portulacea Lam.
科名 Crassulaceae（ベンケイソウ科）
英名 crassula / jade plant
Part of use whole plant
Note 1 —
Note 2 —
注 —

名　称　エンジュ*

他名等　カイヨウ
部位等 葉・サヤ
備　考 花・花蕾・果実は「医」

他名(参考) キフジ（黄藤）
漢字表記・生薬名等 槐（エンジュ）、槐葉（カイヨウ）
Name (Romaji) ENJU*
Other name (s) (Romaji) KAIYÔ
学名 *Sophora japonica* L.*
Styphnolobium japonicum (L.) Schott
科名 Leguminosae（マメ科）
英名 sophora / Japanese sophora / pagoda tree / Japanese pagoda-tree / Chinese scholar-tree
Part of use leaf, pod
Note 1 flower, flower bud and fruit : drug category
Note 2 —
注 —

名　称　エンバク*

他名等　オートムギ／マラカスムギ
部位等 全草
備　考 —

他名(参考) —
漢字表記・生薬名等 燕麦（エンバク）、真烏麦（マカラスムギ）
Name (Romaji) ENBAKU*
Other name (s) (Romaji) ÔTOMUGI／MARAKASUMUGI
学名 *Avena sativa* L.*
科名 Gramineae（イネ科）
英名 oat
Part of use whole plant
Note 1 —
Note 2 MARAKASUMUGI written in the item of "Other names" is incorrect. The correct name is MAKARASUMUGI.
注 「他名等」のマラカスムギの正しい名称はマカラスムギ。

名　称　エンベリア*

他名等 —
部位等 果実
備　考 —

他名(参考) —
漢字表記・生薬名等 白花酸藤果（ハクトウサントウカ：中国名）
Name (Romaji) ENBERIA*
Other name (s) (Romaji) —
学名 *Embelia ribes* Burm. f.*
科名 Myrsinaceae（ヤブコウジ科）
英名 vidanga
Part of use fruit
Note 1 —
Note 2 —
注 —

名　称　エンメイソウ

他名等　クロバナヒキオコシ／ヒキオコシ
部位等 全草
備　考 —

他名(参考) —
漢字表記・生薬名等 延命草（エンメイソウ）、引起（ヒキオコシ）、比木乎古乏（ヒキオコシ）、黒花引起（クロバナヒキオコシ）
Name (Romaji) ENMEISÔ
Other name (s) (Romaji) KUROBANAHIKIOKOSHI／HIKIOKOSHI
学名 *Rabdosia japonica* (Burm. f.) H. Hara（ヒキオコシ）
Isodon japonica (Burm. f.) H. Hara（ヒキオコシ）
Plectranthus trichocarpus Maxim.（クロバナヒキオコシ）
Rabdosia trichocarpa (Maxim.) H. Hara（クロバナヒキオコシ）
科名 Labiatae（シソ科）
英名 Japanese plectranthus
Part of use whole plant
Note 1 —
Note 2 KUROBANAHIKIOKOSHI and HIKIOKOSHI written in the item of "Other names" are different species.
注 「他名等」に記載されているクロバナヒキオコシとヒキオコシは別種。

名　称　**オウギ***

他名等　**キバナオウギ／ナイモウオウギ**
部位等　茎・葉
備　考　根は「医」

他名(参考)　タイツリオウギ（鯛釣黄耆）
漢字表記・生薬名等　黄耆（オウギ）、黄花黄耆（キバナオウギ）、内蒙黄耆（ナイモウオウギ）
Name(Romaji)　ÔGI*
Other name(s) (Romaji)　KIBANAÔGI／NAIMÔÔGI
学名　*Astragalus membranaceus* (Fisch. ex Link) Bunge*（キバナオウギ）
Astragalus mongholicus Bunge（ナイモウオウギ）
Astragalus membranaceus (L.) (Fisch. ex Link) Bunge var. *mongholicus* (Bunge) P.K. Hsiao*（ナイモウオウギ）
科名　Leguminosae（マメ科）
英名　huang qi / astragarus / membranous milkvetch / Mongholian milkvetch
Part of use　stem, leaf
Note 1　root：drug category
Note 2　ÔGI is identical with TÔHOKUÔGI, but their parts of use are different each other. TÔHOKUÔGI is also listed in the item of "Name". KIBANAÔGI and NAIMÔÔGI in the item of "Other names" are different species.
注　オウギは別項のトウホクオウギと同一。但し、「部位等」の記載が異なっている。「他名等」のキバナオウギとナイモウオウギは別種。

名　称　**オウゴン***

他名等　**コガネバナ／コガネヤナギ**
部位等　茎・葉
備　考　根は「医」

他名(参考)　—
漢字表記・生薬名等　黄芩（オウゴン）、黄金花（コガネバナ）、黄金柳（コガネヤナギ）
Name(Romaji)　ÔGON*
Other name(s) (Romaji)　KOGANEBANA／KOGANEYANAGI
学名　*Scutellaria baicalensis* Georgi*
科名　Labiatae（シソ科）
英名　Baikal skullcap / Chinese skullcap / scute
Part of use　stem, leaf
Note 1　root：drug category
Note 2　ÔGON is the name of traditional Japanese herbal medicine and its Japanese names are KOGANEBANA and KOGANEYANAGI.
注　オウゴンは生薬名。

名　称　**オウシュウハンノキ***

他名等　—
部位等　樹皮・葉
備　考　—

他名(参考)　—
漢字表記・生薬名等　欧州榛の木（オウシュウハンノキ）
Name(Romaji)　ÔSHÛHANNOKI*
Other name(s) (Romaji)　—
学名　*Alnus glutinosa* (L.) Gaertn.*
Betula alnus L. var. *glutinosa* L.*
Betula glutinosa (L.) Lam.
科名　Betulaceae（カバノキ科）
英名　alder / black alder / European alder
Part of use　bark, leaf
Note 1　—
Note 2　—
注　—

名　称　**オウセイ***

他名等　**ナルコユリ**
部位等　根茎
備　考　—

他名(参考)　カギクルマバナルコユリ（鍵車葉鳴子百合）
漢字表記・生薬名等　黄精（オウセイ）、鳴子百合（ナルコユリ）
Name(Romaji)　ÔSEI*
Other name(s) (Romaji)　NARUKOYURI
学名　*Polygonatum falcatum* A. Gray（ナルコユリ）
Polygonatum sibiricum F. Delara. ex Redout.*（カギクルマバナルコユリ）
Polygonatum kingianum Collett et Hemsl.
Polygonatum cyrtonema Hua*
科名　Liliaceae（ユリ科）
英名　Huang jing / polygonatum / Siberian Solomon's seal
Part of use　rhizome
Note 1　—
Note 2　ÔSEI is the name of traditional Japanese herbal medicine and its Japanese names are NARUKOYURI and KAGIKURUMABANARUKOYURI.
注　オウセイは生薬名。

名　称　**オウバク***

他名等　キハダ
部位等　葉・実
備　考　樹皮は「医」

他名(参考)　—
漢字表記・生薬名等　黄柏（オウバク）、黄肌（キハダ）
Name(Romaji)　ÔBAKU*
Other name(s) (Romaji)　KIHADA
学名　*Phellodendron amurense* Rupr.*
科名　Rutaceae（ミカン科）
英名　phellodendron / Amur cork tree
Part of use　leaf, fruit
Note 1　bark：drug category
Note 2　ÔBAKU is the name of traditional Japanese herbal medicine and its Japanese name is KIHADA.
注　オウバクは生薬名。

名　称　**オウヤクシ***

他名等　ニガカシュウ
部位等　全草
備　考　—

他名(参考)　カシュウイモ（何首烏芋）
漢字表記・生薬名等　黄薬子（オウヤクシ）、苦何首烏（ニガカシュウ）
Name(Romaji)　ÔYAKUSHI*
Other name(s) (Romaji)　NIGAKASHÛ
学名　*Dioscorea bulbifera* L.*
Dioscorea latifolia Bent.
科名　Dioscoreaceae（ヤマノイモ科）
英名　air potato / aerial yam / hoi / potato yam
Part of use　whole plant
Note 1　—
Note 2　ÔYAKUSHI is the name of traditional Japanese herbal medicine and its Japanese name is NIGA-KASHÛ.
注　オウヤクシは生薬名。

名　称　**オウレン***

他名等　キクバオウレン
部位等　葉
備　考　根茎・ひげ根は「医」

他名(参考)　—
漢字表記・生薬名等　黄連（オウレン）、菊葉黄連（キクバオウレン）
Name(Romaji)　ÔREN*
Other name(s) (Romaji)　KIKUBAÔREN
学名　*Coptis japonica* (Thunb.) Makino*（オウレン）
Coptis chinensis Franch.*
Coptis deltoidea C.Y. Cheng et Hsiao*
Coptis teeta Wall.*
Coptis japonica (Thunb.) Makino var. *japonica*（キクバオウレン）
Coptis japonica (Thunb.) Makino var. *major* (Miq.) Satake（コセリバオウレン）
科名　Ranunculaceae（キンポウゲ科）
英名　coptis / Japanese goldthread / Chinese goldthread / Indian goldthread / Tibetan goldthread
Part of use　leaf
Note 1　rhizome and fibrous root：drug category
Note 2　—
注　—

名　称　**オオイタビ**

他名等　—
部位等　枝・茎・葉
備　考　—

他名(参考)　オウフルギョウ（王不留行）、ドウカンソウ（道灌草）
漢字表記・生薬名等　大崖爬・大木蓮子（オオイタビ）、薜茘（ヘイレイ：中国名）
Name(Romaji)　ÔITABI
Other name(s) (Romaji)　—
学名　*Ficus pumila* L.
Ficus repense hort. non Willd. nec Rottl.
科名　Moraceae（クワ科）
英名　creeping fig / climbing fig / creeping rubber plant
Part of use　branch, stem, leaf
Note 1　—
Note 2　—
注　—

名　称　**オオバコ***

他名等　シャゼンシ／シャゼンソウ／シャゼンヨウ
部位等　全草
備　考　—

他名(参考)　トウドウ（当道）、フイ（芣苡）
漢字表記・生薬名等　大葉子（オオバコ）、種子：車前子（シャゼンシ）、全草：車前草（シャゼンソウ）、葉：車前葉（シャゼンヨウ）
Name(Romaji)　ÔBAKO*

Other name (s) (Romaji)　SHAZENSHI／SHAZENSÔ／SHAZEN'YÔ
学名　*Plantago asiatica* L.*
科名　Plantaginaceae（オオバコ科）
英名　plantain / common plantain / Asian plantain / Asian psyllium
Part of use　whole plant
Note 1　—
Note 2　—
注　—

名　称　**オオハンゴンソウ**

他名等　—
部位等　全草
備　考　—

他名(参考)　—
漢字表記･生薬名等　大反魂草（オオハンゴンソウ）
Name (Romaji)　ÔHANGONSÔ
Other name (s) (Romaji)　—
学名　*Rudbeckia laciniata* L.
科名　Compositae（キク科）
英名　cone flower / cut-leaved coneflower / cut-leaf coneflower / golden glow / gold glow
Part of use　whole plant
Note 1　—
Note 2　—
注　—

名　称　**オオヒレアザミ**

他名等　—
部位等　全草
備　考　—

他名(参考)　ゴロツキアザミ
漢字表記･生薬名等　オオヒレ薊（オオヒレアザミ）
Name (Romaji)　ÔHIREAZAMI
Other name (s) (Romaji)　—
学名　*Onopordon acanthium* L.
科名　Compositae（キク科）
英名　common cotton thistle / Scotch thistle
Part of use　whole plant
Note 1　—
Note 2　—
注　—

名　称　**オオムギ***

他名等　バクガ／Hordeum vulgare
部位等　茎・葉・発芽種子
備　考　—

他名(参考)　カワムギ（皮麦）、ハダカムギ（裸麦）
漢字表記･生薬名等　大麦（オオムギ）、麦芽（バクガ）
Name (Romaji)　ÔMUGI*
Other name (s) (Romaji)　BAKUGA
学名　*Hordeum vulgare* L.*
Hordeum sativum Jessen
科名　Gramineae（イネ科）
英名　barley / malt
Part of use　stem, leaf, germinated seed
Note 1　—
Note 2　Refer to BAKUGA in the item of "Name".
注　別項のバクガを参照。

名　称　**オカオグルマ**

他名等　—
部位等　全草
備　考　—

他名(参考)　—
漢字表記･生薬名等　丘小車（オカオグルマ）、狗舌草（グゼツソウ）
Name (Romaji)　OKAOGURUMA
Other name (s) (Romaji)　—
学名　*Senecio integrifolius* (L.) Clairv. ssp. *fauriei* (Lev. et Vant.) Kitam.
Senecio integrifolius var. *spathulatus* (Miq.) Hara
Senecio fauriei Lev. et Vant.
Senecio aurantiacus var. *spathulatus* Miq.
Tephroseris integrifolia (L.) Holub ssp. *kirilowii* (Turcz. ex DC.) B. Nord.
科名　Compositae（キク科）
英名　ehytlehtivillakko / field fleawort / Japanese senecio
Part of use　whole plant
Note 1　—
Note 2　—
注　—

名　称　**オカヒジキ**

他名等　ミルナ
部位等　茎葉
備　考　—

他名(参考)　オカミル（陸海松、水松）
漢字表記・生薬名等　陸鹿尾菜・岡羊栖菜（オカヒジキ）、海松菜・水松菜（ミルナ）
Name (Romaji)　OKAHIJIKI
Other name (s) (Romaji)　MIRUNA
学名　*Salsola komarovii* Iljin
科名　Chenopodiaceae（アカザ科）
英名　salt-wart / salsola
Part of use　stem, leaf
Note 1　—
Note 2　"茎葉 (stem-leaf)" in the item of "Part of use" written in Japanese should be replaced by "茎・葉 (stem and/or leaf)".
注　「部位等」の茎葉は茎・葉である。

名　称　**オシャグジタケ***

他名等　オシャクシタケ／サヨウ／Cynomorium coccineum
部位等　全草
備　考　—

他名(参考)　オシャクジタケ（鎖陽）
漢字表記・生薬名等　鎖陽（サヨウ）
Name (Romaji)　OSHAGUJITAKE*
Other name (s) (Romaji)　OSHAKUSHITAKE／SAYÔ
学名　*Cynomorium coccineum* L.
　Cynomorium songaricum Rupr.*
科名　Cynomoriaceae（オシャクジタケ科）
英名　cynomorium / so yang
Part of use　whole plant
Note 1　—
Note 2　—
注　—

名　称　**オタネニンジン***

他名等　コウライニンジン／チョウセンニンジン
部位等　果実・根・根茎・葉
備　考　—

他名(参考)　ヤクヨウニンジン（薬用人参）
漢字表記・生薬名等　人参（ニンジン）、御種人参（オタネニンジン）、高麗人参（コウライニンジン）、朝鮮人参（チョウセンニンジン）
Name (Romaji)　OTANENINJIN*
Other name (s) (Romaji)　KÔRAININJIN／CHÔSENNINJIN
学名　*Panax ginseng* C.A. Mey.*
　Panax schinseng T. Nees*
科名　Araliaceae（ウコギ科）
英名　ginseng / Asiatic gingseng / Chinese ginseng / Korean ginseng
Part of use　fruit, root, rhizome, leaf
Note 1　—
Note 2　—
注　—

名　称　**オトギリソウ**

他名等　ショウレンギョウ
部位等　全草
備　考　—

他名(参考)　アオクスリ（青薬）、タカノキズクスリ（鷹の傷薬）、ヤクシソウ（薬師草）
漢字表記・生薬名等　弟切草（オトギリソウ）、小連翹（ショウレンギョウ）
Name (Romaji)　OTOGIRISÔ
Other name (s) (Romaji)　SHÔRENGYÔ
学名　*Hypericum erectum* Thunb.
科名　Guttiferae（オトギリソウ科）
英名　—
Part of use　whole plant
Note 1　—
Note 2　—
注　—

名　称　**オトメアゼア***

他名等　バコパモニエラ
部位等　全草
備　考　—

他名(参考)　—
漢字表記・生薬名等　—
Name (Romaji)　OTOMEAZEA*
Other name (s) (Romaji)　BAKOPAMONIERA
学名　*Bacopa monnieri* (L.) Pennell*
　Herpestis monniera (L.) Kunth*
科名　Scrophulariaceae（ゴマノハグサ科）
英名　bacopa / herb-of-grace / Indian pennywort / water hyssop
Part of use　whole plant

Note 1 —
Note 2 OTOMEAZEA is incorrect. The correct name is OTOMEAZENA.
注 オトメアゼアの正しい名称はオトメアゼナ。

名 称 **オドリコソウ**

他名等 —
部位等 花
備 考 —

他名(参考) —
漢字表記・生薬名等 踊子草（オドリコソウ）
Name(Romaji) ODORIKOSÔ
Other name(s) (Romaji) —
学名 *Lamium album* L. var. *barbatum* (Sieb. et Zucc.) Fr. et Sav.
Lamium barbatum Sieb. et Zucc.
科名 Labiatae（シソ科）
英名 dead nettle / white nettle / archangel / dumb nettle / snowflake
Part of use flower
Note 1 —
Note 2 —
注 —

名 称 **オニサルビア***

他名等 クラリーセージ／Salvia sclarea
部位等 葉
備 考 —

他名(参考) —
漢字表記・生薬名等 —
Name(Romaji) ONISARUBIA*
Other name(s) (Romaji) KURARÎSÊJI
学名 *Salvia sclarea* L.*
科名 Labiatae（シソ科）
英名 clary / clary sage / clary wort / muscatel sage
Part of use leaf
Note 1 —
Note 2 —
注 —

名 称 **オニバス***

他名等 ケツジツ／ミズブキ
部位等 種子
備 考 —

他名(参考) ケイトウ（鶏頭）、カンカイ（雁喙）
漢字表記・生薬名等 芡実（ケツジツ、ケンジツ）、鬼蓮（オニバス）、水蕗（ミズブキ）
Name(Romaji) ONIBASU*
Other name(s) (Romaji) KETSUJITSU／MIZUBUKI
学名 *Euryale ferox* Salisb.*
科名 Nymphaeaceae（スイレン科）
英名 foxnut / euryale / fox nut / gorgon water lily / prickly water-lily / chikin's head
Part of use seed
Note 1 —
Note 2 —
注 —

名 称 **オペルクリナ・タルペタム***

他名等 —
部位等 葉
備 考 —

他名(参考) フウセンヒルガオ（風船昼顔）
漢字表記・生薬名等 —
Name(Romaji) OPERUKURINA・TARUPETAMU*
Other name(s) (Romaji) —
学名 *Operculina turpethum* (L.) Silva Manso*
Ipomoea turpethum (L.) R. Br.*
科名 Convolvulaceae（ヒルガオ科）
英名 Indian jalap / St. Thomas lidpot / trivrit
Part of use leaf
Note 1 —
Note 2 —
注 —

名 称 **オミナエシ***

他名等 ハイショウ／Patrinia scabiosaefolia
部位等 根
備 考 —

他名(参考) キバナハイショウ（黄花敗醤）
漢字表記・生薬名等 女郎花（オミナエシ）、敗醤（ハイショウ）、敗醤根（ハイショウコン）
Name(Romaji) OMINAESHI*
Other name(s) (Romaji) HAISHÔ

学名　*Patrinia scabiosaefolia* Fisch. ex Trevir.*
科名　Valerianaceae（オミナエシ科）
英名　patrinia / goldbaldrian
Part of use　root
Note 1　—
Note 2　HAISHÔ is the name of decontion of dried whole plant of OMINAESHI, but only root is approved here as part of use.
注　ハイショウはオミナエシの全草を乾燥させて煎じたものを指す。但し、本リストでは「部位等」は根とされている。

名　称　オリーブ*

他名等　オリーブ油／オレイフ
部位等　葉・花・果肉油
備　考　—

他名（参考）　—
漢字表記・生薬名等　橄欖（カンラン）
Name (Romaji)　ORÎBU*
Other name(s) (Romaji)　ORÎBU-YU／OREIFU
学名　*Olea europaea* L.*
　　　Olea sativa Hoffmanns. et Link
科名　Oleaceae（モクセイ科）
英名　olive / common olive
Part of use　leaf, flower, fruit oil
Note 1　—
Note 2　—
注　—

名　称　オレンジ*

他名等　オレンジピール
部位等　果実・果皮・蕾
備　考　—

他名（参考）　アマダイダイ（甘橙）、スイートオレンジ
漢字表記・生薬名等　—
Name (Romaji)　ORENJI*
Other name(s) (Romaji)　ORENJIPÎRU
学名　*Citrus sinensis* (L.) Osbeck*
　　　Citrus×aurantium L. var. *sinensis* L.*
科名　Rutaceae（ミカン科）
英名　orange / sweet orange
Part of use　fruit, peel, bud
Note 1　—
Note 2　—
注　—

カ行

名　称　カイコウズ

他名等　—
部位等　花
備　考　—

他名（参考）　マルバデイコ（丸葉梯沽）、ホソバデイコ（細葉梯沽）、アメリカデイコ（亜米利加梯沽）
漢字表記・生薬名等　海紅豆（カイコウズ）、亜米利加梯沽（アメリカデイコ）、エリスリナ
Name (Romaji)　KAIKÔZU
Other name(s) (Romaji)　—
学名　*Erythrina crista-galli* L.
　　　Erythrina pulcherrima Tod.
科名　Leguminosae（マメ科）
英名　common coral tree / cockscomb coral tree / cock-spur coral tree / cry-baby tree
Part of use　flower
Note 1　—
Note 2　—
注　—

名　称　カイソウ＜海草＞

他名等　—
部位等　海中の食用藻類
備　考　カイソウ＜海葱＞属の鱗茎は「医」

他名（参考）　—
漢字表記・生薬名等　海草（カイソウ）
Name (Romaji)　KAISÔ
Other name(s) (Romaji)　—
学名　—
科名　—
英名　seaweed
Part of use　edible seaweed
Note 1　bulb of *Ulginea* Steinh. (sea onion) : drug category
Note 2　—
注　—

名　称　**ガイハク***

他名等　ノビル／ラッキョウ
部位等　鱗茎
備　考　—

他名(参考)　—
漢字表記・生薬名等　薤白（ガイハク）、野蒜（ノビル）、辣韮（ラッキョウ）
Name(Romaji)　GAIHAKU*
Other name(s) (Romaji)　NOBIRU／RAKKYÔ
学名　*Allium chinense* G. Don
Allium macrostemon Bunge*
Allium grayi Regel
Allium bakeri Regel
Allium nipponicum Fr. et Sav.
科名　Liliaceae（ユリ科）
英名　rakkyo / Chinese onion / long-stamen onion / baker's garic
Part of use　bulb
Note 1　—
Note 2　—
注　—

名　称　**ガウクルア**

他名等　アカガウクルア
部位等　全草
備　考　—

他名(参考)　プエラリアミリフィカ
漢字表記・生薬名等　—
Name(Romaji)　GAUKURUA
Other name(s) (Romaji)　AKAGAUKURUA
学名　*Pueraria mirifica* Airy Shaw et Suvatab.（ガウクルア）
Pueraria candollei var. *mirifica*（Airy Shaw et Suvat.）Niyomdham（ガウクルア）
Butea superba Roxb.（アカガウクルア）
科名　Leguminosae（マメ科）
英名　kwakhur / kwao keur / white kwao keur
Part of use　whole plant
Note 1　—
Note 2　GAUKURUA is identical with PUERARIAMIRIFIKA, but their parts of use are different each other. PUERARIAMIRIFIKA is also listed in the item of "Name".
注　ガウクルアは別項のプエラリアミリフィカと同一。但し、「部位等」の記載が異なっている。

名　称　**カガミグサ**

他名等　Ampelopsis japonica
部位等　根
備　考　—

他名(参考)　ビャクレン（白蘞）
漢字表記・生薬名等　鏡草（カガミグサ）、白斂（ビャクレン）
Name(Romaji)　KAGAMIGUSA
Other name(s) (Romaji)　—
学名　*Ampelopsis japonica*（Thunb.）Makino
科名　Vitaceae（ブドウ科）
英名　Japanese ampelopsis
Part of use　root
Note 1　—
Note 2　—
注　—

名　称　**カキ<柿>**

他名等　Diospyros kaki
部位等　渋・葉・果実の宿存がく（ヘタ）
備　考　—

他名(参考)　—
漢字表記・生薬名等　柿（カキ）、柿蔕（シテイ）、柿渋（カキシブ）
Name(Romaji)　KAKI
Other name(s) (Romaji)　—
学名　*Diospyros kaki* Thunb.
科名　Ebenaceae（カキノキ科）
英名　Japanese persimmon / persimmon / sharon fruit / date plum / kaki / kakee / keg fig
Part of use　persimmon tannin, leaf, persistent calyx
Note 1　—
Note 2　—
注　—

名　称　**カキネガラシ***

他名等　ヘッジマスタード／エリシマム
部位等　全草
備　考　—

他名(参考)　—
漢字表記・生薬名等　垣根芥子（カキネガラシ）
Name(Romaji)　KAKINEGARASHI*
Other name(s) (Romaji)　HEJJIMASUTÂDO／ERISHIMAMU

学名　*Sisymbrium officinale* (L.) Scop.*
　　Erysimum officinale L.*
科名　Cruciferae（アブラナ科）
英名　common hedge mustard / bank cress / singer's plant
Part of use　whole plant
Note 1　—
Note 2　—
注　—

名　称　**カシグルミ***

他名等　セイヨウグルミ／ペルシャグルミ
部位等　果実・葉
備　考　—

他名(参考)　チョウセングルミ(朝鮮胡桃)、トウグルミ(唐胡桃)
漢字表記・生薬名等　菓子胡桃（カシグルミ）、西洋胡桃（セイヨウグルミ）
Name (Romaji)　KASHIGURUMI*
Other name(s) (Romaji)　SEIYÔGURUMI／PERUSHA-GURUMI
学名　*Juglans regia* L.*
　　Juglans regia var. *orientis* (Dode) Kitam.
　　Juglans orientis Dode
科名　Juglandaceae（クルミ科）
英名　walnut / common walnut / Madeira nut / English walnut / Persian walnut
Part of use　fruit, leaf
Note 1　—
Note 2　—
注　—

名　称　**カシス***

他名等　クロフサスグリ
部位等　葉
備　考　—

他名(参考)　—
漢字表記・生薬名等　黒房酸塊（クロフサスグリ）
Name (Romaji)　KASHISU*
Other name(s) (Romaji)　KUROFUSASUGURI
学名　*Ribes nigrum* L.*
科名　Saxifragaceae（ユキノシタ科）
英名　black currant / European black currant / common black currant / cassis
Part of use　leaf
Note 1　—
Note 2　KASHISU is identical with KUROSUGURI, but their parts of use are different each other. KUROSUGURI is also listed in the item of "Name".
注　カシスは別項のクロススグリと同一。但し、「部位等」の記載が異なっている。

名　称　**ガジュツ***

他名等　—
部位等　根茎
備　考　—

他名(参考)　ムラサキウコン（紫鬱金）、ホウガジュツ（蓬莪朮）
漢字表記・生薬名等　莪朮・莪蒁（ガジュツ）
Name (Romaji)　GAJUTSU*
Other name(s) (Romaji)　—
学名　*Curcuma zedoaria* (Christm.) Roscoe*
　　Curcuma aeruginosa Roxb.
科名　Zingiberaceae（ショウガ科）
英名　zedoary
Part of use　rhizome
Note 1　—
Note 2　—
注　—

名　称　**カシュトウ**

他名等　カンカトウ／ドカンゾウ
部位等　全草
備　考　—

他名(参考)　—
漢字表記・生薬名等　カシユウトウ（蝦鬚豆）、カンカトウ（干花豆）、ドカンゾウ（土甘草）
Name (Romaji)　KASHUTÔ
Other name(s) (Romaji)　KANKATÔ／DOKANZÔ
学名　*Fordia cauliflora* Hemsl.
　　Millettia cauliflora (Hemsl.) Gagnep.
科名　Leguminosae（マメ科）
英名　shuiluosan
Part of use　whole plant
Note 1　—
Note 2　KASHUTÔ is incorrect. The correct name is KASHUUTÔ.
注　カシュトウではなく、カシユウトウが正しい名称。

名　称　**カツアバ***

他名等　—
部位等　全草
備　考　—

他名(参考)　—
漢字表記・生薬名等　—
Name (Romaji)　KATSUABA*
Other name (s) (Romaji)　—
学名　*Erythroxylum catuaba* A.J. Silva ex Raym.-Hamet*
科名　Erythroxylaceae（コカノキ科）
英名　catuaba / tatuaba / pau da reposta
Part of use　whole plant
Note 1　—
Note 2　Two different trees called "KATSUABA (catuaba)" exist, namely *Trichilia catigua* Adr., Juss. and *Erythroxylum catuaba* A.J. Silva ex Raym.-Hamet. The latter is accepted by the Ministry of Health, Labour and Welfare as "non-drug" category.
注　カツアバと呼ばれる樹木が2種類（*Trichilia catigua* Adr., Juss. 及び*Erythroxylum catuaba* A.J. Silva ex Raym.-Hamet）ある。そのうち「非医」区分として厚生労働省が認めたのは後者である。

名　称　**カッコウアザミ**

他名等　Ageratum conyzoides
部位等　全草
備　考　—

他名(参考)　—
漢字表記・生薬名等　勝紅薊・霍香薊（カッコウアザミ）
Name (Romaji)　KAKKÔAZAMI
Other name (s) (Romaji)　—
学名　*Ageratum conyzoides* L.
科名　Compositae（キク科）
英名　ageratum / floss flow / pussy-foot
Part of use　whole plant
Note 1　—
Note 2　—
注　—

名　称　**カッパリス・マサイカイ**

他名等　バビンロウ／マビンロウ／Capparis masaikai
部位等　種子
備　考　—

他名(参考)　—
漢字表記・生薬名等　マ檳榔（マビンロウ）、バ檳榔（バビンロウ）
Name (Romaji)　KAPPARISU・MASAIKAI
Other name (s) (Romaji)　BABINRÔ／MABINRÔ
学名　*Capparis masaikai* Lévl.
科名　Cappariceae（フウチョウソウ科）
英名　mabinlang
Part of use　seed
Note 1　—
Note 2　—
注　—

名　称　**カニクサ***

他名等　ツルシノブ／Lygodium japonicum
部位等　胞子
備　考　—

他名(参考)　シャミセンズル（三味線蔓）
漢字表記・生薬名等　蟹草（カニクサ）、海金沙・海金砂・金沙藤（カイキンシャ）、蔓葱（ツルシノブ）
Name (Romaji)　KANIKUSA*
Other name (s) (Romaji)　TSURUSHINOBU
学名　*Lygodium japonicum* (Thunb. ex Murr.) Sw.*
科名　Schizaeaceae（マツブサ科）
英名　Japanese climbing fern / climbing fern
Part of use　spore
Note 1　—
Note 2　—
注　—

名　称　**カノコソウ***

他名等　キッソウコン／セイヨウカノコソウ／ワレリア
部位等　根・根茎
備　考　—

他名(参考)　ハルオミナエシ（春女郎花）
漢字表記・生薬名等　鹿子草（カノコソウ）、吉草根（キッソウコン）
Name (Romaji)　KANOKOSÔ*
Other name (s) (Romaji)　KISSÔKON／SEIYÔKANOKOSÔ／WARERIA
学名　*Valeriana fauriei* Briq.（カノコソウ）
Valeriana sambucifolia var. *fauriei* (Briq.) Hara（カノコソウ）
Valeriana officinalis L.*（セイヨウカノコソウ）
科名　Valerianaceae（オミナエシ科）
英名　valerian / garden heliotrope / garden valerian
Part of use　root, rhizome

Note 1　—
Note 2　The correct name of WARERIA written in the item of "Other names" is "WARERIAN".
注　「他名等」のワレリアの正しい名称はワレリアンである。

名　称　**カバノアナタケ***

他名等　—
部位等　菌核
備　考　—

他名(参考)　チャーガ
漢字表記・生薬名等　樺孔茸・樺穴茸（カバノアナタケ）
Name(Romaji)　KABANOANATAKE*
Other name(s) (Romaji)　—
学名　*Inonotus obliquus* (Ach. ex Pers.) Pilát*
Fuscoporia obliqua (Ach. ex Pers.) Aoshima
Boletus obliquus Ach. ex Pers.
Polyporus obliquus (Ach. ex Pers.) Fr.
Fomes obliquus (Ach. ex Pers.) Cooke
Phellinus obliquus (Ach. ex Pers.) Pat.
科名　Hymenochaetaceae（タバコウロコタケ科）
英名　chaga / charga / clinker polypore
Part of use　sclerotium
Note 1　—
Note 2　—
注　—

名　称　**カフン**

他名等　—
部位等　ガマ・ヒメガマ以外の花粉
備　考　ガマ・ヒメガマの花粉は「医」

他名(参考)　—
漢字表記・生薬名等　花粉（カフン）
Name(Romaji)　KAFUN
Other name(s) (Romaji)　—
学名　—
科名　—
英名　pollen
Part of use　pollen except those of *Typha latifolia, Typha angustifolia, Typha angustata*
Note 1　pollen of *Typha latifolia, Typha angustifolia,* and *Typha angustata*：drug category
Note 2　—
注　—

名　称　**カボチャ***

他名等　ナンガニン
部位等　種子・種子油
備　考　—

他名(参考)　トウナス（唐茄子）、ボウブラ、ナンキン（南京）
漢字表記・生薬名等　南瓜仁（ナンガニン）、南瓜子（ナンガシ、ナンカシ）、南瓜・北瓜（カボチャ）
Name(Romaji)　KABOCHA*
Other name(s) (Romaji)　NANGANIN
学名　*Cucurbita pepo* L.*
Cucurbita moschata (Duch. ex Lam.) Duch. ex Poiret.
Cucurbita maxima Duch. ex Lam.*
科名　Cucurbitaceae（ウリ科）
英名　pumpkin / squash / summer squash / marrow / China squash / winter squash
Part of use　seed, seed oil
Note 1　—
Note 2　—
注　—

名　称　**ガマ***

他名等　ヒメガマ
部位等　花粉以外
備　考　花粉（蒲黄）は「医」

他名(参考)　—
漢字表記・生薬名等　蒲（ガマ）、姫蒲（ヒメガマ）、蒲黄（ホオウ）、寛葉香蒲（カンヨウコウホ）、狭葉香蒲（キョウヨウコウホ）
Name(Romaji)　GAMA*
Other name(s) (Romaji)　HIMEGAMA
学名　*Typha latifolia* L.*（ガマ）
Typha angustifolia L.*（ヒメガマ）
Typha angustata Bory et Chaub.*（ヒメガマ）
科名　Typhaceae（ガマ科）
英名　small reedmace / cat tail / bulrush / common cat tail / Cossack asparagus / narrow leaf cat tail / small bulrush
Part of use　whole plant except pollen
Note 1　pollen of *T. latifolia, T. angustifolia,* and *T. angustata*：drug category
Note 2　—
注　—

名　称　**カミツレ***

他名等　カモミール
部位等　小頭花
備　考　―

他名(参考)　カミルレ
漢字表記･生薬名等　加密列（カミツレ）、母菊（ハハギク、ボギク）
Name(Romaji)　KAMITSURE*
Other name(s) (Romaji)　KAMOMÎRU
学名　*Matricaria recutita* L.*
Chamomilla recutita (L.) Rauschert*
Matricaria chamomilla L.*
Matricaria suaveolens L.*
科名　Compositae（キク科）
英名　German chamomile / Hungarian chamomile / true chamomile / chamomile / mayweed / sweet false chamomile
Part of use　small flower
Note 1　―
Note 2　―
注　―

名　称　**カムカム***

他名等　―
部位等　果実
備　考　―

他名(参考)　―
漢字表記･生薬名等　―
Name(Romaji)　KAMUKAMU*
Other name(s) (Romaji)　―
学名　*Myrciaria dubia* (Kunth) McVaugh*
科名　Myrtaceae（フトモモ科）
英名　cumcum / camu-camu
Part of use　fruit
Note 1　―
Note 2　―
注　―

名　称　**ガムググル***

他名等　Commiphora mukul
部位等　樹脂
備　考　その他のコンミフォラ属の全木は「医」

他名(参考)　―
漢字表記･生薬名等　―
Name(Romaji)　GAMUGUGURU*
Other name(s) (Romaji)　―
学名　*Commiphora mukul* (Hook. ex Stocks) Engl.*
Balsamodendron mukul Hook.*
科名　Burseraceae（カンラン科）
英名　gugulipid / gum guggul / guggul / bdellium tree / false myrrh / Indian bdellium tree
Part of use　oleo-gum resin
Note 1　whole tree of *Commiphora* Jacq. other than *C. mukul*：drug category
Note 2　―
注　―

名　称　**カヤツリグサ**

他名等　―
部位等　全草
備　考　―

他名(参考)　―
漢字表記･生薬名等　蚊帳吊草（カヤツリグサ）
Name(Romaji)　KAYATSURIGUSA
Other name(s) (Romaji)　―
学名　*Cyperus microiria* Steud.
科名　Cyperaceae（カヤツリグサ科）
英名　Asian flatsedge / umbrella-sedge
Part of use　whole plant
Note 1　―
Note 2　―
注　―

名　称　**カラスノエンドウ**

他名等　コモンヴィッチ
部位等　全草
備　考　―

他名(参考)　―
漢字表記･生薬名等　烏豌豆（カラスノエンドウ）
Name(Romaji)　KARASUNOENDÔ
Other name(s) (Romaji)　KOMONVITCHI
学名　*Vicia sativa* L. ssp. *nigra* (L.) Ehrh
Vicia angustifolia L.
科名　Leguminosae（マメ科）
英名　winter tares / common vetch / spring vetch
Part of use　whole plant
Note 1　―
Note 2　―
注　―

名　称　カラスムギ*

他名等　ヤエンムギ
部位等　全草
備　考　—

他名(参考)　チャヒキグサ（茶挽草）
漢字表記・生薬名等　烏麦（カラスムギ）、野燕麦（ヤエンムギ）
Name (Romaji)　KARASUMUGI*
Other name(s) (Romaji)　YAENMUGI
学名　*Avena fatua* L.*
科名　Gramineae（イネ科）
英名　oat / oat grass / wild oat
Part of use　whole plant
Note 1　—
Note 2　—
注　—

名　称　カラタチ*

他名等　キコク／Poncirus trifoliata
部位等　果実・果皮・蕾
備　考　—

他名(参考)　—
漢字表記・生薬名等　枳（カラタチ）、枸橘・枳殻（キコク）
Name (Romaji)　KARATACHI*
Other name(s) (Romaji)　KIKOKU
学名　*Poncirus trifoliata* (L.) Rafin.*
Citrus trifoliata L.*
科名　Rutaceae（ミカン科）
英名　gou ju / zhi quiao zhi shi (immature fruit) / trifoliate orange
Part of use　fruit, pericarp, bud
Note 1　—
Note 2　—
注　—

名　称　ガラナ*

他名等　—
部位等　種子
備　考　—

他名(参考)　—
漢字表記・生薬名等　—
Name (Romaji)　GARANA*
Other name(s) (Romaji)　—
学名　*Paullinia cupana* Kunth*
科名　Sapindaceae（ムクロジ科）
英名　guarana / guaraná
Part of use　seed
Note 1　—
Note 2　—
注　—

名　称　カリウスフォレスコリー*

他名等　—
部位等　根
備　考　—

他名(参考)　コレウスフォルスコリー
漢字表記・生薬名等　—
Name (Romaji)　KARIUSUFORESUKORÎ*
Other name(s) (Romaji)　—
学名　*Coleus forskohlii* auct.*
Plectranthus barbatus Andrews*
Coleus barbatus (Andrews) Benth.*
科名　Labiatae（シソ科）
英名　forskohlii
Part of use　root
Note 1　—
Note 2　The general name derived from its scientific name. The better KATAKANA notation of the name would be KOREUSUFORUSKORÎ.
注　名称は学名に基づくカタカナ表記であるが、コレウスフォルスコリーがより近い表記である。

名　称　カルケッハ*

他名等　カルケ／カルケージャ／パッソーラ
部位等　全草
備　考　—

他名(参考)　—
漢字表記・生薬名等　—
Name (Romaji)　KARUKEHHA*
Other name(s) (Romaji)　KARUKE／KARUKÊJA／PASSÔRA
学名　*Baccharis trimera* (Less.) DC.*
Baccharis genistelloides (Lam.) Pers. var. *trimera* (Less.) Baker*
科名　Compositae（キク科）
英名　carqueja / baccharis trimera
Part of use　whole plant
Note 1　—
Note 2　—
注　—

名　称　**ガルシニアカンボジア***

他名等　インディアンデイト／ゴラカ／タマリンド
部位等　果実・果皮・茎・種子・根・葉・花
備　考　—

他名(参考)　—
漢字表記・生薬名等　—
Name (Romaji)　GARUSHINIAKANBOJIA*
Other name (s) (Romaji)　INDIANDEITO／GORAKA／TAMARINDO
学名　*Garcinia cambogia* (Gaertn.) Desr.*
科名　Guttiferae (オトギリソウ科)
英名　citrin / ganboge tree / garcinia / brindall berry / Malabar tamarind / goraka / camboge plant
Part of use　fruit, fruit pericarp, stem, seed, root, leaf, flower
Note 1　—
Note 2　—
注　—

名　称　**ガレガソウ***

他名等　—
部位等　葉
備　考　—

他名(参考)　—
漢字表記・生薬名等　—
Name (Romaji)　GAREGASÔ*
Other name (s) (Romaji)　—
学名　*Galega officinalis* L.*
科名　Leguminosae (マメ科)
英名　goat's rue
Part of use　leaf
Note 1　—
Note 2　—
注　—

名　称　**カロニン***

他名等　オオカラスウリ／キカラスウリ／シナカラスウリ
部位等　果実・種子
備　考　根は「医」

他名(参考)　トウカラスウリ（唐烏瓜）、チョウセンカラスウリ（朝鮮烏瓜）
漢字表記・生薬名等　栝楼仁（カロニン）、大烏瓜（オオカラスウリ）、黄烏瓜（キカラスウリ）、支那烏瓜（シナカラスウリ）
Name (Romaji)　KARONIN*
Other name (s) (Romaji)　ÔKARASUURI／KIKARASUURI／SHINAKARASUURI
学名　*Trichosanthes kirilowii* Maxim.* (シナカラスウリ・トウカラスウリ・チョウセンカラスウリ)
Trichosanthes bracteata Voigt (オオカラスウリ)
Trichosanthes kirilowii Maxim. var. *japonica* (Miq.) Kitam. (キカラスウリ)
Trichosanthes japonica Regel. (キカラスウリ)
科名　Cucurbitaceae (ウリ科)
英名　trichosanthis semen / trichosanthes / Chinese cucumber / Mongolian snakegourd
Part of use　fruit, seed
Note 1　root：drug category
Note 2　—
注　—

名　称　**カワラタケ***

他名等　サルノコシカケ
部位等　子実体
備　考　菌糸体は「医」

他名(参考)　バイキセイ（梅寄生）
漢字表記・生薬名等　瓦茸（カワラタケ）、猿の腰掛（サルノコシカケ）
Name (Romaji)　KAWARATAKE*
Other name (s) (Romaji)　SARUNOKOSHIKAKE
学名　*Trametes versicolor* (L.) Lloyd*
Coriolus versicolor (L.) Quél.*
Boletus versicolor L.
Poria versicolor (L.) Scop.
科名　Polyporaceae (サルノコシカケ科)
英名　Turkey tails / rainbow bracket
Part of use　fruit body
Note 1　mycelium：drug category
Note 2　—
注　—

名　称　**カンカニクジュヨウ**

他名等　Cistanche tubulosa
部位等　肉質茎
備　考　—

他名(参考)　ギョリュウ科ギョリュウ属（タマリクス）植物の根に寄生する植物
漢字表記・生薬名等　管花肉蓯蓉（カンカニクジュヨウ）
Name (Romaji)　KANKANIKUJUYÔ
Other name (s) (Romaji)　—

学名　*Cistanche tubulosa* (Schenk) R. Wight
科名　Orobanchaceae（ハマウツボ科）
英名　—
Part of use　succulent stem
Note 1　—
Note 2　—
注　—

名　称　**カンキョウニン***

他名等　アンズ
部位等　種子
備　考　クキョウニンは「医」

他名(参考)　—
漢字表記･生薬名等　杏子・杏（アンズ)、甘杏仁（カンキョウニン)、南杏（ナンキョウ)、甜杏仁（テンキョウニン：中国名）
Name (Romaji)　KANKYÔNIN*
Other name(s) (Romaji)　ANZU
学名　*Prunus armeniaca* L. var. *ansu* Maxim.（アンズ）
Prunus armeniaca L.*（ホンアンズ）
Armeniaca vulgaris Lam.*（アンズ）
Prunus sibirica L.（モウコアンズ）
科名　Rosaceae（バラ科）
英名　apricot seed (xingren) / apricot / Chinese bitter almond / common apricot
Part of use　seed
Note 1　KUKYÔNIN, seed containing amygdalin more than 2%：drug category
Note 2　—
注　—

名　称　**カンショ***

他名等　サトウキビ
部位等　根
備　考　—

他名(参考)　—
漢字表記･生薬名等　甘蔗（カンショ)、砂糖黍（サトウキビ）
Name (Romaji)　KANSHO*
Other name(s) (Romaji)　SATÔKIBI
学名　*Saccharum officinarum* L.*
科名　Gramineae（イネ科）
英名　sugarcane / noble sugarcane
Part of use　root
Note 1　—
Note 2　—
注　—

名　称　**カンゾウ<甘草>***

他名等　リコライス
部位等　根・ストロン
備　考　—

他名(参考)　—
漢字表記･生薬名等　甘草（カンゾウ）
Name (Romaji)　KANZÔ*
Other name(s) (Romaji)　RIKORAISU
学名　*Glycyrrhiza uralensis* Fisch. ex DC.*
Glycyrrhiza glabra L.*
Glycyrrhiza glandulifera Waldst. et Kit.*
科名　Leguminosae（マメ科）
英名　glycyrrhiza / licorice root / liquorice root / Chinese licorice / licorice / Ural licorice / Russian licorice / Turkish licorice / Spanish licorice
Part of use　root, stolon
Note 1　—
Note 2　—
注　—

名　称　**カンブイ***

他名等　ペドラ・ウマ・カア／ペドラ・ウメカ
部位等　葉
備　考　—

他名(参考)　—
漢字表記･生薬名等　—
Name (Romaji)　KANBUI*
Other name(s) (Romaji)　PEDORA・UMA・KÂ／PEDORA・UMEKA
学名　*Myrcia multiflora* (Lam.) DC.*
Myrcia sphaerocarpa DC.*
科名　Myrtaceae（フトモモ科）
英名　pedra hume / pedra ume caa
Part of use　leaf
Note 1　—
Note 2　—
注　—

名　称　**カンラン***

他名等　Canarium album
部位等　果実
備　考　—

他名(参考)　—
漢字表記・生薬名等　橄欖（カンラン）
Name(Romaji)　KANRAN*
Other name(s)(Romaji)　—
学名　*Canarium album*（Lour.）Raeusch.*
科名　Burseraceae（カンラン科）
英名　Chinese white olive / Chinese olive / white canary tree
Part of use　fruit
Note 1　—
Note 2　—
注　—

名　称　**カンレンボク**

他名等　キジュ
部位等　果実
備　考　—

他名(参考)　—
漢字表記・生薬名等　旱蓮木（カレンボク）、喜樹（キジュ）
Name(Romaji)　KANRENBOKU
Other name(s)(Romaji)　KIJU
学名　*Camptotheca acuminata* Decne.
科名　Nyssaceae（ヌマミズキ科）
英名　xi shu / camptotheca
Part of use　fruit
Note 1　—
Note 2　—
注　—

名　称　**キイチゴ**

他名等　—
部位等　葉
備　考　—

他名(参考)　—
漢字表記・生薬名等　木苺・懸鉤子（キイチゴ）
Name(Romaji)　KIICHIGO
Other name(s)(Romaji)　—
学名　*Rubus* L.
科名　Rosaceae（バラ科）
英名　raspberry / blackberry
Part of use　leaf
Note 1　—
Note 2　—
注　—

名　称　**キキョウ***

他名等　—
部位等　根
備　考　—

他名(参考)　—
漢字表記・生薬名等　桔梗（キキョウ）、桔梗根（キキョウコン）
Name(Romaji)　KIKYÔ*
Other name(s)(Romaji)　—
学名　*Platycodon grandiflorum*（Jacq.）A. DC.*
科名　Campanulaceae（キキョウ科）
英名　bellflower / platycodon / balloon flower / Chinese bellflower / Japanese bellflower
Part of use　root
Note 1　—
Note 2　—
注　—

名　称　**キグ**

他名等　ケンポナシ
部位等　果実・果柄
備　考　—

他名(参考)　—
漢字表記・生薬名等　枳椇（キグ）、玄圃梨（ケンポナシ）
Name(Romaji)　KIGU
Other name(s)(Romaji)　KENPONASHI
学名　*Hovenia dulcis* Thunb.
Hovenia acerba Lindl.
科名　Rhamnaceae（クロウメモドキ科）
英名　hovenia / Japanese raisin-tree / coral tree
Part of use　fruit, pedicle
Note 1　—
Note 2　—
注　—

名　称　**キクイモ***

他名等　—
部位等　塊茎
備　考　—

他名(参考)　—
漢字表記・生薬名等　菊芋（キクイモ）
Name(Romaji)　KIKUIMO*
Other name(s) (Romaji)　—
学名　*Helianthus tuberosus* L.*
科名　Compositae（キク科）
英名　Jerusalem artichoke / sunchoke
Part of use　tuber
Note 1　—
Note 2　—
注　—

名　称　**キクカ***

他名等　キク
部位等　頭花
備　考　—

他名(参考)　—
漢字表記・生薬名等　菊花（キクカ）
Name(Romaji)　KIKUKA*
Other name(s) (Romaji)　KIKU*
学名　*Chrysanthemum*×*morifolium* Ramat.*（キク）
Chrysanthemum indicum L.*（シマカンギク）
Dendranthema grandiflorum (Ramat.) Kitam.*（キク）
Chrysanthemum sinense Sabine*
科名　Compositae（キク科）
英名　chrysanthemum / wild chrysanthemum / florist's chrysanthemum
Part of use　flower
Note 1　—
Note 2　—
注　—

名　称　**キクニガナ***

他名等　チコリー
部位等　根・根の抽出物・葉・花
備　考　—

他名(参考)　—
漢字表記・生薬名等　菊苦菜（キクニガナ）、菊苣（キクキョ）
Name(Romaji)　KIKUNIGANA*
Other name(s) (Romaji)　CHIKORÎ
学名　*Cichorium intybus* L.*
科名　Compositae（キク科）
英名　chicory / succory
Part of use　root, root extract, leaf, flower
Note 1　—
Note 2　—
注　—

名　称　**キクラゲ***

他名等　—
部位等　子実体
備　考　—

他名(参考)　—
漢字表記・生薬名等　木耳（キクラゲ）、槐耳（カイジ）
Name(Romaji)　KIKURAGE*
Other name(s) (Romaji)　—
学名　*Auricularia auricula-judae* (Bull.：Fr.) Wettst.
Auricularia auricula (Hook.) Underw.*
Hirneola auricula-judae (Bull.：Fr.) Berk.
科名　Auriculariaceae（キクラゲ科）
英名　Jew's ear / Judas's ear / wood ear fungus
Part of use　fruit body
Note 1　—
Note 2　—
注　—

名　称　**キダチアロエ**

他名等　—
部位等　葉
備　考　アロエの葉液汁は「医」

他名(参考)　—
漢字表記・生薬名等　木立蘆薈（キダチアロエ）
Name(Romaji)　KIDACHIAROE
Other name(s) (Romaji)　—
学名　*Aloe arborescens* Mill.
科名　Liliaceae（ユリ科）
英名　krantz aloe / candelabra aloe / octopus plant / torch plant
Part of use　leaf
Note 1　juice of aloe leaf：drug category
Note 2　—
注　—

名　称　**キダチキンバイ**

他名等　スイチョウコウ
部位等　全草
備　考　―

他名（参考）　―
漢字表記・生薬名等　木立金梅（キダチキンバイ）、水丁香（スイチョウコウ）
Name (Romaji)　KIDACHIKINBAI
Other name (s) (Romaji)　SUICHÔKÔ
学名　*Ludwigia octovalvis* (Jacq.) P.H. Raven var. *sessiliflora* (Micheli) Shinners
Jussiaea suffruticosa auct. non L.
科名　Onagraceae（アカバナ科）
英名　seedbox
Part of use　whole plant
Note 1　―
Note 2　―
注　―

名　称　**キダチコミカンソウ***

他名等　―
部位等　全草
備　考　―

他名（参考）　―
漢字表記・生薬名等　木立小蜜柑草（キダチコミカンソウ）
Name (Romaji)　KIDACHIKOMIKANSÔ*
Other name (s) (Romaji)　―
学名　*Phyllanthus niruri* L.*
Phyllanthus amarus Schumach.*
Phyllanthus niruri L. ssp. *amarus* (Schumach.) Leandri
Phyllanthus niruri auct. non L.
科名　Euphorbiaceae（トウダイグサ科）
英名　Chanca piedra / phyllanthus / carry-me-seed
Part of use　whole plant
Note 1　―
Note 2　―
注　―

名　称　**キダチハッカ***

他名等　サボリー
部位等　全草
備　考　―

他名（参考）　―
漢字表記・生薬名等　木立薄荷（キダチハッカ）
Name (Romaji)　KIDACHIHAKKA*
Other name (s) (Romaji)　SABORÎ
学名　*Satureja hortensis* L.*
Satureja laxiflora C. Koch
Satureja pachyphylla C. Koch
科名　Labiatae（シソ科）
英名　winter savory / summer savory / annual savory
Part of use　whole plant
Note 1　―
Note 2　―
注　―

名　称　**キヌガサタケ**

他名等　―
部位等　子実体
備　考　―

他名（参考）　コムソウタケ（虚無僧茸）
漢字表記・生薬名等　衣笠茸（キヌガサタケ）
Name (Romaji)　KINUGASATAKE
Other name (s) (Romaji)　―
学名　*Phallus indusiatus* Vent.
Dictyophora indusiata (Vent.) Desv.
科名　Phallaceae（スッポンタケ科）
英名　stinkhorn mushroom / long net stinkhorn / vailed lady
Part of use　fruit body
Note 1　―
Note 2　―
注　―

名　称　**キノア**

他名等　―
部位等　種子・葉
備　考　―

他名（参考）　―
漢字表記・生薬名等　―
Name (Romaji)　KINOA
Other name (s) (Romaji)　―
学名　*Chenopodium quinoa* Willd.
科名　Chenopodiaceae（アカザ科）
英名　quinoa
Part of use　seed, leaf
Note 1　―
Note 2　―
注　―

名　称　キバナアザミ*

他名等　サントリソウ
部位等　全草
備　考　—

他名(参考)　—
漢字表記・生薬名等　黄花薊（キバナアザミ）
Name(Romaji)　KIBANAAZAMI*
Other name(s) (Romaji)　SANTORISÔ
学名　*Cnicus benedictus* L.*
Centaurea benedicta (L.) L.*
Carduus benedictus (L.) Thell.
科名　Compositae（キク科）
英名　blessed thistle / holy thistle
Part of use　whole plant
Note 1　—
Note 2　—
注　—

名　称　キバナシュスラン

他名等　—
部位等　全草
備　考　—

他名(参考)　—
漢字表記・生薬名等　金線蓮（キンセンレン）、黄花繻子蘭（キバナシュスラン）
Name(Romaji)　KIBANASHUSURAN
Other name(s) (Romaji)　—
学名　*Anoectochilus formosanus* Hayata
科名　Orchidaceae（ラン科）
英名　jewel orchid
Part of use　whole plant
Note 1　—
Note 2　KIBANASHUSURAN is identical with KINSENREN, but their parts of use are different each other. KINSENREN is also listed in the item of "Name".
注　キバナシュスランは別項のキンセンレンと同一。但し、「部位等」の記載が異なっている。

名　称　キブネダイオウ

他名等　ネパールサンモ
部位等　根
備　考　—

他名(参考)　—
漢字表記・生薬名等　貴船大黄（キブネダイオウ）
Name(Romaji)　KIBUNEDAIÔ
Other name(s) (Romaji)　NEPÂRUSANMO
学名　*Rumex nepalensis* Spreng. var. *andreaenus* (Makino) Kitam.
科名　Polygonaceae（タデ科）
英名　sheep sorrel
Part of use　root
Note 1　—
Note 2　—
注　—

名　称　ギムネマ*

他名等　—
部位等　葉
備　考　—

他名(参考)　—
漢字表記・生薬名等　匙羹藤（シャカトウ）、武靴糖（ブカトウ）
Name(Romaji)　GIMUNEMA*
Other name(s) (Romaji)　—
学名　*Gymnema sylvestre* (Retz.) R. Br. ex Schult.*
科名　Asclepiadaceae（ガガイモ科）
英名　gymnema / gurmar
Part of use　leaf
Note 1　—
Note 2　GIMUNEMA is identical with BUKATÔ which is the name of traditional Japanese herbal medicine of GIMUNEMA, but their parts of use are different each other. BUKATÔ is also listed in the item of "Name".
注　ギムネマは別項のブカトウと同一。ブカトウはギムネマの生薬名であるが、「部位等」の記載が異なっている。

名　称　キャッサバ*

他名等　タピオカ／マニオク
部位等　塊根・葉
備　考　—

他名(参考)　イモノキ（芋の木）
漢字表記・生薬名等　—
Name(Romaji)　KYASSABA*
Other name(s) (Romaji)　TAPIOKA／MANIOKU
学名　*Manihot esculenta* Crantz.*
Manihot utilissima Pohl.
Janipha manihot (L.) Kunth*
Jatropha manihot L.*

科名　Euphorbiaceae（トウダイグサ科）
英名　manioc / cassava / tapioca / bitter cassava / Brazilian arrow root / manihot
Part of use　root tuber, leaf
Note 1　—
Note 2　—
注　—

名　称　**キャッツクロー***
他名等　—
部位等　全草
備　考　—

他名（参考）　—
漢字表記・生薬名等　—
Name（Romaji）　KYATTSUKURÔ*
Other name(s)（Romaji）　—
学名　*Uncaria tomentosa*（Willd.）DC.*
Uncaria guianensis（Aubl.）J.F. Gmel.
科名　Rubiaceae（アカネ科）
英名　cat's claw / uña-de-gato
Part of use　whole plant
Note 1　—
Note 2　—
注　—

名　称　**キュウセツチャ**
他名等　センリョウ
部位等　全草
備　考　—

他名（参考）　—
漢字表記・生薬名等　九節茶（キュウセツチャ）、千両（センリョウ）、接骨木（セッコツボク）
Name（Romaji）　KYÛSETSUCHA
Other name(s)（Romaji）　SENRYÔ
学名　*Sarcandra glabra*（Thunb.）Nakai
Chloranthus glaber（Thunb.）Makino
Chloranthus monander R. Br. ex Sims
科名　Chloranthaceae（センリョウ科）
英名　sarcandra
Part of use　whole plant
Note 1　—
Note 2　KYÛSETSUCHA is identical with SENRYÔ.
注　キュウセツチャは別項のセンリョウと同一。

名　称　**ギュウハクトウ**
他名等　—
部位等　茎・葉
備　考　—

他名（参考）　テンチャ（甜茶）
漢字表記・生薬名等　牛白藤（ギュウハクトウ）、甜茶（テンチャ）
Name（Romaji）　GYÛHAKUTÔ
Other name(s)（Romaji）　—
学名　*Oldenlandia hedyotidea*（DC.）Hand.-Mazz.
Hedyotis hedyotidea（DC.）Morr.
科名　Rubiaceae（アカネ科）
英名　—
Part of use　stem, leaf
Note 1　—
Note 2　GYÛHAKUTÔ is used for TENCHA（sweet medicinal herbal tea made from tree）. TENCHA is also listed in the item of "Name".
注　ギュウハクトウは別項のテンチャ（樹木から作られる甘い薬草茶）の一種として使用される。

名　称　**ギョウジャニンニク**
他名等　—
部位等　全草
備　考　—

他名（参考）　アイヌネギ（アイヌ葱）
漢字表記・生薬名等　行者葫（ギョウジャニンニク）
Name（Romaji）　GYÔJANINNIKU
Other name(s)（Romaji）　—
学名　*Allium victorialis* L. ssp. *platyphyllum* Hult.
Allium victorialis L. var. *platyphyllum*（Hult.）Makino
科名　Liliaceae（ユリ科）
英名　Alpine leek
Part of use　whole plant
Note 1　—
Note 2　—
注　—

名　称　**キョウチクトウ***
他名等　—
部位等　花
備　考　—

他名（参考）　—

漢字表記･生薬名等　夾竹桃（キョウチクトウ）
Name (Romaji)　KYÔCHIKUTÔ*
Other name (s) (Romaji)　—
学名　*Nerium indicum* Mill.*
Nerium oleander L. var. *indicum* (Mill.) Degener et Greenwell
Nerium odorum Sol.*
科名　Apocynaceae（キョウチクトウ科）
英名　kaner / karavira / oleander / Indian scented oleander / sweet scented oleander
Part of use　flower
Note 1　—
Note 2　—
注　—

名　称　**ギョリュウ**

他名等　—
部位等　全草
備　考　—

他名 (参考)　—
漢字表記･生薬名等　御柳（ギョリュウ）、西河柳（セイカリュウ）、檉柳（テイリュウ）
Name (Romaji)　GYORYÛ
Other name (s) (Romaji)　—
学名　*Tamarix chinensis* Lour.
科名　Tamaricaceae（ギョリュウ科）
英名　Chinese tamarisk
Part of use　whole plant
Note 1　—
Note 2　—
注　—

名　称　**ギョリュウモドキ***

他名等　エリカ／スコッツヘザー
部位等　全草
備　考　—

他名 (参考)　ハイデソウ
漢字表記･生薬名等　御柳擬き（ギョリュウモドキ）
Name (Romaji)　GYORYÛMODOKI*
Other name (s) (Romaji)　ERIKA／SUKOTTSUHEZÂ
学名　*Calluna vulgaris* (L.) Hull*
Erica vulgaris L.
Calluna vulgaris cv. *Sunrise*
科名　Ericaceae（ツツジ科）
英名　heather
Part of use　whole plant
Note 1　—
Note 2　—
注　—

名　称　**キランソウ**

他名等　ジゴクノカマノフタ
部位等　全草
備　考　—

他名 (参考)　—
漢字表記･生薬名等　金蒼小草・金瘡小草（キランソウ）、筋骨草（キンコツソウ）、地獄の釜の蓋（ジゴクノカマノフタ）、白毛夏枯草（ハクモウカゴソウ）
Name (Romaji)　KIRANSÔ
Other name (s) (Romaji)　JIGOKUNOKAMANOFUTA
学名　*Ajuga decumbens* Thunb.
科名　Labiatae（シソ科）
英名　kiransou
Part of use　whole plant
Note 1　—
Note 2　—
注　—

名　称　**キリンケツ***

他名等　キリンケツヤシ
部位等　果実から分泌する紅色樹脂
備　考　—

他名 (参考)　—
漢字表記･生薬名等　麒麟血・麒麟竭（キリンケツ）、麒麟血椰子（キリンケツヤシ）
Name (Romaji)　KIRINKETSU*
Other name (s) (Romaji)　KIRINKETSUYASHI
学名　*Daemonorops draco* (Willd.) Bl.*
科名　Palmae（ヤシ科）
英名　dragon's blood / East Indian dragon's blood / dragon's blood palm
Part of use　red resin secreted from fruit
Note 1　—
Note 2　—
注　—

名　称　**キリンソウ**

他名等　アイゾーン／ホソバノキリンソウ
部位等　全草
備　考　—

他名(参考)　—
漢字表記・生薬名等　黄輪草（キリンソウ)、景天三七（ケイテンサンシチ)
Name (Romaji)　KIRINSÔ
Other name (s) (Romaji)　AIZÔN／HOSOBANOKIRINSÔ
学名　*Sedum aizoon* L.
Sedum aizoon var. *floribundum* Nakai
Sedum kamtschaticum auct. non Fisch.
科名　Crassulaceae（ベンケイソウ科)
英名　yellow sedum
Part of use　whole plant
Note 1　—
Note 2　—
注　—

名　称　**キンカン**

他名等　—
部位等　果実
備　考　—

他名(参考)　—
漢字表記・生薬名等　金柑（キンカン)、金橘（キンキツ)
Name (Romaji)　KINKAN
Other name (s) (Romaji)　—
学名　*Fortunella* Swingle
Fortunella japonica (Thunb.) Swingle
Fortunella margarita (Lour.) Swingle
科名　Rutaceae（ミカン科)
英名　kumquat
Part of use　fruit
Note 1　—
Note 2　—
注　—

名　称　**キンギンカ***

他名等　スイカズラ／ニンドウ
部位等　全草
備　考　—

他名(参考)　—
漢字表記・生薬名等　金銀花（キンギンカ)、忍冬・忍冬藤（ニンドウ：茎及び葉)、吸葛（スイカズラ)
Name (Romaji)　KINGINKA*
Other name (s) (Romaji)　SUIKAZURA／NINDÔ
学名　*Lonicera japonica* Thunb.*
科名　Caprifoliaceae（スイカズラ科)
英名　Japanese honeysuckle
Part of use　whole plant
Note 1　—
Note 2　—
注　—

名　称　**キンシバイ**

他名等　—
部位等　全草
備　考　—

他名(参考)　—
漢字表記・生薬名等　金糸梅（キンシバイ)
Name (Romaji)　KINSHIBAI
Other name (s) (Romaji)　—
学名　*Hypericum patulum* Thunb.
科名　Guttiferae（オトギリソウ科)
英名　—
Part of use　whole plant
Note 1　—
Note 2　—
注　—

名　称　**キンシンサイ***

他名等　ヤブカンゾウ
部位等　花・若芽
備　考　—

他名(参考)　—
漢字表記・生薬名等　金針菜（キンシンサイ)、藪萱草（ヤブカンゾウ)
Name (Romaji)　KINSHINSAI*
Other name (s) (Romaji)　YABUKANZÔ
学名　*Hemerocallis fulva* L. var. *kwanso* Regel*
科名　Liliaceae（ユリ科)
英名　kwanso / orange day lily / golden needle / double tawny day-lily
Part of use　flower, young sprout
Note 1　—
Note 2　—
注　—

名　称　キンセンソウ*

他名等　—
部位等　全草
備　考　—

他名(参考)　—
漢字表記･生薬名等　金銭草（キンセンソウ）
Name(Romaji)　KINSENSÔ*
Other name(s) (Romaji)　—
学名　*Lysimachia christiniae* Hance*
科名　Primulaceae（サクラソウ科）
英名　lysimachia / Christine loosestrife
Part of use　whole plant
Note 1　—
Note 2　—
注　—

名　称　キンセンレン

他名等　—
部位等　葉
備　考　—

他名(参考)　キバナシュスラン（黄花繻子蘭）
漢字表記･生薬名等　金線蓮（キンセンレン）
Name(Romaji)　KINSENREN
Other name(s) (Romaji)　—
学名　*Anoectochilus formosanus* Hayata
科名　Orchidaceae（ラン科）
英名　jewel orchid
Part of use　leaf
Note 1　—
Note 2　KINSENREN is identical with KIBANASHUSURAN, but their parts of use are different each other. KIBANASHUSURAN is also listed in the item of "Name".
注　キンセンレンは別項のキバナシュスランと同一。但し、「部位等」の記載が異なっている。

名　称　ギンネム

他名等　ギンゴウカン
部位等　全草
備　考　—

他名(参考)　—
漢字表記･生薬名等　銀合歓（ギンネム）
Name(Romaji)　GINNEMU
Other name(s) (Romaji)　GINGÔKAN
学名　*Leucaena leucocephala* (Lam.) De Wit
Leucaena glauca (L.) Benth.
Mimosa glauca L.
科名　Leguminosae（マメ科）
英名　lead tree / white popinac / leucaena / wild tamarind
Part of use　whole plant
Note 1　—
Note 2　—
注　—

名　称　キンマ*

他名等　—
部位等　果実・葉
備　考　—

他名(参考)　—
漢字表記･生薬名等　蒟醤（キンマ）
Name(Romaji)　KINMA*
Other name(s) (Romaji)　—
学名　*Piper betle* L.*
科名　Piperaceae（コショウ科）
英名　ikmo / buyo (bisaya) / betel leaf pepper / betel / betel pepper / betel vine / sirih
Part of use　fruit, leaf
Note 1　—
Note 2　—
注　—

名　称　キンミズヒキ*

他名等　センカクソウ／リュウガソウ
部位等　全草
備　考　—

他名(参考)　—
漢字表記･生薬名等　金水引（キンミズヒキ）、竜芽草・竜牙草・龍牙草（リュウガソウ）、仙鶴草（センカクソウ）
Name(Romaji)　KINMIZUHIKI*
Other name(s) (Romaji)　SENKAKUSÔ／RYÛGASÔ
学名　*Agrimonia pilosa* Ledeb.*
科名　Rosaceae（バラ科）
英名　agrimony
Part of use　whole plant
Note 1　—
Note 2　—
注　—

名　称　**キンモクセイ**

他名等　—
部位等　花
備　考　—

他名(参考)　—
漢字表記･生薬名等　金木犀（キンモクセイ）
Name (Romaji)　KINMOKUSEI
Other name(s) (Romaji)　—
学名　*Osmanthus fragrans* Lour. var. *aurantiacus* Makino
科名　Oleaceae（モクセイ科）
英名　fragrant olive / sweet osmanthus / cassia flower / cinnamon flower
Part of use　flower
Note 1　—
Note 2　—
注　—

名　称　**キンレンカ***

他名等　—
部位等　全草
備　考　—

他名(参考)　ノウゼンハレン（凌霄葉蓮）
漢字表記･生薬名等　金蓮花（キンレンカ）
Name (Romaji)　KINRENKA*
Other name(s) (Romaji)　—
学名　*Tropaeolum majus* L.*
科名　Tropaeolaceae（ノウゼンハレン科）
英名　garden nastritium / common nastritium / large Indian cress
Part of use　whole plant
Note 1　—
Note 2　—
注　—

名　称　**グアコ***

他名等　—
部位等　葉
備　考　—

他名(参考)　—
漢字表記･生薬名等　—
Name (Romaji)　GUAKO*
Other name(s) (Romaji)　—
学名　*Mikania guaco* Humb. et Bonpl.*
Mikania amara Willd.
科名　Compositae（キク科）
英名　guaco
Part of use　leaf
Note 1　—
Note 2　—
注　—

名　称　**グアバ***

他名等　バンカ／バンザクロ／バンジロウ／バンセキリュウ
部位等　果実・果皮・葉
備　考　—

他名(参考)　—
漢字表記･生薬名等　蕃石榴（バンジロウ）、蕃果（バンカ）
Name (Romaji)　GUABA*
Other name(s) (Romaji)　BANKA／BANZAKURO／BANJIRÔ／BANSEKIRYÛ
学名　*Psidium guajava* L.*
Psidium pomiferum L.*
Psidium pyriferum L.*
科名　Myrtaceae（フトモモ科）
英名　guava
Part of use　fruit, pericarp, leaf
Note 1　—
Note 2　—
注　—

名　称　**グアヤクノキ***

他名等　ユソウボク
部位等　材部
備　考　—

他名(参考)　—
漢字表記･生薬名等　癒創木（ユソウボク）
Name (Romaji)　GUAYAKUNOKI*
Other name(s) (Romaji)　YUSÔBOKU
学名　*Guaiacum officinale* L.*
科名　Zygophyllaceae（ハマビシ科）
英名　guaiacum / lignum vitae (heart wood) / guaiac (resin)
Part of use　tree
Note 1　—
Note 2　—
注　—

名　称　クガイ*

他名等　ニガヨモギ／ワームウッド
部位等　茎枝
備　考　―

他名(参考)　―
漢字表記・生薬名等　苦艾（ニガヨモギ）、苦蓬（クガイ）
Name(Romaji)　KUGAI*
Other name(s)(Romaji)　NIGAYOMOGI／WÂMUUD-DO
学名　*Artemisia absinthium* L.*
科名　Compositae（キク科）
英名　absinthe / aromoise / wermut / absinthe grande / wermutkraut / wormwood / common wormwood
Part of use　stem, branch
Note 1　―
Note 2　"茎枝（stem-branch）" in the item of "Part of use" written in Japanese should be replaced by "茎・枝（stem and/or branch）"
注　「部位等」の茎枝は茎・枝である。

名　称　クコ*

他名等　クコシ／クコヨウ
部位等　果実・葉
備　考　根皮は「医」

他名(参考)　―
漢字表記・生薬名等　果実：枸杞子（クコシ）、葉：枸杞葉（クコヨウ）、根皮：地骨皮（ジコッピ）
Name(Romaji)　KUKO*
Other name(s)(Romaji)　KUKOSHI／KUKOYÔ
学名　*Lycium barbarum* L.*
Lycium chinense Mill.*
科名　Solanaceae（ナス科）
英名　boxthorn / matrimony vine / Chinese boxthorn / box thorn / lycium / Chinese wolfberry / Chinese matrimony vine / barbary wolfberry
Part of use　fruit, leaf
Note 1　root bark：drug category
Note 2　―
注　―

名　称　クサボケ

他名等　―
部位等　果実
備　考　―

他名(参考)　―
漢字表記・生薬名等　草木瓜（クサボケ）、和木瓜（ワモッカ）
Name(Romaji)　KUSABOKE
Other name(s)(Romaji)　―
学名　*Chaenomeles japonica* (Thunb.) Lindl.
Chaenomeles maulei (T. Moore) Scheid
Pyrus japonica Thunb.
Cydonia japonica (Thunb.) Pers.
科名　Rosaceae（バラ科）
英名　dwarf Japanese quince
Part of use　fruit
Note 1　―
Note 2　―
注　―

名　称　クジチョウ

他名等　―
部位等　全草
備　考　―

他名(参考)　イヌキケマン（イヌ黄華蔓）
漢字表記・生薬名等　苦地丁（クジチョウ）
Name(Romaji)　KUJICHÔ
Other name(s)(Romaji)　―
学名　*Corydalis bungeana* Turcz.
科名　Papaveraceae（ケシ科）
英名　ku di ding
Part of use　whole plant
Note 1　―
Note 2　―
注　―

名　称　クズ*

他名等　―
部位等　種子・葉・花・クズ澱粉・蔓
備　考　根（カッコン）は「医」

他名(参考)　―
漢字表記・生薬名等　葛（クズ）、根：葛根（カッコン）
Name(Romaji)　KUZU*
Other name(s)(Romaji)　―

学名　*Pueraria lobata* (Willd.) Ohwi*
Pueraria thunbergiana (Sieb. et Zucc.) Benth.
Pueraria triloba (Houtt.) Makino
Pueraria montana (Lour.) Merr. var. *lobata* (Willd.) Maesen et S.M. Almeida ex Sanjappa et Predeep*
科名　Leguminosae（マメ科）
英名　kudzu / kudzu-vine
Part of use　seed, leaf, flower, kudzu starch, vine
Note 1　root：drug category
Note 2　Refer to TAIWANSUKU listed in the item of "Name". But TAIWANSUKU is incorrect, the correct name is TAIWANKUZU.
注　別項のタイワンスクを参照。但し、タイワンスクの正しい名称はタイワンクズ。

名　称　**クスノキ***

他名等　—
部位等　葉
備　考　—

他名(参考)　—
漢字表記・生薬名等　楠・樟（クスノキ）、樟樹葉（ショウジュヨウ）
Name (Romaji)　KUSUNOKI*
Other name (s) (Romaji)　—
学名　*Cinnamomum camphora* (L.) J. Presl*
Camphora camphora (L.) H. Karst., nom. illeg.*
Camphora officinalis Nees*
Laurus camphora L.*
科名　Lauraceae（クスノキ科）
英名　camphor tree / camphor
Part of use　leaf
Note 1　—
Note 2　Essential oil of KUSUNOKI is listed as SHÔNÔ in the item of "Name".
注　クスノキの精油は別項のショウノウとして記載されている。

名　称　**グッタペルカ**

他名等　—
部位等　乳液
備　考　—

他名(参考)　ガッタパーチャ、グッタペルカノキ
漢字表記・生薬名等　乳液を固めたものがグッタペルカ
Name (Romaji)　GUTTAPERUKA
Other name (s) (Romaji)　—
学名　*Palaquium gutta* (Hook. f.) Baill.
Isonandra gutta Hook. f.
Dichopsis gutta Benth. et Hook. f.
科名　Sapotaceae（アカテツ科）
英名　gutta-percha
Part of use　latex
Note 1　—
Note 2　GUTTAPERUKA is correctly GUTTAPERUKA-NOKI. GUTTAPERUKA (gutta-percha) obtained from bark of TOCHÛ (*Eucommia ulmoides* Oliv.) is classified in the "drug" category.
注　グッタペルカは、正しくはグッタペルカノキである。トチュウの樹皮より得られるグッタペルカ（樹脂）は「医」リストに区分されている。

名　称　**クマザサ**

他名等　—
部位等　葉
備　考　—

他名(参考)　アタゴザサ（愛宕笹）
漢字表記・生薬名等　隈笹（クマザサ）
Name (Romaji)　KUMAZASA
Other name (s) (Romaji)　—
学名　*Sasa veitchii* (Carr.) Rehd.
Sasa albo-marginata Makino et Shibata
Bambusa veitchii Carr.
科名　Gramineae（イネ科）
英名　tall groundcover
Part of use　leaf
Note 1　—
Note 2　—
注　—

名　称　**クマツヅラ***

他名等　バーベナ／バベンソウ
部位等　全草
備　考　—

他名(参考)　—
漢字表記・生薬名等　馬鞭草（バベンソウ）、熊葛（クマツヅラ）
Name (Romaji)　KUMATSUZURA*
Other name (s) (Romaji)　BÂBENA／BABENSÔ
学名　*Verbena officinalis* L.*
Verbena officinalis L. ssp. *officinalis**
科名　Verbenaceae（クマツズラ科）
英名　fiddlewood / vervain / common vervena / Europe-

an vervain / holy herb
Part of use　whole plant
Note 1　—
Note 2　—
注　—

名　称　**クマヤナギ**

他名等　—
部位等　茎・葉・木部
備　考　—

他名(参考)　—
漢字表記･生薬名等　熊柳（クマヤナギ）
Name(Romaji)　KUMAYANAGI
Other name(s) (Romaji)　—
学名　*Berchemia racemosa* Sieb. et Zucc.
科名　Rhamnaceae（クロウメモドキ科）
英名　—
Part of use　stem, leaf, xylem
Note 1　—
Note 2　—
注　—

名　称　**クミスクチン***

他名等　—
部位等　全草
備　考　—

他名(参考)　ネコノヒゲ、クミス・クチン
漢字表記･生薬名等　猫髭草（ビョウシュソウ、葉はFolia orthosiphonis(Java tea)）
Name(Romaji)　KUMISUKUCHIN*
Other name(s) (Romaji)　—
学名　*Orthosiphon aristatus* (Bl.) Miq.*
Ocimum aristatum Bl.
Ocimum stamineus Benth.
Ocimum spiralis (Lour.) Merr.
Clerodendranthus spicatus Wu et Li
科名　Labiatae（シソ科）
英名　cat's whiskers / Java tea / kumis kucin / kumis kuching
Part of use　whole plant
Note 1　—
Note 2　—
注　—

名　称　**クミン***

他名等　—
部位等　果実
備　考　—

他名(参考)　クミン
漢字表記･生薬名等　孜然芹（コウゼンキン）、馬芹（ウマゼリ）
Name(Romaji)　KUMIN*
Other name(s) (Romaji)　—
学名　*Cuminum cyminum* L.*
科名　Umbelliferae（セリ科）
英名　cumin
Part of use　fruit
Note 1　—
Note 2　—
注　—

名　称　**クラチャイ**

他名等　クンチ
部位等　全草
備　考　—

他名(参考)　—
漢字表記･生薬名等　—
Name(Romaji)　KURACHAI
Other name(s) (Romaji)　KUNCHI
学名　*Boesenbergia pandurata* (Roxb.) Schult.
Kaempferia pandurata Roxb.
Gastrochilus pandulatus (Roxb.) Ridl.
科名　Zingiberaceae（ショウガ科）
英名　Chinese ginger / Chinese key / lesser ginger / temu kunchi / kunchi
Part of use　whole plant
Note 1　—
Note 2　—
注　—

名　称　**グラビオラ***

他名等　サーサップ／トゲバンレイシ／オランダドリアン
部位等　果実
備　考　種子は「医」

他名(参考)　—
漢字表記･生薬名等　棘蕃茘枝（トゲバンレイシ）
Name(Romaji)　GURABIORA*
Other name(s) (Romaji)　SÂSAPPU／TOGEBANREI-

SHI／ORANDADORIAN
学名　*Annona muricata* L.*
科名　Annonaceae（バンレイシ科）
英名　sour-sop / sour apple / guanabana / graviola / sir-sak / nangka blanda / prickly custard apple / durian benggala
Part of use　fruit
Note 1　seed：drug category
Note 2　—
注　—

名　称　**クランベリー***

他名等　ツルコケモモ
部位等　果実・葉
備　考　—

他名(参考)　—
漢字表記･生薬名等　—
Name (Romaji)　KURANBERÎ*
Other name (s) (Romaji)　TSURUKOKEMOMO
学名　*Vaccinium macrocarpon* Ait.*
Oxycoccus macrocarpus (Ait.) Pers.
科名　Ericaceae（ツツジ科）
英名　cranberry / American cranberry / large cranberry / low-bush cranberry
Part of use　fruit, leaf
Note 1　—
Note 2　—
注　—

名　称　**グリーンランドイソツツジ***

他名等　ラブラドールティー*
部位等　全草
備　考　—

他名(参考)　—
漢字表記･生薬名等　—
Name (Romaji)　GURÎNRANDOISOTSUTSUJI
Other name (s) (Romaji)　RABURADÔRUTÎ
学名　*Ledum groenlandicum* Oeder*
Ledum latifolium Jacq.
科名　Ericaceae（ツツジ科）
英名　Labrador tea / bog Labrador tea
Part of use　whole plant
Note 1　—
Note 2　—
注　—

名　称　**グルテン**

他名等　コムギ
部位等　小麦蛋白質の混合物
備　考　—

他名(参考)　—
漢字表記･生薬名等　—
Name (Romaji)　GURUTEN
Other name (s) (Romaji)　KOMUGI
学名　*Triticum sativum* L.
Triticum vulgare Vill.
Triticum aestivum ssp. *vulgare* (Vill.) Mac Key
科名　Gramineae（イネ科）
英名　gluten / wheat / common wheat / bread wheat
Part of use　mixture of wheat protein (gluten)
Note 1　—
Note 2　GURUTEN is the component of KOMUGI. Then scientific names of KOMUGI are listed here.
注　グルテンはコムギの成分名であるので、コムギの学名を記載した。

名　称　**クルマバソウ***

他名等　ウッドラフ
部位等　全草
備　考　—

他名(参考)　—
漢字表記･生薬名等　車葉草（クルマバソウ）
Name (Romaji)　KURUMABASÔ*
Other name (s) (Romaji)　UDDORAFU
学名　*Asperula odorata* L.*
Galium odoratum (L.) Scop.*
科名　Rubiaceae（アカネ科）
英名　sweet woodruff / sweet-scented bedstrow / wood ruff / sweetscented squinacy
Part of use　whole plant
Note 1　—
Note 2　—
注　—

名　称　**グレープフルーツ***

他名等　—
部位等　果実
備　考　—

他名(参考)　—
漢字表記･生薬名等　—

Name (Romaji)　GURÊPUFURÛTSU*
Other name (s) (Romaji)　—
学名　*Citrus×paradisi* Macfad.*
科名　Rutaceae（ミカン科）
英名　grapefruit
Part of use　fruit
Note 1　—
Note 2　—
注　—

名　称　**クローブ***

他名等　—
部位等　花・蕾
備　考　—

他名(参考)　チョウジ（丁子）
漢字表記･生薬名等　丁字（チョウジ)、丁香（チョウコウ）
Name (Romaji)　KURÔBU*
Other name (s) (Romaji)　—
学名　*Syzygium aromaticum* (L.) Merr. et L.M. Perry*
Caryophyllus aromaticus L.*
Eugenia caryophyllata Thunb.*
Eugenia aromatica (L.) Baill. nom. illeg.*
Eugenia caryophyllus (Spreng.) Bullock et S.G. Harrison
科名　Myrtaceae（フトモモ科）
英名　clove
Part of use　flower, bud
Note 1　—
Note 2　KURÔBU is identical with CHÔJI, but their parts of use are different each other. CHÔJI is also listed in the item of “Name”.
注　クローブは別項のチョウジと同一。但し、「部位等」の記載が異なっている。

名　称　**クロガラシ***

他名等　—
部位等　種子
備　考　—

他名(参考)　—
漢字表記･生薬名等　黒芥子（クロガラシ）
Name (Romaji)　KUROGARASHI*
Other name (s) (Romaji)　—
学名　*Brassica nigra* (L.) W.D.J. Koch*
Sinapis erysimoides Roxb.
科名　Cruciferae（アブラナ科）
英名　black mustard / true mustard / brown mustard
Part of use　seed
Note 1　—
Note 2　—
注　—

名　称　**クログルミ***

他名等　—
部位等　成熟果実・葉
備　考　—

他名(参考)　—
漢字表記･生薬名等　黒胡桃（クログルミ）
Name (Romaji)　KUROGURUMI*
Other name (s) (Romaji)　—
学名　*Juglans nigra* L.*
科名　Juglandaceae（クルミ科）
英名　black walnut
Part of use　riped fruit, leaf
Note 1　—
Note 2　—
注　—

名　称　**クロスグリ***

他名等　—
部位等　果実
備　考　—

他名(参考)　クロフサスグリ（黒房酸塊）
漢字表記･生薬名等　黒酸塊（クロスグリ）
Name (Romaji)　KUROSUGURI*
Other name (s) (Romaji)　—
学名　*Ribes nigrum* L.*
科名　Saxifragaceae（ユキノシタ科）
英名　black currant / cassis / European black currant / common black currant
Part of use　fruit
Note 1　—
Note 2　KUROSUGURI is identical with KASHISU, but their parts of use are different each other. KASHISU is also listed in the item of “Name”.
注　クロスグリは別項のカシスと同一。但し、「部位等」の記載が異なる。

名 称 **黒米***

他名等 —
部位等 種子
備 考 —

他名(参考) —
漢字表記・生薬名等 黒米(クロゴメ)
Name(Romaji) KUROGOME*
Other name(s)(Romaji) —
学名 *Oryza sativa* L.*
科名 Gramineae(イネ科)
英名 black rice
Part of use seed
Note 1 —
Note 2 —
注 —

名 称 **クロマメノキ**

他名等 —
部位等 果実
備 考 —

他名(参考) アサマブドウ(浅間葡萄)、ジブドウ(地葡萄)、シラネブドウ(白根葡萄)
漢字表記・生薬名等 黒豆の木・黒豆木(クロマメノキ)
Name(Romaji) KUROMAMENOKI
Other name(s)(Romaji) —
学名 *Vaccinium uliginosum* L.
Vaccinium gaultherioides Bigelow
Vaccinium occidentale A. Gray
Vaccinium uliginosum var. *alpinum* Bigelow
Vaccinium uliginosum L. ssp. *gaultherioides* (Bigelow) S.B. Young
Vaccinium uliginosum var. *microphyllum* Lange
科名 Ericaceae(ツツジ科)
英名 bog bilberry / bog blueberry
Part of use fruit
Note 1 —
Note 2 —
注 —

名 称 **クロヨナ***

他名等 —
部位等 種子
備 考 —

他名(参考) —
漢字表記・生薬名等 水流豆(スイリュウトウ)、九重吹(クロヨナ)
Name(Romaji) KUROYONA*
Other name(s)(Romaji) —
学名 *Pongamia pinnata* (L.) Pierre*
Pongamia glabra Vent.*
Cytisus pinnatus L.
Derris indica (Lam.) Bennett
科名 Leguminosae(マメ科)
英名 pongam / karum tree / poonga-oil tree / Indian beech
Part of use seed
Note 1 —
Note 2 —
注 —

名 称 **クロレラ**

他名等 —
部位等 藻類・エキス
備 考 —

他名(参考) —
漢字表記・生薬名等 —
Name(Romaji) KURORERA
Other name(s)(Romaji) —
学名 *Chlorella* M. Beijerinck
科名 Oocystaceae(オオシスチス科)
英名 chlorella
Part of use algae, algae extract
Note 1 —
Note 2 —
注 —

名 称 **クワ***

他名等 ソウジン/ソウヨウ/マグワ
部位等 葉・花・実(集合果)
備 考 根皮は「医」

他名(参考) トウグワ・カラグワ(唐桑)、シログワ(白桑)、カラヤマグワ(唐山桑)、カントングワ(広東桑)
漢字表記・生薬名等 桑(クワ)、桑椹(ソウジン)、桑葉(ソウヨウ)、真桑(マグワ)、根皮:桑白皮(ソウハクヒ)
Name(Romaji) KUWA*
Other name(s)(Romaji) SÔJIN/SÔYÔ/MAGUWA
学名 *Morus alba* L.*(マグワ・カラヤマグワ)
Morus atropurpurea Roxb.(カントングワ)
科名 Moraceae(クワ科)
英名 mulberry / white mulberry

Part of use　leaf, flower, fruit（sorosis）
Note 1　root bark：drug category
Note 2　Refer to MARUBERÎ listed in the item of "Name". The English name of KUWA is mulberry.
注　別項のマルベリーを参照。クワの英名はマルベリーである。

名　称　クワガタソウ

他名等　—
部位等　根・葉
備　考　—

他名(参考)　—
漢字表記・生薬名等　鍬形草（クワガタソウ）
Name(Romaji)　KUWAGATASÔ
Other name(s)(Romaji)　—
学名　*Veronica miqueliana* Nakai
科名　Scrophulariaceae（ゴマノハグサ科）
英名　brooklime / speedwell
Part of use　root, leaf
Note 1　—
Note 2　—
注　—

名　称　ケイケットウ*

他名等　—
部位等　つる
備　考　—

他名(参考)　ムラサキナツフジ（紫夏藤）、密花豆、白花油麻藤、香花岩豆藤
漢字表記・生薬名等　鶏血藤（ケイケットウ）、昆明鶏血藤（コンメイケイケットウ）、豊城鶏血藤（ホウジョウケイケットウ）
Name(Romaji)　KEIKETTÔ*
Other name(s)(Romaji)　—
学名　*Spatholobus suberectus* Dunn（密花豆）
Millettia reticulata Benth.*（紫夏藤）
Millettia dielsiana Harms ex Diels*（香花岩豆藤）
Mucuna birdwoodiana Tutcher（白花油麻藤）
科名　Leguminosae（マメ科）
英名　spatholobus / Millettia reticulata
Part of use　vine
Note 1　—
Note 2　KEIKETTÔ is the name of traditional Japanese herbal medicine and several different herbs shown in the item of "Scientific name" are called KEIKETTÔ.
注　ケイケットウは生薬名であり、学名に示した数種類の植物がケイケットウと呼ばれている。

名　称　ケイコツソウ

他名等　—
部位等　全草
備　考　—

他名(参考)　シロトウアズキ
漢字表記・生薬名等　鶏骨草（ケイコツソウ）
Name(Romaji)　KEIKOTSUSÔ
Other name(s)(Romaji)　—
学名　*Abrus fruticulosus* Wall. ex Wighte et Arn.
科名　Leguminosae（マメ科）
英名　—
Part of use　whole plant
Note 1　—
Note 2　—
注　—

名　称　ケイシ*

他名等　Cinnamomum cassia
部位等　小枝・若枝
備　考　—

他名(参考)　—
漢字表記・生薬名等　桂枝（ケイシ）、東京肉桂（トンキンニッケイ）、桂（ケイ）
Name(Romaji)　KEISHI*
Other name(s)(Romaji)　—
学名　*Cinnamomum cassia* Presl*
Cinnamomum cassia Blume*
Cinnamomum aromaticum Nees*
科名　Lauraceae（クスノキ科）
英名　cassia / cassia lignea / Chinese cinnamon / cinnamon
Part of use　branch, young branch
Note 1　—
Note 2　KEISHI is identical with KEIHI, but their parts of use are different each other. KEIHI is also listed in the item of "Name".
注　ケイシは別項のケイヒと同一。但し、「部位等」の記載が異なっている。

名　称　**ケイヒ***

他名等　ケイ／シナニッケイ／ニッケイ
部位等　根皮・樹皮
備　考　—

他名(参考)　—
漢字表記・生薬名等　桂皮（ケイヒ）、東京肉桂（トンキンニッケイ）、桂（ケイ）
Name(Romaji)　KEIHI*
Other name(s)(Romaji)　KEI／SHINANIKKEI／NIKKEI
学名　*Cinnamomum cassia* Presl*
Cinnamomum cassia Blume*
Cinnamomum aromaticum Nees*
科名　Lauraceae（クスノキ科）
英名　cassia / cassia lignea / Chinese cinnamon / cinnamon
Part of use　root bark, cortex
Note 1　—
Note 2　KEIHI is identical with KEISHI, but their parts of use are different each other. KEISHI is also listed in the item of "Name".
注　ケイヒは別項のケイシと同一。但し、「部位等」の記載が異なっている。

名　称　**ケール***

他名等　ハゴロモカンラン
部位等　全草
備　考　—

他名(参考)　リョクヨウカンラン（緑葉甘藍）
漢字表記・生薬名等　羽衣甘藍（ハゴロモカンラン）、緑葉甘藍（リョクヨウカンラン）、芥藍（カイラン）
Name(Romaji)　KÊRU*
Other name(s)(Romaji)　HAGOROMOKANRAN
学名　*Brassica oleraceae* L. var. *acephala* DC.*
Brassica alboglabra L.H. Bailey
科名　Cruciferae（アブラナ科）
英名　kale / kail / collards / colewort / tall kale / borecole / Chinese kale
Part of use　whole plant
Note 1　—
Note 2　—
注　—

名　称　**ケシ***

他名等　—
部位等　発芽防止処理した種子・種子油
備　考　発芽防止処理した種子・種子油を除く全草は「医」

他名(参考)　—
漢字表記・生薬名等　芥子（ケシ）
Name(Romaji)　KESHI*
Other name(s)(Romaji)　—
学名　*Papaver somniferum* L.*
科名　Papaveraceae（ケシ科）
英名　garden poppy / poppy / opium poppy / opium
Part of use　seed treated for prevention of germination, seed oil
Note 1　whole plant except seed treated for prevention of germination and seed oil：drug category
Note 2　—
注　—

名　称　**ゲッカビジン**

他名等　ドンカ
部位等　全草
備　考　—

他名(参考)　—
漢字表記・生薬名等　月下美人（ゲッカビジン）、曇花（ドンカ）
Name(Romaji)　GEKKABIJIN
Other name(s)(Romaji)　DONKA
学名　*Epiphyllum oxypetalum* (DC.) Haw.
科名　Cactaceae（サボテン科）
英名　queen of the night / selenicereus / Dutchman's pipe / Dutchman's pipe cactus
Part of use　whole plant
Note 1　—
Note 2　—
注　—

名　称　**ゲッケイジュ**

他名等　ゲッケイヨウ／ベイリーフ／ローレル
部位等　葉
備　考　—

他名(参考)　—
漢字表記・生薬名等　月桂樹（ゲッケイジュ）
Name(Romaji)　GEKKEIJU

Other name(s) (Romaji)　GEKKEIYÔ／BEIRÎFU／RÔRERU
学名　*Laurus nobilis* L.
科名　Lauraceae（クスノキ科）
英名　laurel / bay tree / bay / bay laurel / Grecian laurel / sweet bay / true bay
Part of use　leaf
Note 1　—
Note 2　—
注　—

名　称　**ゲットウ**

他名等　月桃
部位等　葉
備　考　—

他名(参考)　キフゲットウ（黄斑月桃）
漢字表記·生薬名等　アルピニア、砂仁（サンニン）、月桃（ゲットウ）
Name(Romaji)　GETTÔ
Other name(s) (Romaji)　GETTÔ
学名　*Alpinia zerumbet* (Per.) B.L. Burtt et R.M. Sm.
Alpinia speciosa (J.C. Wendl.) K. Schum.
Languas speciosa (J.C. Wendl.) Small
Catinbium speciosum (J.C. Wendl.) Holttum
科名　Zingiberaceae（ショウガ科）
英名　shell ginger / shell flower / pink porcelain lily
Part of use　leaf
Note 1　—
Note 2　—
注　—

名　称　**ケルプ**

他名等　—
部位等　全藻
備　考　—

他名(参考)　—
漢字表記·生薬名等　—
Name(Romaji)　KERUPU
Other name(s) (Romaji)　—
学名　seaweed (Fucaceae, Laminariaceae, Lessoniaceae)
科名　Fucaceae（ヒバマタ科）
Laminariaceae（コンブ科）
Lessoniaceae（レッソニア科）
英名　kelp / bladderwrack / dyer's fucus / red fucus / rock wrack
Part of use　whole seaweed
Note 1　—
Note 2　KERUPU is the name indicating seaweeds such as giant KONBU (tangle).
注　ケルプは大型コンブなどの海藻を指す。

名　称　**ケン**

他名等　—
部位等　種子の核
備　考　—

他名(参考)　ヒユ（莧）
漢字表記·生薬名等　莧（ケン、ヒユ）
Name(Romaji)　KEN
Other name(s) (Romaji)　—
学名　*Amaranthus tricolor* L. ssp. *mangostanus* (L.) Aellen
Amaranthus gangeticus L.
科名　Amaranthaceae（ヒユ科）
英名　ganges amaranth
Part of use　stone
Note 1　—
Note 2　—
注　—

名　称　**ケンケレバ***

他名等　コンブレツム
部位等　葉
備　考　—

他名(参考)　キンケリバ、キンキリバ
漢字表記·生薬名等　—
Name(Romaji)　KENKEREBA*
Other name(s) (Romaji)　KONBURETSUMU
学名　*Combretum micranthum* G. Don.*
Combretum altum Perr.
Combretum floribundum Engle. et Diels
Combretum raimbautii Heck.
科名　Combretaceae（シクンシ科）
英名　kinkeliba / kinkelliba / quinquelibas
Part of use　leaf
Note 1　—
Note 2　—
注　—

名　称　**ゲンチアナ***

他名等　—
部位等　花
備　考　根・根茎は「医」

他名(参考)　—
漢字表記・生薬名等　—
Name(Romaji)　GENCHIANA*
Other name(s) (Romaji)　—
学名　*Gentiana lutea* L.*
科名　Gentianaceae（リンドウ科）
英名　gentian / yellow gentian
Part of use　flower
Note 1　root and rhizome：drug category
Note 2　—
注　—

名　称　**玄米胚芽***

他名等　イネ
部位等　胚芽・胚芽油
備　考　—

他名(参考)　—
漢字表記・生薬名等　玄米胚芽（ゲンマイハイガ）
Name(Romaji)　GENMAIHAIGA*
Other name(s) (Romaji)　INE
学名　*Oryza sativa* L.*
科名　Gramineae（イネ科）
英名　brown rice germ
Part of use　germ, germ oil
Note 1　—
Note 2　—
注　—

名　称　**コウカガンショウ**

他名等　セキレン
部位等　全草
備　考　—

他名(参考)　フチベニベンケイ（縁紅弁慶）、カゲツ（花月）
漢字表記・生薬名等　石蓮（セキレン）、荷花掌（ニカショウ）、玉蓮花（ギョクレンカ）、燕子掌（エンシショウ）、紅花岩松（コウカガンショウ）
Name(Romaji)　KÔKAGANSHÔ
Other name(s) (Romaji)　SEKIREN
学名　*Crassula portulacea* Lam.
科名　Crassulaceae（ベンケイソウ科）
英名　baby Jade / cauliflower ears / Chinese rubber plant / dollar plant / dwarf rubber plant / jade plant / jade tree / Japanese rubber plant
Part of use　whole plant
Note 1　—
Note 2　—
注　—

名　称　**コウキ**

他名等　—
部位等　茎・樹皮・葉
備　考　—

他名(参考)　—
漢字表記・生薬名等　黄杞（コウキ）
Name(Romaji)　KÔKI
Other name(s) (Romaji)　—
学名　*Engelhardtia chrysolepis* Hance
科名　Juglandaceae（クルミ科）
英名　Taiwan engelhardtia
Part of use　stem, bark, leaf
Note 1　—
Note 2　—
注　—

名　称　**コウジュ***

他名等　ナギナタコウジュ
部位等　全草
備　考　—

他名(参考)　—
漢字表記・生薬名等　香需・香茹（コウジュ）、薙刀香需（ナギナタコウジュ）
Name(Romaji)　KÔJU*
Other name(s) (Romaji)　NAGINATAKÔJU
学名　*Elsholtzia ciliata* (Thunb.) Hyl.*
科名　Labiatae（シソ科）
英名　elsholtzia / crested late-summer mint
Part of use　whole plant
Note 1　—
Note 2　—
注　—

名　称　**コウシンコウ***

他名等　コウコウ／コウコウダン
部位等　全草
備　考　—

他名(参考)　サトウボク（沙塘木）、ニオイシタン
漢字表記・生薬名等　降真香（コウシンコウ）、降香（コウコウ）、降香檀（コウコウダン）
Name(Romaji)　KÔSHINKÔ*
Other name(s) (Romaji)　KÔKÔ／KÔKÔDAN
学名　*Dalbergia odorifera* T. Chen*
科名　Leguminosae（マメ科）
英名　fragrant rosewood
Part of use　whole plant
Note 1　—
Note 2　—
注　—

名　称　**コウソウ**

他名等　—
部位等　全藻
備　考　—

他名(参考)　—
漢字表記・生薬名等　紅藻（コウソウ）
Name(Romaji)　KÔSÔ
Other name(s) (Romaji)　—
学名　seaweed（Rhodophyceae）
科名　Families belong to Rhodophyceae（紅藻綱に属する科）
英名　red algae
Part of use　whole seaweed
Note 1　—
Note 2　—
注　—

名　称　**コウホネ**

他名等　—
部位等　茎
備　考　根茎は「医」

他名(参考)　センコツ（川骨）
漢字表記・生薬名等　河骨（コウホネ）
Name(Romaji)　KÔHONE
Other name(s) (Romaji)　—
学名　*Nuphar japonicum* DC.
科名　Nymphaeaceae（スイレン科）
英名　ko-hone
Part of use　stem
Note 1　rhizome：drug category
Note 2　—
注　—

名　称　**酵母**

他名等　**Saccharomycesに属する単細胞生物／トルラ酵母／ビール酵母／Candida utilis**
部位等　菌体
備　考　—

他名(参考)　—
漢字表記・生薬名等　酵母（コウボ）
Name(Romaji)　KÔBO
Other name(s) (Romaji)　—
学名　single-cell organism belongs to *Saccharomyces* Meyen and *Candida utilis* (Henneberg) Lodder et Kreger-wan Rij (Syn. *Torula utilis* (Henneberg) Lodder)
Torula utilis Henneberg
科名　Saccharomycetaceae（サッカロミケス科）
英名　yeast / Torula dried yeast / brewer's yeast / baker yeast
Part of use　fungus body
Note 1　—
Note 2　—
注　—

名　称　**コウモウゴカ**

他名等　**紅毛五加**
部位等　樹皮
備　考　—

他名(参考)　—
漢字表記・生薬名等　広東省では五加皮（ゴカヒ）として用いる。
Name(Romaji)　KÔMÔGOKA
Other name(s) (Romaji)　KÔMÔGOKA
学名　*Acanthopanax giraldii* Harms
Eleutherococcus giraldii (Harms) Nakai
科名　Araliaceae（ウコギ科）
英名　non wu jia
Part of use　bark
Note 1　—
Note 2　—
注　—

名 称 **コオウレン***

他名等 Picrorhiza kurrooa／Picrorhiza scrophulariaeflora
部位等 茎・根茎
備 考 —

他名(参考) コレン（胡蓮）
漢字表記･生薬名等 胡黄蓮（コオウレン）
Name(Romaji) KOÔREN*
Other name(s) (Romaji) —
学名 *Picrorhiza kurrooa* Royle ex Benth.*
Picrorhiza scrophulariiflora Pennell*
Neopicrorhiza sacrophulariiflora (Pennell) D.Y. Hong*
科名 Scrophulariaceae（ゴマノハグサ科）
英名 kutki / katuka / picrorhiza
Part of use stem, rhizome
Note 1 —
Note 2 The correct spelling of *Picrorhiza scrophulariaeflora* written in the item of “Other names” is *Picrorhiza scrophulariiflora.*
注 「他名等」の*Picrorhiza scrophulariaeflora*の正しい綴りは*Picrorhiza scrophulariiflora*。

名 称 **コーヒーノキ***

他名等 アラビアコーヒー
部位等 果実
備 考 —

他名(参考) アラビアコーヒーノキ
漢字表記･生薬名等 —
Name(Romaji) KÔHÎNOKI*
Other name(s) (Romaji) ARABIAKÔHÎ
学名 *Coffea arabica* L.*
科名 Rubiaceae（アカネ科）
英名 Arabian coffee / coffee / common coffee
Part of use fruit
Note 1 —
Note 2 —
注 —

名 称 **コーラ***

他名等 コラ／コラシ／コラノキ
部位等 種子
備 考 —

他名(参考) —
漢字表記･生薬名等 —
Name(Romaji) KÔRA*
Other name(s) (Romaji) KORA／KORASHI／KORA-NOKI
学名 *Cola nitida* (Vent.) Schott et Endl.*
Sterculia nitida Vent.*
Cola acuminata (Brenan) Schott et Endl.*
科名 Sterculiaceae（アオギリ科）
英名 cola / abata cola / bitter cola / bissy nut / kola / gbanja kola
Part of use seed
Note 1 —
Note 2 —
注 —

名 称 **ゴカ***

他名等 ソヨウゴカ／マンシュウウコギ／リンサンゴカ
部位等 根皮・種子・葉・花
備 考 —

他名(参考) ウコギ（五加）、ナンゴカヒ（南五加皮）、ホクゴカヒ（北五加皮）、クロバナカズラ（コウカヒ（香加皮））、エゾウコギ（シゴカ（刺五加））、ゾウヨウゴカ（糙葉五加）
漢字表記･生薬名等 五加（ウコギ）、五加皮（ゴカヒ）、
A. sessiliflorus：南五加皮（ナンゴカヒ）・無梗五加（ムコウゴカ）、
A. senticosus：南五加皮（ナンゴカヒ）・刺五加（シゴカ）、
A. gracilistylus：南五加皮（ナンゴカヒ）
Name(Romaji) GOKA*
Other name(s) (Romaji) SOYÔGOKA／MANSHÛUKOGI／RINSANGOKA
学名 *Eleutherococcus senticosus* (Rupr. et Maxim.) Maxim.（=*Acanthopanax senticosus* (Rupr. et Maxim.) Harms*）（エゾウコギ）
Eleutherococcus sessiliflorus (Rupr. et Maxim.) S.Y. Hu*（=*Acanthopanax sessiliflorus* (Rupr. et Maxim.) Seem)（マンシュウウコギ）
Eleutherococcus gracilistylus (W.W. Sm.) S.Y. Hu（=*Acanthopanax gracilistylus* W.W. Sm.*）（タンナウコギ）
Eleutherococcus henryi Oliv.（=*Acanthopanax henryi* (Oliv.) Harms)（ソヨウゴカ・ゾウヨウゴカ）
Eleutherococcus verticillatus (G. Hoo) H. Ohashi（=*Acanthopanax verticillatus* G. Hoo)（リンサンゴカ）
科名 Araliaceae（ウコギ科）
英名 Eleutherococcus sessiliflorus / stalkless-flower / eleutero / Siberian ginseng / Ussurian thorny / pepper bush / Chinese silk vine

Part of use root bark, seed, leaf, flower
Note 1 —
Note 2 SOYÔGOKA written in the item of "Other names" is incorrect. The correct name is ZÔYÔGOKA. GOKA is deciduous shrubs and belongs to Araliaceae. Its dried root bark is called NANGOKAHI as traditional Japanese herbal medicine and *Eleutherococcus senticosus* is especially called SHIGOKA. KÔKAHI, the dried root bark of *Periploca sepium* Bunge belongs to Asclepiadaceae is called HOKUGOKAHI as traditional Japanese herbal medicine.
注 「他名等」のソヨウゴカはゾウヨウゴカが正しい。
ゴカはウコギ科の落葉低木を指し、乾燥根皮をナンゴカヒ（南五加皮）という。エゾウコギの根皮をシゴカ（刺五加という。
ガガイモ科の*Periploca sepium* Bunge（クロバナカズラ）の乾燥根皮（コウカヒ、香加皮）をホクゴカヒ（北五加皮）という。

名 称 コガネキクラゲ

他名等 Golden Tremella
部位等 子実体
備 考 —

他名（参考） コガネニカワタケ（黄金膠茸）
漢字表記・生薬名等 —
Name (Romaji) KOGANEKIKURAGE
Other name (s) (Romaji) —
学名 *Tremella mesenterica* (Schaeff.) Retz.
Tremella lutescens Pers.
Tremella quercina Pollini
科名 Tremellaceae（シロキクラゲ科）
英名 golden tremella / witches butter / yellow brain
Part of use fruit body
Note 1 —
Note 2 KOGANEKIKURAGE cannot be confirmed. Therefore, KOGANENIKAWATAKE written in the item of "Other names" is taken up here.
注 コガネキクラゲは確認されない。本項では「他名等」のコガネニカワタケとして取り扱った。

名 称 コケモモ*

他名等 —
部位等 果実
備 考 葉は「医」

他名（参考） イワモモ（岩桃）
漢字表記・生薬名等 苔桃（コケモモ）
Name (Romaji) KOKEMOMO*
Other name (s) (Romaji) —
学名 *Vaccinium vitis-idaea* L.*
科名 Ericaceae（ツツジ科）
英名 cowberry / lingonberry / mountain cranberry / foxberry / northern mountain cranberry
Part of use fruit
Note 1 leaf：drug category
Note 2 —
注 —

名 称 コゴメグサ*

他名等 —
部位等 全草
備 考 —

他名（参考） アイブライト
漢字表記・生薬名等 小米草（コゴメグサ）
Name (Romaji) KOGOMEGUSA*
Other name (s) (Romaji) —
学名 *Euphrasia officinalis* L.*
Euphrasia stricta J.P. Wolff ex J.F. Lehm.*
Euphrasia rostkoviana F. Hayne*
科名 Scrophulariaceae（ゴマノハグサ科）
英名 eyebright / drug eyebright
Part of use whole plant
Note 1 —
Note 2 KOGOMEGUSA is identical with AIBURAITO. AIBURAITO is also listed in the item of "Name".
注 コゴメグサは別項のアイブライトと同一。

名 称 コショウ*

他名等 —
部位等 果実
備 考 —

他名（参考） —
漢字表記・生薬名等 胡椒（コショウ）
Name (Romaji) KOSHÔ*
Other name (s) (Romaji) —
学名 *Piper nigrum* L.*
科名 Piperaceae（コショウ科）
英名 pepper / black pepper / common pepper
Part of use fruit
Note 1 —
Note 2 —
注 —

名　称　**コジン***

他名等　タイゲイ
部位等　全草
備　考　—

他名(参考)　ニクジュヨウ（肉蓯蓉、別名：タイゲイ（大芸））、ホンオニク（塩生肉蓯蓉）
漢字表記・生薬名等　大芸（タイゲイ）
Name (Romaji)　KOJIN*
Other name (s) (Romaji)　TAIGEI
学名　*Cistanche deserticola* Ma*
Cistanche salsa (C.A. Mey.) G. Beck*
科名　Orobanchaceae（ハマウツボ科）
英名　broom rape / desert broom rape
Part of use　whole plant
Note 1　—
Note 2　KOJIN cannot be confirmed. Therefore, TAIGEI in the item of "Other names" is taken up here. TAIGEI is identical with NIKUJUYÔ, but their parts of use are different each other. NIKUJUYÔ is also listed in the item of "Name".
注　コジンは確認できない。従って、「他名等」のタイゲイとして取り扱った。
タイゲイは別項のニクジュヨウと同一。 但し、「部位等」の記載が異なっている。

名　称　**コズイシ***

他名等　コエンドロ／コリアンダー
部位等　果実
備　考　—

他名(参考)　—
漢字表記・生薬名等　胡荽子（コズイシ）、香荽（コウサイ）
Name (Romaji)　KOZUISHI*
Other name (s) (Romaji)　KOENDORO／KORIANDÂ
学名　*Coriandrum sativum* L.*
科名　Umbelliferae（セリ科）
英名　coriander / coriander (fruit) / cilantro (leaf) / Chinese parsley / culantro
Part of use　fruit
Note 1　—
Note 2　—
注　—

名　称　**コセンダングサ***

他名等　コシロノセンダングサ
部位等　全草
備　考　—

他名(参考)　—
漢字表記・生薬名等　小栴檀草（コセンダングサ）、金盞銀盤（キンサンギンバン）、小白栴檀草（コシロノセンダングサ）
Name (Romaji)　KOSENDANGUSA*
Other name (s) (Romaji)　KOSHIRONOSENDANGUSA
学名　*Bidens pilosa* L.*
科名　Compositae（キク科）
英名　beggar's ticks / Spanish needles / bur marygold / hairy beggar ticks / black fellows / scented begger ticks
Part of use　whole plant
Note 1　—
Note 2　—
注　—

名　称　**コナスビ**

他名等　—
部位等　果実
備　考　—

他名(参考)　—
漢字表記・生薬名等　小茄子（コナスビ）
Name (Romaji)　KONASUBI
Other name (s) (Romaji)　—
学名　*Lysimachia japonica* Thunb. ex Murray
科名　Primulaceae（サクラソウ科）
英名　Japanese yellow loosestrife / dwarf lysimachia
Part of use　fruit
Note 1　—
Note 2　—
注　—

名　称　**コパイーバ・オフィシナリス***

他名等　Copaifera officinalis
部位等　樹脂
備　考　—

他名(参考)　—
漢字表記・生薬名等　—
Name (Romaji)　KOPAÎBA・OFISHINARISU
Other name (s) (Romaji)　—

学名　*Copaifera officinalis* (Jacq.) L.*
科名　Leguminosae（マメ科）
英名　copaiba / aracaibo copaiba / Venezuela copaiba
Part of use　resin
Note 1　—
Note 2　—
注　—

名　称　**コパイーバ・ラングスドルフィ**

他名等　Copaifera langsdorffii
部位等　樹液
備　考　—

他名(参考)　—
漢字表記・生薬名等　—
Name(Romaji)　KOPAÎBA・RANGUSUDORUFI
Other name(s) (Romaji)　—
学名　*Copaifera langsdorffii* Desf.
科名　Leguminosae（マメ科）
英名　diesel tree / kerosene tree
Part of use　sap (oleoresin)
Note 1　—
Note 2　Sap written in the item of "Part of use" should be replaced by oleoresin.
注　「部位等」の樹液は、樹脂の方が適切である。

名　称　**コハク**

他名等　—
部位等　古代マツ科Pinus属植物樹脂の化合物
備　考　—

他名(参考)　—
漢字表記・生薬名等　松香（ショウコウ）
Name(Romaji)　KOHAKU
Other name(s) (Romaji)　—
学名　*Pinus* L.
科名　Pinaceae（マツ科）
英名　amber / lammer
Part of use　fossil of oleoresin of Pinus L.
Note 1　—
Note 2　"Chemical compound" written in the item of "Part of use" in Japanese should be replaced by "Fossil".
注　「部位等」に記載された古代マツ科Pinus属植物樹脂の化合物は化石の間違い。

名　称　**コフキサルノコシカケ***

他名等　ジュゼツ／バイキセイ
部位等　菌核（菌糸体）
備　考　—

他名(参考)　—
漢字表記・生薬名等　粉吹猿腰掛（コフキサルノコシカケ）、梅寄生（バイキセイ）、樹舌（ジュゼツ）
Name(Romaji)　KOFUKISARUNOKOSHIKAKE*
Other name(s) (Romaji)　JUZETSU／BAIKISEI
学名　*Ganoderma applanatum* (Pers.) Pat.*
Elfvingia applanata (Pers.) P. Karst.
Fomes applanatus (Pers.) Gillet*
Boletus applanatus Pers.
Polyporus applanatus (Pers.) Wall.
Scindalma lipsiense (Batsch) Kuntze
科名　Ganodermataceae（マンネンタケ科）
英名　artist's conk / artist's bracket / flacher lackporling
Part of use　mycelium
Note 1　—
Note 2　—
注　—

名　称　**ゴボウ***

他名等　—
部位等　根・葉
備　考　果実は「医」

他名(参考)　—
漢字表記・生薬名等　牛蒡（ゴボウ）
Name(Romaji)　GOBÔ*
Other name(s) (Romaji)　—
学名　*Arctium lappa* L.*
Lappa major Gaertn.
Lappa edulis Sieb. ex Miq., nom. inval.
科名　Compositae（キク科）
英名　burdock / cockle bur / cockle burr / gobo / great burdock / edible burdock / great but
Part of use　root, leaf
Note 1　fruit (seed)：drug category
Note 2　—
注　—

カ行

名　称　**ゴマ***

他名等　ゴマ油
部位等　種子・種子油・根
備　考　—

他名(参考)　—
漢字表記・生薬名等　胡麻（ゴマ）、胡麻油（ゴマアブラ）
Name(Romaji)　GOMA*
Other name(s) (Romaji)　GOMA-ABURA
学名　*Sesamum indicum* L.*
　　Sesamum orientale L.*
科名　Pedaliaceae（ゴマ科）
英名　sesame / sesame seeds / teel / til / oriental sesame / beni seed / tila
Part of use　seed, seed oil, root
Note 1　—
Note 2　—
注　—

名　称　**コミカンソウ***

他名等　—
部位等　全草
備　考　—

他名(参考)　キツネノチャブクロ
漢字表記・生薬名等　小蜜柑草（コミカンソウ）
Name(Romaji)　KOMIKANSÔ*
Other name(s) (Romaji)　—
学名　*Phyllanthus urinaria* L.*
科名　Euphorbiaceae（トウダイグサ科）
英名　chamber bitter / phyllanthus
Part of use　whole plant
Note 1　—
Note 2　—
注　—

名　称　**コムギ***

他名等　—
部位等　茎・澱粉・葉・胚芽・胚芽油・ふすま
備　考　—

他名(参考)　パンコムギ
漢字表記・生薬名等　小麦（コムギ）
Name(Romaji)　KOMUGI*
Other name(s) (Romaji)　—
学名　*Triticum aestivum* L.*
　　Triticum vulgare Vill.
　　Triticum aestivum ssp. *vulgare*（Vill.）Mac Key
科名　Gramineae（イネ科）
英名　wheat / common wheat
Part of use　stem, starch, leaf, germ, germ oil, bran
Note 1　—
Note 2　—
注　—

名　称　**ゴムノキ**

他名等　—
部位等　全草
備　考　—

他名(参考)　インドゴムノキ
漢字表記・生薬名等　印度膠樹（インドコウジュ）
Name(Romaji)　GOMUNOKI
Other name(s) (Romaji)　—
学名　*Ficus elastica* Roxb. ex Hornem
　　Ficus belgia hort.
　　Ficus rubra hort. non Roth
科名　Moraceae（クワ科）
英名　rubber plant / Assam rubber / Indian rubber tree
Part of use　whole plant
Note 1　—
Note 2　—
注　—

名　称　**コメデンプン***

他名等　イネ
部位等　種子
備　考　—

他名(参考)　コクリュウ（穀粒）
漢字表記・生薬名等　米澱粉（コメデンプン）、粳米（コウベイ）
Name(Romaji)　KOMEDENPUN*
Other name(s) (Romaji)　INE
学名　*Oryza sativa* L.*
科名　Gramineae（イネ科）
英名　rice starch
Part of use　seed
Note 1　—
Note 2　—
注　—

名　称　**コメヌカ***

他名等　イネ
部位等　米糠
備　考　—

他名(参考)　—
漢字表記・生薬名等　米糠（コメヌカ）
Name(Romaji)　KOMENUKA*
Other name(s) (Romaji)　INE
学名　*Oryza sativa* L.*
科名　Gramineae（イネ科）
英名　rice bran (polishings) / rice polishings / rice bran
Part of use　rice bran
Note 1　—
Note 2　—
注　—

名　称　**コリビ**

他名等　—
部位等　茎・根
備　考　—

他名(参考)　—
漢字表記・生薬名等　狐狸尾（コリビ）、兎尾草（トビソウ）
Name(Romaji)　KORIBI
Other name(s) (Romaji)　—
学名　*Uraria lagopodioides* (L.) Desv. ex DC.
科名　Leguminosae（マメ科）
英名　lesser cat's tail
Part of use　stem, root
Note 1　—
Note 2　—
注　—

名　称　**ゴレンシ***

他名等　—
部位等　葉・実
備　考　—

他名(参考)　—
漢字表記・生薬名等　五斂子（ゴレンシ）
Name(Romaji)　GORENSHI*
Other name(s) (Romaji)　—
学名　*Averrhoa carambola* L.*
科名　Oxalidaceae（カタバミ科）
英名　star fruit / carambola
Part of use　leaf, fruit
Note 1　—
Note 2　—
注　—

名　称　**コロハ***

他名等　—
部位等　種子
備　考　—

他名(参考)　—
漢字表記・生薬名等　胡盧巴・胡芦巴（コロハ）
Name(Romaji)　KOROHA*
Other name(s) (Romaji)　—
学名　*Trigonella foenum-graecum* L.*
科名　Leguminosae（マメ科）
英名　fenugreek / fenugrec
Part of use　seed
Note 1　—
Note 2　—
注　—

名　称　**コンブ**

他名等　モエン
部位等　全藻
備　考　—

他名(参考)　—
漢字表記・生薬名等　昆布（コンブ）、海帯（マコンブ）、藻塩（モシオ：海藻からとった塩）
Name(Romaji)　KONBU
Other name(s) (Romaji)　MOEN
学名　seaweed (Laminariaceae)
科名　Laminariaceae（コンブ科）
英名　laminaria / sea tangle / konbu / Japanese kelp / Japanese sea tangle
Part of use　whole seaweed
Note 1　—
Note 2　MOEN written in the item of "Other names" is correctly MOSHIO. MOSHIO is salt obtained from seawater by traditional technique.
注　「他名等」のモエンはモシオである。モシオは伝統的方法で海水から取った塩である。

名　称　**コンフリー***

他名等　**ヒレハリソウ**
部位等　根・葉
備　考　—

他名(参考)　ニットボーン
漢字表記・生薬名等　鰭玻璃草（ヒレハリソウ）
Name (Romaji)　KONFURÎ*
Other name(s) (Romaji)　HIREHARISÔ
学名　*Symphytum officinale* L.*
科名　Boraginaceae（ムラサキ科）
英名　comfrey / common comfrey / healing herb / knitbone / boneset / shop consound
Part of use　root, leaf
Note 1　—
Note 2　—
注　—

サ行

名　称　**サージ***

他名等　**サクリュウカ／ラムノイデス**
部位等　果実・種油
備　考　—

他名(参考)　スナジグミ（砂地茱萸）
漢字表記・生薬名等　沙棘（サージ、シャキョク、サキョウ）、醋柳果（サクリュウカ）
Name (Romaji)　SÂJI*
Other name(s) (Romaji)　SAKURYÛKA／RAMUNOIDESU
学名　*Hippophae rhamnoides* L.*
科名　Elaeagnaceae（グミ科）
英名　serge / sea buckthorn / common sea buckthorn / sallow thorn
Part of use　fruit, seed oil
Note 1　—
Note 2　SÂJI is identical with SAKYÔ, but their parts of use are different each other. SAKYÔ is also listed in the item of “Name”.
注　サージは別項のサキョウと同一。但し、「部位等」の記載が異なっている。

名　称　**サイカチ**

他名等　**ソウカクシ／トウサイカチ**
部位等　樹幹の棘
備　考　—

他名(参考)　—
漢字表記・生薬名等　皂角刺（ソウカクシ：刺（トゲ））、皂莢（ソウキョウ）、唐皂莢（トウサイカチ）
Name (Romaji)　SAIKACHI
Other name(s) (Romaji)　SÔKAKUSHI／TÔSAIKACHI
学名　*Gleditsia japonica* Miq.（サイカチ）
Gleditsia sinensis Lam.（トウサイカチ）
科名　Leguminosae（マメ科）
英名　Japanese honey locust / gleditsia / Chinese honey locust
Part of use　trunk thorn
Note 1　—
Note 2　SAIKACHI is different species from TÔSAIKACHI written in the item of “Other names”.
注　サイカチと「他名等」のトウサイカチは別種。

名　称　**サイコ**

他名等　**ミシマサイコ**
部位等　葉
備　考　根は「医」

他名(参考)　ミナミサイコ（南柴胡）、ベニサイコ（紅柴胡）
漢字表記・生薬名等　柴胡（サイコ）、三島柴胡（ミシマサイコ）
Name (Romaji)　SAIKO
Other name(s) (Romaji)　MISHIMASAIKO
学名　*Bupleurum falcatum* L.
Bupleurum scorzonerifolium Willd. var. *stenophyllum* Nakai
Bupleurum falcatum L. var. *komarowi* Koso-Polj.
科名　Umbelliferae（セリ科）
英名　hare's ear / thorough wax / bupleurum / Chinese thorough wax
Part of use　leaf
Note 1　root：drug category
Note 2　—
注　—

名　称　**サイハイラン**

他名等　トケンラン
部位等　鱗茎
備　考　—

他名(参考)　山慈姑（サンジコ）、毛慈姑（モウジコ）
漢字表記･生薬名等　采配蘭（サイハイラン）、杜鵑蘭（トケンラン）
Name(Romaji)　SAIHAIRAN
Other name(s)(Romaji)　TOKENRAN
学名　*Cremastra appendiculata*（D. Don）Makino
Cremastra variabilis（Bl.）Nakai
Cremastra unguiculata Finet
科名　Orchidaceae（ラン科）
英名　—
Part of use　bulb
Note 1　—
Note 2　—
注　—

名　称　**サキョウ***

他名等　—
部位等　果実
備　考　—

他名(参考)　—
漢字表記･生薬名等　沙棘（サージ、シャキョク、サキョウ）、醋柳果（サクリュウカ）
Name(Romaji)　SAKYÔ*
Other name(s)(Romaji)　—
学名　*Hippophae rhamnoides* L.*
科名　Elaeagnaceae（グミ科）
英名　sea buckthorn / sallow thorn
Part of use　fruit
Note 1　—
Note 2　SAKYÔ is identical with SÂJI, but their parts of use are different each other. SÂJI is also listed in the item of “Name”.
注　サキョウは別項のサージと同一。但し、「部位等」の記載が異なっている。

名　称　**サクラソウ**

他名等　—
部位等　根・葉
備　考　—

他名(参考)　—
漢字表記･生薬名等　桜草（サクラソウ）
Name(Romaji)　SAKURASÔ
Other name(s)(Romaji)　—
学名　*Primula sieboldii* E. Morren
科名　Primulaceae（サクラソウ科）
英名　Siebold’s primrose
Part of use　root, leaf
Note 1　—
Note 2　—
注　—

名　称　**ザクロ***

他名等　サンセキリュウ／セキリュウ／Punica granatum
部位等　果実・果皮・根皮・樹皮・花
備　考　—

他名(参考)　—
漢字表記･生薬名等　石榴・柘榴（ザクロ）、山石榴（サンセキリュウ）、果皮：石榴皮（セキリュウヒ）、根皮：石榴根皮（セキリュウコンピ）
Name(Romaji)　ZAKURO*
Other name(s)(Romaji)　SANSEKIRYÛ／SEKIRYÛ
学名　*Punica granatum* L.*
科名　Punicaceae（ザクロ科）
英名　pomegranate / common pomegranate
Part of use　fruit, pericarp, root bark, bark, flower
Note 1　—
Note 2　—
注　—

名　称　**サゴヤシ**

他名等　—
部位等　茎（髄）
備　考　—

他名(参考)　サグ
漢字表記･生薬名等　サゴ椰子（サゴヤシ）
Name(Romaji)　SAGOYASHI
Other name(s)(Romaji)　—
学名　*Metroxylon sagu* Rottb.（ホンサゴ）
Metroxylon rumphii（Willd.）Mart.（トゲサゴ）
科名　Palmae（ヤシ科）
英名　sago palm / prickly sago palm
Part of use　stem（pith）
Note 1　—
Note 2　—
注　—

名　称　**サッサフラスノキ***

他名等　—
部位等　全草
備　考　—

他名(参考)　—
漢字表記･生薬名等　—
Name(Romaji)　SASSAFURASUNOKI*
Other name(s)(Romaji)　—
学名　*Sassafras albidum* (Nutt.) Nees*
Sassafras officinale T. Nees et C.H. Eberm.*
Sassafras variifolium O. Kuntze
Laurus sassafras L.
科名　Lauraceae (クスノキ科)
英名　sassafras / common sassafras / filé
Part of use　whole plant
Note 1　—
Note 2　—
注　—

名　称　**サトウダイコン***

他名等　ビート
部位等　全草
備　考　—

他名(参考)　—
漢字表記･生薬名等　砂糖大根 (サトウダイコン)
Name(Romaji)　SATÔDAIKON*
Other name(s)(Romaji)　BÎTO
学名　*Beta vulgaris* L.*
Beta vulgaris L. ssp *cicla* (L.) W.D.J. Koch*
科名　Chenopodiaceae (アカザ科)
英名　chard / suger beet / Swiss chard
Part of use　whole plant
Note 1　—
Note 2　—
注　—

名　称　**サフラン***

他名等　—
部位等　柱頭
備　考　—

他名(参考)　—
漢字表記･生薬名等　洎夫藍 (サフラン)、番紅花 (バンコウカ)
Name(Romaji)　SAFURAN*
Other name(s)(Romaji)　—
学名　*Crocus sativus* L.*
科名　Iridaceae (アヤメ科)
英名　saffron / Spanish saffron / true saffron / saffron crocus
Part of use　stigma
Note 1　—
Note 2　—
注　—

名　称　**サボンソウ**

他名等　—
部位等　葉
備　考　—

他名(参考)　シャボンソウ
漢字表記･生薬名等　肥皁草 (中国名)
Name(Romaji)　SABONSÔ
Other name(s)(Romaji)　—
学名　*Saponaria officinalis* L.
科名　Caryophyllaceae (ナデシコ科)
英名　soapwort / bouncing bet / common soapwort / bouncing bess
Part of use　leaf
Note 1　—
Note 2　—
注　—

名　称　**サラシア・レティキュラータ**

他名等　コタラヒム／コタラヒムブツ
部位等　茎・根
備　考　—

他名(参考)　ポンコランチ
漢字表記･生薬名等　—
Name(Romaji)　SARASHIA・RETIKYURÂTA
Other name(s)(Romaji)　KOTARAHIMU／KOTARAHIMUBUTSU
学名　*Salacia reticulata* Wight
科名　Celastraceae (ニシキギ科)
英名　ponkoranti / salacia / kothala himbutu
Part of use　stem, root
Note 1　—
Note 2　—
注　—

名　称　**サラシア・オブロンガ**

他名等　—
部位等　根
備　考　—

他名（参考）　ポンコランチ
漢字表記・生薬名等　—
Name (Romaji)　SARASHIA・OBURONGA
Other name (s) (Romaji)　—
学名　*Salacia oblonga* Wall.
科名　Celastraceae（ニシキギ科）
英名　Tamil-ponkoranti
Part of use　root
Note 1　—
Note 2　—
注　—

名　称　**サラシア・キネンシス**

他名等　—
部位等　茎・根
備　考　—

他名（参考）　—
漢字表記・生薬名等　—
Name (Romaji)　SARASHIA・KINENSHISU
Other name (s) (Romaji)　—
学名　*Salacia chinensis* L.
Salacia prinoides (Willd.) DC.
科名　Celastraceae（ニシキギ科）
英名　Chinese salacia
Part of use　stem, root
Note 1　—
Note 2　—
注　—

名　称　**サルナシ**

他名等　コクワ／シラクチヅル
部位等　果実
備　考　—

他名（参考）　コクワヅル、シラクチカズラ（猿口葛）
漢字表記・生薬名等　猿梨（サルナシ）、山樝（サルナシ）、猿口蔓（シラクチヅル）、猿口葛（シラクチカズラ）
Name (Romaji)　SARUNASHI
Other name (s) (Romaji)　KOKUWA／SHIRAKUCHI-ZURU
学名　*Actinidia arguta* (Sieb. et Zucc.) Planch. ex Miq.
科名　Actinidiaceae（マタタビ科）
英名　tara vine / bower actinidia / yang tao / hardy kiwi / northern kiwi
Part of use　fruit
Note 1　—
Note 2　—
注　—

名　称　**サルビア***

他名等　セージ
部位等　葉
備　考　—

他名（参考）　ヤクヨウセージ（薬用セージ）、ヤクヨウサルビア（薬用サルビア）
漢字表記・生薬名等　薬用サルビア、薬用セージ
Name (Romaji)　SARUBIA*
Other name (s) (Romaji)　SÊJI
学名　*Salvia officinalis* L.*
科名　Labiatae（シソ科）
英名　sage / Dalmatian sage / garden sage / common sage / true sage
Part of use　leaf
Note 1　—
Note 2　—
注　—

名　称　**サンカクトウ**

他名等　—
部位等　外果皮・根皮・種仁
備　考　—

他名（参考）　サントウカク（山桃核）、サンコトウ（山胡桃）、カクトウシュウ（核桃楸）
漢字表記・生薬名等　山核桃（サンカクトウ）
Name (Romaji)　SANKAKUTÔ
Other name (s) (Romaji)　—
学名　*Carya cathayensis* Sarg.
Juglans mandshurica Maxim.
科名　Juglandaceae（クルミ科）
英名　Chinese hickory / Manchurian walnut
Part of use　exocarp, root bark, kernel
Note 1　—
Note 2　—
注　—

名　称　サンキライ*

他名等　**ケナシサルトリイバラ／Smilax glabra**
部位等　葉
備　考　塊茎・根茎は「医」、サンキライ以外のシオデ属の葉・根は「非医」

他名(参考)　ドブクリョウ（土茯苓）、サルサパリラ、サルサコン（サルサ根）、サルトリイバラ（猿捕茨）、シオデ属、サルトリイバラ属
漢字表記・生薬名等　山帰来（サンキライ）、土茯苓（ドブクリョウ）、猿捕茨（サルトリイバラ）、遺糧（イリョウ）、仙遺糧（センイリョウ）、サルサ根
Name (Romaji)　SANKIRAI*
Other name (s) (Romaji)　KENASHISARUTORIIBARA
学名　*Smilax glabra* Roxb.*
科名　Smilacaceae（サルトリイバラ科）
英名　bai bei niu wei cai / Chinese smilax / glabrous greenbrier / cat brier / sarsaparilla
Part of use　leaf
Note 1　tuber and rhizome of *Smilax glabra* Roxb.：drug category,
leaf and root of *Smilax* L. except glabra：non-drug category
Note 2　—
注　—

名　称　サンザシ*

他名等　**オオサンザシ**
部位等　偽実・茎・葉・花
備　考　—

他名(参考)　サンサ（山査、山楂）、オオミサンザシ（大実山査子）、ノサンサ（野山楂）
漢字表記・生薬名等　山査子（サンザシ）、大山査子（オオサンザシ）、大実山査子（オオミサンザシ）
Name (Romaji)　SANZASHI*
Other name (s) (Romaji)　ÔSANZASHI
学名　*Crataegus cuneata* Sieb. et Zucc.*
Crataegus pinnatifida Bunge*
Crataegus pinnatifida Bunge var. *major* N.E. Br.*
科名　Rosaceae（バラ科）
英名　hawthorn (Japanese) / sanzashi / Chinese hawthorn / Nippon hawthorn / northern schanzha / southern schanzha / red hawthorn
Part of use　pseudocarp, stem, leaf, flower
Note 1　—
Note 2　—
注　—

名　称　サンシキスミレ*

他名等　—
部位等　全草
備　考　—

他名(参考)　パンジー
漢字表記・生薬名等　三色菫（サンシキスミレ）
Name (Romaji)　SANSHIKISUMIRE*
Other name (s) (Romaji)　—
学名　*Viola tricolor* L.*
Viola × wittrockiana Hort.
科名　Violaceae（スミレ科）
英名　pansy / European wild pansy / field pansy / garden pansy / heartsease / lady's delight / Johnny-jump-up / miniature pansy
Part of use　whole plant
Note 1　—
Note 2　—
注　—

名　称　サンシシ*

他名等　**クチナシ**
部位等　果実・茎・葉
備　考　—

他名(参考)　スイシシ（水梔子）、コリンクチナシ（小輪梔子）
漢字表記・生薬名等　口無（クチナシ）、梔子（シシ）、山梔（サンシ）、山梔子（サンシシ）
Name (Romaji)　SANSHISHI*
Other name (s) (Romaji)　KUCHINASHI
学名　*Gardenia jasminoides* J. Ellis*
Gardenia augusta Merr.*
Gardenia grandiflora Lour.
Gardenia jasminoides f. *grandiflora* (Lour.) Makino
Gardenia florida L.
科名　Rubiaceae（アカネ科）
英名　zhi zi / gardenia / Cape jasmine / common gardenia
Part of use　fruit, stem, leaf
Note 1　—
Note 2　—
注　—

名　称　**サンシチニンジン***

他名等　デンシチニンジン
部位等　根
備　考　—

他名(参考)　デンサンシチ（田三七）、ニンジンサンシチ（人参三七）、デンシチ（田七）
漢字表記・生薬名等　三七人参（サンシチニンジン）、田七人参（デンシチニンジン）
Name (Romaji)　SANSHICHININJIN*
Other name (s) (Romaji)　DENSHICHININJIN
学名　*Panax notoginseng* (Burkill) F.H. Chen ex C.Y. Wu et K.M. Feng*
Panax pseudoginseng Wall. var. *notoginseng* (Burkill) G. Hoo et C.J. Tseng*
科名　Araliaceae（ウコギ科）
英名　san qi / pseudoginseng / Tienchi ginseng
Part of use　root
Note 1　—
Note 2　—
注　—

名　称　**サンシュユ***

他名等　ハルコガネバナ
部位等　果実
備　考　—

他名(参考)　アキサンゴ（秋珊瑚）、サンユニク（山萸肉）、ユニク（萸肉）
漢字表記・生薬名等　山茱萸（サンシュユ）、春黄金花（ハルコガネバナ）
Name (Romaji)　SANSHUYU*
Other name (s) (Romaji)　HARUKOGANEBANA
学名　*Cornus officinalis* Sieb. et Zucc.*
Macrocarpium officinale (Sieb. et Zucc.) Nakai*
科名　Cornaceae（ミズキ科）
英名　Japanese cornel / dogwood / Asiatic dogwood / Asiatic cornel / Asiatic cornelian cherry
Part of use　fruit
Note 1　—
Note 2　—
注　—

名　称　**サンショウ***

他名等　—
部位等　果実・果皮・根
備　考　—

他名(参考)　—
漢字表記・生薬名等　山椒（サンショウ）
Name (Romaji)　SANSHÔ*
Other name (s) (Romaji)　—
学名　*Zanthoxylum piperitum* (L.) DC.*
科名　Rutaceae（ミカン科）
英名　Japanese pepper / Japanese prickly ash / Sichuan pepper / san sho
Part of use　fruit, peel, root
Note 1　—
Note 2　—
注　—

名　称　**サンショウバラ**

他名等　—
部位等　花
備　考　—

他名(参考)　ハコネバラ（箱根薔薇）
漢字表記・生薬名等　山椒薔薇（サンショウバラ）
Name (Romaji)　SANSHÔBARA
Other name (s) (Romaji)　—
学名　*Rosa hirtula* (Regel) Nakai
Rosa roxburghii Tratt. var. *hirtula* (Regel) Rehder et E.H. Wilson
科名　Rosaceae（バラ科）
英名　rugosa / rugose / shrink
Part of use　flower
Note 1　—
Note 2　—
注　—

名　称　**サンソウニン**

他名等　サネブトナツメ
部位等　種子
備　考　—

他名(参考)　ソウニン（棗仁）、シナナツメ（支那棗）、サンソウ（酸棗）
漢字表記・生薬名等　核太棗（サネブトナツメ）、種子：酸棗仁（サンソウニン）
Name (Romaji)　SANSÔNIN

Other name(s) (Romaji)　SANEBUTONATSUME
学名　*Ziziphus jujuba* Mill. var. *spinosa* (Bunge) Hu ex H.F. Chow
科名　Rhamnaceae（クロウメモドキ科）
英名　jujube / common jujube / Chinese date / Chinese jujube / jujube date
Part of use　seed
Note 1　—
Note 2　SANSÔNIN is the seed of SANEBUTONATSUME used as traditional Japanese herbal medicine. TAISÔ is the riped fruit of NATSUME. TAISÔ is also listed in the item of "Name".
注　サンソウニンは生薬名で、サネブトナツメの種子。別項のタイソウはナツメの成熟果実。

名　称　**サンナ***
他名等　**バンウコン**
部位等　根茎
備　考　—

他名(参考)　—
漢字表記･生薬名等　山奈・三奈（サンナ）、蕃鬱金（バンウコン）
Name (Romaji)　SANNA*
Other name(s) (Romaji)　BAN'UKON
学名　*Kaempferia galanga* L.*
科名　Zingiberaceae（ショウガ科）
英名　galangale / East-Indian galangale / kaempheria galanga / resurrection lily
Part of use　rhizome
Note 1　—
Note 2　—
注　—

名　称　**サンペンズ**
他名等　**カワラケツメイ**
部位等　全草
備　考　—

他名(参考)　コウボウチャ（弘法茶）、リュウキュウカワラケツメイ（琉球河原決明）
漢字表記･生薬名等　山扁豆（サンペンズ）、河原決明（カワラケツメイ）
Name (Romaji)　SANPENZU
Other name(s) (Romaji)　KAWARAKETSUMEI
学名　*Cassia mimosoides* L. ssp. *nomame* (Sieb.) Ohashi
科名　Leguminosae（マメ科）
英名　nomame senna / kawaraketsumei
Part of use　whole plant
Note 1　—
Note 2　—
注　—

名　称　**サンヤク***
他名等　**ナガイモ／ヤマイモコン**
部位等　根茎
備　考　—

他名(参考)　ヤマノイモ（山芋）、ジネンジョウ（自然生）、ショヨ（薯蕷）
漢字表記･生薬名等　山薬（サンヤク）、長芋（ナガイモ）、山芋（ヤマノイモ、サンウ）
Name (Romaji)　SAN'YAKU*
Other name(s) (Romaji)　NAGAIMO／YAMAIMOKON
学名　*Dioscorea opposita* Thunb.（ヤマノイモ）
Dioscorea batatas Decne.*（ナガイモ）
Dioscorea oppositifolia L.*（ヤマノイモ）
Dioscorea japonica Thunb.（ヤマノイモ）
科名　Dioscoreaceae（ヤマノイモ科）
英名　Japanese yam / Chinese yam / cinnamon vine / common yam
Part of use　rhizome
Note 1　—
Note 2　—
注　—

名　称　**シア**
他名等　**シアーバターノキ**
部位等　種子・油
備　考　—

他名(参考)　—
漢字表記･生薬名等　—
Name (Romaji)　SHIA
Other name(s) (Romaji)　SHIÂBATÂNOKI
学名　*Butyrospermum parkii* (G. Don.) Kotschy
Butyrospermum paradoxum (C.F. Gaertn.) Hepper ssp. *parkii* (G. Don.) Hepper
Vitellaria paradoxa C.F. Gaertn.
科名　Sapotaceae（アカテツ科）
英名　shea butter / shea butter tree
Part of use　seed, oil
Note 1　—
Note 2　—
注　—

名　称　**シイタケ***

他名等　—
部位等　菌糸体・子実体
備　考　—

他名(参考)　—
漢字表記・生薬名等　椎茸（シイタケ）
Name(Romaji)　SHÎTAKE*
Other name(s) (Romaji)　—
学名　*Lentinula edodes* (Berk.) Pegler*
Lentinus edodes (Berk.) Singer*
Tricholoma shiitake (J. Schroet.) Lloyd.
Lepiota shiitake (J. Schroet.) Nobuj.
Collybia shiitake J. Schroet.
科名　Omphalotaceae（ツキヨタケ科）
英名　Chinese mushroom / shiitake mushroom / shiitake / Japanese forest mushroom
Part of use　mycelium, fruit body
Note 1　—
Note 2　—
注　—

名　称　**シオデ属**

他名等　サルサ／Smilax属
部位等　葉・サンキライ以外の根
備　考　サンキライ（Smilax glabra）の塊茎・根茎は「医」

他名(参考)　サルトリイバラ属
漢字表記・生薬名等　—
Name(Romaji)　SHIODE-ZOKU
Other name(s) (Romaji)　SARUSA
学名　*Smilax* L.
科名　Smilacaceae（サルトリイバラ科）
英名　green brier / cat brier
Part of use　leaf, root excepting *Smilax glabra*
Note 1　tuber and rhizome of SANKIRAI (*Smilax glabra* Roxb.)：drug category
Note 2　SANKIRAI (*Smilax glabra*) written in the items of "Part of use" and "Note 1" is a species of SHIODE-ZOKU (*Smilax* L.)
注　「部位等」および「備考」に記載されているサンキライはシオデ属（*Smilax* L.）の一種である。

名　称　**シクンシ***

他名等　—
部位等　果実
備　考　—

他名(参考)　リュウキュウシ（留求子）
漢字表記・生薬名等　使君子（シクンシ）
Name(Romaji)　SHIKUNSHI*
Other name(s) (Romaji)　—
学名　*Quisqualis indica* L.*
科名　Combretaceae（シクンシ科）
英名　quisqualis / Rangoon creeper
Part of use　fruit
Note 1　—
Note 2　—
注　—

名　称　**シケイジョテイ**

他名等　—
部位等　葉
備　考　—

他名(参考)　クテイチャ（苦丁茶）、ウンナンクテイチャ（雲南苦丁茶）
漢字表記・生薬名等　紫茎女貞（シケイジョテイ）
Name(Romaji)　SHIKEIJOTEI
Other name(s) (Romaji)　—
学名　*Ligustrum purpurascens* Y.C. Yang.
Ligustrum expansum Rehder
Ligustrum robustum ssp. *chinense* P.S. Green
Ligustrum thibeticum Decne.
科名　Oleaceae（モクセイ科）
英名　—
Part of use　leaf
Note 1　—
Note 2　—
注　—

名　称　**シコウカ***

他名等　ヘンナ
部位等　葉
備　考　—

他名(参考)　ツマクレナイノキ、エジプトイボタノキ（エジプト水蝋樹・疣取木）、ヘナ
漢字表記・生薬名等　指甲花（シコウカ）
Name(Romaji)　SHIKÔKA*

Other name(s) (Romaji)　HENNA
学名　*Lawsonia inermis* L.*
　Lawsonia alba Lam.*
科名　Lythraceae（ミソハギ科）
英名　henna
Part of use　leaf
Note 1　―
Note 2　―
注　―

名　称　**シコクビエ**

他名等　―
部位等　種子
備　考　―

他名(参考)　―
漢字表記・生薬名等　四国稗（シコクビエ）、竜爪稗・龍爪稗（シコクビエ）
Name(Romaji)　SHIKOKUBIE
Other name(s) (Romaji)　―
学名　*Eleusine coracana* (L.) Gaertn.
科名　Gramineae（イネ科）
英名　finger millet
Part of use　seed
Note 1　―
Note 2　―
注　―

名　称　**シシウド***

他名等　Angelica pubescens／Angelica bisserata
部位等　根茎・軟化茎
備　考　ドクカツ（ウド／Aralia cordata）の根茎は「医」

他名(参考)　チョドッカツ（猪独活）、ドッカツ（独活）、トウドッカツ（唐独活）、ウドタラシ
漢字表記・生薬名等　猪独活・香独活（シシウド）
Name(Romaji)　SHISHIUDO*
Other name(s) (Romaji)　―
学名　*Angelica pubescens* Maxim.*
　Angelica biserrata (R.H. Shan et C.Q. Yuan) C.Q. Yuan et R.H. Shan
　Angelica shishiudo Koidz.
科名　Umbelliferae（セリ科）
英名　pubescent angelica
Part of use　rhizome, stem (pubescent)
Note 1　rhizome of *Aralia cordata* Thunb.: drug category
Note 2　―
注　―

名　称　**ジジン**

他名等　―
部位等　全草
備　考　―

他名(参考)　―
漢字表記・生薬名等　地菍・地稔（ジジン：中国名）
Name(Romaji)　JIJIN
Other name(s) (Romaji)　―
学名　*Melastoma dodecandrum* Lour.
科名　Melastomataceae（ノボタン科）
英名　di-niè / twelve stamen melastoma
Part of use　whole plant
Note 1　―
Note 2　―
注　―

名　称　**シソ**

他名等　エゴマ／シソ油
部位等　枝先・種子・種子油・葉
備　考　―

他名(参考)　ジュウネン（十稔）、ハクソ（白蘇）、チリメンジソ（皺紫蘇）
漢字表記・生薬名等　紫蘇（シソ）、荏胡麻（エゴマ）
Name(Romaji)　SHISO
Other name(s) (Romaji)　EGOMA／SHISO-YU
学名　*Perilla frutescens* (L.) Britt. var. *crispa* (Thunb.) Deane（シソ）
　Perilla frutescens (L.) Britt. var. *frutescens*（エゴマ）
　Perilla frutescens (L.) Britt. var. *acuta* Kudo（シソ）
　Perilla frutescens (L.) Britt. var. *japonica* Hara（エゴマ）
　Perilla frutescens (L.) Britt. var. *crispa* (Thunb.) Deane f. crispa (Thunb.) Makino（チリメンジソ）
　Ocimum frutescens L.
科名　Labiatae（シソ科）
英名　beefsteak plant / perilla / shiso
Part of use　spike, seed, seed oil, leaf
Note 1　―
Note 2　―
注　―

名　称　**シセンサンショウ***

他名等　**土山椒**
部位等　根
備　考　—

他名(参考)　カホクサンショウ（華北山椒）、カショウ（花椒、ホアジャオ）、チュウゴクサンショウ（中国山椒）、ショクショウ（蜀椒）、ショウコウ（椒紅）
漢字表記・生薬名等　四川山椒（シセンサンショウ）
Name (Romaji)　SHISENSANSHÔ*
Other name (s) (Romaji)　DOSANSHÔ
学名　*Zanthoxylum bungeanum* Maxim.*
科名　Rutaceae（ミカン科）
英名　Sichuan pepper / Chinese prickly ash
Part of use　root
Note 1　—
Note 2　DOSANSHÔ written in the item of "Other names" cannot be confirmed. The root is written in the item of "Part of use" of SHISENSANSHÔ but the edible part of this herb is pericarp.
SHISENSANSHÔ（*Zanthoxylum bungeanum*）and the Japanese SANSHÔ（*Zanthoxylum pipericum*）are different species but pericarp of Zanthoxylum species sometimes called DOKASHÔ and used as spice.
注「他名等」の土山椒は確認できない。シセンサンショウの「部位等」は根となっているが、食用部位は果皮である。
シセンサンショウは、別項の日本のサンショウと同属異種。一部のサンショウ属の果皮は「土花椒」などと称して、香辛料に使用される例がある。

名　称　**シダレカンバ***

他名等　**ハクカヒ／ユウシカ**
部位等　全草
備　考　—

他名(参考)　ヨーロッパシラカンバ（ヨーロッパ白樺）、オウシュウシラカンバ（欧州白樺）、ベルコーサカンバ、バーチ
漢字表記・生薬名等　枝垂樺（シダレカンバ）、白樺皮（ハクカヒ）
Name (Romaji)　SHIDAREKANBA*
Other name (s) (Romaji)　HAKUKAHI／YÛSHIKA
学名　*Betula pendula* Roth*
Betula verrucosa J.F. Ehrh.*
Betula alba L. sensu Coste
科名　Betulaceae（カバノキ科）
英名　silver birch / white birch / common birch / birch / European white birch / weeping birch
Part of use　whole plant
Note 1　—
Note 2　YÛSHIKA written in the item of "Other names" cannot be confirmed.
注「他名等」のユウシカは確認できない。

名　称　**シタン***

他名等　**インドシタン／Pterocarpus indicus**
部位等　根・樹皮・材
備　考　—

他名(参考)　ヤエヤマシタン（八重山紫檀）
漢字表記・生薬名等　紫檀（シタン）
Name (Romaji)　SHITAN*
Other name (s) (Romaji)　INDOSHITAN
学名　*Pterocarpus indicus* Willd.*
科名　Leguminosae（マメ科）
英名　rosewood / narra / Andaman redwood / Malay padauk
Part of use　root, bark, heart wood
Note 1　—
Note 2　—
注　—

名　称　**ジチョウ***

他名等　—
部位等　全草
備　考　—

他名(参考)　ノジスミレ（野路菫）、シカジチョウ（紫花地丁）、スモウトリバナ
漢字表記・生薬名等　地丁（ジチョウ）
Name (Romaji)　JICHÔ*
Other name (s) (Romaji)　—
学名　*Viola yedoensis* Makino*
Viola mandshurica W. Becker
科名　Violaceae（スミレ科）
英名　Tokyo violet
Part of use　whole plant
Note 1　—
Note 2　JICHÔ is included in SUMIRE, but their parts of use are different each other. SUMIRE is also listed in the item of "Name".
注　ジチョウは別項のスミレに含まれる。但し、「部位等」の記載が異なっている。

名　称　**シナタラノキ***

他名等　ソウボク／Aralia chinensis
部位等　根・根皮・材
備　考　—

他名(参考)　タラノキ（楤木）、タラコンピ（楤根皮）、ソウボクヒ（楤木皮）
漢字表記・生薬名等　楤木（ソウボク）
Name(Romaji)　SHINATARANOKI*
Other name(s)(Romaji)　SÔBOKU
学名　*Aralia chinensis* L.
Aralia elata (Miq.) Seem.*
Aralia mandshurica Rupr. et Maxim.*
Aralia canescens Sieb. et Zucc.
Aralia elata var. *subinermis* Ohwi
科名　Araliaceae（ウコギ科）
英名　Chinese angelica tree / Chinese angelica / angelica tree / Hercules-club tree / devil's walking stick / Japanese aralia
Part of use　root, root bark, heart wood
Note 1　—
Note 2　—
注　—

名　称　**シナノキ**

他名等　—
部位等　全草
備　考　—

他名(参考)　—
漢字表記・生薬名等　科の木・級の木・榀の木・椴（シナノキ）
Name(Romaji)　SHINANOKI
Other name(s)(Romaji)　—
学名　*Tilia japonica* (Miq.) Simonk
科名　Tiliaceae（シナノキ科）
英名　Japanese lime / Japanese linden
Part of use　whole plant
Note 1　—
Note 2　—
注　—

名　称　**シバムギ***

他名等　グラミニス
部位等　根
備　考　—

他名(参考)　ヒメカモジグサ（姫髭草）
漢字表記・生薬名等　芝麦（シバムギ）
Name(Romaji)　SHIBAMUGI*
Other name(s)(Romaji)　GURAMINISU
学名　*Agropyron repens* (L.) P. Beauv.*
Elymus repens (L.) Gould.*
Elytrigia repens (L.) Desv. ex B.D. Jackson*
Triticum repens L.*
科名　Gramineae（イネ科）
英名　couch grass / dog grass / graminis / quack grass / English twitch / triticum / twich grass
Part of use　root
Note 1　—
Note 2　—
注　—

名　称　**ジフ***

他名等　イソボウキ／トンブリ／ホウキギ
部位等　果実・種子・葉
備　考　—

他名(参考)　ニワクサ（爾波久佐）、ネンドウ
漢字表記・生薬名等　地膚（ジフ）、地膚子（ジフシ）、箒木（ホウキギ）、唐鰤子（トンブリ）
Name(Romaji)　JIFU*
Other name(s)(Romaji)　ISOBÔKI／TONBURI／HÔKIGI
学名　*Kochia scoparia* (L.) Schrad.*
Bassia scoparia (L.) A.J. Scott*
Kochia scoparia (L.) Schrad. var. *littorea* (Makino) Kitam.
Kochia scoparia (L.) Schrad. var. *trichophylla* (Stapf) Bailey
科名　Chenopodiaceae（アカザ科）
英名　jif / difu / summer cypress / belvedere / bloom cypress / Belvedere broom goose foot
Part of use　fruit, seed, leaf
Note 1　—
Note 2　—
注　—

名　称　**シマタコノキ***

他名等　アダン
部位等　全草
備　考　—

他名(参考)　リントウ、フイリタコノキ
漢字表記･生薬名等　蛸の木（タコノキ）、露兜樹（ロトウジュ）
Name(Romaji)　SHIMATAKONOKI*
Other name(s) (Romaji)　ADAN
学名　*Pandanus veitchii* hort. Veitch ex M.T. Mast. et T. Moore
Pandanus tectorius Parkins. ex Zucc.*
Pandanus odoratissimus L. f., nom illeg.*
Pandanus tectorius var. *liukiuensis* Warb.
科名　Pandanaceae（タコノキ科）
英名　striped screw pine / veitch screw pine / screw pine / thatch screw pine / hala screw pine / pandan / pandanus palm
Part of use　whole plant
Note 1　—
Note 2　—
注　—

名　称　**シマトウガラシ***

他名等　—
部位等　果実
備　考　—

他名(参考)　コーレーグス（高麗薬）、ラッショウ（辣椒）、バンショウ（蕃椒）
漢字表記･生薬名等　島唐辛子（シマトウガラシ）、唐辛子（トウガラシ）、蕃姜（バンショウ）、辣椒（ラッショウ）
Name(Romaji)　SHIMATÔGARASHI*
Other name(s) (Romaji)　—
学名　*Capsicum frutescens* L.*
Capsicum annuum L. var. *annuum**
Capsicum annuum L. var. *glabriusculum* (Dunal) Heiser et Pickersgill*
Capsicum annuum L. var. *frutescens* (L.) Kuntze
科名　Solanaceae（ナス科）
英名　cayenne pepper / chili pepper / paprika / tabasco pepper / red pepper
Part of use　fruit
Note 1　—
Note 2　—
注　—

名　称　**シャウペデコウロ***

他名等　—
部位等　全草
備　考　—

他名(参考)　—
漢字表記･生薬名等　—
Name(Romaji)　SHAUPEDEKÔRO*
Other name(s) (Romaji)　—
学名　*Echinodorus macrophyllus* (Kunth) Micheli*
Echinodorus macrophyllus ssp. *scaber* (Rataj) R.R. Haynes et Holm-Niels.
Alisma macrophyllum Kunth
科名　Alismataceae（オモダカ科）
英名　chapéau de couro / water plantain
Part of use　whole plant
Note 1　—
Note 2　The correct KATAKANA notation of “chapéau de couro” written in the item of “English name” is SHAPEUDEKÔRO but not SHAUPEDEKÔRO.
注　「英名等」に記載された “chapéau de couro” のカタカナ表記はシャウペデコウロではなく、シャペウデコウロ。

名　称　**シャエンシ***

他名等　—
部位等　種子
備　考　—

他名(参考)　ツルゲンゲ
漢字表記･生薬名等　沙苑子（シャエンシ、サエンシ、サオンシ）、沙苑蒺藜（シャエンシツリ、サエンシツリ）、潼蒺藜（トウシツリ）
Name(Romaji)　SHAENSHI*
Other name(s) (Romaji)　—
学名　*Astragalus complanatus* R. Br. ex Bunge*
Astragalus chinensis L. f.
科名　Leguminosae（マメ科）
英名　flat-stem milkvetch / Chinese milkvetch
Part of use　seed
Note 1　—
Note 2　—
注　—

名　称　**ジャクゼツソウ**

他名等　ノミノフスマ
部位等　葉
備　考　—

他名(参考)　テンホウソウ(天蓬草)、ヒンハンル(濱繁縷)
漢字表記・生薬名等　雀舌草(ジャクゼツソウ)、蚤の衾(ノミノフスマ)
Name(Romaji)　JAKUZETSUSÔ
Other name(s) (Romaji)　NOMINOFUSUMA
学名　*Stellaria alsine* Grim. var. *undulata* (Thunb.) Ohwi
科名　Caryophyllaceae (ナデシコ科)
英名　bog chickweed
Part of use　leaf
Note 1　—
Note 2　—
注　—

名　称　**シャクヤク***

他名等　—
部位等　花
備　考　根は「医」

他名(参考)　セキシャク (赤芍)、ビャクシャク (白芍)
漢字表記・生薬名等　芍薬・芍葯 (シャクヤク)
Name(Romaji)　SHAKUYAKU*
Other name(s) (Romaji)　—
学名　*Paeonia lactiflora* Pall.*
Paeonia albiflora Pall.*
Paeonia veitchii Lynch*
科名　Paeoniaceae (ボタン科)
英名　peony / common garden peony / Chinese peony / red peony / white peony
Part of use　flower
Note 1　root : drug category
Note 2　—
注　—

名　称　**シャジン<沙参>***

他名等　ツリガネニンジン
部位等　根
備　考　シャジン<砂仁>は「医」

他名(参考)　トウシャジン (唐沙参)、マルバノニンジン (丸葉人参)
漢字表記・生薬名等　沙参 (シャジン)、釣鐘人参 (ツリガネニンジン)
Name(Romaji)　SHAJIN*
Other name(s) (Romaji)　TSURIGANENINJIN
学名　*Adenophora tetraphylla* Fisch.*
Adenophora stricta Miq.*
Adenophora hunanensis Nannfeldt
Adenophora triphylla (Thunb. ex Murray) A. DC.*
Adenophora triphylla (Thunb.) A. DC. ssp. *aperticampanulata* Kitam.
科名　Campanulaceae (キキョウ科)
英名　nan sha shen / sha shen / adenophora / lady bells
Part of use　root
Note 1　*Amomum xanthioides* Wall. : drug category
Note 2　—
注　—

名　称　**ジャスミン***

他名等　—
部位等　花
備　考　—

他名(参考)　マツリカ (茉莉花)、モウリンカ (毛輪花)
漢字表記・生薬名等　茉莉花 (マツリカ)、素馨 (ソケイ)
Name(Romaji)　JASUMIN*
Other name(s) (Romaji)　—
学名　*Jasminum grandiflorum* L.*
Jasminum officinale f. *affine* (Royle ex Lindl.) Rehd.
Jasminum sambac (L.) Ait.
Jasminum officinale f. *grandiflorum* (L.) Kobuski
科名　Oleaceae (モクセイ科)
英名　jasmine / Arabian jasmine / poet's jasmine / royal jasmine / Catalonian jasmine / Spanish jasmine
Part of use　flower
Note 1　—
Note 2　—
注　—

名　称　**シャタバリ***

他名等　—
部位等　地下部
備　考　—

他名(参考)　—
漢字表記・生薬名等　—
Name(Romaji)　SHATABARI*
Other name(s) (Romaji)　—
学名　*Asparagus racemosus* Willd.*
科名　Asparagaceae (クサスギカズラ科)
英名　shatavari / Indian asparagus / hundred roots / as-

paragus roots
Part of use　subterranean part
Note 1　—
Note 2　—
注　—

名　称　**ジャトバ***

他名等　オオイナゴマメ
部位等　樹皮
備　考　—

他名(参考)　—
漢字表記･生薬名等　—
Name(Romaji)　JATOBA*
Other name(s) (Romaji)　ÔINAGOMAME
学名　*Hymenaea courbaril* L.*
科名　Leguminosae（マメ科）
英名　jatoba / Brazilian copal / courbaril / lumberjack's tea / West Indian locust
Part of use　bark
Note 1　—
Note 2　—
注　—

名　称　**ジャビャクシ***

他名等　ニオイイガクサ
部位等　全草
備　考　—

他名(参考)　サンコウ（山香）
漢字表記･生薬名等　蛇百子（ジャビャクシ）
Name(Romaji)　JABYAKUSHI*
Other name(s) (Romaji)　NIOIIGAKUSA
学名　*Hyptis suaveolens* (L.) Poit.*
科名　Labiatae（シソ科）
英名　pignut / chia cimarrona / tea bush
Part of use　whole plant
Note 1　—
Note 2　—
注　—

名　称　**ジャワナガコショウ***

他名等　ヒハツ
部位等　果実
備　考　—

他名(参考)　ナガコショウ（長胡椒）、ヒハツモドキ（畢発擬）、サキシマフウトウカズラ（先島風藤葛）
漢字表記･生薬名等　爪哇長胡椒（ジャワナガコショウ）、畢発（ヒハツ）
Name(Romaji)　JAWANAGAKOSHÔ*
Other name(s) (Romaji)　HIHATSU
学名　*Piper retrofractum* Vahl*
*Piper officinalm**
科名　Piperaceae（コショウ科）
英名　Jawa long pepper / Balinese pepper / Bengal pepper / jaborandi pepper / Javanese long pepper
Part of use　fruit
Note 1　—
Note 2　—
注　—

名　称　**ジュウヤク***

他名等　ドクダミ
部位等　地上部
備　考　—

他名(参考)　—
漢字表記･生薬名等　毒痛み（ドクダミ）、十薬・重薬（ジュウヤク）、魚腥草（ギョセイソウ：中国名）、蕺菜（ジュウサイ：中国名）
Name(Romaji)　JÛYAKU*
Other name(s) (Romaji)　DOKUDAMI
学名　*Houttuynia cordata* Thunb.*
科名　Saururaceae（ドクダミ科）
英名　tsi / doku-dami / houttuynia
Part of use　aerial part
Note 1　—
Note 2　—
注　—

名　称　**ジュルベーバ***

他名等　—
部位等　全草
備　考　—

他名(参考)　ジュルベバ
漢字表記･生薬名等　—

Name (Romaji)　JURUBÊBA*
Other name (s) (Romaji)　—
学名　*Solanum paniculatum* L.*
科名　Solanaceae（ナス科）
英名　jurubeba
Part of use　whole plant
Note 1　—
Note 2　—
注　—

名　称　シュロ

他名等　—
部位等　葉
備　考　—

他名（参考）　シュロヨウ（棕櫚葉）
漢字表記・生薬名等　棕櫚・棕梠・棕呂（シュロ）、棕櫚葉（シュロヨウ）、棕櫚皮（シュロヒ）
Name (Romaji)　SHURO
Other name (s) (Romaji)　—
学名　*Trachycarpus fortunei* (Hook.) H. Wendl.
Trachycarpus excelsus (Thunb.) H. Wendl.
Trachycarpus excelsus var. *typicus* Makino
Chamaerops fortunei Hook.
科名　Palmae（ヤシ科）
英名　Chusan palm / windmill palm / hemp palm / Chinese windmill palm
Part of use　leaf
Note 1　—
Note 2　—
注　—

名　称　ショウキョウ*

他名等　カンキョウ／ショウガ
部位等　根茎
備　考　—

他名（参考）　センキョウ（鮮姜）、カンショウキョウ（幹生姜）
漢字表記・生薬名等　生薑・生姜（ショウキョウ）、乾姜（カンキョウ）、生姜（ショウガ）
Name (Romaji)　SHÔKYÔ*
Other name (s) (Romaji)　KANKYÔ／SHÔGA
学名　*Zingiber officinale* Rosc.*
Amomum zingiber L.
科名　Zingiberaceae（ショウガ科）
英名　ginger / Canton ginger / common ginger / true ginger
Part of use　rhizome
Note 1　—
Note 2　—
注　—

名　称　ショウズク*

他名等　カルダモン
部位等　果実
備　考　—

他名（参考）　—
漢字表記・生薬名等　小豆蔲（ショウズク）、白豆蔲（ビャクズク）、白豆蔲殻（ビャクズクカク）、白豆蔲花（ビャクズクカ）
Name (Romaji)　SHÔZUKU*
Other name (s) (Romaji)　KARUDAMON
学名　*Elettaria cardamomum* (L.) Maton var. *cardamomum**
Elettaria cardamomum (L.) var. *miniscula* Burkill*
Elettaria cardamomum L. var. *minus* Watt*
Amomum cardamomum L.
科名　Zingiberaceae（ショウガ科）
英名　cardamom / cardamon / mysore cardamom
Part of use　fruit
Note 1　—
Note 2　SHÔZUKU and BYAKUZUKU are possibly confused with each other in the marketplace. BYAKUZUKU is also listed in the item of "Name".
注　ショウズクと別項のビャクズクは市場では混乱している可能性がある。

名　称　ショウノウ*

他名等　カンフル
部位等　クスノキから得られた精油
備　考　—

他名（参考）　—
漢字表記・生薬名等　樟脳（ショウノウ）
Name (Romaji)　SHÔNÔ*
Other name (s) (Romaji)　KANFURU
学名　*Cinnamomum camphora* (L.) J. Presl*
Camphora camphora (L.) H. Karst., nom. illeg.*
Camphora officinalis Nees*
Laurus camphora L.*
科名　Lauraceae（クスノキ科）
英名　camphor / camphor tree
Part of use　essential oil from camphor tree
Note 1　—
Note 2　Refer to KUSUNOKI listed in the item of

"Name".
注　別項のクスノキを参照。(「部位等」は原リストでは"精"となっているが "精油" に訂正した。)

名　称　**シヨウラン***

他名等　**タイセイ／ホソバタイセイ**
部位等　全草
備　考　—

他名(参考)　マタイセイ（真大青）
漢字表記･生薬名等　松藍（ショウラン)、板藍（バンラン)、板藍根（バンランコン)、大青（タイセイ)、細葉大青（ホソバタイセイ）
Name(Romaji)　SHÔRAN*
Other name(s)(Romaji)　TAISEI／HOSOBATAISEI
学名　*Isatis indigotica* Fortune*
Isatis tinctoria L.*
Isatis canescens DC.
Isatis littoralis Stev.
Isatis taurica Bieb.
科名　Cruciferae（アブラナ科）
英名　woad / isatis / dyer's woad / indigo wood / Chinese indigo
Part of use　whole plant
Note 1　—
Note 2　—
注　—

名　称　**食用ダイオウ**

他名等　**マルバダイオウ**
部位等　葉柄
備　考　—

他名(参考)　—
漢字表記･生薬名等　食用大黄（ショクヨウダイオウ)、丸葉大黄（マルバダイオウ）
Name(Romaji)　SHOKUYÔDAIÔ
Other name(s)(Romaji)　MARUBADAIÔ
学名　*Rheum rhaponticum* hort. non L.
Rheum rhabarbarum L.
Rheum undulatum L.
科名　Polygonaceae（タデ科）
英名　rhubarb / rhapontic rhubarb / pie plant / garden rhubarb / wine plant
Part of use　leafstalk
Note 1　—
Note 2　Refer to DAIÔ listed in the item of "Name".
注　別項のダイオウを参照。

名　称　**食用ホオズキ**

他名等　**プルイノサ**
部位等　果実
備　考　ホオズキの根は「医」

他名(参考)　—
漢字表記･生薬名等　食用鬼灯・食用酸漿（ショクヨウホオズキ）
Name(Romaji)　SHOKUYÔHÔZUKI
Other name(s)(Romaji)　PURUINOSA
学名　*Physalis pruinosa* L.
科名　Solanaceae（ナス科）
英名　strawberry tomato / dwarf Cape gooseberry / husk tomato / ground cherry
Part of use　fruit
Note 1　root of *Physalis alkekengi* L. var. *franchetii* (M.T. Mast.) hort.：drug category
Note 2　—
注　—

名　称　**シラカンバ**

他名等　—
部位等　果実
備　考　—

他名(参考)　シラカバ（白樺）
漢字表記･生薬名等　白樺（シラカバ、シラカンバ）
Name(Romaji)　SHIRAKANBA
Other name(s)(Romaji)　—
学名　*Betula platyphylla* Sukatchev var. *japonica* (Miq.) Hara
Betula alba L. var. *japonica* Miq.
Betula japonica Sieb. non Thunb.
科名　Betulaceae（カバノキ科）
英名　Asian white birch / Japanese white birch
Part of use　fruit
Note 1　—
Note 2　—
注　—

名　称　**シラン***

他名等　—
部位等　花
備　考　—

他名(参考)　—
漢字表記･生薬名等　紫蘭（シラン：シランの球茎を白芨

（ビャッキュウ）という）
Name (Romaji)　SHIRAN*
Other name (s) (Romaji)　—
学名　*Bletilla striata* (Thunb.) Rchb. f.*
科名　Orchidaceae（ラン科）
英名　hyacinth orchid / bletilla / urn orchid / Chinese ground orchid
Part of use　flower
Note 1　—
Note 2　—
注　—

名　称　シリ

他名等　イザヨイバラ
部位等　果実
備　考　—

他名（参考）　トゲナシ（刺梨）
漢字表記・生薬名等　刺梨（シリ、トゲナシ）、十六夜薔薇（イザヨイバラ）
Name (Romaji)　SHIRI
Other name (s) (Romaji)　IZAYOIBARA
学名　*Rosa roxburghii* Tratt.
科名　Rosaceae（バラ科）
英名　chinquapin rose / burr rose / chestnut rose
Part of use　fruit
Note 1　—
Note 2　—
注　—

名　称　シロキクラゲ*

他名等　ハクボクジ
部位等　子実体
備　考　—

他名（参考）　ギンジ（銀茸）
漢字表記・生薬名等　白木耳（シロキクラゲ、ハクボクジ）
Name (Romaji)　SHIROKIKURAGE*
Other name (s) (Romaji)　HAKUBOKUJI
学名　*Tremella fuciformis* Berk.*
Nakaiomyces nipponicus Kobayashi
科名　Tremellaceae（シロキクラゲ科）
英名　tremella / white fungus / white wood ear / silver ear fungs / silver ear
Part of use　fruit body
Note 1　—
Note 2　—
注　—

名　称　シロコヤマモモ*

他名等　—
部位等　樹皮
備　考　—

他名（参考）　シロヤマモモ（白山桃）
漢字表記・生薬名等　白小山桃（シロコヤマモモ）
Name (Romaji)　SHIROKOYAMAMOMO*
Other name (s) (Romaji)　—
学名　*Myrica cerifera* L.*
Myrica carolinensis Mill.
Morella cerifera (L.) Small*
科名　Myricaceae（ヤマモモ科）
英名　southern wax myrtle / southern bayberry / bayberry / candleberry / waxberry / wax myrtle
Part of use　bark
Note 1　—
Note 2　—
注　—

名　称　シンキンソウ*

他名等　ヒカゲノカズラ
部位等　全草
備　考　—

他名（参考）　カゲ（蘿）、セキショウ（石松）、キツネノタスキ（狐の襷）
漢字表記・生薬名等　日陰鬘・日陰蔓（ヒカゲノカズラ）、伸筋草（シンキンソウ）
Name (Romaji)　SHINKINSÔ*
Other name (s) (Romaji)　HIKAGENOKAZURA
学名　*Lycopodium clavatum* L.*
Lycopodium clavatum L. var. *nipponicum* Nakai
科名　Lycopodiaceae（ヒカゲノカズラ科）
英名　common club moss / clubmoss / licopodium / ground pine / running pine / running club moss
Part of use　whole plant
Note 1　—
Note 2　—
注　—

名　称　シントククスノキ

他名等　—
部位等　樹皮
備　考　—

他名（参考）　—

漢字表記･生薬名等　—
Name (Romaji)　SHINTOKUKUSUNOKI
Other name (s) (Romaji)　—
学名　*Cinnamomum sintoc* Bl.
科名　Lauraceae（クスノキ科）
英名　sintok / kulit lawang
Part of use　bark
Note 1　—
Note 2　—
注　—

名　称　**スイートオレンジ***
他名等　—
部位等　果皮
備　考　—

他名(参考)　—
漢字表記･生薬名等　—
Name (Romaji)　SUÎTOORENJI*
Other name (s) (Romaji)　—
学名　*Citrus sinensis* (L.) Osbeck*
Citrus×*aurantium* L. var. *sinensis* L.*
科名　Rutaceae（ミカン科）
英名　sweet orange / orange
Part of use　pericarp
Note 1　—
Note 2　—
注　—

名　称　**ズイカク***
他名等　—
部位等　成熟果核
備　考　—

他名(参考)　ヘンカクボク（扁核木）
漢字表記･生薬名等　蕤核（ズイカク：果肉を除いた果核）、蕤仁（ズイジン：果核の殻を割って取り出した種子）
Name (Romaji)　ZUIKAKU*
Other name (s) (Romaji)　—
学名　*Prinsepia uniflora* Batal.*
科名　Rosaceae（バラ科）
英名　rui ren / prinsepia
Part of use　riped fruit
Note 1　—
Note 2　—
注　—

名　称　**スイバ***
他名等　ヒメスイバ
部位等　茎・葉
備　考　—

他名(参考)　スカンポ（酸模）、スカンボ
漢字表記･生薬名等　蓚・酸葉・酢葉（スイバ）、姫酸葉（ヒメスイバ）
Name (Romaji)　SUIBA*
Other name (s) (Romaji)　HIMESUIBA
学名　*Rumex acetosa* L.*（スイバ）
Rumex acetosella L.*（ヒメスイバ）
科名　Polygonaceae（タデ科）
英名　sheep sorrel / common sorrel / sorrel / garden sorrel / sour grass / sour dock
Part of use　stem, leaf
Note 1　—
Note 2　—
注　—

名　称　**スカルキャップ***
他名等　—
部位等　根以外
備　考　根は「医」

他名(参考)　—
漢字表記･生薬名等　—
Name (Romaji)　SUKARUKYAPPU*
Other name (s) (Romaji)　—
学名　*Scutellaria lateriflora* L.*
科名　Labiatae（シソ科）
英名　scullcap / Virginian skullcap / medweed / blue skullcap
Part of use　whole plant except root
Note 1　root：drug category
Note 2　—
注　—

名　称　**スギナ***
他名等　ツクシ／モンケイ
部位等　栄養茎・胞子茎
備　考　—

他名(参考)　—
漢字表記･生薬名等　杉菜（スギナ）、土筆（ツクシ）、問荊（モンケイ：中国名）
Name (Romaji)　SUGINA*

Other name (s) (Romaji)　TSUKUSHI／MONKEI
学名　*Equisetum arvense* L.*
科名　Equisetaceae（トクサ科）
英名　horsetail / field horsetail / shave grass / shavetail grass / common horsetail
Part of use　stem (horse tail), reproductive shoot
Note 1　—
Note 2　—
注　—

名　称　スグリ*

他名等　—
部位等　実
備　考　—

他名(参考)　セイヨウスグリ（西洋酸塊）、ヨーロッパスグリ（ヨーロッパ酸塊）、オオスグリ（大酸塊）
漢字表記･生薬名等　酸塊（スグリ）
Name (Romaji)　SUGURI*
Other name (s) (Romaji)　—
学名　*Ribes sinanense* F. Maek.（スグリ）
Ribes formosana Hayata var. *sinanense* (F. Maek.) Kitam.（スグリ）
Ribes grossularia L.*（セイヨウスグリ）
Ribes uva-crispa L.*（セイヨウスグリ）
科名　Saxifragaceae（ユキノシタ科）
英名　gooseberry / European gooseberry / cat berry / English gooseberry
Part of use　fruit
Note 1　—
Note 2　The scientific names of SEIYÔSUGURI (*Ribes grossularia* and *Ribes uva-crispa*) are included here.
注　学名にセイヨウスグリを含めた。

名　称　ステビア*

他名等　—
部位等　葉
備　考　—

他名(参考)　アマハステビア（甘葉ステビア）
漢字表記･生薬名等　ステビア葉
Name (Romaji)　SUTEBIA*
Other name (s) (Romaji)　—
学名　*Stevia rebaudiana* (Bertoni) Hemsl.*
Eupatorium rebaudianum Bertoni*
科名　Compositae（キク科）
英名　stevia / candy leaf / Paraguayan sweet herb / sweet leaf
Part of use　leaf
Note 1　—
Note 2　—
注　—

名　称　ストローブ*

他名等　ストローブマツ
部位等　全木
備　考　—

他名(参考)　—
漢字表記･生薬名等　北美喬松（ホクビキョウショウ：中国名）
Name (Romaji)　SUTORÔBU*
Other name (s) (Romaji)　SUTORÔBUMATSU
学名　*Pinus strobus* L.*
科名　Pinaceae（マツ科）
英名　strobe / white pine / eastern white pine / weymouth pine
Part of use　whole tree
Note 1　—
Note 2　—
注　—

名　称　スピルリナ*

他名等　—
部位等　全藻
備　考　—

他名(参考)　アルスロスピラ（オルソスピラ）属の藍藻
漢字表記･生薬名等　—
Name (Romaji)　SUPIRURINA*
Other name (s) (Romaji)　—
学名　algae (*Spirulina* P. Fischer)
Spirulina platensis (Gomont) Geitler*
(=*Arthrospira platensis* (Nordst.) Gomont*)
Spirulina maxima (Setchell et Gardener) Geitler*
(=*Arthrospira maxima* Setchell et Gardener*)
科名　Oscillatoriaceae（ユレモ科）
英名　spirulina
Part of use　whole algae
Note 1　—
Note 2　—
注　—

名　称　**スペアミント***

他名等　オランダハッカ／ミドリハッカ
部位等　全草
備　考　—

他名(参考)　スペアミント油
漢字表記・生薬名等　緑薄荷（ミドリハッカ）、留蘭香（リュウランコウ：中国名）
Name(Romaji)　SUPEAMINTO*
Other name(s)(Romaji)　ORANDAHAKKA／MIDORIHAKKA
学名　*Mentha spicata* L.*
Mentha viridis L.*
Mentha longifolia auct. non (L.) Huds.
Mentha nilaca auct. non Juss. et Jacq.
科名　Labiatae（シソ科）
英名　spearmint / spearminth / green minth / common green minth / lamb minth
Part of use　whole plant
Note 1　—
Note 2　—
注　—

名　称　**スマ***

他名等　パフィア／ブラジルニンジン
部位等　根
備　考　—

他名(参考)　アマゾンジンセン
漢字表記・生薬名等　—
Name(Romaji)　SUMA*
Other name(s)(Romaji)　PAFIA／BURAJIRUNINJIN
学名　*Pfaffia glomerata* (Spreng.) Pedersen
Pfaffia paniculata (Mart.) Kuntze*
科名　Amaranthaceae（ヒユ科）
英名　suma / pfaffia / Brazilian ginseng
Part of use　root
Note 1　—
Note 2　—
注　—

名　称　**スマック***

他名等　ジビジビ
部位等　果実
備　考　—

他名(参考)　ヌルデ（白膠木）、エンフシ（塩麩子：ヌルデの果実の生薬名）
漢字表記・生薬名等　塩麩子（エンフシ）
Name(Romaji)　SUMAKKU*
Other name(s)(Romaji)　JIBIJIBI
学名　*Rhus coriaria* L.*（スマック）
Rhus chinensis Mill.*（スマック）
Rhus japonica L.（スマック）
Rhus javanica L.（スマック）
Caesalpinia coriaria (Jacq.) Willd.（ジビジビ）
Poinciana coriaria Jacq.（ジビジビ）
科名　スマック：Anacardiaceae（ウルシ科）
ジビジビ：Leguminosae（マメ科）
英名　sumac / Sicilian sumac / Chinese sumac / tanner's sumac / nut gall tree / divi-divi
Part of use　fruit
Note 1　—
Note 2　SUMAKKU and JIBIJIBI are different species. SUMAKKU is the common name of herbs belonging to Anacardiaceae but JIBIJIBI is the common name of *Caesalpinia coriata* belonging to Leguminosae. NURUDE is a species of SUMAKKU and also listed in the item of "Name".
注　スマックとジビジビは別種。スマックはウルシ科植物の総称であるのに対し、ジビジビはマメ科の*Caesalpinia coriata*を指す。別項のヌルデはスマックの一種。

名　称　**スミレ***

他名等　—
部位等　花
備　考　—

他名(参考)　ノジスミレ（野路菫）、ニオイスミレ（匂菫）
漢字表記・生薬名等　菫（スミレ）、紫花地丁（シカジチョウ）、地丁（ジチョウ）、紫地丁（シジチョウ）
Name(Romaji)　SUMIRE*
Other name(s)(Romaji)　—
学名　*Viola* L.
Viola yedoensis Makino*
Viola mandshurica W. Becker
Viola odorata L.*
Viola tricolor L.*
科名　Violaceae（スミレ科）
英名　viola / violet / sweet violet / English violet / garden violet / sweet blue violet / wild pansy / heartsease / Johnny-jump up / European wild pansy
Part of use　flower
Note 1　—
Note 2　SUMIRE includes JICHÔ and NIOISUMIRE, but their parts of use are different one another. JICHÔ

and NIOISUMIRE are also listed in the items of "Name".

注　スミレは別項のジチョウ及びニオイスミレを含む。但し、「部位等」の記載が異なっている。

名　称　**スリムアマランス***

他名等　アラマンサス・ハイブリダス
部位等　種子
備　考　—

他名(参考)　—
漢字表記・生薬名等　—
Name (Romaji)　SURIMUAMARANSU*
Other name (s) (Romaji)　ARAMANSASU・HAIBURIDASU
学名　*Amaranthus hypochondriacus* L.
Amaranthus hybridus L.*
Amaranthus frumentaceus Buch.-Ham.
科名　Amaranthaceae（ヒユ科）
英名　amaranth / amaranthus / slim amaranth / smooth amaranth / green amaranth / pigweed
Part of use　seed
Note 1　—
Note 2　—
注　—

名　称　**ズルカマラ***

他名等　—
部位等　茎
備　考　—

他名(参考)　ツルナス（蔓茄子）、クカ（苦茄）、センネンフランシン（千年不爛心）
漢字表記・生薬名等　ズルカマラ枝（茎）
Name (Romaji)　ZURUKAMARA*
Other name (s) (Romaji)　—
学名　*Solanum dulcamara* L.*
科名　Solanaceae（ナス科）
英名　bitter nightshade / bittersweet / climbing nightshade / dulcamara
Part of use　stem
Note 1　—
Note 2　—
注　—

名　称　**セイセンリュウ**

他名等　—
部位等　葉
備　考　—

他名(参考)　—
漢字表記・生薬名等　青銭柳（センセンリュウ）
Name (Romaji)　SEISENRYÛ
Other name (s) (Romaji)　—
学名　*Cyclocarya paliurus* (Batal.) Iljin.
科名　Juglandaceae（クルミ科）
英名　—
Part of use　leaf
Note 1　—
Note 2　—
注　—

名　称　**セイタカカナビキソウ**

他名等　ヤカンゾウ
部位等　全草
備　考　—

他名(参考)　シマカナビキソウ（島金引草）
漢字表記・生薬名等　野甘草（ヤカンゾウ）
Name (Romaji)　SEITAKAKANABIKISÔ
Other name (s) (Romaji)　YAKANZÔ
学名　*Scoparia dulcis* L.
Scoparia temata Forsk.
科名　Scrophulariaceae（ゴマノハグサ科）
英名　vassourinha / escobilla / piqu pichana / canchara-gua / beet broomwart / sweet broomwart / sweet broomweet
Part of use　whole plant
Note 1　—
Note 2　—
注　—

名　称　**セイタカミロバラン***

他名等　—
部位等　全草
備　考　—

他名(参考)　ベレリカミロバラン
漢字表記・生薬名等　鞞醯勒果（vibhitaka）
Name (Romaji)　SEITAKAMIROBARAN*
Other name (s) (Romaji)　—
学名　*Terminalia bellirica* (Gaertn.) Roxb.

Terminalia bellerica (Gaertn.) Roxb.*
科名　Combretaceae（シクンシ科）
英名　bahira / bilhitak / bahera / baheda / vibhidhaka / belleric myrobalan / beleric myrobalan / belliric myrobalan / vibhitaka
Part of use　whole plant
Note 1　―
Note 2　SEITAKAMIROBARAN is identical with TÂMINARIA・BERIRIKA, but their parts of use are different each other. TÂMINARIA・BERIRIKA is also listed in the item of "Name".
注　セイタカミロバランは別項のターミナリア・ベリリカと同一。但し、「部位等」の記載が異なっている。

名　称　**セイヒ**

他名等　**オオベニミカン**
部位等　未熟果実
備　考　―

他名(参考)　ウンシュウミカン（温州蜜柑）、ベニミカン（紅蜜柑）、フクキツ（福橘）
漢字表記・生薬名等　青皮（セイヒ）、大紅蜜柑（オオベニミカン）
Name(Romaji)　SEIHI
Other name(s) (Romaji)　ÔBENIMIKAN
学名　*Citrus tangerina* hort. ex T. Tanaka
Citrus unshiu Marcow.
Citrus reticulata var. *unshiu* (Marcow.) Hu
科名　Rutaceae（ミカン科）
英名　dancy tangerine / green tangerine peel / Satsuma mandarin / Satsuma tangerin
Part of use　unriped fruit
Note 1　―
Note 2　―
注　―

名　称　**セイヨウアカネ***

他名等　―
部位等　根
備　考　―

他名(参考)　―
漢字表記・生薬名等　西洋茜（セイヨウアカネ）
Name(Romaji)　SEIYÔAKANE*
Other name(s) (Romaji)　―
学名　*Rubia tinctorum* L.*
科名　Rubiaceae（アカネ科）
英名　madder / common madder / dyer's madder / European madder
Part of use　root
Note 1　―
Note 2　―
注　―

名　称　**セイヨウイラクサ***

他名等　―
部位等　全草
備　考　―

他名(参考)　―
漢字表記・生薬名等　西洋蕁草・西洋刺草（セイヨウイラクサ）
Name(Romaji)　SEIYÔIRAKUSA*
Other name(s) (Romaji)　―
学名　*Urtica dioica* L.
Urtica dioica L. ssp. *dioica**
科名　Urticaceae（イラクサ科）
英名　common nettle / common stinging nettle / stinging nettle / nettle
Part of use　whole plant
Note 1　―
Note 2　―
注　―

名　称　**セイヨウエビラハギ***

他名等　**メリロート**
部位等　全草
備　考　―

他名(参考)　シナガワハギ（品川萩）、ソウモクセイ（草木犀）
漢字表記・生薬名等　西洋箙萩（セイヨウエビラハギ）、品川萩（シナガワハギ）
Name(Romaji)　SEIYÔEBIRAHAGI*
Other name(s) (Romaji)　MERIRÔTO
学名　*Melilotus officinalis* (L.) Pall.*
Melilotus suaveolens Ledeb.
科名　Leguminosae（マメ科）
英名　melilot / field melilot / yellow sweet clover / yellow melilot / melist / Daghestan sweet clover
Part of use　whole plant
Note 1　―
Note 2　―
注　―

名　称　**セイヨウオオバコ***

他名等　**オニオオバコ**
部位等　全草
備　考　—

他名(参考)　ヨウシュオオバコ（洋種大葉子）
漢字表記・生薬名等　西洋大葉子（セイヨウオオバコ）、鬼大葉子（オニオオバコ）
Name(Romaji)　SEIYÔÔBAKO*
Other name(s) (Romaji)　ONIÔBAKO
学名　*Plantago major* L.*
科名　Plantaginaceae（オオバコ科）
英名　plantain / broadleaf plantain / common plantain / greater plantain / cart-track plant / white-man's foot / round leaf plantain / waybread / American plantain / rat tail plantain / dog tail / green plantain
Part of use　whole plant
Note 1　—
Note 2　—
注　—

名　称　**セイヨウオトギリソウ***

他名等　**セントジョンズワート／ヒペリクムソウ**
部位等　全草
備　考　—

他名(参考)　セイヨウオトギリ（西洋弟切）、カンヨウレンギョウ（貫葉連翹）
漢字表記・生薬名等　西洋弟切草（セイヨウオトギリソウ）
Name(Romaji)　SEIYÔOTOGIRISÔ*
Other name(s) (Romaji)　SENTOJONZUWÂTO／HIPERIKUMUSÔ
学名　*Hypericum perforatum* L.*
科名　Guttiferae（オトギリソウ科）
英名　St. John's wort / common St. John's wort
Part of use　whole plant
Note 1　—
Note 2　—
注　—

名　称　**セイヨウキイチゴ***

他名等　**セイヨウヤブイチゴ**
部位等　果実・葉
備　考　—

他名(参考)　ヨーロッパキイチゴ、エゾキイチゴ（蝦夷木苺）
漢字表記・生薬名等　西洋木苺（セイヨウキイチゴ）、西洋藪苺（セイヨウヤブイチゴ）
Name(Romaji)　SEIYÔKIICHIGO*
Other name(s) (Romaji)　SEIYÔYABUICHIGO
学名　*Rubus idaeus* L.（セイヨウキイチゴ）
Rubus strigosus Michx.*（セイヨウキイチゴ）
Rubus fruticosus L.*（セイヨウヤブイチゴ）
科名　Rosaceae（バラ科）
英名　bramble / blackberry / shrubby blackberry / European raspberry / red raspberry / wild raspberry / European red raspberry / American raspberry / European blackberry
Part of use　fruit, leaf
Note 1　—
Note 2　SEIYÔKIICHIGO is identical with RAZUBERÎ and both of them are included in KIICHIGO. *Rubus fruticosus*, one of the scientific names of SEIYÔKIICHIGO is also written in the item of "Scientific name" of BURAKKUBERÎ.
RAZUBERÎ, KIICHIGO and BURAKKUBERÎ are also listed in the items of "Name".
注　セイヨウキイチゴは別項のラズベリーと同一であり、両者は別項のキイチゴに含まれる。
本ハーブの学名に記載した*Rubus fruticosus*はブラックベリーの一種としても記載されている。

名　称　**セイヨウキンミズヒキ***

他名等　**アグリモニー／アグリモニア**
部位等　全草
備　考　—

他名(参考)　—
漢字表記・生薬名等　西洋金水引（セイヨウキンミズヒキ）
Name(Romaji)　SEIYÔKINMIZUHIKI*
Other name(s) (Romaji)　AGURIMONÎ／AGURIMONIA
学名　*Agrimonia eupatoria* L.*
科名　Rosaceae（バラ科）
英名　agrimony / church steeples
Part of use　whole plant
Note 1　—
Note 2　—
注　—

名　称　**セイヨウサクラソウ***

他名等　—
部位等　根
備　考　—

他名(参考)　キバナノクリンザクラ（黄花の九輪桜）
漢字表記・生薬名等　西洋桜草（セイヨウサクラソウ）
Name(Romaji)　SEIYÔSAKURASÔ*
Other name(s)(Romaji)　—
学名　*Primula veris* L.*
Primula officinalis Hill.
科名　Primulaceae（サクラソウ科）
英名　cowslip / paigle
Part of use　root
Note 1　—
Note 2　—
注　—

名　称　**セイヨウサンザシ***

他名等　Crataegus oxyacantha／Crataegus laevigata／Crataegus monogyna
部位等　果実・葉
備　考　—

他名(参考)　—
漢字表記・生薬名等　西洋山査子（セイヨウサンザシ）
Name(Romaji)　SEIYÔSANZASHI*
Other name(s)(Romaji)　—
学名　*Crataegus oxyacantha* L.*
Crataegus laevigata (Poir.) DC.*
Crataegus monogyna Jacq.*
科名　Rosaceae（バラ科）
英名　hawthorn / May tree / May flower / English hawthorn / May bush / white thorn / one-seed hawthorn / hedge-row thorn / quick-set thorn
Part of use　fruit, leaf
Note 1　—
Note 2　—
注　—

名　称　**セイヨウシナノキ***

他名等　—
部位等　果実・樹皮・葉・花
備　考　—

他名(参考)　セイヨウボダイジュ（西洋菩提樹）
漢字表記・生薬名等　西洋科の木・西洋級の木・西洋榀の木（セイヨウシナノキ）
Name(Romaji)　SEIYÔSHINANOKI*
Other name(s)(Romaji)　—
学名　*Tilia×europaea* L.*
Tilia×vulgaris Hayne*
Tilia intermedia DC.
科名　Tiliaceae（シナノキ科）
英名　common lime / linden / European linden / European lime tree / tilia
Part of use　fruit, bark, leaf, flower
Note 1　—
Note 2　SEIYÔSHINANOKI is identical with TIYÛRU but their parts of use are different each other. TIYÛRU is also listed in the item of "Name".
注　セイヨウシナノキと別項のティユールは同一。但し、「部位等」の記載が異なっている。

名　称　**セイヨウシロヤナギ***

他名等　ホワイトウイロー
部位等　全草
備　考　—

他名(参考)　—
漢字表記・生薬名等　西洋白柳（セイヨウシロヤナギ）
Name(Romaji)　SEIYÔSHIROYANAGI*
Other name(s)(Romaji)　HOWAITOUIRÔ
学名　*Salix alba* L.*
Salix aurea Salisb.
科名　Salicaceae（ヤナギ科）
英名　golden willow / white willow / European willow / goat willow / common willow
Part of use　whole plant
Note 1　—
Note 2　—
注　—

名　称　**セイヨウスモモ***

他名等　プルーン
部位等　果実・果実エキス
備　考　—

他名(参考)　ヨーロッパスモモ
漢字表記・生薬名等　西洋酸桃（セイヨウスモモ）
Name(Romaji)　SEIYÔSUMOMO*
Other name(s)(Romaji)　PURÛN
学名　*Prunus domestica* L.*
科名　Rosaceae（バラ科）
英名　plum / prune / common plum / garden plum / Eu-

ropean plum
Part of use　fruit, fruit extract
Note 1　—
Note 2　—
注　—

名　称　セイヨウタンポポ*

他名等　—
部位等　根・葉
備　考　—

他名(参考)　—
漢字表記・生薬名等　西洋蒲公英（セイヨウタンポポ）
Name(Romaji)　SEIYÔTANPOPO*
Other name(s) (Romaji)　—
学名　*Taraxacum officinale* Weber ex F.H. Wigg.*
Taraxacum dens-leonis Desf.*
Taraxacum vulgare (Lam.) Schrank*
科名　Compositae（キク科）
英名　dandelion / common dandelion / lion's tooth
Part of use　root, leaf
Note 1　—
Note 2　Refer to HOKÔEIKON listed in the item of "Name".
注　別項のホコウエイコンを参照。

名　称　セイヨウトチノキ*

他名等　—
部位等　樹皮・葉・花・芽
備　考　種子は「医」

他名(参考)　ウマグリ（馬栗）、マロニエ、ヨウシュトチノキ（洋種橡）
漢字表記・生薬名等　西洋栃・西洋橡（セイヨウトチノキ）
Name(Romaji)　SEIYÔTOCHINOKI*
Other name(s) (Romaji)　—
学名　*Aesculus hippocastanum* L.*
科名　Hippocastanaceae（トチノキ科）
英名　horse chestnut / common horse chestnut / European horse chestnut / marronnier
Part of use　bark, leaf, flower, sprout
Note 1　seed：drug category
Note 2　—
注　—

名　称　セイヨウトネリコ*

他名等　オウシュウトネリコ
部位等　全草
備　考　—

他名(参考)　—
漢字表記・生薬名等　西洋梣（セイヨウトネリコ）、欧州梣（オウシュウトネリコ）
Name(Romaji)　SEIYÔTONERIKO*
Other name(s) (Romaji)　ÔSHÛTONERIKO
学名　*Fraxinus excelsior* L.*
科名　Oleaceae（モクセイ科）
英名　European ash / ash / common ash
Part of use　whole plant
Note 1　—
Note 2　—
注　—

名　称　セイヨウナツユキソウ*

他名等　—
部位等　全草
備　考　—

他名(参考)　—
漢字表記・生薬名等　西洋夏雪草（セイヨウナツユキソウ）
Name(Romaji)　SEIYÔNATSUYUKISÔ*
Other name(s) (Romaji)　—
学名　*Filipendula ulmaria* (L.) Maxim.*
Spiraea ulmaria L.*
科名　Rosaceae（バラ科）
英名　meadowsweet / queen-of-the-meadow / meadow-sweety / European meadowsweet
Part of use　whole plant
Note 1　—
Note 2　—
注　—

名　称　セイヨウニワトコ*

他名等　エルダー
部位等　茎・葉・花
備　考　—

他名(参考)　—
漢字表記・生薬名等　西洋接骨木（セイヨウニワトコ）、西洋庭常（セイヨウニワトコ）
Name(Romaji)　SEIYÔNIWATOKO*
Other name(s) (Romaji)　ERUDÂ

学名　*Sambucus nigra* L.*
科名　Caprifoliaceae（スイカズラ科）
英名　bourtree / European elder / black elder / European black elder
Part of use　stem, leaf, flower
Note 1　—
Note 2　—
注　—

名　称　セイヨウニンジンボク*

他名等　イタリアニンジンボク
部位等　全草
備　考　—

他名(参考)　—
漢字表記・生薬名等　西洋人参木（セイヨウニンボク）
Name(Romaji)　SEIYÔNINJINBOKU*
Other name(s) (Romaji)　ITARIANINJINBOKU
学名　*Vitex agnus-castus* L.*
科名　Verbenaceae（クマツヅラ科）
英名　chaste tree / agnus-castus / chasteberry / monk's pepper tree / hemp tree / Indian-spice / sage tree / wild pepper
Part of use　whole plant
Note 1　—
Note 2　—
注　—

名　称　セイヨウネズ*

他名等　セイヨウビャクシン
部位等　全草
備　考　—

他名(参考)　トショウ（杜松）、ヨウシュネズ（洋種杜松）
漢字表記・生薬名等　西洋杜松（セイヨウネズ）、西洋柏槇（セイヨウビャクシン）
Name(Romaji)　SEIYÔNEZU*
Other name(s) (Romaji)　SEIYÔBYAKUSHIN
学名　*Juniperus communis* L.*
科名　Cupressaceae（ヒノキ科）
英名　juniper / common juniper
Part of use　whole plant
Note 1　—
Note 2　—
注　—

名　称　セイヨウノコギリソウ*

他名等　ヤロー
部位等　全草
備　考　—

他名(参考)　—
漢字表記・生薬名等　西洋蓍草（セイヨウシソウ）、西洋鋸草（セイヨウノコギリソウ）
Name(Romaji)　SEIYÔNOKOGIRISÔ*
Other name(s) (Romaji)　YARÔ
学名　*Achillea millefolium* L.*
Achillea millefolium L. var. *occidentalis* DC.*
Achillea lanulosa Nutt.*
科名　Compositae（キク科）
英名　yarrow / milfoil / common yarrow / nose-bleed / sanguinary / thousand-seal yarrow / western yarrow
Part of use　whole plant
Note 1　—
Note 2　—
注　—

名　称　セイヨウハッカ*

他名等　ペパーミント
部位等　全草
備　考　—

他名(参考)　ハッカヨウ（薄荷葉）
漢字表記・生薬名等　西洋薄荷（セイヨウハッカ）
Name(Romaji)　SEIYÔHAKKA*
Other name(s) (Romaji)　PEPÂMINTO
学名　*Mentha*×*piperita* L.*
科名　Labiatae（シソ科）
英名　peppermint
Part of use　whole plant
Note 1　—
Note 2　Refer to HAKKA and MINTO listed in the items of "Name". SEIYÔHAKKA is one of the s pecies of MINTO (*Mentha* L.), but their parts of use are different each other.
注　別項のハッカ及びミントを参照。セイヨウハッカはミント（ハッカ属）に含まれるが、「部位等」の記載が異なっている。

名　称　**セイヨウヒイラギ**

他名等　—
部位等　花
備　考　—

他名(参考)　ヒイラギモチ（柊黐）
漢字表記・生薬名等　西洋柊（セイヨウヒイラギ）
Name(Romaji)　SEIYÔHÎRAGI
Other name(s) (Romaji)　—
学名　*Ilex aquifolium* L.
科名　Aquifoliaceae（モチノキ科）
英名　English holly / European holly / Oregon holly / common holly
Part of use　flower
Note 1　—
Note 2　—
注　—

名　称　**セイヨウヒメスノキ***

他名等　—
部位等　果実・葉
備　考　—

他名(参考)　ビルベリー
漢字表記・生薬名等　西洋姫臼の木（セイヨウヒメスノキ）
Name(Romaji)　SEIYÔHIMESUNOKI*
Other name(s) (Romaji)　—
学名　*Vaccinium myrtillus* L.*
科名　Ericaceae（ツツジ科）
英名　bilberry / European blueberry / huckleberry / whortleberry / lowbush blueberry
Part of use　fruit, leaf
Note 1　—
Note 2　SEIYÔHIMESUNOKI is identical with BIRUBERÎ. BIRUBERÎ is also listed in the item of "Name".
注　セイヨウヒメスノキは別項のビルベリーと同一。

名　称　**セイヨウマツタケ**

他名等　シャンピニオン／ツクリタケ
部位等　子実体
備　考　—

他名(参考)　ハラタケ（原茸）、セイヨウキノコ（西洋茸）
漢字表記・生薬名等　西洋松茸（セイヨウマツタケ）、作茸（ツクリタケ）
Name(Romaji)　SEIYÔMATSUTAKE
Other name(s) (Romaji)　SHANPINION／TSUKURITAKE
学名　*Agaricus bisporus* (J.E. Lange) Imbach
科名　Agaricaceae（ハラタケ科）
英名　brown mushroom / common mushroom / champignon
Part of use　fruit body
Note 1　—
Note 2　—
注　—

名　称　**セイヨウミザクラ***

他名等　—
部位等　果実・葉
備　考　—

他名(参考)　カンカオウトウ（甘果桜桃）
漢字表記・生薬名等　西洋実桜（セイヨウミザクラ）
Name(Romaji)　SEIYÔMIZAKURA*
Other name(s) (Romaji)　—
学名　*Prunus avium* (L.) L.*
Cerasus avium (L.) Moench*
Cerasus sylvestris Lund.
Cerasus nigra Mill.
科名　Rosaceae（バラ科）
英名　bird cherry / mazzard cherry / sweet cherry / gean
Part of use　fruit, leaf
Note 1　—
Note 2　—
注　—

名　称　**セイヨウメギ***

他名等　—
部位等　全草
備　考　—

他名(参考)　ショウバク（小檗）
漢字表記・生薬名等　西洋目木（セイヨウメギ）
Name(Romaji)　SEIYÔMEGI*
Other name(s) (Romaji)　—
学名　*Berberis vulgaris* L.*
科名　Berberidaceae（メギ科）
英名　barberry / European barberry / common barberry / jaundice berry / pirage
Part of use　whole plant
Note 1　—
Note 2　—
注　—

名　称　**セキイ***

他名等　ヒトツバ／Pyrrosia lingua／Pyrrosia grandisimus／Pyrrosia pelislosus／Pyrrosia hastata
部位等　全草
備　考　—

他名(参考)　イワオモダカ（岩沢潟、岩面高：P. hastata）
漢字表記・生薬名等　石韋（セキイ）、一ツ葉（ヒトツバ）
Name(Romaji)　SEKII*
Other name(s) (Romaji)　HITOTSUBA
学名　*Pyrrosia lingua* (Thunb.) Farw.*
Pyrrosia hastata (Thunb.) Ching
Pyrrosia tricuspis (Swartz) Tagawa
科名　Polpodiaceae（ウラボシ科）
英名　felt fern / tongue fern / Japanese felt fern / pyrrosia
Part of use　whole plant
Note 1　—
Note 2　Neither *Pyrrosia grandisimus* nor *Pyrrosia pelislosus* listed in the item of “Other names” can be confirmed.
注　「他名等」の*Pyrrosia grandisimus*及び*Pyrrosia pelislosus*は確認できない。

名　称　**セキコウジュ**

他名等　—
部位等　全草
備　考　—

他名(参考)　ホソバヤマジソ（細葉山紫蘇）、セキコウジュウ（石香菜）
漢字表記・生薬名等　石香薷（セキコウジュ）
Name(Romaji)　SEKIKÔJU
Other name(s) (Romaji)　—
学名　*Mosla chinensis* Maxim.
科名　Labiatae（シソ科）
英名　—
Part of use　whole plant
Note 1　—
Note 2　There is an information that the experience of using SEKIKÔJU as traditional Japanese harebal medicine is well known but the history of dietary use in Japan does not exist. (Reference：The Collaborative Reference Database of National Diet Library in Japan, February, 2012)
注　セキコウジュは生薬としての使用経験はあるが、日本における食経験情報は得られていないという情報がある。(国会図書館レファレンス協同データベース、2012年2月現在)。

名　称　**セキショウ***

他名等　—
部位等　茎
備　考　根茎は「医」

他名(参考)　セキショウブ（石菖蒲）、ショウブ（菖蒲）
漢字表記・生薬名等　石菖（セキショウ）
Name(Romaji)　SEKISHÔ*
Other name(s) (Romaji)　—
学名　*Acorus gramineus* Sol. ex Aiton*
Acorus tatarinowii Schott*
科名　Araceae（サトイモ科）
英名　grass-leaf sweet flag / grass-leaf calamus / Japanese sweet flag / dwarf sedge / Japanese rush / grassy-leaved sweet flag
Part of use　stem
Note 1　rhizome：drug category
Note 2　—
注　—

名　称　**セキショウモ**

他名等　クソウ／セイヨウセキショウモ
部位等　全草
備　考　—

他名(参考)　ヘラモ（篦藻）、コウガイモ（笄藻）
漢字表記・生薬名等　石菖藻（セキショウモ）、苦草（クソウ）、西洋石菖藻（セイヨウセキショウモ）
Name(Romaji)　SEKISHÔMO
Other name(s) (Romaji)　KUSÔ／SEIYÔSEKISHÔMO
学名　*Vallisneria natans* (Lour.) Hara
Vallisneria asiatica Miki
Vallisneria spiralis L.
Vallisneria gigantea Graebn.
Vallisneria denseserrulata Makino
Physkium natans Lour.
科名　Hydrocharitaceae（トチカガミ科）
英名　giant vallis / tape grass / eelgrass
Part of use　whole plant
Note 1　—
Note 2　—
注　—

名　称　セキヨウ

他名等　**ソロバンノキ／ハノキ／ハンノキ**
部位等　全草
備　考　―

他名(参考)　―
漢字表記･生薬名等　赤楊（セキヨウ）、榛木（ハンノキ）
Name (Romaji)　SEKIYÔ
Other name(s) (Romaji)　SOROBANNOKI／HANOKI／HANNOKI
学名　*Alnus japonica* (Thunb.) Steud.
Betula japonica Thunb.
科名　Betulaceae（カバノキ科）
英名　Japanese alder / alder
Part of use　whole plant
Note 1　―
Note 2　―
注　―

名　称　セッコツボク*

他名等　**ニワトコ**
部位等　茎・葉・花
備　考　―

他名(参考)　トウニワトコ（接骨木）
漢字表記･生薬名等　接骨木（セッコツボク）、茎：接骨木（セッコツボク）、根：接骨木根（セッコツボクコン）、花：接骨木花（セッコツボクカ）、葉及び若枝：接骨木葉（セッコツボクヨウ）、庭常（ニワトコ）
Name (Romaji)　SEKKOTSUBOKU*
Other name(s) (Romaji)　NIWATOKO
学名　*Sambucus racemosa* L. ssp. *sieboldiana* (Miq.) Hara
Sambucus sieboldiana Blume ex Graebn.
Sambucus williamsii Hance*
科名　Caprifoliaceae（スイカズラ科）
英名　European red elder / red-barried elder
Part of use　stem, leaf, flower
Note 1　―
Note 2　―
注　―

名　称　セツレンカ

他名等　―
部位等　全草
備　考　―

他名(参考)　メントウセツレンカ（綿頭雪蓮花）、ダイホウセツレンカ（大苞雪蓮花）、スイボセツレンカ（水母雪蓮花）
漢字表記･生薬名等　雪蓮（セツレン）、雪蓮花（セツレンカ）、綿頭雪蓮花（メントウセツレンカ：*Saussurea laniceps*）、大苞雪蓮花（ダイホウセツレンカ：*Saussurea involucrata*）、スイボセツレンカ（水母雪蓮花：*Saussurea medusa*）
Name (Romaji)　SETSURENKA
Other name(s) (Romaji)　―
学名　*Saussurea involucrata* (Kar. et Kir.) Sch. Bip.
Saussurea laniceps Hand.-Mazz.
Saussurea medusa Maxim.
科名　Compositae（キク科）
英名　herb of snow lotus
Part of use　whole plant
Note 1　―
Note 2　―
注　―

名　称　ゼニアオイ*

他名等　**マロー**
部位等　葉・花
備　考　―

他名(参考)　ゼニバアオイ（銭葉葵）、ウスベニアオイ（薄紅葵）、マロウ
漢字表記･生薬名等　銭葵（ゼニアオイ）、薄紅葵（ウスベニアオイ）、錦葵葉（キンキヨウ）、錦葵花（キンキカ）
Name (Romaji)　ZENIAOI*
Other name(s) (Romaji)　MARÔ
学名　*Malva sylvestris* L.*
Malva sylvestris L. var. *mauritiana* (L.) Boiss.
Malva mauritiana L.
Malva neglecta Wallr.*
科名　Malvaceae（アオイ科）
英名　common mallow / blue mallow / high mallow / tall mallow / cheeses / tree mallow / dwarf mallow / malva
Part of use　leaf, flower
Note 1　―
Note 2　ZENIAOI is identical with USUBENIAOI. USUBENIAOI is also listed in the item of “Name”.
注　ゼニアオイは別項のウスベニアオイと同一。

名　称　セルピウムソウ*

他名等　**テイムス・セルピウム**
部位等　全草
備　考　—

他名（参考）　イブキジャコウソウ（伊吹麝香草）、ヒャクリコウ（百里香）
漢字表記・生薬名等　伊吹麝香草（イブキジャコウソウ）、百里香（ヒャクリコウ）
Name (Romaji)　SERUPIUMUSÔ*
Other name (s) (Romaji)　TEIMUSU・SERUPIUMU
学名　*Thymus serpyllum* L.*
Thymus serpyllum L. ssp. *quinquecostatus* (Celak.) Kitam.
Thymus quinquecostatus Celak.
科名　Labiatae（シソ科）
英名　wild thyme / creeping thyme / mother-of-thyme / lemon thyme
Part of use　whole plant
Note 1　—
Note 2　SERUPIUMUSÔ is identical with IBUKIJAKÔSÔ, but their parts of use are different each other. IBUKIJAKÔSÔ is also listed in the item of "Name".
注　セルピウムソウは別項のイブキジャコウソウと同一。但し、「部位等」の記載が異なっている。

名　称　セロリ*

他名等　**オランダミツバ／セルリー**
部位等　種子
備　考　—

他名（参考）　マツバゼリ（松葉芹）、キヨマサニンジン（清正人参）
漢字表記・生薬名等　芹菜（チンサイ）、オランダ三葉（オランダミツバ）
Name (Romaji)　SERORI*
Other name (s) (Romaji)　ORANDAMITSUBA／SERURÎ
学名　*Apium graveolens* L. var. *dulce* (Mill.) Pers.*
科名　Umbelliferae（セリ科）
英名　celery / wild celery
Part of use　seed
Note 1　—
Note 2　—
注　—

名　称　センキュウ*

他名等　—
部位等　葉
備　考　根茎は「医」

他名（参考）　—
漢字表記・生薬名等　川芎（センキュウ）、川窮（センキュウ）、芎窮（センキュウ）、撫芎（ブキュウ）
Name (Romaji)　SENKYÛ*
Other name (s) (Romaji)　—
学名　*Cnidium officinale* Makino*
Ligusticum ibukiense Yabe*
Ligusticum chuanxiong Hort.*
科名　Umbelliferae（セリ科）
英名　marsh parsely
Part of use　leaf
Note 1　rhizome：drug category
Note 2　—
注　—

名　称　センザンリュウ

他名等　**ウチワドコロ**
部位等　全草
備　考　—

他名（参考）　コウモリドコロ（蝙蝠野老）
漢字表記・生薬名等　穿山竜（センザンリュウ）、団扇野老（ウチワドコロ）
Name (Romaji)　SENZANRYÛ
Other name (s) (Romaji)　UCHIWADOKORO
学名　*Dioscorea nipponica* Makino
科名　Dioscoreaceae（ヤマノイモ科）
英名　chuanlong yam / uchiwadokoro
Part of use　whole plant
Note 1　—
Note 2　—
注　—

名　称　センシンレン*

他名等　—
部位等　葉
備　考　—

他名（参考）　イチケンキ（一見喜）
漢字表記・生薬名等　穿心蓮（センシンレン）
Name (Romaji)　SENSHINREN*
Other name (s) (Romaji)　—

学名　*Andrographis paniculata* (Burm. f.) Nees*
科名　Acanthaceae（キツネノマゴ科）
英名　chiretta / chuan xin lian / kalmegh / kirata / andrographis / creat / green chiretta / Indian chiretta
Part of use　leaf
Note 1　—
Note 2　—
注　—

名　称　センソウ＜仙草＞*

他名等　リョウフンソウ
部位等　全草
備　考　センソウ＜茜草＞の根は「医」

他名(参考)　—
漢字表記･生薬名等　仙草（センソウ）、涼粉草（リョウフンソウ）
Name (Romaji)　SENSÔ*
Other name (s) (Romaji)　RYÔFUNSÔ
学名　*Mesona chinensis* Benth.*
Mesona procumbens Hemsl.
科名　Labiatae（シソ科）
英名　mesona / Chinese mesona
Part of use　whole plant
Note 1　root of *Rubia akane* Nakai (=*Rubia cordifolia* L.) : drug category
Note 2　—
注　—

名　称　センソウトウ*

他名等　—
部位等　全草
備　考　—

他名(参考)　トウゲシバ（峠芝）
漢字表記･生薬名等　千層塔（センソウトウ）
Name (Romaji)　SENSÔTÔ*
Other name (s) (Romaji)　—
学名　*Lycopodium serratum* Thunb.
Huperzia serrata (Thunb.) Rothm.*
Urostachys serratus (Thunb.) Herter
科名　Lycopodiaceae（ヒカゲノカズラ科）
英名　—
Part of use　whole plant
Note 1　—
Note 2　—
注　—

名　称　センタウリウムソウ*

他名等　Centaurium minus
部位等　全草
備　考　—

他名(参考)　ベニバナセンブリ（紅花千振）
漢字表記･生薬名等　紅花千振（ベニバナセンブリ）
Name (Romaji)　SENTAURIUMUSÔ*
Other name (s) (Romaji)　—
学名　*Centaurium minus* auct. non Moench
Centaurium erythreae Raf.*
Centaurium umbellatum Gilib.
Erythraea centaurium Pers.
科名　Gentianaceae（リンドウ科）
英名　common centaury / European centaury / centaury / bitter herb
Part of use　whole plant
Note 1　—
Note 2　—
注　—

名　称　センダン*

他名等　クレン／トキワセンダン／Melia azedarach
部位等　葉
備　考　センダン（Melia azedarach）及びトウセンダン（Melia toosendan）の果実・樹皮は「医」

他名(参考)　センレン（川楝）
漢字表記･生薬名等　栴檀（センダン）、苦楝（クレン）
Name (Romaji)　SENDAN*
Other name (s) (Romaji)　KUREN／TOKIWASENDAN
学名　*Melia azedarach* L.*（センダン）
Melia toosendan Sieb. et Zucc.*（トウセンダン）
Melia japonica G. Don
Melia azedarach var. *japonica* (G. Don) Makino
Melia dubia Cav.
Melia azedarach var. *azedarach*
科名　Meliaceae（センダン科）
英名　bead tree / melia / China berry / China tree / pagoda tree / Persian lilac / pride-of-India / pride-of-China
Part of use　leaf
Note 1　fruit and bark of *Melia azedarach* L. and *Melia toosendan* Sieb. et Zucc. : drug category
Note 2　—
注　—

名　称　**センナ***

他名等　—
部位等　茎
備　考　果実・小葉・葉柄・葉軸は「医」

他名(参考)　ホソバセンナ（狭葉番瀉）、チンネベリ・センナ（Tinnevelly senna）
漢字表記・生薬名等　番瀉葉（バンシャヨウ）
Name (Romaji)　SENNA*
Other name (s) (Romaji)　—
学名　*Cassia angustifolia* Vahl*（ホソバセンナ）
Cassia acutifolia Delile*（チンネベリ・センナ）
Senna alexandrina Mill.*
Senna angustifolia (Vahl) Batka*
科名　Leguminosae（マメ科）
英名　senna / Alexandrian senna / Indian senna / Tinnevelly senna / true senna
Part of use　stem
Note 1　fruit, microphyll, petiole and rachis : drug category
Note 2　—
注　—

名　称　**センボウ***

他名等　キンバイザサ
部位等　根茎
備　考　—

他名(参考)　—
漢字表記・生薬名等　仙茅（センボウ）、金梅笹（キンバイザサ）
Name (Romaji)　SENBÔ*
Other name (s) (Romaji)　KINBAIZASA
学名　*Curculigo orchioides* Gaertn.*
Curculigo ensifolia R. Br.
科名　Hypoxidaceae（キンバイザサ科）
英名　curculigo / golden eye grass / weevil-wort
Part of use　rhizome
Note 1　—
Note 2　—
注　—

名　称　**センリコウ**

他名等　タイキンギク
部位等　全草
備　考　—

他名(参考)　ユキミギク（雪見菊）
漢字表記・生薬名等　千里光（センリコウ）、堆金菊（タイキンギク）
Name (Romaji)　SENRIKÔ
Other name (s) (Romaji)　TAIKINGIKU
学名　*Senecio scandens* Buch.-Ham. ex D. Don
Senecio wightianus DC. ex Wight
科名　Compositae（キク科）
英名　charlatan ivy
Part of use　whole plant
Note 1　—
Note 2　—
注　—

名　称　**センリョウ**

他名等　腫節風／竹節草／草珊瑚
部位等　全株
備　考　—

他名(参考)　—
漢字表記・生薬名等　仙寥・千両（センリョウ）、実千両（ミセンリョウ）
Name (Romaji)　SENRYÔ
Other name (s) (Romaji)　SHUSETSUFÛ／CHIKUSETSUSÔ／KUSASANGO
学名　*Sarcandra glabra* (Thunb.) Nakai
Ardisia glabra Thunb.
Chloranthus monander R. Br. ex Sims
Chloranthus glaber (Thunb.) Makino
科名　Chloranthaceae（センリョウ科）
英名　chloranthus
Part of use　whole plant
Note 1　—
Note 2　ZENKABU written in the item of "Part of use" in Japanese possibly be translated a "whole roots" but it was translated as "whole plat" shown in the item of "Part of use" in English.
SENRYÔ is identical with KYÛSETSUCHA.
注　「部位等」の全株は全草と訳した。
センリョウは別項のキュウセツチャと同一。

名　称　**ソウジュヨウ***

他名等　ハマウツボ／Orobanche coerulescens
部位等　茎
備　考　—

他名(参考)　—
漢字表記·生薬名等　草蓯蓉（ソウジュヨウ）、浜靫（ハマウツボ）
Name (Romaji)　SÔJUYÔ*
Other name (s) (Romaji)　HAMAUTSUBO
学名　*Orobanche coerulescens* Steph.*
科名　Orobancaceae（ハマウツボ科）
英名　skyblue bloomrape / orobanche
Part of use　stem
Note 1　—
Note 2　—
注　—

名　称　**ソゴウコウ***

他名等　—
部位等　分泌樹脂
備　考　—

他名(参考)　—
漢字表記·生薬名等　蘇合香（ソゴウコウ）
Name (Romaji)　SOGÔKÔ*
Other name (s) (Romaji)　—
学名　*Liquidambar orientalis* Mill.*
科名　Hamamelidaceae（マンサク科）
英名　Chinese liquidambar / oriental sweet gum / styrax / formosan sweet gum
Part of use　resin
Note 1　—
Note 2　—
注　—

名　称　**ソクハクヨウ***

他名等　コノテガシワ
部位等　枝・葉
備　考　—

他名(参考)　ハクシジン（柏子仁）
漢字表記·生薬名等　側柏葉（ソクハクヨウ）、児手柏（コノテガシワ）
Name (Romaji)　SOKUHAKUYÔ*
Other name (s) (Romaji)　KONOTEGASHIWA
学名　*Platycladus orientalis* (L.) Franco*
Thuja orientalis L.*
Biota orientalis (L.) Endl.*
科名　Cupressaceae（ヒノキ科）
英名　oriental arborvitae / Chinese arborvitae
Part of use　branch, leaf
Note 1　—
Note 2　SOKUHAKUYÔ is identical with HAKUSHIJIN, but their parts of use are different each other. HAKUSHIJIN is listed in the item of "Name" in the "drug" category list and its part of use is seed. Therefore, seed of SOKUHAKUYÔ is forbidden to use as food.
注　ソクハクヨウは別項のハクシジンと同一。ハクシジンは「医」リストに区分されており、その「部位等」は種子とされている。従って、ソクハクヨウの種子は食品に使用することができない。

名　称　**ソバ***

他名等　キョウバク／ソバミツ／Fagopyrum esulentum
部位等　種子・花から集めた蜂蜜・茎・葉
備　考　—

他名(参考)　—
漢字表記·生薬名等　蕎麦・蕎麥（ソバ、キョウバク）、蕎麦密（ソバミツ）
Name (Romaji)　SOBA*
Other name (s) (Romaji)　KYÔBAKU／SOBAMITSU
学名　*Fagopyrum esculentum* Moench*
Fagopyrum vulgare Nees
Fagopyrum sagittatum Gilib.
Polygonum fagopyrum L.
科名　*Polygonaceae*（タデ科）
英名　brank / buckwheat / notch-seeded buckwheat
Part of use　seed, honey from buckwheat flower, stem, leaf
Note 1　—
Note 2　—
注　—

タ行

名　称　ターミナリア・ベリリカ*

他名等　Terminalia bellirica
部位等　完熟果実
備　考　—

他名(参考)　—
漢字表記・生薬名等　鞞醯勒果（vibhitaka）
Name(Romaji)　TÂMINARIA・BERIRIKA*
Other name(s)(Romaji)　—
学名　*Terminalia bellirica* (Gaertn.) Roxb.
Terminalia bellerica (Gaertn.) Roxb.*
科名　Combretaceae（シクンシ科）
英名　bahira / bilhitak / bahera / baheda / vibhidhaka / belleric myrobalan / beleric myrobalan / belliric myrobalan / vibhitaka
Part of use　riped fruit
Note 1　—
Note 2　TÂMINARIA・BERIRIKA is identical with SEITAKAMIROBARAN, but their parts of use are different each other. SEITAKAMIROBARAN is also listed in the item of "Name".
注　ターミナリア・ベリリカは別項のセイタカミロバランと同一。但し、「部位等」の記載が異なっている。

名　称　ダイウイキョウ*

他名等　スターアニス
部位等　果実
備　考　—

他名(参考)　トウシキミ（唐樒）、ハッカクウイキョウ（八角茴香）
漢字表記・生薬名等　大茴香（ダイウイキョウ）
Name(Romaji)　DAIUIKYÔ*
Other name(s)(Romaji)　SUTÂANISU
学名　*Illicium verum* Hook. f.*
科名　Illiciaceae（シキミ科）
英名　ba jiao hui xian / star anise / Chinese star anise
Part of use　fruit
Note 1　—
Note 2　—
注　—

名　称　ダイオウ*

他名等　ヤクヨウダイオウ／ルバーブ
部位等　葉
備　考　根茎は「医」

他名(参考)　ショクヨウダイオウ（食用大黄）、マルバダイオウ（丸葉大黄）、ショウヨウダイオウ（掌葉大黄）、タングートダイオウ（唐古特大黄）、カラダイオウ（唐大黄）
漢字表記・生薬名等　大黄（ダイオウ）、薬用大黄（ヤクヨウダイオウ）
Name(Romaji)　DAIÔ*
Other name(s)(Romaji)　YAKUYÔDAIÔ／RUBÂBU
学名　*Rheum* L.
Rheum palmatum L.*（ショウヨウダイオウ）
Rheum palmatum L. var. *tanguticum* Maxim. ex Regel*（タングートダイオウ）
Rheum officinale Baill.*（ヤクヨウダイオウ）
Rheum rhaponticum L.（ショクヨウダイオウ）
Rheum rhabarbarum L.（カラダイオウ）
科名　Polygonaceae（タデ科）
英名　rhubarb / Chinese rhubarb / Turkey rhubarb / medicinal rhubarb / East Indian rhubarb / rhapontic rhubarb / pie-plant / garden rhubarb
Part of use　leaf
Note 1　rhizome：drug category
Note 2　Refer to SHOKUYÔDAIÔ listed in the item of "Name".
注　別項の食用ダイオウを参照。

名　称　ダイケットウ

他名等　—
部位等　茎
備　考　—

他名(参考)　コウトウ（紅藤）
漢字表記・生薬名等　大血藤（ダイケットウ）
Name(Romaji)　DAIKETTÔ
Other name(s)(Romaji)　—
学名　*Sargentodoxa cuneata* (Oliv.) Rehd. et Wils.
Holboellia cuneata Oliv.
科名　Sargentodoxaceae（サルゲントドクサ科）
英名　—
Part of use　stem
Note 1　—
Note 2　—
注　—

名　称　**ダイコンソウ**

他名等　スイヨウバイ
部位等　全草
備　考　—

他名(参考)　—
漢字表記・生薬名等　大根草（ダイコンソウ）、水楊梅（スイヨウバイ）
Name (Romaji)　DAIKONSÔ
Other name(s) (Romaji)　SUIYÔBAI
学名　*Geum japonicum* Thunb.
科名　Rosaceae（バラ科）
英名　Japanese avens
Part of use　whole plant
Note 1　—
Note 2　—
注　—

名　称　**タイシジン***

他名等　ワダソウ
部位等　塊根
備　考　—

他名(参考)　ガイジシン（孩児参）、イヨウカハンロウ（異葉仮繁縷）
漢字表記・生薬名等　太子参（タイシジン）、和田草（ワダソウ）
Name (Romaji)　TAISHIJIN*
Other name(s) (Romaji)　WADASÔ
学名　*Pseudostellaria heterophylla* (Miq.) Pax ex Pax et Hoffm.*
科名　Caryophyllaceae（ナデシコ科）
英名　tai zi shen / pseudostellaria / lesser ginseng / prince ginseng
Part of use　root tuber
Note 1　—
Note 2　—
注　—

名　称　**ダイズ***

他名等　コクダイズ／ダイズオウケン／ダイズ油
部位等　種子・種子油・種皮・葉・花・大豆の特殊発酵品
備　考　—

他名(参考)　—
漢字表記・生薬名等　大豆（ダイズ）、黒大豆（コクダイズ）、大豆黄巻（ダイズオウケン）、香豉（コウシ：大豆種子の発酵品）、豆豉（ズシ、トウシ：大豆種子の発酵品）
Name (Romaji)　DAIZU*
Other name(s) (Romaji)　KOKUDAIZU／DAIZUÔKEN／DAIZU-YU
学名　*Glycine max* (L.) Merr.*
Phaseolus max L.
科名　Leguminosae（マメ科）
英名　soybean / soja bean / soya bean
Part of use　seed, seed oil, seed coat, leaf, flower, fermented soybean
Note 1　—
Note 2　—
注　—

名　称　**タイソウ***

他名等　ナツメ
部位等　果実・種子・葉
備　考　—

他名(参考)　コウソウ（紅棗）
漢字表記・生薬名等　大棗（タイソウ）、棗・夏芽（ナツメ）、種子：酸棗仁（サンソウニン）
Name (Romaji)　TAISÔ*
Other name(s) (Romaji)　NATSUME
学名　*Ziziphus jujuba* Mill.*
Ziziphus jujuba Mill. var. *inermis* (Bunge) Rehd.
Ziziphus vulgaris Lam.*
Ziziphus vulgaris Lam. var. *spinosa* Bunge
Ziziphus zizyphus (L.) H. Karst.
Ziziphus sativa Gaertn.
科名　Rhamnaceae（クロウメモドキ科）
英名　jujube / Chinese date / Chinese jujube / jujube date / sour date / sour jujube
Part of use　fruit, seed, leaf
Note 1　—
Note 2　TAISÔ is riped fruit of NATSUME used as traditional Japanese herbal medicie. SANSÔNIN is seed of SANEBUTONATSUME. SANSÔNIN is also listed in the item of "Name".
注　タイソウは生薬名で、ナツメの成熟果実。別項のサンソウニンはサネブトナツメの種子。

名　称　ダイダイ*

他名等　キジツ／キコク／トウヒ／Citrus aurantium
部位等　果実・果皮・蕾・花
備　考　—

他名(参考)　カボス（臭橙）、カブス（蚊無須）、サントウ（酸橙）
漢字表記・生薬名等　代々・橙（ダイダイ）、枳実（キジツ）、枳殻（キコク）、橙皮（トウヒ）
Name (Romaji)　DAIDAI*
Other name(s) (Romaji)　KIJITSU／KIKOKU／TÔHI
学名　*Citrus aurantium* L.*
科名　Rutaceae（ミカン科）
英名　sour orange / bitter orange / bigarade / marmalade orange / seville orange
Part of use　fruit, pericarp, bud, flower
Note 1　—
Note 2　—
注　—

名　称　タイワンスク*

他名等　—
部位等　枝・茎
備　考　—

他名(参考)　—
漢字表記・生薬名等　台湾葛・越南葛藤（タイワンクズ）
Name (Romaji)　TAIWANSUKU*
Other name(s) (Romaji)　—
学名　*Pueraria montana* (Lour.) Merr.
Pueraria montana (Lour.) Merr. var. *chinense* Maesen et S.M. Almeida*
Pueraria montana (Lour.) Merr. var. *lobata* (Willd.) Maesen et S.M. Almeida ex Sanjappa et Predeep*
Pueraria thomsonii Benth.*
科名　Leguminosae（マメ科）
英名　kudzu
Part of use　branch, stem
Note 1　—
Note 2　TAIWANSUKU is incorrect. The correct name is TAIWANKUZU. Refer to KUZU listed in the item of "Name".
注　タイワンスクの正しい名称はタイワンクズ。別項のクズを参照。

名　称　タイワンテイカカズラ

他名等　—
部位等　果実
備　考　—

他名(参考)　ラクセキ（絡石）、トウキョウチクトウ（唐夾竹桃）、トウテイカカズラ（唐定家葛（蔓））
漢字表記・生薬名等　台湾定家葛（蔓）（タイワンテイカカズラ）、絡石（ラクセキ）
Name (Romaji)　TAIWANTEIKAKAZURA
Other name(s) (Romaji)　—
学名　*Trachelospermum jasminoides* (Lindl.) Lem.
科名　Apocynaceae（キョウチクトウ科）
英名　confederate jasmine / star jasmine / Malayan jasmin
Part of use　fruit
Note 1　—
Note 2　—
注　—

名　称　タウコギ*

他名等　—
部位等　全草
備　考　—

他名(参考)　ロウハソウ（狼把草）
漢字表記・生薬名等　田五加木（タウコギ）
Name (Romaji)　TAUKOGI*
Other name(s) (Romaji)　—
学名　*Bidens tripartita* L.*
Bidens comosa (A. Gray) Wieg.
Bidens acuta (Wieg.) Britt.
科名　Compositae（キク科）
英名　tickseed / swamp tickseed / swamp marigold / three-lobe beggar ticks
Part of use　whole plant
Note 1　—
Note 2　—
注　—

名　称　タカサゴギク*

他名等　—
部位等　全草
備　考　—

他名(参考)　ガイノウコウ（艾納香）、ガイヘン（艾片）
漢字表記・生薬名等　高砂菊（タカサゴギク）、艾納香（ガ

イノウコウ）
Name (Romaji)　TAKASAGOGIKU*
Other name (s) (Romaji)　—
学名　*Blumea balsamifera* (L.) DC.*
科名　Compositae（キク科）
英名　Nagi camphor tree / Ngai camphor plant
Part of use　whole plant
Note 1　—
Note 2　—
注　—

名　称　タカサブロウ*

他名等　カンレンソウ
部位等　全草
備　考　—

他名(参考)　ボクカンレン（墨旱蓮）、レイチョウ（鱧腸）
漢字表記・生薬名等　高三郎（タカサブロウ）、旱蓮草（カンレンソウ）
Name (Romaji)　TAKASABURÔ*
Other name (s) (Romaji)　KANRENSÔ
学名　*Eclipta prostrata* (L.) L.*
Eclipta alba L. Hassk.*
Eclipta erecta L.
科名　Compositae（キク科）
英名　han lian cao / eclipta / false daisy
Part of use　whole plant
Note 1　—
Note 2　—
注　—

名　称　タガヤサン

他名等　テツトウボク
部位等　全草
備　考　—

他名(参考)　コクシンジュ（黒心樹）
漢字表記・生薬名等　鉄刀木（タガヤサン、テツトウボク）
Name (Romaji)　TAGAYASAN
Other name (s) (Romaji)　TETSUTÔBOKU
学名　*Cassia siamea* Lam.
Cassia florida Vahl
Senna siamea H.S. Irwin et Barneby
科名　Leguminosae（マメ科）
英名　kassod tree / Bombay black wood / siamese cassia / siamese senna / rosewood
Part of use　whole plant
Note 1　—
Note 2　—
注　—

名　称　タケ類

他名等　タケノコ
部位等　若芽
備　考　—

他名(参考)　モウソウチク（孟宗竹：通常、日本のタケノコを指す）、マダケ（真竹）、カンチク（寒竹）、ハチク（淡竹）、ネマガリタケ（根曲竹、根曲がり竹）
漢字表記・生薬名等　竹の子・筍（タケノコ）
Name (Romaji)　TAKE-RUI
Other name (s) (Romaji)　TAKENOKO
学名　*Phyllostachys* Sieb. et Zucc.（マダケ属）
Bambusa Schreb.（ホウライチク属）
Phyllostachys pubescens Mazel（モウソウチク）
Phyllostachys heterocycla (Carr.) Mitf.（モウソウチク）
Phyllostachys heterocycla var. *pubescens* (Mazel) Ohwi（モウソウチク）
科名　Gramineae（イネ科）
英名　bamboo / bamboo shoot
Part of use　sprout
Note 1　—
Note 2　—
注　—

名　称　タコノアシ

他名等　カンコウソウ／Penthorum chinense
部位等　茎・葉
備　考　—

他名(参考)　—
漢字表記・生薬名等　蛸の足（タコノアシ）
Name (Romaji)　TAKONOASHI
Other name (s) (Romaji)　KANKÔSÔ
学名　*Penthorum chinense* Pursh
科名　Penthoraceae（タコノアシ科）（ベンケイソウ科：Crassulaceaeあるいはユキノシタ科：Saxifragaceaeに分類されることもある）
英名　—
Part of use　stem, leaf
Note 1　—
Note 2　—
注　—

名　称　タチアオイ*

他名等　—
部位等　茎葉・種子・根・花
備　考　—

他名(参考)　ハナアオイ（花葵）
漢字表記・生薬名等　立葵（タチアオイ）
Name(Romaji)　TACHIAOI*
Other name(s)(Romaji)　—
学名　*Althaea rosea* (L.) Cav.*
Alcea rosea L.*
科名　Malvaceae（アオイ科）
英名　hollyhock / holly hock / golden holly hock / rose mallow
Part of use　stem, leaf, seed, root, flower
Note 1　—
Note 2　"茎葉 (stem-leaf)" in the item of "Part of use" written in Japanese should be replaced by "茎・葉 (stem and leaf)".
注　「部位等」の茎葉は「茎_葉」である。

名　称　タチジャコウソウ*

他名等　タイム
部位等　全草
備　考　—

他名(参考)　キダチヒャクリコウ（木立百里香）
漢字表記・生薬名等　立麝香草（タチジャコウソウ）、麝香草（ジャコウソウ）、木立百里香（キダチヒャクリコウ）
Name(Romaji)　TACHIJAKÔSÔ*
Other name(s)(Romaji)　TAIMU
学名　*Thymus vulgaris* L.*
科名　Labiatae（シソ科）
英名　thyme / common thyme / garden thyme
Part of use　whole plant
Note 1　—
Note 2　—
注　—

名　称　タチバナ

他名等　Citrus tachibana
部位等　葉・果皮
備　考　—

他名(参考)　ヤマトタチバナ（大和橘）、ニッポンタチバナ（日本橘）
漢字表記・生薬名等　橘（タチバナ）、多知波奈（タチバナ）
Name(Romaji)　TACHIBANA
Other name(s)(Romaji)　—
学名　*Citrus tachibana* (Makino) T. Tanaka
科名　Rutaceae（ミカン科）
英名　tachibana mandarin / tachibana orange
Part of use　leaf, pericarp
Note 1　—
Note 2　—
注　—

名　称　タチバナアデク*

他名等　スリナムチェリー／ブラジルチェリー
部位等　果実・葉
備　考　—

他名(参考)　—
漢字表記・生薬名等　橘アデク（タチバナアデク）
Name(Romaji)　TACHIBANAADEKU*
Other name(s)(Romaji)　SURINAMUCHERÎ／BURAJIRUCHERÎ
学名　*Eugenia uniflora* L.*
Eugenia michelii Lam.*
科名　Myrtaceae（フトモモ科）
英名　Brazilian cherry / cayenne cherry / Surinam cherry / pitanga
Part of use　fruit, leaf
Note 1　—
Note 2　—
注　—

名　称　ダッタンソバ

他名等　—
部位等　全草
備　考　—

他名(参考)　ニガソバ（苦蕎麦）
漢字表記・生薬名等　韃靼蕎麦（ダッタンソバ）
Name(Romaji)　DATTANSOBA
Other name(s)(Romaji)　—
学名　*Fagopyrum tataricum* (L.) Gaertn.
科名　Polygonaceae（タデ科）
英名　Tartarian buckwheat / tartary buckwheat / Indian buckwheat / Indian wheat / Kangra buckwheat
Part of use　whole plant
Note 1　—
Note 2　—
注　—

名　称　**タデアイ***

他名等　—
部位等　根
備　考　—

他名(参考)　アイ（藍）
漢字表記・生薬名等　蓼藍（タデアイ、リョウラン）、藍（アイ）
Name(Romaji)　TADEAI*
Other name(s)(Romaji)　—
学名　*Polygonum tinctorium* Lour.*
Persicaria tinctoria (Lour.) H. Gross
科名　Polygonaceae（タデ科）
英名　Chinese indigo / polygonum indigo
Part of use　root
Note 1　—
Note 2　—
注　—

名　称　**タベブイア***

他名等　タヒボ
部位等　樹皮・葉
備　考　—

他名(参考)　インペティギノサ、イペ、イペロッショ、ラパチョ
漢字表記・生薬名等　—
Name(Romaji)　TABEBUIA*
Other name(s)(Romaji)　TAHIBO
学名　*Tabebuia impetiginosa* (Mart. ex DC.) Standl.*
Tabebuia avellanedae Lorentz ex Griseb.*
Tabebuia heptaphylla (Vell.) Toledo*
Tecoma impetiginosa Mart. ex DC.*
科名　Bignoniaceae（ノウゼンカズラ科）
英名　taheebo tree / pau d'arco / ipe roxo / lapacho / taheebo
Part of use　bark, leaf
Note 1　—
Note 2　TABEBUIA is identical with both of INPETIGINOSA and PAUDARUKO. But parts of use of INPETIGINOSA is different form those of other two species. The former is whole plant and the latter is bark and leaf, but bark and／or leaf of these trees are commonly used.
注　タベブイアは別項のインペティギノサ及びパウダルコと同一。インペティギノサの「部位等」は全草であるが、タベブイア及びパウダルコは樹皮・葉とされている。通常は樹皮と葉が用いられる。

名　称　**タモギタケ**

他名等　—
部位等　子実体
備　考　—

他名(参考)　ニレタケ（楡茸）、タモキノコ（タモ茸）
漢字表記・生薬名等　楡木茸（タモギタケ）
Name(Romaji)　TAMOGITAKE
Other name(s)(Romaji)　—
学名　*Pleurotus cornucopiae* var. *citrinopileatus* (Singer) Ohira
Pleurotus citrinopileatus Singer
Pleurotus cornucopiae citrinopileatus (Singer) O. Hilber
科名　Pleurotaceae（ヒラタケ科）
英名　golden oyster mushroom / tamogitake
Part of use　fruit body
Note 1　—
Note 2　—
注　—

名　称　**タラノキ***

他名等　Aralia elata
部位等　葉・芽・根皮・樹皮
備　考　—

他名(参考)　—
漢字表記・生薬名等　楤木・桜木（タラノキ、ソウボク）、楤根皮（タラコンピ）、楤木皮（タラボクヒ）、刺老鴉（シロウア）
Name(Romaji)　TARANOKI*
Other name(s)(Romaji)　—
学名　*Aralia elata* (Miq.) Seem.*
Aralia mandshurica Rupr. et Maxim.*
科名　Araliaceae（ウコギ科）
英名　devil's-walking-stick / Japanese aralia / angelica tree / Chinese angelica tree / Japanese angelica tree / Hercules-club
Part of use　leaf, sprout, root bark, bark
Note 1　—
Note 2　—
注　—

名　称　**タラヨウ**

他名等　クテイチャ
部位等　葉
備　考　—

他名(参考)　—
漢字表記・生薬名等　多羅葉・大場冬青（タラヨウ：*Ilex latifolia*）、苦丁茶（クテイチャ）
Name(Romaji)　TARAYÔ
Other name(s)(Romaji)　KUTEICHA
学名　*Ilex latifolia* Thunb.
Ilex kudingcha C.J. Tseng
科名　Aquifoliaceae（モチノキ科）
英名　ku ding cha / luster-leaf holly / tarajo / tarajo holly
Part of use　leaf
Note 1　—
Note 2　For making herbal tea, KUTEICHA written in the item of "Other names"is made from leaves of TARAYÔ or HÎRAGIMOCHI.
注　「他名等」のクテイチャとしては、タラヨウの葉以外にヒイラギモチ（*Ilex cornuta*）の葉を用いる場合もある。

名　称　**タンジン***

他名等　—
部位等　葉
備　考　根は「医」

他名(参考)　セキジン（赤参）、レッドセージ
漢字表記・生薬名等　丹参（タンジン）
Name(Romaji)　TANJIN*
Other name(s)(Romaji)　—
学名　*Salvia miltiorrhiza* Bunge*
科名　Labiatae（シソ科）
英名　dan shen / Chinese salvia / Chinese sage / red-root sage
Part of use　leaf
Note 1　root：drug category
Note 2　—
注　—

名　称　**タンチクヨウ***

他名等　ササクサ
部位等　全草
備　考　—

他名(参考)　—
漢字表記・生薬名等　淡竹葉（タンチクヨウ）、笹草（ササクサ）
Name(Romaji)　TANCHIKUYÔ*
Other name(s)(Romaji)　SASAKUSA
学名　*Lophatherum gracile* Brongn.*
科名　Gramineae（イネ科）
英名　dan zhu ye / lophatherum
Part of use　whole plant
Note 1　—
Note 2　—
注　—

名　称　**タンテイヒホウ**

他名等　トウサンサイシン
部位等　全草
備　考　—

他名(参考)　エゾムカシヨモギ（蝦夷昔蓬）
漢字表記・生薬名等　短葶飛蓬（タンテイヒホウ）、灯盞細辛（トウサンサイシン）、灯盞花（トウサンカ）
Name(Romaji)　TANTEIHIHÔ
Other name(s)(Romaji)　TÔSANSAISHIN
学名　*Erigeron breviscapus* (Vant.) Hand.-Mazz.
科名　Compositae（キク科）
英名　—
Part of use　whole plant
Note 1　—
Note 2　—
注　—

名　称　**チア***

他名等　—
部位等　全草
備　考　—

他名(参考)　—
漢字表記・生薬名等　—
Name(Romaji)　CHIA*
Other name(s)(Romaji)　—
学名　*Salvia hispanica* L.*
科名　Labiatae（シソ科）

英名　chia / Spanish sage
Part of use　whole plant
Note 1　—
Note 2　—
注　—

名　称　**チクレキ**

他名等　**タンチク**
部位等　ハチクの茎を火で炙って流れた液汁
備　考　—

他名(参考)　—
漢字表記・生薬名等　竹瀝（チクレキ）、淡竹（タンチク）
Name (Romaji)　CHIKUREKI
Other name (s) (Romaji)　TANCHIKU
学名　*Phyllostachys nigra* (Lodd.) Munro var. *henonis* (Bean) Stapf
Phyllostachys henonis Bean
科名　Gramineae（イネ科）
英名　giant reed / henon bamboo / black bamboo
Part of use　extract from Henon bamboo stem by broiling
Note 1　—
Note 2　—
注　—

名　称　**チシマザサ**

他名等　**ネマガリタケ**
部位等　葉・幼茎
備　考　—

他名(参考)　—
漢字表記・生薬名等　千島笹（チシマザサ）、根曲竹（ネマガリタケ）
Name (Romaji)　CHISHIMAZASA
Other name (s) (Romaji)　NEMAGARITAKE
学名　*Sasa kurilensis* (Rupr.) Makino et Shibata
Arundinaria kurilensis Rupr.
科名　Gramineae（イネ科）
英名　Chishima zasa
Part of use　leaf, sprout
Note 1　—
Note 2　—
注　—

名　称　**チシマルリソウ**

他名等　—
部位等　全草
備　考　—

他名(参考)　—
漢字表記・生薬名等　千島瑠璃草（チシマルリソウ）
Name (Romaji)　CHISHIMARURISÔ
Other name (s) (Romaji)　—
学名　*Mertensia pterocarpa* (Turcz.) Tatew. et Ohwi
科名　Boraginaceae（ムラサキ科）
英名　Virginia bluebells
Part of use　whole plant
Note 1　—
Note 2　—
注　—

名　称　**チャ***

他名等　**アッサムチャ／プーアルチャ／フジチャ／リョクチャ**
部位等　茎・葉・葉の精油・花（蕾を含む）
備　考　—

他名(参考)　—
漢字表記・生薬名等　茶（チャ）、普洱茶（フジチャ：プーアル茶）、緑茶（リョクチャ）
Name (Romaji)　CHA*
Other name (s) (Romaji)　ASSAMUCHA／PÛARUCHA／FUJICHA／RYOKUCHA
学名　*Camellia sinensis* (L.) O. Kuntze*
Thea sinensis L.*
Camellia thea Link
Camellia sinensis (L.) O. Kunze var. *assamica* (J.W. Mast.) Kitam.
科名　Theaceae（ツバキ科）
英名　black tea / Chinese tea / green tea / pu'ercha / Assam tea
Part of use　stem, leaf, essential oil from leaf, flower (including bud)
Note 1　—
Note 2　Refer to HAKUCHA listed in the item of "Name".
注　別項のハクチャを参照。

名　称　**チャービル***

他名等　—
部位等　葉
備　考　—

他名(参考)　—
漢字表記・生薬名等　—
Name(Romaji)　CHÂBIRU*
Other name(s)(Romaji)　—
学名　*Anthriscus cerefolium* (L.) Hoffm.*
Scandix cerefolium L.
Chaerofolium cerefolium (L.) Schinz.
科名　Umbelliferae (セリ科)
英名　chervil / garden chervil / salad chervil / leaf chervil
Part of use　leaf
Note 1　—
Note 2　—
注　—

名　称　**チャデブグレ***

他名等　—
部位等　全草
備　考　—

他名(参考)　—
漢字表記・生薬名等　—
Name(Romaji)　CHADEBUGURE*
Other name(s)(Romaji)　—
学名　*Cordia salicifolia* Cham.*
Cordia ecalyculata Vell.*
Cordia digynia Vell.
Cordia coffeoides Warm
科名　Boraginaceae (ムラサキ科)
英名　chá de bugre / cafe do mato / cafe de bugre
Part of use　whole plant
Note 1　—
Note 2　—
注　—

名　称　**チャボトケイソウ***

他名等　—
部位等　果実・根・葉・花
備　考　—

他名(参考)　—
漢字表記・生薬名等　矮鶏時計草(チャボトケイソウ)
Name(Romaji)　CHABOTOKEISÔ*
Other name(s)(Romaji)　—
学名　*Passiflora incarnata* L.*
科名　Passifloraceae (トケイソウ科)
英名　passionflower / apricot vine / May pop / wild passionflower / May apple / purple passion flower
Part of use　fruit, root, leaf, flower
Note 1　—
Note 2　CHABOTOKEISÔ is included in TOKEISÔ. TOKEISÔ is also listed in the item of "Name" but the parts of use are different each other.
注　チャボトケイソウは別項のトケイソウに含まれるが、「部位等」の記載が異なっている。

名　称　**チョウトウコウ***

他名等　カギカズラ/コウトウ
部位等　葉
備　考　とげは「医」

他名(参考)　チョウトウコウ(釣藤鉤)、チョウトウ(釣藤)、トウカギカズラ(唐鉤葛)、カチョウトウ(華釣藤)
漢字表記・生薬名等　釣藤鉤(チョウトウコウ)、鉤葛(カギカズラ)、鉤藤(コウトウ)
Name(Romaji)　CHÔTÔKÔ*
Other name(s)(Romaji)　KAGIKAZURA/KÔTÔ
学名　*Uncaria rhynchophylla* (Miq.) Jacks.* (カギカズラ)
Uncaria sinensis (Oliv.) Havil.
科名　Rubiaceae (アカネ科)
英名　uncaria stem / uncaria ryunchophylla / gambir
Part of use　leaf
Note 1　thorn : drug category
Note 2　—
注　—

名　称　**チョウジ***

他名等　クローブ/チョウコウ/チョウジ油
部位等　花蕾・葉の精油
備　考　—

他名(参考)　—
漢字表記・生薬名等　丁子(チョウジ)、丁香(チョウコウ)、丁子油(チョウジユ)
Name(Romaji)　CHÔJI*
Other name(s)(Romaji)　KURÔBU/CHÔKÔ/CHÔJI-YU
学名　*Syzygium aromaticum* (L.) Merr. et L.M. Perry*
Eugenia aromatica (L.) Baill. nom. illeg.*
Eugenia caryophyllata Thunb.*

Caryophyllus aromaticus L.*
Eugenia caryophyllus (Spreng.) Bullock et S.G. Harrison
科名　Myrtaceae（フトモモ科）
英名　clove / clove tree
Part of use　flower bud, essential oil from leaf
Note 1　—
Note 2　CHÔJI is identical with KURÔBU, but their parts of use are different each other. CHÔJI is also listed in the item of "Name".
注　チョウジは別項のクローブと同一。但し、「部位等」の記載が異なる。

名　称　チョウセンアザミ*

他名等　アーティチョーク
部位等　茎・根・葉・頭花の総苞・花床
備　考　—

他名(参考)　—
漢字表記･生薬名等　朝鮮薊（チョウセンアザミ）
Name (Romaji)　CHÔSEN'AZAMI*
Other name (s) (Romaji)　ÂTICHÔKU
学名　*Cynara scolymus* L.*
科名　Compositae（キク科）
英名　artichoke / cynara / globe artichoke
Part of use　stem, root, leaf, involucre, receptacle
Note 1　—
Note 2　—
注　—

名　称　チョウマメ*

他名等　Clitoria ternatea
部位等　花
備　考　—

他名(参考)　パイプマメ
漢字表記･生薬名等　蝶豆（チョウマメ）
Name (Romaji)　CHÔMAME*
Other name (s) (Romaji)　—
学名　*Clitoria ternatea* L.*
科名　Leguminosae（マメ科）
英名　butterfly pea / Asian pigeon wings / kordofan pea
Part of use　flower
Note 1　—
Note 2　—
注　—

名　称　チンピ*

他名等　ウンシュウミカン
部位等　果皮
備　考　—

他名(参考)　マンダリン
漢字表記･生薬名等　陳皮（チンピ）、温州蜜柑（ウンシュウミカン）
Name (Romaji)　CHINPI*
Other name (s) (Romaji)　UNSHÛMIKAN
学名　*Citrus unshiu* Marcow.
Citrus reticulata Blanco *'Satsuma'* *
Citrus reticulata var. *unshiu* (Marcow.) Hu
科名　Rutaceae（ミカン科）
英名　chen pi / tangerine / red tangerin / mandarine / mandarine orange / Satsuma orange / Unshiu orange
Part of use　pericarp
Note 1　—
Note 2　—
注　—

名　称　ツウダツボク

他名等　カミヤツデ
部位等　樹皮
備　考　—

他名(参考)　—
漢字表記･生薬名等　通脱木（ツウダツボク）、通草（ツウソウ）、大通草（ダイツウソウ）、紙八手（カミヤツデ）
Name (Romaji)　TSÛDATSUBOKU
Other name (s) (Romaji)　KAMIYATSUDE
学名　*Tetrapanax papyriferum* (Hook.) K. Koch
Tetrapanax papyrifera (Hook.) K. Koch
Tetrapanax papyriferus (Hook.) K. Koch
Tetrapanax papyrifer (Hook.) K. Koch
Aralia papyrifera Hook.
Fatsia papyrifera Benth. et Hook. f.
科名　Araliaceae（ウコギ科）
英名　rice paper plant / Chinese rice paper plant
Part of use　bark
Note 1　—
Note 2　—
注　—

名　称　**ツキミソウ油**

他名等　ツキミソウ
部位等　種子の油
備　考　—

他名(参考)　ツキミグサ（月見草）
漢字表記･生薬名等　月見草油（ツキミソウユ）、月見草（ツキミソウ）
Name(Romaji)　TSUKIMISÔ-ABURA
Other name(s)(Romaji)　TSUKIMISÔ
学名　*Oenothera tetraptera* Cav.
科名　Onagraceae（アカバナ科）
英名　fourwing evening primrose
Part of use　seed oil
Note 1　—
Note 2　—
注　—

名　称　**ツチアケビ**

他名等　ドツウソウ
部位等　果実
備　考　—

他名(参考)　—
漢字表記･生薬名等　土木通・土通草（ツチアケビ）、土通草（ドツウソウ：乾燥果実）
Name(Romaji)　TSUCHIAKEBI
Other name(s)(Romaji)　DOTSÛSÔ
学名　*Galeola septentrionalis* Reichb. f.
科名　Orchidaceae（ラン科）
英名　—
Part of use　fruit
Note 1　—
Note 2　—
注　—

名　称　**ツノマタゴケ***

他名等　オークモス
部位等　樹枝状地衣
備　考　—

他名(参考)　—
漢字表記･生薬名等　角叉苔（ツノマタゴケ）
Name(Romaji)　TSUNOMATAGOKE*
Other name(s)(Romaji)　ÔKUMOSU
学名　*Evernia prunastri* (L.) Ach.*
科名　Usneaceae（サルオガセ科）
英名　ring lichen / oak moss / oakmoss
Part of use　branch like lichen
Note 1　—
Note 2　—
注　—

名　称　**ツバキ**

他名等　—
部位等　種子・葉・花
備　考　—

他名(参考)　ヤブツバキ（藪椿）、サンチャ（山茶）、サンチャカ（山茶花）、ベニサンチャ（紅山茶）
漢字表記･生薬名等　椿（ツバキ）
Name(Romaji)　TSUBAKI
Other name(s)(Romaji)　—
学名　*Camellia japonica* L.
Camellia japonica L. var. *hortensis* Makino
科名　Theaceae（ツバキ科）
英名　common camellia / rose camellia
Part of use　seed, leaf, flower
Note 1　—
Note 2　—
注　—

名　称　**ツボクサ***

他名等　ゴツコーラ／セキセツソウ／レンセンソウ
部位等　全草
備　考　—

他名(参考)　—
漢字表記･生薬名等　壺草・坪草（ツボクサ）、全草：連銭草（レンセンソウ）、積雪草（セキセツソウ）
Name(Romaji)　TSUBOKUSA*
Other name(s)(Romaji)　GOTSUKÔRA／SEKISETSUSÔ／RENSENSÔ
学名　*Centella asiatica* (L.) Urban*
Hydrocotyle asiatica L.*
科名　Umbelliferae（セリ科）
英名　gotu kola / Asiatic pennywort / Indian pennywort
Part of use　whole plant
Note 1　—
Note 2　—
注　—

名　称　**ツユクサ**

他名等　—
部位等　若芽
備　考　—

他名(参考)　アオバナ（青花）、ボウシバナ（帽子花）、オウセキソウ（鴨跖草）
漢字表記･生薬名等　露草（ツユクサ）
Name(Romaji)　TSUYUKUSA
Other name(s)(Romaji)　—
学名　*Commelina communis* L.
科名　Commelinaceae（ツユクサ科）
英名　day flower / Asiatic day flower
Part of use　sprout
Note 1　—
Note 2　—
注　—

名　称　**ツリガネダケ**

他名等　—
部位等　子実体
備　考　—

他名(参考)　—
漢字表記･生薬名等　釣鐘茸（ツリガネタケ）
Name(Romaji)　TSURIGANEDAKE
Other name(s)(Romaji)　—
学名　*Fomes fomentarius* (L.) J. Kickx f.
Agaricus fomentarius (L.) Lam.
Boletus fomentarius L.
Elfvingiella fomentaria (L.) Murrill
Placodes fomentarius (L.) Quél.
Ungulina fomentaria (L.) Pat.
科名　Polyporaceae（サルノコシカケ科）
英名　tinder fungus / hoof fungus / tinder conk / tinder polypore / true tinder polypore / ice man fungus
Part of use　fruit body
Note 1　—
Note 2　—
注　—

名　称　**ツルドクダミ***

他名等　—
部位等　茎・葉
備　考　塊根は「医」

他名(参考)　シュウ（首烏）、カシュウ（何首烏：乾燥した塊根）、ヤコウトウ（夜交藤）、シュウトウ（首烏藤）
漢字表記･生薬名等　蔓戢・蔓毒痛（ツルドクダミ）
Name(Romaji)　TSURUDOKUDAMI*
Other name(s)(Romaji)　—
学名　*Polygonum multiflorum* Thunb.*
Pleuropterus multiflorus (Thunb.) Turcz. ex Nakai
Pleuropterus cordatus Turcz.
Fallopia multiflora (Thunb.) Haraldson
科名　Polygonaceae（タデ科）
英名　fo-ti / fleeceflower
Part of use　stem, leaf
Note 1　tuberous root：drug category
Note 2　—
注　—

名　称　**ツルナ**

他名等　ハマジシャ／バンキョウ
部位等　全草
備　考　—

他名(参考)　ハマナ（浜菜）
漢字表記･生薬名等　蔓菜（ツルナ）、浜千舎（ハマジシャ）、浜千佐（ハマジシャ）、番杏（バンキョウ）
Name(Romaji)　TSURUNA
Other name(s)(Romaji)　HAMAJISHA／BANKYÔ
学名　*Tetragonia tetragonoides* (Pall.) O. Kuntze
Tetragonia expansa Thunb. ex J. Murr.
科名　Aizoaceae（ハマミズナ科（ツルナ科））
英名　Warrigal greens / New Zealand ice plant / New Zealand spinach
Part of use　whole plant
Note 1　—
Note 2　—
注　—

名　称　**ツルニンジン**

他名等　ジイソブ
部位等　全草
備　考　—

他名(参考)　ヨウニュウ（洋乳）
漢字表記･生薬名等　蔓人参（ツルニンジン）、党参（トウジン）、爺雀斑・爺蕎（ジイソブ）
Name(Romaji)　TSURUNINJIN
Other name(s)(Romaji)　JÎSOBU
学名　*Codonopsis lanceolata* (Sieb. et Zucc.) Trautv.
科名　Campanulaceae（キキョウ科）

英名　Asian bonnet bellflower / todok
Part of use　whole plant
Note 1　—
Note 2　—
注　—

名　称　**ツルマンネングサ***

他名等　**石指甲**
部位等　全草
備　考　—

他名(参考)　ホコウケイテン（圃行景天）、スイボンソウ（垂盆草）
漢字表記・生薬名等　蔓万年草（ツルマンネングサ）、石指甲（セキシコウ）
Name(Romaji)　TSURUMANNENGUSA*
Other name(s) (Romaji)　SEKISHIKÔ
学名　*Sedum sarmentosum* Bunge*
科名　Crassulaceae（ベンケイソウ科）
英名　sedum / stringy stone crop
Part of use　whole plant
Note 1　—
Note 2　—
注　—

名　称　**ツルムラサキ***

他名等　—
部位等　全草
備　考　—

他名(参考)　ラクキ（落葵）
漢字表記・生薬名等　蔓紫（ツルムラサキ）
Name(Romaji)　TSURUMURASAKI*
Other name(s) (Romaji)　—
学名　*Basella rubra* L.*
Basella alba L. *'Rubra'* *
科名　Basellaceae（ツルムラサキ科）
英名　Malabar spinach / Malabar nightshade / red vine spinach / Ceylon spinach / Indian spinach
Part of use　whole plant
Note 1　—
Note 2　—
注　—

名　称　**ティユール***

他名等　—
部位等　葉
備　考　—

他名(参考)　セイヨウシナノキ（西洋科の木）
漢字表記・生薬名等　西洋菩提樹（セイヨウボダイジュ）、西洋科の木（セイヨウシナノキ）
Name(Romaji)　TIYÛRU*
Other name(s) (Romaji)　—
学名　*Tilia*×*europaea* L.*
Tilia×*vulgaris* Hayne*
Tilia×*intermedia* DC.
科名　Tiliaceae（シナノキ科）
英名　tilia / common lime / European lime / common linden / linden / European linden
Part of use　leaf
Note 1　—
Note 2　TIYÛRU is identical with SEIYÔSHINANOKI, but parts of use are different each other. SEIYÔSHINANOKI is also listed in the item of "Name".
注　ティユールは別項のセイヨウシナノキと同一。但し、「部位等」の記載が異なっている。

名　称　**テガタチドリ**

他名等　**チドリソウ／シュショウジン**
部位等　根
備　考　—

他名(参考)　—
漢字表記・生薬名等　手形千鳥（テガタチドリ）、千鳥草（チドリソウ）、手掌参（シュショウジン）
Name(Romaji)　TEGATACHIDORI
Other name(s) (Romaji)　CHIDORISÔ／SHUSHÔJIN
学名　*Gymnadenia conopsea* (L.) R. Br.
科名　Orchidaceae（ラン科）
英名　fragrant orchid
Part of use　root
Note 1　—
Note 2　—
注　—

名　称　**デカルピス・ハミルトニー**

他名等　—
部位等　根茎
備　考　—

他名(参考)　—
漢字表記・生薬名等　—
Name (Romaji)　DEKARUPISU・HAMIRUTONÎ
Other name (s) (Romaji)　—
学名　*Decalepis hamiltonii* Wight et Arn.
科名　Ascepidaceae（ガガイモ科）
英名　swallowroot
Part of use　rhizome
Note 1　—
Note 2　—
注　—

名　称　**デビルズクロー***

他名等　—
部位等　全草
備　考　—

他名(参考)　—
漢字表記・生薬名等　—
Name (Romaji)　DEBIRUZUKURÔ*
Other name (s) (Romaji)　—
学名　*Harpagophytum procumbens* (Burch.) DC. ex Meisn.*
科名　Pedaliaceae（ゴマ科）
英名　grapple plant / devil's claw
Part of use　whole plant
Note 1　—
Note 2　—
注　—

名　称　**デュナリエラ***

他名等　**ドナリエラ／ドナリエラ油**
部位等　全藻・圧搾油
備　考　—

他名(参考)　シオヒゲムシ（*Dunaliella salina*）
漢字表記・生薬名等　—
Name (Romaji)　DYUNARIERA*
Other name (s) (Romaji)　DONARIERA／DONARI-ERA-YU
学名　*Dunaliella bardawil* Ben-Amotz et Avron
Dunaliella salina (Dunal) Teodor.*
科名　Dunaliellaceae（ドナリエラ科）
英名　dunaliella
Part of use　whole algae, squeezed oil
Note 1　—
Note 2　—
注　—

名　称　**テングサ***

他名等　**カンテン**
部位等　全草
備　考　—

他名(参考)　セッカサイ（石花菜）、トコロテン（心太）
漢字表記・生薬名等　天草（テングサ）、寒天（カンテン）
Name (Romaji)　TENGUSA*
Other name (s) (Romaji)　KANTEN
学名　seaweed (Gelidiaceae)
Gelidium amansii (J.V. Lamouroux) J.V. Lamouroux*（マクサ）
Gelidium subcostatum Okamura（ヒラクサ）
科名　Gelidiaceae（テングサ科）
英名　agar / Ameircan agar / agar-agar
Part of use　whole seaweed
Note 1　—
Note 2　—
注　—

名　称　**テンジクオウ***

他名等　**マダケ／青皮竹**
部位等　茎
備　考　—

他名(参考)　チクオウ（竹黄）、テンチクオウ（天竹黄）、ジクオウ（竺黄）、大節竹
漢字表記・生薬名等　天竺黄（テンジクオウ）、大節竹（*Indosasa crassiflora*）
Name (Romaji)　TENJIKUÔ*
Other name (s) (Romaji)　MADAKE／SEIHICHIKU
学名　*Bambusa textilis* McClure*（青皮竹）
Phyllostachys bambusoides Sieb. et Zucc.（真竹）
Indosasa crassiflora McClure（大節竹）
科名　Gramineae（イネ科）
英名　madake / giant timber bamboo / Japanese timber bamboo
Part of use　stem
Note 1　—
Note 2　—
注　—

名　称　テンチャ*

他名等　タスイカ／タスイセキカヨウ
部位等　葉
備　考　—

他名(参考)　テンヨウケンコウシ（甜葉懸鉤子）
漢字表記・生薬名等　甜茶（テンチャ）、多穂柯（タスイカ）、多穂石柯葉（タスイセキカヨウ）
Name (Romaji)　TENCHA*
Other name (s) (Romaji)　TASUIKA／TASUISEKIKAYÔ
学名　*Rubus suavissimus* S.K. Lee*（テンヨウケンコウシ）
Lithocarpus polystachyus（Wall. ex A. DC.）Rehder（タスイカ）
科名　*Rubus suavissimus*：Rosaceae（バラ科）
Lithocarpus polystachyus：Fagaceae（ブナ科）
英名　Chinese blackberry / sweet tea
Part of use　leaf
Note 1　—
Note 2　TENCHA is sweet herbal tea made of tree. Several kinds of trees can be the ingredient for TENCHA. TASUIKA is one of them, and GYÛHAKUTÔ (Rubiacae) or YAKUSHIMAAJISAI that is also called DOJÔZAN (Saxifragaceae) is also used for the tea. TEN'YÔKENKÔSHI (*Rubus sauvissimus*, Rosaceae) is especially attracting the attention in Japan. GYÛHAKUTÔ and YAKUSHIMAAJISAI are also listed in the items of “Name”.
注　テンチャは樹木から作られる甘い薬草茶で、数種のハーブが使用される。タスイカはその一つで、その他に別項のギュウハクトウ（アカネ科）、あるいはヤクシマアジサイ（＝ドジョウザン、ユキノシタ科）も用いられる。日本ではテンヨウケンコウシ（甜葉懸鉤子, *Rubus suavissimus*, バラ科）がテンチャとして注目されている。

名　称　テンモンドウ*

他名等　クサスギカズラ
部位等　種子・葉・花
備　考　根は「医」

他名(参考)　テンドウ（天冬）
漢字表記・生薬名等　天門冬（テンモンドウ）、草杉蔓（クサスギカズラ）
Name (Romaji)　TENMONDÔ*
Other name (s) (Romaji)　KUSASUGIKAZURA
学名　*Asparagus cochinchinensis* (Lour.) Merr.*
Asparagus lucidus Lindle.
科名　Liliaceae（ユリ科）
英名　Chinese asparagus
Part of use　seed, leaf, flower
Note 1　root：drug category
Note 2　—
注　—

名　称　トウガシ*

他名等　トウガニン／トウガン／ハクガ
部位等　果実
備　考　種子は「医」

他名(参考)　ハクカシ（白瓜子）、カモウリ（氈瓜）、チョウセンウリ（朝鮮瓜）
漢字表記・生薬名等　冬瓜子（トウガシ）、冬瓜仁（トウガニン）、冬瓜（トウガン）、白瓜（ハクカ）
Name (Romaji)　TÔGASHI*
Other name (s) (Romaji)　TÔGANIN／TÔGAN／HAKUGA
学名　*Benincasa hispida* (Thunb.) Cogn.*
Benincasa cerifera Savi*
Benincasa cerifera Savi. f. *emarginata* K. Kimura et Sugiyama
Cucurbita hispida Thunb.
科名　Cucurbitaceae（ウリ科）
英名　wax gourd / white gourd / white pumpkin / winter melon
Part of use　fruit
Note 1　seed：drug category
Note 2　—
注　—

名　称　トウガラシ*

他名等　—
部位等　果実・果皮
備　考　—

他名(参考)　—
漢字表記・生薬名等　唐辛子（トウガラシ）、蕃椒（バンショウ）、辣椒（ラッショウ）
Name (Romaji)　TÔGARASHI*
Other name (s) (Romaji)　—
学名　*Capsicum annuum* L.
Capsicum frutescens L.*
科名　Solanaceae（ナス科）
英名　capsicum / cayenne / cayenne pepper / chili pepper / paprika / red pepper / tabasco pepper
Part of use　fruit, peel
Note 1　—

タ行

Note 2　—
注　—

名　称　**トウキ***

他名等　**オニノダケ／カラトウキ**
部位等　葉
備　考　根は「医」

他名(参考)　ホッカイトウキ（北海当帰）
漢字表記･生薬名等　当帰（トウキ）、唐当帰（カラトウキ）
Name(Romaji)　TÔKI*
Other name(s) (Romaji)　ONINODAKE／KARATÔKI
学名　*Angelica acutiloba* (Sieb. et Zucc.) Kitag.（トウキ）
Ligusticum acutiloba Sieb. et Zucc.（トウキ）
Angelica acutiloba (Sieb. et Zucc.) Kitag. var. *sugiyamae* Hikino（ホッカイトウキ）
Angelica gigas Nakai（オニノダケ）
Angelica sinensis (Oliv.) Diels*（カラトウキ）
Angelica polymorpha Maxim. var. *sinensis* Oliv.*（カラトウキ）
科名　Umbelliferae（セリ科）
英名　dong quai / Chinese angelica / tang kuai
Part of use　leaf
Note 1　root：drug category
Note 2　—
注　—

名　称　**トウキシ***

他名等　**フユアオイ**
部位等　種子・葉
備　考　—

他名(参考)　キシ（葵子）、ケイジツ（苘実）、ケイマ（苘麻）、イチビ（苘麻）、ボウマ（苘麻）、キリアサ（桐麻）、カンアオイ（寒葵）
漢字表記･生薬名等　冬葵子（トウキシ）、冬葵（フユアオイ）
Name(Romaji)　TÔKISHI*
Other name(s) (Romaji)　FUYUAOI
学名　*Malva verticillata* L.*
Abutilon theophrasti Medik.
Abutilon avicennae Gaertn.
科名　Malvaceae（アオイ科）
英名　China jute / mallow / butter print / curled mallow / Chinese jute / Indian mallow / pie maker / velvet leaf / button weed
Part of use　seed, leaf
Note 1　—
Note 2　Nowadays it is said that all of TÔKISHI sold in China is KEIMASHI, seed of ICHIBI. ICHIBI is also listed in the item of "Name".
注　今日の中国でトウキシ（冬葵子）として売られているのは、すべてケイマシ（イチビの種子）であるという。イチビは別項に記載されている。

名　称　**トウキンセンカ***

他名等　**キンセンカ／マリーゴールド**
部位等　花
備　考　—

他名(参考)　キンセンキク（金盞菊）
漢字表記･生薬名等　唐金盞花（トウキンセンカ）、金盞花（キンセンカ）
Name(Romaji)　TÔKINSENKA*
Other name(s) (Romaji)　KINSENKA／MARÎGÔRUDO
学名　*Calendula officinalis* L.*
科名　Compositae（キク科）
英名　calendula / marigold / pot marigold / common marigold
Part of use　flower
Note 1　—
Note 2　—
注　—

名　称　**トウチャ**

他名等　**茶葡萄／藤茶／Ampelopsis grossedentata／Ampelopsis cantoniensis var. grossedentata**
部位等　茎・葉
備　考　—

他名(参考)　ウドカズラ（独活葛）
漢字表記･生薬名等　藤茶（トウチャ）
Name(Romaji)　TÔCHA
Other name(s) (Romaji)　CHABUDÔ／TÔCHA
学名　*Ampelopsis grossedentata* (Hand.-Mazz.) W.T. Wang
Ampelopsis cantoniensis var. *grossedentata* (Hook. et Aln.) Planch.（ウドカズラ）
Ampelopsis leeoides (Maxim.) Planch.（ウドカズラ）
科名　Vitaceae（ブドウ科）
英名　tocha
Part of use　stem, leaf
Note 1　—
Note 2　—
注　—

名　称　**トウチュウカソウ***

他名等　ホクチュウソウ
部位等　全草
備　考　—

他名(参考)　フユムシナツクサタケ（冬虫夏草菌）、チュウソウ（虫草）
漢字表記・生薬名等　冬虫夏草（トウチュウカソウ）
Name(Romaji)　TÔCHÛKASÔ*
Other name(s)(Romaji)　HOKUCHÛSÔ
学名　*Cordyceps sinensis* (Berk.) Sacc.*
科名　Clavicipitaceae（バッカクキン科）
英名　cordyceps / Chinese caterpillar fungus
Part of use　whole plant
Note 1　—
Note 2　—
注　—

名　称　**トウホクオウギ***

他名等　—
部位等　花
備　考　—

他名(参考)　タイツリオウギ（鯛釣黄耆）、マクキョウオウギ（膜莢黄芪：バクキョウコウキ）
漢字表記・生薬名等　東北黄耆（トウホクオウギ）、黄花黄耆（キバナオウギ）
Name(Romaji)　TÔHOKUÔGI*
Other name(s)(Romaji)　—
学名　*Astragalus membranaceus* (Fisch.) Bunge*
科名　Leguminosae（マメ科）
英名　membranaceus milk-vetch
Part of use　flower
Note 1　—
Note 2　TÔHOKUÔGI is identical with ÔGI, but their parts of use are different each other. ÔGI is also listed in the item of "Name".
注　トウホクオウギは別項のオウギと同一。但し、「部位等」の記載が異なっている。

名　称　**トウモロコシ***

他名等　トウキビ／トウモロコシ油／ナンバンキビ／Zea mays
部位等　種子油・澱粉・花柱・柱頭
備　考　—

他名(参考)　トウムギ（唐麦）
漢字表記・生薬名等　玉蜀黍（トウモロコシ）、唐黍（トウキビ）、南蛮黍（ナンバンキビ）、南蠻毛（ナンバンモウ、ナンバンゲ）
Name(Romaji)　TÔMOROKOSHI*
Other name(s)(Romaji)　TÔKIBI／TÔMOROKOSHI-YU／NANBANKIBI
学名　*Zea mays* L.*
科名　Gramineae（イネ科）
英名　field corn / makai / sweet corn / corn / cornsilk / maize / guinea wheat / Indian corn mealies / Turkey wheat
Part of use　seed oil, starch, style, stigma
Note 1　—
Note 2　—
注　—

名　称　**ドオウレン**

他名等　クサノオウ／ハックツサイ
部位等　全草
備　考　—

他名(参考)　イボクサ（疣草）、タムシグサ（タムシ草）、ヒゼングサ（皮癬草）
漢字表記・生薬名等　土黄連（ドオウレン）、草の黄・瘡の王・草王（クサノオウ）、白屈菜（ハックツサイ）
Name(Romaji)　DOÔREN
Other name(s)(Romaji)　KUSANOÔ／HAKKUTSUSAI
学名　*Chelidonium majus* L. var. *asiaticum* (Hara) Ohwi
科名　Papaveraceae（ケシ科）
英名　celandine / greater celandine
Part of use　whole plant
Note 1　—
Note 2　—
注　—

名　称　**トーメンティル***

他名等　タチキジムシロ／チシエンコン
部位等　根茎
備　考　—

他名(参考)　—
漢字表記・生薬名等　立雉莚・立雉蓆（タチキジムシロ）
Name(Romaji)　TÔMENTIRU*
Other name(s)(Romaji)　TACHIKIJIMUSHIRO／CHISHIENKON
学名　*Potentilla tormentilla* Stokes*
Potentilla erecta (L.) Raeusch.*
科名　Rosaceae（バラ科）

タ行

英名　tormentil / common tormentil / cinquefoil / erect cinquefoil / ewe daisy / bloodroot / redroot / tormentilla
Part of use　rhizome
Note 1　—
Note 2　CHISIENKON listed in the item of "Other names" cannot be confirmed.
注　「他名等」のチシエンコンは確認できない。

名　称　**トキンソウ**

他名等　ガフショクソウ
部位等　全草
備　考　—

他名(参考)　タネヒリグサ、ハナヒリグサ
漢字表記・生薬名等　吐金草（トキンソウ）、鵝不食草・鵞不食草（ガフショクソウ）
Name (Romaji)　TOKINSÔ
Other name (s) (Romaji)　GAFUSHOKUSÔ
学名　*Centipeda minima* (L.) A. Br. et Aschers.
Centipeda orbicularis Lour.
科名　Compositae（キク科）
英名　Spreading sneeze weed
Part of use　whole plant
Note 1　—
Note 2　—
注　—

名　称　**トケイソウ***

他名等　パッションフラワー
部位等　果実・茎・葉・花
備　考　—

他名(参考)　—
漢字表記・生薬名等　時計草（トケイソウ）
Name (Romaji)　TOKEISÔ*
Other name (s) (Romaji)　PASSHONFURAWÂ
学名　*Passiflora caerulea* L.*（トケイソウ）
Passiflora edulis Sims*（パッションフルーツ）
Passiflora incarnata L.*（チャボトケイソウ）
Passiflora trifasciata Lem.（ムラサキフイリバトケイソウ）
科名　Passifloraceae（トケイソウ科）
英名　*P. caerulea*：blue passionflower / blue crown passionflower
P. edulis：purple granadilla / purple passionflower / passion fruit
P. incarnata：May pop / May apple / apricot vine / wild passionflower
Part of use　fruit, stem, leaf, flower
Note 1　—
Note 2　CHABOTOKEISÔ is one of the species of TOKEISÔ, but their parts of use are different each other. CHABOTOKEISÔ is also listed in the item of "Name".
注　別項のチャボトケイソウはトケイソウの一種であるが、「部位等」の記載が異なっている。

名　称　**トショウ**

他名等　トショウジツ／ネズ
部位等　全草
備　考　—

他名(参考)　ネズミサシ（鼠刺）、トショウシ（杜松子）、ムロ・ムロノキ（回香樹、天木香樹、榁、榁樫、室乃樹）
漢字表記・生薬名等　杜松（トショウ、ネズ）、杜松実（トショウジツ）
Name (Romaji)　TOSHÔ
Other name (s) (Romaji)　TOSHÔJITSU／NEZU
学名　*Juniperus rigida* Sieb. et Zucc.
科名　Cupressaceae（ヒノキ科）
英名　needle juniper
Part of use　whole plant
Note 1　—
Note 2　—
注　—

名　称　**トチノキ**

他名等　—
部位等　種子・樹皮
備　考　セイヨウトチノキの種子は「医」

他名(参考)　—
漢字表記・生薬名等　栃・橡（トチノキ）
Name (Romaji)　TOCHINOKI
Other name (s) (Romaji)　—
学名　*Aesculus turbinata* Bl.
科名　Hippocastanaceae（トチノキ科）
英名　buckeye / Japanese horse chestnut
Part of use　bark, seed
Note 1　seed of *Aesculus hippocastanum* L.：drug category
Note 2　—
注　—

名　称　**トチュウ***

他名等　—
部位等　果実・葉・葉柄・木部
備　考　樹皮は「医」

他名(参考)　—
漢字表記・生薬名等　杜仲（トチュウ）
Name(Romaji)　TOCHŪ*
Other name(s) (Romaji)　—
学名　*Eucommia ulmoides* Oliv.*
科名　Eucommiaceae（トチュウ科）
英名　eucommia / Chinese gutta percha / Chinese rubber tree / hardy rubber tree
Part of use　fruit, leaf, petiole, xylem
Note 1　bark : drug category
Note 2　—
注　—

名　称　**トックリイチゴ**

他名等　**Rubus coreanus**
部位等　完熟偽果
備　考　—

他名(参考)　覆盆子（フクボンシ）
漢字表記・生薬名等　徳利苺（トックリイチゴ）
Name(Romaji)　TOKKURIICHIGO
Other name(s) (Romaji)　—
学名　*Rubus coreanus* Miq.
Rubus tokkura Sieb.
科名　Rosaceae（バラ科）
英名　Korean bramble / Korean black raspberry
Part of use　riped pseudocarp
Note 1　—
Note 2　—
注　—

名　称　**ドッグローズ***

他名等　—
部位等　果実・葉・花
備　考　—

他名(参考)　カニナバラ
漢字表記・生薬名等　実：ローズヒップ（rose hip）
Name(Romaji)　DOGGURÔZU*
Other name(s) (Romaji)　—
学名　*Rosa canina* L.*
科名　Rosaceae（バラ科）
英名　dog rose / dog brier / brier rose / brier bush
Part of use　fruit, leaf, flower
Note 1　—
Note 2　The scientific name of DOGGURÔZU is the same with RÔZUHIPPU. RÔZUHIPPU is also listed in the item of "Name" and it the fruit of rose, but the fruit and pseudocarp of *Rosa multiflora* are classified in the "drug" category.
注　ドッグローズの学名は別項のローズヒップと同一。ローズヒップはバラの果実。但し、ノイバラの偽果・果実は「医」に分類されている。

名　称　**トマト***

他名等　—
部位等　果実
備　考　—

他名(参考)　トウシ（唐柿）、バンカ（蕃茄）、アカナス（赤伽子）、コガネウリ（小金瓜）
漢字表記・生薬名等　—
Name(Romaji)　TOMATO*
Other name(s) (Romaji)　—
学名　*Lycopersicon esculentum* Mill.*
Lycopersicon lycopersicum (L.) H. Karst., nom. rej.*
Solanum lycopersicum L.*
科名　Solanaceae（ナス科）
英名　tomato / gold apple / love apple
Part of use　fruit
Note 1　—
Note 2　—
注　—

名　称　**トラガント***

他名等　**Astragalus gummifer又はその同属植物(Leguminosae)の幹から得た分泌物**
部位等　樹脂
備　考　—

他名(参考)　—
漢字表記・生薬名等　—
Name(Romaji)　TORAGANTO*
Other name(s) (Romaji)　—
学名　*Astragalus gummifer* Labill.*
科名　Leguminosae（マメ科）
英名　gum tragacanth (The standardized common name of the dried, gummy exudate of the stems of *A. gummifer*.) / tragacanth milkvetch / goat thorn

bush
Part of use　resin
Note 1　—
Note 2　—
注　—

名　称　**トロロアオイ**

他名等　Abelmoschus manihot
部位等　花
備　考　—

他名(参考)　クサダモ、トロロ
漢字表記・生薬名等　黄蜀葵（トロロアオイ、オウショッキ）
Name(Romaji)　TOROROAOI
Other name(s) (Romaji)　—
学名　*Abelmoschus manihot* (L.) Medik.
Hibiscus manihot L.
Hibiscus japonicus Miq.
科名　Malvaceae（アオイ科）
英名　sunset hibiscus / sunset muskmallow / manioc hibiscus / aibika
Part of use　flower
Note 1　—
Note 2　—
注　—

ナ行

名　称　**ナガエカサ**

他名等　トンカット・アリ
部位等　根
備　考　—

他名(参考)　—
漢字表記・生薬名等　—
Name(Romaji)　NAGAEKASA
Other name(s) (Romaji)　TONKATTO・ARI
学名　*Eurycoma longifolia* Jack
科名　Simaroubaceae（ニガキ科）
英名　tongkat Ali / Malaysian ginseng / Ali's walking stick / eurycoma / long Jack / longjack / Ali's umbrella
Part of use　root
Note 1　—
Note 2　—
注　—

名　称　**ナギイカダ***

他名等　—
部位等　根
備　考　—

他名(参考)　—
漢字表記・生薬名等　仮葉樹（ナギイカダ）
Name(Romaji)　NAGIIKADA*
Other name(s) (Romaji)　—
学名　*Ruscus aculeatus* L.*
科名　Liliaceae（ユリ科）
英名　butcher's broom / box holly / Jew's myrtle
Part of use　root
Note 1　—
Note 2　—
注　—

名　称　**ナズナ***

他名等　ペンペングサ
部位等　全草
備　考　—

他名(参考)　シャミセングサ（三味線草）
漢字表記・生薬名等　薺・撫菜（ナズナ）、薺菜（セイサイ）
Name(Romaji)　NAZUNA*
Other name(s) (Romaji)　PENPENGUSA
学名　*Capsella bursa-pastoris* (L.) Medik.*
科名　Cruciferae（アブラナ科）
英名　shepherd's purse / capsell / mother's heart
Part of use　whole plant
Note 1　—
Note 2　—
注　—

名　称　**ナタネ油***

他名等　ナタネ
部位等　種子油
備　考　—

他名(参考)　ナノハナ（菜の花）、アブラナ（油菜）
漢字表記・生薬名等　菜種油（ナタネアブラ）、菜種（ナタネ）
Name(Romaji)　NATANE-ABURA*
Other name(s) (Romaji)　NATANE
学名　*Brassica campestris* L. ssp. *napus* (L.) Hook. f. et Anders. var. *nippo-oleifera* Makino
Brassica campestris L.*

Brassica napus L.
Brassica rapa L. var. *rapa**
科名 Cruciferae（アブラナ科）
英名 rape oil / turnip / rape seed / Chinese colza / field mustard
Part of use seed oil
Note 1 —
Note 2 —
注 —

名 称 **ナツシロギク***
他名等 フィーバーフュー
部位等 全草
備 考 —

他名(参考) —
漢字表記・生薬名等 夏白菊（ナツシロギク）
Name(Romaji) NATSUSHIROGIKU*
Other name(s) (Romaji) FÎBÂFYÛ
学名 *Tanacetum parthenium* (L.) Sch. Bip.*
Chrysanthemum parthenium (L.) Bernh.*
Pyrethrum parthenium Sm.
Matricaria parthenium L.
科名 Compositae（キク科）
英名 feverfew / wild chamomile
Part of use whole plant
Note 1 —
Note 2 —
注 —

名 称 **ナットウ***
他名等 ナットウ菌
部位等 納豆菌の発酵ろ液
備 考 —

他名(参考) ズシ（豆鼓）、クキ（鼓）、タントウシ（淡豆鼓）、コウシ（香鼓）、タンシ（淡鼓）、ダイズシ（大豆鼓）
漢字表記・生薬名等 納豆（ナットウ）、納豆菌（ナットウキン）
Name(Romaji) NATTÔ*
Other name(s) (Romaji) NATTÔ-KIN
学名 *Bacillus subtilis* var. *natto*
Glycine max (L.) Merr.* (fermented with *Bacillus natto*)
Phaseolus max L.
Soya max (L.) Piper
Dolichos soya L.
Glycine gracilis Skvortsov (fermented with *Bacillus natto*)（マンシュウダイズ）
科名 Bacillaceae（バシルス科）
Leguminosae（マメ科）
英名 natto
Part of use fermented soybean with *Bacillus subtilis* var. *natto*
Note 1 —
Note 2 —
注 —

名 称 **ナツミカン**
他名等 キジツ／キコク／トウヒ／Citrus natsudaidai
部位等 果実・果皮・蕾
備 考 —

他名(参考) ナツカン（夏柑）、ナツダイダイ（夏橙）、ナツガワ（夏皮）
漢字表記・生薬名等 夏蜜柑（ナツミカン）、枳実（キジツ）、枳殻（キコク）、橙皮（トウヒ）
Name(Romaji) NATSUMIKAN
Other name(s) (Romaji) KIJITSU／KIKOKU／TÔHI
学名 *Citrus natsudaidai* Hayata
科名 Rutaceae（ミカン科）
英名 natsumikan / natsudaidai / Watson pomelo / Japanese summer orange
Part of use fruit, pericarp, bud
Note 1 —
Note 2 —
注 —

名 称 **ナツメヤシ***
他名等 —
部位等 果実・葉
備 考 —

他名(参考) センショウボク（戦捷木）、ムロウシ（無漏子）
漢字表記・生薬名等 棗椰子（ナツメヤシ）
Name(Romaji) NATSUMEYASHI*
Other name(s) (Romaji) —
学名 *Phoenix dactylifera* L.*
科名 Palmae（ヤシ科）
英名 date / date palm / date tree / common date palm / edible date
Part of use fruit, leaf
Note 1 —
Note 2 —
注 —

名　称　**ナナカマド**

他名等　—
部位等　種子・樹皮
備　考　—

他名(参考)　オオナナカマド（大七竈）、エゾナナカマド（蝦夷七竈）
漢字表記・生薬名等　七竈（ナナカマド）
Name (Romaji)　NANAKAMADO
Other name (s) (Romaji)　—
学名　*Sorbus commixta* Hedl.
Sorbus commixta Hedl. var. *sachalinensis* Koidz.
科名　Rosaceae（バラ科）
英名　Japanese mountain ash / Japanese rowan
Part of use　seed, bark
Note 1　—
Note 2　—
注　—

名　称　**ナベナ***

他名等　**センゾクダン／ゾクダン／Dipsacus japonica／Dipsacus asperoides／Dipsacus asper**
部位等　根
備　考　—

他名(参考)　トウナベナ（川続断）
漢字表記・生薬名等　鍋菜（ナベナ）、続断（ゾクダン、ナベナ）、川続断（センゾクダン、トウナベナ）
Name (Romaji)　NABENA*
Other name (s) (Romaji)　SENZOKUDAN／ZOKUDAN
学名　*Dipsacus japonicus* Miq.*（ナベナ）
Dipsacus asperoides C.Y. Cheng et T.M. Ai（トウナベナ）
Dipsacus asper Wall.*（トウナベナ）
Dipsacus asper auct.*（トウナベナ）
科名　Dipsacaceae（マツムシソウ科）
英名　Sichuan teasel（トウナベナ） / Sichuan dipsacus（トウナベナ） / Japanese teasel（ナベナ） / Japanese dipsacus（ナベナ）
Part of use　root
Note 1　—
Note 2　*Dipsacus japonica* written in the item of "Other names" should be replaced by *Dipsacus japonicus*.
注　「他名等」の*Dipsacus japonica*は*Dipsacus japonicus*である。

名　称　**ナンキョウ***

他名等　**コウズク**
部位等　果実・根
備　考　—

他名(参考)　ダイリョウキョウ（大良姜）、ナンキョウソウ
漢字表記・生薬名等　紅豆蔻（コウズク）
Name (Romaji)　NANKYÔ*
Other name (s) (Romaji)　KÔZUKU
学名　*Alpinia galanga* (L.) Sw.*
Maranta galanga L.*
Languas galanga (L.) Stuntz
科名　Zingiberaceae（ショウガ科）
英名　greater galangal / galanga / Java galanga / Siamese galanga
Part of use　fruit, root
Note 1　—
Note 2　—
注　—

名　称　**ナンサンソウ**

他名等　**ゴガンカジュヒ／チャンチンモドキ**
部位等　果核・果実・樹皮
備　考　—

他名(参考)　カナメノキ（要木）
漢字表記・生薬名等　南酸棗（ナンサンソウ）、五眼果樹皮（ゴガンカジュヒ）、香椿擬（チャンチンモドキ）
Name (Romaji)　NANSANSÔ
Other name (s) (Romaji)　GOGANKAJUHI／CHANCHINMODOKI
学名　*Choerospondias axillaris* (Roxb.) B.L. Burtt et A.W. Hill
Choerospondias axillaris (Roxb.) B.L. Burtt et A.W. Hill var. *japonica* (Ohwi) Ohwi
科名　Anacardiaceae（ウルシ科）
英名　xuyencoc / Nepari hog plum
Part of use　fruit nucleus, fruit, bark
Note 1　—
Note 2　—
注　—

名　称　**ナンショウヤマイモ**

他名等　—
部位等　根茎
備　考　—

他名(参考)　不明
漢字表記・生薬名等　不明
Name(Romaji)　NANSHÔYAMAIMO
Other name(s) (Romaji)　—
学名　不明
科名　Dioscoreaceae (?) (ヤマノイモ科 (?))
英名　不明
Part of use　rhizome
Note 1　—
Note 2　NANSHÔYAMAIMO cannot be confirmed.
注　ナンショウヤマイモは確認できない。

名　称　**ナンヨウアブラギリ***

他名等　**タイワンアブラギリ**
部位等　葉
備　考　—

他名(参考)　ジャトロファ、ヤトロファ、マフウジュ（麻瘋樹）、モッカセイ（木花生）
漢字表記・生薬名等　南洋油桐（ナンヨウアブラギリ）、台湾油桐（タイワンアブラギリ）
Name(Romaji)　NAN'YÔABURAGIRI*
Other name(s) (Romaji)　TAIWAN'ABURAGIRI
学名　*Jatropha curcas* L.*
科名　Euphorbiaceae (トウダイグサ科)
英名　physic nut / Barbados nut / purging nut / pignon d'inde / kuikui pake
Part of use　leaf
Note 1　—
Note 2　—
注　—

名　称　**ニオイスミレ***

他名等　—
部位等　全草
備　考　—

他名(参考)　バイオレット
漢字表記・生薬名等　匂菫（ニオイスミレ）
Name(Romaji)　NIOISUMIRE*
Other name(s) (Romaji)　—
学名　*Viola odorata* L.*
科名　Violaceae (スミレ科)
英名　sweet violet / English violet / garden violet / sweet blue violet / florist's violet
Part of use　whole plant
Note 1　—
Note 2　NIOISUMIRE is one of the species of SUMIRE, but the parts of use are different each other. SUMIRE is also listed in the item of "Name".
注　ニオイスミレは別項のスミレに含まれる。

名　称　**ニガウリ***

他名等　**ツルレイシ／Momordica charantia**
部位等　果実・根・葉
備　考　—

他名(参考)　バンシュウレイシ（晩秋茘枝）、ゴーヤー、ゴーヤ、ゴーラ、ニガゴリ、ニガゴイ、ニガウイ、トーグリ
漢字表記・生薬名等　苦瓜（ニガウリ）、蔓茘枝（ツルレイシ）、苦瓜子（クカシ）
Name(Romaji)　NIGAURI*
Other name(s) (Romaji)　TSURUREISHI
学名　*Momordica charantia* L.*
Momordica charantia L. var. *pavel* Crantz.
科名　Cucurbitaceae (ウリ科)
英名　bitter cucumber / bitter melon / African cucamber / balsam pear / bitter gourd / la-kwa
Part of use　fruit, root, leaf
Note 1　—
Note 2　—
注　—

名　称　**ニクジュヨウ***

他名等　**オニク／キムラタケ／ホンオニク／Cistanche salsa／Boschniakia rossica (=Boschniakia glabra)**
部位等　肉質茎
備　考　—

他名(参考)　タイゲイ（大芸）、タイウン（大雲）
漢字表記・生薬名等　肉蓯蓉（ニクジュヨウ）、御肉（オニク）、塩生肉蓯蓉（ホンオニク）、金精茸（キムラタケ、キンマラタケ）
Name(Romaji)　NIKUJUYÔ*
Other name(s) (Romaji)　ONIKU／KIMURATAKE／HON'ONIKU
学名　*Cistanche salsa* (C.A. Mey.) G. Beck* (ホンオニク)
Boschniakia rossica (Cham. et Schltdl.) B. Fedtsch.*

（オニク、キムラタケ）
Boschniakia glabra C.A. Mey. ex Bong.（オニク、キムラタケ）
科名 Orobanchaceae（ハマウツボ科）
英名 poque（オニク）/ broomrape（ホンオニク）
Part of use succulent stem
Note 1 —
Note 2 *Boschniakia rossica* written in the item of "Other names" is ONIKU（=KIMURATAKE）. ONIKU is used as a substitute for NIKUJUYÔ and it is called as WANIKUJUYÔ.
注 「他名等」の*Boschniakia rossica*はオニク（=キムラタケ）である。ニクジュヨウの代用品として使用され、ワニクジュヨウと呼ばれる。

名　称 **ニクズク***

他名等 ナツメグ
部位等 種子
備　考 —

他名(参考) —
漢字表記・生薬名等 種子：肉豆蔲（ニクズク；nutmeg）、仮種皮：肉豆蔲花（ニクズクカ；mace）
Name(Romaji) NIKUZUKU*
Other name(s)(Romaji) NATSUMEGU
学名 *Myristica fragrans* Houtt.*
Myristica moschata Thunb.*
Myristica officinalis L. f.*
Myristica aromatica Lam.
科名 Myristicaceae（ニクズク科）
英名 noix muscade / nuez moscada / nutmeg / mace / common nutmeg / banda nutmeg
Part of use seed
Note 1 —
Note 2 —
注 —

名　称 **ニシキギ**

他名等 —
部位等 全草
備　考 —

他名(参考) エイボウ（衛矛）、キセン（鬼箭）、キセンウ（鬼箭羽）、ヤハズニシキギ（矢筈錦木）、アオハダニシキギ（青肌錦木、青膚錦木）、オオバニシキギ（大葉錦木）
漢字表記・生薬名等 錦木（ニシキギ）
Name(Romaji) NISHIKIGI
Other name(s)(Romaji) —
学名 *Euonymus alatus*（Thunb.）Sieb. f. *alatus*
Euonymus alatus（Thunb.）Sieb.
科名 Celastraceae（ニシキギ科）
英名 winged spindle tree
Part of use whole plant
Note 1 —
Note 2 —
注 —

名　称 **ニトベギク**

他名等 —
部位等 全草
備　考 —

他名(参考) —
漢字表記・生薬名等 腫柄菊（ニトベギク）、新渡戸菊（ニトベギク）
Name(Romaji) NITOBEGIKU
Other name(s)(Romaji) —
学名 *Tithonia diversifolia*（Hemsl.）A. Gray
科名 Compositae（キク科）
英名 tree marigold / Mexican sunflower
Part of use whole plant
Note 1 —
Note 2 —
注 —

名　称 **乳酸菌**

他名等 Lactobacillus属／Streptococcus属
部位等 菌体
備　考 —

他名(参考) —
漢字表記・生薬名等 —
Name(Romaji) NYÛSAN-KIN
Other name(s)(Romaji) —
学名 *Lactobacillus* Beijerinck（Biosafety level 1に限る）
Streptococcus Rosenback（Biosafety level 1に限る）
科名 Lactobacillaceae（ラクトバシルス科）
英名 acidophilus / lactic acid bacilli / lactic acid bacteria / lactic acid bacterium / lactic bacteria / lactobacillus / leuconostoc
Part of use fungus body
Note 1 —
Note 2 ASHIDOFIRUSU-KIN is icluded in NYÛSAN-KIN. ASHIDOFIRUSU-KIN is also listed in the item of "Name".

注　別項のアシドフィルス菌は乳酸菌に含まれる。

名　称　**ニョテイ***

他名等　ジョテイシ／タマツバキ／トウネズミモチ／ネズミモチ／Ligustrum japonicum／Ligustrum lucidum
部位等　葉・種子・果実
備　考　—

他名（参考）　—
漢字表記・生薬名等　Ligustrum lucidumの干した果実：女貞（ニョテイ、ジョテイ）・女貞子（ニョテイシ、ジョテイシ）
鼠黐（ネズミモチ）、唐鼠黐（トウネズミモチ）、玉椿（タマツバキ）
Name (Romaji)　NYOTEI*
Other name(s) (Romaji)　JOTEISHI／TAMATSUBAKI／TÔNEZUMIMOCHI／NEZUMIMOCHI
学名　*Ligustrum lucidum* W.T. Aiton*（ニョテイ、ジョテイ、トウネズミモチ）
Ligustrum japonicum Thunb.*（タマツバキ、ネズミモチ）
科名　Oleaceae（モクセイ科）
英名　*Ligustrum lucidum*：Chinese privet / glossy privet
Ligustrum japonicum：Japanese privet
Part of use　leaf, seed, fruit
Note 1　—
Note 2　—
注　—

名　称　**ニラ***

他名等　キュウサイシ／コミラ／リーキ
部位等　種子
備　考　—

他名（参考）　フタモジ（二文字）、ミラ（弥良）
漢字表記・生薬名等　韮・韭（ニラ）、韮菜子（キュウサイシ）、韮子（キュウシ）、古美良（コミラ）
Name (Romaji)　NIRA*
Other name(s) (Romaji)　KYÛSAISHI／KOMIRA／RÎKI
学名　*Allium tuberosum* Rottl. ex Spreng.*
科名　Liliaceae（ユリ科）
英名　Chinese chive / garlic chive / oriental garlic
Part of use　seed
Note 1　—
Note 2　—
注　—

名　称　**ニレ**

他名等　—
部位等　根皮
備　考　—

他名（参考）　ハルニレ（春楡）、アキニレ（秋楡）、クロニレ（黒楡）
漢字表記・生薬名等　楡（ニレ）
Name (Romaji)　NIRE
Other name(s) (Romaji)　—
学名　*Ulmus davidiana* Planch. var. *japonica* (Rehd.) Nakai（ニレ、ハルニレ）
Ulmus japonica (Rehd.) Sarg.（ニレ、ハルニレ）
Ulmus parvifolia Jacq.（アキニレ）
科名　Ulmaceae（ニレ科）
英名　elm / Japanese elm（ハルニレ）/ Chinese elm（アキニレ）
Part of use　root bark
Note 1　—
Note 2　—
注　—

名　称　**ニンジン***

他名等　ニンジン油
部位等　根・根の圧搾油
備　考　—

他名（参考）　セリニンジン（芹人参）、ナニンジン（菜人参）、ハタニンジン（畑人参）
漢字表記・生薬名等　人参（ニンジン）、人参油（ニンジンユ）
Name (Romaji)　NINJIN*
Other name(s) (Romaji)　NINJIN-YU
学名　*Daucus carota* L. ssp. *sativus* (Hoffm.) Arcang.*
科名　Umbelliferae（セリ科）
英名　carrot / carrot oil
Part of use　root, compressed root oil
Note 1　—
Note 2　—
注　—

名　称　**ニンジンボク**

他名等　タイワンニンジンボク
部位等　全草
備　考　—

他名（参考）　—

ナ行

漢字表記・生薬名等　人参木（ニンジンボク）、台湾人参木（タイワンニンジンボク）
ニンジンボク：牡荊（ボケイ）、牡荊子（ボケイシ）
タイワンニンジンボク：荘荊（ソウケイ）、荊条（ケイジョウ）
Name (Romaji)　NINJINBOKU
Other name (s) (Romaji)　TAIWANNINJINBOKU
学名　*Vitex negundo* L. var. *cannabifolia* (Sieb. et Zucc.) Hand.-Mazz.（ニンジンボク）
Vitex cannabifolia Sieb. et Zucc.（ニンジンボク）
Vitex negundo L. var. *negundo*（タイワンニンジンボク）
科名　Verbenaceae（クマツヅラ科）
英名　Chinese chaste tree / Indian privet / five leaved chaste tree / horse shoe vitex / huan jing（黄荊）
Part of use　whole plant
Note 1　—
Note 2　—
注　—

名　称　**ニンニク***

他名等　オオニンニク／ダイサン
部位等　鱗茎
備　考　—

他名（参考）　コサン（胡蒜）、コ（葫）、タイサン（大蒜）、オオビル（大蒜）
漢字表記・生薬名等　葫・忍辱（ニンニク）、大蒜（オオニンニク、ダイサン）
Name (Romaji)　NINNIKU*
Other name (s) (Romaji)　ÔNINNIKU／DAISAN
学名　*Allium sativum* L.*
Allium sativum L. f. *pekinense* Makino
Allium sativum L. var. *japonicum* Kitam.
Allium sativum L. var. *pekinense* (Prokh.) F. Maek.
科名　Liliaceae（ユリ科）
英名　garlic
Part of use　bulb
Note 1　—
Note 2　—
注　—

名　称　**ヌルデ***

他名等　ゴバイシ／Rhus javanica
部位等　嚢状虫癭
備　考　—

他名（参考）　フシノキ（附子木）、キブシ（木附子）、フシ（付子）、ブシ（附子）
漢字表記・生薬名等　白膠木・塩麸木（ヌルデ）、五倍子（ゴバイシ、フシ）
Name (Romaji)　NURUDE*
Other name (s) (Romaji)　GOBAISHI
学名　*Rhus javanica* L.
Rhus japonica L.
Rhus chinensis Mill.*
科名　Anacardiaceae（ウルシ科）
英名　Japanese sumac / Chinese sumac
ゴバイシ（GOBAISHI）：gall nut / smac gall nut / Japanese gall / call nut
Part of use　acidiate insect gall
Note 1　—
Note 2　The part of use is acidiate insect gall on the leaf of NURUDE that is made by *Schlechtendaria chinensis* Bell. (=*Melaphis chinensis* (Bell.) Baker) of Aphidiae parasitizing on the young sprout or leaf of NURUDE.
注　ヌルデの若芽や葉上にアブラムシ科（Aphidiae）のヌルデシロアブラムシ*Schlechtendaria chinensis* Bell.（=*Melaphis chinensis* (Bell.) Baker）が寄生し、その刺激によって葉上に生成した嚢状虫癭。

名　称　**ネギ***

他名等　ソウジツ／ソウシ／Allium fistulosum
部位等　種子
備　考　—

他名（参考）　ネブカ（根深）、ヒトモジ（一文字、比止毛之）、タイソウ（大葱）、ソウハク（葱白）
漢字表記・生薬名等　葱（ネギ）、葱実（ソウジツ）、葱子（ソウシ）
Name (Romaji)　NEGI*
Other name (s) (Romaji)　SÔJITSU／SÔSHI
学名　*Allium fistulosum* L.*
Allium bouddhae Debeaux
科名　Alliaceae（ネギ科）
英名　Welsh onion / cibol / stone leek / spring onion / Japanese bunching onion / Spanish onion / two-bladed onion
Part of use　seed
Note 1　—
Note 2　—
注　—

名　称　**ネバリミソハギ***

他名等　セッテ・サングリアス
部位等　全草
備　考　—

他名(参考)　—
漢字表記・生薬名等　粘禊萩（ネバリミソハギ）
Name (Romaji)　NEBARIMISOHAGI*
Other name (s) (Romaji)　SETTE・SANGURIASU
学名　*Cuphea carthagenensis* (Jacq.) J.F. Macbr.*
Cuphea balsamona Cham. et Schltdl.*
Cuphea cartagensis (Jacq.) J.F. Macbr.
Parsonia balsamona (Cham. et Schlecht.) Arth.
科名　Lythraceae（ミソハギ科）
英名　Colombian waxweed / sete sangrias
Part of use　whole plant
Note 1　—
Note 2　—
注　—

名　称　**ネムノキ***

他名等　ゴウカンヒ／ネムノハナ
部位等　樹皮・花
備　考　—

他名(参考)　ネム・ネブ（合歓）、ゴウカンカ（合歓花）
漢字表記・生薬名等　合歓木（ネムノキ）、合歓皮（ゴウカンヒ）、合歓花（ゴウカンカ）
Name (Romaji)　NEMUNOKI*
Other name (s) (Romaji)　GÔKANHI／NEMUNOHANA
学名　*Albizia julibrissin* Durazz.*
Acacia julibrissin (Durazz.) Willd.
Mimosa nemu Poir.
科名　Leguminosae（マメ科）
英名　mimosa / silk tree / mimosa tree / pink siris / Persian silk tree
Part of use　bark, flower
Note 1　—
Note 2　—
注　—

名　称　**ノアザミ***

他名等　タイケイ／Cirsium nipponense／Cirsium spicatum／Cirsium japonicumとその近縁種
部位等　根
備　考　—

他名(参考)　Cirsium spicatum：ヤマアザミ、オニアザミ、オオアザミ
漢字表記・生薬名等　野薊（ノアザミ）、大薊（タイケイ）、小薊（ショウケイ）
Name (Romaji)　NOAZAMI*
Other name (s) (Romaji)　TAIKEI
学名　*Cirsium japonicum* Fisch. ex DC.*（ノアザミ）and it's closely related species
Cirsium borealinipponense Kitam.（オニアザミ）
Cirsium spicatum (Maxim.) Matsum.（マアザミ）
科名　Compositae（キク科）
英名　Japanese thistle
Part of use　root
Note 1　—
Note 2　—
注　—

名　称　**ノゲイトウ***

他名等　セイショウ
部位等　種子
備　考　—

他名(参考)　ケイトウ（鶏頭）
漢字表記・生薬名等　野鶏頭（ノゲイトウ）、青葙（セイショウ、セイソウ）、青葙子（セイショウシ、セイソウシ）
Name (Romaji)　NOGEITÔ*
Other name (s) (Romaji)　SEISHÔ
学名　*Celosia argentea* L.*
Celosia argentea L. var. *cristata* (L.) Kuntze*
科名　Amaranthaceae（ヒユ科）
英名　common cockscomb / ockscomb / feather cockscomb / quail grass / crested cockscomb
Part of use　seed
Note 1　—
Note 2　—
注　—

名　称　**ノゲシ***

他名等　—
部位等　茎・葉・花
備　考　—

他名（参考）　ケシアザミ（芥子薊）、ハルノゲシ（春野芥子）、クキョサイ（苦苣菜）
漢字表記・生薬名等　野芥子（ノゲシ）
Name (Romaji)　NOGESHI*
Other name (s) (Romaji)　—
学名　*Sonchus oleraceus* L.*
科名　Compositae（キク科）
英名　sow thistle / common sow thistle / milk thistle
Part of use　stem, leaf, flower
Note 1　—
Note 2　—
注　—

名　称　**ノコギリヤシ***

他名等　ノコギリパルメット
部位等　果実
備　考　—

他名（参考）　—
漢字表記・生薬名等　鋸椰子（ノコギリヤシ）
Name (Romaji)　NOKOGIRIYASHI*
Other name (s) (Romaji)　NOKOGIRIPARUMETTO
学名　*Serenoa repens* (W. Bartram) Small*
Serenoa serrulata (Michx.) G. Nichols*
Sabal serrulata (Michx.) Nutt. ex Schult. et Schult. f.*
科名　Palmae（ヤシ科）
英名　saw palmetto / sabal palm / scrub palmetto
Part of use　fruit
Note 1　—
Note 2　—
注　—

名　称　**ノブドウ**

他名等　—
部位等　茎・根・葉・実
備　考　—

他名（参考）　—
漢字表記・生薬名等　野葡萄（ノブドウ）、蛇葡萄（ジャブドウ）、蛇葡萄根（ジャブドウコン）
Name (Romaji)　NOBUDÔ
Other name (s) (Romaji)　—
学名　*Ampelopsis glandulosa* (Wall.) Momiyama var. *heterophylla* (Thunb.) Momiyama
Ampelopsis brevipedunculata (Maxim.) Trautv.
Cissus brevipedunculata Maxim.
Ampelopsis brevipedunculata (Maxim.) Trautv. var. *heterophylla* (Thunb.) Hara
科名　Vitaceae（ブドウ科）
英名　porcelain vine / porcelain berry
Part of use　stem, root, leaf, fruit
Note 1　—
Note 2　—
注　—

ハ行

名　称　**バアソブ**

他名等　Codonopsis ussuriensis
部位等　根
備　考　—

他名（参考）　—
漢字表記・生薬名等　婆蕎・婆雀斑（バアソブ）
Name (Romaji)　BAASOBU
Other name (s) (Romaji)　—
学名　*Codonopsis ussuriensis* (Rupr. et Maxim.) Hemsl.
科名　Campanulaceae（キキョウ科）
英名　ba-sob
Part of use　root
Note 1　—
Note 2　—
注　—

名　称　**ハイゴショウ**

他名等　—
部位等　果実
備　考　—

他名（参考）　—
漢字表記・生薬名等　這胡椒（ハイゴショウ）
Name (Romaji)　HAIGOSHÔ
Other name (s) (Romaji)　—
学名　*Piper sarmentosum* Roxb.
科名　Piperaceae（コショウ科）
英名　false kava / wild pepper / wild betel
Part of use　fruit

Note 1 —
Note 2 —
注 —

名 称 **パイナップル***

他名等 **パイナップル加工品**
部位等 果実
備 考 パパインは「医」

他名(参考) アナナス
漢字表記・生薬名等 鳳梨（パイナップル、ホウリ）
Name (Romaji) PAINAPPURU*
Other name (s) (Romaji) PAINAPPURUKAKÔHIN
学名 *Ananas comosus* (L.) Merr.*
Ananas ananas (L.) Voss*
Bromelia ananas L.*
Bromelia comosus L.*
Ananas sativus Schult. f.
科名 Bromeliaceae（パイナップル科）
英名 pineapple tree / pineapple
Part of use fruit
Note 1 papain：drug category
Note 2 —
注 —

名 称 **ハイビスカス***

他名等 —
部位等 果実・萼
備 考 —

他名(参考) ブッソウゲ（仏桑華、仏桑花）、ロゼル、ローゼル、ロゼリソウ（ロゼリ草）
漢字表記・生薬名等 紅槿（コウキン、ベニムクゲ）
Name (Romaji) HAIBISUKASU*
Other name (s) (Romaji) —
学名 *Hibiscus rosa-sinensis* L.*（ブッソウゲ）
Hibiscus sabdariffa L.*（ロゼル）
Hibiscus chinensis Hort., p.p., non Roxb.
科名 Malvaceae（アオイ科）
英名 *H. rosa-sinensis*：hibiscus / rose of China / shoe flower / roselle / China rose / Chinese hibiscus / rose of sharon
H. sabdariffa：Jamaica sorrel / Guinea sorrel / Florida cranberry
Part of use fruit, calyx
Note 1 —
Note 2 The Japanese name of the herbs commonly called HAIBISUKASU is BUSSÔGE. BUSSÔGE is also listed in the item of "Name" as FUSSÔGE.
注 一般にハイビスカスと呼ばれているハーブの和名はブッソウゲである。ブッソウゲは別項にフッソウゲとして記載されている。

名 称 **パウダルコ***

他名等 **アクアインカー／イペ**
部位等 樹皮・葉
備 考 —

他名(参考) —
漢字表記・生薬名等 —
Name (Romaji) PAUDARUKO*
Other name (s) (Romaji) AKUAINKÂ／IPE
学名 *Tabebuia impetiginosa* (Mart. ex DC.) Standl.*
Tabebuia avellanedae Lorentz et Griseb.*
Tabebuia heptaphylla (Vell.) Toledo*
Tecoma impetiginosa Mart. ex DC.*
科名 Bignoniaceae（ノウゼンカズラ科）
英名 pau d'arco / ipe roxo / lapacho / taheebo / trumpet tree
Part of use bark, leaf
Note 1 —
Note 2 PAUDARUKO is identical with both of INPETIGINOSA and TABEBUIA. But parts of use of INPETIGINOSA is different from those of other two species. The former is whole plant and the latter is bark and leaf, but bark and/or leaf of these trees are commonly used.
注 パウダルコは別項のインペティギノサ及びタベブイアと同一。インペティギノサの「部位等」は全草であるが、タベブイア及びパウダルコは樹皮・葉とされている。通常は樹皮と葉が用いられる。

名 称 **バオバブ**

他名等 **アフリカバオバブ**
部位等 果実
備 考 —

他名(参考) —
漢字表記・生薬名等 —
Name (Romaji) BAOBABU
Other name (s) (Romaji) AFURIKABAOBABU
学名 *Adansonia digitata* L.
Adansonia baobab Gaertn.
Adansonia bahobab L.
Adansonia situla Spreng.
Adansonia somalensis Chiov.

Adansonia sphaerocarpa A. Chev.
科名 Bombacaceae（パンヤ科）
英名 African baobab / dead rat tree / monkey bread tree / baobab of Mahajanga / cream tartar tree / Ethiopian sour bread / sour gourd
Part of use fruit
Note 1 —
Note 2 —
注 —

名 称 ハカマウラボシ*
他名等 骨砕補
部位等 根茎
備 考 —

他名(参考) —
漢字表記・生薬名等 袴裏星（ハカマウラボシ）、骨砕補（コツサイホ）、候姜（コウキョウ）、申姜（シンキョウ）、毛姜（モウキョウ）
Name (Romaji) HAKAMAURABOSHI*
Other name (s) (Romaji) KOTSUSAIHO
学名 *Drynaria fortunei* (Kunze ex Mett.) J. Sm.*
科名 Polypodiaceae（ウラボシ科）
英名 Drynaria / Gu-Sui-Bu / oak-leaved fern
Part of use rhizome
Note 1 —
Note 2 —
注 —

名 称 バクガ*
他名等 —
部位等 発芽種子
備 考 —

他名(参考) ロクジョウオオムギ（六条大麦）、ニジョウオオムギ（二条大麦）
漢字表記・生薬名等 麦芽（バクガ）
Name (Romaji) BAKUGA*
Other name (s) (Romaji) —
学名 *Hordeum vulgare* L.*
Hordeum vulgare L. var. *hexastichon* Aschers.（ロクジョウオオムギ）
Hordeum vulgare L. var. *distichon* (L.) Hook. f.（ニジョウオオムギ）
科名 Gramineae（イネ科）
英名 malt / barley
Part of use germinating seed
Note 1 —
Note 2 BAKUGA is also listed in the item of "Other names" of ÔMUGI.
注 バクガはオオムギの「他名等」にも記載されている。

名 称 ハクチャ*
他名等 —
部位等 葉
備 考 —

他名(参考) —
漢字表記・生薬名等 白茶（ハクチャ、シロチャ）
Name (Romaji) HAKUCHA*
Other name (s) (Romaji) —
学名 *Camellia sinensis* (L.) O. Kuntze*
Thea sinensis L.*
Camellia thea Link
科名 Theaceae（ツバキ科）
英名 Chinese tea / whtie tea
Part of use leaf
Note 1 —
Note 2 HAKUCHA is distinctive Chinese tea made from lightly fermented leaves of *Camelia sinensis.* HAKUGÔGINSHIN, HAKUBOTAN and JUBI are known as the main types of HAKUCHA.
注 白茶は中国独特の半発酵茶。主なもの：白毫銀針（ハクゴウギンシン）、白牡丹（ハクボタン）、寿眉（ジュビ）など。

名 称 ハクトウスギ
他名等 ウンナンコウトウスギ
部位等 心材
備 考 樹皮・葉は「医」

他名(参考) ハクトウサン（白豆杉）、コウトウサン（紅豆杉）
漢字表記・生薬名等 白豆杉（ハクトウサン、ハクトウスギ）、雲南紅豆杉（ウンナンコウトウサン、ウンナンコウトウスギ）
Name (Romaji) HAKUTÔSUGI
Other name (s) (Romaji) UNNANKÔTÔSUGI
学名 *Pseudotaxus chienii* (W.C. Cheng) W.C. Cheng（ハクトウスギ）
Taxus yunnanensis W.C. Cheng et L.K. Fu（ウンナンコウトウスギ）
Taxus wallichiana Zucc. var. *wallichiana*（ウンナンコウトウスギ）
科名 Taxaceae（イチイ科）
英名 *P. chienii*：white berry yew

T. yunnanensis：Himalayan yew
Part of use　heart wood
Note 1　bark and leaf：drug category
Note 2　—
注　—

名　称　**ハクヒショウ**

他名等　ハクショウトウ
部位等　球果
備　考　—

他名(参考)　シロマツ（白松）、ハクショウ（白松）、サンコノマツ（三鈷松）、シロカワマツ（白皮松）
漢字表記・生薬名等　白皮松（ハクヒショウ）
Name(Romaji)　HAKUHISHÔ
Other name(s) (Romaji)　HAKUSHÔTÔ
学名　*Pinus bungeana* Zucc. ex Endl.
科名　Pinaceae（マツ科）
英名　lace-bark pine / Bunge's pine / white bark pine
Part of use　cone
Note 1　—
Note 2　—
注　—

名　称　**ハコベ***

他名等　—
部位等　全草
備　考　—

他名(参考)　コハコベ（小繁縷）、ヒヨコグサ（雛草）、スズメグサ（雀草）、ハコベラ（繁縷）
漢字表記・生薬名等　繁縷・蘩蔞（ハコベ）
Name(Romaji)　HAKOBE*
Other name(s) (Romaji)　—
学名　*Stellaria media*（L.）Vill.*
科名　Caryophyllaceae（ナデシコ科）
英名　chickweed / common chickweed / chickwort / starwort
Part of use　whole plant
Note 1　—
Note 2　—
注　—

名　称　**ハゴロモソウ***

他名等　—
部位等　全草
備　考　—

他名(参考)　ハゴロモグサ（羽衣草）
漢字表記・生薬名等　羽衣草（ハゴロモソウ）
Name(Romaji)　HAGOROMOSÔ*
Other name(s) (Romaji)　—
学名　*Alchemilla vulgaris* auct. non L.*（ハゴロモソウ）
　　Alchemilla xanthochlora Rothm.*（ハゴロモソウ）
科名　Rosaceae（バラ科）
英名　lady's mantle
Part of use　whole plant
Note 1　—
Note 2　—
注　—

名　称　**バシカン***

他名等　スベリヒユ
部位等　全草
備　考　—

他名(参考)　—
漢字表記・生薬名等　馬歯莧（バシケン）、滑莧（スベリヒユ）
Name(Romaji)　BASHIKAN*
Other name(s) (Romaji)　SUBERIHIYU
学名　*Portulaca oleracea* L.*
科名　Portulacaceae（スベリヒユ科）
英名　green purslane / common purslane / pusley / purslane
Part of use　whole plant
Note 1　—
Note 2　BASHIKAN is the name of traditional Chinese medicine and its Japanese name is SUBERIHIYU. But BASHIKAN is incorrect and its correct name is BASHIKEN.
注　バシカンは中薬名であり、和名はスベリヒユである。またバシカンではなくバシケン（馬歯莧）" が正しい。

ハ行

名　称　**バショウ***

他名等　—
部位等　全草
備　考　—

他名(参考)　—
漢字表記・生薬名等　芭蕉（バショウ）
Name(Romaji)　BASHÔ*
Other name(s)(Romaji)　—
学名　*Musa basjoo* Sieb. et Zucc.*
科名　Musaceae（バショウ科）
英名　Japanese banana
Part of use　whole plant
Note 1　—
Note 2　—
注　—

名　称　**ハス***

他名等　**レンカ／レンコン／レンジツ／レンニク／レンヨウ**
部位等　雄しべ・果実・根茎・種子・葉・花柄・花蕾
備　考　—

他名(参考)　—
漢字表記・生薬名等　蓮（ハス）、蓮花（レンカ）、蓮根（レンコン）、蓮実（レンジツ）、蓮肉（レンニク）、蓮葉（レンヨウ）、蓮子（レンシ）、蓮子心（レンシシン）、石蓮子（セキレンシ）、荷葉（カヨウ）
Name(Romaji)　HASU*
Other name(s)(Romaji)　RENKA／RENKON／RENJITSU／RENNIKU／REN'YÔ
学名　*Nelumbo nucifera* Gaertn.*
Nelumbium speciosum Willd.*
Nymphaea nelumbo L.*
Nelumbium nelumbo (L.) Druce
科名　Nelumbonaceae（ハス科）
英名　Indian lotus / sacred lotus / East Indian lotus / oriental lotus / Hindu lotus / Egyptian lotus / Chinese water lily
Part of use　stamen, fruit, rhizome, seed, leaf, peduncle bud
Note 1　—
Note 2　—
注　—

名　称　**パセリ***

他名等　**パセリ油**
部位等　種子油・根・葉
備　考　—

他名(参考)　オランダゼリ（和蘭芹）
漢字表記・生薬名等　旱芹菜（パセリ）
Name(Romaji)　PASERI*
Other name(s)(Romaji)　PASERI-ABURA
学名　*Petroselinum crispum* (Mill.) Nym. ex A.W. Hill*
Petroselinum sativum Hoffm.*
Petroselinum hortense Hoffm.
Apium petroselinum L.
科名　Umbelliferae（セリ科）
英名　parsley / curly parsley
Part of use　seed oil, root, leaf
Note 1　—
Note 2　—
注　—

名　称　**バターナット***

他名等　—
部位等　種子・種子油
備　考　—

他名(参考)　—
漢字表記・生薬名等　—
Name(Romaji)　BATÂNATTO*
Other name(s)(Romaji)　—
学名　*Juglans cinerea* L.*
Wallia cinerea (L.) Alef.
科名　Juglandaceae（クルミ科）
英名　butternut / white walnut / lemon walnut / oilnut
Part of use　seed, seed oil
Note 1　—
Note 2　—
注　—

名　称　**パタデバカ***

他名等　**ウシノツメ**
部位等　葉
備　考　—

他名(参考)　—
漢字表記・生薬名等　—
Name(Romaji)　PATADEBAKA*
Other name(s)(Romaji)　USHINOTSUME

学名　*Bauhinia fortificata* Link*
Bauhinia divaricata L.*
科名　Leguminosae（マメ科）
英名　pata-de-vaca / Bauhinia divaricata / cow's foot
Part of use　leaf
Note 1　—
Note 2　—
注　—

MINTO (*Mentha* L.). But the parts of use are different each other. SEIYÔHAKKA and MINTO are also listed in the items of "Name".
注　ハッカ及び別項のセイヨウハッカは別項のミント（ハッカ属）に含まれる。但し、使用部位の記載が異なっている。

名　称　**ハチミツ**
他名等　—
部位等　トウヨウミツバチ等が巣に集めた甘味物
備　考　—
他名（参考）　—
漢字表記・生薬名等　蜂蜜（ハチミツ）
Name (Romaji)　HACHIMITSU
Other name (s) (Romaji)　—
学名　—
科名　—
英名　honey
Part of use　sweet sticky substance accumulated in hives by bees such as *Apis indica* Radoszkowski
Note 1　—
Note 2　—
注　—

名　称　**ハッカクレイシ**
他名等　—
部位等　全草
備　考　—
他名（参考）　—
漢字表記・生薬名等　白鶴霊芝（ハッカクレイシ）
Name (Romaji)　HAKKAKUREISHI
Other name (s) (Romaji)　—
学名　*Rhinacanthus nasutus* (L.) Kurz
Justicia nasuta L.
Pseuderanthemum connatum Lindau
Rhinacanthus communis Nees
科名　Acanthaceae（キツネノマゴ科）
英名　snake jasmine
Part of use　whole plant
Note 1　—
Note 2　—
注　—

名　称　**ハッカ***
他名等　—
部位等　葉
備　考　—
他名（参考）　イエハッカ（家薄荷）
漢字表記・生薬名等　薄荷（ハッカ）
Name (Romaji)　HAKKA*
Other name (s) (Romaji)　—
学名　*Mentha arvensis* L. var. *piperascens* Malinv. ex Holmes*
Mentha canadensis L.*
Mentha haplocalyx Briq.*
Mentha haplocalyx Briq. var. *piperascens* (Malinv.) Wu et Li
科名　Labiatae（シソ科）
英名　corn mint / Chinese mint / Japanese mint / common mint / field mint / wild mint
Part of use　leaf
Note 1　—
Note 2　HAKKA and SEIYÔHAKKA are included in

名　称　**ハックルベリー**
他名等　—
部位等　果実・葉
備　考　—
他名（参考）　—
漢字表記・生薬名等　—
Name (Romaji)　HAKKURUBERÎ
Other name (s) (Romaji)　—
学名　*Gaylussacia* Kunth
科名　Ericaceae（ツツジ科）
英名　huckleberry
Part of use　fruit, leaf
Note 1　—
Note 2　—
注　—

ハ行

名　称　**ハッショウマメ**

他名等　**ビロウドマメ**
部位等　全草
備　考　—

他名（参考）　—
漢字表記・生薬名等　八升豆（ハッショウマメ）
Name（Romaji）　HASSHÔMAME
Other name（s）（Romaji）　BIRÔDOMAME
学名　*Mucuna pruriens*（L.）DC. var. *utilis*（Wall ex Wight）Burk.
科名　Leguminosae（マメ科）
英名　velvet bean / cowitch / buffalo bean / cawage
Part of use　whole plant
Note 1　—
Note 2　—
注　—

名　称　**ハトムギ***

他名等　**ジュズダマ／ヨクイニン／ヨクベイ**
部位等　種子・種子エキス・種子油
備　考　—

他名（参考）　センコク（川穀）
漢字表記・生薬名等　鳩麦（ハトムギ）、数珠玉（ジュズダマ）、薏苡仁（ヨクイニン）、薏米（ヨクベイ）
Name（Romaji）　HATOMUGI*
Other name（s）（Romaji）　JUZUDAMA／YOKUININ／YOKUBEI
学名　*Coix lacryma-jobi* L. var. *ma-yuen*（Roman.）Stapf*（ハトムギ）
Coix ma-yuen Roman.（ハトムギ）
Coix lacryma-jobi L.*（ジュズダマ）
科名　Gramineae（イネ科）
英名　Job's tears / Chinese pearl barley / coix
Part of use　seed, seed extract, seed oil
Note 1　—
Note 2　—
注　—

名　称　**ハナシュクシャ**

他名等　**キョウカ**
部位等　花から得られた精油
備　考　—

他名（参考）　—
漢字表記・生薬名等　花縮砂（ハナシュクシャ）、姜花（キョウカ）
Name（Romaji）　HANASHUKUSHA
Other name（s）（Romaji）　KYÔKA
学名　*Hedychium coronarium* J. König
科名　Zingiberaceae（ショウガ科）
英名　white garland-lily / garland flower / ginger lily / common ginger lily / butterfly ginger / butterfly lily / cinnamon jasmine
Part of use　essential oil from flower
Note 1　—
Note 2　—
注　—

名　称　**バナナ**

他名等　**Musa acuminate（Cavendish種）**
部位等　成熟した果実の果皮
備　考　—

他名（参考）　タイワンバナナ（台湾バナナ）、ミバショウ（実芭蕉）
漢字表記・生薬名等　—
Name（Romaji）　BANANA
Other name（s）（Romaji）　—
学名　*Musa acuminata* Colla
科名　Musaceae（バショウ科）
英名　banana / dwarf Cavendish / giant Cavendish
Part of use　pericarp of riped fruit
Note 1　—
Note 2　*Musa acuminate* listed in the item of "Other names" is incorrect. The correct name is *Musa acumitata.*
注　「他名等」の*Musa acuminate*は*Musa acuminata*が正しい。

名　称　**バナバ**

他名等　**オオバナサルスベリ**
部位等　全木
備　考　—

他名（参考）　ジャワザクラ（ジャワ桜）
漢字表記・生薬名等　大花百日紅（オオバナサルスベリ）、大花猿滑（オオバナサルスベリ）
Name（Romaji）　BANABA
Other name（s）（Romaji）　ÔBANASARUSUBERI
学名　*Lagerstroemia speciosa*（L.）Pers.
Lagerstroemia flos-reginae Retz.
科名　Lythraceae（ミソハギ科）
英名　banaba / pride-of-India / queen's crape myrtle /

rose of India
Part of use　whole tree
Note 1　—
Note 2　—
注　—

名　称　**ハナビシソウ***

他名等　—
部位等　全草
備　考　—

他名(参考)　キンエイカ（金英花）
漢字表記・生薬名等　花菱草（ハナビシソウ）
Name(Romaji)　HANABISHISÔ*
Other name(s)(Romaji)　—
学名　*Eschscholzia californica* Cham.*
科名　Papaveraceae（ケシ科）
英名　California poppy / common Californian poppy
Part of use　whole plant
Note 1　—
Note 2　—
注　—

名　称　**ハナビラタケ**

他名等　—
部位等　子実体
備　考　—

他名(参考)　—
漢字表記・生薬名等　花弁茸（ハナビラタケ）
Name(Romaji)　HANABIRATAKE
Other name(s)(Romaji)　—
学名　*Sparassis crispa* (Wulfen) Fr.
Sparassis latifolia Y.C. Dai et Zheng Wang
Manina crispa Scop.
Masseola crispa (Wulfen) Kuntze
Clavaria crispa Wulfen
科名　Sparassidaceae（ハナビラタケ科）
英名　cauliflower mushroom / couliflower fungus / wood cauliflower
Part of use　fruit body
Note 1　—
Note 2　—
注　—

名　称　**ハネセンナ***

他名等　—
部位等　全草
備　考　—

他名(参考)　タイヨウトウ（対葉豆）
漢字表記・生薬名等　—
Name(Romaji)　HANESENNA*
Other name(s)(Romaji)　—
学名　*Cassia alata* L.*
Senna alata (L.) Roxb.*
Herpetica alata (L.) Raf.
科名　Leguminosae（マメ科）
英名　ringworm senna / ringworm cassia / candle bush / candlestick senna / Christmas-candle / empress candle plant / impetigo bush / golden candle
Part of use　whole plant
Note 1　—
Note 2　—
注　—

名　称　**パパイヤ***

他名等　チチウリ／モクカ
部位等　種子・葉・花
備　考　パパインは「医」

他名(参考)　バンモッカ（番木瓜）、バンカジュ（番瓜樹）、マンジュマイ（万寿瓜）、マンジュカ（万寿果）
漢字表記・生薬名等　乳瓜（チチウリ）、木瓜（モクカ）
Name(Romaji)　PAPAIYA*
Other name(s)(Romaji)　CHICHIURI／MOKUKA
学名　*Carica papaya* L.*
科名　Caricaceae（パパイア科）
英名　papaya / pawpaw / papaw / melon tree / common papaw
Part of use　seed, leaf, flower
Note 1　papain : drug category
Note 2　Papaya in KATAKANA is generally transcripted as PAPAIA in the Japanese dictionaries. Caricaceae, the family name is also transcripted as PAPAIA-KA in KATAKANA.
注　パパイヤは通常、辞書等ではパパイアと表記される。また、科名も通常、パパイア科と表記される。

名　称　**ハハコグサ**

他名等　オギョウ／ゴギョウ／ソキクソウ
部位等　全草
備　考　—

他名(参考)　モチバナ（餅花）、モチヨモギ（餅艾）
漢字表記･生薬名等　母子草（ハハコグサ）、御行（ゴギョウ、オギョウ）、鼠麹草（ソキクソウ）
Name(Romaji)　HAHAKOGUSA
Other name(s)(Romaji)　OGYÔ／GOGYÔ／SOKIKUSÔ
学名　*Gnaphalium affine* D. Don
Pseudognaphalium affine（D. Don）Anderb.
Gnaphalium luteoalbum L. ssp. *affine*（D. Don）Koster
Pseudognaphalium luteoalbum（L.）Hillard et B.L. Burtt ssp. *affine*（D. Don）Hillard et B.L. Burtt
科名　Compositae（キク科）
英名　cudweed / Jersey cudweed
Part of use　whole plant
Note 1　—
Note 2　—
注　—

名　称　**ハブソウ***

他名等　—
部位等　全草
備　考　—

他名(参考)　オオハブソウ、クサセンナ、ハブ茶
漢字表記･生薬名等　波布草（ハブソウ）、望江南（ボウコウナン）
Name(Romaji)　HABUSÔ*
Other name(s)(Romaji)　—
学名　*Senna occidentalis*（L.）Link.*
Cassia occidentalis L.
Cassia torosa auct. non Cav.
科名　Leguminosae（マメ科）
英名　coffee senna / foetid cassia / stinking weed / styptic weed / nigro caffee
Part of use　whole plant
Note 1　—
Note 2　—
注　—

名　称　**ハマゼリ**

他名等　—
部位等　全草（果実を除く）
備　考　—

他名(参考)　ハマニンジン（浜人参）
漢字表記･生薬名等　浜芹（ハマゼリ）
Name(Romaji)　HAMAZERI
Other name(s)(Romaji)　—
学名　*Cnidium japonicum* Miq.
科名　Umbelliferae（セリ科）
英名　—
Part of use　whole plant except fruit
Note 1　—
Note 2　—
注　—

名　称　**ハマナス***

他名等　ハマナシ
部位等　果実・花
備　考　—

他名(参考)　マイカイカ（玫瑰花）
漢字表記･生薬名等　浜茄子（ハマナス）、浜梨（ハマナシ）、玫瑰（マイカイ、バイカイ）
Name(Romaji)　HAMANASU*
Other name(s)(Romaji)　HAMANASHI
学名　*Rosa rugosa* Thunb.*
Rosa rugosa var. *ferox*（Lawrance）C.A. Mey.
Rosa rugosa var. *thunbergiana* C.A. Mey.
Rosa ferox Lawrance
Rosa kamtschatica Vent. var. *ferox*（Lawrance）Geel
科名　Rosaceae（バラ科）
英名　rugose rose / Japanese rose / ramanas rose / Turkestan rose
Part of use　fruit, flower
Note 1　—
Note 2　—
注　—

名　称　**ハマボウフウ***

他名等　—
部位等　根・根茎・種子・若芽
備　考　—

他名(参考)　ハマスガナ（波未須加奈）、ハマニガナ（波

未爾加奈)、ヤオヤボウフウ（八百屋防風）
漢字表記・生薬名等　浜防風（ハマボウフウ)、根：防風（ボウフウ)、北沙参（ホクシャジン、bei sha shen）
Name (Romaji)　HAMABÔFÛ*
Other name (s) (Romaji)　—
学名　*Glehnia littoralis* Fr. Schm. ex Miq.*
Phellopteris littoralis Benth.
科名　Umbelliferae（セリ科）
英名　bei sha shen / glehnia / American silvertop / beach silvertop
Part of use　root, rhizome, seed, sprout
Note 1　—
Note 2　—
注　—

名　称　**ハマメリス***

他名等　Hamamelis virginiana
部位等　葉
備　考　—

他名(参考)　—
漢字表記・生薬名等　アメリカ満作・アメリカ万作（アメリカマンサク）
Name (Romaji)　HAMAMERISU*
Other name (s) (Romaji)　—
学名　*Hamamelis virginiana* L.*
科名　Hamamelidaceae（マンサク科）
英名　witch hazel
Part of use　leaf
Note 1　—
Note 2　HAMAMERISU in the item of "Name" is the KATAKANA notation of genus name, "*Hamamelis*", and it does not indicate a particular herb. AMERIKAMANSAKU which is the Japanese name of *Hamamelis virginiana* is appropriate to be used for this item.
注　「名称」のハマメリスは属名の*Hamamelis*のカタカナ表記であり、固有のハーブを示す名称ではない。本名称としては*Hamamelis virginiana*の和名であるアメリカマンサクが適切である。

名　称　**バラ**

他名等　バラ科植物
部位等　果実・葉・花
備　考　エイジツは「医」

他名(参考)　—
漢字表記・生薬名等　薔薇（バラ）
Name (Romaji)　BARA
Other name (s) (Romaji)　BARA-KA SHOKUBUTSU
学名　*Rosa* L.（バラ属）
科名　Rosaceae（バラ科）
英名　rose / brier
Part of use　fruit, leaf, flower
Note 1　fruit and pseudocarp of *Rosa multiflora* Thunb.：drug category
Note 2　Rosaceae is in the item of "Other names" but "BARA-ZOKU（*Rosa* L.)" is listed in the item of "Scientific name".
注　「他名等」にバラ科植物と記載されているが、学名は「バラ属」とした。

名　称　**パラミツ**

他名等　ジャック
部位等　果実・種子・葉・花
備　考　—

他名(参考)　ジャックフルーツ、ナンカ（南果)、ナガミパンノキ（長実パンの木）
漢字表記・生薬名等　波羅密・菠蘿蜜（パラミツ)、婆羅蜜樹（パラミツジュ）
Name (Romaji)　PARAMITSU
Other name (s) (Romaji)　JAKKU
学名　*Artocarpus heterophyllus* Lam.
Artocarpus integrifolius auct. non L. f.
Artocarpus nanca Noranha
Artocarpus maxima Blanco
Artocarpus integra auct. non（Thunb.）Merril
科名　Moraceae（クワ科）
英名　Jack fruit / Jack / Jack tree
Part of use　fruit, seed, leaf, flower
Note 1　—
Note 2　—
注　—

名　称　**バラン**

他名等　—
部位等　葉
備　考　—

他名(参考)　ハラン（葉蘭)、バレン、ヒトツバ、ヒロハ
漢字表記・生薬名等　葉蘭（ハラン、バラン)、蜘蛛抱蛋（チチュウホウタン）
Name (Romaji)　BARAN
Other name (s) (Romaji)　—
学名　*Aspidistra elatior* Blume

Plectogyne elatior hort.
Aspidistra punctata Lindl.
Aspidistra elatior Blume var. *albomaculata* Hook.
Plectogyne variegata Link.

科名　Liliaceae（ユリ科）
英名　cast iron plant / barroom plant
Part of use　leaf
Note 1　—
Note 2　BARAN is commonly called HARAN.
注　バラン（葉蘭）は通常ハランと呼ばれる。

名　称　ハルウコン*

他名等　**アロマティカ**
部位等　根茎
備　考　—

他名(参考)　—
漢字表記・生薬名等　春鬱金（ハルウコン）、薑黄・姜黄（キョウオウ）
Name (Romaji)　HARUUKON*
Other name (s) (Romaji)　AROMATIKA
学名　*Curcuma aromatica* Salisb.*
科名　Zingiberaceae（ショウガ科）
英名　yujin / wild turmeric / yellow zedoary / yellow ginger
Part of use　rhizome
Note 1　—
Note 2　—
注　—

名　称　バレイショ*

他名等　**バレイショデンプン**
部位等　塊茎
備　考　—

他名(参考)　ジャガタライモ（ジャガタラ芋）、ジャガイモ（ジャガ芋）、キンカイモ（金柑芋）、ニドイモ（二度芋）、サンドイモ（三度芋）、アップラ、アンプラ、カンプラ
漢字表記・生薬名等　馬鈴薯（バレイショ）、馬鈴薯澱粉（バレイショデンプン）
Name (Romaji)　BAREISHO*
Other name (s) (Romaji)　BAREISHODENPUN
学名　*Solanum tuberosum* L.*
科名　Solanaceae（ナス科）
英名　potato / Irish potato / potatoe
Part of use　tuber
Note 1　—
Note 2　—
注　—

名　称　パロアッスル

他名等　—
部位等　全草
備　考　—

他名(参考)　アカミノキ
漢字表記・生薬名等　—
Name (Romaji)　PAROASSURU
Other name (s) (Romaji)　—
学名　*Haematoxylum campechianum* L.
Haematoxylon campechianum L.
Cymbosepalum baroni Baker
Cymbosepalum baronii Baker
科名　Leguminosae（マメ科）
英名　palo azul / logwood / longwood / bloodwoodtree / campeche wood / palo negro
Part of use　whole plant
Note 1　—
Note 2　PAROASSURU (palo azul) approved by the Ministry of Health, Labour and Welfare is *Haematoxylum campechianum* L. (Leguminosae), but *Eysenharditia polystachya* (Ortega) Sarg. (Leguminosae) is another herb that is also called palo azul. The synonymes are as follows：
① *Dalea fruticosa* G. Don
② *Eysenhardtia amorphoides* Kunth
③ *Psoralea fruticosa* Sesse et Moc.
④ *Psoralea stipularis* Sesse et Moc.
⑤ *Varennea polystachya* (Ortega) DC.
⑥ *Viborquia polystachya* Ortega

注　厚生労働省が認めたパロアッスル（palo azul）は、マメ科の*Haematoxylum campechianum* L.であるが、その他にパロアッスルと呼ばれるマメ科の*Eysenhardtia polystachya* (Ortega) Sarg.もある。その異名は以下の通りである。
① *Dalea fruticosa* G. Don
② *Eysenhardtia amorphoides* Kunth
③ *Psoralea fruticosa* Sesse et Moc.
④ *Psoralea stipularis* Sesse et Moc.
⑤ *Varennea polystachya* (Ortega) DC.
⑥ *Viborquia polystachya* Ortega

名　称　**ハンゲショウ**

他名等　**カタシログサ／三白草**
部位等　茎・葉
備　考　—

他名(参考)　オシロイカケ（白粉掛け）、ハンゲグサ（半夏草）
漢字表記･生薬名等　半夏生・半化粧（ハンゲショウ）、片白草（カタシログサ）、三白草（ミツシロソウ）
Name (Romaji)　HANGESHÔ
Other name (s) (Romaji)　KATASHIROGUSA／MITSUJIROGUSA
学名　*Saururus chinensis* (Lour.) Baill.
科名　Saururaceae（ドクダミ科）
英名　lizard's tail / Chinese lizardtail / oriental lizardtail
Part of use　stem, leaf
Note 1　—
Note 2　—
注　—

名　称　**ハンシレン***

他名等　**—**
部位等　全草
備　考　—

他名(参考)　—
漢字表記･生薬名等　半枝蓮（ハンシレン）
Name (Romaji)　HANSHIREN*
Other name (s) (Romaji)　—
学名　*Scutellaria barbata* D. Don*
科名　Labiatae（シソ科）
英名　barbed skullcap / maddog desert scullcap / barbat skullcap / skute barbata
Part of use　whole plant
Note 1　—
Note 2　—
注　—

名　称　**ハンダイカイ**

他名等　**バクダイ**
部位等　果実・種子
備　考　—

他名(参考)　ハクジュ（伯樹、柏樹）、ハンタイカイ（胖大海）
漢字表記･生薬名等　胖大海（ハンダイカイ）、莫大（バクダイ）、莫大海（バクダイカイ）
Name (Romaji)　HANDAIKAI
Other name (s) (Romaji)　BAKUDAI
学名　*Sterculia lychnophora* Hance
Sterculia scaphigera Wall. ex G. Don
Scaphium scaphigerum (G. Don) Guib.
Scaphium wallichii Schott et Endl.
Scaphium affine Pierre
科名　Sterculiaceae（アオギリ科）
英名　malva nut
Part of use　fruit, seed
Note 1　—
Note 2　—
注　—

名　称　**ヒイラギメギ***

他名等　**オレゴンブドウ**
部位等　全草
備　考　—

他名(参考)　—
漢字表記･生薬名等　柊目木（ヒイラギメギ）
Name (Romaji)　HÎRAGIMEGI*
Other name (s) (Romaji)　OREGONBUDÔ
学名　*Mahonia aquifolium* (Pursh) Nutt.*
Berberis aquifolium Pursh*
科名　Berberidaceae（メギ科）
英名　Oregon grape / Oregongrape / holly-leaf barberry / mountain grape / Oregon grapeholly / Oregon barberry
Part of use　whole plant
Note 1　—
Note 2　—
注　—

名　称　**ヒイラギモチ**

他名等　**クコツ**
部位等　果実・樹皮・根・葉
備　考　—

他名(参考)　シナヒイラギ（支那柊）、ヒイラギモドキ（柊擬き）、ヤバネヒイラギモチ（矢羽柊黐）、クテイチャ（苦丁茶）
漢字表記･生薬名等　柊黐（ヒイラギモチ）、枸骨（クコツ）
Name (Romaji)　HÎRAGIMOCHI
Other name (s) (Romaji)　KUKOTSU
学名　*Ilex cornuta* Lindl. ex Paxt.
科名　Aquifoliaceae（モチノキ科）
英名　horned holly / Chinese holly

Part of use　fruit, bark, root, leaf
Note 1　—
Note 2　—
注　—

名　称　**ヒカゲミズ***

他名等　—
部位等　根
備　考　—

他名(参考)　—
漢字表記・生薬名等　墻草（ショウソウ）
Name(Romaji)　HIKAGEMIZU*
Other name(s) (Romaji)　—
学名　*Parietaria micrantha* Ledeb.
Parietaria diffusa Mert. et W.D.J. Koch*
Parietaria judaica L.*
科名　Urticaceae（イラクサ科）
英名　pellitory of the wall / spreading pellitory / sticky weed
Part of use　root
Note 1　—
Note 2　—
注　—

名　称　**ヒジツ**

他名等　カヤ
部位等　果実
備　考　—

他名(参考)　シナガヤ（支那榧）
漢字表記・生薬名等　榧実（ヒジツ）、榧子（ヒシ）、榧（カヤ）
Name(Romaji)　HIJITSU
Other name(s) (Romaji)　KAYA
学名　*Torreya grandis* Forst.（シナガヤ）
Torreya nucifera (L.) Sieb. et Zucc.（カヤ）
Taxus nucifera L.（カヤ）
科名　Taxaceae（イチイ科）
英名　*T. grandis*：Chinese torreya
T. nucifera：Japanese torreya / Japanese plum yew / Japanese nut meg tree / kaya
Part of use　fruit
Note 1　—
Note 2　—
注　—

名　称　**ヒシノミ**

他名等　ヒシ
部位等　果実
備　考　—

他名(参考)　ヒメビシ（姫菱）、メビシ（雌菱）、オニビシ（鬼菱）
漢字表記・生薬名等　菱の実（ヒシノミ）、菱実（リョウジツ）、菱（ヒシ）
Name(Romaji)　HISHINOMI
Other name(s) (Romaji)　HISHI
学名　*Trapa japonica* Flerow（ヒシ）
Trapa bispinosa Roxb. var. *iinumai* Nakano（ヒシ）
Trapa natans L.（オニビシ）
Trapa japonica Flerow var. *rubeola* (Makino) Ohwi（メビシ）
Trapa incisa Sieb et Zucc.（ヒメビシ）
Trapa natans L. var. *rubeola* Makino（メビシ）
科名　Trapaceae（ヒシ科）
英名　*T. japonica*：water chestnut
T. natans：European water chestnut
Part of use　fruit
Note 1　—
Note 2　The name of this tree is not HISHINOMI but HISHI. HISHINOMI means the fruit of HISHI.
注　名称はヒシノミではなく、ヒシである。

名　称　**ビジョザクラ**

他名等　—
部位等　全草
備　考　—

他名(参考)　ハナガサ（花笠）、サクラシバ（桜芝）、バーベナ
漢字表記・生薬名等　美女桜（ビジョザクラ）
Name(Romaji)　BIJOZAKURA
Other name(s) (Romaji)　—
学名　*Verbena*×*hybrida* Voss
Verbena×*hortensis* hort. Vilm.
科名　Verbenaceae（クマツヅラ科）
英名　florist's verbena / common garden verbena / garden verbena
Part of use　whole plant
Note 1　—
Note 2　—
注　—

名　称　ヒソップ*

他名等　ヤナギハッカ
部位等　全草
備　考　—

他名(参考)　—
漢字表記・生薬名等　柳薄荷（ヤナギハッカ）
Name (Romaji)　HISOPPU*
Other name (s) (Romaji)　YANAGIHAKKA
学名　*Hyssopus officinalis* L.*
科名　Labiatae（シソ科）
英名　hyssop
Part of use　whole plant
Note 1　—
Note 2　—
注　—

名　称　ヒナギク*

他名等　エンメイギク
部位等　全草
備　考　—

他名(参考)　チョウメイギク（長命菊）、デイジー
漢字表記・生薬名等　雛菊（ヒナギク）、延命菊（エンメイギク）
Name (Romaji)　HINAGIKU*
Other name (s) (Romaji)　ENMEIGIKU
学名　*Bellis perennis* L.*
科名　Compositae（キク科）
英名　garden daisy / common daisy / true daisy / English daisy
Part of use　whole plant
Note 1　—
Note 2　—
注　—

名　称　ヒナゲシ*

他名等　グビジンソウ／レイシュンカ
部位等　花
備　考　—

他名(参考)　コクリコ（雛罌粟）、シャーレーポピー（shirley poppy）
漢字表記・生薬名等　雛芥子（ヒナゲシ）、虞美人草（グビジンソウ）、麗春花（レイシュンカ）
Name (Romaji)　HINAGESHI*
Other name (s) (Romaji)　GUBIJINSÔ／REISHUNKA
学名　*Papaver rhoeas* L.*
科名　Papaveraceae（ケシ科）
英名　field poppy / corn poppy / Flanders poppy / red weed / cup rose / knap bottle
Part of use　flower
Note 1　—
Note 2　—
注　—

名　称　ヒノキ

他名等　—
部位等　枝・材・葉
備　考　—

他名(参考)　マキ（真木）
漢字表記・生薬名等　檜・桧（ヒノキ）
Name (Romaji)　HINOKI
Other name (s) (Romaji)　—
学名　*Chamaecyparis obtusa* (Sieb. et Zucc.) Sieb. et Zucc. ex Endl.
科名　Cupressaceae（ヒノキ科）
英名　Japanese cypress / hinoki / hinoki false cypress / hinoki cypress / Japanese false cypress
Part of use　branch, wood, leaf
Note 1　—
Note 2　—
注　—

名　称　ヒバマタ*

他名等　—
部位等　全藻
備　考　—

他名(参考)　—
漢字表記・生薬名等　桧葉叉（ヒバマタ）
Name (Romaji)　HIBAMATA*
Other name (s) (Romaji)　—
学名　*Fucus vesiculosus* L.*（ブラダーラック）
Fucus evanescens C. Agardh*（ヒバマタ）
Fucus distichus ssp. *evanescens* (C. Agardh) H.T. Powell（ヒバマタ）
科名　Fucaceae（ヒバマタ科）
英名　*F. evanescens*：fucus / flat wrack / rockweed / *F. vesiculosus*：bladder wrack / bladderwrack / black tang
Part of use　whole seaweed
Note 1　—
Note 2　—

注　—

名　称　**ビフィズス菌**

他名等　Bifidobacterium属
部位等　菌体
備　考　—

他名(参考)　—
漢字表記･生薬名等　—
Name (Romaji)　BIFIZUSU-KIN
Other name(s) (Romaji)　—
学名　*Bifidobacterium*（乳製品、ヒト腸管由来、Biosafety level 1に限る）
科名　Bifidobacteriaceae（ビフィドバクテリウム科）
英名　Bifidobacterium
Part of use　fungus body
Note 1　—
Note 2　—
注　—

名　称　**ヒマラヤニンジン**

他名等　—
部位等　根茎
備　考　—

他名(参考)　ウヨウサンシチ（羽葉三七）、ウヨウチクセツジン（羽葉竹節参）
漢字表記･生薬名等　—
Name (Romaji)　HIMARAYANINJIN
Other name(s) (Romaji)　—
学名　*Panax pseudoginseng* Wall. ssp. *himalaicus* H. Hara
Panax bipinnatifidus Seem.
Panax pseudoginseng Wall. var. *bipinnatifidus* (Seem.) Li.
科名　Araliaceae（ウコギ科）
英名　Himalayan panax
Part of use　rhizome
Note 1　—
Note 2　—
注　—

名　称　**ヒマワリ***

他名等　ニチリンソウ／ヒグルマ／ヒマワリ油
部位等　種子・種子油・葉・花
備　考　—

他名(参考)　—
漢字表記･生薬名等　向日葵（ヒマワリ）、日輪草（ニチリンソウ）、日車（ヒグルマ）
Name (Romaji)　HIMAWARI*
Other name(s) (Romaji)　NICHIRINSÔ／HIGURUMA／HIMAWARI-YU
学名　*Helianthus annuus* L.*
科名　Compositae（キク科）
英名　sunflower / common garden sunflower / common sunflower / mirasol
Part of use　seed, seed oil, leaf, flower
Note 1　—
Note 2　—
注　—

名　称　**ヒメウイキョウ***

他名等　イノンド／キャラウェイ／ジラシ
部位等　果実・種子
備　考　—

他名(参考)　カツズイシ（葛縷子）
漢字表記･生薬名等　姫茴香（ヒメウイキョウ）、蒔蘿子（ジラシ）、葛縷子（カツズイシ）
Name (Romaji)　HIMEUIKYÔ*
Other name(s) (Romaji)　INONDO／KYARAWEI／JIRASHI
学名　*Carum carvi* L.*
Apium carvi (L.) Crantz.
科名　Umbelliferae（セリ科）
英名　caraway
Part of use　fruit, seed
Note 1　—
Note 2　—
注　—

名　称　**ヒメジョオン***

他名等　デイジー
部位等　全草
備　考　—

他名(参考)　イチネンホウ（一年蓬）
漢字表記･生薬名等　姫女菀（ヒメジョオン）

Name (Romaji)　HIMEJOON*
Other name (s) (Romaji)　DEIJÎ
学名　*Erigeron annuus* (L.) Pers.*
Stenactis annuus (L.) Cass.
Phalacroloma annuum (L.) Dumort.
科名　Compositae (キク科)
英名　daisy / fleabane / annual fleabane / daisy fleabane / eastern daisy fleabane / erigeron
Part of use　whole plant
Note 1　—
Note 2　—
注　—

名　称　**ヒメツルニチニチソウ***
他名等　—
部位等　全草
備　考　—

他名(参考)　ショウマンチョウシュンカ（小蔓長春花）
漢字表記・生薬名等　姫蔓日々草（ヒメツルニチニチソウ）
Name (Romaji)　HIMETSURUNICHINICHISÔ*
Other name (s) (Romaji)　—
学名　*Vinca minor* L.*
科名　Apocynaceae (キョウチクトウ科)
英名　common periwinkle / lesser periwinkle / running myrtle / myrtle
Part of use　whole plant
Note 1　—
Note 2　—
注　—

名　称　**ビャクズク***
他名等　—
部位等　果実
備　考　—

他名(参考)　ショウズク（小豆蔻）、カルダモン、タコツ（多骨）、ハクズク（白豆蔻）、ビャック（白蔻）
漢字表記・生薬名等　白豆蔻（ビャクズク）、爪哇白豆蔻（ジャワビャクズク＝*Amomum compactum*）、白豆蔻殻（ビャクズクカク）
Name (Romaji)　BYAKUZUKU*
Other name (s) (Romaji)　—
学名　*Amomum cardamomum* L.
Amomum compactum Sol. ex Maton*
Amomum keplaga Sprag. et Burk.
Amomum kravanh Pierre ex Gagnep.*
科名　Zingiberaceae (ショウガ科)
英名　Chinese cardamom / Chinese cardamon / round cardamom / round cardamon / Java cardamom / Java cardamon / Siam cardamom / Siam cardamon / white fruit amomum
Part of use　fruit
Note 1　—
Note 2　BYAKUZUKU and SHÔZUKU are possibly confused with each other in the marketplace. SHÔZUKU is also listed in the item of "Name".
注　ビャクズク別項のショウズクは市場では混乱している可能性がある。

名　称　**ヒョウタン***
他名等　—
部位等　果肉・葉
備　考　—

他名(参考)　—
漢字表記・生薬名等　瓢箪（ヒョウタン）、葫蘆（コロ）
Name (Romaji)　HYÔTAN*
Other name (s) (Romaji)　—
学名　*Lagenaria siceraria* (Molina) Standl. var. *siceraria*
Lagenaria siceraria (Molina) Standl. var. *gourda* (Ser.) Hara
Lagenaria leucantha Rusby var. *gourda* Makino
Cucurbita lagenaria (L.) L.*
Lagenaria leucantha Rusby*
Lagenaria vulgaris Ser.*
科名　Cucurbitaceae (ウリ科)
英名　bottle gourd / calabash
Part of use　sarcocarp, leaf
Note 1　—
Note 2　Refer to FUKUBE and YÛGAO. Both of FUKUBE and YÛGAO are also listed in the item of "Name".
注　別項のフクベ及びユウガオを参照。

名　称　**ヒヨドリジョウゴ**
他名等　ハクエイ／ハクモウトウ
部位等　全草
備　考　—

他名(参考)　ホロシ（保呂之）
漢字表記・生薬名等　蜀羊泉（ショクヨウセン、ヒヨドリジョウゴ）、鵯上戸（ヒヨドリジョウゴ）、白英（ハクエイ）、白毛藤（ハクモウトウ）
Name (Romaji)　HIYODORIJÔGO
Other name (s) (Romaji)　HAKUEI／HAKUMÔTÔ

学名　*Solanum lyratum* Thunb.
Solanum dulcamara var. *lyratum* (Thunb.) Sieb. et Zucc.
Solanum dulcamara var. *pubescens* Blume
科名　Solanaceae（ナス科）
英名　bitter sweet / bitter nightshade / climbing nightshade / dulcamara
Part of use　whole plant
Note 1　—
Note 2　Caution：HIYODORIJÔGO contains toxic alkaloid, solanine, in the whole plant.
注　全草に有毒アルカロイドであるソラニンを含有するため注意を要する。

名　称　**ヒルガオ**

他名等　—
部位等　全草
備　考　—

他名(参考)　—
漢字表記・生薬名等　昼顔（ヒルガオ）
Name(Romaji)　HIRUGAO
Other name(s) (Romaji)　—
学名　*Calystegia japonica* Choisy
科名　Convolvulaceae（ヒルガオ科）
英名　Japanese bindweed / bindweed
Part of use　whole plant
Note 1　—
Note 2　—
注　—

名　称　**ビルベリー***

他名等　—
部位等　果実・葉
備　考　—

他名(参考)　セイヨウスノキ（西洋酢の木）、ホワートルベリー（whortleberry）、ウィンベリー（winberry）、ブレーベリー（blaeberry）、ヨーロッパブルーベリー（European blueberry）
漢字表記・生薬名等　—
Name(Romaji)　BIRUBERÎ*
Other name(s) (Romaji)　—
学名　*Vaccinium myrtillus* L.*
科名　Ericaceae（ツツジ科）
英名　bilberry / European blueberry / huckleberry / whortleberry / European lowbush blueberry
Part of use　fruit, leaf
Note 1　—
Note 2　BIRUBERÎ is identical with SEIYÔHIMESUNOKI. SEIYÔHIMESUNOKI is also listed in the item of "Name".
注　ビルベリーは別項のセイヨウヒメスノキと同一。

名　称　**ビルマネム***

他名等　Albizia lebbeck
部位等　樹皮
備　考　—

他名(参考)　オオバネム（大葉合歓）
漢字表記・生薬名等　ビルマ合歓（ビルマネム）、緬甸合歓（ビルマネム）
Name(Romaji)　BIRUMANEMU*
Other name(s) (Romaji)　—
学名　*Albizia lebbeck* (L.) Benth.*
科名　Leguminosae（マメ科）
英名　lebbeck tree / woman's tangue tree / Siris tree / East Indian walnut
Part of use　bark
Note 1　—
Note 2　—
注　—

名　称　**ビロウドモウズイカ***

他名等　マレイン
部位等　茎・葉・花
備　考　—

他名(参考)　ニワタバコ（庭煙草）、モウズイカ（毛蕊花）
漢字表記・生薬名等　天鵞絨毛蕊花（ビロウドモウズイカ）
Name(Romaji)　BIRÔDOMÔZUIKA*
Other name(s) (Romaji)　MAREIN
学名　*Verbascum thapsus* L.*
科名　Scrophulariaceae（ゴマノハグサ科）
英名　great mullein / mullein / common mullein / candlewick / Adam's flannel / blanket leaf / flannel plant / hag taper / Jacob's staff / shepherd's club / torches / Aaron's rod / flannel leaf / velvet plant
Part of use　stem, leaf, flower
Note 1　—
Note 2　—
注　—

名　称　ビワ*

他名等　—
部位等　種子・樹皮・葉
備　考　—

他名（参考）　—
漢字表記・生薬名等　枇杷（ビワ）、枇杷葉（ビワヨウ）、枇杷核（ビワカク）、枇杷木白皮（ビワボクハクヒ）、枇杷葉露（ビワヨウロ）
Name (Romaji)　BIWA*
Other name (s) (Romaji)　—
学名　*Eriobotrya japonica* (Thunb.) Lindl.*
Mespilus japonica Thunb.
科名　Rosaceae（バラ科）
英名　Japanese medlar / loquat / Japanese plum / Japanese loquat
Part of use　seed, bark, leaf
Note 1　—
Note 2　—
注　—

名　称　ビンロウジ*

他名等　ビンロウ
部位等　種子
備　考　果皮は「医」

他名（参考）　ビンロウヤシ（檳榔椰子）
漢字表記・生薬名等　檳榔（ビンロウ）、種子：檳榔子（ビンロウジ）、果皮：大腹皮（ダイフクヒ）
Name (Romaji)　BINRÔJI*
Other name (s) (Romaji)　BINRÔ
学名　*Areca catechu* L.*
科名　Palmae（ヤシ科）
英名　betel nut / areca nut / betel palm nut / betelnut palm / areca nut palm / catechu / pinang
Part of use　seed
Note 1　pericarp：drug category
Note 2　—
注　—

名　称　フーディア・ゴードニー

他名等　—
部位等　地上部
備　考　—

他名（参考）　レイハイカク（麗盃閣）
漢字表記・生薬名等　麗盃閣（レイハイカク）
Name (Romaji)　FÛDIA・GÔDONÎ
Other name (s) (Romaji)　—
学名　*Hoodia gordonii* (Masson) Sweet ex Decne.
Gonostemon gordonii Sweet
Monothylaceum gordonii G. Don
Stapelia gordonii Masson
科名　Asclepiadaceae（ガガイモ科）
英名　hoodia / hoodia cuctus / wild ghaap / South African desert cactus
Part of use　aerial part
Note 1　—
Note 2　—
注　—

名　称　フウトウカズラ*

他名等　カイフウトウ
部位等　茎
備　考　—

他名（参考）　フウトウ（風藤）
漢字表記・生薬名等　風藤葛（フウトウカズラ）、海風藤（カイフウトウ）
Name (Romaji)　FÛTÔKAZURA*
Other name (s) (Romaji)　KAIFÛTÔ
学名　*Piper kadsura* (Choisy) Ohwi*
Piper futokadsura Sieb.*
科名　Piperaceae（コショウ科）
英名　Japanese pepper / kadsura pepper
Part of use　vine
Note 1　—
Note 2　—
注　—

名　称　プエラリアミリフィカ

他名等　—
部位等　貯蔵根
備　考　—

他名（参考）　プエラリア
漢字表記・生薬名等　—
Name (Romaji)　PUERARIAMIRIFIKA
Other name (s) (Romaji)　—
学名　*Pueraria mirifica* Airy Shaw et Suvatab.（ガウクルア）
Pueraria candollei var. *mirifica* (Airy Shaw et Suvat.) Niyomdham（ガウクルア）
Butea superba Roxb.（アカガウクルア）
科名　Leguminosae（マメ科）

ハ行

英名　red kwaao khruea / kwao krua / white kwao keur
Part of use　storage root
Note 1　—
Note 2　PUERARIAMIRIFIKA is identical with GAUKURUA, but their parts of use are different each other. GAUKURUA is also listed in the item of "Name".
注　プエラリアミリフィカは別項のガウクルアと同一。但し、「部位等」の記載が異なっている。

名　称　**ブカトウ***

他名等　—
部位等　根・葉
備　考　—

他名(参考)　—
漢字表記・生薬名等　武靴糖（ブカトウ）、貲蘘藤（シャカトウ、シコウトウ）
Name(Romaji)　BUKATÔ*
Other name(s)(Romaji)　—
学名　*Gymnema sylvestre* (Retz.) R. Br. ex Schult.*
科名　Asclepiadaceae（ガガイモ科）
英名　gymnema / gurmar
Part of use　root, leaf
Note 1　—
Note 2　BUKATÔ is identical with GIMUNEMA. BUKATÔ is the name of traditional Japanese herbal medicine, but their parts of use are different each other. GIMUNEMA is also listed in the item of "Name".
注　ブカトウは別項のギムネマと同一。ブカトウはギムネマの生薬名であるが、「部位等」の記載が異なっている。

名　称　**フキタンポポ***

他名等　カントウヨウ／フキノトウ
部位等　葉・幼若花茎
備　考　花蕾は「医」

他名(参考)　カトウ（顆凍）、トケイ（莵奚）、タクゴ（橐吾）、コシュ（虎鬚）、テイトウ（氐冬）、サントウ（鑚涷）
漢字表記・生薬名等　蕗蒲公英（フキタンポポ）、葉：款冬葉（カントウヨウ）、幼若花茎：款冬花（カントウカ）、蕗の薹
Name(Romaji)　FUKITANPOPO*
Other name(s)(Romaji)　KANTÔYÔ／FUKINOTÔ
学名　*Tussilago farfara* L.*
科名　Compositae（キク科）
英名　coltsfoot
Part of use　leaf, juvenile flower stalk
Note 1　flower bud：drug category
Note 2　—
注　—

名　称　**フクベ**

他名等　—
部位等　果実・葉
備　考　—

他名(参考)　—
漢字表記・生薬名等　瓢（フクベ、ヒサゴ）、瓠（フクベ）
Name(Romaji)　FUKUBE
Other name(s)(Romaji)　—
学名　*Lagenaria siceraria* (Molina) Standl. var. *depressa* (Ser.) Hara
Lagenaria leucantha Rusby var. *depressa* (Ser.) Makino
Lagenaria vulgaris Ser. var. *depressa* Ser.
科名　Cucurbitaceae（ウリ科）
英名　bottle gourd / calabash gourd
Part of use　fruit, leaf
Note 1　—
Note 2　Refer to HYÔTAN and YÛGAO. These herbs are also listed in the item of "Name".
注　別項のヒョウタンとユウガオを参照。

名　称　**フジ**

他名等　—
部位等　茎（フジコブ菌が寄生し生じた瘤以外）
備　考　フジコブ菌が寄生し生じた瘤は「医」

他名(参考)　ノダフジ（野田藤）
漢字表記・生薬名等　藤（フジ）
Name(Romaji)　FUJI
Other name(s)(Romaji)　—
学名　*Wisteria floribunda* (Willd.) DC.
科名　Leguminosae（マメ科）
英名　Japanese wisteria
Part of use　stem except knob being parasitic with *Erwinia herbicola* pv. *milletiae*
Note 1　knob being parasitic with *Erwinia herbicola* pv. *milletiae*：drug category
Note 2　—
注　—

名 称 **ブシュカン***

他名等 **コウエン／シトロン**
部位等 果実・花
備 考 —

他名(参考) テブシュカン（手仏手柑）、ブシュコウエン（仏手香櫞）、ブシュ（佛手、仏手）
漢字表記・生薬名等 佛手柑・仏手柑（ブシュカン）、香櫞（コウエン）
Name (Romaji) BUSHUKAN*
Other name (s) (Romaji) KÔEN／SHITORON
学名 *Citrus medica* L. var. *sarcodactylis* (Hoola van Nooten) Swingle*
科名 Rutaceae（ミカン科）
英名 flesh finger citron / fingered citoron / Buddha's hand citron
Part of use fruit, flower
Note 1 —
Note 2 —
注 —

名 称 **フタバムグサ***

他名等 **ハッカジャセツソウ**
部位等 全草
備 考 —

他名(参考) —
漢字表記・生薬名等 双葉葎（フタバムグラ）、百花蛇舌草（ビャッカジャゼツソウ、ハクカジャゼツソウ）
Name (Romaji) FUTABAMUGUSA*
Other name (s) (Romaji) HAKKAJASETSUSÔ
学名 *Oldenlandia diffusa* (Willd.) Roxb.*
Hedyotis diffusa Willd.*
科名 Rubiaceae（アカネ科）
英名 hedyotis / star violet
Part of use whole plant
Note 1 —
Note 2 FUTABAMUGUSA is incorrect. The correct name is FUTABAMUGURA. HAKKAJAZETSUSÔ in the item of “Other names” is incorrect. The correct name is BYAKKAJAZETSUSÔ.
注 フタバムグサの正しい名称はフタバムグラ。「別名等」のハッカジャセツソウはビャッカジャゼツソウ。

名 称 **フダンソウ**

他名等 **トウジシャ**
部位等 葉
備 考 —

他名(参考) トウチシャ（唐萵苣）
漢字表記・生薬名等 不断草（フダンソウ）、唐萵苣（トウジシャ）
Name (Romaji) FUDANSÔ
Other name (s) (Romaji) TÔJISHA
学名 *Beta vulgaris* L. var. *cicla* (L.) K. Koch
Beta cicla (L.) L.
Beta hortensis Mill.
科名 Chenopodiaceae（アカザ科）
英名 Swiss chard / spinach beet / leaf beet / chard
Part of use leaf
Note 1 —
Note 2 —
注 —

名 称 **ブッコ***

他名等 —
部位等 葉
備 考 —

他名(参考) ブチュ、ブック、ブッコノキ、ラウンド・ブック
漢字表記・生薬名等 —
Name (Romaji) BUKKO*
Other name (s) (Romaji) —
学名 *Barosma betulina* (P.J. Berg.) Bartl. et H.L. Wendl.*
Agathosma betulina (P.J. Berg.) Pillans*
科名 Rutaceae（ミカン科）
英名 buchu / bookoo / round buchu / short buchu / buku / bucco
Part of use leaf
Note 1 —
Note 2 The name of BUKKO may be derived from the general name, buchu or bookoo which are listed in the item of “English name, etc.” Their pronunciations may be BUCHU or BÛKÛ.
注 名称のブッコは一般名のbuchuあるいはbookooに由来するものと思われる。ブチュ、ブークーとも発音される。

ハ行

名　称　ブッシュティー*

他名等　—
部位等　全草
備　考　—

他名(参考)　ルイボス
漢字表記･生薬名等　—
Name(Romaji)　BUSSHUTÎ*
Other name(s) (Romaji)　—
学名　*Aspalathus linearis* (Burm. f.) R. Dahlgren*
科名　Leguminosae（マメ科）
英名　rooibos / bush tea / redbush tea / South African red tea / red tea
Part of use　whole plant
Note 1　—
Note 2　BUSSHUTÎ is the tea made from leaves of RUIBOSU. RUIBOSU is also listed in the item of "Name". Refer to RUIBOSU listed in the item of "Name".
注　ブッシュティーは別項のルイボスの葉を用いたお茶である。別項のルイボスを参照。

名　称　フッソウゲ*

他名等　—
部位等　花
備　考　—

他名(参考)　リュウキュウムクゲ（琉球木槿）、フソウゲ（扶桑花）、シュキン（朱槿）、ソウキン（桑槿）、ハイビスカス
漢字表記･生薬名等　仏桑花（ブッソウゲ）
Name(Romaji)　FUSSÔGE*
Other name(s) (Romaji)　—
学名　*Hibiscus rosa-sinensis* L.*
科名　Malvaceae（アオイ科）
英名　hibiscus / rosell / rose of China / shoe flower / China rose / Chinese hibiscus / rose-of-sharon / blacking plant / Hawaiian hibiscus
Part of use　flower
Note 1　—
Note 2　Refer to HAIBISUKASU. HAIBISUKASU is also listed in the item of "Name". FUSSÔGE is also called BUSSÔGE.
注　別項のハイビスカスを参照。フッソウゲはブッソウゲとも呼ばれる。

名　称　ブドウ*

他名等　—
部位等　茎・種子・種皮・葉・花
備　考　—

他名(参考)　—
漢字表記･生薬名等　葡萄（ブドウ）
Name(Romaji)　BUDÔ*
Other name(s) (Romaji)　—
学名　*Vitis* L.
Vitis vinifera L.*
科名　Vitaceae（ブドウ科）
英名　grape / wine grape / European grape / vine / grape vine
Part of use　vine, seed, seed coat, leaf, flower
Note 1　—
Note 2　—
注　—

名　称　ブラッククミン*

他名等　ニゲラ
部位等　全草
備　考　—

他名(参考)　クロタネソウ（黒種草）
漢字表記･生薬名等　—
Name(Romaji)　BURAKKUKUMIN*
Other name(s) (Romaji)　NIGERA
学名　*Nigella damascena* L.*（ニゲラ、クロタネソウ）
Nigella sativa L.*（ブラッククミン）
Nigella indica Roxb. ex Flem.（ブラッククミン）
科名　Ranunculaceae（キンポウゲ科）
英名　*N. damascena*：Love-in-a-mist / deril-in-a-bush / wild fennel / fennel flower
N. sativa：nigella / black cumin / small fennel / nutmeg flower / Roman coriander
Part of use　whole plant
Note 1　—
Note 2　BURAKKUKUMIN and NIGERA written in the item of "Other names" are different species.
注　ブラッククミンと「他名等」のニゲラは別種。

名　称　**ブラックコホッシュ***

他名等　ラケモサ
部位等　全草
備　考　—

他名(参考)　アメリカショウマ（アメリカ升麻）
漢字表記・生薬名等　—
Name (Romaji)　BURAKKUKOHOSSHU*
Other name(s) (Romaji)　RAKEMOSA
学名　*Cimicifuga racemosa* (L.) Nutt.*
Actaea racemosa (Nutt.) L.*
Cimicifuga racemosa (L.) Nutt. var. *cordifolia* (Pursh) A. Gray
Cimicifuga cordifolia Pursh
科名　Ranunculaceae（キンポウゲ科）
英名　black cohosh / black bugbane / black snakeroot / rheumatism weed / fairly canndle
Part of use　whole plant
Note 1　—
Note 2　—
注　—

名　称　**ブラックジンジャー**

他名等　Kaempferia parviflora
部位等　根茎
備　考　—

他名(参考)　クロショウガ（黒生姜）、クロウコン（黒鬱金）、クラチャイ・ダム
漢字表記・生薬名等　—
Name (Romaji)　BURAKKUJINJÂ
Other name(s) (Romaji)　—
学名　*Kaempferia parviflora* Wall. ex Baker
Kaempferia rubromarginata (S.Q. Tong) R.J. Searle
Stahlianthus rubromarginatus S.Q. Tong
科名　Zingiberaceae（ショウガ科）
英名　black galingale / krachaidam / krachaidum / kra chai dam / krachai dam
Part of use　rhizome
Note 1　—
Note 2　—
注　—

名　称　**ブラックプラム***

他名等　ポルトガルプラム／パープルプラム
部位等　果実
備　考　—

他名(参考)　—
漢字表記・生薬名等　—
Name (Romaji)　BURAKKUPURAMU*
Other name(s) (Romaji)　PORUTOGARUPURAMU／PÂPURUPURAMU
学名　*Syzygium cumini* (L.) Skeels*
Syzygium jambolana (Lam.) DC.*
Eugenia cumini (L.) Druce
Eugenia jambolana Lam.*
Eugenia obtusifolia Roxb.
Myrtus cumini L.
科名　Myrtaceae（フトモモ科）
英名　black plum / purple plum / Java plum / jambolan plum / jambolan / jambolang / Portugues plum / jambool / jambul
Part of use　fruit
Note 1　—
Note 2　BURAKKUPURAMU is identical with MURASAKIFUTOMOMO. MURASAKIFUTOMOMO is also listed in the item of "Name".
注　ブラックプラムと別項のムラサキフトモモは同一。但し、「部位等」の記載が異なっている。

名　称　**ブラックベリー***

他名等　—
部位等　果実
備　考　—

他名(参考)　北米、ヨーロッパ原産の多くのキイチゴ属の種が、ブラックベリーの名前で呼ばれる。
漢字表記・生薬名等　—
Name (Romaji)　BURAKKUBERÎ*
Other name(s) (Romaji)　—
学名　*Rubus fruticosus* L.*（セイヨウヤブイチゴ）
Rubus laciniatus Willd.（キレハブラックベリー）
Rubus ulmiformis Schott
Rubus allegheniensis T.C. Porter（クロミキイチゴ）
Rubus argutus Link（オニクロイチゴ）
Rubus ursinus Cham. et Schlecht.（クロイチゴ）
科名　Rosaceae（バラ科）
英名　blackberry
Part of use　fruit
Note 1　—
Note 2　Many species are included in BURAKKUBERÎ.

Therefore, scientific names of representative species are described here. *Rubus fruticosus* is also listed as a scientific name of SEIYÔKIICHIGO.
注　ブラックベリーは多種あるため、本項では代表的な種の学名をあげた。*Rubus fruticosus*は別項のセイヨウキイチゴの学名としても記載されている。

名　称　ブラックルート*
他名等　アメリカクガイソウ
部位等　全草
備　考　—

他名(参考)　—
漢字表記・生薬名等　アメリカ九蓋草(アメリカクガイソウ)
Name (Romaji)　BURAKKURÛTO*
Other name (s) (Romaji)　AMERIKAKUGAISÔ
学名　*Veronicastrum virginicum* (L.) Farw.*
Leptandra virginica (L.) Nutt.*
Veronica virginica L.
科名　Plantaginaceae (オオバコ科 (以前はゴマノハグサ科))
英名　black root / blackroot / culver's root / culver's physic
Part of use　whole plant
Note 1　—
Note 2　—
注　—

名　称　フランスカイガンショウ*
他名等　オニマツ／カイガンショウ
部位等　樹皮・樹皮エキス
備　考　—

他名(参考)　カイガンマツ (海岸松)、フツコクカイガンショウ (仏国海岸松)
漢字表記・生薬名等　仏国海岸松 (フランスカイガンショウ)、仏蘭西海岸松 (フランスカイガンショウ)、鬼松 (オニマツ)、海岸松 (カイガンショウ)
Name (Romaji)　FURANSUKAIGANSHÔ*
Other name (s) (Romaji)　ONIMATSU／KAIGANSHÔ
学名　*Pinus pinaster* Ait.*
Pinus maritima Poir.*
科名　Pinaceae (マツ科)
英名　maritime pine / cluster pine
Part of use　bark, bark extract
Note 1　—
Note 2　—
注　—

名　称　プランタゴ・オバタ*
他名等　サイリウム・ハスク
部位等　種子・種皮
備　考　—

他名(参考)　インドオオバコ (印度大葉子)
漢字表記・生薬名等　—
Name (Romaji)　PURANTAGO・OBATA*
Other name (s) (Romaji)　SAIRIUMU・HASUKU
学名　*Plantago ovata* Forssk.* (プランタゴ・オバタ)
Plantago ispaghula Roxb. ex Fleming* (プランタゴ・オバタ)
Plantago psyllium L.* (エダウチオオバコ)
科名　Plantaginaceae (オオバコ科)
英名　Indian plantain / psyllium husk / blond psyllium / Indian psyllium / ispaghula / ipsagol / sand plantain
Part of use　seed, seed coat
Note 1　—
Note 2　—
注　—

名　称　ブリオニア*
他名等　—
部位等　全草
備　考　—

他名(参考)　—
漢字表記・生薬名等　—
Name (Romaji)　BURIONIA*
Other name (s) (Romaji)　—
学名　*Bryonia dioica* Jacq.*
Bryonia cretica L. ssp. *dioica* (Jacq.) Tutin*
科名　Cucurbitaceae (ウリ科)
英名　bryony / briony / red bryony
Part of use　whole plant
Note 1　—
Note 2　—
注　—

名　称　ブルーベリー*
他名等　—
部位等　果実
備　考　—

他名(参考)　ヌマスノキ (沼酢の木)、アメリカスノキ (アメリカ酢の木)
漢字表記・生薬名等　—

Name (Romaji)　BURÛBERÎ*
Other name (s) (Romaji)　—
学名　*Vaccinium angustifolium* Ait.*（ローブッシュ・ブルーベリー）
Vaccinium corymbosum L.*（ハイブッシュ・ブルーベリー）
Vaccinium australe Small（ハイブッシュ・ブルーベリー）
科名　Ericaceae（ツツジ科）
英名　blueberry / lowbush blueberry / highbush blueberry / giant whortleberry / late sweet blueberry / low sweet blueberry / sweet hurts / swamp blueberry / whortleberry
Part of use　fruit
Note 1　—
Note 2　—
注　—

名　称　プルット

他名等　—
部位等　葉
備　考　—

他名(参考)　コブミカン（瘤蜜柑）、スワンギ
漢字表記・生薬名等　瘤蜜柑（コブミカン）
Name (Romaji)　PURUTTO
Other name (s) (Romaji)　—
学名　*Citrus hystrix* DC.
Citrus papeda Miq.
Papeda rumphii Hassk.
科名　Rutaceae（ミカン科）
英名　leech lime / purut / Kaffir lime / Makrud lime / swangi / Mauritius papeda / Ichang lime / porcupine orange
Part of use　leaf
Note 1　—
Note 2　PURUTTO derives from the general name in the countries of origin such as Indonesia and Malaysia. The Japanese general name is KOBUMIKAN.
注　プルットはインドネシア、マレーシア等の原産地の名称であり、和名はコブミカンである。

名　称　ブンタン

他名等　ザボン／ボンタン
部位等　果実・種子
備　考　—

他名(参考)　ウチムラサキ（内紫）、ジャガタラカン、ジャボン
漢字表記・生薬名等　文旦（ブンタン）、朱欒（サボン）
Name (Romaji)　BUNTAN
Other name (s) (Romaji)　ZABON／BONTAN
学名　*Citrus grandis* (L.) Osbeck
Citrus maxima (Burm.) Merr.
科名　Rutaceae（ミカン科）
英名　pumelo / pummelo / pomelo / pommelo / pomelmous / shaddock
Part of use　fruit, seed
Note 1　—
Note 2　—
注　—

名　称　ペグアセンヤク*

他名等　—
部位等　心材の水性エキス
備　考　—

他名(参考)　アセンヤクノキ（阿仙薬木）、ペグノキ、カテキュ
漢字表記・生薬名等　芯材の濃縮物：ペグ阿仙薬（ペグアセンヤク）、樹脂：アラビアゴム
Name (Romaji)　PEGUASEN'YAKU*
Other name (s) (Romaji)　—
学名　*Acacia catechu* (L. f.) Willd.*
Mimosa catechu L. f.
科名　Leguminosae（マメ科）
英名　catechu / cutch tree / black cutch / pegu cutch
Part of use　aqueous extract of heart wood
Note 1　—
Note 2　PEGUASEN'YAKU　is not a herbal namc and it means the aqueous extract obtained from the heart wood of ASEN'YAKUNOKI.
注　ペグアセンヤクは植物名ではなくアセンヤクノキの心材から得られた水性エキスをいう。

名　称　**ヘチマ***

他名等　シカラク
部位等　果実・果実繊維・茎・葉
備　考　—

他名（参考）　—
漢字表記・生薬名等　糸瓜（ヘチマ）、成熟果実の繊維：糸瓜絡（シカラク）、果皮：糸瓜皮（シカヒ）、花：糸瓜花（シカカ）、根：糸瓜根（シカコン）、茎：糸瓜藤（シカトウ）、種子：糸瓜子（シカシ）
Name (Romaji)　HECHIMA*
Other name (s) (Romaji)　SHIKARAKU
学名　*Luffa cylindrica* (L.) M. Roem.*
Luffa aegyptiaca Mill.*
Luffa cylindrica auct. non. M.J. Roem.
Momordica cylindrica L.
Momordica luffa L.
科名　Cucurbitaceae（ウリ科）
英名　smooth loofah / luffa / sponge gourd / loofah / dishrag gourd / dishcloth gourd
Part of use　fruit, fruit fiber, stem, leaf
Note 1　—
Note 2　—
注　—

名　称　**ベニコウジ***

他名等　—
部位等　麹米
備　考　—

他名（参考）　—
漢字表記・生薬名等　紅麹（ベニコウジ）
Name (Romaji)　BENIKÔJI*
Other name (s) (Romaji)　—
学名　*Monascus purpureus* Went.*
Monascus albidus K. Sato
Monascus anka K. Sato
Monascus vini Savul. et Hulea
Monascus rubiginosus K. Sato
Monascus major K. Sato
科名　Monascaceae（ベニコウジカビ科）
英名　red yeast rice / red rice / red leaven / beni-koji (Japanese) / hung-chu / hong qu / angkak / zhitai (Chinese) / red yeast / ang-khak
Part of use　rice koji
Note 1　—
Note 2　—
注　—

名　称　**ベニバナ***

他名等　コウカ／サフラワー／ベニバナ油／Carthamus tinctorius
部位等　管状花・種子油・種子
備　考　—

他名（参考）　クレノアイ（呉藍、九礼乃阿井、紅藍）、スエツムハナ（末摘花）、カラクレナイ（韓呉藍）
漢字表記・生薬名等　紅花（ベニバナ、コウカ）
Name (Romaji)　BENIBANA*
Other name (s) (Romaji)　KÔKA／SAFURAWÂ／BENI-BANA-YU
学名　*Carthamus tinctorius* L.*
科名　Compositae（キク科）
英名　safflower / false saffron / bastard saffron / saffron thistle
Part of use　tubal flower, seed oil, seed
Note 1　—
Note 2　—
注　—

名　称　**ベニバナボロギク**

他名等　ナンヨウギク
部位等　全草
備　考　—

他名（参考）　—
漢字表記・生薬名等　紅花襤褸菊（ベニバナボロギク）、南洋菊（ナンヨウギク）
Name (Romaji)　BENIBANABOROGIKU
Other name (s) (Romaji)　NAN'YÔGIKU
学名　*Crassocephalum crepidioides* (Benth.) S. Moore
科名　Compositae（キク科）
英名　fireweed / ebolo / thickhead / redflower / ragleaf
Part of use　whole plant
Note 1　—
Note 2　—
注　—

名　称　**ペピーノ**

他名等　メロンペア／Solanum muricatum
部位等　果実
備　考　—

他名（参考）　ペピノ
漢字表記・生薬名等　—
Name (Romaji)　PEPÎNO

Other name (s) (Romaji) MERONPEA
学名 *Solanum muricatum* L'Hér. ex Ait.
科名 Solanaceae（ナス科）
英名 pepino / melon pear / melon shurub / pear melon / pepino morade / pepino dulce
Part of use fruit
Note 1 —
Note 2 —
注 —

名 称 **ヘラオオバコ***
他名等 —
部位等 全草
備 考 —

他名(参考) —
漢字表記・生薬名等 箆大葉子（ヘラオオバコ）
Name (Romaji) HERAÔBAKO*
Other name (s) (Romaji) —
学名 *Plantago lanceolata* L.*
科名 Plantaginaceae（オオバコ科）
英名 ribwort plantain / Eglish plantain / lance-leaf plantain / narrow-leaf plantain / ribgrass / buckhorn / ripplegrass
Part of use whole plant
Note 1 —
Note 2 —
注 —

名 称 **ヘリクリサム・イタリカム**
他名等 カレープラント
部位等 全草
備 考 —

他名(参考) —
漢字表記・生薬名等 —
Name (Romaji) HERIKURISAMU・ITARIKAMU
Other name (s) (Romaji) KARÊPURANTO
学名 *Helichrysum italicum* (Roth) G. Don
Helichrysum angustifolium ssp. *italicum* (Roth) Briq. et Cavill.
Gnaphalium angustifolium Lam.
Helichrysum angustifolium (Lam.) DC.
Helichrysum serotinum Boiss
科名 Compositae（キク科）
英名 curry plant / immortelle / everlasting / Helichrysum
Part of use whole plant
Note 1 —
Note 2 —
注 —

名 称 **ヘルニアリアソウ***
他名等 —
部位等 全草
備 考 —

他名(参考) コゴメビユ（治疝草）
漢字表記・生薬名等 治疝草（ココメビユ）
Name (Romaji) HERUNIARIASÔ*
Other name (s) (Romaji) —
学名 *Herniaria glabra* L.*
科名 Caryophyllaceae（ナデシコ科）
英名 rupture wort / herniary breastwort
Part of use whole plant
Note 1 —
Note 2 HERUNIARIASÔ cannot be confirmed. Therfore *Herniaria glabra* of which general name is KOGOMEBIYU is listed here. *Hernia hirsta* is also used in the purpose same as *Hernia glabra* but this herb is not listed.
注 ヘルニアリアソウは確認できない。本項では*Herniaria glabra*とした。一般名はコゴメビユである。*Herniaria hirsuta* L.も*Herniariga glabra*と同様の目的で使用されるが、本項では取り上げなかった。

名 称 **ベルノキ***
他名等 —
部位等 成熟果実
備 考 —

他名(参考) ベンガルカラタチ（ベンガル枳）、インドカラタチ（印度枳）、バエルフルーツ
漢字表記・生薬名等 —
Name (Romaji) BERUNOKI*
Other name (s) (Romaji) —
学名 *Aegle marmelos* (L.) Correa ex Roxb.*
Belou marmelos W.F. Wight
科名 Rutaceae（ミカン科）
英名 golden apple / bell tree / Bengal quince / bael fruit / stone apple / Indian bael / Bengal fruit
Part of use riped fruit
Note 1 —
Note 2 BERUNOKI is identical with INDOKARATACHI.
注 ベルノキは別項のインドカラタチと同一。

ハ行

名　称　**ヘンズ***

他名等　フジマメ
部位等　種子・種皮・根・葉・花・つる
備　考　—

他名(参考)　ビャクヘンズ(白扁豆)、ハクヘンズ(白扁豆)、センゴクマメ（千石豆)、アジマメ（味豆)
漢字表記･生薬名等　扁豆（ヘンズ)、藤豆（フジマメ)、白扁豆（ビャクヘンズ)
Name (Romaji)　HENZU*
Other name (s) (Romaji)　FUJIMAME
学名　*Dolichos lablab* L.*
Lablab purpureus (L.) Sweet*
Dolichos purpureus L.
Lablab niger Medik.
科名　Leguminosae（マメ科）
英名　Indian bean / hyacinth bean / bonavist / bonavista bean / Egyptian bean / lubia bean / seim bean / lablab bean
Part of use　seed, seed coat, root, leaf, flower, vine
Note 1　—
Note 2　FUJIMAME is also listed in the item of "Other names" of INGENMAME, but FUJIMAME and INGENMAME are different species.
注　フジマメはインゲンマメの「他名等」にも記載されているが、フジマメとインゲンマメは別種である。

名　称　**ヘンルーダ***

他名等　—
部位等　種子
備　考　—

他名(参考)　ウンコウ（芸香)、シュウソウ（臭草)、ルー(Rue)、ヘンルウダ
漢字表記･生薬名等　芸香（ウンコウ）
Name (Romaji)　HENRÛDA*
Other name (s) (Romaji)　—
学名　*Ruta graveolens* L.*
科名　Rutaceae（ミカン科）
英名　rue / common rue / herb of grace
Part of use　seed
Note 1　—
Note 2　—
注　—

名　称　**ボウシュウボク***

他名等　コウスイボク／レモンバーベナ
部位等　葉
備　考　—

他名(参考)　—
漢字表記･生薬名等　防臭木（ボウシュウボク)、香水木（コウスイボク）
Name (Romaji)　BÔSHÛBOKU*
Other name (s) (Romaji)　KÔSUIBOKU／REMONBÂBENA
学名　*Lippia citriodora* (Ort. ex Pers.) H.B.K.*
Aloysia citriodora Palau*
Aloysia triphylla (L'Hér.) Britton*
Verbena triphylla L'Hér.
Verbena citriodora (Lam.) Cav.
科名　Verbenaceae（クマツヅラ科）
英名　lemmon verbena / verbena / lemon scented verbena
Part of use　leaf
Note 1　—
Note 2　—
注　—

名　称　**ホウセンカ***

他名等　—
部位等　全草（種子を除く）
備　考　種子は「医」

他名(参考)　ツマクレナイ（爪紅)、ツマベニ（爪紅)、センシソウ（染指草)、トウコツソウ（透骨草)、ホウセン（鳳仙）
漢字表記･生薬名等　鳳仙花（ホウセンカ)、種子：急性子（キュウセイシ）
Name (Romaji)　HÔSENKA*
Other name (s) (Romaji)　—
学名　*Impatiens balsamina* L.*
科名　Balsaminaceae（ツリフネソウ科）
英名　impatiens / jewelweed / garden balsam / rose balsam / alegria / belen
Part of use　whole plant except seed
Note 1　seed：drug category
Note 2　—
注　—

名　称　**ホークウィード***

他名等　ミヤマコウゾウリナ
部位等　全草
備　考　—

他名（参考）　ケミヤマコウゾリナ（毛深山顔剃菜、毛深山髪剃菜）
漢字表記・生薬名等　深山顔剃菜（ミヤマコウゾリナ）、深山髪剃菜（ミヤマコウゾリナ）、毛深山顔剃菜（ケミヤマコウゾリナ）、毛深山髪剃菜（ケミヤマコウゾリナ）
Name（Romaji）　HÔKUWÎDO*
Other name(s)（Romaji）　MIYAMAKÔZOURINA
学名　*Hieracium pilosella* L.*（ケミヤマコウゾリナ）
Hieracium japonicum Franch. et Sav.（ミヤマコウゾリナ）
科名　Compositae（キク科）
英名　hawkweed / mouse ear hawkweed
Part of use　whole plant
Note 1　—
Note 2　HÔKUWÎDO (hawkweed) is the English name indicating the Hieracium genus. MIYAMAKÔZOURINA listed in the item of “Other names” is incorrect. The correct name is MIYAMAKÔZORINA.
注　ホークウィードはミヤマコウゾリナ属の属名を指す英語名である。「他名等」のミヤマコウゾウリナの正しい名称はミヤマコウゾリナである。

名　称　**ボケ***

他名等　—
部位等　果実
備　考　—

他名（参考）　カラボケ（唐木瓜）、カンボケ（寒木瓜）、チョウシュンボケ（長春木瓜）、ヒボケ（緋木瓜）、シロボケ（白木瓜）、ヨドボケ（淀木瓜）、モケ（母計）
漢字表記・生薬名等　木瓜（ボケ）
Name（Romaji）　BOKE*
Other name(s)（Romaji）　—
学名　*Chaenomeles speciosa* (Sweet) Nakai*
Chaenomeles cardinalis (Carriére) Nakai
Chaenomeles lagenaria (Loisel.) Koidz.*
Cydonia japonica Loisel. non (Thunb.) Pers.
Cydonia speciosa f. *eburnea* (Carriére) Hara
Malus japonica Andr.
科名　Rosaceae（バラ科）
英名　larry / moron / flowering quince / lesser flowering quince / Japanese quince
Part of use　fruit
Note 1　—
Note 2　—
注　—

名　称　**ホコウエイコン***

他名等　タンポポ
部位等　根・根茎
備　考　—

他名（参考）　セイヨウタンポポ（西洋蒲公英）
漢字表記・生薬名等　全草：蒲公英（ホコウエイ）、根：蒲公英根（ホコウエイコン）
Name（Romaji）　HOKÔEIKON*
Other name(s)（Romaji）　TANPOPO
学名　*Taraxacum* Weber（タンポポ属）
Taraxacum platycarpum Dahlst.（タンポポ）
Taraxacum japonicum Koidz.（カンサイタンポポ）
Taraxacum officinale Weber ex F.H. Wigg.*（セイヨウタンポポ）
Taraxacum vulgare (Lam.) Schrank*（セイヨウタンポポ）
Taraxacum dens-leonis Desf.*（エゾタンポポ）
科名　Compositae（キク科）
英名　dandelion / lion's tooth / Chinese dandelion
Part of use　root, rhizome
Note 1　—
Note 2　SEIYÔTANPOPO is icluded in here. Refer to SEIYÔTANPOPO listed in the item of “Name”.
注　セイヨウタンポポも学名の項に記載した。別項の西洋タンポポを参照。

名　称　**ホコツシ***

他名等　オランダビユ
部位等　果実
備　考　—

他名（参考）　ハコシ（破故紙）、ハゴシ（婆固脂）
漢字表記・生薬名等　補骨脂（ホコツシ）、和蘭莧（オランダビユ）
Name（Romaji）　HOKOTSUSHI*
Other name(s)（Romaji）　ORANDABIYU
学名　*Psoralea corylifolia* L.*
Cullen corylifolia (L.) Medik.*
科名　Leguminosae（マメ科）
英名　bu gu zhi / psoralea / Malaytea scurfpea / scurfy pea
Part of use　fruit

Note 1　—
Note 2　—
注　—

名　称　ボスウェリア・セラータ*

他名等　インド乳香／Boswellia serrata
部位等　樹脂
備　考　その他のボスウェリア属の全木は「医」

他名(参考)　—
漢字表記・生薬名等　乳香樹（ニュウコウジュ）
Name(Romaji)　BOSUWERIA・SERÂTA*
Other name(s) (Romaji)　INDONYÛKÔ
学名　*Boswellia serrata* Roxb.*
科名　Burseraceae（カンラン科）
英名　Indian olibanum / Indian frankincense / frankincense
Part of use　resin
Note 1　whole tree of *Boswellia* Roxb. other than *Boswellia serrata*：drug category
Note 2　—
注　—

名　称　ボダイジュ*

他名等　ナツボダイジュ／フユボダイジュ／ボダイジュミツ
部位等　果実・花・花の蜜
備　考　—

他名(参考)　フユボダイジュ（冬菩提樹）：コバノシナノキ（小葉菩提樹）
ナツボダイジュ（夏菩提樹）：オオバボダイジュ（大葉菩提樹）
漢字表記・生薬名等　菩提樹（ボダイジュ）、冬菩提樹（フユボダイジュ）、夏菩提樹（ナツボダイジュ）
Name(Romaji)　BODAIJU*
Other name(s) (Romaji)　NATSUBODAIJU／FUYUBODAIJU／BODAIJUMITSU
学名　*Tilia miqueliana* Maxim.（ボダイジュ）
Tilia platyphyllos Scop.*（ナツボダイジュ）
Tilia grandifolia Ehrh.（ナツボダイジュ）
Tilia cordata Mill.*（フユボダイジュ）
Tilia ulmifolia Scop.（フユボダイジュ）
Tilia parvifolia Ehrh.（フユボダイジュ）
科名　Tiliaceae（シナノキ科）
英名　*T. miqueliana*：linden / lime tree
T. cordata：small leaved European linden / small leaf lime tree
T. grandifolia：large leaved linden
Part of use　fruit, flower, necter
Note 1　—
Note 2　—
注　—

名　称　ボタン*

他名等　—
部位等　葉・花
備　考　根皮は「医」

他名(参考)　フウキソウ（富貴草）、カオウ（花王）、ヒャッカオウ（百花王）、フカミグサ（深見草）、ナトリソウ（名取草）、ハツカグサ（二十日草、廿日草）、ヨロイグサ（鎧草）、テンコウコクショク（天香国色）、ボウタン（牡丹）、ボウタングサ（牡丹草）
漢字表記・生薬名等　牡丹（ボタン）
Name(Romaji)　BOTAN*
Other name(s) (Romaji)　—
学名　*Paeonia suffruticosa* Andr.*
Paeonia moutan Sims*
Paeonia arborea Donn ex K. Koch
科名　Paeoniaceae（ボタン科）
英名　tree peony / Japanese tree peony / Moutan peony / mountain peony
Part of use　leaf, flower
Note 1　root bark：drug category
Note 2　—
注　—

名　称　ボタンボウフウ

他名等　Peucedanum japonicum
部位等　茎・葉・根・根茎
備　考　—

他名(参考)　チョウメイソウ（長命草）、サクナ、チョーミーグサ（沖縄：長命草）、ナガイキグサ（長生き草）、ショクヨウボウフウ（食用防風）
漢字表記・生薬名等　牡丹防風（ボタンボウフウ）
Name(Romaji)　BOTANBÔFÛ
Other name(s) (Romaji)　—
学名　*Peucedanum japonicum* Thunb.
科名　Umbelliferae（セリ科）
英名　—
Part of use　stem, leaf, root, rhizome
Note 1　—
Note 2　—
注　—

名　称　**ホップ***

他名等　ヒシュカ
部位等　球果
備　考　—

他名(参考)　セイヨウカラハナソウ（西洋唐花草）
漢字表記･生薬名等　忽布（ホップ）、啤酒花（ヒシュカ）
Name (Romaji)　HOPPU*
Other name (s) (Romaji)　HISHUKA
学名　*Humulus lupulus* L.*
科名　Cannabidaceae（アサ科）
英名　hop / hops / European hop / common hop
Part of use　cone
Note 1　—
Note 2　—
注　—

名　称　**ホホバ***

他名等　—
部位等　種子・種子油
備　考　—

他名(参考)　—
漢字表記･生薬名等　—
Name (Romaji)　HOHOBA*
Other name (s) (Romaji)　—
学名　*Simmondsia chinensis* (Link) C.K. Schneid.*
Simmondsia californica Nutt.*
科名　Simmondsiaceae（シモンジア科）
英名　jojoba / goat nut
Part of use　seed, seed oil
Note 1　—
Note 2　—
注　—

名　称　**ポリポディウム・レウコトモス**

他名等　Polypodium leucotomos
部位等　葉・茎
備　考　—

他名(参考)　ダイオウウラボシ（大王裏星）
漢字表記･生薬名等　—
Name (Romaji)　PORIPODIUMU・REUKOTOMOSU
Other name (s) (Romaji)　—
学名　*Polypodium leucotomos*
Polypodium leucatomos Poir.
Polypodium aureum L.
Phlebodium aureum (L.) J. Sm.
Phlebodium decumanum (Willd.) J. Sm.
科名　Polypodiaceae（ウラボシ科）
英名　golden polypody / golden serpent / cabbage palm fern / gold foot fern / hare foot fern / rabbit foot fern
Part of use　leaf, stem
Note 1　—
Note 2　The scientific name is *Polypodium leucatomos* Poir. according to the International Plant Name Index (IPNI).
注　The international Plant Name Index (IPNI) によれば学名は*Polypodium leucatomos* Poir. である。

名　称　**ボルド***

他名等　—
部位等　葉
備　考　—

他名(参考)　—
漢字表記･生薬名等　—
Name (Romaji)　BORUDO*
Other name (s) (Romaji)　—
学名　*Peumus boldus* Molina*
Boldu boldus (Mol.) Lyons
科名　Monimiaceae（モニミア科）
英名　boldo
Part of use　leaf
Note 1　—
Note 2　—
注　—

名　称　**ボロホ**

他名等　—
部位等　果実・果皮・種子
備　考　—

他名(参考)　—
漢字表記･生薬名等　—
Name (Romaji)　BOROHO
Other name (s) (Romaji)　—
学名　*Borojoa patinoi* Cuatrec.
科名　Rubiaceae（アカネ科）
英名　borojó / burijo / burojó
Part of use　fruit, pericarp, seed
Note 1　—
Note 2　—
注　—

名　称　**ホワイトセージ***

他名等　—
部位等　葉
備　考　—

他名(参考)　—
漢字表記・生薬名等　—
Name(Romaji)　HOWAITOSÊJI*
Other name(s) (Romaji)　—
学名　*Salvia apiana* Jeps.*
科名　Labiatae（シソ科）
英名　white sage / California white sage / greasewood
Part of use　leaf
Note 1　—
Note 2　—
注　—

マ行

名　称　**マアザミ**

他名等　—
部位等　葉
備　考　—

他名(参考)　—
漢字表記・生薬名等　真薊（マアザミ）
Name(Romaji)　MAAZAMI
Other name(s) (Romaji)　—
学名　*Cirsium yezoense*（Maxim.）Makino
科名　Compositae（キク科）
英名　—
Part of use　leaf
Note 1　—
Note 2　—
注　—

名　称　**マーシュ**

他名等　—
部位等　全草
備　考　—

他名(参考)　ノヂシャ（野苣）
漢字表記・生薬名等　（マーシュ：mâche）
Name(Romaji)　MÂSHU
Other name(s) (Romaji)　—
学名　*Valerianella locusta*（L.）Laterr.
Valerianella olitoria（L.）Pollich
科名　Valerianaceae（オミナエシ科）
英名　lamb's lettuce / corn salad / common corn salad / European corn salad
Part of use　whole plant
Note 1　—
Note 2　—
注　—

名　称　**マイタケ***

他名等　シロマイタケ
部位等　子実体
備　考　—

他名(参考)　—
漢字表記・生薬名等　舞茸（マイタケ）、白舞茸（シロマイタケ）
Name(Romaji)　MAITAKE*
Other name(s) (Romaji)　SHIROMAITAKE
学名　*Grifola frondosa* (Dicks.：Fr.) S.F. Gray*（マイタケ）
Polyporus frondosus（Dicks.：Fr.）Fr.*（マイタケ）
Cladodendron frondosus（Dicks.：Fr.）Lázaro Ibiza（マイタケ）
Grifola albicans Imaz.（シロマイタケ）
科名　Polyporaceae（サルノコシカケ科）
英名　grifola frondosa / maitake mashrooms / dancing mushroom / hen of the woods / ram's head / sheep's head
Part of use　fruit body
Note 1　—
Note 2　—
注　—

名　称　**マイテン**

他名等　—
部位等　全草
備　考　—

他名(参考)　—
漢字表記・生薬名等　—
Name(Romaji)　MAITEN
Other name(s) (Romaji)　—
学名　*Maytenus boaria* Mol.
Maytenus chilensis DC.
Celastrus maytenus Willd.
科名　Celastraceae（ニシキギ科）
英名　mayten / mayten tree

Part of use　whole plant
Note 1　—
Note 2　—
注　—

名　称　**マカ***

他名等　マカマカ
部位等　根
備　考　—

他名（参考）　—
漢字表記・生薬名等　—
Name (Romaji)　MAKA*
Other name(s) (Romaji)　MAKAMAKA
学名　*Lepidium meyenii* Walp.*
　　Lepidium peruvianum G. Chacón de Popovici
科名　Cruciferae（アブラナ科）
英名　Peruvian ginseng / maca / macamaca
Part of use　root
Note 1　—
Note 2　—
注　—

名　称　**マキバクサギ**

他名等　タイセイヨウ／ロヘンソウ
部位等　枝・葉
備　考　—

他名（参考）　—
漢字表記・生薬名等　マキバ臭木（マキバクサギ）、大青（タイセイ）、路辺青（ロヘンセイ）
Name (Romaji)　MAKIBAKUSAGI
Other name(s) (Romaji)　TAISEIYÔ／ROHENSÔ
学名　*Clerodendrum cyrtophyllum* Turcz.
科名　Verbenaceae（クマツヅラ科）
英名　—
Part of use　branch, leaf
Note 1　—
Note 2　ROHENSÔ listed in the item of "Other names" is incorrect. The correct name is ROHENSEI.
注　「他名等」のロヘンソウの正しい名称はロヘンセイ（路辺青）である。

名　称　**マコモ**

他名等　—
部位等　葉
備　考　—

他名（参考）　—
漢字表記・生薬名等　菰（マコモ）
Name (Romaji)　MAKOMO
Other name(s) (Romaji)　—
学名　*Zizania latifolia* (Griseb.) Turcz. ex Stapf
　　Zizania caduciflora (Turcz.) Hand.-Mazz.
　　Zizania aquatica auct. japon., non L.
科名　Gramineae（イネ科）
英名　Indian wild rice / Manchurian water rice / Manchurian wild rice / Manchurian zizania / water bamboo
Part of use　leaf
Note 1　—
Note 2　—
注　—

名　称　**マチコ***

他名等　—
部位等　茎・葉
備　考　—

他名（参考）　—
漢字表記・生薬名等　—
Name (Romaji)　MACHIKO*
Other name(s) (Romaji)　—
学名　*Piper aduncum* L.*
　　Piper angustifolium Ruiz et Pav.
　　Piper celtidifolium Kunth
　　Piper elongatum Vahl
科名　Piperaceae（コショウ科）
英名　matico / spiked pepper
Part of use　stem, leaf
Note 1　—
Note 2　MACHIKO (matico) is the Spanish general name and the English general name is "spiked pepper".
注　マチコはスペイン語の一般名（matico）であり、英語名はspiked pepperである。

名　称　**マツ**

他名等　**カイショウシ／ショウボクヒ／マツノミ／マツバ／マツヤニ**
部位等　殻・殻皮・種子・樹脂・葉・樹皮
備　考　—

他名（参考）　—
漢字表記・生薬名等　松（マツ）、海松子（カイショウシ）、松木皮（ショウボクヒ）、松の実（マツノミ）、松葉（ショウヨウ、マツバ）、松脂（ショウシ、マツヤニ）
Name (Romaji)　MATSU
Other name (s) (Romaji)　KAISHÔSHI／SHÔBOKUHI／MATSUNOMI／MATSUBA／MATSUYANI
学名　*Pinus* L.
科名　Pinaceae（マツ科）
英名　pine / pine tree
Part of use　theca, rhytidome, seed, resin, leaf, bark
Note 1　—
Note 2　—
注　—

名　称　**マツタケ**

他名等　—
部位等　子実体
備　考　—

他名（参考）　—
漢字表記・生薬名等　松茸（マツタケ）
Name (Romaji)　MATSUTAKE
Other name (s) (Romaji)　—
学名　*Tricholoma matsutake* (S. Ito et S. Imai) Singer
科名　Tricholomataceae（キシメジ科）
英名　matsutake mushroom
Part of use　fruit body
Note 1　—
Note 2　—
注　—

名　称　**マテ***

他名等　—
部位等　葉
備　考　—

他名（参考）　—
漢字表記・生薬名等　マテ茶（マテチャ）
Name (Romaji)　MATE*
Other name (s) (Romaji)　—
学名　*Ilex paraguariensis* A. St.-Hil.*
科名　Aquifoliaceae（モチノキ科）
英名　mate / maté / Brazilian tea / yarba maté / Paraguay tea / Paraguayan tea
Part of use　leaf
Note 1　—
Note 2　—
注　—

名　称　**マヨラナ***

他名等　**ハナハッカ／マジョラム**
部位等　葉
備　考　—

他名（参考）　マージョラム
漢字表記・生薬名等　花薄荷（ハナハッカ）
Name (Romaji)　MAYORANA*
Other name (s) (Romaji)　HANAHAKKA／MAJORAMU
学名　*Origanum majorana* L.*
Origanum dubium Boiss.
Majorana hortensis Moench
科名　Labiatae（シソ科）
英名　origanum / sweet marjoram
Part of use　leaf
Note 1　—
Note 2　—
注　—

名　称　**マリアアザミ***

他名等　**オオアザミ**
部位等　全草
備　考　—

他名（参考）　—
漢字表記・生薬名等　マリア薊（マリアアザミ）、大薊（オオアザミ）
Name (Romaji)　MARIAAZAMI*
Other name (s) (Romaji)　ÔAZAMI
学名　*Silybum marianum* (L.) Gaertn.*
科名　Compositae（キク科）
英名　lady's thistle / milk thistle / blessed milk thistle / blessed thistle / our lady's milk thistle / St. Mary's thistle / bull thistle / gundagai thistle / variegated thistle / Mary's thistle / holy thistle
Part of use　whole plant
Note 1　—
Note 2　—

注　—

名　称　**マルバハッカ***

他名等　ニガハッカ
部位等　全草
備　考　—

他名(参考)　—
漢字表記･生薬名等　丸葉薄荷（マルバハッカ）、苦薄荷（ニガハッカ）
Name (Romaji)　MARUBAHAKKA*
Other name (s) (Romaji)　NIGAHAKKA
学名　*Marrubium vulgare* L.*
科名　Labiatae（シソ科）
英名　horehound / common horehound / white horehound
Part of use　whole plant
Note 1　—
Note 2　—
注　—

名　称　**マルベリー***

他名等　—
部位等　小梢・葉
備　考　—

他名(参考)　*M. alba*：マグワ（真桑）、トウグワ（唐桑）、唐山桑（カラヤマグワ）、シログワ（白桑）
M. bombycis：ヤマグワ（山桑）、クワ（桑）、ノグワ（野桑）
漢字表記･生薬名等　葉：桑葉（ソウヨウ）、根：桑白皮（ソウハクヒ）、桑根（ソウコン）、実：桑椹子（ソウジンシ）
Name (Romaji)　MARUBERÎ*
Other name (s) (Romaji)　—
学名　*Morus alba* L.*（マグワ、カラヤマグワ）
Morus bombycis Koidz.（ヤマグワ、クワ）
Morus alba L. var. *stylosa* Bur.（ヤマグワ、クワ）
Morus japonica Bailey non. Sieb.（ヤマグワ、クワ）
Morus australis Poir.（ヤマグワ、クワ）
科名　Moraceae（クワ科）
英名　*M. Alba*：white mulberry / Russian mulberry / silkworm mulberry
M. bombycis：shima guwa / yama guwa / wild Korean mulberry
Part of use　twing, leaf
Note 1　—
Note 2　Refer to KUWA. KUWA is also listed in the item of "Name".
注　別項のクワを参照。

名　称　**マンゴー***

他名等　—
部位等　果実・葉
備　考　—

他名(参考)　—
漢字表記･生薬名等　檬果（モウカ）、杧果・芒果（ボウカ）、菴羅（アンラ）、菴摩羅（アンマラ）
Name (Romaji)　MANGÔ*
Other name (s) (Romaji)　—
学名　*Mangifera indica* L.*
Mangifera mekongensis anon.
科名　Anacardiaceae（ウルシ科）
英名　mango / common mango / Indian mango
Part of use　fruit, leaf
Note 1　—
Note 2　—
注　—

名　称　**マンゴージンジャー***

他名等　Curcuma amada
部位等　根茎
備　考　—

他名(参考)　—
漢字表記･生薬名等　—
Name (Romaji)　MANGÔJINJÂ*
Other name (s) (Romaji)　—
学名　*Curcuma amada* Roxb.*
科名　Zingiberaceae（ショウガ科）
英名　mango ginger
Part of use　rhizome
Note 1　—
Note 2　—
注　—

名　称　**マンゴスチン***

他名等　Garcinia mangostana
部位等　果皮
備　考　—

他名(参考)　—
漢字表記･生薬名等　—

Name (Romaji)　MANGOSUCHIN*
Other name (s) (Romaji)　—
学名　*Garcinia mangostana* L.*
科名　Guttiferae（オトギリソウ科）
英名　mangsteen / mangosteen / purple mangosteen / king's fruit / mangostan
Part of use　pericarp
Note 1　—
Note 2　—
注　—

名　称　マンダリン*

他名等　—
部位等　果実
備　考　—

他名（参考）　ポンカン（椪柑、凸柑）
漢字表記・生薬名等　椪柑・凸柑（ポンカン）
Name (Romaji)　MANDARIN*
Other name (s) (Romaji)　—
学名　*Citrus reticulata* Blanco*
科名　Rutaceae（ミカン科）
英名　tangerine / tangerine orange / mandarin / mandarin orange / mandarine orange / red tangeline / Satsuma orange / culate mandarin / Swatow orange
Part of use　fruit
Note 1　—
Note 2　—
注　—

名　称　ミソハギ

他名等　—
部位等　全草
備　考　—

他名（参考）　ボンバナ（盆花）、ショウリョウバナ（精霊花）
漢字表記・生薬名等　禊萩（ミソハギ）
Name (Romaji)　MISOHAGI
Other name (s) (Romaji)　—
学名　*Lythrum anceps* (Koehne) Makino
Lythrum salicaria L. ssp. *anceps* (Kohene) H. Hara
Lythrum virgatum Miq. non L.
科名　Lythraceae（ミソハギ科）
英名　spiked loosestrife / purple loosestrife / black blood / miso-hagi / bon-bana
Part of use　whole plant
Note 1　—
Note 2　—
注　—

名　称　ミチヤナギ*

他名等　—
部位等　全草
備　考　—

他名（参考）　—
漢字表記・生薬名等　路柳・道柳（ミチヤナギ）、庭柳（ニワヤナギ）、扁蓄（ヘンチク、ニワヤナギ）
Name (Romaji)　MICHIYANAGI*
Other name (s) (Romaji)　—
学名　*Polygonum aviculare* L.*
科名　Polygonaceae（タデ科）
英名　knotgrass / knotweed / doorweed / English knotgrass / common knotgrass / erect knotgrass / prostrate knotweed
Part of use　whole plant
Note 1　—
Note 2　—
注　—

名　称　ミモザアカシア

他名等　—
部位等　全草
備　考　—

他名（参考）　フサアカシア（房アカシア）
漢字表記・生薬名等　—
Name (Romaji)　MIMOZAAKASHIA
Other name (s) (Romaji)　—
学名　*Acacia dealbata* Link
Acacia decurrens (Wendl. f.) Willd. var. *dealbata* (Link) F.J. Muell.
Acacia decurrens var. *dealbata* (Link) F.J. Muell.
科名　Leguminosae（マメ科）
英名　silver wattle / mimosa
Part of use　whole plant
Note 1　—
Note 2　—
注　—

名　称　**ミヤコグサ**

他名等　—
部位等　全草
備　考　—

他名(参考)　—
漢字表記・生薬名等　都草（ミヤコグサ）
Name(Romaji)　MIYAKOGUSA
Other name(s) (Romaji)　—
学名　*Lotus corniculatus* L. var. *japonicus* Regel
科名　Leguminosae（マメ科）
英名　bird's-foot-trefoil / common bird's-foot-trefoil
Part of use　whole plant
Note 1　—
Note 2　—
注　—

名　称　**ミント**

他名等　—
部位等　葉
備　考　—

他名(参考)　ハッカ属
漢字表記・生薬名等　—
Name(Romaji)　MINTO
Other name(s) (Romaji)　—
学名　*Mentha* L.
科名　Labiatae（シソ科）
英名　mint
Part of use　leaf
Note 1　—
Note 2　SEIYÔHAKKA and HAKKA are included in MINTO (*Mentha* L.) but the parts of use are different among these herbs. SEIYÔHAKKA and HAKKA are also listed in the item of "Name".
注　別項のセイヨウハッカ及びハッカはミント（ハッカ属）に含まれる。但し、「部位等」の記載が異なっている。

名　称　**ムイラプアマ***

他名等　—
部位等　根以外
備　考　根は「医」

他名(参考)　—
漢字表記・生薬名等　—
Name(Romaji)　MUIRAPUAMA*
Other name(s) (Romaji)　—
学名　*Ptychopetalum olacoides* Benth.*
Ptychopetalum uncinatum Anselmino*
科名　Olacaceae（ボロボロノキ科）
英名　muira puama
Part of use　whole plant except root
Note 1　root：drug category
Note 2　Two kinds of trees called MUIRAPUAMA exist in Brazil. The tree known medicinal use, etc. is *Ptycopetalum olacoides* Benth.
Liriosma ovata Miers is another species called MUIRAPUAMA but this is completely different from *P. olacoides* including its components.
注　ムイラプアマと呼ばれるブラジル原産の樹木が２種類ある。薬用等の目的で使用されるのは*Ptycopetalum olacoides* Benth.である。
Liriosma ovata Miersもムイラプアマと呼ばれるが、成分も含めて*P. olacoides*とは全く異なる。

名　称　**ムカンシ**

他名等　ムクロジ
部位等　果肉
備　考　—

他名(参考)　—
漢字表記・生薬名等　無患子（ムカンシ、ムクロジ）、無久呂之（ムクロジ）
Name(Romaji)　MUKANSHI
Other name(s) (Romaji)　MUKUROJI
学名　*Sapindus mukorossi* Gaertn.
科名　Sapindaceae（ムクロジ科）
英名　Chinese soapberry / Kashmir soapberry / mukuroji / North Indian soapnut / reetha / washing nut / soapnut tree
Part of use　sarcocarp
Note 1　—
Note 2　MUKANSHI is the name of traditional Chinese medicine. The Japanese name is MUKURO or MUKUROJI.
注　ムカンシは中薬名である。和名はムクロ、あるいはムクロジである。

名　称　**ムラサキセンブリ**

他名等　—
部位等　全草
備　考　—

他名(参考)　—
漢字表記・生薬名等　紫千振（ムラサキセンブリ）

Name (Romaji)　MURASAKISENBURI
Other name (s) (Romaji)　—
学名　*Swertia pseudochinensis* H. Hara
　Ophelia pseudochinensis (Hara) Toyokuni
科名　Gentianaceae（リンドウ科）
英名　—
Part of use　whole plant
Note 1　—
Note 2　—
注　—

名　称　ムラサキフトモモ*

他名等　ジャンブル／Syzygium cumini
部位等　種子
備　考　—

他名(参考)　ヨウミャクアデク（葉脈アデク）、メシゲラック、ムレザキフトモモ
漢字表記・生薬名等　紫蒲桃（ムラサキフトモモ）
Name (Romaji)　MURASAKIFUTOMOMO*
Other name (s) (Romaji)　JANBURU
学名　*Syzygium cumini* (L.) Skeels*
　Syzygium jambolana (Lam.) DC.*
　Eugenia cumini (L.) Druce
　Eugenia jambolana Lam.*
　Eugenia obtusifolia Roxb.
　Myrtus cumini L.
科名　Mitaceae（フトモモ科）
英名　Java plum / jambolan / jaman / jambolan plum / jambolang / black plum / jambool / jambu
Part of use　seed
Note 1　—
Note 2　MURASAKIFUTOMOMO is identical with BURAKKUPURAMU, but parts of use are different each other. BURAKKUPURAMU is also listed in the item of "Name".
注　ムラサキフトモモは別項のブラックプラムと同一。但し、「部位等」の記載が異なっている。

名　称　メグサハッカ*

他名等　—
部位等　葉
備　考　—

他名(参考)　ペニーローヤルミント、フリーミント（flea mint）
漢字表記・生薬名等　目草薄荷（メグサハッカ）
Name (Romaji)　MEGUSAHAKKA*
Other name (s) (Romaji)　—
学名　*Mentha pulegium* L.*
科名　Labiatae（シソ科）
英名　pennyroyal / European pennyroyal / pudding grass / flea mint
Part of use　leaf
Note 1　—
Note 2　—
注　—

名　称　メグスリノキ

他名等　—
部位等　枝・樹皮・葉
備　考　—

他名(参考)　チョウジャノキ（長者木）、センリガンノキ（千里眼木）、ミツバナ（三ツ花）、ミツバハナ（三葉花木）
漢字表記・生薬名等　目薬木（メグスリノキ）
Name (Romaji)　MEGUSURINOKI
Other name (s) (Romaji)　—
学名　*Acer nikoense* (Miq.) Maxim.
　Acer maximowiczianum Miq.
科名　Aceraceae（カエデ科）
英名　Nikko maple
Part of use　branch, bark, leaf
Note 1　—
Note 2　—
注　—

名　称　メシマコブ

他名等　—
部位等　子実体・菌糸体
備　考　—

他名(参考)　ソウオウ（桑黄）
漢字表記・生薬名等　女島瘤（メシマコブ）
Name (Romaji)　MESHIMAKOBU
Other name (s) (Romaji)　—
学名　*Phellinus linteus* (Berk. et M.A. Curtis) Teng
　Inonotus linteus (Berk. et M.A. Curtis) Teixeira
科名　Hymenochaetaceae（タバコウロコタケ科）
英名　meshimacobu (Japanese) / song gen (Chinese) / sanghwang (Korean)
Part of use　fruit body, mycelium
Note 1　—
Note 2　—
注　—

名　称　**メナモミ**

他名等　キケン／キレンソウ／ツクシメナモミ／Siegesbeckia pubescens／Siegesbeckia orientalis
部位等　茎・葉
備　考　—

他名（参考）　—
漢字表記・生薬名等　豨薟揉み・豨生揉（メナモミ）、豨薟（キレン）
Name (Romaji)　MENAMOMI
Other name (s) (Romaji)　KIKEN／KIRENSÔ／TSUKUSHIMENAMOMI
学名　*Siegesbeckia pubescens* (Makino) Makino
Siegesbeckia orientalis L. ssp. *pubescens* (Makino) Kitam ex H. Koyama
科名　Compositae（キク科）
英名　siegesbeckia / holy herb / common St. Paul's wort
Part of use　stem, leaf
Note 1　—
Note 2　—
注　—

名　称　**メボウキ***

他名等　アルファバーカ／バジリコ／バジル
部位等　全草
備　考　—

他名（参考）　アルファバカ（alfavaca）
漢字表記・生薬名等　目箒（メボウキ）、全草：羅勒（ラロク）、佩蘭（ハイラン）、果実：羅勒子（ラロクシ）
Name (Romaji)　MEBÔKI*
Other name (s) (Romaji)　ARUFABÂKA／BAJIRIKO／BAJIRU
学名　*Ocimum basilicum* L.*
Ocimum basilicum var. *glabratum* Benth.
Ocimum basilicum var. *majus* Benth.
科名　Labiatae（シソ科）
英名　common basil / basil / garden basil / sweet basil
Part of use　whole plant
Note 1　—
Note 2　—
注　—

名　称　**メマツヨイグサ***

他名等　オオマツヨイグサ／マツヨイグサ
部位等　全草
備　考　—

他名（参考）　ツキミソウ（月見草）、ヨイマチグサ（宵待草）
漢字表記・生薬名等　雌待宵草（メマツヨイグサ）、大待宵草（オオマツヨイグサ）、待宵草（マツヨイグサ）
Name (Romaji)　MEMATSUYOIGUSA*
Other name (s) (Romaji)　ÔMATSUYOIGUSA／MATSUYOIGUSA
学名　*Oenothera biennis* L.*（メマツヨイグサ）
Onagra biennis (L.) Scop.（メマツヨイグサ）
Oenothera erythrosepala Borb.（オオマツヨイグサ）
Oenothera lamarckiana de Vries non Ser.（オオマツヨイグサ）
Oenothera stricta Ledeb. ex Link（マツヨイグサ）
Oenothera odorata Jacq.（マツヨイグサ）
科名　Onagraceae（アカバナ科）
英名　*O. biennis*：evening primrose / common evening primrose / German rampion
O. erythrosepala：large flowered evening primrose
O. odorata：sundrops / evening primrose
Part of use　whole plant
Note 1　—
Note 2　MEMATSUYOIGUSA, ÔMATSUYOIGUSA and MATSUYOIGUSA are different species one another.
注　メマツヨイグサ、オオマツヨイグサ、マツヨイグサはそれぞれ別種。

名　称　**メラレウカ***

他名等　ティートリー油
部位等　精油
備　考　—

他名（参考）　—
漢字表記・生薬名等　—
Name (Romaji)　MERAREUKA*
Other name (s) (Romaji)　TÎTORÎ-YU
学名　*Melaleuca alternifolia* (Maiden et Betche) Cheel*
科名　Myrtaceae（フトモモ科）
英名　tea tree / narrow leaf paperbark / narrow leaf tea tree / narrow leaf ti tree / ti tree
Part of use　essential oil
Note 1　—
Note 2　MERAREUKA is the name of Melaleuca genus. The general English name is TÎTORÎ (tea tree).
注　メラレウカは属名であり、英語の一般名はティートリーである。

名　称　メリッサ*

他名等　コウスイハッカ／セイヨヤマハッカ／レモンバーム
部位等　葉
備　考　—

他名(参考)　—
漢字表記・生薬名等　西洋山薄荷（セイヨウヤマハッカ）
Name (Romaji)　MERISSA*
Other name (s) (Romaji)　KÔSUIHAKKA／SEIYOYA-MAHAKKA／REMONBÂMU
学名　*Melissa officinalis* L.*
科名　Labiatae（シソ科）
英名　lemon balm / common balm / sweet balm / balm / bee balm / melissa / melissa balm
Part of use　leaf
Note 1　—
Note 2　SEIYOYAMAHAKKA written in the item of "Other names" is incorrect. The correct name is SEIYÔYAMAHAKKA.
注　「他名等」のセイヨヤマハッカの正しい名称はセイヨウヤマハッカである。

名　称　メロン*

他名等　—
部位等　果実
備　考　—

他名(参考)　—
漢字表記・生薬名等　甜瓜（メロン）
Name (Romaji)　MERON*
Other name (s) (Romaji)　—
学名　*Cucumis melo* L.*
科名　Cucurbitaceae（ウリ科）
英名　melon / muskmelon
Part of use　fruit
Note 1　—
Note 2　—
注　—

名　称　メンジツ油*

他名等　—
部位等　種子油
備　考　—

他名(参考)　—
漢字表記・生薬名等　綿実油（メンジツユ）
Name (Romaji)　MENJITSU-YU*
Other name (s) (Romaji)　—
学名　*Gossypium* L.（ワタ属）
Gossypium herbaceum L.*（シロバナワタ）
Gossypium hirsutum L.*（リクチメン）
科名　Malvaceae（アオイ科）
英名　cottonseed oil
Part of use　seed oil
Note 1　—
Note 2　—
注　—

名　称　モクテンリョウ

他名等　マタタビ
部位等　果実・虫癭
備　考　—

他名(参考)　—
漢字表記・生薬名等　枝・葉：木天蓼（モクテンリョウ）、果実の虫癭：木天蓼子（モクテンリョウシ）、又旅（マタタビ）
Name (Romaji)　MOKUTENRYÔ
Other name (s) (Romaji)　MATATABI
学名　*Actinidia polygama* (Sieb. et Zucc.) Planch. ex Maxim.
Trocostigma polygama Sieb. et Zucc.
科名　Actinidiaceae（マタタビ科）
英名　silver vine / cat powder
Part of use　fruit, insect gall
Note 1　—
Note 2　—
注　—

名　称　モッカ*

他名等　カリン
部位等　偽果
備　考　—

他名(参考)　モッカ（ボケ）：ボケ（木瓜）、マボケ（真木瓜）、カラボケ（唐木瓜）、カンボケ（寒木瓜）、チョ

ウシュンボケ（長春木瓜）、ヒボケ（緋木瓜）、モケ（木瓜）、ヨドボケ（淀木瓜）
カリン：アンランジュ（安蘭樹）、カラナシ（唐梨、加良奈志）、キボケ（木木瓜）、メイサ（榠樝）、コウヒモッカ（光皮木瓜）

漢字表記・生薬名等 木瓜（モッカ、ボケ）、花梨（カリン）

Name (Romaji) MOKKA*

Other name (s) (Romaji) KARIN

学名 *Chaenomeles speciosa* (Sweet) Nakai*（モッカ、ボケ）
Chaenomeles lagenaria (Loisel.) Koidz.*（モッカ、ボケ）
Cydonia speciosa Sweet（モッカ、ボケ）
Pseudocydonia sinensis (Thouin) C.K. Schnied.（カリン）
Chaenomeles sinensis (Thouin) Koehne（カリン）
Cydonia sinensis (Dum.-Cours.) Thouin（カリン）

科名 Rosaceae（バラ科）

英名 *C. speciosa*：flower quince / Japanese quince
C. sinensis：Chisese quince

Part of use pseudocarp

Note 1 —

Note 2 MOKKA and KARIN written in the item of "Other names" are different each other but a fruit of KARIN is marketed as that of MOKKA in the Japanese market because the fruit of KARIN is defined as MOKKA by the Standards of Natural Drugs Not Listed in the Japanese Pharmacopoeia. It would be better to use BOKE, a synonym of MOKKA, as the name here in order to avoid the above cofusion with MOKKA and KARIN.

注 モッカとカリンは別種。しかし、日本薬局方外生薬規格において、カリンの果実を木瓜として規定しているため、現在、日本の市場で木瓜として流通しているのは、実は榠樝（めいさ、カリン）である。 このような混乱をさけるため、名称にはモッカではなく、その異名のボケを使用したほうが良いと思われる。

名 称 モッショクシ*

他名等 ガラエ
部位等 虫癭
備 考 —

他名(参考) —

漢字表記・生薬名等 没食子（モッショクシ）

Name (Romaji) MOSSHOKUSHI*

Other name (s) (Romaji) GARAE

学名 An excerescence on *Quercus lusitanica*, Lamarck (*Quercus infectoria* Olivier*), caused by the punctures and deposited ova of *Cynips gallae tinctoriae* Olivier.-(U. S. P.).（タマバチ科インクフシバチの幼虫の腺分泌物により、ブナ科の没食子樹（*Quercus infectoria* Olivier*）の若芽や稚枝に生じた虫瘤）

科名 Fagaceae（ブナ科）

英名 Aleppo galls / galls / galla tinctoria / galla halepense / galla levantica / galla quercina

Part of use insect gall

Note 1 —

Note 2 It is not MOSSHOKUSHI, a tree belongs to Fagaceae but the excrescence made by gall wasp is approved as a "non-drug" ingredient. Therefore explanation of the insect gall is written in the item of "Scientific name" but the family name of MOSSHOKUSHI, Fagaceae is listed here.

注 「非医」成分として許可されているのはモッショクシではなく、その虫癭であることから、学名にはその旨を記載した。但し、科名はモッショクシが属するブナ科とした。

名 称 モミジヒルガオ

他名等 五爪竜
部位等 全草
備 考 —

他名(参考) タイワンアサガオ（台湾朝顔）、モミジバヒルガオ（紅葉葉昼顔）、モミジバアサガオ（紅葉葉朝顔）

漢字表記・生薬名等 紅葉昼顔（モミジヒルガオ）、五爪龍（ゴソウリュウ）、五爪金龍（ゴソウキンリュウ）、番仔藤

Name (Romaji) MOMIJIHIRUGAO

Other name (s) (Romaji) GOSÔRYÛ

学名 *Ipomoea cairica* (L.) Sweet
Ipomoea palmata Forssk.
Ipomoea heptaphylla Voigt
Ipomoea pulchella Roth

科名 Convolvulaceae（ヒルガオ科）

英名 mile a minute vine / mile a minute / Cairo morning glory / coastal morning glory / five leaf morning glory / railroad creeper / railway creeper

Part of use whole plant

Note 1 —

Note 2 —

注 —

名　称　**モモ***

他名等　—
部位等　葉・花
備　考　種子（トウニン）は「医」

他名(参考)　—
漢字表記・生薬名等　桃（モモ）
Name (Romaji)　MOMO*
Other name (s) (Romaji)　—
学名　*Prunus persica* (L.) Batsch.*
　Prunus vulgaris Mill.*
　Amygdalus persica L.*
　Persica vulgaris
　Prunus persica var. *persica*
　Prunus persica var. *vulgaris* (Mill.) Maxim.
科名　Rosaceae（バラ科）
英名　peach / common peach
Part of use　leaf, flower
Note 1　seed：drug category
Note 2　—
注　—

名　称　**モモタマナ***

他名等　—
部位等　樹皮・実
備　考　—

他名(参考)　コバテイシ（枯葉手樹）、シマボウ
漢字表記・生薬名等　桃玉名（モモタマナ）
Name (Romaji)　MOMOTAMANA*
Other name (s) (Romaji)　—
学名　*Terminalia catappa* L.*
　Phytolacca javanica Osbeck
科名　Combretaceae（シクンシ科）
英名　tropcial almond / arjuna / country almond / marabal almond / sea almond / Indian almond / false kamani / olive bark tree
Part of use　bark, fruit
Note 1　—
Note 2　—
注　—

名　称　**モリアザミ**

他名等　ヤマゴボウ／Cirsium dipsacolepis
部位等　根
備　考　Phytolacca esculentaの根は「医」

他名(参考)　ゴボウアザミ（牛蒡薊）、キクゴボウ（菊牛蒡）、サンペイゴボウ（三瓶牛蒡）、ヤマゴボウ（山牛蒡）
漢字表記・生薬名等　森薊（モリアザミ）
Name (Romaji)　MORIAZAMI
Other name (s) (Romaji)　YAMAGOBÔ
学名　*Cirsium dipsacolepis* (Maxim.) Matsum.
　Cnicus dipsacolepis Maxim.
科名　Compositae（キク科）
英名　—
Part of use　root
Note 1　root of *Phytolacca esculenta* van Houtte：drug category
Note 2　CAUTION：MORIAZAMI is a herb belonging to *Circium* Mill. Its root is sometimes called YAMAGOBÔ and used as food. Another YAMAGOBÔ, *Phytolacca esculenta* van Houtte belonging to *Phytolacca* L. is a toxic herb because large amount of potassium nitrate and an alkaloide, chynanchotoxin are included in its root. The latter YAMAGOBÔ is called SHÔRIKU as the traditional Japanese herbal medicine and it is classified into drug category.
注　モリアザミの根はヤマゴボウと呼ばれ食用にされるが、本植物はアザミ属である。ヤマゴボウ属のヤマゴボウ（*Phytolacca esculenta* van Houtte）の根には多量の硝酸カリウムとアルカロイドのキナンコトキシン（chynanchotoxin）が含まれており、有毒である。後者は「医」に分類されており、生薬名は商陸である。

名　称　**モリシマアカシア**

他名等　Acacia mearnsii
部位等　樹皮
備　考　—

他名(参考)　コクケイジュ（黒荊樹）
漢字表記・生薬名等　mollissimaアカシア（モリシマアカシア）
Name (Romaji)　MORISHIMAAKASIA
Other name (s) (Romaji)　—
学名　*Acacia mearnsii* De Wild.
　Acacia mollissima auct. non Willd.
　Acacia decurrens var. *mollis* Lindl.
科名　Leguminosae（マメ科）

英名　black wattle / green wattle / late black wattle / tan wattle
Part of use　bark
Note 1　―
Note 2　―
注　―

名　称　**モロヘイヤ**

他名等　**タイワンツナソ**
部位等　葉
備　考　―

他名(参考)　シマツナソ（縞綱麻）、ナガミツナソ（長実綱麻）、ジュート
漢字表記・生薬名等　台湾綱麻（タイワンツナソ）
Name(Romaji)　MOROHEIYA
Other name(s) (Romaji)　TAIWANTSUNASO
学名　*Corchorus olitorius* L.
Corchorus catharticus Blanco
Corchorus decemangularis Roxb.
Corchorus lobatus Wildem.
Corchorus quinqueloclaris Moench
科名　Tiliaceae（シナノキ科）
英名　mulukhiyah / Jew's mallow / nalta jute / tossa jute
Part of use　leaf
Note 1　―
Note 2　―
注　―

ヤ行

名　称　**ヤーコン**

他名等　**アンデスポテト**
部位等　塊根・茎・葉
備　考　―

他名(参考)　―
漢字表記・生薬名等　―
Name(Romaji)　YÂKON
Other name(s) (Romaji)　ANDESUPOTETO
学名　*Smallanthus sonchifolius* (Poepp. et Endl.) H. Rob.
Polymnia sonchifolia Poepp. et Endl.
Polymnia edulis Wedd.
科名　Compositae（キク科）
英名　yacon / yacon strawberry / yakon / earth apple
Part of use　root tuber, stem, leaf
Note 1　―
Note 2　ANDESUPOTETO in the item of "Other names" is sometimes confused with Andes potato belonging to Solanaceae.
注　アンデスポテトは、その名称のためにアンデスのジャガイモ（ナス科）と混同されることがある。

名　称　**ヤエヤマアオキ***

他名等　**インディアンマルベリー／ノニ**
部位等　果実・種子・葉
備　考　―

他名(参考)　ヤマベアオキ（ヤマベ青木）、アカダマノキ（赤玉の木）、オオマツカサノキ
漢字表記・生薬名等　八重山青木（ヤエヤマアオキ）
Name(Romaji)　YAEYAMAAOKI*
Other name(s) (Romaji)　INDIANMARUBERÎ／NONI
学名　*Morinda citrifolia* L.*
科名　Rubiaceae（アカネ科）
英名　noni / canary wood / cheesefruit / great morinda / rotten cheesefruit / painkiller / Indian mulberry
Part of use　fruit, seed, leaf
Note 1　―
Note 2　―
注　―

名　称　**ヤクシマアジサイ**

他名等　**ドジョウザン／ロウレンシュウキュウ**
部位等　根・葉
備　考　―

他名(参考)　―
漢字表記・生薬名等　屋久島紫陽花（ヤクシマアジサイ）
以下は甜茶の１種である（ヤクシマアジサイも甜茶の１種に用いられる）。
・土常山（ドジョウザン）：*Hydrangea serrata* (Thunb. ex Murray) Ser. var. *thumbergii* (Sieb.) H. Ohba
・臘蓮繍球（ロウレンシュウキュウ）：*Hydrangea aspara* ssp. *strigosa*
Name(Romaji)　YAKUSHIMAAJISAI
Other name(s) (Romaji)　DOJÔZAN／RÔRENSHÛKYÛ
学名　*Hydrangea grosseserrata* Engl.
Hydrangea angustipetala Hayata
科名　Saxifragaceae（ユキノシタ科）
英名　―
Part of use　root, leaf

Note 1　—
Note 2　—
注　—

名　称　**ヤグルマギク***

他名等　—
部位等　花
備　考　—

他名(参考)　ヤグルマソウ（矢車草）
漢字表記･生薬名等　矢車菊（ヤグルマギク）
Name(Romaji)　YAGURUMAGIKU*
Other name(s) (Romaji)　—
学名　*Centaurea cyanus* L.*
　　Cyanus segetum Hill
科名　Compositae（キク科）
英名　cornflower / blue bottle / blaver / blue poppy / bluebonnet / brushes / corn pinks / hurtsickle / timbles / witch's bell / bachelor's button / cyani
Part of use　flower
Note 1　—
Note 2　—
注　—

名　称　**ヤグルマハッカ***

他名等　ホースミント
部位等　葉
備　考　—

他名(参考)　—
漢字表記･生薬名等　矢車薄荷（ヤグルマハッカ）
Name(Romaji)　YAGURUMAHAKKA*
Other name(s) (Romaji)　HÔSUMINTO
学名　*Monarda fistulosa* L.*
科名　Labiatae（シソ科）
英名　wild bergamot / wild bergamot beebalm / beebalm / horse mint / oswego tea / purple beebalm
Part of use　leaf
Note 1　—
Note 2　—
注　—

名　称　**ヤシ***

他名等　ココヤシ／ヤシ油
部位等　種子油・樹皮・葉・花
備　考　—

他名(参考)　ホンヤシ（本椰子）、ココナッツ
漢字表記･生薬名等　椰子（ヤシ）、古古椰子（ココヤシ）、椰子油（ヤシユ）
Name(Romaji)　YASHI*
Other name(s) (Romaji)　KOKOYASHI／YASHI-YU
学名　*Cocos nucifera* L.*
科名　Palmae（ヤシ科）
英名　coconut / coconut palm / copra
Part of use　seed oil, bark, leaf, flower
Note 1　—
Note 2　—
注　—

名　称　**ヤシャビシャク**

他名等　—
部位等　実
備　考　—

他名(参考)　テンノウメ（天の梅）、テンバイ（天梅）
漢字表記･生薬名等　夜叉柄杓（ヤシャビシャク）
Name(Romaji)　YASHABISHAKU
Other name(s) (Romaji)　—
学名　*Ribes ambiguum* Maxim.
科名　Grossulariaceae（スグリ科）
英名　—
Part of use　fruit
Note 1　—
Note 2　—
注　—

名　称　**ヤチダモ**

他名等　—
部位等　葉
備　考　—

他名(参考)　タモ（梻）、オオバトネリコ（大葉梣）
漢字表記･生薬名等　谷地梻（ヤチダモ）
Name(Romaji)　YACHIDAMO
Other name(s) (Romaji)　—
学名　*Fraxinus mandshurica* Rupr.
　　Fraxinus mandshurica Rupr. var. *japonica* Maxim.
科名　Oleaceae（モクセイ科）

英名　Japanese ash / Manchurian ash
Part of use　leaf
Note 1　—
Note 2　—
注　—

名　称　**ヤナギ**

他名等　—
部位等　全木
備　考　—

他名(参考)　ゴールデンウィロー
漢字表記・生薬名等　—
Name(Romaji)　YANAGI
Other name(s) (Romaji)　—
学名　*Salix vitellina* L.
　Salix alba L. ssp. *vitellina* (L.) Schübl. et G. Martens
　Salix alba L. var. *vitellina* (L.) Stokes
科名　Salicaceae（ヤナギ科）
英名　golden willow
Part of use　whole tree
Note 1　—
Note 2　Various Salix species (YANAGI) exists. Golden willow is written here as one of the species. Refer to SEIYÔSHIROYANAGI in the item of "Name".
注　ヤナギは多種存在する。例として*Salix vitellina*（英名Golden willow）を記載した。セイヨウシロヤナギの項も参照のこと。

名　称　**ヤナギラン***

他名等　ファイアウィード
部位等　葉
備　考　—

他名(参考)　—
漢字表記・生薬名等　柳蘭（ヤナギラン）
Name(Romaji)　YANAGIRAN*
Other name(s) (Romaji)　FAIAWÎDO
学名　*Chamerion angustifolium* (L.) Holub*
　Epilobium angustifolium L.*
　Chamaenerion angustifolium (L.) Scop.*
　Chamerion angustifolium (L.) Holub ssp. *angustifolium*
　Chamerion angustifolium ssp. *circumvagum*（ウスゲヤナギラン）
科名　Onagraceae（アカバナ科）
英名　fireweed / French willow / great willowherb / rosebay willowherb
Part of use　leaf
Note 1　—
Note 2　—
注　—

名　称　**ヤハズツノマタ***

他名等　アイリッシュモス
部位等　全藻
備　考　—

他名(参考)　トチャカ
漢字表記・生薬名等　ヤハズ角叉（ヤハズツノマタ）
Name(Romaji)　YAHAZUTSUNOMATA*
Other name(s) (Romaji)　AIRISSHUMOSU
学名　*Chondrus crispus* Stackh.*
科名　Gigartinaceae（スギノリ科）
英名　carrageen moss / Irish moss / carrageen / carageen
Part of use　whole seaweed
Note 1　—
Note 2　—
注　—

名　称　**ヤブタバコ**

他名等　Carpesium abrotanoides
部位等　茎・根・葉・果実
備　考　—

他名(参考)　テンメイセイ（天名精）、カクシツ（鶴虱）
漢字表記・生薬名等　藪煙草（ヤブタバコ）、葉・茎・根：天名精（テンメイセイ）、果実：鶴虱（カクシツ）
Name(Romaji)　YABUTABAKO
Other name(s) (Romaji)　—
学名　*Carpesium abrotanoides* L.
科名　Compositae（キク科）
英名　—
Part of use　stem, root, leaf, fruit
Note 1　—
Note 2　—
注　—

名　称　ヤマウルシ

他名等　—
部位等　若芽
備　考　—

他名(参考)　—
漢字表記・生薬名等　山漆（ヤマウルシ）
Name (Romaji)　YAMAURUSHI
Other name(s) (Romaji)　—
学名　*Rhus trichocarpa* Miq.
Toxicodendron trichocarpum (Miq.) Kuntze
科名　Anacardiaceae（ウルシ科）
英名　—
Part of use　sprout
Note 1　—
Note 2　—
注　—

名　称　ヤマノイモ属

他名等　—
部位等　根茎
備　考　—

他名(参考)　ジネンジョウ（自然生）、ジネンショ（自然薯）、ヤマイモ（山芋）、ショヨ（薯蕷）
漢字表記・生薬名等　山の芋（ヤマノイモ）、山芋（ヤマノイモ）、山薬（サンヤク）
Name (Romaji)　YAMANOIMO-ZOKU
Other name(s) (Romaji)　—
学名　*Dioscorea* L.
科名　Dioscoreaceae（ヤマノイモ科）
英名　yam
Part of use　rhizome
Note 1　—
Note 2　—
注　—

名　称　ヤマハハコ*

他名等　—
部位等　若芽
備　考　—

他名(参考)　—
漢字表記・生薬名等　山母子（ヤマハハコ）
Name (Romaji)　YAMAHAHAKO*
Other name(s) (Romaji)　—
学名　*Anaphalis margaritacea* (L.) Benth. et Hook. f.*
科名　Compositae（キク科）
英名　pearly everlasting / life everlasting / western pearly everlasting
Part of use　sprout
Note 1　—
Note 2　—
注　—

名　称　ヤマハマナス*

他名等　シバイカ
部位等　果実
備　考　—

他名(参考)　カラフトイバラ（樺太茨）
漢字表記・生薬名等　山浜梨・山浜茄子（ヤマハマナス）
Name (Romaji)　YAMAHAMANASU*
Other name(s) (Romaji)　SHIBAIKA
学名　*Rosa davurica* Pall.*
科名　Rosaceae（バラ科）
英名　rose / Amur rose
Part of use　fruit
Note 1　—
Note 2　—
注　—

名　称　ヤマブキ

他名等　—
部位等　実
備　考　—

他名(参考)　—
漢字表記・生薬名等　山吹（ヤマブキ）
Name (Romaji)　YAMABUKI
Other name(s) (Romaji)　—
学名　*Kerria japonica* (L.) DC.
科名　Rosaceae（バラ科）
英名　Japanese rose / Japanese kerria / Japanese globe-flower / Jew's mallow / kerria
Part of use　fruit
Note 1　—
Note 2　—
注　—

名　称　**ヤマブシタケ**

他名等　—
部位等　子実体
備　考　—

他名(参考)　ウサギタケ、ハリセンボン（針千本）、ジョウコタケ（上戸茸）
漢字表記・生薬名等　山伏茸（ヤマブシタケ）、猴頭菇（ホウトウクウ）
Name (Romaji)　YAMABUSHITAKE
Other name (s) (Romaji)　—
学名　*Hericium erinaceus* (Bull.) Pers.
Hericium erinaceum (Bull. : Fr.) Pers.
Dryodon erinaceus (Bull.) P. Karst.
Hydnum erinaceus Bull.
Clavaria erinaceus (Bull.) Paulet
Steccherinum quercinum Gray
科名　Hericiaceae（サンゴハリタケ科）
英名　bear's-head / monkey head mushroom / lion head mushroom / lion's mane mushroom / bearded tooth mushroom（アゴヒゲハリタケ） / hedgehog mushroom（ハリネズミタケ） / bearded hedgehog mushroom（アゴヒゲハリネズミタケ） / pom pom mushroom（ポンポンタケ）
Part of use　fruit body
Note 1　—
Note 2　—
注　—

名　称　**ヤマブドウ**

他名等　—
部位等　葉・実
備　考　—

他名(参考)　—
漢字表記・生薬名等　山葡萄（ヤマブドウ）
Name (Romaji)　YAMABUDÔ
Other name (s) (Romaji)　—
学名　*Vitis coignetiae* Pulliat ex Planch.
科名　Vitaceae（ブドウ科）
英名　crimson glory vine
Part of use　leaf, fruit
Note 1　—
Note 2　—
注　—

名　称　**ヤマモモ**

他名等　ヨウバイヒ／Myrica rubra
部位等　樹皮
備　考　—

他名(参考)　ヨウバイ（楊梅）、ユスラ（山桜桃）
漢字表記・生薬名等　山桃（ヤマモモ）、実：楊梅（ヨウバイ）、樹皮：楊梅皮（ヨウバイヒ）
Name (Romaji)　YAMAMOMO
Other name (s) (Romaji)　YÔBAIHI
学名　*Myrica rubra* Sieb. et Zucc.
Morella rubra Lour.
科名　Myricaceae（ヤマモモ科）
英名　yama momo / Chinese arbutus / Chinese strawberry tree / wax myrtle / bayberry
Part of use　bark
Note 1　—
Note 2　—
注　—

名　称　**ユウガオ***

他名等　コシ
部位等　果肉・葉・若芽
備　考　—

他名(参考)　カンピョウ（干瓢）、カンコ（甘瓠）
漢字表記・生薬名等　夕顔（ユウガオ）、果実：瓠子（コシ）、種子：瓠子子（コシシ）
Name (Romaji)　YÛGAO*
Other name (s) (Romaji)　KOSHI
学名　*Lagenaria siceraria* (Molina) Standl.*
Lagenaria siceraria var. *hispida* (Thunb.) Hara
Cucumis hispida Thunb.
Lagenaria siceraria var. *clavata* Ser.
Lagenaria leucantha var. *clavata* Makino
科名　Cucurbitaceae（ウリ科）
英名　moonflower gourd / white flowered gourd / bottle gourd / calabash gourd
Part of use　sarcocarp, leaf, sprout
Note 1　—
Note 2　Refer to HYÔTAN and FUKUBE. These herbs are also listed in the item of "Name".
注　別項のヒョウタンとフクベを参照。

名　称　**ユーカリ***

他名等　**ユーカリノキ／ユーカリ油**
部位等　葉・精油
備　考　—

他名(参考)　—
漢字表記･生薬名等　桉葉（アンヨウ）
Name(Romaji)　YÛKARI*
Other name(s) (Romaji)　YÛKARINOKI／YÛKARI-YU
学名　*Eucalyptus globulus* Labill.*
科名　Myrtaceae（フトモモ科）
英名　eucalyptus / blue gum / southern blue gum / Tasmanian blue gum / southern blue gum / Victorian blue gum
Part of use　leaf, essential oil
Note 1　—
Note 2　—
注　—

名　称　**ユキチャ**

他名等　**ムシゴケ**
部位等　全草
備　考　—

他名(参考)　ジチャ（地茶）、タイハクチャ（太白茶）
漢字表記･生薬名等　雪茶（ユキチャ、セッチャ）、虫苔（ムシゴケ）
Name(Romaji)　YUKICHA
Other name(s) (Romaji)　MUSHIGOKE
学名　*Thamnolia vermicularis* (Sw.) Ach. ex Schaer
科名　Usneaceae（サルオガセ科）
英名　whiteworm lichen / white worm lichen
Part of use　whole plant
Note 1　—
Note 2　—
注　—

名　称　**ユズ**

他名等　**トウシ**
部位等　果実・種子
備　考　—

他名(参考)　ホンユ（本柚）、ホンユズ（本柚子）、ユノス（柚子）、ユジツ（柚実）
漢字表記･生薬名等　柚（ユズ）、柚子（ユズ）、香橙（コウトウ）、橙子（トウシ）、果皮：橙子皮（トウシヒ）
Name(Romaji)　YUZU
Other name(s) (Romaji)　TÔSHI
学名　*Citrus junos* Sieb. ex Tanaka
科名　Rutaceae（ミカン科）
英名　yuzu
Part of use　fruit, seed
Note 1　—
Note 2　—
注　—

名　称　**ユズリハ**

他名等　**コウジョウボク**
部位等　全草
備　考　—

他名(参考)　—
漢字表記･生薬名等　楪（ユズリハ）、譲葉（ユズリハ）、交譲木（コウジョウボク）
Name(Romaji)　YUZURIHA
Other name(s) (Romaji)　KÔJÔBOKU
学名　*Daphniphyllum macropodum* Miq.
Daphniphyllum himalense (Benth.) Muell. Arg. ssp. *macropodum* (Miq.) Huang
科名　Daphniphyllaceae（ユズリハ科）
英名　—
Part of use　whole plant
Note 1　—
Note 2　—
注　—

名　称　**ユッカ**

他名等　**キミガヨラン**
部位等　根
備　考　—

他名(参考)　—
漢字表記･生薬名等　君が代蘭（キミガヨラン）
Name(Romaji)　YUKKA
Other name(s) (Romaji)　KIMIGAYORAN
学名　*Yucca recurvifolia* Salisb.
Yucca gloriosa var. *tristis* Carrière
Yucca gloriosa var. *recurvifolia* (Salisb.) Engelm.
科名　Asparagaceae（クサスギカズラ科）（Agavaceae（リュウゼツラン科））
英名　yucca / cure leaf yucca / pendulous yucca / weeping yucca
Part of use　root
Note 1　—
Note 2　—

注 —

名 称 **ユリ***

他名等 オニユリ／ビャクゴウ
部位等 花・鱗茎
備 考 —

他名(参考) ハカタユリ（博多百合）、ホソバユリ（細葉百合）
漢字表記・生薬名等 百合（ユリ、ビャクゴウ）、鬼百合（オニユリ）
Name (Romaji) YURI*
Other name (s) (Romaji) ONIYURI／BYAKUGÔ
学名 *Lilium lancifolium* Thunb.*（オニユリ）
Lilium brownii F.E. Br. ex Miellez*（ハカタユリ）
Lilium brownii F.E. Br. ex Miellez var. *viridulum* Baker*（ハカタユリ）
Lilium pumilum DC.*（ホソバユリ）
科名 Liliaceae（ユリ科）
英名 *L. lancifolium*：lily / tiger lily
L. brownii：true tiger lily / Brown's lily
L. pumilum：coral lily
Part of use flower, bulb
Note 1 —
Note 2 —
注 —

名 称 **ヨウシュカンボク**

他名等 —
部位等 全草
備 考 —

他名(参考) セイヨウカンボク（西洋肝木）
漢字表記・生薬名等 洋種肝木（ヨウシュカンボク）
Name (Romaji) YÔSHUKANBOKU
Other name (s) (Romaji) —
学名 *Viburnum opulus* L. var. *opulus*
Viburnum opulus f. *nanum*（I. David）Zabel
Viburnum opulus f. *xanthocarpum*（Endl.）Rehder
科名 Caprifoliaceae（スイカズラ科）
英名 cranberry bush / crampbark / guelder rose / high bush cranberry / European cranberry bush / rose elder / whitten tree / snow ballbush
Part of use whole plant
Note 1 —
Note 2 —
注 —

名 称 **ヨウテイ***

他名等 ギシギシ／ナカバギシギシ
部位等 根
備 考 —

他名(参考) ウマスイバ（馬酸葉）、ウシグサ（牛草）、イヌスイバ（犬酸葉）、ジゴクノネ（地獄の根）、ギシギシダイオウ（羊蹄大黄）
漢字表記・生薬名等 羊蹄（ヨウテイ）、羊蹄（ギシギシ）、長葉羊蹄（ナガバギシギシ）、羊蹄根（ヨウテイコン）
Name (Romaji) YÔTEI*
Other name (s) (Romaji) GISHIGISHI／NAKABAGI-SHIGISHI
学名 *Rumex japonicus* Houtt.（ギシギシ）
Rumex crispus L. ssp. *japonicus*（Houtt.）Kitam.（ギシギシ）
Rumex crispus L. ssp. *crispus*（ナガバギシギシ）
Rumex crispus L.*（ナガバギシギシ）
科名 Polygonaceae（タデ科）
英名 dock / curly dock / curled dock / yellow dock / sour dock
Part of use root
Note 1 —
Note 2 NAKABAGISHIGISHI written in the item of "Other names" is incorrect. The correct name is NAGABAGISHIGISHI.
注 「他名等」のナカバギシギシの正しい名称はナガバギシギシである。

名 称 **ヨーロッパソクズ***

他名等 —
部位等 全草
備 考 —

他名(参考) —
漢字表記・生薬名等 ヨーロッパ蒴藋（ヨーロッパソクズ）
Name (Romaji) YÔROPPASOKUZU*
Other name (s) (Romaji) —
学名 *Sambucus ebulus* L.*
科名 Caprifoliaceae（スイカズラ科）
英名 dwarf elder / Danewort / wallwort / European dwarf elder
Part of use whole plant
Note 1 —
Note 2 —
注 —

名　称　**ヨカンシ***

他名等　**アンマロク／ユカン**
部位等　果実・樹皮・根・葉
備　考　—

他名(参考)　アムラ（amla）
漢字表記・生薬名等　余甘子（ヨカンシ）、乾燥した果実：庵摩勒（アンマロク）、油柑（ユカン）、葉：油柑葉（ユカンヨウ）、樹皮：油柑枝（ユカンシ）、油柑木皮（ユカンボクヒ）
Name(Romaji)　YOKANSHI*
Other name(s) (Romaji)　ANMAROKU／YUKAN
学名　*Phyllanthus emblica* L.*
Emblica officinalis Gaertn.
Milobalanus embilica Burn.
科名　Euphorbiaceae（トウダイグサ科）
英名　amla / emblic / emblic myrobalan / Indian gooseberry
Part of use　fruit, bark, root, leaf
Note 1　—
Note 2　—
注　—

名　称　**ヨモギ***

他名等　**ガイヨウ／モグサ**
部位等　枝先・葉
備　考　—

他名(参考)　カズザキヨモギ（数咲き蓬）、エゾヨモギ（蝦夷蓬）、モチグサ（餅草）
漢字表記・生薬名等　蓬（ヨモギ）、艾葉（ガイヨウ）、野艾・艾（モグサ）
Name(Romaji)　YOMOGI*
Other name(s) (Romaji)　GAIYÔ／MOGUSA
学名　*Artemisia princeps* Pamp.（ヨモギ）
Artemisia indica Willd. var. *maximowiczii* (Nakai) H. Hara（ヨモギ）
Artemisia montana (Nakai) Pamp.（ヤマヨモギ、オオヨモギ、エゾヨモギ）
Artemisia vulgaris L. var. *vulgatissima* Bess.*（ヤマヨモギ、オオヨモギ、エゾヨモギ）
科名　Compositae（キク科）
英名　Japanese mugwort / yomogi
Part of use　top of branch, leaf
Note 1　—
Note 2　—
注　—

名　称　**ヨモギギク***

他名等　**タンジー**
部位等　全草
備　考　—

他名(参考)　エゾヨモギギク（蝦夷蓬菊）
漢字表記・生薬名等　蓬菊（ヨモギギク）
Name(Romaji)　YOMOGIGIKU*
Other name(s) (Romaji)　TANJÎ
学名　*Tanacetum vulgare* L.*
Chrysanthemum vulgare (L.) Bernh.*
Tanacetum boreale Fisch. ex DC.
科名　Compositae（キク科）
英名　tansy / common tansy / golden buttons
Part of use　whole plant
Note 1　—
Note 2　—
注　—

ラ行

名　称　**ライガン***

他名等　**チクリョウ／モクレンシ／ライシ／ライジツ**
部位等　乾燥した菌核
備　考　—

他名(参考)　ライガンキン（雷丸菌）、チクレイシ（竹鈴芝）
漢字表記・生薬名等　雷丸（ライガン）、竹苓（チクリョウ）、雷実（ライジツ）、雷矢（ライシ）、木連子（モクレンシ）
Name(Romaji)　RAIGAN*
Other name(s) (Romaji)　CHIKURYÔ／MOKURENSHI／RAISHI／RAIJITSU
学名　*Polyporus mylittae* Cooke et Massee*
Laccocephalum mylittae (Cooke et Massee) Núñez et Ryvarden
Omphalia lapidescens Schroet.
科名　Polyporaceae（サルノコシカケ科）
英名　polyporus mylittae / native bread / blackfellow's bread / thunder ball
Part of use　dried sclerotium
Note 1　—
Note 2　RAIGAN is the dried sclerotium of *Polyporus mylittae* paracitizing in bamboo rhizome. It is also called CHIKURYÔ. Refer to TAKE-RUI regarding bamboo. TAKE-RUI is also listed in the item of "Name".

注　ライガン（雷丸）とは、竹の根茎に寄生するライガンの乾燥菌核をいう。竹苓（チクリョウ）とも呼ばれる。タケについては別項のタケ類を参照。

名　称　**ライフクシ***

他名等　ダイコン
部位等　種子
備　考　—

他名（参考）　ロフク（蘆菔）、ラフク（蘿菔）、シロダイコン（白大根）
漢字表記・生薬名等　莱菔子（ライフクシ）、大根（ダイコン）
Name (Romaji)　RAIFUKUSHI*
Other name (s) (Romaji)　DAIKON
学名　*Raphanus sativus* L.*
Raphanus sativus L. var. *hortensis* Backer f. *acanthiformis* Makino
Raphanus sativus L. var. *longipinnatus* L.H. Bailey
科名　Cruciferae（アブラナ科）
英名　radish / Japanese white radish / Chinese radish / giant white radish / mooli / radis oriental / true daikon
Part of use　seed
Note 1　—
Note 2　—
注　—

名　称　**ライムギ***

他名等　—
部位等　茎・葉
備　考　—

他名（参考）　クロムギ（黒麦）、ライ
漢字表記・生薬名等　ライ麦（ライムギ）
Name (Romaji)　RAIMUGI*
Other name (s) (Romaji)　—
学名　*Secale cereale* L.*
Secale cereale L. ssp. *cereale*
科名　Gramineae（イネ科）
英名　rye / cereal rye
Part of use　stem, leaf
Note 1　—
Note 2　—
注　—

名　称　**ラカンカ***

他名等　—
部位等　果実
備　考　—

他名（参考）　—
漢字表記・生薬名等　羅漢果（ラカンカ）
Name (Romaji)　RAKANKA*
Other name (s) (Romaji)　—
学名　*Momordica grosvenorii* Swingle*
Siraitia grosvenorii (Swingle) C. Jeffrey ex A.M. Lu et Zhi Y. Zhang*
Thladiantha grosvenorii (Swingle) C. Jeffrey*
科名　Cucurbitaceae（ウリ科）
英名　—
Part of use　fruit
Note 1　—
Note 2　—
注　—

名　称　**ラスグラブラ***

他名等　—
部位等　根皮
備　考　—

他名（参考）　—
漢字表記・生薬名等　—
Name (Romaji)　RASUGURABURA*
Other name (s) (Romaji)　—
学名　*Rhus glabra* L.*
Rhus glabra var. *cismontana* (Greene) Cockerell
Rhus cismontana Greene
科名　Anacardiaceae（ウルシ科）
英名　smooth sumac / vinegar tree / vinegar bush / scarlet sumac / scarlet sumach / red sumac / upland sumach
Part of use　root bark
Note 1　—
Note 2　RASUGURABURA is not confirmed but it is thought to be *Rhus glabra* native to north America and one of the Rhus species of Anacardiaceae. The KATAKANA notation is preferably “RUSU・GURABURA”.
注　ラスグラブラの名称は確認できないが、ウルシ科ヌルデ属の北米原産の低木、*Rhus glabra* L. と思われる。名称のカタカナ記述は、“ルス・グラブラ”の方が良い。

名　称　**ラズベリー***

他名等　—
部位等　果実・葉
備　考　—

他名(参考)　エゾキイチゴ（蝦夷木苺）、ヨーロッパキイチゴ（ヨーロッパ木苺）、フクボンシ（覆盆子）、フランボワーズ
漢字表記・生薬名等　覆盆子（フクボンシ）
Name (Romaji)　RAZUBERÎ*
Other name (s) (Romaji)　—
学名　*Rubus idaeus* L.（セイヨウキイチゴ）
Rubus strigosus Michx.*（セイヨウキイチゴ）
科名　Rosaceae（バラ科）
英名　raspberry / European red raspberry / American red raspberry / red raspberry
Part of use　fruit, leaf
Note 1　—
Note 2　RAZUBERÎ is identical with SEIYÔKIICHIGO. SEIYÔKIICHIGO is also listed in the item of "Name".
注　ラズベリーは別項のセイヨウキイチゴと同一。

名　称　**ラッカセイ***

他名等　ナンキンマメ
部位等　種子
備　考　—

他名(参考)　地豆（ジマメ）、ピーナッツ
漢字表記・生薬名等　落花生（ラッカセイ）、南京豆（ナンキンマメ）
Name (Romaji)　RAKKASEI*
Other name (s) (Romaji)　NANKINMAME
学名　*Arachis hypogaea* L.*
科名　Leguminosae（マメ科）
英名　peanut / ground nut / goober / earth nut / grass nut / monkey nut / pindar / Spanish peanut / Valencia peanut
Part of use　seed
Note 1　—
Note 2　—
注　—

名　称　**ラフマ**

他名等　コウマ
部位等　全草
備　考　—

他名(参考)　トウバシクルモン（紅麻）、オショロソウ（忍路草）
漢字表記・生薬名等　羅布麻（ラフマ）、紅麻（コウマ）
Name (Romaji)　RAFUMA
Other name (s) (Romaji)　KÔMA
学名　*Apocynum venetum* L.
Trachomitum venetum (L.) Woodson
科名　Apocynaceae（キョウチクトウ科）
英名　dogbane / kendyr
Part of use　whole plant
Note 1　—
Note 2　—
注　—

名　称　**ラベンサラ**

他名等　—
部位等　葉
備　考　—

他名(参考)　—
漢字表記・生薬名等　—
Name (Romaji)　RABENSARA
Other name (s) (Romaji)　—
学名　*Ravensara aromatica* J.F. Gmel.
科名　Lauraceae（クスノキ科）
英名　Madagascar clove / clove nutmeg / Madagascar nutmeg
Part of use　leaf
Note 1　—
Note 2　An specific herb cannot be identified by RABENSARA as it is the name of genus. *Ravensara aromatica* or *Ravensara anisata* is seemed to be used for aromatherapy but there is information on the latter herb that it should not be used because of including carcinogenic compound. Therefore, the former is listed here.
注　ラベンサラは属名のため、種が特定できない。アロマテラピーでは、*Ravensara aromatica*と*R. anisata*が用いられるようだが、後者には発がん性物質が含まれているため、使用すべきではないとの解説も見受けられる。従って、本書では前者の学名を採用した。

名 称 ラベンダー*

他名等 —
部位等 花
備 考 —

他名(参考) クンイソウ（薫衣草）
漢字表記・生薬名等 ラベンダー油
Name (Romaji) RABENDÂ*
Other name (s) (Romaji) —
学名 *Lavandula* L.（ラベンダー属）
Lavandula angustifolia Mill.*（トゥルー・ラベンダー、コモン・ラベンダー）
Lavandula dentata L.*（デンタータ・ラベンダー）
Lavandula×intermedia Emeric ex Loisel.*（ラバンジン）
Lavandula latifolia Medik.*（スパイク・ラベンダー）
Lavandula stoechas L.*（フレンチ・ラベンダー）
科名 Labiatae（シソ科）
英名 lavender / common lavender / true lavender / English lavender / lavandin / Duch lavender / French lavender / topped lavender / spike lavender
Part of use flower
Note 1 —
Note 2 —
注 —

名 称 ランブータン

他名等 —
部位等 果実
備 考 —

他名(参考) —
漢字表記・生薬名等 紅毛丹、韶子（ショウシ）、毛龍眼
Name (Romaji) RANBÛTAN
Other name (s) (Romaji) —
学名 *Nephelium lappaceum* L.
Euphoria nephelium DC.
Dimocarpus crinita Lour.
科名 Sapindaceae（ムクロジ科）
英名 rambutan / ramboota
Part of use fruit
Note 1 —
Note 2 —
注 —

名 称 リュウガン*

他名等 —
部位等 果肉・仮種皮・花
備 考 —

他名(参考) リョウガン（龍眼）
漢字表記・生薬名等 竜眼・龍眼（リュウガン）、桂圓（ケイエン）、圓眼（エンガン）、亜茘枝（アレイシ）、果肉：竜眼肉（リュウガンニク）、桂圓肉（ケイエンニク）、果皮：竜眼殻（リュウガンカク）、種子：竜眼核（リュウガンカク）
Name (Romaji) RYÛGAN*
Other name (s) (Romaji) —
学名 *Dimocarpus longan* Lour.*
Euphoria longana Lam.*
Euphoria longan (Lour.) Steud.*
Nephelium longana (Lam.) Camb.*
Nephelium longan (Lour.) Hook.*
科名 Sapindaceae（ムクロジ科）
英名 longan / lungan / dragon's eye
Part of use sarcocarp, arillate, flower
Note 1 —
Note 2 —
注 —

名 称 リュウキド*

他名等 —
部位等 全草
備 考 —

他名(参考) —
漢字表記・生薬名等 劉寄奴（リュウキド）、奇蒿（キコウ、*Artemisia anomala*、キク科）、陰行草（ヒキヨモギ、*Siphonostegia chinensis*、ゴマノハグサ科）、蔞蒿・水蒿（タカヨモギ、*Artemisia selengensis*、キク科）
Name (Romaji) RYÛKIDO*
Other name (s) (Romaji) —
学名 *Artemisia anomala* S. Moore*（アルテミシア・アノマラ、奇蒿）
Siphonostegia chinensis Benth.（ヒキヨモギ）
Artemisia selengensis Turcz. ex Besser（タカヨモギ）
科名 Compositae（キク科）
Scrophulariaceae（ゴマノハグサ科）
英名 diverse wormwood
Part of use whole plant
Note 1 —
Note 2 RYÛKIDO is the name of traditional Japanese herbal medicine and three different kinds of herbs

are used as RYÛKIDO, namely *Artemisia anomala*, *Siphonostagia chinensis* and *Artemisia selengensis*. Their Japanese names are KIKÔ, HIKIYOMOGI and TAKAYOMOGI, respectively.

注 リュウキドは生薬名であり、これに用いられる植物は３種ある。すなわち、*Artemisia anomala*（奇蒿）、*Siphonostegia chinensis*（ヒキヨモギ）、及び*Artemisia selengensis*（タカヨモギ）である。

名　称　リュウキュウアイ*

他名等　—
部位等　枝・葉
備　考　—

他名(参考)　バラン（馬藍）
漢字表記・生薬名等　琉球藍（リュウキュウアイ）
Name (Romaji)　RYÛKYÛAI*
Other name(s) (Romaji)　—
学名　*Strobilanthes cusia* (Nees) Kuntze*
Baphicacanthus cusia (Nees) Bremek.*
Strobilanthes flaccidifolia Nees
科名　Acanthaceae（キツネノマゴ科）
英名　strobilanthus cusia / baphicacanthus cusia / rum / Assam indigo / cone head
Part of use　branch, leaf
Note 1　—
Note 2　—
注　—

名　称　リュウノウ*

他名等　Dryobalanops aromatica
部位等　樹皮
備　考　—

他名(参考)　リュウノウジュ（竜脳樹）、ボルネオショウノウ（ボルネオ樟脳）
漢字表記・生薬名等　竜脳（リュウノウ）
Name (Romaji)　RYÛNÔ*
Other name(s) (Romaji)　—
学名　*Dryobalanops aromatica* C.F. Gaertn.*
Dryobalanops sumatrensis (J.F. Gmel.) Kosterm.*
Laurus sumatrensis J.F. Gmel.
科名　Dipterocarpaceae（フタバガキ科）
英名　Borneo camphor / Malay camphor / Sumatra camphor
Part of use　bark
Note 1　—
Note 2　—
注　—

名　称　リョウショウカ

他名等　ノウゼンカズラ
部位等　花
備　考　—

他名(参考)　ノウショウ・ノショウ（凌霄）、シイ（紫葳）
漢字表記・生薬名等　凌霄花（リョウショウカ、ノウゼンカズラ）
Name (Romaji)　RYÔSHÔKA
Other name(s) (Romaji)　NÔZENKAZURA
学名　*Campsis grandiflora* (Thunb.) K. Schum.
Bignonia chinensis Lam.
Campsis chinensis (Lam.) Voss
科名　Bignoniaceae（ノウゼンカズラ科）
英名　trumpet creeper / Chinese trumpet creeper / Chinese trumpet flower
Part of use　flower
Note 1　—
Note 2　—
注　—

名　称　リョクトウ*

他名等　ブンドウ
部位等　種子・花
備　考　—

他名(参考)　ヤエナリ（八重生）、アオアズキ（青小豆）
漢字表記・生薬名等　緑豆（リョクトウ）、文豆（ブンドウ）
Name (Romaji)　RYOKUTÔ*
Other name(s) (Romaji)　BUNDÔ
学名　*Vigna radiata* (L.) R. Wilczek*
Phaseolus radiatus L.*
科名　Leguminosae（マメ科）
英名　mung bean / green gram / celera bean / golden gram
Part of use　seed, flower
Note 1　—
Note 2　—
注　—

名　称　**リンゴ酢**

他名等　リンゴ
部位等　汁液発酵の食用酢
備　考　—

他名(参考)　セイヨウリンゴ（西洋林檎）
漢字表記・生薬名等　林檎酢（リンゴズ）
Name (Romaji)　RINGO-SU
Other name(s) (Romaji)　RINGO
学名　*Malus pumila* Mill.
Malus pumila Mill. var. *domestica* (Borkh.) C.K. Schneid.
Malus domestica Borkh.
Pyrus pumila (Mill.) K. Koch
科名　Rosaceae（バラ科）
英名　apple vinegar / apple cider vinegar / apple / cultivated apple
Part of use　vinegar made from fermented apple juice
Note 1　—
Note 2　RINGO-SU is the vinegar made from apple juice. Therefore, the scientific name, family name and other information on apple are described here.
注　リンゴ酢はリンゴの発酵食用酢であるので、本項ではリンゴの学名・科名等を記載した。

名　称　**ルイボス***

他名等　—
部位等　葉
備　考　—

他名(参考)　—
漢字表記・生薬名等　—
Name (Romaji)　RUIBOSU*
Other name(s) (Romaji)　—
学名　*Aspalathus linearis* (Burm. f.) R. Dahlgren*
Aspalathus contaminatus auct.
Borbonia pinifolia Marloth
科名　Leguminosae（マメ科）
英名　rooibos / rooibos tea
Part of use　leaf
Note 1　—
Note 2　Refer to BUSSHUTÎ listed in the item of "Name". BUSSHUTÎ is the tea made of the leaf of RUIBOSU.
注　別項のブッシュティーを参照。ブッシュティーはルイボスの葉を用いたお茶である。

名　称　**ルリジシャ***

他名等　ボラゴソウ／ボレイジ
部位等　葉・花
備　考　—

他名(参考)　ボリジ、ボラージ、スターフラワー、ルリジサ（瑠璃苣）
漢字表記・生薬名等　瑠璃苣（ルリジシャ）
Name (Romaji)　RURIJISHA*
Other name(s) (Romaji)　BORAGOSÔ／BOREIJI
学名　*Borago officinalis* L.*
科名　Boraginaceae（ムラサキ科）
英名　borage / common borage / beebread / beeplant / starflower / taleflower / cooltankard / talewort
Part of use　leaf, flower
Note 1　—
Note 2　—
注　—

名　称　**ルリハコベ***

他名等　—
部位等　全草
備　考　—

他名(参考)　—
漢字表記・生薬名等　瑠璃繁縷（ルリハコベ）
Name (Romaji)　RURIHAKOBE*
Other name(s) (Romaji)　—
学名　*Anagallis arvensis* L.*
Anagallis arvensis L. f. *coerulea* (Schreb.) Baumg.
Anagallis coerulea Schreb.
科名　Primulacea（サクラソウ科）
英名　scarlet pimpernel / common pimpernel / blue pimpernel / scarlet pimpernel / poor man's wealther-glass / crue all
Part of use　whole plant
Note 1　—
Note 2　—
注　—

名　称　**ルリヒエンソウ***

他名等　ラークスパー
部位等　全草
備　考　—

他名(参考)　モウコン（毛茛）、ブルースプレー
漢字表記・生薬名等　瑠璃飛燕草（ルリヒエンソウ）

Name (Romaji)　RURIHIENSÔ*
Other name (s) (Romaji)　RÂKUSUPÂ
学名　*Consolida regalis* Gray*
Delphinium consolida L.*
科名　Ranunculaceae（キンポウゲ科）
英名　forking larkspur / branching larkspur / field larkspur
Part of use　whole plant
Note 1　—
Note 2　—
注　—

学名　*Litchi chinensis* Sonn.*
Nephelium litchi Cambess.
科名　Sapindaceae（ムクロジ科）
英名　litchi / leechee / lichi / lychee
Part of use　fruit, seed
Note 1　—
Note 2　"REISHIKAKU／枝核" written in the item of "Other names" is correctly "REISHIKAKU／茘枝核".
注　「他名等」の "レイシカク／枝核" は " レイシカク／茘枝核" である。

名　称　レイシ<霊芝>*

他名等　マンネンタケ／ロッカクレイシ
部位等　子実体
備　考　—

他名(参考)　レイシソウ（霊芝草）、カドデタケ（門出茸）、ヒジリタケ（聖茸）、マゴジャクシ（孫杓子）、シソウ（芝草）
漢字表記・生薬名等　霊芝（レイシ）、万年茸（マンネンタケ）、鹿角霊芝（ロッカクレイシ）、紫芝（シシバ）
Name (Romaji)　REISHI*
Other name (s) (Romaji)　MANNENTAKE／ROKKAKU-REISHI
学名　*Ganoderma lucidum* (Curtis) P. Karst.*（マンネンタケ）
Ganoderma lucidum (Leyss. ex Fr.) Karst.*（マンネンタケ）
Ganoderma neo-japonicum Imazeki（マゴジャクシ）
科名　Ganodermataceae（マンネンタケ科）
英名　reishi / reishi mushroom / ganoderma
Part of use　fruit body
Note 1　—
Note 2　—
注　—

名　称　レイシ<茘枝>*

他名等　レイシカク／枝核
部位等　果実・種子
備　考　—

他名(参考)　ライチー
漢字表記・生薬名等　茘枝（レイシ）、種子：茘枝核（レイシカク）
Name (Romaji)　REISHI*
Other name (s) (Romaji)　REISHIKAKU

名　称　レオヌルスソウ*

他名等　—
部位等　全草
備　考　—

他名(参考)　メハジキ（目弾）、ホソバメハジキ（細葉目弾）、モミジバキセワタ（紅葉着せ綿）、ヤクモソウ（益母草）
漢字表記・生薬名等　益母草（ヤクモソウ）、細葉益母草（ホソバヤクモソウ）、目弾（メハジキ）、細葉目弾（ホソバメハジキ）、紅葉着せ綿（モミジバキセワタ）、メハジキの種子：茺蔚子（ジュウイシ）
Name (Romaji)　REONURUSUSÔ*
Other name (s) (Romaji)　—
学名　*Leonurus japonicus* Houtt.*（メハジキ）
Leonurus artemisia (Lour.) S.Y. Hu*（メハジキ）
Leonurus sibiricus auct. non L.（メハジキ）
Leonurus heterophyllus Sweet*（メハジキ）
Leonurus sibiricus L.*（ホソバメハジキ）
Leonurus cardiaca L.*（モミジバキセワタ）
科名　Labiatae（シソ科）
英名　motherwort / common motherwort / Siberian motherwort / Chinese motherwort
Part of use　whole plant
Note 1　—
Note 2　—
注　—

名　称　レモングラス*

他名等　レモンソウ
部位等　茎・葉
備　考　—

他名(参考)　—
漢字表記・生薬名等　香茅（コウボウ）
Name (Romaji)　REMONGURASU*

Other name (s) (Romaji)　REMONSÔ
学名　*Cymbopogon citratus* (DC.) Stapf*
　　Andropogon citratus DC.*
科名　Gramineae (イネ科)
英名　lemongrass / West Indian lemongrass / fever grass
Part of use　stem, leaf
Note 1　—
Note 2　—
注　—

名　称　**レモンタイム***

他名等　—
部位等　葉
備　考　—

他名(参考)　—
漢字表記・生薬名等　—
Name (Romaji)　REMONTAIMU*
Other name (s) (Romaji)　—
学名　*Thymus serpyllum* L. ssp. *citriodorum* Pers.
　　Thymus×*citriodorus* (Pers.) Schreb. ex Schweigg et Körte*
科名　Labiatae (シソ科)
英名　lemon thyme
Part of use　leaf
Note 1　—
Note 2　—
注　—

名　称　**レモンマートル**

他名等　—
部位等　葉
備　考　—

他名(参考)　—
漢字表記・生薬名等　—
Name (Romaji)　REMONMÂTORU
Other name (s) (Romaji)　—
学名　*Backhousia citriodra* F. Muell.
科名　Myrtaceae (フトモモ科)
英名　lemon myrtle / Australian lemon myrtle / lemon ironwood / lemon scent backhousia / lemon scent myrtle / lemon scent vervena / sweet vervena myrtle / sweet vervena tree
Part of use　leaf
Note 1　—
Note 2　—
注　—

名　称　**レンギョウ***

他名等　連翹
部位等　葉
備　考　果実は「医」

他名(参考)　レンギョウウツギ（連翹空木）
漢字表記・生薬名等　連翹（レンギョウ）
Name (Romaji)　RENGYÔ*
Other name (s) (Romaji)　RENGYÔ
学名　*Forsythia suspensa* (Thunb.) Vahl*
　　Rangium suspensum (Thunb.) Ohwi
科名　Oleaceae (モクセイ科)
英名　forsythia / golden bell / golden bell tree / weeping forsythia / weeping goldenbells / goldenbells
Part of use　leaf
Note 1　fruit：drug category
Note 2　—
注　—

名　称　**レンゲソウ**

他名等　—
部位等　地上部
備　考　—

他名(参考)　レンゲ（蓮華）、ゲンゲ（紫雲英、翹揺）、ゲゲバナ（五形花）、コウカサイ（紅花菜）
漢字表記・生薬名等　蓮華草（レンゲソウ）、紅花菜（コウカサイ）
Name (Romaji)　RENGESÔ
Other name (s) (Romaji)　—
学名　*Astragalus sinicus* L.
　　Astragalus lotoides Lam.
　　Hedysarum japonicum Basin.
科名　Leguminosae (マメ科)
英名　Chinese milk vetch / milk vetch / renge
Part of use　aerial part
Note 1　—
Note 2　—
注　—

名　称　**レンセンソウ**

他名等　カキドオシ
部位等　全草
備　考　—

他名(参考)　セキセツソウ（積雪草）、カントリソウ（疳取草）、バテイソウ（馬蹄草）

漢字表記･生薬名等　連銭草（レンセンソウ)、積雪草（セキセツソウ)、垣通し・籬通（カキドオシ）
Name(Romaji)　RENSENSÔ
Other name(s)(Romaji)　KAKIDÔSHI
学名　*Glechoma hederacea* L. ssp. *grandis* (A. Gray) H. Hara
Glechoma hederacea L. var. *grandis* (A. Gray) Kudo
Glechoma grandis (A. Gray) Kuprian.
科名　Labiatae（シソ科）
英名　ground ivy / alehoof / field balm / gill over the ground / runaway robin
Part of use　whole plant
Note 1　—
Note 2　RENSENSÔ is the name of traditional Japanese herbal medicin and KAKIDÔSHI is the Japanese general name.
注　レンセンソウは生薬名であり、和名はカキドオシである。

名　称　**レンリソウ**

他名等　—
部位等　豆果・若芽
備　考　—

他名(参考)　ハマエンドウ(浜豌豆)、ノエンドウ(野豌豆)
漢字表記･生薬名等　連理草（レンリソウ）
Name(Romaji)　RENRISÔ
Other name(s)(Romaji)　—
学名　*Lathyrus quinquenervius* (Miq.) Litv.（レンリソウ）
Vicia quinquenervia Miq.（レンリソウ）
Lathyrus japonicus Willd.（ハマエンドウ、ノエンドウ）
Pisum maritimum L.（ハマエンドウ、ノエンドウ）
科名　Leguminosae（マメ科）
英名　*L. quinquenervius*：vetchling
L. japonicus：sea pea / seaside pea / beach pea
Part of use　legume, sprout
Note 1　—
Note 2　—
注　—

名　称　**ローズヒップ***

他名等　—
部位等　果実・果皮・茎・花
備　考　—

他名(参考)　—
漢字表記･生薬名等　—
Name(Romaji)　RÔZUHIPPU*
Other name(s)(Romaji)　—
学名　*Rosa canina* L.*
Rosa lutetiana Léman
科名　Rosaceae（バラ科）
英名　rose hip / brier rose / common briar / briar bush / dog rose
Part of use　fruit, pericarp, stem, flower
Note 1　—
Note 2　The scientific name of RÔZUHIPPU is the same with DOGGURÔZU. DOGGURÔZU is also listed in the item of “Name”. RÔZUHIPPU is the fruit of rose but the fruit and pseudocarp of *Rosa multiflora* are classified in the “drug” category.
注　ローズヒップは別項のドッグローズと同一。ローズヒップはバラの果実。但し、ノイバラの偽果・果実は「医」に分類されている。

名　称　**ローズマリー***

他名等　マンネンロウ
部位等　葉
備　考　—

他名(参考)　—
漢字表記･生薬名等　万年朗（マンネンロウ)、迷迭香（メイテツコウ）
Name(Romaji)　RÔZUMARÎ*
Other name(s)(Romaji)　MANNENRÔ
学名　*Rosmarinus officinalis* L.*
Rosmarinus officinalis var. *prostratus* hort.
科名　Labiatae（シソ科）
英名　rosemary / romero
Part of use　leaf
Note 1　—
Note 2　—
注　—

名　称　**ローマカミツレ***

他名等　—
部位等　頭状花
備　考　—

他名(参考)　ローマンカモミール、ローマカミルレ
漢字表記･生薬名等　ローマ加密列（ローマカミツレ）
Name(Romaji)　RÔMAKAMITSURE*
Other name(s)(Romaji)　—
学名　*Chamaemelum nobile* (L.) All.*

Anthemis nobilis L.*
Ormenis nobilis (L.) J. Gay ex Coss. et Germ.
科名 Compositae（キク科）
英名 chamomile / common chamomile / Roman chamomile / corn chamomile / English chamomile / garden chamomile / noble chamomile / Russian chamomile / sweet chamomile
Part of use capitate flower
Note 1 —
Note 2 —
注 —

名　称 **ロベージ***

他名等 **レビスチクム**
部位等 全草
備　考 —

他名(参考) ラベージ、ラビッジ、ラベッジ、オウトウキ（欧当帰）
漢字表記・生薬名等 —
Name (Romaji) ROBÊJI*
Other name (s) (Romaji) REBISUCHIKUMU
学名 *Levisticum officinale* W.D.J. Koch*
Angelica levisticum Baill.
科名 Umbelliferae（セリ科）
英名 lovage / garden lovage / lovage angelica / American lovage
Part of use whole plant
Note 1 —
Note 2 —
注 —

ワ行

名　称 **ワイルドチェリー***

他名等 **ワイルドブラックチェリー**
部位等 樹皮
備　考 —

他名(参考) アメリカクロミザクラ（アメリカ黒実桜）
漢字表記・生薬名等 —
Name (Romaji) WAIRUDOCHERÎ*
Other name (s) (Romaji) WAIRUDOBURAKKUCHERÎ
学名 *Prunus serotina* Ehrh.*
科名 Rosaceae（バラ科）
英名 rum cherry / wild cherry / wild black cherry / black cherry / mountain black cherry / black chokecherry / black choke / American wild cherry / American bird cherry
Part of use bark
Note 1 —
Note 2 —
注 —

名　称 **ワイルドレタス***

他名等 **ワイルドカナダレタス**
部位等 茎・葉
備　考 —

他名(参考) —
漢字表記・生薬名等 —
Name (Romaji) WAIRUDORETASU*
Other name (s) (Romaji) WAIRUDOKANADARETASU
学名 *Lactuca virosa* L.*
科名 Compositae（キク科）
英名 great lettuce / wild lettuce / bitter lettuce / lettuce opium / laitue vireuse / opium lettuce / poisonous lettuce / poor man's opium
Part of use stem, leaf
Note 1 —
Note 2 —
注 —

名　称 **ワサビダイコン***

他名等 —
部位等 根
備　考 —

他名(参考) ホースラディッシュ、ルホール、レホール、セイヨウワサビ（西洋山葵）、ウマワサビ（馬山葵）、ウマダイコン（馬大根）、アイヌワサビ
漢字表記・生薬名等 山葵大根（ワサビダイコン）、西洋山葵（セイヨウワサビ）
Name (Romaji) WASABIDAIKON*
Other name (s) (Romaji) —
学名 *Armoracia rusticana* P. Gaertn., B. Mey. et Schreb.*
Armoracia lapathifolia Gilib. ex Usteri*
Cochlearia armoracia L.
Nasturtium armoracia (L.) Fr.
Radicula armoracia (L.) B.L. Rob.
Rorippa armoracia (L.) Hitchc.
科名 Cruciferae（アブラナ科）

英名 horseradish / horse radish / red cole
Part of use root
Note 1 —
Note 2 —
注 —

名　称 **ワレモコウ***

他名等 チユ／Sanguisorba officialis
部位等 根・根茎
備　考 —

他名(参考) ジユ（地楡）
漢字表記・生薬名等 吾亦紅・吾木香（ワレモコウ）、地楡（チユ）
Name (Romaji) WAREMOKÔ*
Other name(s) (Romaji) CHIYU
学名 *Sanguisorba officinalis* L.*
Poterium officinale（L.）A. Gray
Sanguisorba polygama F. Nyl.
科名 Rosaceae（バラ科）
英名 great burnet / garden burnet / burnet bloodwort / salad burnet / sanguisorba
Part of use root, rhizome
Note 1 —
Note 2 —
注 —

2．動物由来物等

2. Substances originated in animals

網掛け部分：網掛け部分には「名称」、「他名等」、「部位等」、「備考」の４項目が含まれる。これらの項目は食薬区分リストの表記に準拠し、そのまま一切の変更を加えずに記載した。

注１）「名称」及び「他名等」の欄については、生薬名、一般名及び起源動物名、該当する部位等を記載している。

注２）リストに掲載されている成分本質（原材料）のうち、該当する部位について、「部位等」の欄に記載している。

注３）他の部位が別のリストに掲載されている場合等、その取扱いが紛らわしいものについては、備考欄にその旨記載している。

注４）備考欄の「医」は「専ら医薬品として使用される成分本質（原材料）リスト」に掲載されていることを示す。

Shaded section：The shaded section consists of four items：Name, Other name(s), Part of use, and Remarks. These items are shown exactly as recorded in the food and drug classification lists without any changes having been made whatsoever.

1) The “Name” and “Other name(s)” entries include the crude drug name, common name, and source animal name, and the relevant part of use.
2) Of the ingredients (raw materials) included in the list, the relevant part used is included in the “Part of use” entry.
3) Where other parts are included in other lists, notes are entered in the “Remarks” column if there could be any confusion over the handling.
4) Where the “Remarks” column shows “drug (医)”, the substance is included in the “List of ingredients (raw materials) used exclusively for drugs”.

動物由来等の原材料の見方
(Notation of a substance originated in animal(s).)

名　称 他名等 部位等 備　考	**Name** **Other name(s)** **Part of Use** **Remarks**	食薬区分リストの記載事項とその内容。 The shaded section consists of the following four items which are exactly shown as recorded in the food and drug classification lists without any changes.
他名(参考)	食薬区分リストには載っていないが、実際に使用されている名称。 **Other name(s) (for reference)**：Names in actual use but not recorded in the food and drug classification list.	
漢字表記・生薬名等	「名称」「他名等」の漢字表記と読み。それらの生薬、漢方等における名称の漢字表記と読み。 **Kanji notation and crude drug name**：The kanji notations of "Name" and "Other name(s)" along with the names (kanji) used in crude drug and/or Kampo medicine (traditional Japanese medicine), etc.	
Name (Romaji)	「名称」のローマ字表記。 Roman alphabet (romaji) of the "Name" in the food and drug classification list.	
Other name(s) (Romaji)	「他名等」のローマ字表記。 Roman alphabet (romaji) of the "Other name(s)" in the food and drug classification list.	
学名 科名 英名	**Scientific name(s)** **Family name** **English name(s)**	「名称」または「他名等」の学名、科名、英名。 Scientific name(s), Family name and English name(s) of the "Name" or "Other name(s)".
Part of use	「部位等」の英訳。 English translation of the "Part of use" in the food and drug classification list.	
Note 1	「備考」の英訳。 English translation of the content of "Remarks" in the food and drug classification list.	
Note 2	下記「注」の英訳。 English translation of "Note (注)" in the last item.	
注	食薬区分リストの記載事項についての補足情報等。 **Note**：Comments or supplementary information on the content of the food and drug classification records are given.	

ア行

名　称　アキョウ

他名等　ウシ／ラバ／ロバ
部位等　皮膚を水で煮て製したにかわ
備　考　—

他名(参考)　デンチキョウ（傳致膠）、ロヒキョウ（驢皮膠）
漢字表記・生薬名等　阿膠（アキョウ）
Name (Romaji)　AKYÔ
Other name (s) (Romaji)　USHI／RABA／ROBA
学名　*Bos taurus* L.（ウシ、ウシ科）
Equus asinus L.（ラバ、ウマ科）
Equus caballus×*Equus asinus*（ロバ、ウマ科）
科名　Bovidae（ウシ科）
Equidae（ウマ科）
英名　donkey-hide gelatin
Part of use　glue obtained from skin with boiled water
Note 1　—
Note 2　—
注　—

名　称　アザラシ

他名等　—
部位等　油
備　考　—

他名(参考)　ゴマフアザラシ（胡麻斑海豹）、タテゴトアザラシ（竪琴海豹）、トッカリ
漢字表記・生薬名等　海豹（アザラシ）
Name (Romaji)　AZARASHI
Other name (s) (Romaji)　—
学名　*Phoca vitulina* L.（ゴマフアザラシ）
Pagophilus groenlandicus Erxleben（タテゴトアザラシ）
Phoca groenlandica Erxleben（タテゴトアザラシ）
科名　Phocidae（アザラシ科）
英名　harp seal / earless seal / common Arctic seal
Part of use　fat
Note 1　—
Note 2　—
注　—

名　称　アズマニシキガイ

他名等　—
部位等　貝肉
備　考　—

他名(参考)　—
漢字表記・生薬名等　吾妻錦貝・東錦貝（アズマニシキガイ）
Name (Romaji)　AZUMANISHIKIGAI
Other name (s) (Romaji)　—
学名　*Chlamys farreri nipponensis* Kuroda
Chlamys farreri Jones et Preston
科名　Pectinidae（イタヤガイ科）
英名　farrer's scallop / Chlamys farreri
Part of use　shellfish meat
Note 1　—
Note 2　—
注　—

名　称　アリ

他名等　アリノコ
部位等　アリ・アリの子
備　考　—

他名(参考)　ギコクタシアリ（擬黒多刺蟻）、クロアリ（黒蟻）、オオクロアリ（大黒蟻）
漢字表記・生薬名等　—
Name (Romaji)　ARI
Other name (s) (Romaji)　ARINOKO
学名　*Polyrhachis vicina* Roger
科名　Formicidae（アリ科）
英名　ant / Chinese black ant
Part of use　ant, ant pupae
Note 1　—
Note 2　—
注　—

名　称　アワビ

他名等　セキケツメイ
部位等　殻
備　考　—

他名(参考)　センリコウ（千里光）、エゾアワビ（蝦夷鮑）、クロアワビ（黒鮑）、マダカアワビ（目高鮑）
漢字表記・生薬名等　石決明（セキケツメイ）、鮑（アワビ）
Name (Romaji)　AWABI
Other name (s) (Romaji)　SEKIKETSUMEI

学名　*Haliotis diversicolor* Reeve（ザッショクアワビ）
Haliotis gigantea Gmelin（メガイアワビ）
Haliotis discus hannai Ino（エゾアワビ）
Haliotis discus Reeve（クロアワビ）
Haliotis madaka Habe（マダカアワビ）
科名　Haliotidae（ミミガイ科）
英名　sea-ear shell / ear shell / abalone / Japanese abalone
Part of use　shell
Note 1　—
Note 2　—
注　—

名　称　**イカ**

他名等　**イカスミ／ウゾクコツ／コウイカ**
部位等　イカの墨・甲骨
備　考　—

他名(参考)　ハリイカ（針烏賊）、マイカ（真烏賊）、スミイカ（墨烏賊）
漢字表記・生薬名等　烏賊墨（イカスミ）、烏賊骨（ウゾクコツ）、海螵蛸（カイヒョウショウ）、甲烏賊（コウイカ）
Name(Romaji)　IKA
Other name(s) (Romaji)　IKASUMI／UZOKUKOTSU／KÔIKA
学名　*Sepia esculenta* Hoyle（コウイカ）
科名　Sepiidae（コウイカ科）
英名　squid / cuttlefish / golden cuttlefish
Part of use　squid ink, oracle bones
Note 1　—
Note 2　—
注　—

名　称　**イワシ**

他名等　**サーディンペプチド**
部位等　油・タンパク質
備　考　—

他名(参考)　ナナツボシ（七つ星）、ウルメ（潤目）
漢字表記・生薬名等　鰯（イワシ）、真鰯（マイワシ）、潤目鰯（ウルメイワシ）、片口鰯（カタクチイワシ）
Name(Romaji)　IWASHI
Other name(s) (Romaji)　SÂDINPEPUCHIDO
学名　*Sardinops melanostictus* Temminck et Schlegel（マイワシ、ニシン科）
Sardinops sagax Jenyns（マイワシ、ニシン科）
Etrumeus teres DeKey（ウルメイワシ、ニシン科）
Engraulis japonica Houttuyn（カタクチイワシ、カタクチイワシ科）
Engraulis japonicus Temminck et Schlegel（カタクチイワシ、カタクチイワシ科）
科名　Culpeidae（ニシン科）
Engraulidae（カタクチイワシ科）
英名　*Sardinops sagax*：Japanese sardine / Japanese pilchard
Etrumeus teres：red eye round herrings / round herrings
Engraulis japonicus：Japanese anchovy
Part of use　fat, protein
Note 1　—
Note 2　—
注　—

名　称　**陰茎**

他名等　**ウシ／ウマ／トラ／ヒツジ／ブタ／ヘビ**
部位等　陰茎・睾丸
備　考　イヌ・オットセイ・シカの陰茎・睾丸は「医」

他名(参考)　—
漢字表記・生薬名等　牯牛卵嚢、馬茎（バケイ）、豚卵（トンラン）、虎鞭（コベン）、蛇鞭（ジャベン）
Name(Romaji)　INKEI
Other name(s) (Romaji)　USHI／UMA／TORA／HITSUJI／BUTA／HEBI
学名　*Bos taurus* L.（ウシ、ウシ科）
Equus caballus L.（ウマ、ウマ科）
Panthera tigris L.（トラ、ネコ科）
Ovis aries L.（ヒツジ、ウシ科）
Sus scrofa L.（ブタ、イノシシ科）
Serpentes L.（ヘビ、ヘビ亜目）
科名　Bovidae（ウシ科）
Equidae（ウマ科）
Felidae（ネコ科）
Suidae（イノシシ科）
Serpentes（ヘビ亜目）
英名　penis or testis of bovine, horse, sheep, swine, tiger or serpent
Part of use　penis, testis
Note 1　penis and testis of dog, seal and deer：drug category
Note 2　International trade of tigers is completely prohibited because tigers are included in the Appendix I of CITES (Convention on International Trade in Endangered Species of Wild Fauna and Flora).
注　トラは、ワシントン条約附属書Ⅰに含まれ、全面的に商取引が禁止されている。

名　称　**ウコッケイ**

他名等　—
部位等　血液・卵・内臓・肉
備　考　—

他名(参考)　ニワトリ
漢字表記・生薬名等　烏骨鶏（ウコッケイ）
Name (Romaji)　UKOKKEI
Other name (s) (Romaji)　—
学名　*Gallus gallus* L.
科名　Phasianidae（キジ科）
英名　chicken / bantam / silky fowl
Part of use　blood, egg, internal organ, meat
Note 1　—
Note 2　—
注　—

名　称　**ウナギ**

他名等　ヤツメウナギ
部位等　全体
備　考　—

他名(参考)　カワヤツメ
漢字表記・生薬名等　鰻（ウナギ）、八目鰻（ヤツメウナギ）
Name (Romaji)　UNAGI
Other name (s) (Romaji)　YATSUMEUNAGI
学名　*Anguilla japonica* Temminck et Schlegel（ウナギ、ウナギ科）
Anguilla remifera Jordan et Evermann（ウナギ、ウナギ科）
Lethenteron camtschaticum Tilesius（ヤツメウナギ、ヤツメウナギ科）
Lethenteron japonicum Martens（ヤツメウナギ、ヤツメウナギ科）
科名　Anguillidae（ウナギ科）
Petromyzontidae（ヤツメウナギ科）
英名　*Anguilla japonica*：Japanese eel
Lethenteron camtshaticum：arctic lamprey / lamprey
Part of use　whole body
Note 1　—
Note 2　—
注　—

名　称　**オオトカゲ**

他名等　—
部位等　全体
備　考　—

他名(参考)　—
漢字表記・生薬名等　大蜥蜴（オオトカゲ）
Name (Romaji)　ÔTOKAGE
Other name (s) (Romaji)　—
学名　*Varanidae* Hardwicke et Gray（オオトカゲ科）
科名　Varanidae（オオトカゲ科）
英名　monitor lizard
Part of use　whole body
Note 1　—
Note 2　This species is included in the Appendix II of CITES (Convention on International Trade in Endangered Species of Wild Fauna and Flora).
注　本種はワシントン条約附属書 II に指定されている。

名　称　**オオヤモリ**

他名等　ゴウカイ／Gekko gecko
部位等　内臓を除いた全身
備　考　—

他名(参考)　トッケイヤモリ（トッケイ守宮）、トッケイ
漢字表記・生薬名等　大守宮（オオヤモリ）、蛤蚧（ゴウカイ）
Name (Romaji)　ÔYAMORI
Other name (s) (Romaji)　GÔKAI
学名　*Gekko gecko* L.
科名　Gekkonidae（ヤモリ科）
英名　Tokay gecko / Tokay gekko
Part of use　whole body excepting internal organs
Note 1　—
Note 2　—
注　—

名　称　**オットセイ**

他名等　カロペプタイド
部位等　骨格筋抽出物
備　考　陰茎・睾丸は「医」

他名(参考)　キタオットセイ（北膃肭臍）
漢字表記・生薬名等　膃肭臍（オットセイ）
Name (Romaji)　OTTOSEI
Other name (s) (Romaji)　KAROPEPUTAIDO
学名　*Callorhinus ursinus* L.

科名　Otariidae（アシカ科）
英名　northern fur seal
Part of use　skeletal muscle
Note 1　penis and testis：drug category
Note 2　—
注　—

カ行

名　称　**カイエン**

他名等　**イトマキヒトデ**
部位等　全体
備　考　—

他名(参考)　—
漢字表記・生薬名等　海燕（カイエン）、糸巻海星・糸巻人手（イトマキヒトデ）
Name(Romaji)　KAIEN
Other name(s)(Romaji)　ITOMAKIHITODE
学名　*Patiria pectinifera* Müller et Troschel
Asterina pectinifera Müller et Troschel
Asteriscus pectinifera Müller et Troschel
科名　Asterinidae（イトマキヒトデ科）
英名　starfish
Part of use　whole body
Note 1　—
Note 2　—
注　—

名　称　**カイコ**

他名等　**カサンガ／ゲンサンガ**
部位等　蛹・死んだ幼虫・成虫・糞便・繭・幼虫の抜殻・卵殻
備　考　—

他名(参考)　カイコガ（蚕蛾）
漢字表記・生薬名等　蚕（カイコ）、原蚕蛾（ゲンサンガ）、原蚕子（ゲンサンシ）、原蚕沙（ゲンサンシャ）、白殭蚕・白姜蚕（ビャッキョウサン）、僵蚕・姜蚕（キョウサン）
Name(Romaji)　KAIKO
Other name(s)(Romaji)　KASANGA／GENSANGA
学名　*Bombyx mori* L.
科名　Bombycidae（カイコガ科）
英名　silk moth / silkworm
Part of use　pupa, dead larva, imago, fece, cocoon, cast-off skin of larva, shell
Note 1　—
Note 2　—
注　—

名　称　**カイバ**

他名等　**タツノオトシゴ**
部位等　全体
備　考　—

他名(参考)　オオウミウマ（克氏海馬）、イバラタツ（刺海馬、茨竜）、ダイカイバ（大海馬）、クロウミウマ（黒海馬）、三斑海馬
漢字表記・生薬名等　海馬（カイバ）、竜の落とし子（タツノオトシゴ）
Name(Romaji)　KAIBA
Other name(s)(Romaji)　TATSUNOOTOSHIGO
学名　*Hippocampus kelloggi* Jordan et Snyder（オオウミウマ）
Hippocampus histrix Kaup（イバラタツ）
Hippocampus kuda Bleeker（クロウミウマ）
Hippocampus trimaculatus Leach（三斑海馬）
Hippocampus coronatus Temminck et Schlegel（タツノオトシゴ）
科名　Syngnathidae（ヨウジウオ科）
英名　seahorse / spotted seahorse
Part of use　whole body
Note 1　—
Note 2　Seahorse is included in the Appendix II of CITES (Convention on International Trade in Endangered Species of Wild Fauna and Flora).
注　タツノオトシゴはワシントン条約附属書IIに含まれる。

名　称　**カイリュウ**

他名等　**ギカイリュウ／センカイリュウ／チョウカイリュウ／トゲヨウジ**
部位等　全体
備　考　—

他名(参考)　ギカイリュウ、トゲヨウジ（擬海竜）、センカイリュウ（尖海竜）、チョウカイリュウ（刁海竜）
漢字表記・生薬名等　海竜（カイリュウ）、擬海龍・擬海竜（ギカイリュウ）
Name(Romaji)　KAIRYÛ
Other name(s)(Romaji)　GIKAIRYÛ／SENKAIRYÛ／CHÔKAIRYÛ／TOGEYÔJI
学名　*Syngnathoides biaculeatus* Bloch（トゲヨウジ）

Syngnathus acus L.（センカイリュウ）
Solegnathus hardwickii Gray（チョウカイリュウ）
Solenognathus hardwickii Gray（チョウカイリュウ）

科名 Syngnathidae（ヨウジウオ科）

英名 seaweed pipefish / pallid seahorse / Hardwicke's pipefish / great pipefish / longnosed pipefish

Part of use whole body

Note 1 —

Note 2 "*Solenognathus hardwickii* Gray" listed as the fourth scientific name is the misspelling and its correct generic name is "Solegnathus". The misspelled scientific name is listed here because it is sometimes used.

注 *Solenognathus hardwickii* Gray（4番目の学名）はミススペルであるが、本学名が使用されることもあるので掲載した。

名称 カキ＜牡蛎＞

他名等 マガキ／ボレイ
部位等 貝殻・貝肉・貝肉エキス
備考 —

他名（参考） イワガキ（岩牡蠣）、スミノエガキ（住之江牡蠣）、イタボガキ（板甫牡蠣）、シカメガキ

漢字表記・生薬名等 牡蛎（カキ、ボレイ）、真牡蠣（マガキ）

Name (Romaji) KAKI

Other name (s) (Romaji) MAGAKI／BOREI

学名 *Ostrea gigas* Thunb.
Crassostrea gigas Thunb.

科名 Ostreidae（イタボガキ科）

英名 oyster shell / giant cupped oyster / giant oyster / giant Pacific oyster / immigrant oyster / Japanese oyster / Pacific cupped oyster

Part of use seashell, shellfish meat, shellfish meat extract

Note 1 —

Note 2 —

注 —

名称 カギュウマツ

他名等 カタツムリ
部位等 腹足類の乾燥粉末
備考 —

他名（参考） オナジマイマイ（同蝸牛）、デンデンムシ

漢字表記・生薬名等 蝸牛（カギュウ、カタツムリ）

Name (Romaji) KAGYÛMATSU

Other name (s) (Romaji) KATATSUMURI

学名 *Bradybaena similaris* Ferussac

科名 Bradybaenidae（オナジマイマイ科）

英名 land snail / Asian trampsnail

Part of use dried powder of gastropod

Note 1 —

Note 2 KAGYÛMATSU consists of two words, namely KAGYÛ for land snail and MATSU for dry powder.

注 カギュウマツ（名称）はカギュウ末である。

名称 核酸

他名等 DNA／RNA
部位等 —
備考 —

他名（参考） —

漢字表記・生薬名等 —

Name (Romaji) KAKUSAN

Other name (s) (Romaji) —

学名 —

科名 —

英名 nucleic acid

Part of use —

Note 1 —

Note 2 —

注 —

名称 カツオ

他名等 かつお節／かつお節オリゴペプチド
部位等 魚乾燥物
備考 —

他名（参考） —

漢字表記・生薬名等 鰹（カツオ）、鰹節（カツオブシ）

Name (Romaji) KATSUO

Other name (s) (Romaji) KATSUOBUSHI／KATSUOBUSHIORIGOPEPUCHIDO

学名 *Katsuwonus pelamis* L.

科名 Scombridae（サバ科）

英名 bonito / skipjack tuna / Oceanic bonito / dried bonito

Part of use jerked meat

Note 1 —

Note 2 —

注 —

名　称　**カニ**

他名等　—
部位等　甲羅
備　考　—

他名(参考)　(例) ズワイガニ（楚蟹、津和井蟹、松葉蟹）
漢字表記・生薬名等　蟹（カニ）
Name (Romaji)　KANI
Other name (s) (Romaji)　—
学名　*Brachyura* L.（短尾下目（カニ下目））
　　(e.g. *Chionoecetes opilio* O. Fabricius（ズワイガニ））
科名　Brachyura（タンビカ目（短尾下目））
英名　crab
Part of use　shell
Note 1　—
Note 2　—
注　—

名　称　**カメ**

他名等　**ウミガメ**
部位等　全体
備　考　—

他名(参考)　—
漢字表記・生薬名等　亀（カメ）、海亀（ウミガメ）
Name (Romaji)　KAME
Other name (s) (Romaji)　UMIGAME
学名　*Testudines* L.（カメ目）
科名　Testudines（カメ目）
英名　testudines / turtle / sea turtle / marine turtle
Part of use　whole body
Note 1　—
Note 2　Sea turtles such as hawksbill are included in the Appendix I of CITES (Convention on International Trade in Endangered Species of Wild Fauna and Flora).
注　タイマイ等ウミガメはワシントン条約付属書Ⅰに含まれる。

名　称　**カメムシ**

他名等　**九香虫**
部位等　全体
備　考　—

他名(参考)　ツマキクロカメムシ（ツマキクロ亀虫）
漢字表記・生薬名等　椿像（カメムシ）、亀虫（カメムシ）、九香虫（キュウコウチュウ）
Name (Romaji)　KAMEMUSHI
Other name (s) (Romaji)　KYÛKÔCHÛ
学名　*Aspongopus chinensis* Dallas
　　Coridius chinensis Dallas
科名　Pentatomidae（カメムシ科）
英名　stink bug / bugs
Part of use　whole body
Note 1　—
Note 2　—
注　—

名　称　**肝臓**

他名等　**ウシ／トリ／ブタ**
部位等　ウシ・トリ・ブタの肝臓・エキス
備　考　—

他名(参考)　—
漢字表記・生薬名等　牛肝（ギュウカン）、鶏肝（ケイカン）
Name (Romaji)　KANZÔ
Other name (s) (Romaji)　USHI／TORI／BUTA
学名　*Bos taurus* L.（ウシ、ウシ科）
　　Gallus gallus L.（ニワトリ、キジ科）
　　Sus scrofa L.（ブタ、イノシシ科）
科名　Bovidae（ウシ科）
　　Phasianidae（キジ科）
　　Suidae（イノシシ科）
英名　liver
Part of use　liver of bovine, fowl and swine, and their liver extract
Note 1　—
Note 2　—
注　—

名　称　**肝油**

他名等　—
部位等　タラ等魚類肝臓の脂肪油
備　考　—

他名(参考)　マダラ（真鱈）、スケトウダラ（介党鱈）、コマイ（氷下魚）
漢字表記・生薬名等　肝油（カンユ）
Name (Romaji)　KAN'YU
Other name (s) (Romaji)　—
学名　*Gadus macrocephalus* Tilesius（マダラ）
　　Theragra chalcogramma Pallas（スケトウダラ）
　　Eleginus gracilis Tilesius（コマイ）
科名　Gadidae（タラ科）
英名　cod liver oil of :

Gadus macrocephalus；Pacific cod
Theragra chalcogramma；Alaska pollock / bigeye / walleye pollock
Eleginus gracilis；saffron cod
Part of use　liver fatty oil of pollacks and other fishes
Note 1　—
Note 2　—
注　—

名　称　**魚油**
他名等　—
部位等　イワシ等の精製油
備　考　—

他名(参考)　マイワシ（真鰯)、ウルメイワシ（潤鰯)、カタクチイワシ（片口鰯）
漢字表記・生薬名等　魚油（ギョユ）
Name(Romaji)　GYOYU
Other name(s) (Romaji)　—
学名　*Sardinops sagax* Jenyns（マイワシ、ニシン科）
Sardinops melanostictus Temminck et Schlegel（マイワシ、ニシン科）
Etrumeus teres DeKay（ウルメイワシ、ニシン科）
Engraulis japonicus Temminck et Schlegel（カタクチイワシ、カタクチイワシ科）
科名　Clupeidae（ニシン科）
Engraulidae（カタクチイワシ科）
英名　Fish oil of：
Sardinops sagax；California pilchard / Japanese pilchard / Pacific sardine
Etrumeus teres；red-eye round herring / round herring
Engraulis japonicus；Japanese anchovy
Part of use　purified fish oil of sardine and others
Note 1　—
Note 2　—
注　—

名　称　**血液**
他名等　**ウシ／シカ／ブタ**
部位等　ウシ・シカ・ブタの血液・血漿
備　考　ヒト血液は「医」

他名(参考)　—
漢字表記・生薬名等　牛血、鹿血、猪血
Name(Romaji)　KETSUEKI
Other name(s) (Romaji)　USHI／SHIKA／BUTA
学名　*Bos taurus* L.（ウシ、ウシ科）
Cervus elaphus L.（シカ、シカ科）
Sus scrofa L.（ブタ、イノシシ科）
科名　Bovidae（ウシ科）
Cervidae（シカ科）
Suidae（イノシシ科）
英名　blood of bovine, red deer or swine
Part of use　blood or plasma of bovine, deer or swine
Note 1　human blood：drug category
Note 2　—
注　—

名　称　**ゴウシマ**
他名等　**アカガエル**
部位等　アカガエルの輸卵管
備　考　—

他名(参考)　—
漢字表記・生薬名等　哈士蟆（ゴウシマ)、雪蛤・雪哈（セツゴウ）
Name(Romaji)　GÔSHIMA
Other name(s) (Romaji)　AKAGAERU
学名　*Rana chensinensis* David（中国林蛙）
Rana temporaria chinensis（中国林蛙）
Rana amurensis Boulenger（黒竜江林蛙）
科名　Ranidae（アカガエル科）
英名　Chinese brown frog / Inkiapo frog / Far Eastern wood frog / Asiatic wood frog / Asiatic grass frog / true frogs / Siberian tree frog / Siberian wood frog / Amur brown frog
Part of use　Fallopian tube of ranid
Note 1　—
Note 2　—
注　—

名　称　**骨髄**
他名等　**ウシ**
部位等　ウシ骨髄
備　考　ヒト骨髄は「医」

他名(参考)　—
漢字表記・生薬名等　牛髄
Name(Romaji)　KOTSUZUI
Other name(s) (Romaji)　USHI
学名　*Bos taurus* L.
科名　Bovidae（ウシ科）
英名　bone marrow of bovine
Part of use　bone marrow of bovine
Note 1　human bone marrow：drug category

Note 2 —
注 —

名 称 **骨粉**

他名等 —
部位等 ウシ・魚類等の骨の粉末
備 考 —

他名(参考) —
漢字表記・生薬名等 —
Name(Romaji) KOPPUN
Other name(s)(Romaji) —
学名 *Bos taurus* L.
科名 Bovidae(ウシ科)
英名 powdered bones of bovine or fishes
Part of use bone powder of bovine or fishes
Note 1 —
Note 2 —
注 —

名 称 **コブラ**

他名等 インドコブラ/フィリピンコブラ
部位等 全体
備 考 —

他名(参考) メガネヘビ(眼鏡蛇)
漢字表記・生薬名等 —
Name(Romaji) KOBURA
Other name(s)(Romaji) INDOKOBURA/FIRIPINKOBURA
学名 *Naja naja* L.(インドコブラ)
Naja philippinensis Taylor(フィリピンコブラ)
科名 Elapidae(コブラ科)
英名 Indian cobra / Philippine cobra
Part of use whole body
Note 1 —
Note 2 *Naja naja* L. and *Naja philippinensis* Taylor are included in the Appendix II of CITES (Convention on International Trade in Endangered Species of Wild Fauna and Flora).
注 コブラはワシントン条約附属書IIに含まれる。

名 称 **コンドロイチン加水分解二糖**

他名等 —
部位等 海洋性微生物の生産するグリコサミノグリカンの分解物
備 考 —

他名(参考) —
漢字表記・生薬名等 —
Name(Romaji) KONDOROICHINKASUIBUNKAINITÔ
Other name(s)(Romaji) —
学名 *Pseudomonas* Migula(シュードモナス属)
科名 Pseudomonadaceae(シュードモナス科)
英名 disaccharide from hydrolysed chondroitin
Part of use degradation products of glycosaminoglycan produced by marine microbe
Note 1 —
Note 2 —
注 —

サ行

名 称 **サソリ**

他名等 キョクトウサソリ
部位等 食塩水に入れ殺して乾燥したもの
備 考 —

他名(参考) —
漢字表記・生薬名等 蝎(サソリ)、全蝎(ゼンカツ)、極東蠍(キョクトウサソリ)
Name(Romaji) SASORI
Other name(s)(Romaji) KYOKUTÔSASORI
学名 *Mesobuthus martensii* Karsch
Buthus martensii Karsch
科名 Buthidae(トクササソリ科)
英名 Chinese scorpion / Manchurian scorpion
Part of use dried scorpion killed by soaking in salt water
Note 1 —
Note 2 —
注 —

名　称　**サメ**

他名等　サメナンコツ／フカヒレ
部位等　軟骨・ヒレ・ヒレのエキス
備　考　—

他名（参考）　（例）ヨシキリザメ（葦切鮫）
漢字表記・生薬名等　鮫（サメ）、鮫軟骨（サメナンコツ）、鱶鰭（フカヒレ）
Name（Romaji）　SAME
Other name(s)（Romaji）　SAMENANKOTSU／FUKAHIRE
学名　*Elasmobranchii* Bonaparte
(e.g. *Prionace glauca* L.（ヨシキリザメ））
科名　Elasmobranchii（バンサイ亜綱（板鰓亜綱））
英名　shark
Part of use　cartilage, fin, fin extract
Note 1　—
Note 2　—
注　—

名　称　**サンゴ**

他名等　—
部位等　—
備　考　—

他名（参考）　沖縄サンゴ、風化造礁サンゴ、コーラルサンゴ
漢字表記・生薬名等　珊瑚（サンゴ）
Name（Romaji）　SANGO
Other name(s)（Romaji）　—
学名　*Coralliidae* Lamouroux（サンゴ科）
科名　Coralliidae（サンゴ科）
英名　coral（coral from Okinawa / weathered hermatypic coral）
Part of use　—
Note 1　—
Note 2　—
注　—

名　称　**角**

他名等　サンバー／トナカイ／ニューカレドニアジカ／ファロージカ／ベルベット
部位等　シカ等の成熟した角・袋角・幼角
備　考　レイヨウカク・ロクジョウは「医」

他名（参考）　スイロク（水鹿、サンバー）、ルサジカ（ルサ鹿、ニューカレドニア鹿）、ダマジカ（ダマ鹿、ファロー鹿）
漢字表記・生薬名等　—
Name（Romaji）　TSUNO
Other name(s)（Romaji）　SANBÂ／TONAKAI／NYÛKAREDONIAJIKA／FARÔJIKA／BERUBETTO
学名　*Rusa unicolor* Kerr（サンバー）
Rangifer tarandus L.（トナカイ）
Rusa timorensis de Blainville（ニューカレドニアジカ）
Dama dama L.（ファロージカ）
科名　Cervidae（シカ科）
英名　antlers or velvet of sambar, reindeer（caribou）, rusa deer or fallow deer
Part of use　matured antlers, velvet and immatured antlers
Note 1　Antelopis Cornu（horn of *Saiga tatarica* L. and *Gazalla subgutturos*a G-Ldenstaedt）and Cervi Parvum Cornu（pilose antler of *Cervus*（Cervus）*elaphus* L. var. *xanthopygus* Milne-Edwards and *Cervus*（Sika）*nippon* Temminck var. *mantchuricus* Swinhoe）：drug category
Note 2　—
注　—

名　称　**シジミ**

他名等　マシジミ／ヤマトシジミ
部位等　貝肉・貝肉エキス
備　考　—

他名（参考）　—
漢字表記・生薬名等　蜆（シジミ）、真蜆（マシジミ）、大和蜆（ヤマトシジミ）
Name（Romaji）　SHIJIMI
Other name(s)（Romaji）　MASHIJIMI／YAMATOSHIJIMI
学名　*Corbicula leana* Prime（マシジミ）
Corbicula japonica Primc（ヤマトシジミ）
科名　Corbiculidae（シジミ科）
英名　fresh water clam / Asian clam / shijimi clam
Part of use　shellfish meat, shellfish meat extract
Note 1　—
Note 2　It is known that shellfish poison may be detected in shijimi clam.
注　シジミは貝毒を含むことがあると知られている。

名　称　シャチュウ

他名等　サツマゴキブリ
部位等　全虫
備　考　—

他名(参考)　ジベツ（地鼈）（虫）、ドベツ（土鼈）（虫）、ドゲン（土元）、ジヒチュウ（地卑虫）、カハチュウ（蚵蚾虫）
漢字表記・生薬名等　䗪虫（シャチュウ）、金辺土鼈、薩摩蜚蠊（サツマゴキブリ）
Name(Romaji)　SHACHÛ
Other name(s) (Romaji)　SATSUMAGOKIBURI
学名　*Opisthoplatia orientalis* Burmeister（サツマゴキブリ、ブラベルスゴキブリ科）
Eupolyphaga sinensis Walker（シナゴキブリ、ゴキブリ科）
科名　Blaberidae（ブラベルスゴキブリ科）
Blattidae（ゴキブリ科）
英名　cockroach / roaches
Part of use　whole insect body
Note 1　—
Note 2　—
注　—

名　称　心臓

他名等　ウシ／ウマ
部位等　ウシ・ウマの心臓
備　考　—

他名(参考)　ハツ
漢字表記・生薬名等　—
Name(Romaji)　SHINZÔ
Other name(s) (Romaji)　USHI／UMA
学名　*Bos taurus* L.（ウシ、ウシ科）
Equus caballus L.（ウマ、ウマ科）
科名　Bovidae（ウシ科）
Equidae（ウマ科）
英名　heart of bovine or horse
Part of use　heart of bovine or horse
Note 1　—
Note 2　—
注　—

名　称　スクアラミン

他名等　—
部位等　サメの肝臓
備　考　—

他名(参考)　—
漢字表記・生薬名等　—
Name(Romaji)　SUKUARAMIN
Other name(s) (Romaji)　—
学名　*Elasmobranchii* Bonaparte
（e.g. *Squalus acanthias* L.（アブラツノザメ））
科名　Elasmobranchii（バンサイ亜綱（板鰓亜綱））
英名　shark liver squalamine
Part of use　shark liver
Note 1　—
Note 2　Squalamine is an aminosterol compound.
注　スクアラミンはアミノステロール化合物の一種。

名　称　スッポン

他名等　シナスッポン／ベッコウ
部位等　血液・卵・内臓・肉・背甲・腹甲
備　考　—

他名(参考)　—
漢字表記・生薬名等　鼈（スッポン）、支那鼈（シナスッポン）、鼈甲（ベッコウ）、土鼈甲・土別甲（ドベッコウ）
Name(Romaji)　SUPPON
Other name(s) (Romaji)　SHINASUPPON／BEKKÔ
学名　*Pelodiscus sinensis* Wiegmann（シナスッポン）
Amyda sinensis Wiegmann（シナスッポン）
Amyda japonica Temminck et Schlegel（スッポン）
科名　Trionychidae（スッポン科）
英名　Chinese softshell turtle
Part of use　blood, egg, viscera, meat, upper shell, lower shell
Note 1　—
Note 2　—
注　—

名　称　精巣

他名等　シラコ
部位等　食用魚類の精巣
備　考　—

他名(参考)　サケ（鮭）、シロザケ（白鮭）、タラ（鱈）の精巣（タチ、キク、キクワタ、クモコ）

漢字表記・生薬名等　精巣（セイソウ）、白子（シラコ）
Name (Romaji)　SEISÔ
Other name (s) (Romaji)　SHIRAKO
学名　testis of edible fish (e.g. Salmonidae, Gadidae)
科名　—
英名　—
Part of use　testicle of edible fish
Note 1　—
Note 2　—
注　—

名　称　**ソウヒョウショウ**

他名等　カマキリ
部位等　カマキリの卵鞘
備　考　—

他名(参考)　オオカマキリ（大刀蜋、団螵蛸）、コカマキリ（小刀蜋、黒螵蛸）、ウスバカマキリ（薄翅螗螂）、ハラビロカマキリ（巨斧螗螂）
漢字表記・生薬名等　桑螵蛸（ソウヒョウショウ）、螗螂・螳螂・鎌切（カマキリ）
Name (Romaji)　SÔHYÔSHÔ
Other name (s) (Romaji)　KAMAKIRI
学名　*Tenodera sinensis* Saussure（オオカマキリ）
Paratenodera sinensis Saussure（オオカマキリ）
Statilia maculata Thunb.（コカマキリ）
Mantis religiosa L.（ウスバカマキリ）
Hierodula patellifera Serv.（ハラビロカマキリ）
科名　Mantidae（カマキリ科）
英名　mantis / praying mantis / mantids / Chinese praying mantis
Part of use　mantis ootheca
Note 1　—
Note 2　—
注　—

タ行

名　称　**胎盤**

他名等　ウシ／ヒツジ／ブタ
部位等　ウシ・ヒツジ・ブタの胎盤
備　考　ヒト胎盤は「医」

他名(参考)　プラセンタ
漢字表記・生薬名等　—
Name (Romaji)　TAIBAN
Other name (s) (Romaji)　USHI／HITSUJI／BUTA
学名　*Bos taurus* L.（ウシ、ウシ科）
Ovis aries L.（ヒツジ、ウシ科）
Sus scrofa L.（ブタ、イノシシ科）
科名　Bovidae（ウシ科）
Suidae（イノシシ科）
英名　placenta
Part of use　placenta of bovine, sheep or swine
Note 1　human placenta : drug category
Note 2　—
注　—

名　称　**胆嚢**

他名等　—
部位等　コイ・ヘビの胆嚢
備　考　ウシ・クマ・ブタの胆汁・胆嚢は「医」

他名(参考)　—
漢字表記・生薬名等　鯉魚胆（リギョタン）、鯉胆（リタン）、蝮蛇胆（フクダタン）、蛇胆（ジャタン）
Name (Romaji)　TANNÔ
Other name (s) (Romaji)　—
学名　*Cyprinus carpio* L.（コイ、コイ科）
Serpentes L.（ヘビ亜目）
(e.g. *Gloydius blomhoffii* Boie（ニホンマムシ、クサリヘビ科）、*Agkistrodon halys* Pallas（マムシ、クサリヘビ科））
科名　Cyprinidae（コイ科）
Serpentes（ヘビ亜目）
英名　gallbladder of carp or mamushi
Part of use　gallbladder of carp or snake
Note 1　bile and gallbladder of bovine, bear and swine : drug category
Note 2　—
注　—

名　称　**チンジュ**

他名等　アコヤガイ／シンジュ
部位等　外套膜組織中の顆粒物・真珠・貝肉
備　考　—

他名(参考)　クロチョウガイ（黒蝶貝）、カワシンジュガイ（川真珠貝）、シナカラスガイ（支那烏貝）、他
漢字表記・生薬名等　珍珠（チンジュ）、真珠（シンジュ）、阿古屋貝（アコヤガイ）
Name (Romaji)　CHINJU
Other name (s) (Romaji)　AKOYAGAI／SHINJU
学名　*Pinctada fucata martensii* Dunker（アコヤガイ、ウ

グイスガイ科）
Pinctada margaritifera L.（クロチョウガイ、ウグイスガイ科）
Margaritifera margaritifera L.（カワシンジュガイ、カワシンジュガイ科）
Cristaria plicata Leach（シナカラスガイ、イシガイ科）

科名 Pteriidae（ウグイスガイ科）
Margaritiferidae（カワシンジュガイ科）
Unionidae（イシガイ科）

英名 pearl oyster / Japanese pearl oyster / Akoya pearl oyster / black-lip oyster

Part of use granule of pallium membrane, pearl, shellfish meat

Note 1 —

Note 2 —

注 —

名　称 **ツバメ巣**

他名等 —
部位等 ツバメの巣
備　考 —

他名（参考） ジャワアナツバメ、オオアナツバメ

漢字表記・生薬名等 燕窩（エンカ）、穴燕（アナツバメ）

Name（Romaji） TSUBAMESU

Other name（s）（Romaji） —

学名 *Aerodramus fuciphagus* Thunb.（ジャワアナツバメ）
Aerodramus maximus Hume（オオアナツバメ）

科名 Apodidae（アマツバメ科）

英名 *Aerodramus fuciphagus*：edible nest swiftlet / white-nest swiftlet
Aerodramus maximus：black nest swiftlet

Part of use swallow's nest

Note 1 —

Note 2 —

注 —

ナ行

名　称 **軟骨**

他名等 —
部位等 爬虫類・哺乳類の軟骨抽出物
備　考 —

他名（参考） —

漢字表記・生薬名等 —

Name（Romaji） NANKOTSU

Other name（s）（Romaji） —

学名 *Reptilia* Laurenti（爬虫綱）
Mammalia L.（哺乳綱）

科名 —

英名 cartilage of reptilia or mammalia

Part of use reptilian and mammalian cartilage extract

Note 1 —

Note 2 —

注 —

名　称 **ニホンヤモリ**

他名等 ヘキコ／Gekko japonicus
部位等 全体
備　考 —

他名（参考） —

漢字表記・生薬名等 壁虎（ヘキコ）、日本守宮（ニホンヤモリ）

Name（Romaji） NIHON'YAMORI

Other name（s）（Romaji） HEKIKO

学名 *Gekko japonicus* Schlegel

科名 Gekkonidae（ヤモリ科）

英名 Schlegel's Japanese gecko

Part of use whole body

Note 1 —

Note 2 —

注 —

名　称　**ニワトリ**

他名等　ケイナイキン
部位等　胃の内壁
備　考　—

他名(参考)　—
漢字表記・生薬名等　鶏内金（ケイナイキン）
Name(Romaji)　NIWATORI
Other name(s) (Romaji)　KEINAIKIN
学名　*Gallus gallus* L.
科名　Phasianidae（キジ科）
英名　stomach lining of chicken
Part of use　stomach lining
Note 1　—
Note 2　—
注　—

名　称　**乳汁**

他名等　バニュウ
部位等　ウマの乳汁
備　考　—

他名(参考)　—
漢字表記・生薬名等　馬乳（バニュウ）
Name(Romaji)　NYÛJÛ
Other name(s) (Romaji)　BANYÛ
学名　*Equus caballus* L.
科名　Equidae（ウマ科）
英名　mare's milk
Part of use　horse milk
Note 1　—
Note 2　—
注　—

ハ行

名　称　**ハチ**

他名等　ハチノコ
部位等　ハチの幼虫
備　考　—

他名(参考)　ヘボ（地蜂（黒雀蜂）の子）、ジバチ（地蜂）、タカブ、スガレ、クロスズメバチ（黒雀蜂、黒胡蜂）、キイロスズメバチ（黄色雀蜂）、オオスズメバチ（大雀蜂）
漢字表記・生薬名等　蜂の子（ハチノコ）
Name(Romaji)　HACHI
Other name(s) (Romaji)　HACHINOKO
学名　*Vespula flaviceps* Smith（クロスズメバチ、スズメバチ科）
Vespa simillima xanthoptera Cameron（キイロスズメバチ、スズメバチ科）
Vespa mandarinia japonica Radoszkowski（オオスズメバチ、スズメバチ科）
Apis mellifera L.（ミツバチ、ミツバチ科）
科名　Vespidae（スズメバチ科）
Apidae（ミツバチ科）
英名　wasp larva / honeybee larva / Japanese hornet larva / Japanese yellow hornet larva
Part of use　bee larva
Note 1　—
Note 2　—
注　—

名　称　**ハブ**

他名等　ヒメハブ
部位等　全体
備　考　—

他名(参考)　—
漢字表記・生薬名等　姫波布・姫飯匙倩（ヒメハブ）
Name(Romaji)　HABU
Other name(s) (Romaji)　HIMEHABU
学名　*Ovophis okinavensis* Boulenger
Trimeresurus okinavensis Boulenger
Lachesis okinavensis Boulenger
科名　Viperadae（クサリヘビ科）
英名　dwarf lancehead snake / Okinawa pitviper
Part of use　whole body
Note 1　—
Note 2　—
注　—

名　称　**ヒル**

他名等　ウマビル／スイテツ／チスイビル／チャイロビル
部位等　全体
備　考　—

他名(参考)　—
漢字表記・生薬名等　水蛭（スイテツ）、寛水蛭・長條水蛭（ウマビル）
Name(Romaji)　HIRU
Other name(s) (Romaji)　UMABIRU／SUITETSU／

CHISUIBIRU／CHAIROBIRU
学名　*Whitmania pigra* Whitman（ウマビル）
Whitmania acranulata Whitman（チャイロビル）
Hirudo nipponica Whitman（チスイビル）
科名　Hirudinidae（ヒルド科）
英名　leech / segmented worm
Part of use　whole body
Note 1　—
Note 2　—
注　—

名　称　**ヒレイケチョウガイ**

他名等　Hyriopsis cumingii
部位等　貝殻
備　考　—

他名(参考)　湖水真珠（コスイシンジュ)、三角帆貝
漢字表記･生薬名等　ひれ池蝶貝（ヒレイケチョウガイ）
Name(Romaji)　HIREIKECHÔGAI
Other name(s) (Romaji)　—
学名　*Hyriopsis cumingii* Lea
Hyriopsis goliath Rolle
Unio cumingii Lea
科名　Unionidae（イシガイ科）
英名　triangle sail mussel
Part of use　seashell
Note 1　—
Note 2　—
注　—

名　称　**フグノクロヤキ**

他名等　フグ／マフグ
部位等　フグの黒焼
備　考　—

他名(参考)　—
漢字表記･生薬名等　河豚（フグ)、真河豚（マフグ）
Name(Romaji)　FUGUNOKUROYAKI
Other name(s) (Romaji)　FUGU／MAFUGU
学名　*Takifugu porphyreus* Temminck et Schlegel
科名　Tetraodontidae（フグ科）
英名　purple puffer / globe fish
Part of use　charred blowfish
Note 1　—
Note 2　—
注　—

名　称　**ヘビ**

他名等　アオマダラウミヘビ／アマガサヘビ／エラブウミヘビ／ガラガラヘビ／ヒャッポダ
部位等　全体
備　考　蛇毒は「医」

他名(参考)　タイワンアマガサ（台湾雨傘)、ゴホダ（五歩蛇）
漢字表記･生薬名等　白花蛇（ビャッカダ)、蛇婆、永良部海蛇（エラブウミヘビ)、青斑海蛇（アオマダラウミヘビ)、雨傘蛇（アマガサヘビ)、百歩蛇（ヒャッポダ）
Name(Romaji)　HEBI
Other name(s) (Romaji)　AOMADARAUMIHEBI／AMAGASAHEBI／ERABUUMIHEBI／GARAGARAHEBI／HYAPPODA
学名　*Laticauda colubrina* Schneider（アオマダラウミヘビ、コブラ科）
Laticauda semifasciata Reinwardt（エラブウミヘビ、コブラ科）
Bungarus multicinctus Blyth（アマガサヘビ、コブラ科）
Deinagkistrodon acutus Günther（ヒャッポダ、クサリヘビ科）
Crotalus L.（ガラガラヘビ属、クサリヘビ科）
科名　Elapidae（コブラ科）
Viperidae（クサリヘビ科）
英名　*L. colubrina*：yellow lipped sea krait
L. semifasciata：Erabu black banded sea krait / broad banded blue sea snake
B. multicinctus：Many banded krait
D. acutus：Hundred pace snake / Chinese moccasin / rattlesnake
Crotalus L.：rattlesnake
Part of use　whole body
Note 1　snake toxin：drug category
Note 2　—
注　—

マ行

名　称　**マムシ**

他名等　ハンビ／フクダ
部位等　全体
備　考　—

他名(参考)　ニホンマムシ（日本蝮)、アカマムシ（赤蝮）

漢字表記・生薬名等　反鼻（ハンピ）、蝮蛇（フクダ）
Name (Romaji)　MAMUSHI
Other name (s) (Romaji)　HANBI／FUKUDA
学名　*Gloydius blomhoffii* Boie
Gloydius halys Pallas
科名　Viperidae（クサリヘビ科）
英名　Japanese mamushi / mamushi / mamushi pit viper / Nihon mamushi
Part of use　whole body
Note 1　—
Note 2　—
注　—

名　称　**ミツロウ**

他名等　—
部位等　ハチが分泌するロウ質
備　考　—

他名（参考）　—
漢字表記・生薬名等　蜜蝋（ミツロウ）
Name (Romaji)　MITSURÔ
Other name (s) (Romaji)　—
学名　*Apis mellifera* L.
科名　Apidae（ミツバチ科）
英名　beeswax
Part of use　wax secreted by bee
Note 1　—
Note 2　—
注　—

名　称　**ミドリイガイ**

他名等　—
部位等　貝肉
備　考　—

他名（参考）　—
漢字表記・生薬名等　緑貽貝（ミドリイガイ）
Name (Romaji)　MIDORIIGAI
Other name (s) (Romaji)　—
学名　*Perna viridis* L.
Mytilus viridis L.
科名　Mytilidae（イガイ科）
英名　Asian green mussel / green-lipped mussel
Part of use　shellfish meat
Note 1　—
Note 2　*Mytilus galloprovincialis* Lamarck is a close relative of *Mytilus viridis* L. and known as moule (Mediterranean mussel).
注　近縁種のムラサキイガイはムール貝。

ラ行

名　称　**卵黄油**

他名等　—
部位等　卵黄の油
備　考　—

他名（参考）　ランユ（卵油）
漢字表記・生薬名等　—
Name (Romaji)　RAN'ÔYU
Other name (s) (Romaji)　—
学名　*Gallus gallus* L.
科名　Phasianidae（キジ科）
英名　egg yolk oil
Part of use　egg yolk oil
Note 1　—
Note 2　—
注　—

名　称　**卵殻**

他名等　—
部位等　卵殻
備　考　—

他名（参考）　—
漢字表記・生薬名等　—
Name (Romaji)　RANKAKU
Other name (s) (Romaji)　—
学名　*Gallus gallus* L.
科名　Phasianidae（キジ科）
英名　egg shell
Part of use　egg shell
Note 1　—
Note 2　—
注　—

名　称　**リュウシツ**

他名等　ケンゴロウ
部位等　全虫
備　考　—

他名（参考）　スイキシ（水亀子）、スイベッチュウ（水鼈中）、

サンセイリュウシツ（三星龍虱）、オウヘンダイリュウシツ（黄辺大龍虱）

漢字表記・生薬名等　龍虱（リュウシツ）、源五郎（ゲンゴロウ）

Name (Romaji)　RYÛSHITSU

Other name (s) (Romaji)　KENGORÔ

学名　*Cybister tripunctatus orientalis* Gschwendtner（コガタノゲンゴロウ）

Cybister tripunctatus lateralis Fabricus（コガタノゲンゴロウ）

科名　Dytiscidae（ゲンゴロウ科）

英名　predaceous diving beetle

Part of use　whole insect body

Note 1　—

Note 2　—

注　—

名　称　**ローヤルゼリー**

他名等　—

部位等　メスバチの咽頭腺分泌物

備　考　—

他名(参考)　オウニュウ（王乳）

漢字表記・生薬名等　—

Name (Romaji)　RÔYARUZERÎ

Other name (s) (Romaji)　—

学名　*Apis mellifera* L.

科名　Apidae（ミツバチ科）

英名　royal jelly

Part of use　pharingeal glands secretion of female bee

Note 1　—

Note 2　—

注　—

3．その他（化学物質等）

3. Other substances (chemicals, vitamins and minerals, etc.)

網掛け部分：網掛け部分には「名称」、「他名等」、「部位等」、「備考」の４項目が含まれる。これらの項目は食薬区分リストの表記に準拠し、そのまま一切の変更を加えずに記載した。

注１）リストに掲載されている成分本質（原材料）のうち、該当する部位について、「部位等」の欄に記載している。

注２）他の部位が別のリストに掲載されている場合等、その取扱いが紛らわしいものについては、備考欄にその旨記載している。

注３）備考欄の「医」は「専ら医薬品として使用される成分本質（原材料）リスト」に掲載されていることを示す。

Shaded section：The shaded section consists of four items：Name, Other name(s), Part of use, and Remarks. These items are shown exactly as recorded in the food and drug classification lists without any changes having been made whatsoever.

1) Of the ingredients (raw materials) included in the list, the relevant part used is included in the "Part of use" entry.
2) Where other parts are included in other lists, notes are entered in the "Remarks" column if there could be any confusion over the handling.
3) Where the "Remarks" column shows "drug (医)", the substance is included in the "List of ingredients (raw materials) used exclusively for drugs".

その他（化学物質等）の原材料の見方
(Notation of a substance (chemical(s), vitamin(s) and mineral(s), etc.)

名　称 他名等 部位等 備　考	**Name** **Other name(s)** **Part of Use** **Remarks**	食薬区分リストの記載事項とその内容。 The shaded section consists of the following four items which are exactly shown as recorded in the food and drug classification lists without any changes.
Name	成分の英名 English name of the ingredient.	
Other name(s)	「他名等」の英名 The English translation of "Other name(s)".	
IUPAC Name		
CAS No.		
Synonyms		
分子式	**Molecular formula**	
特性・カテゴリー	**Properties and category**	
Note 1	「部位等」及び「備考」の英訳 English translation of "Part of use" and the content of "Remarks" in the food and drug classification list.	
Note 2	下記「注」の英訳。 English translation of "Note (注)" in the last item.	
注	食品衛生法による本成分の取り扱い、その他補足情報等 **Note**：The handling of each ingredient in the non-drug list according to the Food Sanitation Act is given here. Other comments or supplementary information on the content of the food and drug classification records are also given.	
構造式	**The structural formula**	

ア行

名　称　**亜鉛**

他名等　—
部位等　—
備　考　—

Name　Zinc
Other name(s)　—
IUPAC Name　zinc
CAS No.　7440-66-6
Synonyms　—
元素記号　Zn
特性・カテゴリー　ミネラル／Mineral
Note 1　—
Note 2　Fall under the category of designated food additive.
注　指定添加物に該当する。

名　称　**アスタキサンチン**

他名等　—
部位等　ヘマトコッカス藻の主成分
備　考　ヘマトコッカス藻は「非医」

Name　Astaxanthin
Other name(s)　—
IUPAC Name　6-hydroxy-3-[(1E,3E,5E,7E,9E,11E,13E,15E,17E)-18-(4-hydroxy-2,6,6-trimethyl-3-oxocyclohexen-1-yl)-3,7,12,16-tetramethyloctadeca-1,3,5,7,9,11,13,15,17-nonaenyl]-2,4,4-trimethylcyclohex-2-en-1-one
CAS No.　472-61-7
Synonyms　Astaxanthine / Ovoester / 3,3'-Dihydroxy-beta-carotene-4,4'-dione
分子式　$C_{40}H_{52}O_4$
特性・カテゴリー　カロテノイド／Carotenoid
Note 1　*Haematococus pulvialis*：non-drug category
Note 2　Fall under the category of existing food additive. Generally treated as a component of "*Haematococcus* algae color" as an existing food additive, however, note that this substance may have the possibility to be treated as an undesignated food additive which has not been designated based on the Food Sanitation Act.
注　既存添加物に該当する。通常は、既存添加物に該当するが、食品衛生法に基づく指定がなされていない未指定の食品添加物に該当する場合もあるので注意すること。

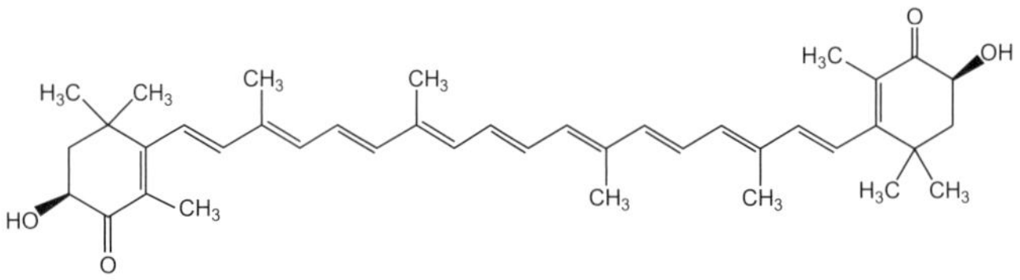

名　称　**アスパラギン**

他名等　—
部位等　—
備　考　—

Name　Asparagine
Other name(s)　—
IUPAC Name　(2S)-2,4-diamino-4-oxobutanoic acid
CAS No.　70-47-3
Synonyms　L-Asparagine / Aspartamic acid / (S)-Asparagine / Agedoite / Altheine / Asparamide / Asparagine acid / Crystal VI / (-)-Asparagine
分子式　$C_4H_8N_2O_3$
特性・カテゴリー　アミノ酸／Amino acid
Note 1　—
Note 2　Fall under the category of existing food additive.
注　既存添加物に該当する。

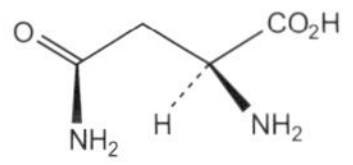

名　称　**アスパラギン酸**

他名等　—
部位等　—
備　考　—

Name　Aspartic acid
Other name(s)　—
IUPAC Name　(2S)-2-aminobutanedioic acid
CAS No.　56-84-8
Synonyms　L-Aspartic acid / Asparagic acid / H-Asp-OH / L-Asparaginic acid / Asparaginic acid / L-Asparagic acid / Aspatofort / (2S)-Aspartic acid
分子式　$C_4H_7NO_4$
特性・カテゴリー　アミノ酸／Amino acid

Note 1　—

Note 2　Fall under the categories of designated food additive and existing food additive.

注　指定添加物及び既存添加物に該当する。

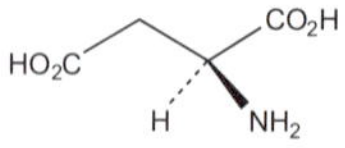

名　称　5-アミノレブリン酸リン酸塩

他名等　5-Aminolevulinic acid・phosphate

部位等　光合成細菌（ロドバクター・セファロイデス）の生成したもの

備　考　—

Name　5-Aminolevulinic acid・phosphate

Other name(s)　5-Aminolevulinic acid・phosphate

IUPAC Name　5-amino-4-oxopentanoic acid (Free acid)

CAS No.　106-60-5 (Free acid)

Synonyms　5-Amino-4-oxopentanoic acid / phosphate / delta-Aminolevulinic acid phosphate

分子式　H_3O_4P・$C_5H_9NO_3$

特性･カテゴリー　アミノ酸の一種。フリー体はヘム及びクロロフィル生合成時のテトラピロールの前駆物質。／Natural amino acid phosphate. Free acid is the precursor of tetrapyrroles in the biosynthesis of chlorophyll and heme.

Note 1　—

Note 2　Seek the judgement by the Ministry of Health, Labour and Welfare before using whether the substance will be fall under the category of food additive.

注　使用に先立ち、食品添加物に該当するか否かの判断を厚生労働省より受ける必要がある。

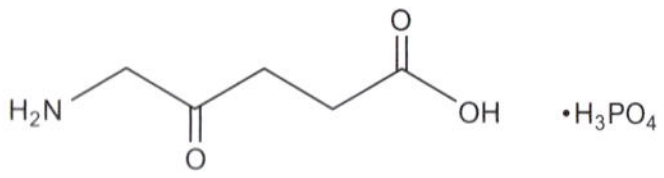

名　称　アラニン

他名等　—

部位等　—

備　考　—

Name　Alanine

Other name(s)　—

IUPAC Name　(2S)-2-aminopropanoic acid

CAS No.　56-41-7

Synonyms　L-Alanine / (S)-Alanine / L-2-Aminopropionic acid / L-alpha-Alanine / 2-Aminopropionic acid / L-(+)-Alanine / (S)-2-Aminopropanoic acid

分子式　$C_3H_7NO_2$

特性･カテゴリー　アミノ酸／Amino acid

Note 1　—

Note 2　Fall under the categories of designated food additive and existing food additive.

注　指定添加物及び既存添加物に該当する。

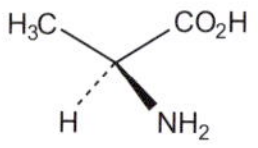

名　称　アリシン

他名等　—

部位等　—

備　考　ニンニクの成分

Name　Allicin

Other name(s)　—

IUPAC Name　3-prop-2-enylsulfinylsulfanylprop-1-ene

CAS No.　539-86-6

Synonyms　Diallyl thiosulfinate / Diallyldisulfid-S-oxid / Thio-2-propene-1-sulfinic acid S-allyl ester

分子式　$C_6H_{10}OS_2$

特性･カテゴリー　植物成分／Botanical constituent

Note 1　Constituent of garlic

Note 2　Seek the judgement by the Ministry of Health, Labour and Welfare before using whether the substance will be fall under the category of food additive.

注　使用に先立ち、食品添加物に該当するか否かの判断を厚生労働省より受ける必要がある。

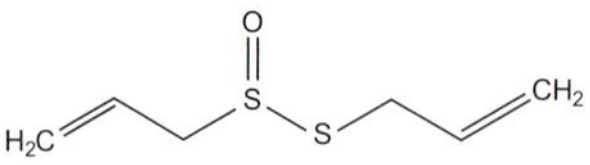

名　称　アルブミン

他名等　—

部位等　—

備　考　—

Name　Albumin

Other name(s)　—

IUPAC Name —

CAS No. Egg albumin, Ovalbumin：9006-59-1
alpha-Lactalbumin：12585-12-5
Serum albumin：9048-46-8

Synonyms Egg albumin（卵白アルブミン）/ Ovalbumin（オバルブミン）/ Milk albumin（乳アルブミン）/ alpha-Lactalbumin（alpha-ラクトアルブミン）

分子式 —

特性・カテゴリー タンパク質／Protein

Note 1 —

Note 2 Treated as a substance which is generally provided for eating or drinking as a food and which is also used as a food additive.

注 一般に食品として飲食に供される物であって添加物として使用されるものとして取り扱われる。

名　称　アントシアニジン

他名等 —

部位等 —

備　考 —

Name Anthocyanidin

Other name(s) —

IUPAC Name 2-phenylchromenium（アントシアニン（Anthocyanins）は2-phenylchromenylium）

CAS No. —

Synonyms —

分子式 構造式参照／See chemical structures

特性・カテゴリー 植物成分（ポリフェノール）。植物に広く存在する色素成分、通常は配糖体として存在する。／Botanical constituent (polyphenol). Anthocyanidins are common plant pigments. They are the sugar-free counterparts of anthocyanins based on the flavylium ion or 2-phenylchromenylium

Note 1 —

Note 2 Seek the judgement by the Ministry of Health, Labour and Welfare before using whether the substance will be fall under the category of food additive.

注 使用に先立ち、食品添加物に該当するか否かの判断を厚生労働省より受ける必要がある。

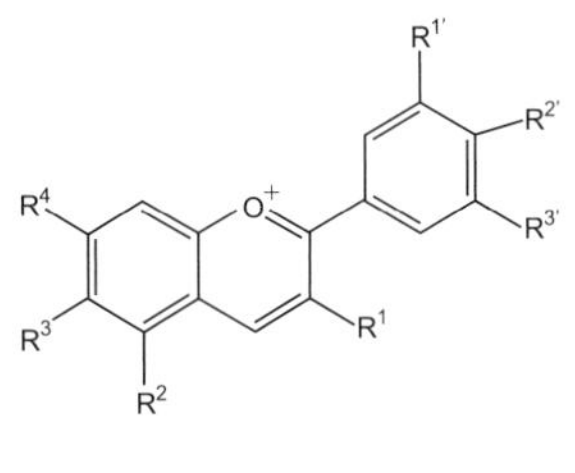

アントシアニジン	R1'	R2'	R3'	R1	R2	R3	R4
オーランチニジン	H	OH	H	OH	OH	OH	OH
シアニジン	OH	OH	H	OH	OH	H	OH
デルフィニジン	OH	OH	OH	OH	OH	H	OH
ヨーロピニジン	OCH_3	OH	OH	OH	OCH_3	H	OH
ルテオリニジン	OH	OH	H	H	OH	H	OH
ペラルゴニジン	H	OH	H	OH	OH	H	OH
マルビジン	OCH_3	OH	OCH_3	OH	OH	H	OH
ペオニジン	OCH_3	OH	H	OH	OH	H	OH
ペチュニジン	OH	OH	OCH_3	OH	OH	H	OH
ロシニジン	OCH_3	OH	H	OH	OH	H	OCH_3

名　称　イオウ

他名等　メチルサリフォニルメタン

部位等 —

備　考 —

Name Sulfur

Other name(s) Methylsulfonylmethane

IUPAC Name methylsulfonylmethane

CAS No. Sulfur：7704-34-9
Methylsulfonylmethane：67-71-0

Synonyms Methyl sulfone / Sulfonylbismethane / Dimethyl sulphone

元素記号 Sulfur：S

分子式 Methylsulfonylmethane：$C_2H_6O_2S$

特性・カテゴリー イオウ：ミネラル／Sulfur：Mineral
メチルサリフォニルメタン：有機イオウ化合物／Methylsulfonylmethane：Organosulfur substance

Note 1 —

Note 2 Seek the judgement by the Ministry of Health, Labour and Welfare before using whether the substance will be fall under the category of food additive but methlsulfonylmethane is excepted.
Methlsulfonylmethane is treated as a substance which is generally provided for eating or drinking as a food and which is also used as a food additive.

注 使用に先立ち、食品添加物に該当するか否かの判断を厚生労働省より受ける必要がある（但し、メチルサリフォニルメタンを除く）。
メチルサリフォニルメタンは、一般に食品として飲食に供される物であって添加物として使用されるものとして取り扱われる。

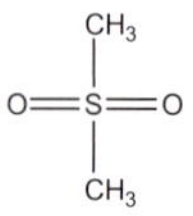

Methylsulfonylmethane

名　称　イコサペント酸＜EPA＞

他名等　EPA／エイコサペンタエン酸
部位等　—
備　考　—

Name　Icosapentaenoic acid＜EPA＞
Other name (s)　EPA / Eicosapentaenoic acid
IUPAC Name　(5E,8E,11E,14E,17E)-icosa-5,8,11,14,17-pentaenoic acid
CAS No.　10417-94-4
Synonyms　Icosa-5,8,11,14,17-Pentaenoic acid / Timnodonic acid
分子式　$C_{20}H_{30}O_2$
特性・カテゴリー　多価不飽和脂肪酸／Polyunsatulated fatty acid
Note 1　—
Note 2　Treated as a substance which is generally provided for eating or drinking as a food and which is also used as a food additive.
注　一般に食品として飲食に供される物であって添加物として使用されるものとして取り扱われる。

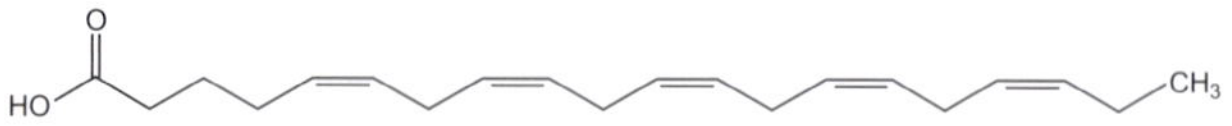

名　称　イソフラキシジン

他名等　—
部位等　—
備　考　—

Name　Isofraxidin
Other name (s)　—
IUPAC Name　7-hydroxy-6,8-dimethoxychromen-2-one
CAS No.　486-21-5
Synonyms　Phytodolor / 6,8-Dimethoxyumbelliferone / 7-Hydroxy-6,8-dimethoxy-2*H*-1-benzopyran-2-one
分子式　$C_{11}H_{10}O_5$
特性・カテゴリー　植物成分（クマリン）／Botanical constituent (Coumarin)
Note 1　—
Note 2　Seek the judgement by the Ministry of Health, Labour and Welfare before using whether the substance will be fall under the category of food additive.
注　使用に先立ち、食品添加物に該当するか否かの判断を厚生労働省より受ける必要がある。

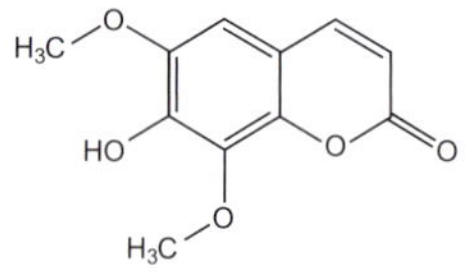

名　称　イソロイシン

他名等　—
部位等　—
備　考　—

Name　Isoleucine
Other name (s)　—
IUPAC Name　(2S,3S)-2-amino-3-methylpentanoic acid
CAS No.　73-32-5
Synonyms　L-Isoleucine / (S)-Isoleucine / (S,S)-Isoleucine / 2S,3S-Isoleucine / erythro-L-Isoleucine / 2-Amino-3-methylvaleric acid
分子式　$C_6H_{13}NO_2$
特性・カテゴリー　アミノ酸／Amino acid
Note 1　—
Note 2　Fall under the category of designated food additive.
注　指定添加物に該当する

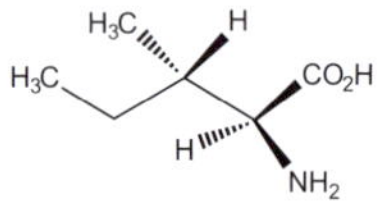

名　称　イヌリン

他名等　—
部位等　—
備　考　—

Name　Inulin
Other name (s)　—
IUPAC Name　(2R,3R,4S,5S,6R)-2-[(2S,3S,4S,5R)-2-[[(2R,3S,4S,5R)-2-[[(2R,3S,4S,5R)-2-[[(2R,3S,4S,5R)-2-[[(2R,3S,4S,5R)-2-[[(2R,3S,4S,5R)-2-[[(2R,3S,4S,5R)-2-[[(2R,3S,4S,5R)-2-[[(2R,3S,4S,5R)-2-[[(2R,3S,4S,5R)

-2-[[(2R,3S,4S,5R)-3,4-dihydroxy-2,5-bis(hydroxymethyl)oxolan-2-yl]oxymethyl]-3,4-dihydroxy-5-(hydroxymethyl)oxolan-2-yl]oxy-6-(hydroxymethyl)oxane-3,4,5-triol

CAS No. 9005-80-5

Synonyms Dahlin / Alantin / Alant starch / Inulin from Jerusalem artichokes

分子式 $C_{228}H_{382}O_{191}$

特性・カテゴリー 多糖類／Polysaccharide

Note 1 —

Note 2 Treated as a substance which is generally provided for eating or drinking as a food and which is also used as a food additive.

注 一般に食品として飲食に供される物であって添加物として使用されるものとして取り扱われる。

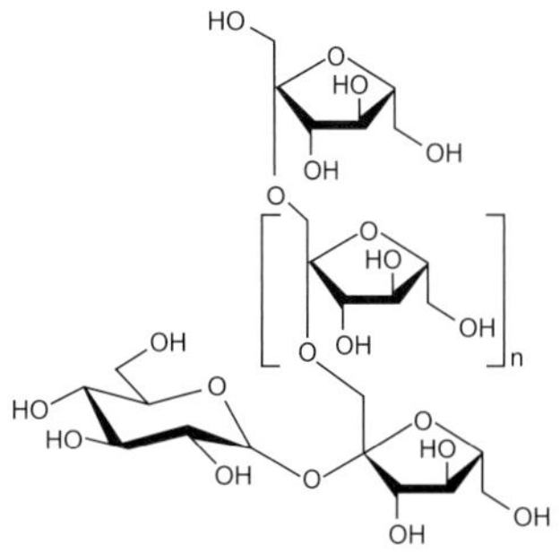

名　称　イノシトール

他名等 フィチン

部位等 —

備　考 —

Name Inositol

Other name(s) Phytin

IUPAC Name cyclohexane-1,2,3,4,5,6-hexol

CAS No. 87-89-8

Synonyms myo-Inositol / meso-Inositol / scyllo-Inositol / muco-Inositol / allo-Inositol / i-Inositol / epi-Inositol

分子式 $C_6H_{12}O_6$

特性・カテゴリー 単糖類／Monosaccharide

Note 1 —

Note 2 Fall under the category of existing food additive including d-chiro-Inositol.

注 既存添加物に該当する（d-キロイノシトールを含む）。

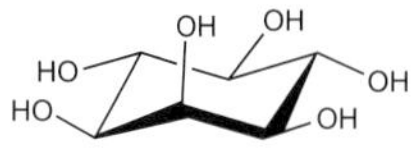

名　称　雲母

他名等　—
部位等　—
備　考　—

Name　Mica
Other name(s)　—
IUPAC Name　—
CAS No.　—
Synonyms　Isinglass
分子式　—
特性・カテゴリー　鉱物／Mineral, silicate (phyllosilicate)
Note 1　—
Note 2　Seek the judgement by the Ministry of Health, Labour and Welfare before using whether the substance will be fall under the category of food additive.
注　使用に先立ち、食品添加物に該当するか否かの判断を厚生労働省より受ける必要がある。

名　称　sn-グリセロ(3)ホスホコリン

他名等　L-α-グリセリルホスホリルコリン／sn-Glycero(3)phosphocholine
部位等　—
備　考　—

Name　sn-Glycero-3-phosphocholine
Other name(s)　L-alpha-Glycerylphosphorylcholine / sn-Glycero(3)phosphocholine
IUPAC Name　[(2R)-2,3-dihydroxypropyl]2-(trimethylazaniumyl)ethyl phosphate
CAS No.　28319-77-9
Synonyms　Glycero-3-phosphocholine / L-alpha-Glycerylphosphorylcholine / Choline alfoscerate
分子式　$C_8H_{20}NO_6P$
特性・カテゴリー　リン脂質／Phospholipid
Note 1　—
Note 2　Seek the judgement by the Ministry of Health, Labour and Welfare before using whether the substance will be fall under the category of food additive.
注　使用に先立ち、食品添加物に該当するか否かの判断を厚生労働省より受ける必要がある。

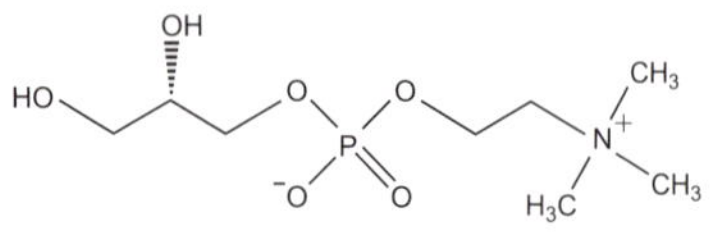

名　称　N-アセチルグルコサミン

他名等　—
部位等　—
備　考　—

Name　N-Acetylglucosamine
Other name(s)　—
IUPAC Name　N-[(2R,3R,4R,5S,6R)-2,4,5-trihydroxy-6-(hydroxymethyl)oxan-3-yl]acetamide
CAS No.　7512-17-6
Synonyms　N-Acetyl-D-glucosamine / N-Acetyl-beta-D-glucosamine / 2-Acetamido-2-deoxy-D-glucose
分子式　$C_8H_{15}NO_6$
特性・カテゴリー　単糖類／Monosaccharide
Note 1　—
Note 2　Seek the judgement by the Ministry of Health, Labour and Welfare before using whether the substance will be fall under the category of food additive.
注　使用に先立ち、食品添加物に該当するか否かの判断を厚生労働省より受ける必要がある。

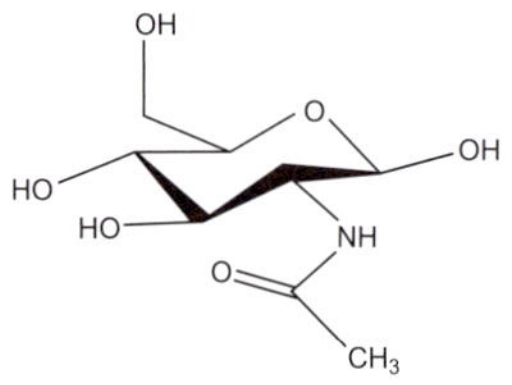

名　称　L-カルニチン

他名等　—
部位等　—
備　考　—

Name　L-Carnitine
Other name(s)　—
IUPAC Name　(3R)-3-hydroxy-4-(trimethylazaniumyl)butanoate
CAS No.　541-15-1
Synonyms　Levocarnitine / Vitamin B_T / Carnitor / (-)-Carnitine / Karnitin / (R)-Carnitine / (-)-L-Carnitine
分子式　$C_7H_{15}NO_3$
特性・カテゴリー　生理活性物質（アミノ酸代謝産物）／Bioactive substance (Amino acid metabolite)
Note 1　—
Note 2　Treated as a substance which is generally provided for eating or drinking as a food and which is

also used as a food additive.

注　一般に食品として飲食に供される物であって添加物として使用されるものとして取り扱われる。

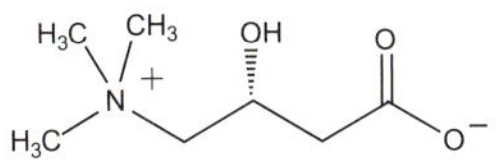

名　称　**L-シトルリン**

他名等　L-Citrulline

部位等　—

備　考　—

Name　L-Citrulline

Other name(s)　—

IUPAC Name　(2S)-2-amino-5-(carbamoylamino)pentanoic acid

CAS No.　372-75-8

Synonyms　Sitrulline / delta-Ureidonorvaline / N5-Carbamoyl-L-ornithine / L-Cytrulline / N5-(Aminocarbonyl)ornithine

分子式　$C_6H_{13}N_3O_3$

特性・カテゴリー　アミノ酸／Amino acid

Note 1　—

Note 2　Treated as a substance which is generally provided for eating or drinking as a food and which is also used as a food additive.

注　一般に食品として飲食に供される物であって添加物として使用されるものとして取り扱われる。

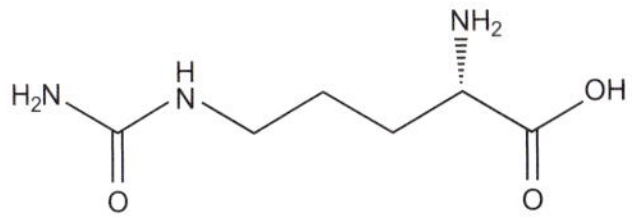

名　称　**オクタコサノール**

他名等　—

部位等　—

備　考　—

Name　Octacosanol

Other name(s)　—

IUPAC Name　octacosan-1-ol

CAS No.　557-61-9

Synonyms　1-Octacosanol / Montanyl alcohol / Octacosyl alcohol / Cluytyl alcohol / n-Octacosanol

分子式　$C_{28}H_{58}O$

特性・カテゴリー　高級脂肪族アルコール／Higher fatty alcohol

Note 1　—

Note 2　Seek the judgement by the Ministry of Health, Labour and Welfare before using whether the substance will be fall under the category of food additive.

注　使用に先立ち、食品添加物に該当するか否かの判断を厚生労働省より受ける必要がある。

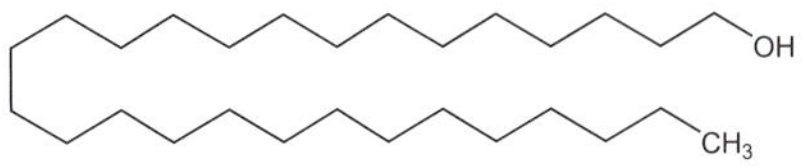

名　称　**オリゴ糖**

他名等　オリゴ配糖体

部位等　—

備　考　—

Name　Oligosaccharide

Other name(s)　Oligoglycoside

IUPAC Name　—

CAS No.　—

Synonyms　ex) Glucose glycoside

分子式　—

特性・カテゴリー　小糖類／Oligosaccharide

Note 1　—

Note 2　Treated as a substance which is generally provided for eating or drinking as a food and which is also used as a food additive.
General term of saccharide polymers containing a small number (typically three to ten) of monosaccharide.

注　一般に食品として飲食に供される物であって添加物として使用されるものとして取り扱われる。
単糖類が3～10個程度結合した糖類の総称。

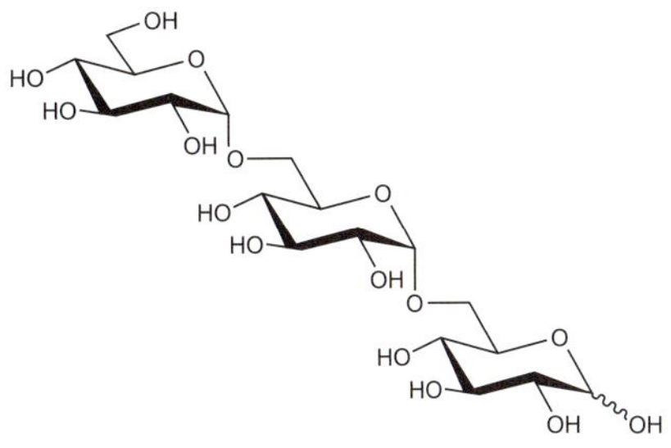

Isomaltotriose

※オリゴ糖の例としてイソマルトオリゴ糖であるイソマルトトリオースの構造式を示す。

名　称　**オルニチン**

他名等　—
部位等　—
備　考　—

Name　Ornithine
Other name(s)　—
IUPAC Name　(2S)-2,5-diaminopentanoic acid
CAS No.　70-26-8
Synonyms　L-Ornithine / (S)-Ornithine / (S)-2,5-Diaminopentanoic acid
分子式　$C_5H_{12}N_2O_2$
特性・カテゴリー　アミノ酸／Amino acid
Note 1　—
Note 2　Treated as a substance which is generally provided for eating or drinking as a food and which is also used as a food additive.
注　一般に食品として飲食に供される物であって添加物として使用されるものとして取り扱われる。

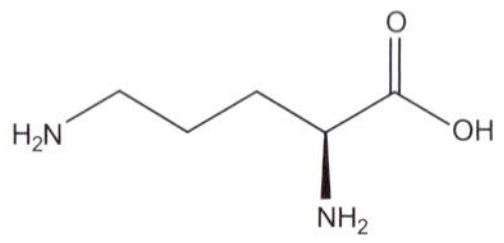

名　称　**オロト酸**

他名等　Orotic acid／1,2,3,6-tetrahydro-2,6-dioxo-4-pyrimidinecarboxylic acid
部位等　—
備　考　フリー体、カリウム塩、マグネシウム塩に限る

Name　Orotic acid
Other name(s)　Orotic acid / 1,2,3,6-tetrahydro-2,6-dioxo-4-pyrimidinecarboxylic acid
IUPAC Name　2,4-dioxo-1*H*-pyrimidine-6-carboxylic acid
CAS No.　65-86-1
Synonyms　6-Carboxyuracil / Orodin / Oropur / Orotonin / Oroturic / Orotyl / Whey factor / Uracil-6-carboxylic acid
分子式　$C_5H_4N_2O_4$
特性・カテゴリー　生理活性物質／Bioactive substance
Note 1　limited to free body, potassium salt and magnesium salt
Note 2　Seek the judgement by the Ministry of Health, Labour and Welfare before using whether the substance will be fall under the category of food additive. A pyrimidine precursor in animals.
注　使用に先立ち、食品添加物に該当するか否かの判断を厚生労働省より受ける必要がある。
動物におけるピリミジンの前駆物質。

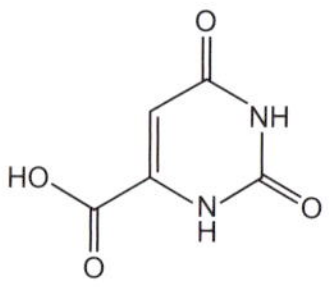

カ行

名　称　**カテキン**

他名等　カテキン酸
部位等　—
備　考　緑茶の成分

Name　Catechin
Other name(s)　Catechinic acid
IUPAC Name　(2R,3S)-2-(3,4-dihydroxyphenyl)-3,4-dihydro-2*H*-chromene-3,5,7-triol
CAS No.　154-23-4
Synonyms　Catechinic acid / (+)-Catechin / Catechuic acid / Catergen / Cyanidanol
分子式　$C_{15}H_{14}O_6$
特性・カテゴリー　高等植物に含まれるフラボノイド成分／Flavonoid found primarily in higher woody plants
Note 1　Green tea component
Note 2　Fall under the category of existing food additive.
注　既存添加物に該当する。

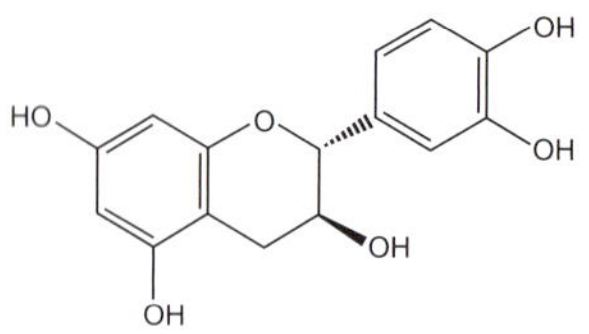

名　称　**果糖**

他名等　—
部位等　—
備　考　—

Name　Fructose
Other name(s)　—
IUPAC Name　(3S,4R,5R)-1,3,4,5,6-pentahydroxyhexan-

2-one

CAS No. 57-48-7

Synonyms Arabino-Hexulose / Furucton / Nevulose / Fruit sugar / D-Fructose / D(−)-Fructose

分子式 $C_6H_{12}O_6$

特性・カテゴリー 単糖類／Monosaccharide

Note 1 —

Note 2 Treated as a substance which is generally provided for eating or drinking as a food and which is also used as a food additive.

注 一般に食品として飲食に供される物であって添加物として使用されるものとして取り扱われる。

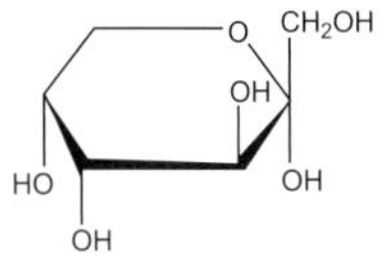

α-D-フルクトピラノース

名 称 カフェイン

他名等 —
部位等 —
備 考 —

Name Caffeine

Other name(s) —

IUPAC Name 1,3,7-trimethylpurine-2,6-dione

CAS No. 58-08-2

Synonyms Guaranine / Thein / Methyltheobromine / Cafeina / Koffein / Mateina / Alert-pep / Cafipel

分子式 $C_8H_{10}N_4O_2$

特性・カテゴリー 生理活性物質(植物成分、アルカロイド)／Bioactive substance (Botanical consutituent, alkaloid)

Note 1 —

Note 2 Fall under the category of existing food additive. Natural alkaloid found in tea leaves and coffee beans, etc.

注 既存添加物に該当する。
茶葉、コーヒー豆などに含まれる天然のアルカロイド。

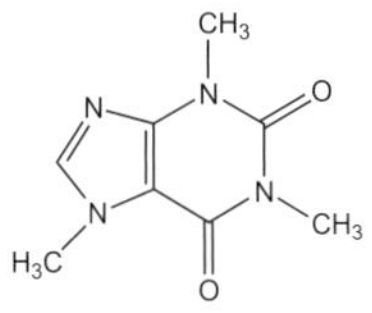

名 称 カラギーナン

他名等 —
部位等 —
備 考 天草の成分

Name Carrageenan

Other name(s) —

IUPAC Name [(2R,3S,4R,5R,6S)-6-[[(1R,3S,4R,5R,8S)-3,4-dihydroxy-2,6-dioxabicyclo[3.2.1]octan-8-yl]oxy]-4-[[(1R,3R,4R,5R,8S)-8-[(2S,3R,4R,5R,6R)-3,4-dihydroxy-6-(hydroxymethyl)-5-sulfonatooxyoxan-2-yl]oxy-4-hydroxy-2,6-dioxabicyclo[3.2.1]octan-3-yl]oxy]-5-hydroxy-2-(hydroxymethyl)oxan-3-yl]sulfate

CAS No. Carrageenan：9000-07-1
kappa-Carrageenan：11114-20-8
iota-Carrageenan：9062-07-1
lambda-Carrageenan：9064-57-7

Synonyms kappa-Carrageenan / iota-Carrageenan / lambda Carrageenan

分子式 kappa-Carrageenan：$(C_{12}H_{17}O_{12}S)_n$
iota-Carrageenan：$(C_{12}H_{18}O_9)_n$
lambda-Carrageenan：$(C_{12}H_{17}O_{19}S_3)_n$

特性・カテゴリー 直鎖含硫多糖類／Linear sulfated polysaccharide

Note 1 Constituent of Gelidiaceae (red seaweeds)

Note 2 Fall under the category of existing food additive. Sulfated polysaccharoide extracted from red algae.

注 既存添加物に該当する。
海藻（紅藻）から抽出される多糖類の硫化物。

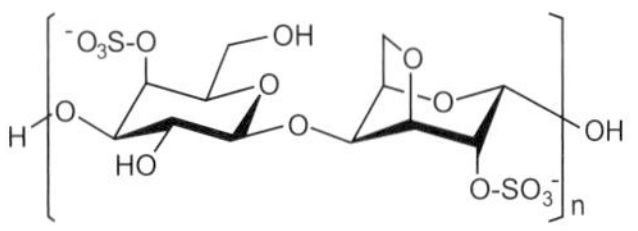

iota-carrageenan

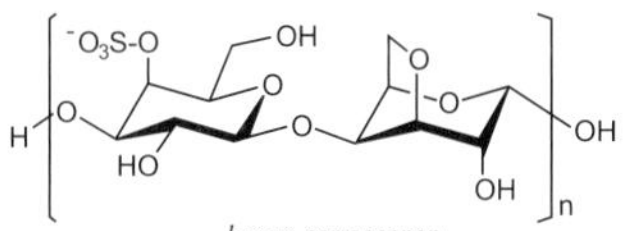

kappa-carrageenan

MW=100,000~150,000

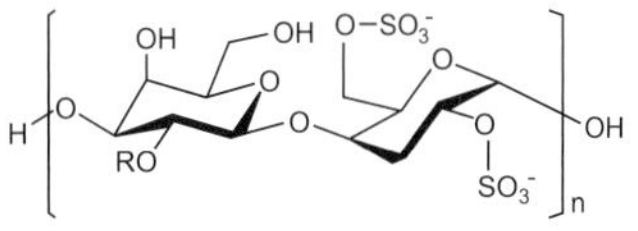

R=H(30%), SO_3^-(70%)

lambda -carrageenan

名　称　**カリウム**

他名等　—
部位等　—
備　考　—

Name　Potassium
Other name(s)　—
IUPAC Name　potassium(1+)
CAS No.　7440-09-7
Synonyms　—
元素記号　K
特性・カテゴリー　ミネラル／Mineral
Note 1　—
Note 2　Fall under the categories of designated food additive and existing food additive. Obtained as a salt in practice.
注　指定添加物及び既存添加物に該当する。
　実際には塩として供給される。

名　称　**カルシウム**

他名等　炭酸カルシウム
部位等　—
備　考　—

Name　Calcium
Other name(s)　Calcium carbonate
IUPAC Name　Calcium：calcium(2+)
　Calcium carbonate：carcium carbonate
CAS No.　Calcium：7440-70-2
　Calcium carbonate：471-34-1
Synonyms　Calcium carbonate：Limestone / Marble / Chalk / Aragonite / Calcite / Precipitated calcium carbonate / Neoanticid / Aeromatt / Agstone
元素記号　Ca
分子式　Calcium carbonate：$CaCO_3$, $CCaO_3$
特性・カテゴリー　ミネラル／Mineral
Note 1　—
Note 2　Fall under the categories of designated food additive and existing food additive.
注　指定添加物及び既存添加物に該当する。

名　称　**カロチン**

他名等　—
部位等　—
備　考　—

Name　Carotene
Other name(s)　—
IUPAC Name
　beta-Carotene：1,3,3-trimethyl-2-[(1E,3E,5E,7E,9E,11E,13E,15E,17E)-3,7,12,16-tetramethyl-18-(2,6,6-trimethylcyclohexen-1-yl)octadeca-1,3,5,7,9,11,13,15,17-nonaenyl]cyclohexene
　alpha-Carotene：1,3,3-trimethyl-2-[(1E,3E,5E,7E,9E,11E,13E,15E,17E)-3,7,12,16-tetramethyl-18-(2,6,6-trimethylcyclohex-2-en-1-yl)octadeca-1,3,5,7,9,11,13,15,17-nonaenyl]cyclohexene
CAS No.　alpha-Carotene：7488-99-5
　beta-Carotene：7235-40-7
　gamma-Carotene：472-93-5
　delta-Carotene：472-92-4
Synonyms　alpha-Carotene / beta-Carotene / gamma-Carotene / delta-Carotene / Carotenes
分子式　$C_{40}H_{56}$
特性・カテゴリー　カロテノイド、ビタミンAの前駆体／Carotenoid that is a precursor of vitamin A.
Note 1　—
Note 2　Fall under the category of existing food additive. See “beta-Caroten” in this list.
注　既存添加物に該当する。
　ベータカロチンの項を参照。

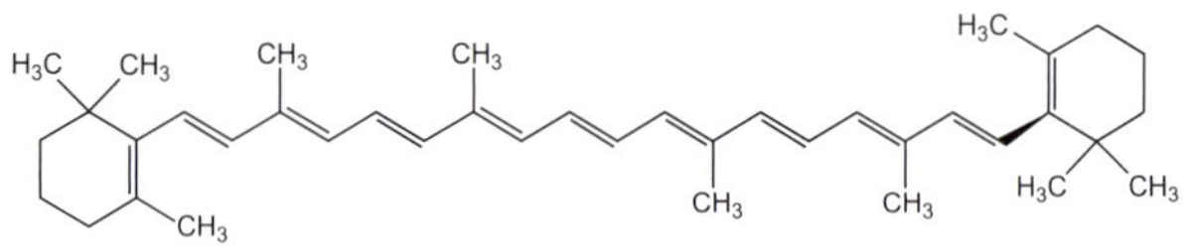

β-Caroten

名　称　**還元麦芽糖**

他名等　—
部位等　—
備　考　—

Name　Reduced maltose
Other name(s)　—
IUPAC Name　—
CAS No.　Maltitol：585-88-6
Synonyms　Maltitol / Maltisorb / Malbit / Maltit / Amalti syrup / 4-*O*-alpha-D-Glucopyranosyl-D-sorbitol / 4-*O*-alpha-D-Glucopyranosyl-D-glucitol
分子式　Maltitol：$C_{12}H_{24}O_{11}$
特性・カテゴリー　2糖類、糖アルコール／Disaccharide, sugar alcohol
Note 1　—
Note 2　Treated as a substance which is generally pro-

vided for eating or drinking as a food and which is also used as a food additive.

注　一般に食品として飲食に供される物であって添加物として使用されるものとして取り扱われる。

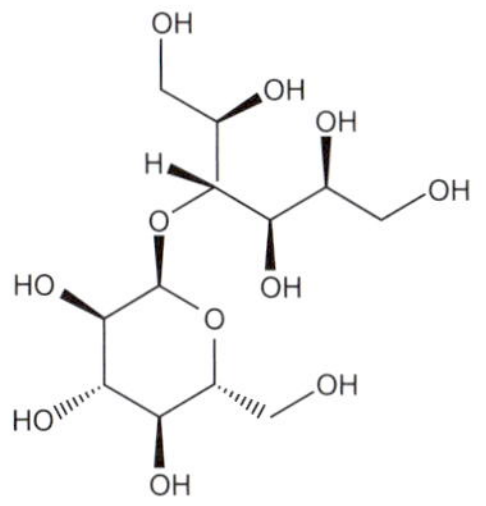

名　称　**環状重合乳酸**

他名等　—
部位等　—
備　考　—

Name　Cyclic polylactate（CPL）
Other name(s)　—
IUPAC Name　—
CAS No.　Poly（L-lactic acid）：33135-50-1
Synonyms　—
分子式　$(C_3H_4O_2)n$
特性・カテゴリー　（乳酸オリゴマー／Lactic acid oligomer）
Note 1　—
Note 2　Seek the judgement excepting lactic acid oligomer by the Ministry of Health, Labour and Welfare before using whether the substance will be fall under the category of food additive. Lactic acid oligomer is treated as a substance which is generally provided for eating or drinking as a food and which is also used as a food additive.

注　使用に先立ち、食品添加物に該当するか否かの判断を厚生労働省より受ける必要がある（但し、乳酸オリゴマーを除く）。
乳酸オリゴマーは、一般に食品として飲食に供される物であって添加物として使用されるものとして取り扱われる。

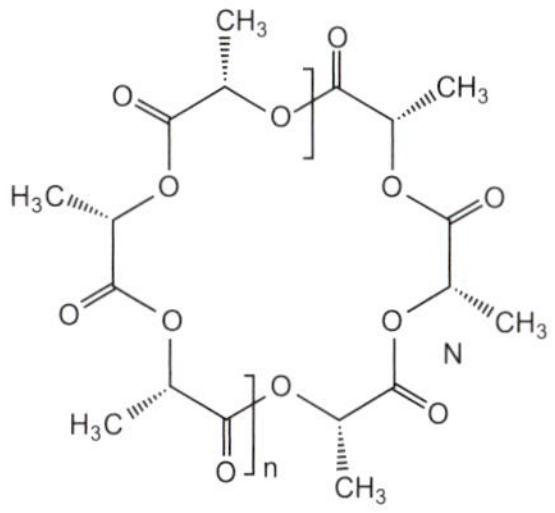

n = 1 - 17

名　称　**岩石粉**

他名等　—
部位等　—
備　考　—

Name　Rock powder
Other name(s)　—
IUPAC Name　—
CAS No.　—
Synonyms　—
分子式　—
特性・カテゴリー　鉱 物／Mixture of mainly inorganic salts
Note 1　—
Note 2　Fall under the category of existing food additive. In geology, a rock is a naturally occurring solid aggregate of one or more minerals or mineraloids. (“Rock（geology）” by Wikipedia)

注　既存添加物に該当する。
鉱物や岩石の破片、ガラス（結晶でないもの）、化石、生物由来の有機物などの集合体（混合物）である。

名　称　**γ-アミノ酪酸**

他名等　ギャバ
部位等　—
備　考　—

Name　gamma-Aminobutyric acid
Other name(s)　GABA
IUPAC Name　4-aminobutanoic acid
CAS No.　56-12-2
Synonyms　4-Aminobutyric acid / Piperidic acid / Piperidinic acid / Aminalon / Gaballon / Gammalon / Mielogen
分子式　$C_4H_9NO_2$
特性・カテゴリー　アミノ酸／Amino acid
Note 1　—
Note 2　Treated as a substance which is generally provided for eating or drinking as a food and which is also used as a food additive.

注　一般に食品として飲食に供される物であって添加物として使用されるものとして取り扱われる。

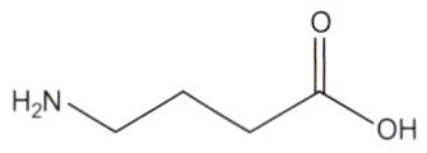

名　称　キシリトール

他名等　—
部位等　—
備　考　—

Name　Xylitol
Other name(s)　—
IUPAC Name　(2S,4R)-pentane-1,2,3,4,5-pentol
CAS No.　87-99-0
Synonyms　Adonitol / D-Xylitol / Ribitol / Eutrit / Klinit / Xylite / Xyliton / D-Ribitol / Xylite (sugar)
分子式　$C_5H_{12}O_5$
特性・カテゴリー　糖アルコール／Sugar alcohol
Note 1　—
Note 2　Fall under the category of designated food additive.
注　指定添加物に該当する。

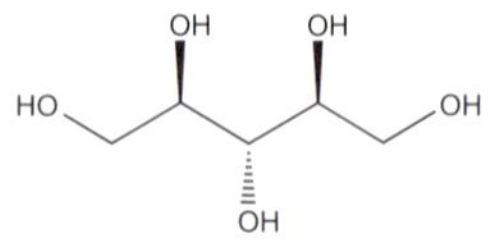

名　称　キチン

他名等　—
部位等　—
備　考　—

Name　Chitin
Other name(s)　—
IUPAC Name　N-[(2R)-2,4,5-trihydroxy-6-(hydroxymethyl)oxan-3-yl]acetamide
CAS No.　1398-61-4
Synonyms　Poly(N-acetyl-1,4-beta-D-glucopyranosamine) / N-acetyl-D-hexosaminides
分子式　$(C_8H_{13}NO_5)_n$
特性・カテゴリー　含窒素ムコ多糖類／Mucopolysaccharide containing nitrogen
Note 1　—
Note 2　Fall under the category of existing food additive.
注　既存添加物に該当する。

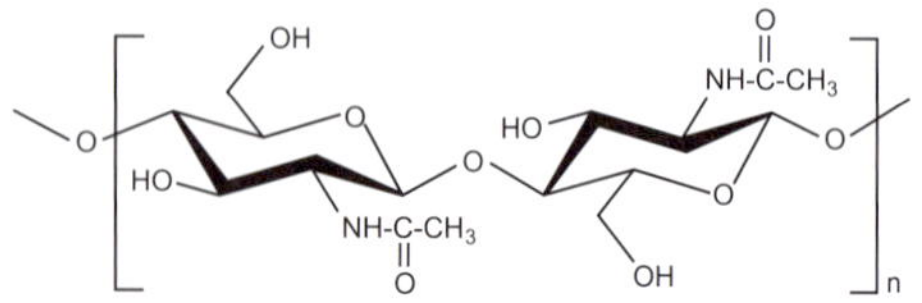

MW >1,000,000
n>5,000

名　称　キトサン

他名等　—
部位等　—
備　考　—

Name　Chitosan
Other name(s)　—
IUPAC Name　methyl N-[(2S,3R,4R,5S,6R)-5-[(2S,3R,4R,5S,6R)-3-amino-5-[(2S,3R,4R,5S,6R)-3-amino-5-[(2S,3R,4R,5S,6R)-3-amino-5-[(2S,3R,4R,5S,6R)-3-amino-5-[(2S,3R,4R,5S,6R)-3-amino-5-[(2S,3R,4R,5S,6R)-3-amino-4,5-dihydroxy-6-(hydroxymethyl)oxan-2-yl]oxy-4-hydroxy-6-(hydroxymethyl)oxan-2-yl]oxy-4-hydroxy-6-(hydroxymethyl)oxan-2-yl]oxy-4-hydroxy-6-(hydroxymethyl)oxan-2-yl]oxy-4-hydroxy-6-(hydroxymethyl)oxan-2-yl]oxy-4-hydroxy-6-(hydroxymethyl)oxan-2-yl]oxy-2-[(2R,3S,4R,5R,6S)-5-amino-6-[(2R,3S,4R,5R,6R)-5-amino-4,6-dihydroxy-2-(hydroxymethyl)oxan-3-yl]oxy-4-hydroxy-2-(hydroxymethyl)oxan-3-yl]oxy-4-hydroxy-6-(hydroxymethyl)oxan-3-yl]carbamate
CAS No.　9012-76-4
Synonyms　Deacetylchitin / Poliglusam / Chicol / Flonac C / Flonac N / Sea Cure Plus / Kytex H / Kytex M / Sea Cure F
分子式　$(C_6H_{11}NO_4)_n$
特性・カテゴリー　多糖類／Polysaccharide
Note 1　—
Note 2　Fall under the category of existing food additive.
注　既存添加物に該当する。

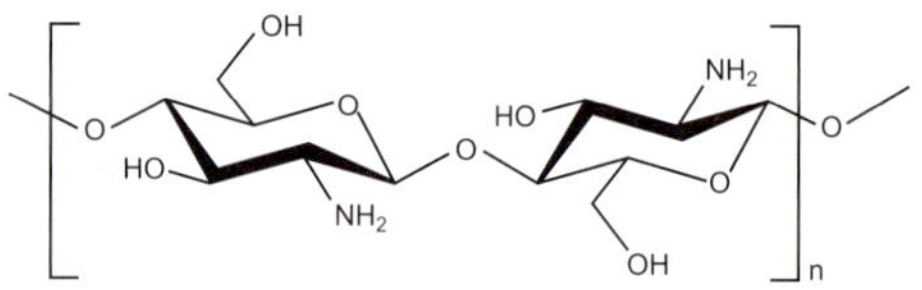

MW=10,000~1,000,000
n=50~5,000

名　称　キトサンオリゴ糖

他名等　—
部位等　—
備　考　—

Name　Chitosan oligosaccharide
Other name(s)　—
IUPAC Name　ex) Chitosan oligosaccharide lactate : (2R,3S,4R,5R,6S)-5-amino-6-[(2R,3S,4R,5R,6R)

-5-amino-4,6-dihydroxy-2-(hydroxymethyl)oxan-3-yl]oxy-2-(hydroxymethyl)oxane-3,4-diol

CAS No. ex) Chitosan oligosaccharide lactate：148411-57-8

Synonyms —

分子式 ex) Chitosan oligosaccharide lactate：$(C_6H_{11}NO_4)_{2\text{-}20}$

特性・カテゴリー キトサンのオリゴマー／Chitosan oligomers

Note 1 —

Note 2 Seek the judgement by the Ministry of Health, Labour and Welfare before using whether the substance will be fall under the category of food additive.

Sufficient data are not found.

注 使用に先立ち、食品添加物に該当するか否かの判断を厚生労働省より受ける必要がある。

十分な資料が見当たらない。

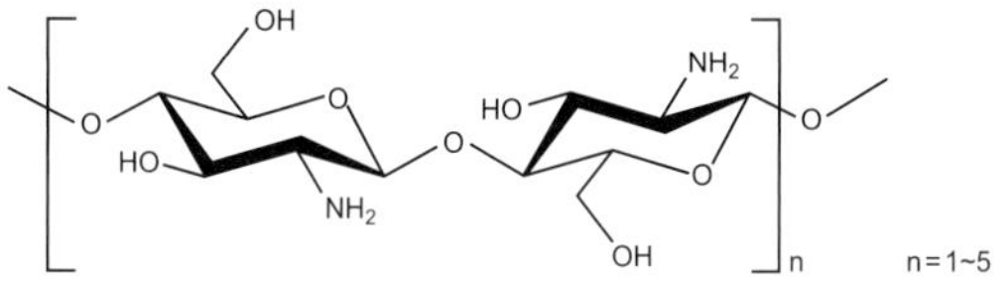

名 称 **絹**

他名等 シルク

部位等 —

備 考 —

Name Silk

Other name(s) Silk

IUPAC Name —

CAS No. Fibroins：9007-76-5

Synonyms Silk protein

分子式 —

特性・カテゴリー フィブロイン（繊維状タンパク質）／Fibroin (Fibrous protein)

Note 1 —

Note 2 Seek the judgement by the Ministry of Health, Labour and Welfare before using whether the substance will be fall under the category of food additive, but silk protein is excepted.

Silk protein is treated as a substance which is generally provided for eating or drinking as a food and which is also used as a food additive.

注 使用に先立ち、食品添加物に該当するか否かの判断を厚生労働省より受ける必要がある（但し、絹タンパクを除く）。

絹タンパクは「一般に食品として飲食に供される物であって添加物として使用されるもの」として取り扱われる。

名 称 **金**

他名等 —

部位等 —

備 考 —

Name Gold

Other name(s) —

IUPAC Name gold

CAS No. 7440-57-5

Synonyms —

元素記号 Au

特性・カテゴリー ミネラル／Mineral

Note 1 —

Note 2 Fall under the category of existing food additive.

注 既存添加物に該当する。

名 称 **グアガム**

他名等 —

部位等 —

備 考 —

Name Guar gum

Other name(s) —

IUPAC Name —

CAS No. 9000-30-0

Synonyms Guaran / Gum cyamopsis

分子式 —

特性・カテゴリー 多糖類／Polysaccharide

Note 1 —

Note 2 Fall under the category of existing food additive. The powdered endosperms of *Cyamopsis tetragonolobus* (L.) Taub.

注 既存添加物に該当する。

Cyamopsis tetragonolobus (L.) Taub. の内胚乳を粉末にしたもの。

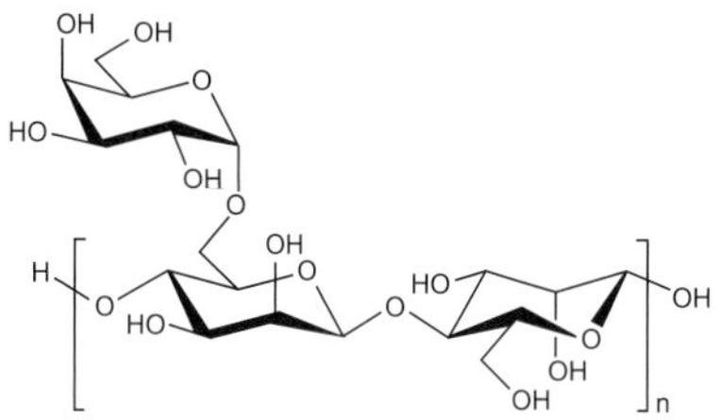

名　称　クエン酸

他名等　クエン酸マグネシウム
部位等　—
備　考　—

Name　Citric acid
Other name(s)　Magnesium citrate
IUPAC Name
Citric acid：2-hydroxypropane-1,2,3-tricarboxylic acid
Magnesium citrate：trimagnesium；2-hydroxypropane-1,2,3-tricarboxylate
CAS No.　Citric acid：77-92-9
Magnesium citrate：7779-25-1, 3344-18-1
Synonyms
Citric acid：Citro / Citrate / Aciletten / Citretten / Chemfill / Hydrocerol A / Anhydrous citric acid / 3-carboxy-3-hydroxypentanedioic acid / 2-hydroxy-1,2,3-propanetricarboxylic acid
Magnesium citrate：Trimagnesium dicitrate / Trimagnesium citrate
分子式　Citric acid：$C_6H_8O_7$
Magnisium citrate：$C_{12}H_{10}Mg_3O_{14}$
特性・カテゴリー　有機酸／Organic acid
Note 1　—
Note 2　Fall under the category of designated food additive.
注　指定添加物に該当する。

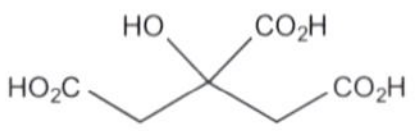

名　称　グリシン

他名等　—
部位等　—
備　考　—

Name　Glycine
Other name(s)　—
IUPAC Name　glycine
CAS No.　56-40-6
Synonyms　Aminoacetic acid / Glycocoll / Glycolixir / Aminoethanoic acid / Glicoamin / Glycosthene / Aciport / Padil
分子式　$C_2H_5NO_2$
特性・カテゴリー　アミノ酸／Amino acid
Note 1　—
Note 2　Fall under the category of designated food additive.
注　指定添加物に該当する。

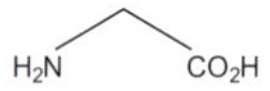

名　称　グリセリン

他名等　—
部位等　—
備　考　—

Name　Glycerine
Other name(s)　—
IUPAC Name　propane-1,2,3-triol
CAS No.　56-81-5
Synonyms　Glycerol / Glycerin / 1,2,3-Propanetriol / Glyceritol / Glycyl alcohol / Trihydroxypropane / Propanetriol / Osmoglyn / 1,2,3-trihydroxypropane
分子式　$C_3H_8O_3$
特性・カテゴリー　3価糖アルコール／Trihydroxy sugar alcohol
Note 1　—
Note 2　Fall under the category of designated food additive.
注　指定添加物に該当する。

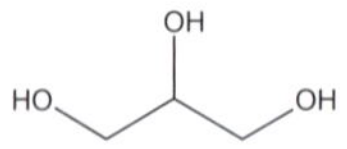

名　称　クルクミン

他名等　—
部位等　—
備　考　ウコン由来色素

Name　Curcumin
Other name(s)　—
IUPAC Name　(1E,6E)-1,7-bis(4-hydroxy-3-methoxyphenyl)hepta-1,6-diene-3,5-dione
CAS No.　458-37-7
Synonyms　Diferuloylmethane / Natural yellow 3 / Turmeric yellow / Turmeric / Kacha haldi / Gelbwurz / Curcuma / Haldar / Souchet
分子式　$C_{21}H_{20}O_6$
特性・カテゴリー　植物成分（ポリフェノール）／Botanical constituent (Polyphenol)

Note 1　Turmeric pigment

Note 2　Fall under the category of existing food additive.

注　既存添加物に該当する。

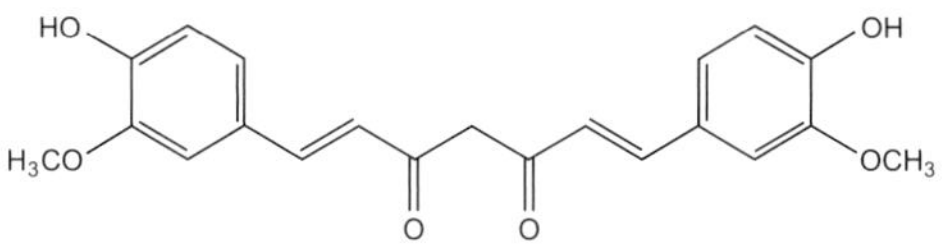

名　称　グルコサミン塩酸塩

他名等　—
部位等　—
備　考　—

Name　Glucosamine hydrochloride

Other name(s)　—

IUPAC Name　(2R,3R,4S,5R)-2-amino-3,4,5,6-tetrahydroxyhexanal;hydrochloride

CAS No.　66-84-2

Synonyms　Cosamin / D-(+)-Glucosamine hydrochloride / 2-Amino-2-deoxy-D-glucosamine / Chitosamine hydrochloride

分子式　$C_6H_{14}ClNO_5$

特性・カテゴリー　アミノ糖／Amino sugar

Note 1　—

Note 2　Fall under the categories of designated food additive and existing food additive.

注　指定添加物及び既存添加物に該当する。

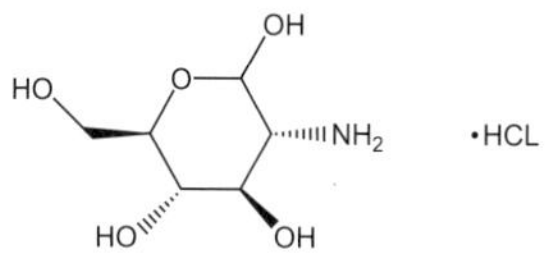

名　称　グルコマンナン

他名等　—
部位等　—
備　考　コンニャク等の複合多糖類

Name　Glucomannan

Other name(s)　—

IUPAC Name　(2S,3S,4S,5S,6R)-2-[(2R,3S,4R,5R,6S)-6-[(2R,3S,4R,5S,6S)-4,5-dihydroxy-2-(hydroxymethyl)-6-[(2R,4R,5S,6R)-4,5,6-trihydroxy-2-(hydroxymethyl)oxan-3-yl]oxyoxan-3-yl]oxy-4,5-dihydroxy-2-(hydroxymethyl)oxan-3-yl]oxy-6-(hydroxymethyl)oxane-3,4,5-triol

CAS No.　76081-94-2

Synonyms　Glucomannoglycan / (1-6)-alpha-Glucomannan

分子式　$C_{24}H_{42}O_{21}$

特性・カテゴリー　複合多糖類／Heteropolysaccharide

Note 1　Heteropolysaccharide contained in konjac

Note 2　Treated as a substance which is generally provided for eating or drinking as a food and which is also used as a food additive.
The chemical structural formula of konjac glucomannan is shown.

注　一般に食品として飲食に供される物であって添加物として使用されるものとして取り扱われる。
コンニャクグルコマンナンの構造式を示す。

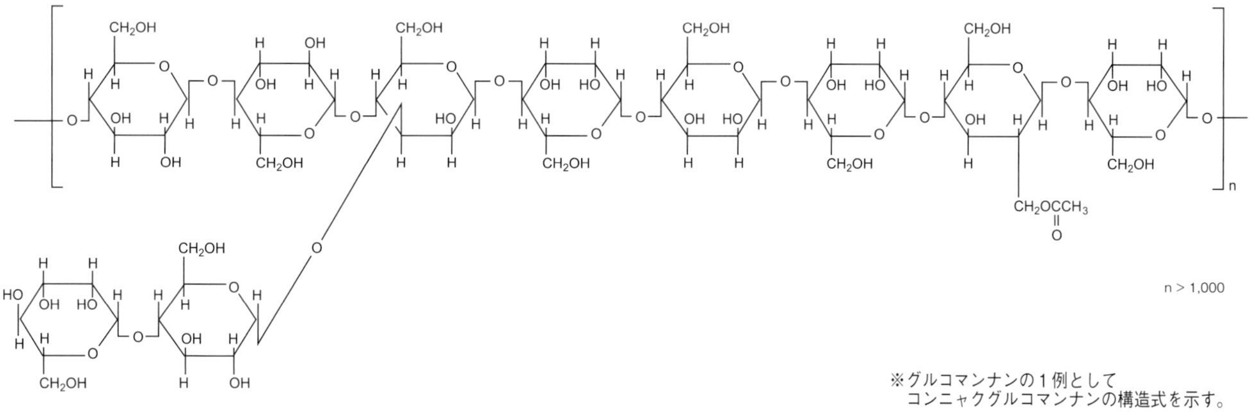

※グルコマンナンの1例として
コンニャクグルコマンナンの構造式を示す。

名　称　グルコン酸亜鉛

他名等　—
部位等　—
備　考　—

Name　Zinc gluconate
Other name(s)　—
IUPAC Name　zinc;2,3,4,5,6-pentahydroxyhexanoate
CAS No.　4468-02-4
Synonyms　bis(D-Gluconato-kappaO1,kappaO2)Zinc / Rubozine / BioZn-AAS / Zinc D-gluconate(1：2) / Zinc bis(D-gluconate-O1,O2)
分子式　$C_{12}H_{22}O_{14}Zn$
特性・カテゴリー　ミネラル／Mineral
Note 1　—
Note 2　Fall under the category of designated food additive.
注　指定添加物に該当する。

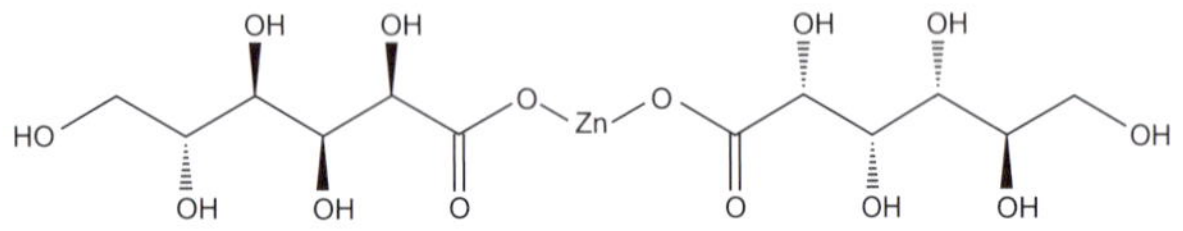

名　称　グルコン酸鉄

他名等　—
部位等　—
備　考　—

Name　Ferrous gluconate
Other name(s)　—
IUPAC Name　iron;(2R,3S,4R,5R)-2,3,4,5,6-pentahydroxyhexanoic acid
CAS No.　299-29-6
Synonyms　Iron(2+)bis[(2R,3S,4R,5R)-2,3,4,5,6-pentahydroxyhexanoate]
分子式　$C_{12}H_{22}FeO_{14}$
特性・カテゴリー　ミネラル／Mineral
Note 1　—
Note 2　Fall under the category of designated food additive.
注　指定添加物に該当する。

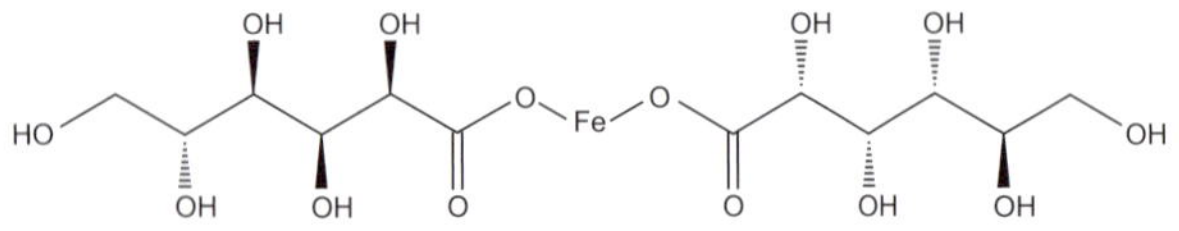

名　称　グルタミン

他名等　—
部位等　—
備　考　—

Name　Glutamine
Other name(s)　—
IUPAC Name　(2S)-2,5-diamino-5-oxopentanoic acid
CAS No.　56-85-9
Synonyms　L-Glutamine / Levoglutamide / Cebrogen / Glavamin / Stimulina / Glumin / Levoglutamid / Glutamic acid amide / L-(+)-Glutamine
分子式　$C_5H_{10}N_2O_3$
特性・カテゴリー　アミノ酸／Amino acid
Note 1　—
Note 2　Fall under the category of existing food additive.
注　既存添加物に該当する

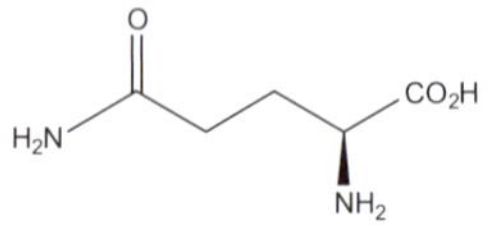

名　称　グルタミン酸

他名等　—
部位等　—
備　考　—

Name　Glutamic acid
Other name(s)　—
IUPAC Name　(2S)-2-aminopentanedioic acid
CAS No.　56-86-0
Synonyms　L-Glutamic acid / L-Glutamate / Glutacid / Glutamicol / Glutamidex / Glutaminol / Glutaton / Aciglut / Glusate / Glutaminic acid
分子式　$C_5H_9NO_4$
特性・カテゴリー　アミノ酸／Amino acid
Note 1　—
Note 2　Fall under the category of designated food additive.
注　指定添加物に該当する

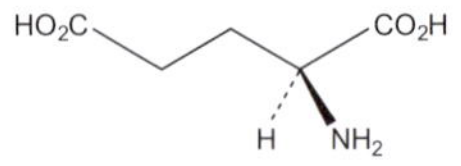

名　称　クレアチン

他名等　—
部位等　—
備　考　—

Name　Creatine
Other name(s)　—
IUPAC Name　2-[carbamimidoyl(methyl)amino]acetic acid
CAS No.　57-00-1
Synonyms　Creatin / Kreatin / Krebiozon / N-Amidinosarcosine / N-Methyl-N-guanylglycine / Pyrolysate / (alpha-Methylguanido)acetic acid
分子式　$C_4H_9N_3O_2$
特性・カテゴリー　有機酸／Organic acid
Note 1　—
Note 2　Treated as a substance which is generally provided for eating or drinking as a food and which is also used as a food additive.
注　一般に食品として飲食に供される物であって添加物として使用されるものとして取り扱われる。

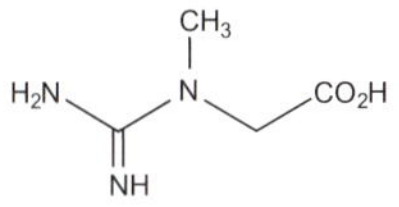

名　称　クレアチン・エチルエステル塩酸塩

他名等　Ethyl *N*-(aminoiminomethyl)-*N*-methylglycine Hydrochloride
部位等　—
備　考　—

Name　Creatine ethyl ester hydrochloride
Other name(s)　Ethyl *N*-(aminoiminomethyl)-*N*-methylglycine hydrochloride
IUPAC Name　ethyl 2-[carbamimidoyl(methyl)amino]acetate;hydrochloride
CAS No.　15366-32-2
Synonyms　Creatine ethyl ester HCl(P)
分子式　$C_6H_{14}ClN_3O_2$
特性・カテゴリー　有機酸エステル／Organic acid ester
Note 1　—
Note 2　Seek the judgement by the Ministry of Health, Labour and Welfare before using whether the substance will be fall under the category of food additive.
注　使用に先立ち、食品添加物に該当するか否かの判断を厚生労働省より受ける必要がある。

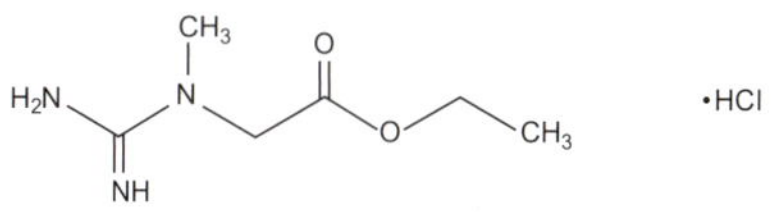

名　称　クロム（Ⅲ）

他名等　—
部位等　—
備　考　—

Name　Chromium（Ⅲ）
Other name(s)　—
IUPAC Name　chromium(3+)
CAS No.　7440-47-3
Synonyms　Chromium(Ⅲ) ion / Chromic ion / Chromium (3+) ions / Chromium ion (Cr^{3+})
元素記号　Cr^{3+}
特性・カテゴリー　ミネラル／Mineral
Note 1　—
Note 2　Before using, it is necessary to be designated as a new food additive based on the article 10 of the Food Sanitation Act.
注　使用に先立ち、新たに食品添加物の指定を受ける必要がある。

名　称　クロロフィル

他名等　—
部位等　—
備　考　葉緑体中の緑色色素

Name　Chlorophyll
Other name(s)　—
IUPAC Name　—
CAS No.　Chlorophyll：1406-65-1
Chlorophyll a：479-61-8, 42617-16-3
Synonyms　Chlorophyll a / Chlorofolin / Chlorofyl / Chlorophyl / Chlorophylls / Chromule / Deodophyll
分子式　Chlorophyll a：$C_{55}H_{72}MgN_4O_5$
特性・カテゴリー　植物成分及び微生物（シアノバクテリア）成分／Botanical constituent or constituent of cyanobacteria
Note 1　Green pigment in chloroplast
Note 2　Fall under the category of existing food additive.
注　既存添加物に該当する。

カ行

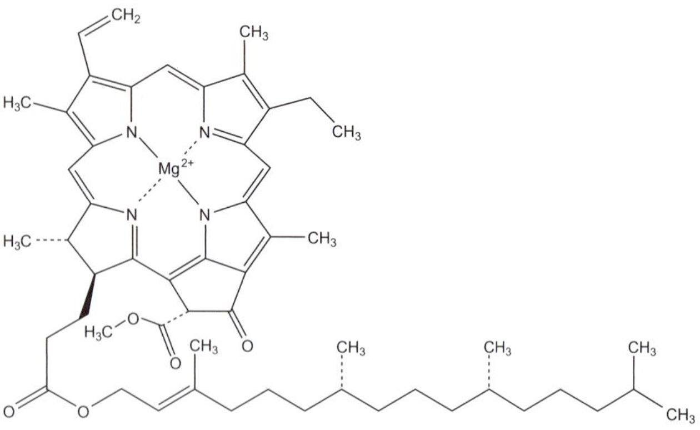

※クロロフィルはa～fの総称である。
その1例としてクロロフィルaの構造式を示す。

名　称　ケイ素

他名等　酸化ケイ素
部位等　—
備　考　—

Name　Silicon
Other name(s)　Dioxosilane
IUPAC Name
Silicon：silicon
Silicon dioxide：dioxosilane
CAS No.　Silicon：7440-21-3
Silicon dioxide：7631-86-9
Synonyms
Silicon：Silane / Silicon tetrahydride / Monosilane / Silicone / Silicon metal / Silicon dust
Silicon dioxide：Silica / Sand / Diatomaceous earth / Diatomaceous silica / Cristobalite / Silicon (Ⅳ) oxide / Infusorial earth
元素記号　Silicon：Si
分子式　Silicon dioxide：SiO_2, O_2Si
特性･カテゴリー　ミネラル／Mineral
Note 1　—
Note 2　Fall under the category of designated food additive.
注　指定添加物に該当する。

名　称　ケルセチン

他名等　—
部位等　—
備　考　—

Name　Quercetin
Other name(s)　—
IUPAC Name　2-(3,4-dihydroxyphenyl)-3,5,7-trihydroxychromen-4-one
CAS No.　117-39-5
Synonyms　Meletin / Sophoretin / Xanthaurine / Quercetine / Quercetol / Quercitin / Quertine / Flavin meletin
分子式　$C_{15}H_{10}O_7$
特性･カテゴリー　植物成分（フラボノイド）／Botanical constituent (Flavonoid)
Note 1　—
Note 2　Fall under the category of existing food additive.
注　既存添加物に該当する。

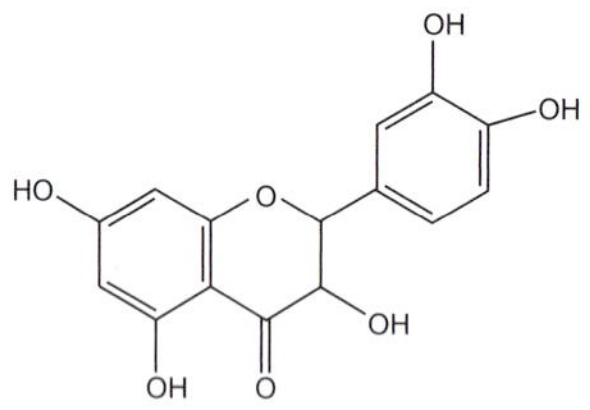

名　称　ゲルマニウム

他名等　無機ゲルマニウム／有機ゲルマニウム
部位等　—
備　考　—

Name　Germanium
Other name(s)　Inorganic germanium / Organic germanium
IUPAC Name　germanium
CAS No.　7440-56-4
Synonyms　Germanium element / Germide / Ge(4+) / Germanio
元素記号　Ge / Ge^{4+}
特性･カテゴリー　ミネラル／Mineral
Note 1　—
Note 2　Treated as a substance which is generally provided for eating or drinking as a food and which is also used as a food additive.
Serious adverse events by inorganic germanium have occurred.
注　一般に食品として飲食に供される物であって添加物として使用されるものとして取り扱われる。
無機ゲルマニウムによる重篤な有害事象が知られている。

名　称　コエンザイムA

他名等　—
部位等　—
備　考　—

Name　Coenzyme A
Other name (s)　—
IUPAC Name　[[(2R,3S,4R,5R)-5-(6-aminopurin-9-yl)-4-hydroxy-3-phosphonooxyoxolan-2-yl]methoxy-hydroxyphosphoryl] [(3R)-3-hydroxy-2,2-dimethyl-4-oxo-4-[[3-oxo-3-(2-sulfanylethylamino)propyl]amino]butyl]hydrogen phosphate
CAS No.　85-61-0
Synonyms　CoASH / Aluzime / Coalip / Co-enzyme-A / HS-CoA / Co-A-SH / CoA
分子式　$C_{21}H_{36}N_7O_{16}P_3S$
特性・カテゴリー　生理活性物質／Bioactive substance
Note 1　—
Note 2　Seek the judgement by the Ministry of Health, Labour and Welfare before using whether the substance will be fall under the category of food additive.
注　使用に先立ち、食品添加物に該当するか否かの判断を厚生労働省より受ける必要がある。

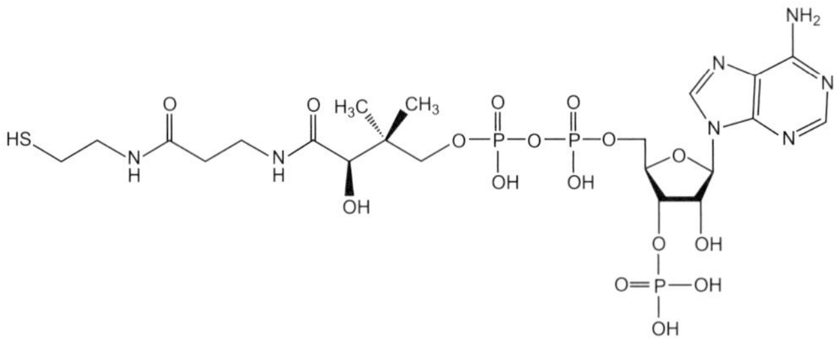

名　称　コエンザイムQ10

他名等　ユビキノン
部位等　—
備　考　—

Name　Coenzyme Q_{10}
Other name (s)　Ubiquinone
IUPAC Name　2-[(2E,6E,10E,14E,18E,22E,26E,30E,34E)-3,7,11,15,19,23,27,31,35,39-decamethyltetraconta-2,6,10,14,18,22,26,30,34,38-decaenyl]-5,6-dimethoxy-3-methylcyclohexa-2,5-diene-1,4-dione
CAS No.　303-98-0
Synonyms　Ubidecarenone / Ubiquinone 50 / Ubiquinone-10 / Neuquinon / CoQ_{10} / Emitolon / Heartcin / Inokiten
分子式　$C_{59}H_{90}O_4$
特性・カテゴリー　生理活性物質／Bioactive substance
Note 1　—
Note 2　Treated as a substance which is generally provided for eating or drinking as a food and which is also used as a food additive.
注　一般に食品として飲食に供される物であって添加物として使用されるものとして取り扱われる。

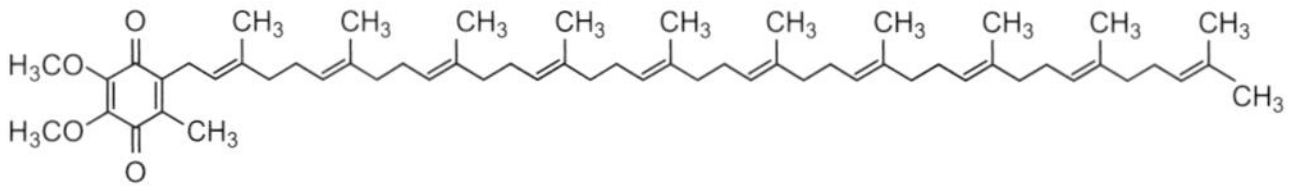

名　称　コラーゲン

他名等　—
部位等　—
備　考　—

Name　Collagen
Other name (s)　—
IUPAC Name　ex) Collagen (Type I) : [2-[[(2S)-2-[[(2S)-2-[[2-[[(2S)-2-[[(2S)-2-[[2-[[(2S)-6-amino-2-[[(2S)-2-[[2-[[(2S,4R)-4-hydroxypyrrolidine-2-carbonyl]amino]acetyl]amino]hexanoyl]amino]-5,6-ditritiohexanoyl]amino]acetyl]amino]-3-(4*H*-imidazol-4-yl)propanoyl]amino]-5-(diaminomethylideneamino)pentanoyl]amino]acetyl]amino]-3-phenylpropanoyl]amino]-3-hydroxypropanoyl]amino]acetyl] (2S)-2-[(2-aminoacetyl)amino]-4-methylpentanoate
CAS No.　Collagen (Type I) : 9007-34-5
Synonyms　Ossein
分子式　Collagen (Type I) : $C_{57}H_{91}O_{16}$
特性・カテゴリー　タンパク質（コラーゲン）／Protein (Collagen)
Note 1　—
Note 2　Treated as a substance which is generally provided for eating or drinking as a food and which is also used as a food additive.
注　一般に食品として飲食に供される物であって添加物として使用されるものとして取り扱われる。

カ行

名　称　コリン安定化オルトケイ酸

他名等　Choline-stabilised orthosilicic acid
部位等　—
備　考　—

Name　Choline-stabilised orthosilicic acid
Other name(s)　Choline-stabilised orthosilicic acid
IUPAC Name　—
CAS No.　7440-21-3
Synonyms　ch-OSA
分子式　Orthosilicic acid：$Si(OH)_4$
Choline chlorid：$[HOCH_2CH_2N^+(CH_3)_3]Cl^-$
特性・カテゴリー　ミネラル（ケイ素供給物質）／Mineral (Source of silicon)
Note 1　—
Note 2　Seek the judgement by the Ministry of Health, Labour and Welfare before using whether the substance will be fall under the category of food additive.
Mixture of orthosilicic acid and choline chlorid.
注　使用に先立ち、食品添加物に該当するか否かの判断を厚生労働省より受ける必要がある。
オルトケイ酸と塩化コリンの混合物。

名　称　コンドロイチン硫酸

他名等　—
部位等　—
備　考　—

Name　Chondroitin sulfate
Other name(s)　—
IUPAC Name　(2S,3S,4S,5R,6R)-6-[(2R,3R,4R,5R,6R)-3-acetamido-2,5-dihydroxy-6-sulfooxyoxan-4-yl]oxy-3,4,5-trihydroxyoxane-2-carboxylic acid
CAS No.　9007-28-7
Synonyms　Mucopolysaccharide / Chondroitinsulfate
分子式　$(C_{14}H_{21}NO_{14}S)_n$
特性・カテゴリー　多糖類（ムコ多糖類）／Polysaccharide (Mucopolysaccharide)
Note 1　—
Note 2　Treated as a substance which is generally provided for eating or drinking as a food and which is also used as a food additive.
注　一般に食品として飲食に供される物であって添加物として使用されるものとして取り扱われる。

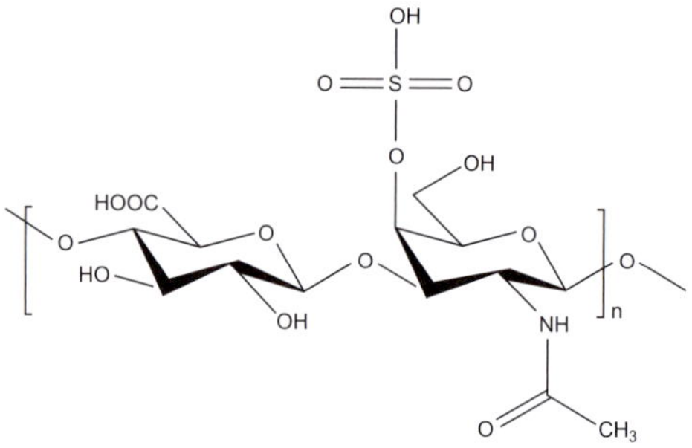

※コンドロイチン硫酸は硫酸基の結合位置が数種類ある。
その1例としてコンドロイチン硫酸Aの構造式を示す。
通常は、タンパク質と結合している。

名　称　コンドロムコタンパク

他名等　—
部位等　—
備　考　—

Name　Chondromucoprotein
Other name(s)　—
IUPAC Name　—
CAS No.　—
Synonyms　—
分子式　—
特性・カテゴリー　プロテオグリカン（コンドロイチン硫酸とムコタンパクの共重合体）／Proteoglycan (Copolymer of a mucoprotein and chondroitin sulfates)
Note 1　—
Note 2　Seek the judgement by the Ministry of Health, Labour and Welfare before using whether the substance will be fall under the category of food additive.
注　使用に先立ち、食品添加物に該当するか否かの判断を厚生労働省より受ける必要がある。

サ行

名　称　サポニン

他名等　大豆サポニン
部位等　—
備　考　—

Name　Saponin
Other name(s)　Soy saponins
IUPAC Name　ex) Soy saponin I：(2S,3S,4S,5R,6R)-6-

[[(3S,4S,4aR,6aR,6bS,8aR,9R,12aS,14aR,14bR)-9-hydroxy-4-(hydroxymethyl)-4,6a,6b,8a,11,11,14b-heptamethyl-1,2,3,4a,5,6,7,8,9,10,12,12a,14,14a-tetradecahydropicen-3-yl]oxy]-5-[(2S,3R,4S,5R,6R)-4,5-dihydroxy-6-(hydroxymethyl)-3-[(2S,3R,4R,5R,6S)-3,4,5-trihydroxy-6-methyloxan-2-yl]oxyoxan-2-yl]oxy-3,4-dihydroxyoxane-2-carboxylic acid

CAS No. ex) Soy saponin I：51330-27-9

Synonyms ex) Soy saponin I：Soyasaponin I / Soyasaponin Bb

分子式 ex) Soy saponin I：$C_{48}H_{78}O_{18}$

特性・カテゴリー 植物成分（トリテルペン配糖体あるいはステロイド配糖体）／Botanical consutituent (Triterpene glycoside or steroid glycoside)

Note 1 —

Note 2 Fall under the category of existing food additive. The chemical structural formula of Soy saponin I is shown as an example of saponin.

注 既存添加物に該当する。
例としてSoy saponin Iの構造式を示す。

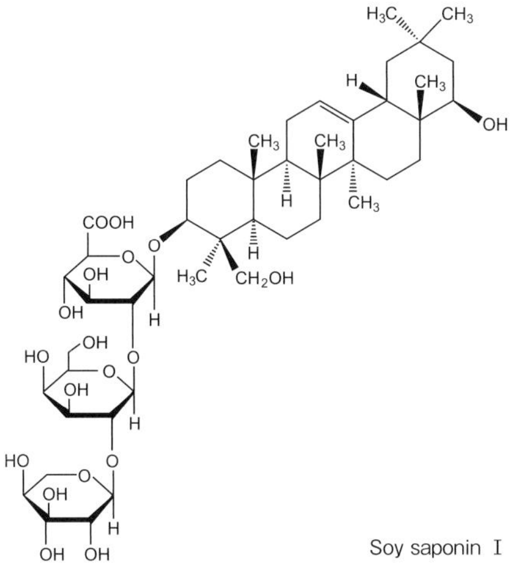

Soy saponin I

※サポニンは、トリテルペンやステロイド骨格に糖類が結合した化合物の総称である。ダイズサポニンは数種類存在する。その1例として大豆サポニンIの構造式を示す。

名 称 シスタチオン

他名等 —

部位等 —

備 考 マムシの成分

Name "Cystationine" would be correct name, though "Cystatione" is in the name column in Japanese.

Other name(s) —

IUPAC Name 2-amino-4-(2-amino-2-carboxyethyl)sulfanylbutanoic acid

CAS No. Cystathionine：56-88-2

Synonyms DL-Cystathionine / DL-Allocystathionine / dl, dl-Allo-cystathionine / L-(+)-Cystathionine

分子式 Cystathionine：$C_7H_{14}N_2O_4S$

特性・カテゴリー 含硫アミノ酸中間代謝物／Intermediate metabolite of sulfur amino acid

Note 1 Constituent of Crotalinae (pit viper)

Note 2 Seek the judgement by the Ministry of Health, Labour and Welfare before using whether the substance will be fall under the category of food additive.
"Cystation" was not detected. The correct substance name would be "Cystationine", though "Cystation" is in the name column in Japanese.

注 使用に先立ち、食品添加物に該当するか否かの判断を厚生労働省より受ける必要がある。
シスタチオンという物質は検索されない。名称はシスタチオニン（Cystationine）の間違いと思われる。

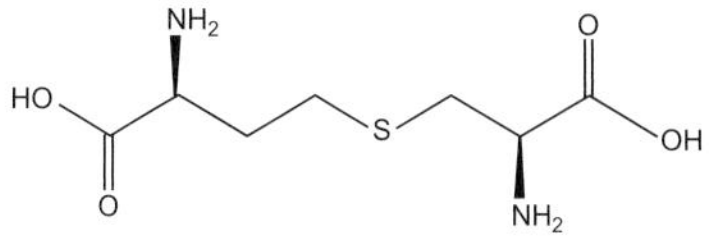

名 称 シスチン

他名等 —

部位等 —

備 考 —

Name Cystine

Other name(s) —

IUPAC Name (2R)-2-amino-3-[[(2R)-2-amino-2-carboxyethyl]disulfanyl]propanoic acid

CAS No. 56-89-3

Synonyms L-Cystine / Cystine acid / L-Cystin / Cysteine disulfide / Dicysteine / Oxidized L-cysteine / Cystin / L-Dicysteine / beta,beta'-Dithiodialanine

分子式 $C_6H_{12}N_2O_4S_2$

特性・カテゴリー アミノ酸／Amino acid

Note 1 —

Note 2 Fall under the category of existing food additive.

注 既存添加物に該当する。

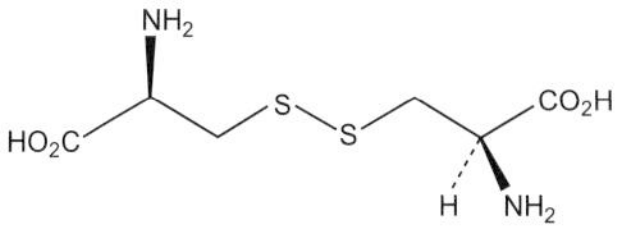

名　称　システイン

他名等　—
部位等　—
備　考　—

Name　Cysteine
Other name(s)　—
IUPAC Name　(2R)-2-amino-3-sulfanylpropanoic acid
CAS No.　52-90-4
Synonyms　L-Cysteine / Half-cystine / Thioserine / Cystein / (R)-Cysteine / L-(+)-Cysteine / beta-Mercaptoalanine / Half cystine
分子式　$C_3H_7NO_2S$
特性・カテゴリー　アミノ酸／Amino acid
Note 1　—
Note 2　Fall under the category of designated food additive.
注　指定添加物に該当する。

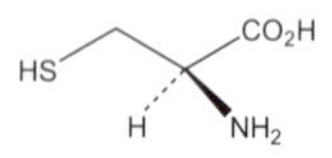

名　称　脂肪酸

他名等　—
部位等　—
備　考　—

Name　Fatty acid
Other name(s)　—
IUPAC Name　—
CAS No.　—
Synonyms　—
分子式　—
特性・カテゴリー　脂肪酸／Fatty acid
Note 1　—
Note 2　Fall under the categories of designated food additive and existing food additive.
注　指定添加物及び既存添加物に該当する。

名　称　酒石酸

他名等　—
部位等　—
備　考　—

Name　Tartaric acid
Other name(s)　—
IUPAC Name
DL-tartaric acid：2,3-dihydroxybutanedioic acid
L-(+)-tartaric acid：(2R,3R)-2,3-dihydroxybutanedioic acid
D-(−)-tartaric acid：(2S,3S)-2,3-dihydroxybutanedioic acid
CAS No.　DL-Tartaric acid：133-37-9
L-(+)-Tartaric acid：87-69-4
D-(−)-Tartaric acid：147-71-7
Synonyms　DL-Tartaric acid / L-(+)-Tartaric acid / D-(−)-Tartaric acid
分子式　$C_4H_6O_6$
特性・カテゴリー　有機酸／Organic acid
Note 1　—
Note 2　Fall under the category of designated food additive.
注　指定添加物に該当する。

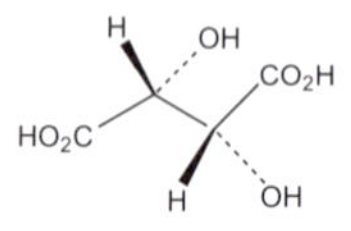

名　称　植物性酵素・果汁酵素

他名等　—
部位等　植物体又は果実の液汁から得られる酵素
備　考　パパイン・ブロメライン等消化酵素は「医」

Name　Plant enzyme, Fruit enzyme
Other name(s)　—
IUPAC Name　—
CAS No.　—
Synonyms　—
分子式　—
特性・カテゴリー　植物成分（酵素）／Botanical constituent (Enzyme)
Note 1　Digestive enzymes such as papain and bromelain：drug category
Note 2　Fall under the category of existing food additive.
注　既存添加物に該当する。

名　称　植物性ステロール

他名等　—
部位等　—
備　考　—

Name　Phytosterol
Other name(s)　—
IUPAC Name
　ex) Sitosterol：(3S,8S,9S,10R,13R,14S,17R)-17-[(2R,5R)-5-ethyl-6-methylheptan-2-yl]-10,13-dimethyl-2,3,4,7,8,9,11,12,14,15,16,17-dodecahydro-1H-cyclopenta[a]phenanthren-3-ol
　Campesterol：(3S,8S,9S,10R,13R,14S,17R)-17-[(2R,5R)-5,6-dimethylheptan-2-yl]-10,13-dimethyl-2,3,4,7,8,9,11,12,14,15,16,17-dodecahydro-1H-cyclopenta[a]phenanthren-3-ol
　Stigmasterol：(3S,8S,9S,10R,13R,14S,17R)-17-[(E,2R,5S)-5-ethyl-6-methylhept-3-en-2-yl]-10,13-dimethyl-2,3,4,7,8,9,11,12,14,15,16,17-dodecahydro-1H-cyclopenta[a]phenanthren-3-ol
CAS No.　ex) Sitosterol：83-46-5
　Campesterol：474-62-4
　Stigmasterol：83-48-7
Synonyms　Plant sterol
分子式　ex) Sitosterol：$C_{29}H_{50}O$
　Campesterol：$C_{28}H_{48}O$
　Stigmasterol：$C_{29}H_{48}O$
特性・カテゴリー　植物成分（ステロール）／Botanical constituent (Sterol)
Note 1　—
Note 2　Fall under the category of existing food additive.
注　既存添加物に該当する。

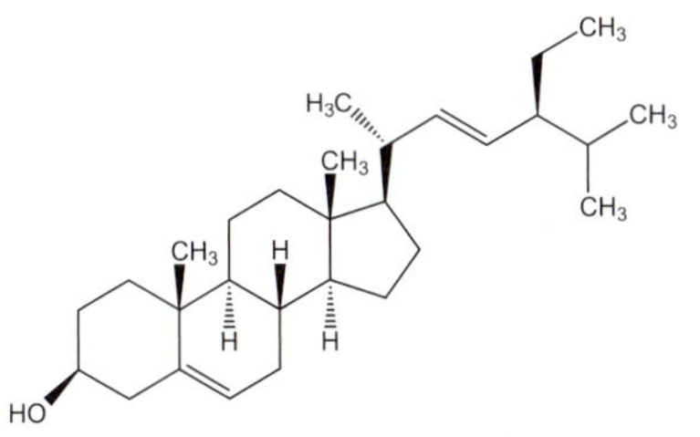

※植物ステロールは、植物に含まれるステロール類の総称である。
その一例としてスティグマステロールの構造式を示す。

名　称　植物繊維

他名等　—
部位等　—
備　考　—

Name　Vegetable fiber
Other name(s)　—
IUPAC Name　—
CAS No.　—
Synonyms　—
分子式　—
特性・カテゴリー　食物繊維／Dietary fiber
Note 1　—
Note 2　Treated as a substance which is generally provided for eating or drinking as a food and which is also used as a food additive.
注　一般に食品として飲食に供される物であって添加物として使用されるものとして取り扱われる。

名　称　食物繊維

他名等　—
部位等　—
備　考　—

Name　Dietary fiber
Other name(s)　—
IUPAC Name　—
CAS No.　—
Synonyms　—
分子式　—
特性・カテゴリー　食物繊維／Dietary fiber
Note 1　—
Note 2　Treated as a substance which is generally provided for eating or drinking as a food and which is also used as a food additive.
注　一般に食品として飲食に供される物であって添加物として使用されるものとして取り扱われる。

名　称　スーパーオキシドディスムターゼ＜SOD＞

他名等　SOD
部位等　—
備　考　—

Name　Superoxide dismutase (SOD)
Other name(s)　SOD
IUPAC Name　—

CAS No.　9054-89-1
Synonyms　SOD-3 / hrSOD / Cuprein / Orgotein / Ontosein / Ormetein / Palosein / Cu/Zn SOD / Sudismase
分子式　—
特性・カテゴリー　酵素／Enzyme
Note 1　—
Note 2　Seek the judgement by the Ministry of Health, Labour and Welfare before using whether the substance will be fall under the category of food additive.
注　使用に先立ち、食品添加物に該当するか否かの判断を厚生労働省より受ける必要がある。

名　称　**スクワレン**

他名等　—
部位等　—
備　考　—

Name　Squalene
Other name(s)　—
IUPAC Name　(6E,10E,14E,18E)-2,6,10,15,19,23-hexamethyltetracosa-2,6,10,14,18,22-hexaene
CAS No.　111-02-4
Synonyms　trans-Squalene / (E,E,E,E)-Squalene / 2,6,10,15,19,23-Hexamethyltetracosa-2,6,10,14,18,22-hexaene / Supraene
分子式　$C_{30}H_{50}$
特性・カテゴリー　高度不飽和炭化水素／Highly unsaturated hydrocarbon
Note 1　—
Note 2　Seek the judgement by the Ministry of Health, Labour and Welfare before using whether the substance will be fall under the category of food additive.
注　使用に先立ち、食品添加物に該当するか否かの判断を厚生労働省より受ける必要がある。

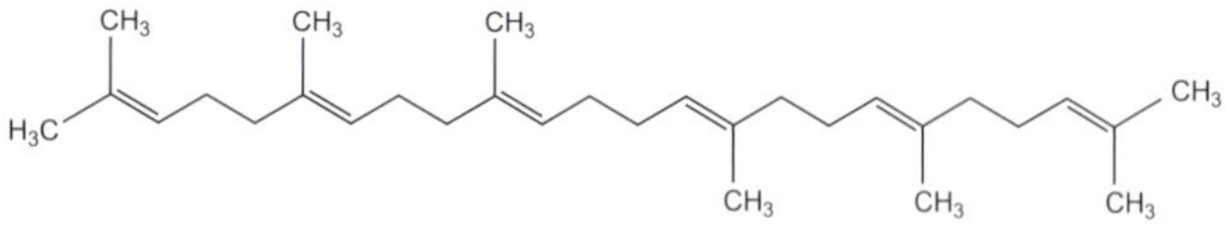

名　称　**炭焼の乾留水**

他名等　—
部位等　—
備　考　—

Name　Charcoal dry distilled water
Other name(s)　—
IUPAC Name　—
CAS No.　Pyroligneous acid：8030-97-5
Synonyms　Wood vinegar / Pyroligneous vinegar / Pyroligneous acid / Mokusaku wood vinegar
分子式　—
特性・カテゴリー　木酢液／Mokusaku wood vinegar
Note 1　—
Note 2　Seek the judgement by the Ministry of Health, Labour and Welfare before using whether the substance will be fall under the category of food additive.
注　使用に先立ち、食品添加物に該当するか否かの判断を厚生労働省より受ける必要がある。

名　称　**石膏**

他名等　—
部位等　—
備　考　鉱石

Name　Gypsum
Other name(s)　—
IUPAC Name　calcium;sulfate
CAS No.　7778-18-9
Synonyms　Calcium sulfate / Anhydrous gypsum / Drierite
分子式　$CaSO_4$, CaO_4S
特性・カテゴリー　ミネラル／Mineral
Note 1　Mineral (Ore)
Note 2　Seek the judgement by the Ministry of Health, Labour and Welfare before using whether the substance will be fall under the category of food additive.
注　使用に先立ち、食品添加物に該当するか否かの判断を厚生労働省より受ける必要がある。

名　称　ゼラチン

他名等　—
部位等　—
備　考　—

Name　Gelatin
Other name(s)　—
IUPAC Name　—
CAS No.　9000-70-8
Synonyms　—
分子式　—
特性・カテゴリー　タンパク質（コラーゲンの加水分解物）／Protein (Collagen hydrolysate)
Note 1　—
Note 2　Treated as a substance which is generally provided for eating or drinking as a food and which is also used as a food additive.
注　一般に食品として飲食に供される物であって添加物として使用されるものとして取り扱われる。

名　称　セラミド

他名等　—
部位等　—
備　考　—

Name　Ceramide
Other name(s)　—
IUPAC Name　ex) N-palmitoylsphingosine (C16 Ceramide) : N-[(E)-1,3-dihydroxyoctadec-4-en-2-yl]hexadecanamide
CAS No.　ex) N-palmitoylsphingosine (C16 Ceramide) : 4201-58-5
Synonyms　ex) N-palmitoylsphingosine (C16 Ceramide) : N-Palmitoyl 4-sphingenine / Palmitoyl ceramide
分子式　ex) N-palmitoylsphingosine (C16 Ceramide) : $C_{34}H_{67}NO_3$
特性・カテゴリー　リン脂質（スフィンゴ脂質）／Phospholipid (Sphingolipid)
Note 1　—
Note 2　Seek the judgement by the Ministry of Health, Labour and Welfare before using whether the substance will be fall under the category of food additive.
A ceraimide is composed of sphingosine and fatty acid. The chemical structural formula of a ceramide is depending on a fatty acid combined. Here, palmitic acid is taken up as an example.
注　使用に先立ち、食品添加物に該当するか否かの判断を厚生労働省より受ける必要がある。
セラミドはスフィンゴシンと脂肪酸がアミド結合したものであり、結合する脂肪酸によって構造が異なる。ここではパルミチン酸によって構造式を代表させた。

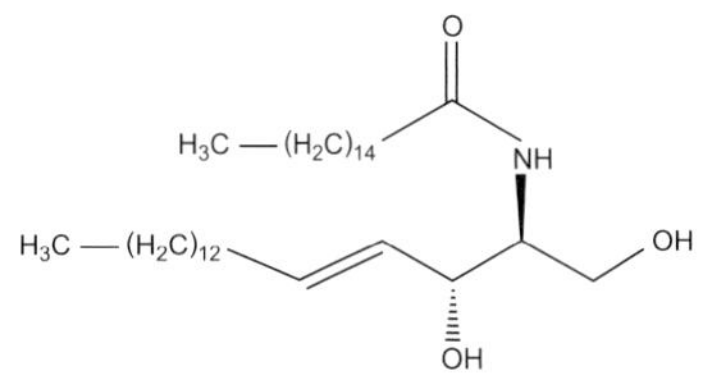

名　称　セリン

他名等　—
部位等　—
備　考　—

Name　Serine
Other name(s)　—
IUPAC Name　serine
CAS No.　L-isomer : 56-45-1
D-isomer : 312-84-5
DL-form : 302-84-1
Synonyms　beta-Hydroxyalanine / (S)-Serine / L-Serine / L-3-Hydroxy-alanine / 2-Amino-3-hydroxypropionic acid
分子式　$C_3H_7NO_3$
特性・カテゴリー　アミノ酸／Amino acid
Note 1　—
Note 2　Fall under the category of existing food additive.
注　既存添加物に該当する。

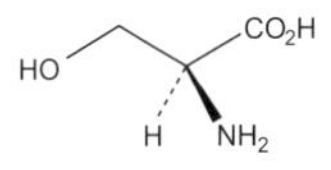

名　称　セレン

他名等　—
部位等　—
備　考　—

Name　Selenium
Other name(s)　—
IUPAC Name　selenium
CAS No.　7782-49-2
Synonyms　Selen / Selenium atom
元素記号　Se

特性・カテゴリー　ミネラル／Mineral
Note 1　—
Note 2　Before using, it is necessary to be designated as a new food additive based on the article 10 of the Food Sanitation Act.
注　使用に先立ち、新たに食品添加物の指定を受ける必要がある。

タ行

名　称　タルク

他名等　—
部位等　—
備　考　—

Name　Talc
Other name(s)　—
IUPAC Name　trimagnesium;dioxido(oxo)silane;hydroxy-oxido-oxosilane
CAS No.　14807-96-6
Synonyms　Steatite / Mussolinite / Agalite
分子式　$Mg_3Si_4O_{10}(OH)_2$, $H_2Mg_3O_{12}Si_4$
特性・カテゴリー　ミネラル／Mineral
Note 1　—
Note 2　Fall under the category of existing food additive.
注　既存添加物に該当する。

名　称　チオクト酸

他名等　α-リポ酸
部位等　—
備　考　—

Name　Thioctic acid
Other name(s)　alpha-Lipoic acid
IUPAC Name　(R)-5-(1,2-dithiolan-3-yl)pentanoic acid
CAS No.　(R)-(+)-alpha Lipoic acid：1200-22-2
(±)-alpha-Lipoic acid：62-46-4
DL-form：1077-28-7
Synonyms　Lipoic acid / Thioctacid
分子式　$C_8H_{14}O_2S_2$
特性・カテゴリー　生理活性物質／Bioactive substance
Note 1　—
Note 2　Treated as a substance which is generally provided for eating or drinking as a food and which is also used as a food additive.
注　一般に食品として飲食に供される物であって添加物として使用されるものとして取り扱われる。

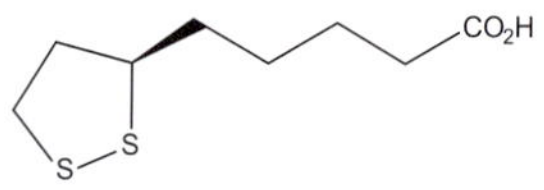

名　称　チロシン

他名等　—
部位等　—
備　考　—

Name　Tyrosine
Other name(s)　—
IUPAC Name　(2S)-2-amino-3-(4-hydroxyphenyl)propanoic acid
CAS No.　60-18-4
Synonyms　L-Tyrosine / 4-Hydroxy-L-phenylalanine / beta-(*p*-Hydroxyphenyl)alanine
分子式　$C_9H_{11}NO_3$
特性・カテゴリー　アミノ酸／Amino acid
Note 1　—
Note 2　Fall under the category of existing food additive.
注　既存添加物に該当する。

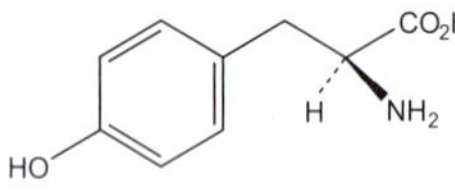

名　称　D-chiro-イノシトール

他名等　—
部位等　—
備　考　—

Name　D-chiro-Inositol
Other name(s)　—
IUPAC Name　cis-1,2,4-trans-3,5,6-cyclohexanehexol
CAS No.　643-12-9
Synonyms　D-(+)-chiro-Inositol / 1,2,4/3,5,6-Hexahydroxycyclohexene / DCI
分子式　$C_6H_{12}O_6$
特性・カテゴリー　単糖類／Monosaccharide
Note 1　—
Note 2　Fall under the category of existing food additive.
注　既存添加物に該当する。

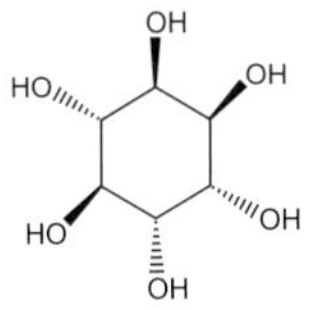

名　称　**デキストリン**

他名等　—
部位等　—
備　考　—

Name　Dextrin
Other name(s)　—
IUPAC Name　(3R,4S,5S,6R)-2-[(2R,3S,4R,5R)-4,5-dihydroxy-2-(hydroxymethyl)-6-[(2R,3S,4R,5R,6S)-4,5,6-trihydroxy-2-(hydroxymethyl)oxan-3-yl]oxyoxan-3-yl]oxy-6-(hydroxymethyl)oxane-3,4,5-triol
CAS No.　9004-53-9
Synonyms　Caloreen / Dextrine / Dextrins
分子式　$(C_6H_{10}O_5)n$
特性・カテゴリー　多糖類／Polysaccharide
Note 1　—
Note 2　Treated as a substance which is generally provided for eating or drinking as a food and which is also used as a food additive.
注　一般に食品として飲食に供される物であって添加物として使用されるものとして取り扱われる。

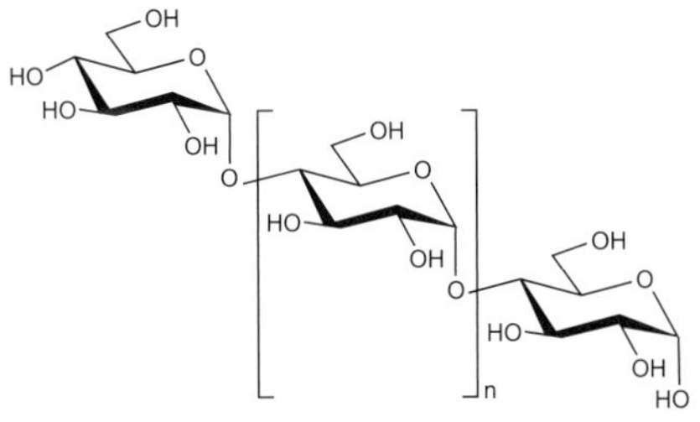

n=10~100

※デキストリンは、デンプンをグルコースに分解する途中で得られる中間生成物の総称である。
分子量約1万のものをアミロデキストリン、
分子量約7,000のものをエリスロデキストリン、
分子量約4,000のものをアクロデキストリンと呼ぶ。

名　称　**鉄**

他名等　—
部位等　—
備　考　—

Name　Iron
Other name(s)　—
IUPAC Name　iron
CAS No.　7439-89-6
Synonyms　Ferrum / Ferrous iron
元素記号　Fe
特性・カテゴリー　ミネラル／Mineral
Note 1　—
Note 2　Fall under the categories of designated food additive and existing food additive.
注　指定添加物及び既存添加物に該当する。

名　称　**鉄クロロフィリンナトリウム**

他名等　—
部位等　—
備　考　—

Name　Sodium iron chlorophyllin
Other name(s)　—
IUPAC Name　Disodium;3-[20-(carboxylatomethyl)-18-(dioxidomethylidene)-8-ethenyl-13-ethyl-3,7,12,17-tetramethyl-2,3-dihydroporphyrin-23-id-2-yl]propanoate;hydron;iron(2+)
CAS No.　—
Synonyms　Disodium;3-[18-(dioxidomethylidene)-8-ethenyl-13-ethyl-3,7,12,17-tetramethyl-20-(2-oxido-2-oxoethyl)-2,3-dihydroporphyrin-23-id-2-yl]propanoate;hydron;iron(2+)
分子式　$C_{34}H_{32}FeN_4Na_2O_6$
特性・カテゴリー　ミネラル／Mineral
Note 1　—
Note 2　Fall under the category of designated food additive.
注　指定添加物に該当する。

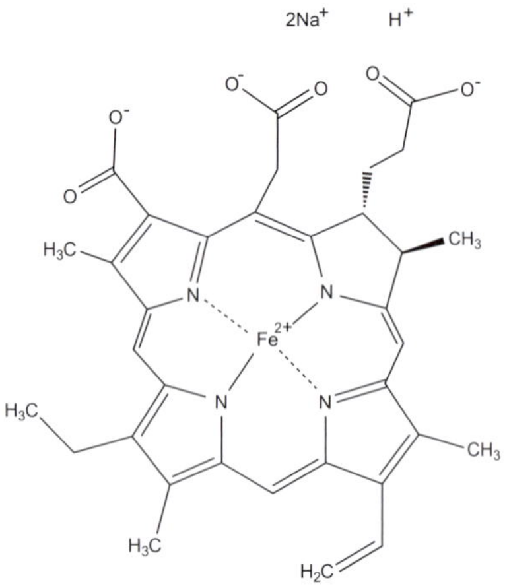

名　称　銅

他名等　—
部位等　—
備　考　—

Name　Copper
Other name(s)　—
IUPAC Name　copper
CAS No.　7440-50-8
Synonyms　Cuprum
元素記号　Cu
特性・カテゴリー　ミネラル／Mineral
Note 1　—
Note 2　Fall under the categories of designated food additive and existing food additive.
注　指定添加物及び既存添加物に該当する。

名　称　ドコサヘキサエン酸<DHA>

他名等　DHA
部位等　—
備　考　—

Name　Docosahexaenoic acid (DHA)
Other name(s)　DHA
IUPAC Name　(4Z,7Z,10Z,13Z,16Z,19Z)-docosa-4,7,10,13,16,19-hexaenoic acid
CAS No.　6217-54-5
Synonyms　cis-4,7,10,13,16,19-Docosahexaenoic acid / Doconexent / Cervonic acid
分子式　$C_{22}H_{32}O_2$
特性・カテゴリー　高度不飽和脂肪酸／Higher poylunsaturated fatty acid
Note 1　—
Note 2　Treated as a substance which is generally provided for eating or drinking as a food and which is also used as a food additive.
注　一般に食品として飲食に供される物であって添加物として使用されるものとして取り扱われる。

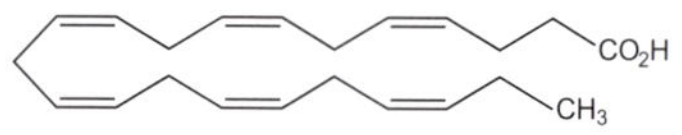

名　称　トコトリエノール

他名等　—
部位等　—
備　考　ビタミンE関連物質

Name　Tocotrienol
Other name(s)　—
IUPAC Name　ex) alpha-Tocotrienol : (2R)-2,5,7,8-tetramethyl-2-[(3E,7E)-4,8,12-trimethyltrideca-3,7,11-trienyl]-3,4-dihydrochromen-6-ol
CAS No.　ex) alpha-Tocotrienol : 58864-81-6
Synonyms　ex) alpha-Tocotrienol : D-alpha-Tocotrienol / (2R,3'E,7'E)-alpha-Tocotrienol
分子式　ex) alpha-Tocotrienol : $C_{29}H_{44}O_2$
特性・カテゴリー　ビタミンE関連物質／Vitamin E related substance
Note 1　Vitamin E related substance
Note 2　Fall under the category of existing food additive. See "Vitamin E" in this list.
注　既存添加物に該当する。
ビタミンEの項を参照。

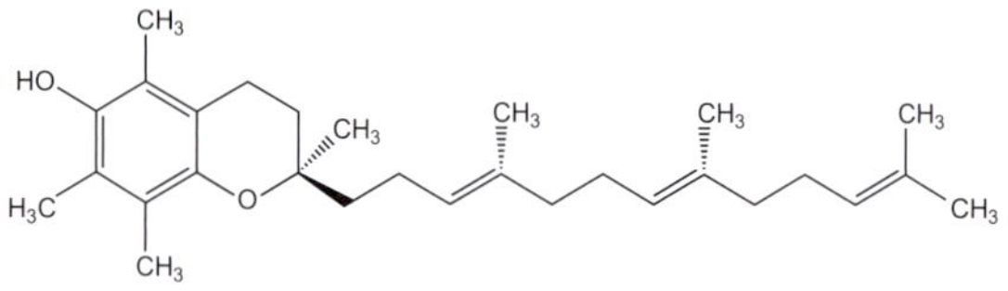

α-Tocotrienol

名　称　trans-レスベラトロール

他名等　*E*-レスベラトロール
部位等　—
備　考　—

Name　trans-Resveratrol
Other name(s)　*E*-Resveratrol
IUPAC Name　5-[(E)-2-(4-hydroxyphenyl)ethenyl]benzene-1,3-diol

CAS No. 501-36-0
Synonyms Resveratrol / 3,4',5-Stilbenetriol / 3,4',5-Trihydroxystilbene / Resvida
分子式 $C_{14}H_{12}O_3$
特性・カテゴリー 植物成分（ポリフェノール）／Botanical constituent (Polyphenol)
Note 1 —
Note 2 Seek the judgement by the Ministry of Health, Labour and Welfare before using whether the substance will be fall under the category of food additive.
注 使用に先立ち、食品添加物に該当するか否かの判断を厚生労働省より受ける必要がある。

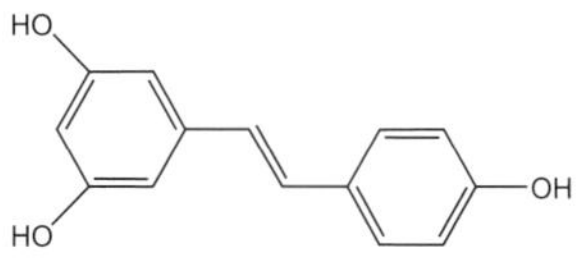

名 称 **ドロマイト鉱石**

他名等 —
部位等 —
備 考 —

Name Dolomite
Other name(s) —
IUPAC Name calcium ; magnesium ; dicarbonate
CAS No. 16389-88-1
Synonyms Pearlspar / Taraspite / Carbonic acid / Calcium magnesium salt (2 : 1 : 1) / Dolomite (CaMg $(CO_3)_2$)
分子式 $Ca \cdot Mg(CO_3)_2$, C_2CaMgO_6
特性・カテゴリー ミネラル／Mineral
Note 1 —
Note 2 Treated as a substance which is generally provided for eating or drinking as a food and which is also used as a food additive.
注 一般に食品として飲食に供される物であって添加物として使用されるものとして取り扱われる。

名 称 **トリプトファン**

他名等 —
部位等 —
備 考 —

Name Tryptophan
Other name(s) —
IUPAC Name (2S)-2-amino-3-(1*H*-indol-3-yl)propanoic acid
CAS No. 73-22-3
Synonyms L-Tryptophan / Indole-3-alanine / Tryptophane / Trofan / Triptacin
分子式 $C_{11}H_{12}N_2O_2$
特性・カテゴリー アミノ酸／Amino acid
Note 1 —
Note 2 Fall under the category of designated food additive.
注 指定添加物に該当する。

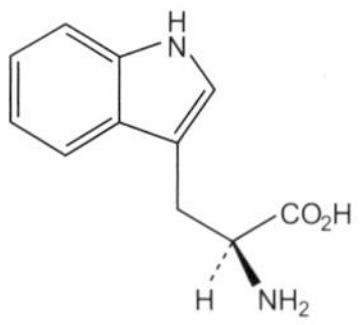

名 称 **トレオニン**

他名等 —
部位等 —
備 考 —

Name Threonine
Other name(s) —
IUPAC Name (2S,3R)-2-amino-3-hydroxybutanoic acid
CAS No. 72-19-5
Synonyms L-Threonine / L-(-)-Threonine / 2-Amino-3-hydroxybutyric acid
分子式 $C_4H_9NO_3$
特性・カテゴリー アミノ酸／Amino acid
Note 1 —
Note 2 Fall under the category of designated food additive.
注 指定添加物に該当する。

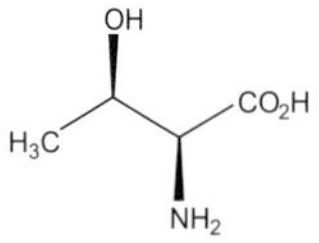

名 称 トレハロース

他名等 —
部位等 —
備 考 菌体をリゾチーム処理したものの抽出物

Name Trehalose
Other name(s) —
IUPAC Name (2R,3S,4S,5R,6R)-2-(hydroxymethyl)-6-[(2R,3R,4S,5S,6R)-3,4,5-trihydroxy-6-(hydroxymethyl)oxan-2-yl]oxyoxane-3,4,5-triol
CAS No. 99-20-7
Synonyms alpha, alpha-Trehalose / D-Trehalose / alpha-D-Trehalose / alpha-D-Glucopyranosyl-alpha-D-glucopyranoside
分子式 $C_{12}H_{22}O_{11}$
特性・カテゴリー 二糖類／Disaccharide
Note 1 Extract from lysozyme-treated mycelium
Note 2 Fall under the category of existing food additive.
注 既存添加物に該当する。

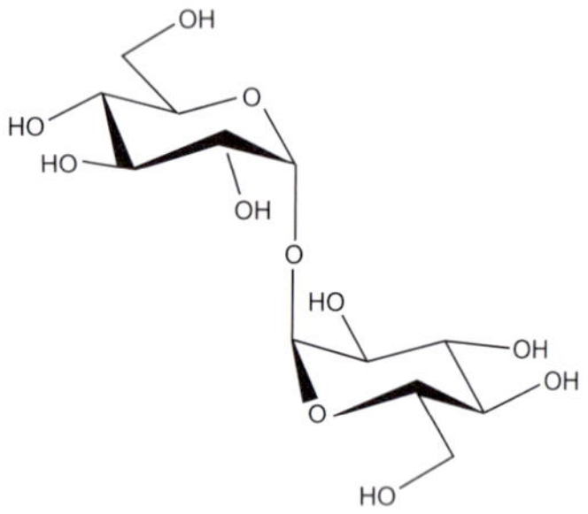

ナ行

名 称 ナイアシン

他名等 ニコチン酸
部位等 —
備 考 —

Name Niacin
Other name(s) Nicotinic acid
IUPAC Name pyridine-3-carboxylic acid
CAS No. 59-67-6
Synonyms 3-Pyridinecarboxylic acid / Apelagrin / Pellagrin
分子式 $C_6H_5NO_2$
特性・カテゴリー ビタミン／Vitamin
Note 1 —
Note 2 Fall under the category of designated food additive.
注 指定添加物に該当する。

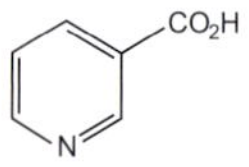

名 称 乳清

他名等 —
部位等 —
備 考 —

Name Whey
Other name(s) —
IUPAC Name —
CAS No. —
Synonyms —
分子式 —
特性・カテゴリー 乳由来水溶性成分／Watery part of milk separated from the coagulable part or curd
Note 1 —
Note 2 Treated as a substance which is generally provided for eating or drinking as a food and which is also used as a food additive.
注 一般に食品として飲食に供される物であって添加物として使用されるものとして取り扱われる。

名 称 乳糖

他名等 —
部位等 —
備 考 —

Name Lactose
Other name(s) —
IUPAC Name (2R,3R,4S,5R,6S)-2-(hydroxymethyl)-6-[(2R,3S,4R,5R,6R)-4,5,6-trihydroxy-2-(hydroxymethyl)oxan-3-yl]oxyoxane-3,4,5-triol
CAS No. 63-42-3
Synonyms 4-O-beta-D-Galactopyranosyl-beta-D-glucopyranose / Lactin / beta-D-Lactose
分子式 $C_{12}H_{22}O_{11}$
特性・カテゴリー 二糖類／Disaccharide
Note 1 —
Note 2 Treated as a substance which is generally provided for eating or drinking as a food and which is also used as a food additive.

注　一般に食品として飲食に供される物であって添加物として使用されるものとして取り扱われる。

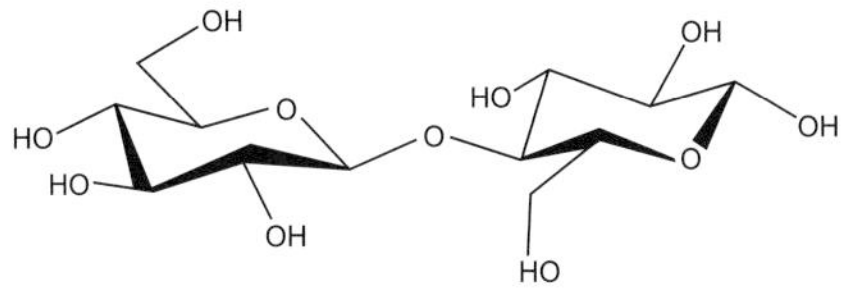

ハ行

名　称　麦飯石

他名等　—
部位等　—
備　考　—

Name　Maifan stone
Other name(s)　—
IUPAC Name　—
CAS No.　—
Synonyms　—
分子式　—
特性・カテゴリー　ミネラル／Mineral
Note 1　—
Note 2　Fall under the category of existing food additive. The pronunciation of this ingredienteis "BAKU-HANSEKI".
A kind of granite porphyry or quartz porphyry.
注　既存添加物に該当する。
麦飯石の発音は「バクハンセキ」。Granite porphyry（花崗斑岩），Quartz porphyry（石英斑岩）の一種。
組織はSiO_2:71.23%，Al_2O_3:14.21%，Fe_2O_3（contein FeO）:3.23%，MgO:3.22%，CaO:3.18%，Na_2O:1.88%，K_2O:1.82%，TiO_2:0.36%，P_2O_5:0.22%，MnO:0.02%，etc.:0.63%

名　称　バリン

他名等　—
部位等　—
備　考　—

Name　Valine
Other name(s)　—
IUPAC Name　(2S)-2-amino-3-methylbutanoic acid
CAS No.　72-18-4
Synonyms　L-Valine / 2-Amino-3-methylbutyric acid / (S)-2-Amino-3-methylbutyric acid / (S)-2-Amino-3-methylbutanoic acid
分子式　$C_5H_{11}NO_2$
特性・カテゴリー　ビタミン／Vitamin
Note 1　—
Note 2　Fall under the category of designated food additive.
注　指定添加物に該当する。

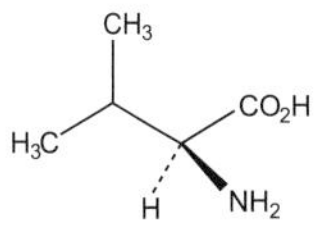

名　称　パントテン酸

他名等　パントテン酸カルシウム
部位等　—
備　考　—

Name　Pantothenic acid
Other name(s)　Calcium pantothenate
IUPAC Name
Pantothenic acid：3-[[(2R)-2,4-dihydroxy-3,3-dimethylbutanoyl]amino]propanoic acid
Calcium pantothenate：calcium;3-[[(2R)-2,4-dihydroxy-3,3-dimethylbutanoyl]amino]propanoate
CAS No.　Pantothenic acid：79-83-4
Calcium pantothenate：137-08-6
Synonyms
Pantothenic acid：Vitamin B_5 / Pantothenate / D-Pantothenic acid
Calcium pantothenate：Calcium D-pantothenate
分子式　Pantothenic acid：$C_9H_{17}NO_5$
Calcium pantothenate：$C_{18}H_{32}CaN_2O_{10}$
特性・カテゴリー　ビタミン／Vitamin
Note 1　—
Note 2　Fall under the category of designated food additive.
注　指定添加物に該当する。

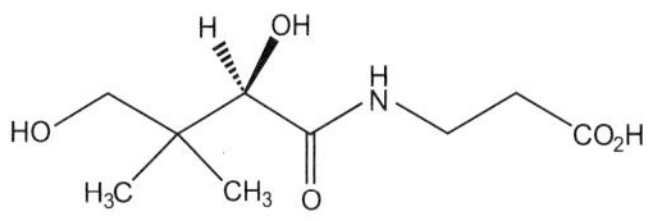

名　称　ヒアルロン酸

他名等　―
部位等　―
備　考　―

Name　Hyaluronic acid
Other name(s)　―
IUPAC Name　6-[3-acetamido-2-[6-[3-acetamido-2,5-dihydroxy-6-(hydroxymethyl)oxan-4-yl]oxy-2-carboxy-4,5-dihydroxyoxan-3-yl]oxy-5-hydroxy-6-(hydroxymethyl)oxan-4-yl]oxy-3,4,5-trihydroxyoxane-2-carboxylic acid
CAS No.　9004-61-9
Synonyms　beta-D-Glucopyranuronosyl-(1->3)-(3xi)-2-(acetylamino)-2-deoxy-beta-D-ribo-hexopyranosyl-(1->4)-beta-D-glucopyranuronosyl-(1->3)-(3xi)-2-(acetylamino)-2-deoxy-beta-D-ribo-hexopyranose
分子式　$(C_{14}H_{21}NO_{11})_n$
特性・カテゴリー　多糖類／Polysaccharide
Note 1　―
Note 2　Fall under the category of existing food additive.
注　既存添加物に該当する。

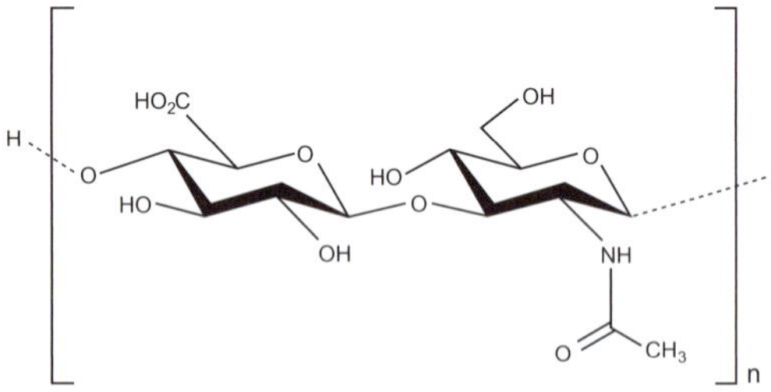

MW > 1,000,000

名　称　ビオチン

他名等　ビタミンH
部位等　―
備　考　―

Name　Biotin
Other name(s)　Vitamin H
IUPAC Name　5-[(3aS,4S,6aR)-2-oxo-1,3,3a,4,6,6a-hexahydrothieno[3,4-d]imidazol-4-yl]pentanoic acid
CAS No.　58-85-5
Synonyms　d-Biotin / Coenzyme R / Vitamin B_7
分子式　$C_{10}H_{16}N_2O_3S$
特性・カテゴリー　ビタミン／Vitamin
Note 1　―
Note 2　Fall under the category of designated food additive.
注　指定添加物に該当する。

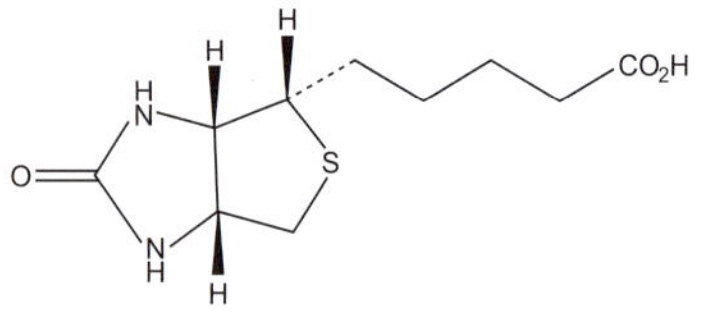

名　称　ピコリン酸クロム

他名等　クロミウムピコリネート
部位等　―
備　考　―

Name　Chromium picolinate
Other name(s)　Chromium tripicolinate
IUPAC Name　chromium(3+);pyridine-2-carboxylate
CAS No.　14639-25-9
Synonyms　Chromium(Ⅲ)trispicolinate / Chromium(Ⅲ) picolinate
分子式　$C_{18}H_{12}CrN_3O_6$
特性・カテゴリー　ミネラル／Mineral
Note 1　―
Note 2　Before using, it is necessary to be designated as a new food additive based on the article 10 of the Food Sanitation Act.
注　使用に先立ち、新たに食品添加物の指定を受ける必要がある。

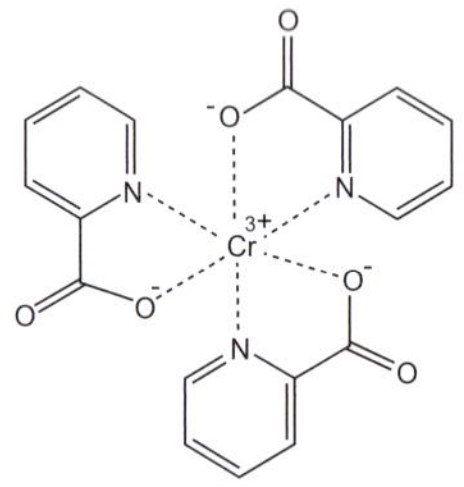

名　称　ヒスチジン

他名等　―
部位等　―
備　考　―

Name　Histidine
Other name(s)　―
IUPAC Name　(2S)-2-amino-3-(1*H*-imidazol-5-yl)propanoic acid

CAS No.　71-00-1

Synonyms　L-Histidine / Glyoxaline-5-alanine / (S)-4-(2-Amino-2-carboxyethyl) imidazole

分子式　$C_6H_9N_3O_2$

特性・カテゴリー　アミノ酸／Amino acid

Note 1　—

Note 2　Fall under the categories of designated food additive and existing food additive.

注　指定添加物及び既存添加物に該当する。

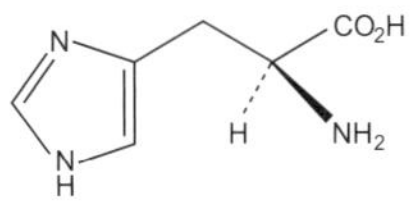

名　称　**ビス-3-ヒドロキシ-3-メチルブチレートモノハイドレート**

他名等　Bis (3-hydroxy-3-methylbutyrate) monohydrate ／3-Hydroxy-3-methylbutyric acid<HMB>

部位等　—

備　考　—

Name　bis (3-Hydroxy-3-methylbutyrate) monohydrate

Other name (s)　bis (3-Hydroxy-3-methylbutyrate) monohydrate / 3-Hydroxy-3-methylbutyric acid, (HMB)

IUPAC Name　3-hydroxy-3-methylbutanoic acid

CAS No.　625-08-1

Synonyms　3-Hydroxyisovaleric acid / HMB / beta-Hydroxyisovaleric acid / 3-Hydroxyisovaleric acid / beta-Hydroxy-beta-methylbutylate

分子式　$C_5H_{10}O_3$

特性・カテゴリー　ロイシンの代謝物／Leucine metabolite

Note 1　—

Note 2　Seek the judgement by the Ministry of Health, Labour and Welfare before using whether the substance will be fall under the category of food additive.

注　使用に先立ち、食品添加物に該当するか否かの判断を厚生労働省より受ける必要がある。

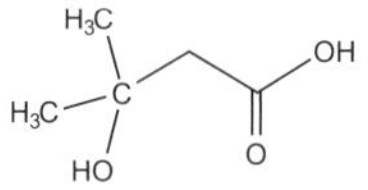

名　称　**ピロロキノリンキノンニナトリウム塩**

他名等　—

部位等　—

備　考　—

Name　Pyrroloquinoline quinone disodium salt

Other name (s)　—

IUPAC Name　disodium;9-carboxy-4,5-dioxo-1*H*-pyrrolo[2,3-*f*] quinoline-2,7-dicarboxylate

CAS No.　122628-50-0

Synonyms　Methoxatin disodium salt

分子式　$C_{14}H_4N_2Na_2O_8$

特性・カテゴリー　補酵素／Coenzyme

Note 1　—

Note 2　Seek the judgement by the Ministry of Health, Labour and Welfare before using whether the substance will be fall under the category of food additive.

注　使用に先立ち、食品添加物に該当するか否かの判断を厚生労働省より受ける必要がある。

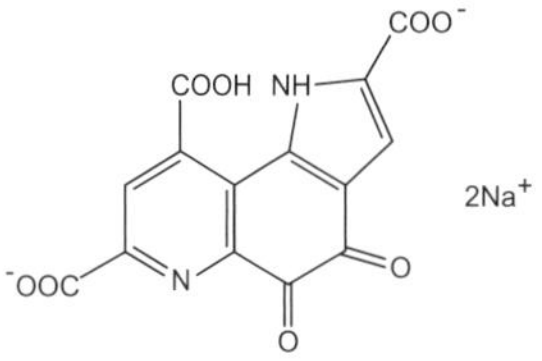

名　称　**ビタミンA**

他名等　レチノール

部位等　—

備　考　—

Name　Vitamin A

Other name (s)　Retinol

IUPAC Name　Retinol : (2E,4E,6E,8E)-3,7-dimethyl-9-(2,6,6-trimethylcyclohexen-1-yl) nona-2,4,6,8-tetraen-1-ol

CAS No.　68-26-8

Synonyms　all-trans-Retinol / Vitamin A_1 / Alphalin / Axerophthol / Oleovitamin A

分子式　$C_{20}H_{30}O$

特性・カテゴリー　ビタミン／Vitamin

Note 1　—

Note 2　Fall under the category of designated food additive.

注　指定添加物に該当する。

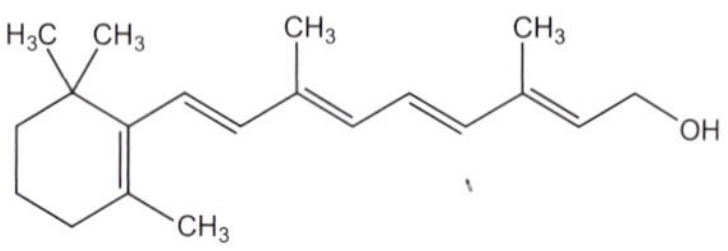

名　称　ビタミンB1

他名等　チアミン
部位等　—
備　考　—

Name　Vitamin B_1
Other name(s)　Thiamine
IUPAC Name　2-[3-[(4-amino-2-methylpyrimidin-5-yl)methyl]-4-methyl-1,3-thiazol-3-ium-5-yl]ethanol
CAS No.　59-43-8
Synonyms　Aneurin / Thiadoxine / Antiberiberi factor / Vitaneuron / Betaxin / Biamine / Bewon
分子式　$C_{12}H_{17}N_4OS^+$
特性・カテゴリー　ビタミン／Vitamin
Note 1　—
Note 2　Fall under the category of designated food additive.
注　指定添加物に該当する。

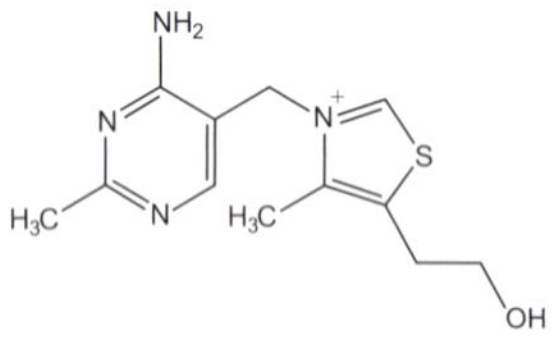

名　称　ビタミンB12

他名等　シアノコバラミン
部位等　—
備　考　—

Name　Vitamin B_{12}
Other name(s)　Cyanocobalamin
IUPAC Name　cobalt(3+);[(2R,3S,4R,5S)-5-(5,6-dimethylbenzimidazol-1-yl)-4-hydroxy-2-(hydroxymethyl)oxolan-3-yl] [(2R)-1-[3-[(1R,2R,3R,5Z,7S,10Z,12S,13S,15Z,17S,18S,19R)-2,13,18-tris(2-amino-2-oxoethyl)-7,12,17-tris(3-amino-3-oxopropyl)-3,5,8,8,13,15,18,19-octamethyl-2,7,12,17-tetrahydro-1*H*-corrin-24-id-3-yl]propanoylamino]propan-2-yl]phosphate;cyanide
CAS No.　68-19-9
Synonyms　Cobalamin / Crystamine / Berubigen / Cobavite / Cycobemin
分子式　$C_{63}H_{88}CoN_{14}O_{14}P$
特性・カテゴリー　ビタミン／Vitamin
Note 1　—
Note 2　Fall under the category of existing food additive.
注　既存添加物に該当する。

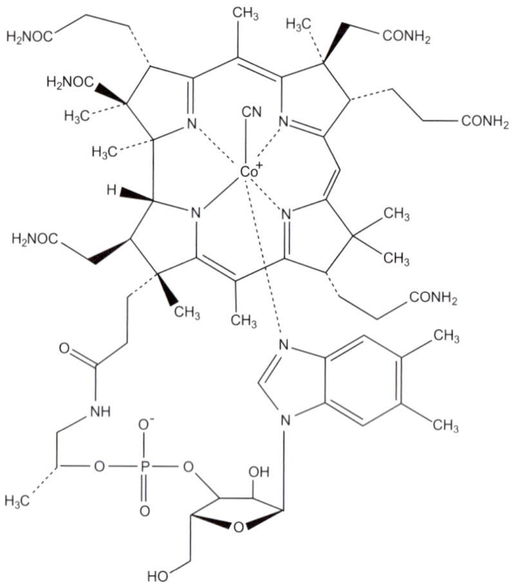

名　称　ビタミンB2

他名等　リボフラビン
部位等　—
備　考　—

Name　Vitamin B_2
Other name(s)　Riboflavin
IUPAC Name　7,8-dimethyl-10-[(2S,3S,4R)-2,3,4,5-tetrahydroxypentyl]benzo[g]pteridine-2,4-dione
CAS No.　83-88-5
Synonyms　Lactoflavin / Vitamin G / Beflavin
分子式　$C_{17}H_{20}N_4O_6$
特性・カテゴリー　ビタミン／Vitamin
Note 1　—
Note 2　Fall under the category of designated food additive.
注　指定添加物に該当する。

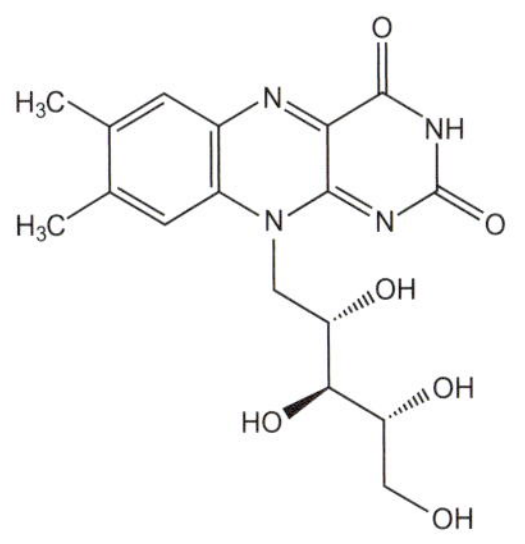

名　称　ビタミンB6

他名等　ピリドキシン
部位等　—
備　考　—

Name　Vitamin B_6
Other name(s)　Pyridoxine
IUPAC Name　4,5-bis(hydroxymethyl)-2-methylpyridin-3-ol
CAS No.　Pyridoxine hydrochloride：58-56-0
Synonyms　Pyridoxol / Pyridoxin
分子式　$C_8H_{11}NO_3$
特性・カテゴリー　ビタミン／Vitamin
Note 1　—
Note 2　Fall under the category of designated food additive. Pyridoxine, pyridoxal and pyridoxamine are known as vitamin B_6. Pyridoxine hydrochloride is in the designated food additives list.
注　指定添加物に該当する。
ビタミンB_6にはピリドキシン、ピリドキサール、ピリドキサミンがあるが、指定添加物リストに掲載されているのはピリドキシン塩酸塩である。

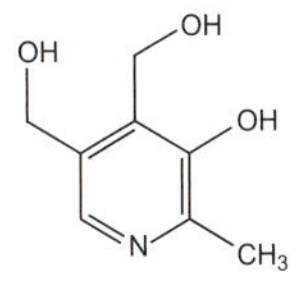

pyridoxine

名　称　ビタミンC

他名等　アスコルビン酸
部位等　—
備　考　—

Name　Vitamin C
Other name(s)　Ascorbic acid
IUPAC Name　(2R)-2-[(1S)-1,2-dihydroxyethyl]-3,4-dihydroxy-2*H*-furan-5-one
CAS No.　50-81-7
Synonyms　L-Ascorbic acid / Ascorbate / Ascoltin
分子式　$C_6H_8O_6$
特性・カテゴリー　ビタミン／Vitamin
Note 1　—
Note 2　Fall under the category of designated food additive.
注　指定添加物に該当する。

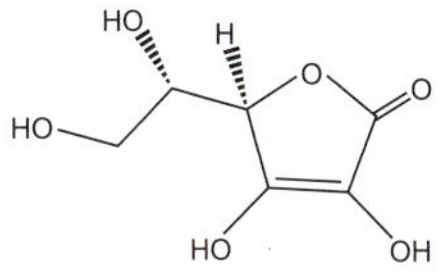

名　称　ビタミンD

他名等　カルシフェロール
部位等　—
備　考　—

Name　Vitamin D
Other name(s)　Calciferol
IUPAC Name
Vitamin D_3：(1S,3Z)-3-[(2E)-2-[(1R,3aS,7aR)-7a-methyl-1-[(2R)-6-methylheptan-2-yl]-2,3,3a,5,6,7-hexahydro-1*H*-inden-4-ylidene]ethylidene]-4-methylidenecyclohexan-1-ol
Vitamin D_2：(1S,3Z)-3-[(2E)-2-[(1R,3aS,7aR)-1-[(E,2R,5R)-5,6-dimethylhept-3-en-2-yl]-7a-methyl-2,3,3a,5,6,7-hexahydro-1*H*-inden-4-ylidene]ethylidene]-4-methylidenecyclohexan-1-ol
CAS No.　Vitamin D_3：67-97-0
Vitamin D_2：50-14-6
Synonyms
Vitamin D_3：Calciol / Colecalciferol
Vitamin D_2：Ergocalciferol / Calciferol
分子式　Vitamin D_3：$C_{27}H_{44}O$
Vitamin D_2：$C_{28}H_{44}O$
特性・カテゴリー　ビタミン／Vitamin
Note 1　—
Note 2　Fall under the categories of designated food additive.
注　指定添加物に該当する。

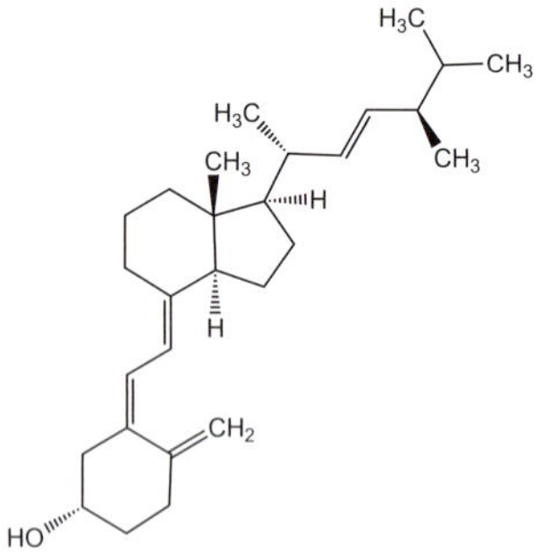

Vitamin D_2

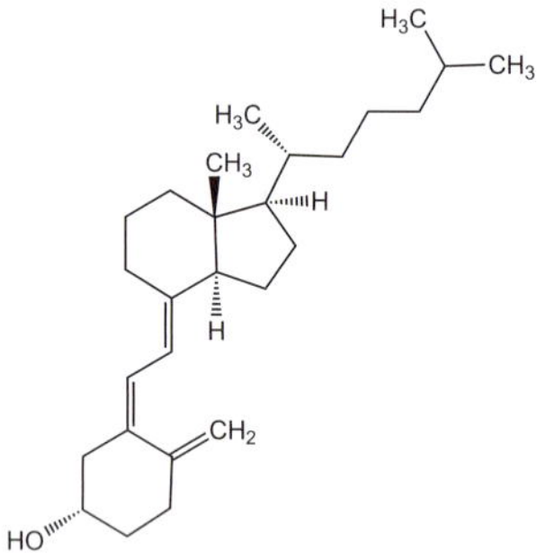

Vitamin D_3

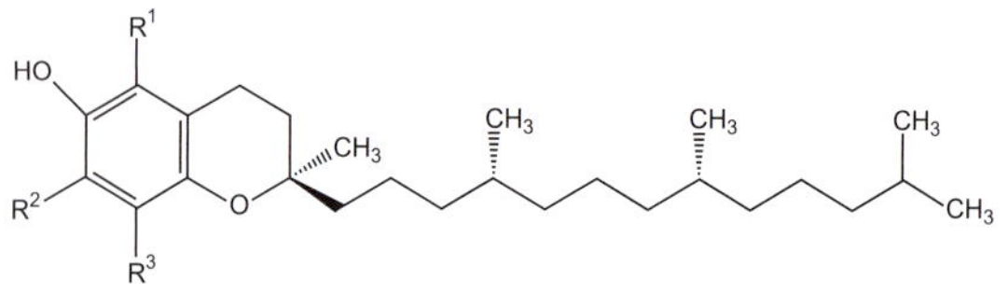

Tocopherol

※ビタミンEは同属体としてトコフェロールとトコトリエノールが存在する。
ここでは、トコフェロールの構造式を示す。

	R^1	R^2	R^3
α	CH_3	CH_3	CH_3
β	CH_3	H	CH_3
γ	H	CH_3	CH_3
δ	H	H	CH_3

名　称　ビタミンE

他名等　トコフェロール
部位等　—
備　考　—

Name　Vitamin E
Other name(s)　Tocopherol
IUPAC Name
alpha-Tocopherol：(2R)-2,5,7,8-tetramethyl-2-[(4R,8R)-4,8,12-trimethyltridecyl]-3,4-dihydrochromen-6-ol
dl-alpha-Tocopherol：2,5,7,8-tetramethyl-2-(4,8,12-trimethyltridecyl)-3,4-dihydrochromen-6-ol
CAS No.　alpha-Tocopherol：59-02-9
dl-alpha-Tocopherol：10191-41-0
Natural vitamine E：1406-18-4
Synonyms　alpha-Tochopherol
分子式　$C_{29}H_{50}O_2$
特性・カテゴリー　ビタミン／Vitamin
Note 1　—
Note 2　Fall under the categories of designated food additive and existing food additive. See “tocotrienol”, the vitamin E homologue in this list.
注　指定添加物及び既存添加物に該当する。
トコトリエノール（ビタミンE同族体）の項を参照。

名　称　ビタミンK

他名等　フィトナジオン／メナジオン
部位等　—
備　考　—

Name　Vitamin K
Other name(s)　Phytonadione / Menadione
IUPAC Name
Vitamin K_1(Phytonadione)：2-methyl-3-[(E,7R,11R)-3,7,11,15-tetramethylhexadec-2-enyl]naphthalene-1,4-dione
Vitamin K_2(Menaquinone-4)：2-methyl-3-[(2E,6E,10E)-3,7,11,15-tetramethylhexadeca-2,6,10,14-tetraenyl]naphthalene-1,4-dione
Vitamin K_2(Menaquinone-7)：2-[(2E,6E,10E,14E,18E,22E)-3,7,11,15,19,23,27-heptamethyloctacosa-2,6,10,14,18,22,26-heptaenyl]-3-methylnaphthalene-1,4-dione
CAS No.　Vitamin K_1(Phytonadione)：84-80-0
Vitamin K_2 (Menaquinone-4)：863-61-6
Vitamin K_2 (Menaquinone-7)：2124-57-4
Synonyms
Vitamin K_1(Phytonadione)：Phylloquinone / Phytonadion
Vitamin K_2(Menaquinone-4)：Menatetrenone / Menaquinone 4 / Kefton-2
Vitamin K_2 (Menaquinone-7)：Menaquinone 7 / Vitamin K_2(35)
分子式　Vitamin K_1(Phytonadione)：$C_{31}H_{46}O_2$
Vitamin K_2 (Menaquinone-4)：$C_{31}H_{40}O_2$
Vitamin K_2 (Menaquinone-7)：$C_{46}H_{64}O_2$
特性・カテゴリー　ビタミン／Vitamin
Note 1　—

Note 2 Vitamin K_2 (Menaquinone) falls under the category of existing food additive.
Before using, Phytonadione (V.K_1) and Menadione (V.K_3) are necessary to be designated as new food additives based on the article 10 of the Food Sanitation Act. Menadione (V.K_3) is used for neither drug nor food because of its toxicity.

注 ビタミンK_2（メナキノン）は既存添加物に該当する。
フィトナジオン（V.K_1）及びメナジオン（V.K_3）は使用に先立ち、新たに食品添加物としての指定を受ける必要がある。
Menadione（V.K_3）は毒性があるため医薬品、食品には使用されない。

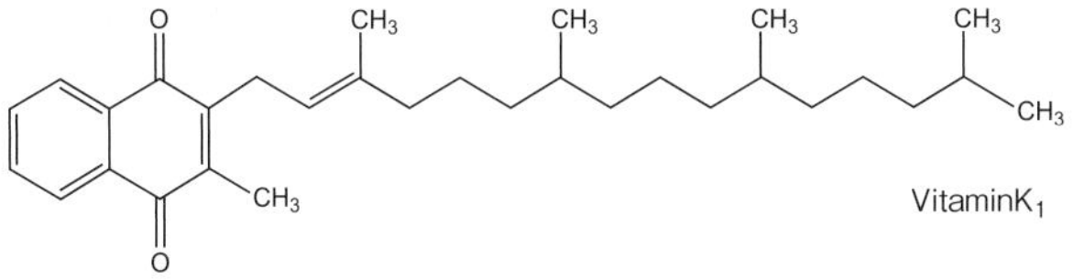

VitaminK1

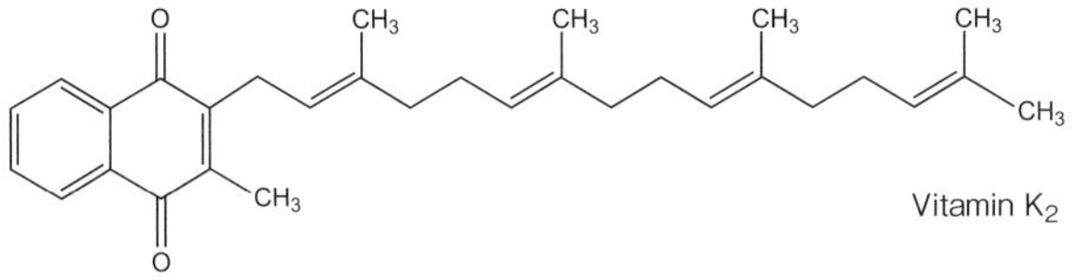

Vitamin K2

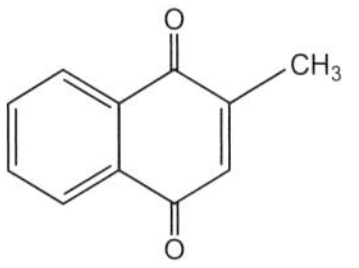

Vitamin K3

名　称　4-ヒドロキシプロリン

他名等　—
部位等　—
備　考　—

Name　4-Hydroxyproline
Other name(s)　—
IUPAC Name　(2S,4R)-4-hydroxypyrrolidine-2-carboxylic acid
CAS No.　51-35-4
Synonyms　L-4-Hydroxyproline / L-Hydroxyproline / trans-4-Hydroxy-L-proline / Hydroxy-L-proline
分子式　$C_5H_9NO_3$
特性・カテゴリー　アミノ酸／Amino acid
Note 1　—
Note 2　Fall under the category of existing food additive.

注　既存添加物に該当する。

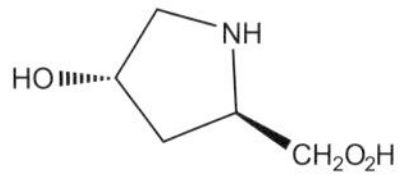

名　称　ヒドロキシリシン

他名等　—
部位等　—
備　考　—

Name　Hydroxylysine
Other name(s)　—
IUPAC Name　(2S,5R)-2,6-diamino-5-hydroxyhexanoic acid
CAS No.　28902-93-4
Synonyms　L-Hydroxylysine / 2,6-Diamino-5-hydroxyhexanoic acid / 5-Hydroxylysine
分子式　$C_6H_{14}N_2O_3$
特性・カテゴリー　アミノ酸／Amino acid
Note 1　—
Note 2　Seek the judgement by the Ministry of Health, Labour and Welfare before using whether the substance will be fall under the category of food additive.

注　使用に先立ち、食品添加物に該当するか否かの判断を厚生労働省より受ける必要がある。

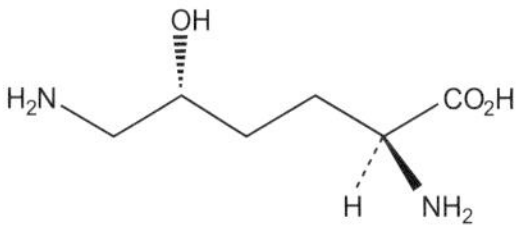

名　称　フィコシアニン

他名等　—
部位等　—
備　考　—

Name　Phycocyanins
Other name(s)　—
IUPAC Name　—
CAS No.　—
Synonyms　C-Phycocyanin / R-Phycocyanin
分子式　C-Phycocyanin from *Spirulina* spp.：11016-15-2
特性・カテゴリー　フィコビリタンパク質／Phycobiliproteins
Note 1　—

Note 2　Fall under the category of existing food additive. Phycocyanins are the photosynthetic pigments (chromoprotein) included in blue-green algae. The chemical structural formula of Phycocyanobilin is shown.

注　既存添加物に該当する。
藍藻類に含まれる光合成色素（色素タンパク）。フィコシアノビリンの構造式を示す。

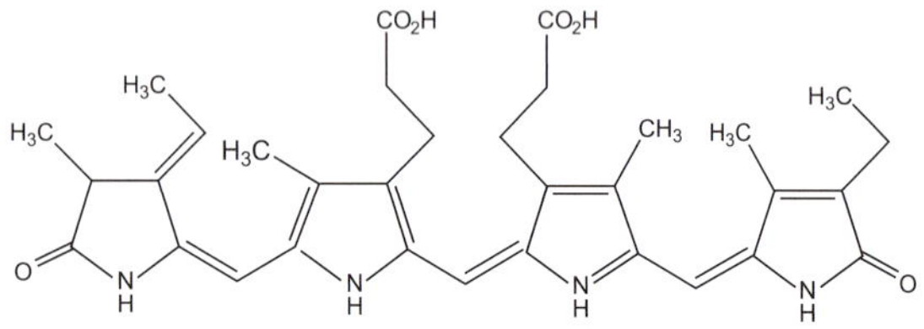

Phycocyanobiline

名　称　**フェニルアラニン**

他名等　—
部位等　—
備　考　—

Name　Phenylalanine
Other name(s)　—
IUPAC Name　(2S)-2-amino-3-phenylpropanoic acid
CAS No.　63-91-2
Synonyms　L-Phenylalanine / 3-Phenyl-L-alanine / beta-Phenyl-L-alanine
分子式　$C_9H_{11}NO_2$
特性・カテゴリー　アミノ酸／Amino acid
Note 1　—
Note 2　Fall under the category of designated food additive.
注　指定添加物に該当する。

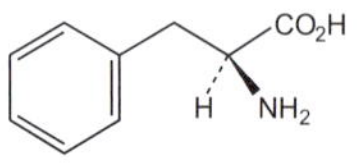

名　称　**フェリチン鉄**

他名等　—
部位等　—
備　考　—

Name　Ferritin-Fe
Other name(s)　—
IUPAC Name　—
CAS No.　9007-73-2 (Ferritin)
Synonyms　—
分子式　—
特性・カテゴリー　鉄－貯蔵タンパク／Iron strage protein
Note 1　—
Note 2　Fall under the category of existing food additive.
注　既存添加物に該当する。

名　称　**フェルラ酸**

他名等　3-(4-Hydroxy-3-methoxyphenyl)-2-propenoic acid
部位等　—
備　考　—

Name　Ferulic acid
Other name(s)　3-(4-Hydroxy-3-methoxyphenyl)-2-propenoic acid
IUPAC Name　(E)-3-(4-hydroxy-3-methoxyphenyl)prop-2-enoic acid
CAS No.　1135-24-6
Synonyms　trans-Ferulic Acid / 4-Hydroxy-3-methoxycinnamic acid / Ferulate / (E)-Ferulic acid / 3-(4-Hydroxy-3-methoxyphenyl)-2-propenoic acid
分子式　$C_{10}H_{10}O_4$
特性・カテゴリー　植物成分（主に細胞壁に分布）／Botanical constituent mainly found in cell wall
Note 1　—
Note 2　Generally fall under the category of existing food additive, however it should be noted that this substance may have a possibility to be treated as an undesignated food additive which has not been designated based on the Food Sanitation Act.
注　通常は既存添加物に該当するが、食品衛生法に基づく指定がなされていない未指定の食品添加物に該当する場合もあるので留意すること。

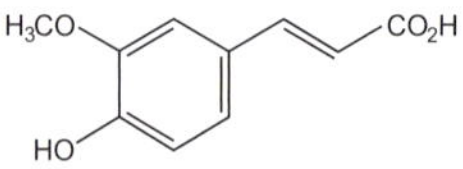

名　称　**フッ素**

他名等　—
部位等　—
備　考　—

Name　Fluorine

Other name(s) —
IUPAC Name molecular fluorine
CAS No. 7782-41-4
Synonyms Fluor / Bifluoriden
元素記号 F
特性・カテゴリー ミネラル(ハロゲン)/Mineral (Halogen)
Note 1 —
Note 2 Before using, it is necessary to be designated as a new food additive based on the article 10 of the Food Sanitation Act.
注 使用に先立ち、新たに食品添加物の指定を受ける必要がある。

名 称 フルボ酸

他名等 —
部位等 —
備 考 —

Name Fulvic acid
Other name(s) —
IUPAC Name 3,7,8-trihydroxy-3-methyl-10-oxo-1,4-dihydropyrano[4,3-*b*]chromene-9-carboxylic acid
CAS No. 479-66-3
Synonyms 1*H*,3*H*-Pyrano(4,3-b)(1)benzopyran-9-carboxylic acid
分子式 $C_{14}H_{12}O_8$
特性・カテゴリー 腐植物質のうち酸によって沈殿しない無定形高分子有機酸。土壌や天然水中に広く分布している。/Natural organic polymer that can be extracted from hums found in soil, sediment, or aquatic environments.
Note 1 —
Note 2 Treated as a substance which is generally provided for eating or drinking as a food and which is also used as a food additive.
注 一般に食品として飲食に供される物であって添加物として使用されるものとして取り扱われる。

名 称 プルラン

他名等 —
部位等 —
備 考 非消化吸収性の多糖類

Name Pullulan
Other name(s) —
IUPAC Name —
CAS No. 9057-02-7
Synonyms Pururan
分子式 $[(C_6H_{10}O_5)_n]_m$
特性・カテゴリー 難消化性多糖類/Indigestible polysaccharide
Note 1 Non-digestible and non-absorbable polysaccharide
Note 2 Fall under the category of existing food additive.
注 既存添加物に該当する。

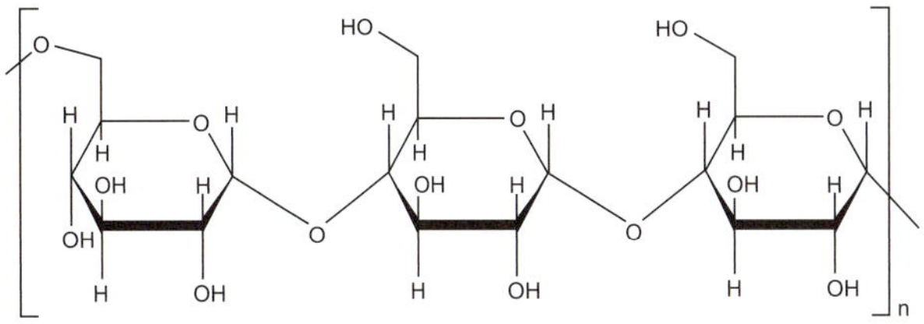

名 称 プロアントシアニジン

他名等 —
部位等 —
備 考 —

Name Proanthocyanidin
Other name(s) —
IUPAC Name ex) Proanthocyanidin A:(3R)-2-(3,5-dihydroxy-4-methoxyphenyl)-8-[(2R,3R,4R)-3,5,7-trihydroxy-2-(4-hydroxyphenyl)-3,4-dihydro-2*H*-chromen-4-yl]-3,4-dihydro-2*H*-chromene-3,5,7-triol
CAS No. 18206-61-6
Synonyms Proanthocyanidins / Proanthocyanidin A / Polyhydroxyflavan-3-ol
分子式 Proanthocyanidin (dimer):$C_{31}H_{28}O_{12}$
特性・カテゴリー 植物成分(ポリフェノール)/Botanical constituent (Polyphenol)
Note 1 —
Note 2 Fall under the category of existing food additive.
注 既存添加物に該当する。

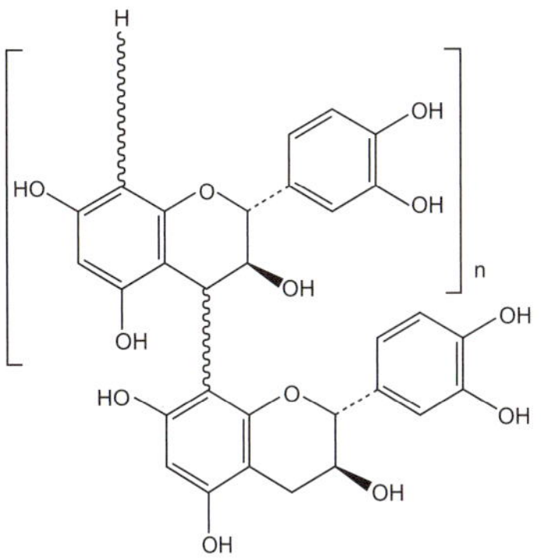

名　称　**プロポリス**

他名等　—
部位等　—
備　考　—

Name　Propolis
Other name(s)　—
IUPAC Name　—
CAS No.　—
Synonyms　Bee glue / Bee propolis / Beeswax acid / Hive dross / Propolis balsam / Propolis resin / Propolis wax
分子式　—
特性・カテゴリー　樹脂様物質（蜂ヤニ）／Resin-like material (Beeswax)
Note 1　—
Note 2　Fall under the category of existing food additive.
注　既存添加物に該当する。

名　称　**プロリン**

他名等　—
部位等　—
備　考　—

Name　Proline
Other name(s)　—
IUPAC Name　(2S)-pyrrolidine-2-carboxylic acid
CAS No.　147-85-3
Synonyms　L-Proline / L-(-)-Proline / (-)-Proline
分子式　$C_5H_9NO_2$
特性・カテゴリー　アミノ酸／Amino acid
Note 1　—
Note 2　Fall under the category of existing food additive.
注　既存添加物に該当する。

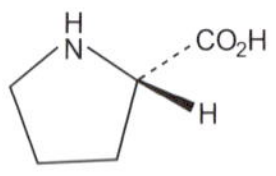

名　称　**ベータカロチン**

他名等　—
部位等　—
備　考　—

Name　beta-Carotene
Other name(s)　—
IUPAC Name　1,3,3-trimethyl-2-[(1E,3E,5E,7E,9E,11E,13E,15E,17E)-3,7,12,16-tetramethyl-18-(2,6,6-trimethylcyclohexen-1-yl)octadeca-1,3,5,7,9,11,13,15,17-nonaenyl]cyclohexene
CAS No.　7235-40-7
Synonyms　beta Carotene / Solatene / Carotaben / Provitamin A / all-trans-beta-Carotene / Provatene
分子式　$C_{40}H_{56}$
特性・カテゴリー　ビタミンAの前駆体／Precursor of vitamin A
Note 1　—
Note 2　Fall under the category of designated food additive.
注　指定添加物に該当する。

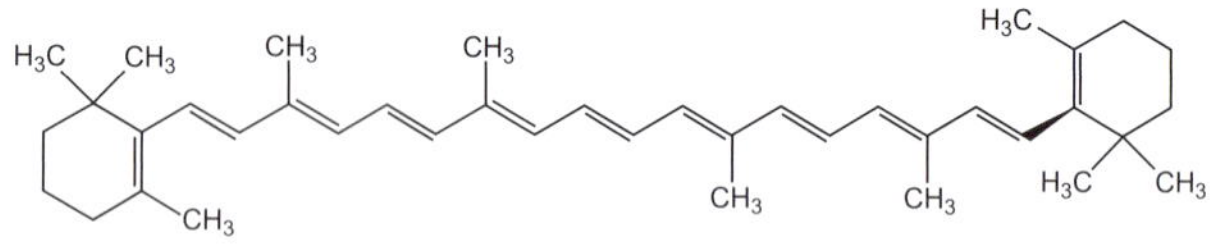

名　称　**ヘスペリジン**

他名等　—
部位等　—
備　考　—

Name　Hesperidin
Other name(s)　—
IUPAC Name　(2S)-5-hydroxy-2-(3-hydroxy-4-methoxyphenyl)-7-[(2S,3R,4S,5S,6R)-3,4,5-trihydroxy-6-[[(2R,3R,4R,5R,6S)-3,4,5-trihydroxy-6-methyloxan-2-yl]oxymethyl]oxan-2-yl]oxy-2,3-dihydrochromen-4-one
CAS No.　520-26-3
Synonyms　Hesperidine / Cirantin / Hesperetin-7-rutinoside / Hesperetin-7-rhamnoglucoside / Hesperidoside / Hesper bitabs / Hesperidine-rutinoside
分子式　$C_{28}H_{34}O_{15}$
特性・カテゴリー　柑橘類に含まれる主要なフラボノイド／Predominant flavonoid in citrus fruits
Note 1　—
Note 2　Fall under the category of existing food additive.
注　既存添加物に該当する。

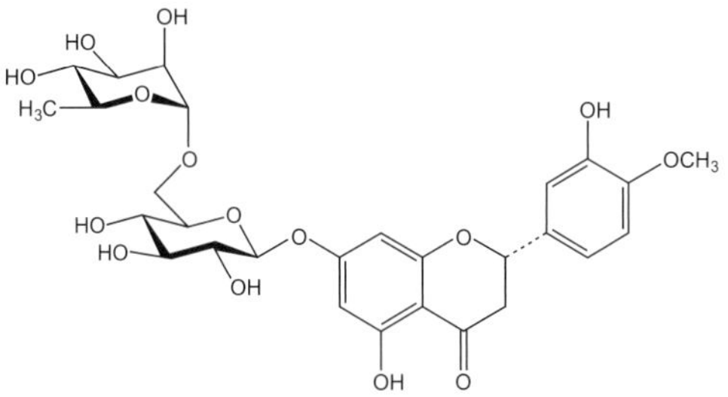

名　称　ヘマトコッカス藻色素

他名等　—

部位等　—

備　考　—

Name　Pigment in *Haematococcus* algae

Other name(s)　—

IUPAC Name　ex) Astaxanthine：6-hydroxy-3-[(1E,3E,5E,7E,9E,11E,13E,15E,17E)-18-(4-hydroxy-2,6,6-trimethyl-3-oxocyclohexen-1-yl)-3,7,12,16-tetramethyloctadeca-1,3,5,7,9,11,13,15,17-nonaenyl]-2,4,4-trimethylcyclohex-2-en-1-one

CAS No.　ex) Astaxanthine：472-61-7

Synonyms　ex) Astaxanthine：Astaxanthin / Ovoester

分子式　ex) Astaxanthine：$C_{40}H_{52}O_4$

特性・カテゴリー　植物成分（カロテノイド）／Botanical constituent (Carotenoid)

Note 1　—

Note 2　Fall under the category of existing food additive. *Haematococcus pluvialis* is mainly used.

注　既存添加物に該当する。主に*Haematococcus pluvialis*が用いられる。

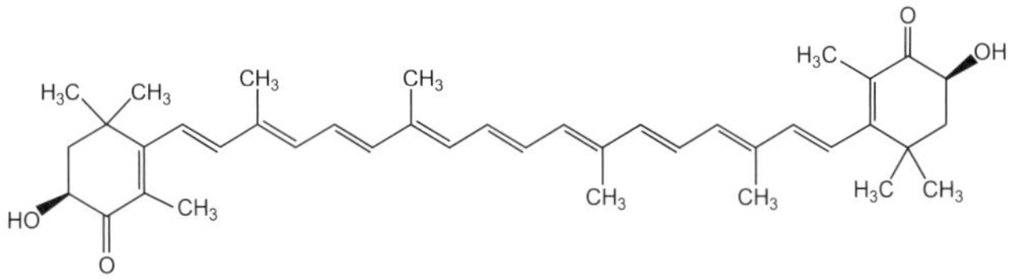

Astaxanthin

※ヘマトコッカス藻の主成分はアスタキサンチンであるため、ここではアスタキサンチンの構造式を示す。

名　称　ヘム鉄

他名等　—

部位等　—

備　考　—

Name　Heme iron

Other name(s)　—

IUPAC Name　3-[18-(2-carboxyethyl)-8,13-bis(ethenyl)-3,7,12,17-tetramethylporphyrin-21,24-diid-2-yl]propanoic acid；iron(2+)

CAS No.　ex) Heme b：14875-96-8

Synonyms　Hemin / Protoheme / Haem / Ferrous protoheme Ⅸ / Heme b / Ferroprotoporphyrin / Hematin

分子式　ex) Heme b：$C_{34}H_{32}FeO_4N_4$

特性・カテゴリー　ヘモグロビン、チトクロムなどの構成要素／Constituent of hemoglobins, cytochromes and others

Note 1　—

Note 2　Fall under the category of existing food additive.

注　既存添加物に該当する。

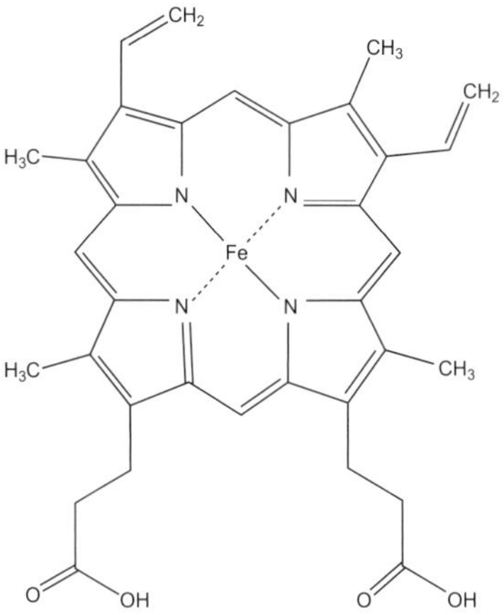

名　称　ホスファチジルセリン

他名等　—

部位等　—

備　考　リン脂質

Name　Phosphatidylserine

Other name(s)　—

IUPAC Name　(2S)-2-amino-3-[(2-butanoyloxy-3-propanoyloxypropoxy)-hydroxyphosphoryl]oxypropanoic acid

CAS No.　8002-43-5

Synonyms　PSF / Phosphatidyl-L-serine / L-1-Phosphatidylserine / O3-Phosphatidyl-L-serine / 3-*O*-sn-Phosphatidyl-L-serine / 1,2-Diacyl-sn-glycerol 3-phospho-L-serine

分子式 $C_{13}H_{24}NO_{10}P$

特性･カテゴリー 植物、動物、微生物に広く含まれるリン脂質（レシチンの一種）／Phospholipid distributed widely among animals, plants and microorganisms. (A kind of Lecithins)

Note 1 Phospholipid

Note 2 Treated as a substance which is generally provided for eating or drinking as a food and which is also used as a food additive.

注 一般に食品として飲食に供される物であって添加物として使用されるものとして取り扱われる。

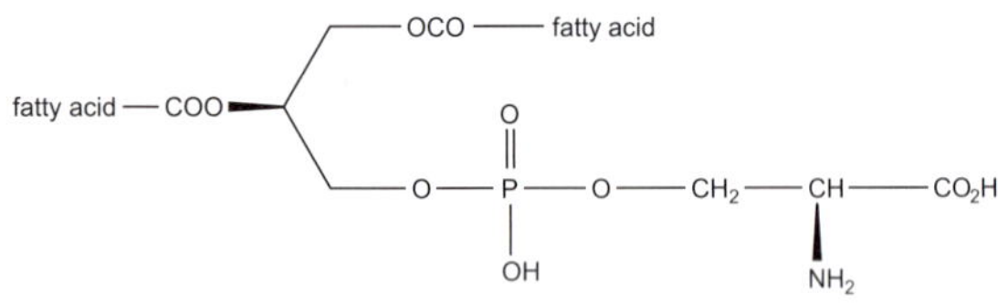

マ行

名　称　マグネシウム

他名等 —
部位等 —
備　考 —

Name Magnesium
Other name(s) —
IUPAC Name magnesium
CAS No. 7439-95-4
Synonyms —
元素記号 Mg
特性･カテゴリー ミネラル／Mineral
Note 1 —
Note 2 Fall under the category of existing food additive.
注 既存添加物に該当する。

名　称　マンガン

他名等 —
部位等 —
備　考 —

Name Manganese
Other name(s) —
IUPAC Name manganese
CAS No. 7439-96-5
Synonyms —
元素記号 Mn
特性･カテゴリー ミネラル／Mineral
Note 1 —
Note 2 Before using, it is necessary to be designated as a new food additive based on the article 10 of the Food Sanitation Act.
注 使用に先立ち、新たに食品添加物の指定を受ける必要がある。

名　称　ムコ多糖類

他名等 —
部位等 —
備　考 —

Name Mucopolysaccharide
Other name(s) —
IUPAC Name —
CAS No. 94945-04-7
Synonyms Glycosaminoglycans
分子式 —
特性･カテゴリー 多糖類（ムコ多糖類）／Polysaccharide (Mucopolysaccharide)
Note 1 —
Note 2 Fall under the category of existing food additive.
注 既存添加物に該当する。

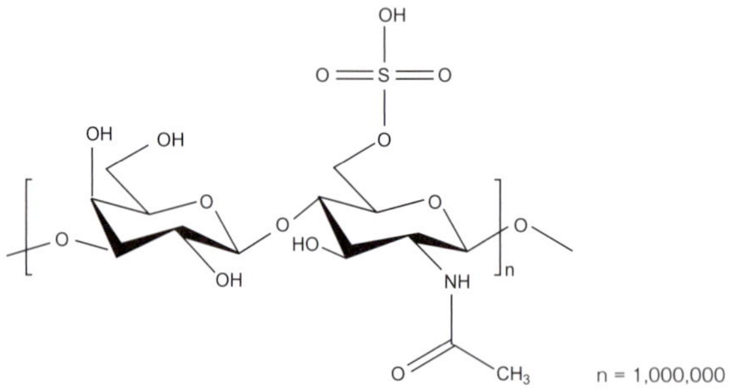

Keratan sulfate

※ムコ多糖類とは、アミノ酸を有する多糖の総称であり、代表的なムコ多糖にコンドロイチン硫酸、ヒアルロン酸、ケラタン硫酸がある。ここでは、ケラタン硫酸の構造式を示す。

名　称　**メチオニン**

他名等　—
部位等　—
備　考　—

Name　Methionine
Other name(s)　—
IUPAC Name　(2S)-2-amino-4-methylsulfanylbutanoic acid
CAS No.　63-68-3
Synonyms　L-Methionine / Cymethion / L-(-)-Methionine / Liquimeth
分子式　$C_5H_{11}NO_2S$
特性・カテゴリー　アミノ酸／Amino acid
Note 1　—
Note 2　Fall under the category of designated food additive.
注　指定添加物に該当する。

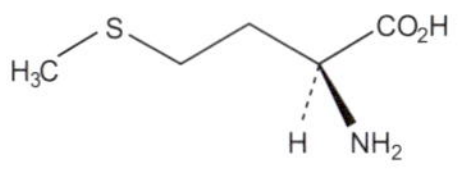

名　称　**木灰**

他名等　—
部位等　—
備　考　—

Name　Wood ash
Other name(s)　—
IUPAC Name　—
CAS No.　—
Synonyms　—
分子式　—
特性・カテゴリー　木を燃焼させた後の灰／Residue powder left after the combustion of wood
Note 1　—
Note 2　Fall under the category of existing food additive.
注　既存添加物に該当する。

名　称　**モリブデン**

他名等　—
部位等　—
備　考　—

Name　Molybdenum
Other name(s)　—
IUPAC Name　molybdenum
CAS No.　7439-98-7
Synonyms　—
元素記号　Mo
特性・カテゴリー　ミネラル／Mineral
Note 1　—
Note 2　Before using, it is necessary to be designated as a new food additive based on the article 10 of the Food Sanitation Act.
注　使用に先立ち、新たに食品添加物の指定を受ける必要がある。

ヤ行

名　称　**葉酸**

他名等　ビタミンM
部位等　—
備　考　—

Name　Folic acid
Other name(s)　Vitamin M
IUPAC Name　(2S)-2-[[4-[(2-amino-4-oxo-1*H*-pteridin-6-yl)methylamino]benzoyl]amino]pentanedioic acid
CAS No.　59-30-3
Synonyms　Folate / Folvite / Folacin / Pteroylglutamic acid
分子式　$C_{19}H_{19}N_7O_6$
特性・カテゴリー　ビタミン／Vitamin
Note 1　—
Note 2　Fall under the category of designated food additive.
注　指定添加物に該当する。

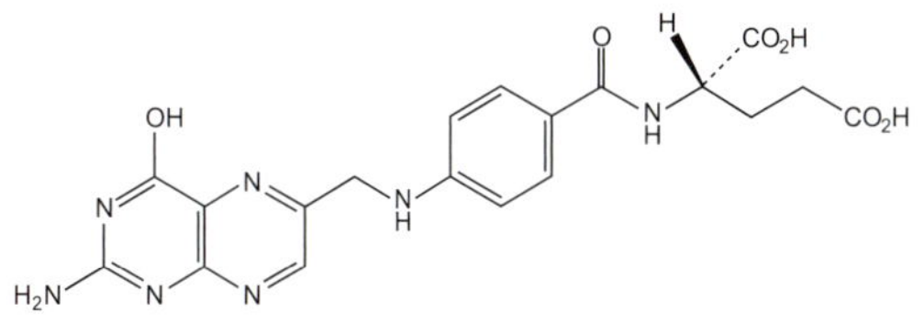

名　称　ヨウ素

他名等　—
部位等　—
備　考　—

Name　Iodine
Other name(s)　—
IUPAC Name　molecular iodine
CAS No.　7553-56-2
Synonyms　—
元素記号　I
特性・カテゴリー　ミネラル／Mineral
Note 1　—
Note 2　Before using, it is necessary to be designated as a new food additive based on the article 10 of the Food Sanitation Act.
注　使用に先立ち、新たに食品添加物の指定を受ける必要がある。

ラ行

名　称　ラクトフェリン

他名等　—
部位等　—
備　考　—

Name　Lactoferrin
Other name(s)　—
IUPAC Name　—
CAS No.　146897-68-9
Synonyms　Lactotransferrin (LTF)
分子式　—
特性・カテゴリー　乳タンパク／Multifunctional protein of the transferrin family
Note 1　—
Note 2　Fall under the category of existing food additive. Lactoferrin is a globular glycoprotein.
注　既存添加物に該当する。
ラクトフェリンは球状の糖タンパクである。

名　称　リグナン

他名等　樹脂アルコール／レジノール
部位等　—
備　考　—

Name　Lignans
Other name(s)　Resin alcohol / Resinols
IUPAC Name　ethyl 6,7-dimethoxy-3-methyl-4-oxo-1-(3,4,5-trimethoxyphenyl)-2,3-dihydro-1*H*-naphthalene-2-carboxylate
CAS No.　6549-68-4
Synonyms　Ethyl 6,7-dimethoxy-3-methyl-4-oxo-1-(3,4,5-trimethoxyphenyl)-1,2,3,4-tetrahydronaphthalene-2-carboxylate
分子式　$C_{25}H_{30}O_8$
特性・カテゴリー　植物成分（ケイヒ酸重合体）／Botanical consutituent (Cinnamic acid polymer)
Note 1　—
Note 2　Seek the judgement by the Ministry of Health, Labour and Welfare before using whether the substance will be fall under the category of food additive. The chemical structural formula of sesamin is shown as an example of lignans.
注　使用に先立ち、食品添加物に該当するか否かの判断を厚生労働省より受ける必要がある。例としてセサミンの構造式を示す。

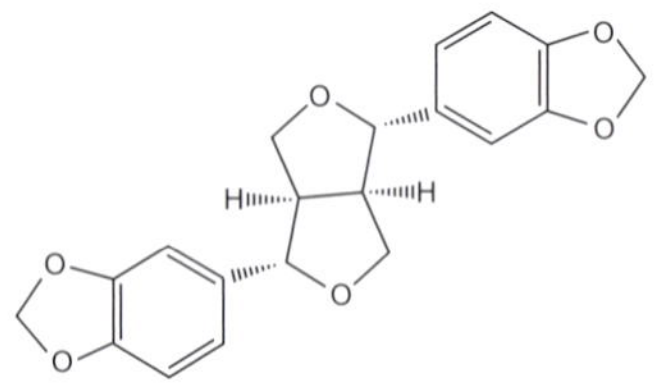

Sesamin

名　称　リジン

他名等　—
部位等　—
備　考　—

Name　Lysine
Other name(s)　—
IUPAC Name　(2S)-2,6-diaminohexanoic acid
CAS No.　56-87-1
Synonyms　L-Lysine / Lysine acid / Aminutrin
分子式　$C_6H_{14}N_2O_2$
特性・カテゴリー　アミノ酸／Amino acid

Note 1 —
Note 2 Fall under the category of existing food additive.
注 既存添加物に該当する。

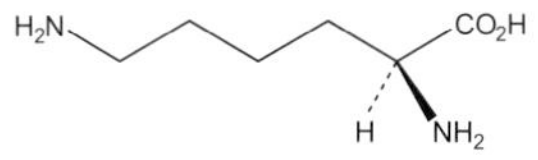

名 称 リノール酸

他名等 —
部位等 —
備 考 —

Name Linoleic acid
Other name(s) —
IUPAC Name (9Z,12Z)-octadeca-9,12-dienoic acid
CAS No. 60-33-3
Synonyms Linolic acid / Linoleate / cis,cis-9,12-Octadecadienoic acid
分子式 $C_{18}H_{32}O_2$
特性・カテゴリー 高度不飽和脂肪酸／Polyunsaturated fatty acid
Note 1 —
Note 2 Treated as a substance which is generally provided for eating or drinking as a food and which is also used as a food additive.
注 一般に食品として飲食に供される物であって添加物として使用されるものとして取り扱われる。

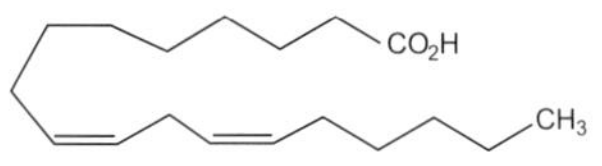

名 称 リノレン酸

他名等 —
部位等 —
備 考 —

Name Linolenic acid
Other name(s) —
IUPAC Name (9Z,12Z,15Z)-octadeca-9,12,15-trienoic acid
CAS No. 463-40-1
Synonyms alpha-Linolenic acid / Linolenate / alpha-Linolenate / 9,12,15-Octadecatrienoic acid
分子式 $C_{18}H_{30}O_2$
特性・カテゴリー 高度不飽和脂肪酸／Polyunsaturated fatty acid
Note 1 —
Note 2 Treated as a substance which is generally provided for eating or drinking as a food and which is also used as a food additive.
注 一般に食品として飲食に供される物であって添加物として使用されるものとして取り扱われる。

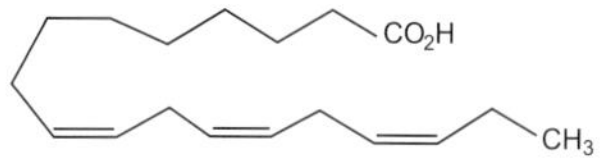

名 称 流動パラフィン

他名等 —
部位等 —
備 考 —

Name Liquid paraffin
Other name(s) —
IUPAC Name —
CAS No. 8012-95-1
Synonyms Paraffinum liquidum / Nujol / Medicinal paraffin / Saxol / Albolene / Glymol / Mineral oil / Paraffin oil / White mineral oil
分子式 C_nH_{2N+2}
特性・カテゴリー 精製白色鉱油／Purified white mineral oil
Note 1 —
Note 2 Fall under the category of existing food additive.
注 既存添加物に該当する。

名 称 リン

他名等 —
部位等 —
備 考 —

Name Phosphorus
Other name(s) —
IUPAC Name phosphane
CAS No. 7723-14-0
Synonyms Phosphorus cation / Phosphine / Phosphane / Phosphorus trihydride
元素記号 P
特性・カテゴリー ミネラル／Mineral
Note 1 —
Note 2 Before using, it is necessary to be designated as a new food additive based on the article 10 of the

Food Sanitation Act.

注 使用に先立ち、新たに食品添加物の指定を受ける必要がある。

名 称 ルチン

他名等 —

部位等 —

備 考 —

Name Rutin

Other name(s) —

IUPAC Name 2-(3,4-dihydroxyphenyl)-5,7-dihydroxy-3-[(2S,3R,4S,5S,6R)-3,4,5-trihydroxy-6-[[(2R,3R,4R,5R,6S)-3,4,5-trihydroxy-6-methyloxan-2-yl]oxymethyl]oxan-2-yl]oxychromen-4-one

CAS No. 153-18-4

Synonyms Quercetin 3-rutinoside / Bioflavonoid / Rutoside / Birutan / Sophorin / Eldrin / Rutin trihydrate

分子式 $C_{27}H_{30}O_{16}$

特性・カテゴリー 植物成分（フラボノイド）／Botanical constituent (Flavonoid)

Note 1 —

Note 2 Fall under the category of existing food additive.

注 既存添加物に該当する。

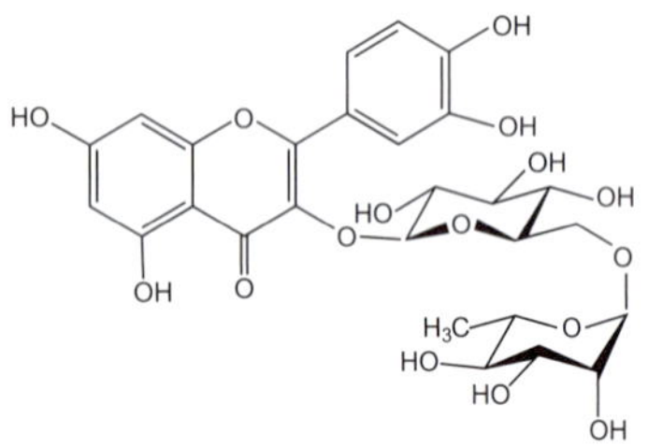

名 称 ルテイン

他名等 —

部位等 —

備 考 カロテノイドの一種

Name Lutein

Other name(s) —

IUPAC Name 4-[(1E,3E,5E,7E,9E,11E,13E,15E,17E)-18-(4-Hydroxy-2,6,6-trimethylcyclohex-2-en-1-yl)-3,7,12,16-tetramethyloctadeca-1,3,5,7,9,11,13,15,17-nonaenyl]-3,5,5-trimethylcyclohex-3-en-1-ol

CAS No. 127-40-2

Synonyms trans-Lutein / Carotenoid / Phylloxanthin / Luteine / Xanthophyll / all-trans-Xanthophyll / Vegitable luteol

分子式 $C_{40}H_{56}O_2$

特性・カテゴリー 植物成分（カロテノイド）／Botanical constituent(Carotenoid)

Note 1 One of Carotenoids

Note 2 Fall under the category of existing food additive.

注 既存添加物に該当する。

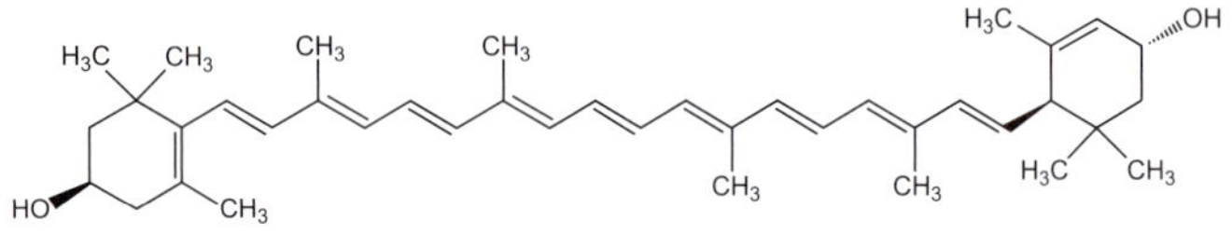

名 称 レシチン

他名等 大豆レシチン／ホスファチジルコリン／卵黄レシチン

部位等 —

備 考 —

Name Lecithin

Other name(s) Soybean lecithin / Phosphatidylcholine / Egg yolk lecithin

IUPAC Name [(2R)-3-hexadecanoyloxy-2-[(9E,12E)-octadeca-9,12-dienoyl]oxypropyl]2-(trimethylazaniumyl)ethyl phosphate

CAS No. 8002-43-5 (Lecithin)

Synonyms L-alpha-Lecithin / 3-sn-Phosphatidylcholine / L-alpha-Phosphatidylcholine solution

分子式 Soy bean Lecithin：$C_{12}H_{24}NO_7P$

Egg yolk lecithin：$C_{42}H_{80}NO_8P$

特性・カテゴリー リン脂質／Phospholipid

Note 1 —

Note 2 Fall under the category of existing food additive.

注 既存添加物に該当する。

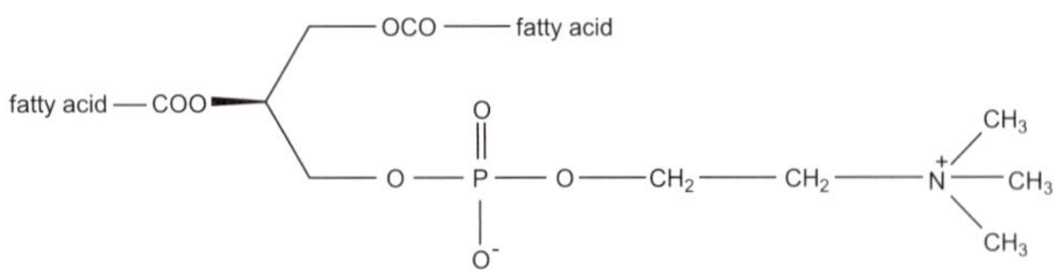

名　称　ロイシン

他名等　—
部位等　—
備　考　—

Name　Leucine
Other name(s)　—
IUPAC Name　(2S)-2-amino-4-methylpentanoic acid
CAS No.　61-90-5
Synonyms　L-Leucine / (S)-Leucine / (S)-2-Amino-4-methylpentanoic acid / Leucinum / L-alpha-Aminoisocaproic acid
分子式　$C_6H_{13}NO_2$
特性・カテゴリー　アミノ酸／Amino acid
Note 1　—
Note 2　Fall under the category of existing food additive.
注　既存添加物に該当する。

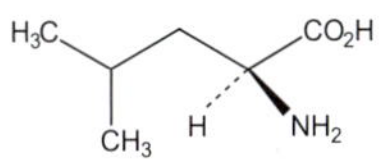

第2部 「医」リスト
[専ら医薬品として使用される成分本質（原材料）リスト]

Part 2 Drug List
(List of ingredients (raw materials) used exclusively for drugs)

1．植物由来物等
Substances originated in plants

2．動物由来物等
Substances originated in animals

3．その他（化学物質等）
Other substances (chemicals, vitamins and minerals, etc.)

1．植物由来物等

1. Substances originated in plants

網掛け部分：網掛け部分には「名称」、「他名等」、「部位等」、「備考」の４項目が含まれる。これらの項目は食薬区分リストの表記に準拠し、そのまま一切の変更を加えずに記載した。

注１）「名称」及び「他名等」の欄については、生薬名、一般名及び起源植物等を記載している。

注２）リストに掲載されている成分本質（原材料）のうち、該当する部位について、「部位等」の欄に記載している。

注３）他の部位が別のリストに掲載されている場合等、その取扱いが紛らわしいものについては、備考欄にその旨記載している。

注４）備考欄の「非医」は「医薬品的効能効果を標ぼうしない限り医薬品と判断しない成分本質（原材料）リスト」に掲載されていることを示す。

Shaded section：The shaded section consists of four items：Name, Other name(s), Part of use, and Remarks. These items are shown exactly as recorded in the food and drug classification lists without any changes having been made whatsoever.

1) The "Name" and "Other name(s)" entries include the crude drug name, common name, source plant, and other names.
2) Of the ingredients (raw materials) included in the list, the relevant part used is included in the "Part of use" entry.
3) Where other parts are included in other lists, notes are entered in the "Remarks" column if there could be any confusion over the handling.
4) Where the "Remarks" column shows "non-drug (非医)", the substance is included in the "List of ingredients (raw materials) not deemed drugs unless claiming medicinal efficacy".

植物由来等の原材料の見方
(Notation of a substance originated in plant(s).)

名　称 **他名等** **部位等** **備　考**	**Name** **Other name(s)** **Part of Use** **Remarks**	食薬区分リストの記載事項とその内容。 The shaded section consists of the following four items which are exactly shown as recorded in the food and drug classification lists without any changes.

他名(参考)

食薬区分リストには載っていないが、実際に使用されている名称。
Other name(s) (for reference)：Names in actual use but not recorded in the food and drug classification list.

漢字表記・生薬名等

「名称」「他名等」の漢字表記と読み。それらの生薬、漢方等における名称の漢字表記と読み。
Kanji notation and crude drug name：The kanji notations of "Name" and "Other name (s)" along with the names (kanji) used in crude drug and/or Kampo medicine (traditional Japanese medicine), etc.

Name (Romaji)

「名称」のローマ字表記。
Roman alphabet (romaji) of the "Name" in the food and drug classification list.

Other name(s) (Romaji)

「他名等」のローマ字表記。
Roman alphabet (romaji) of the "Other name(s)" in the food and drug classification list.

学名 **科名** **英名**	**Scientific name(s)** **Family name** **English name(s)**	「名称」または「他名等」の学名、科名、英名。 Scientific name(s), Family name and English name(s) of the "Name" or "Other name(s)".

Part of use

「部位等」の英訳。
English translation of the "Part of use" in the food and drug classification list.

Note 1

「備考」の英訳。
English translation of the content of "Remarks" in the food and drug classification list.

Note 2

下記「注」の英訳。
English translation of "Note (注)" in the last item.

注

食薬区分リストの記載事項についての補足情報等。
Note：Comments or supplementary information on the content of the food and drug classification records are given.

＊印：本書に掲載した学名が "*Herbs of Commerce* (2nd Ed. by American Herbal Products Association)" に収載されている場合は、当該「学名」と「名称」、「Name(Romaji)」表記に＊印を付した（ただし、植物の「非医」と「医」リストに限る）。

Asterisk (*)：If a scientific name given in this publication is recorded in *Herbs of Commerce* (2nd Ed. by American Herbal Products Association), it is marked with an asterisk (*)."Name"and its Romanized name are also asterisked.

ア行

名　称　**アラビアチャノキ***

他名等　—
部位等　葉
備　考　—

他名(参考)　—
漢字表記･生薬名等　—
Name(Romaji)　ARABIACHANOKI*
Other name(s) (Romaji)　—
学名　*Catha edulis* (Vahl) Forsk. ex Endl.*
　　Celastrus edulis Vahl*
科名　Cerastraceae（ニシキギ科）
英名　khat / Arabian tea / Abyssinian tea
Part of use　leaf
Note 1　—
Note 2　—
注　—

名　称　**アルニカ***

他名等　—
部位等　全草
備　考　—

他名(参考)　—
漢字表記･生薬名等　—
Name(Romaji)　ARUNIKA*
Other name(s) (Romaji)　—
学名　*Arnica montana* L.*
科名　Compositae（キク科）
英名　arnica / European arnica / leopard's bane / mountain tabaco
Part of use　whole plant
Note 1　—
Note 2　—
注　—

名　称　**アロエ***

他名等　キュラソー・アロエ／ケープ・アロエ
部位等　葉の液汁
備　考　根・葉肉は「非医」、キダチアロエの葉は「非医」

他名(参考)　—
漢字表記･生薬名等　蘆薈（ロカイ）
Name(Romaji)　AROE*
Other name(s) (Romaji)　KYURASÔ・AROE／KÊPU・AROE
学名　*Aloe ferox* Mill.*
　　Aloe africana Mill.
　　Aloe spicata Baker*
　　Aloe barbadensis Mill.*
科名　Liliaceae（ユリ科）
英名　aloe vera / cape aloe / aloealoe / barbados aloe / curaçao aloe
Part of use　juice of leaf
Note 1　root, inner leaf gel：non-drug category
　　leaf of *Aloe arborescens* Mill.：non-drug category
Note 2　—
注　—

名　称　**イチイ**

他名等　アララギ
部位等　枝・心材・葉
備　考　果実は「非医」

他名(参考)　—
漢字表記･生薬名等　一位葉（イチイヨウ)、枝杉（アララギ）
Name(Romaji)　ICHII*
Other name(s) (Romaji)　ARARAGI
学名　*Taxus cuspidata* Sieb. et Zucc.
科名　Taxaceae（イチイ科）
英名　Japanese yew / pyramidal yew
Part of use　branch, heart wood, leaf
Note 1　fruit：non-drug category
Note 2　—
注　—

名　称　**イヌサフラン***

他名等　—
部位等　種子
備　考　—

他名(参考)　—

漢字表記・生薬名等　コルヒクム子
Name (Romaji)　INUSAFURAN*
Other name (s) (Romaji)　—
学名　*Colchicum autumnale* L.*
科名　Liliaceae（ユリ科）
英名　colchicum / autumn crocus / meadow saffron
Part of use　seed
Note 1　—
Note 2　—
注　—

名　称　イリス*

他名等　—
部位等　根茎
備　考　—

他名(参考)　—
漢字表記・生薬名等　イリス根（イリスコン）
Name (Romaji)　IRISU*
Other name (s) (Romaji)　—
学名　*Iris florentina* L.
Iris germanica L. var. *florentina* Dykes*
科名　Iridaceae（アヤメ科）
英名　orris / irris / Frorentine
Part of use　rhizome
Note 1　—
Note 2　—
注　—

名　称　イレイセン*

他名等　シナボタンヅル
部位等　根・根茎
備　考　葉は「非医」

他名(参考)　—
漢字表記・生薬名等　威霊仙（イレイセン）、支那牡丹蔓（シナボタンヅル）
Name (Romaji)　IREISEN*
Other name (s) (Romaji)　SHINABOTANZURU
学名　*Clematis chinensis* Osbeck*
Clematis mandshurica Rupr.
Clematis hexapetala Pall.
Clematis uncinata Champ. ex Benth.
科名　Ranunculaceae（キンポウゲ科）
英名　Chinese clematis
Part of use　root, rhizome
Note 1　leaf：non-drug category
Note 2　—
注　—

名　称　インチンコウ*

他名等　カワラヨモギ
部位等　花穂・帯花全草
備　考　—

他名(参考)　—
漢字表記・生薬名等　茵蔯蒿（インチンコウ）、河原艾（カワラヨモギ）
Name (Romaji)　INCHINKÔ*
Other name (s) (Romaji)　KAWARAYOMOGI
学名　*Artemisia capillaris* Thunb.*
科名　Compositae（キク科）
英名　yin-chen wormwood / capillaris / capillary artemisia
Part of use　spica, flowering whole plant
Note 1　—
Note 2　—
注　—

名　称　インドサルサ*

他名等　—
部位等　根
備　考　—

他名(参考)　—
漢字表記・生薬名等　—
Name (Romaji)　INDOSARUSA*
Other name (s) (Romaji)　—
学名　*Hemidesmus indicus* (L.) W.T. Aiton*
Periploca indica L.*
科名　Ascrepiadaceae（ガガイモ科）
英名　Hemidesmus indicus / Indian sarsaparilla / East Indian sarsaparilla
Part of use　root
Note 1　—
Note 2　—
注　—

名　称　インドジャボク属*

他名等　インドジャボク／ラウオルフィア
部位等　根・根茎
備　考　—

他名(参考)　—

漢字表記・生薬名等　印度蛇木（インドジャボク）
Name (Romaji)　INDOJABOKU-ZOKU*
Other name (s) (Romaji)　INDOJABOKU／RAUORUFIA
学名　*Rauvolfia* L.
Rauvolfia serpentina (L.) Benth. ex Kurz*
Rauvolfia vomitoria Afzel.
科名　Apocynaceae（キョウチクトウ科）
英名　rauwolfia / Indian snakeroot / serpentine wood
Part of use　root, rhizome
Note 1　—
Note 2　—
注　—

名　称　**インヨウカク***

他名等　イカリソウ
部位等　全草
備　考　—

他名（参考）　—
漢字表記・生薬名等　淫羊藿（インヨウカク）、千金両（センキンリョウ）、仙霊脾（センレイヒ）、碇草・錨草（イカリソウ）
Name (Romaji)　IN'YÔKAKU*
Other name (s) (Romaji)　IKARISÔ
学名　*Epimedium grandiflorum* C. Morr. var. *thunbergianum* Nakai*（イカリソウ）
Epimedium koreanum Nakai*（キバナイカリソウ）
Epimedium sagittatum Maxim.*（ホザキイカリソウ）
※「注」参照（See "Note 2"）
科名　Berberidaceae（メギ科）
英名　barrenwort
Part of use　whole plant
Note 1　—
Note 2　The aerial parts of *E. pubescens* Maxim., *E. brevicornu* Maxim., *E. wushanense*, *E. samperviens* Nakai (TOKIWAIKARISÔ) are used as IN'YÔKAKU (IKARISÔ). (Ref.：The Japanese Pharmacopoeia 16th Edition)
注　インヨウカク（イカリソウ）としては、他に*E. pubescens* Maxim., *E. brevicornu* Maxim., *E. wushanense*, *E. samperviens* Nakai（トキワイカリソウ）の地上部がある（第十六改正日本薬局方）。

名　称　**ウィザニア***

他名等　アシュワガンダ
部位等　全草
備　考　—

他名（参考）　—
漢字表記・生薬名等　—
Name (Romaji)　WIZANIA*
Other name (s) (Romaji)　ASHUWAGANDA
学名　*Withania somnifera* (L.) Dunal*
科名　Solanaceae（ナス科）
英名　ashwaganda / winter cherry / withania
Part of use　whole plant
Note 1　—
Note 2　—
注　—

名　称　**ウマノスズクサ属**

他名等　—
部位等　全草
備　考　—

他名（参考）　—
漢字表記・生薬名等　広防已（コウボウイ）、関木通（カンモクツウ）
Name (Romaji)　UMANOSUZUKUSA-ZOKU
Other name (s) (Romaji)　—
学名　*Aristolochia* L.
科名　Aristrochiaceae（ウマノスズクサ科）
英名　Birthwort (Chinese birthwort)
Part of use　whole plant
Note 1　—
Note 2　—
注　—

名　称　**ウヤク***

他名等　テンダイウヤク
部位等　根
備　考　葉・実は「非医」

他名（参考）　—
漢字表記・生薬名等　烏薬（ウヤク）、天台烏薬（テンダイウヤク）
Name (Romaji)　UYAKU*
Other name (s) (Romaji)　TENDAIUYAKU
学名　*Lindera strychnifolia* (Sieb. et Zucc.) F. Vill.*
Lindera aggregata (Sims) Kosterm.*

科名　Lauraceae（クスノキ科）
英名　lindera / black medicine / Chinese allspice
Part of use　root
Note 1　leaf, fruit：non-drug category
Note 2　—
注　—

名　称　**ウワウルシ***

他名等　クマコケモモ
部位等　葉
備　考　—

他名(参考)　—
漢字表記・生薬名等　ウワウルシ、熊苔桃（クマコケモモ）
Name(Romaji)　UWAURUSHI*
Other name(s)(Romaji)　KUMAKOKEMOMO
学名　*Arctostaphylos uva-ursi* (L.) Spreng.*
科名　Ericaceae（ツツジ科）
英名　uva-ursi / bearberry
Part of use　leaf
Note 1　—
Note 2　—
注　—

名　称　**ウンカロアポ***

他名等　—
部位等　根
備　考　—

他名(参考)　—
漢字表記・生薬名等　—
Name(Romaji)　UNKAROAPO*
Other name(s)(Romaji)　—
学名　*Pelargonium reniforme* Curt.*
　　Pelargonium sidoides DC.
科名　Geraniaceae（フウロソウ科）
英名　Pelargonium reniforme / rooirabas / Umckaloabo
Part of use　root
Note 1　—
Note 2　—
注　—

名　称　**エイジツ***

他名等　ノイバラ
部位等　果実・偽果
備　考　—

他名(参考)　—
漢字表記・生薬名等　営実（エイジツ）、ノイバラ（野茨）
Name(Romaji)　EIJITSU*
Other name(s)(Romaji)　NOIBARA
学名　*Rosa multiflora* Thunb. ex Murray*
科名　Rosaceae（バラ科）
英名　multiflora rose / baby rose / bramble rose / rambler rose
Part of use　fruit, pseudocarp
Note 1　—
Note 2　—
注　—

名　称　**エニシダ***

他名等　—
部位等　枝・葉
備　考　花は「非医」

他名(参考)　—
漢字表記・生薬名等　金雀枝（エニシダ）
Name(Romaji)　ENISHIDA*
Other name(s)(Romaji)　—
学名　*Cytisus scoparius* (L.) Link*
　　Sarothamnus scoparius (L.) Wimm. ex W.D.J. Koch*
　　Spartium scoparium L.*
科名　Leguminosae（マメ科）
英名　Scotch broom / broom / scoparium
Part of use　branch, leaf
Note 1　flower：non-drug category
Note 2　—
注　—

名　称　**エンゴサク***

他名等　エゾエンゴサク
部位等　塊茎
備　考　—

他名(参考)　—
漢字表記・生薬名等　延胡索（エンゴサク）、蝦夷延胡索（エゾエンゴサク）
Name(Romaji)　ENGOSAKU*

Other name(s) (Romaji)　EZOENGOSAKU
学名　*Corydalis turtschaninovii* Bess. f. *yanhusuo* Y.H. Chou et C.C. Hsu*
Corydalis ambigua Cham. et Schlecht.*
Corydalis yanhusuo W.T. Wang*
科名　Papaveraceae（ケシ科）
英名　Corydalis yanhusuo / Corydalis ambigua / Chinese fumewort
Part of use　tuber
Note 1　—
Note 2　—
注　—

名　称　**エンジュ***

他名等　**カイカ／カイカク**
部位等　花・花蕾・果実
備　考　葉・サヤは「非医」

他名(参考)　—
漢字表記・生薬名等　槐（エンジュ、カイ）、槐花（カイカ）、槐角（カイカク）
Name(Romaji)　ENJU*
Other name(s) (Romaji)　KAIKA／KAIKAKU
学名　*Sophora japonica* L.*
科名　Leguminosae（マメ科）
英名　Japanese sophora / Chinese scholar tree / Japanese pagoda / pagoda tree
Part of use　flower, bud, fruit
Note 1　leaf, hull：non-drug category
Note 2　—
注　—

名　称　**オウカコウ***

他名等　**クソニンジン**
部位等　帯果・帯花枝葉
備　考　—

他名(参考)　—
漢字表記・生薬名等　—
Name(Romaji)　ÔKAKÔ*
Other name(s) (Romaji)　KUSONINJIN
学名　*Artemisia annua* L.*
科名　Compositaea（キク科）
英名　sweet wormwood / annual wormwood / sweet Annie
Part of use　branch and leaf with fruit or flower
Note 1　—
Note 2　—
注　—

名　称　**オウカシ***

他名等　—
部位等　根・葉
備　考　—

他名(参考)　マルバキンゴジカ（丸葉金午時花）、ウスバキンゴジカ（薄葉金午時花）、キュウケツソウ（吸血草）
漢字表記・生薬名等　黄花仔（オウカシ）
Name(Romaji)　ÔKASHI*
Other name(s) (Romaji)　—
学名　*Sida cordifolia* L.*（マルバキンゴジカ）
Sida mysorensis Wight et Arn.（ウスバキンゴジカ）
科名　Malvaceae（アオイ科）
英名　country mallow / flannel sida / flannelweed / heart leaf sida
Part of use　root, leaf
Note 1　—
Note 2　—
注　—

名　称　**オウカボ***

他名等　**キンゴジカ**
部位等　全草
備　考　—

他名(参考)　—
漢字表記・生薬名等　黄花母（オウカボ）、黄花稔（オウカボ）、金午時花（キンゴジカ）
Name(Romaji)　ÔKABO*
Other name(s) (Romaji)　KINGOJIKA
学名　*Sida rhombifolia* L.*
科名　Malvaceae（アオイ科）
英名　arrow-leaf-sida / arrowleaf sida / broomjue sida / common sida / Cuban jute / Quban jute / paddy lucerne / Queensland hemp / sida retusa / sida weed / teaweed
Part of use　whole plant
Note 1　—
Note 2　—
注　—

名　称　**オウギ***

他名等　キバナオウギ／ナイモウオウギ
部位等　根
備　考　茎・葉は「非医」

他名(参考)　—
漢字表記・生薬名等　黄耆（オウギ）、黄花黄耆（キバナオウギ）、内蒙黄耆（ナイモウオウギ）
Name(Romaji)　ÔGI*
Other name(s) (Romaji)　KIBANAÔGI／NAIMÔÔGI
学名　*Astragalus membranaceus* (Fisch. ex Link) Bunge*（キバナオウギ）
Astragalus mongholicus Bunge*（ナイモウオウギ）
Astragalus membranaceus (L.) (Fisch. ex Link) Bunge var. *mongholicus* (Bunge) P.K. Hsiao*（ナイモウオウギ）
科名　Leguminosae（マメ科）
英名　astragalus / membranous milkvetch / Mongolian milkvetch
Part of use　root
Note 1　stem, leaf : non-drug category
Note 2　—
注　—

名　称　**オウゴン***

他名等　コガネバナ／コガネヤナギ
部位等　根
備　考　茎・葉は「非医」

他名(参考)　タツナミソウ（立浪草）
漢字表記・生薬名等　黄芩（オウゴン）、黄金花（コガネバナ）、黄金柳（コガネヤナギ）
Name(Romaji)　ÔGON*
Other name(s) (Romaji)　KOGANEBANA／KOGANE-YANAGI
学名　*Scutellaria baicalensis* Georgi*
科名　Labiatae（シソ科）
英名　Chinese skullcap / Baikal skullcap / scute
Part of use　root
Note 1　stem, leaf : non-drug category
Note 2　—
注　—

名　称　**オウバク***

他名等　キハダ
部位等　樹皮
備　考　葉・実は「非医」

他名(参考)　—
漢字表記・生薬名等　黄柏（オウバク）、黄肌（キハダ）
Name(Romaji)　ÔBAKU*
Other name(s) (Romaji)　KIHADA
学名　*Phellodendron amurense* Rupr.*（キハダ）
Phellodendron chinense C.K. Schneid.*（シナキハダ）
Phellodendron amurense Rupr. var. *sachalinense* F. Schmidt（ヒロハノキハダ）
※「注」参照（See "Note 2"）
科名　Rutaceae（ミカン科）
英名　phellodendron / Amur cork tree
Part of use　bark
Note 1　leaf, fruit : non-drug category
Note 2　Bark removed cortex of *P. amurense* Rupr.var. *japonicum* (Maxim.) Ohwi (ÔBANOKIHADA), *P. amurense* Rupr. var. *lavallei* (Dode) Sprague (MIYAMAKIHADA) are used as ÔBAKU. (Ref. : The Japanese Pharmacopoeia 16th Eedition)
注　オウバクとしては、他に*P. amurense* Rupr. var. *japonicum* (Maxim.) Ohwi（オオバノキハダ）、*P. amurense* Rupr. var. *lavallei* (Dode) Sprague（ミヤマキハダ）の周皮を除いた樹皮がある（第十六改正日本薬局方）。

名　称　**オウヒ**

他名等　ヤマザクラ
部位等　樹皮
備　考　—

他名(参考)　—
漢字表記・生薬名等　桜皮（オウヒ）、山桜（ヤマザクラ）
Name(Romaji)　ÔHI
Other name(s) (Romaji)　YAMAZAKURA
学名　*Prunus jamasakura* Sieb. ex Koidz.（ヤマザクラ）
Prunus verecunda (Koidz.) Koehne（カスミザクラ）
科名　Rosaceae（バラ科）
英名　Japanese mountain cherry / yama zakra / hill cherry
Part of use　cortex
Note 1　—
Note 2　—
注　—

名　称　オウレン*

他名等　キクバオウレン
部位等　根茎・ひげ根
備　考　葉は「非医」

他名(参考)　小芹葉黄蓮（コセリバオウレン）、毛黄蓮（モウオウレン）
漢字表記・生薬名等　黄蓮（オウレン）、菊葉黄連（キクバオウレン）
Name (Romaji)　ÔREN*
Other name(s) (Romaji)　KIKUBAÔREN
学名　*Coptis japonica* (Thunb.) Makino*（オウレン）
Coptis chinensis Franch.*（オウレン）
Coptis deltoidea C.Y. Cheng et Hsiao*（オウレン）
Coptis teeta Wall.*（オウレン）
Coptis japonica (Thunb.) Makino var. *japonica*（キクバオウレン）
Coptis japonica (Thunb.) Makino var. *major* (Miq.) Satake（コセリバオウレン）
科名　Ranunculaceae（キンポウゲ科）
英名　coptis / Japanese goldthread / Chinese goldthread / Indian goldthread / Tibetan goldthread
Part of use　rhizome, fibrous root
Note 1　leaf : non-drug category
Note 2　ÔREN is identical with MÔÔREN, but their parts of use are different each other. MÔÔREN is also listed in the item of "Name". Leaf of ÔREN is classified in the "non-drug" category.
注　オウレンは別項のモウオウレンと同一。但し、「部位等」の記載が異なっている。オウレンの葉は「非医」とされている。

名　称　オシダ*

他名等　—
部位等　根茎・葉基
備　考　—

他名(参考)　メンマコン（綿馬根）
漢字表記・生薬名等　貫衆（カンジュウ）、綿馬根（メンマコン）、雄羊歯（オシダ）
Name (Romaji)　OSHIDA*
Other name(s) (Romaji)　—
学名　*Dryopteris crassirhizoma* Nakai*（オシダ）
Dryopteris filix-mas (L.) Schott*（セイヨウオシダ）
Aspidium filix-mas (L.) Sw.*
科名　Dryopteridaceae（オシダ科）
英名　shield fern / male fern / Japanese male fern / crown wood fern
Part of use　rhizome, leaf base
Note 1　—
Note 2　—
注　—

名　称　オノニス*

他名等　—
部位等　根・根茎
備　考　—

他名(参考)　—
漢字表記・生薬名等　オノニス根（オノニスコン）
Name (Romaji)　ONONISU*
Other name(s) (Romaji)　—
学名　*Ononis spinosa* L.*
Ononis campestris W.D.J. Koch et Ziz*
科名　Leguminosae（マメ科）
英名　restharrow / spiny restharrow / thorny restharrow
Part of use　root, rhizome
Note 1　—
Note 2　—
注　—

名　称　オモト

他名等　—
部位等　根茎
備　考　—

他名(参考)　—
漢字表記・生薬名等　万年青（オモト）
Name (Romaji)　OMOTO*
Other name(s) (Romaji)　—
学名　*Rohdea japonica* (Thunb.) Roth
科名　Liliaceae（ユリ科）
英名　Japanese Rohdea / lily of China / sacred lily of China
Part of use　rhizome
Note 1　—
Note 2　—
注　—

名　称　オンジ*

他名等　イトヒメハギ
部位等　根
備　考　—

他名(参考)　—

漢字表記・生薬名等　遠志（オンジ）、糸姫萩（イトヒメハギ）
Name (Romaji)　ONJI*
Other name (s) (Romaji)　ITOHIMEHAGI
学名　*Polygala tenuifolia* Willd.*
科名　Polygalaceae（ヒメハギ科）
英名　polygala / thin leaf polygala
Part of use　root
Note 1　—
Note 2　—
注　—

カ行

名　称　カイソウ<海葱>属*

他名等　—
部位等　鱗茎
備　考　カイソウ<海草>の全藻は「非医」

他名（参考）　—
漢字表記・生薬名等　海葱（カイソウ）
Name (Romaji)　KAISÔ-ZOKU*
Other name (s) (Romaji)　—
学名　*Urginea* Steinh.
Urginea maritima (L.) Baker*
Urginea scilla Steinh.
Scilla maritima L.*
Drimia maritima (L.) Stearn*
科名　Liliaceae（ユリ科）
英名　sea onion
Part of use　bulb
Note 1　whole algae of sea weed：non-drug category
Note 2　—
注　—

名　称　カイトウヒ*

他名等　—
部位等　樹皮
備　考　—

他名（参考）　デイゴ（梯梧）、デイコ（梯枯）、エリスリナ
漢字表記・生薬名等　海桐皮（カイトウヒ）
Name (Romaji)　KAITÔHI*
Other name (s) (Romaji)　—
学名　*Erythrina variegata* L.*
Erythrina indica Lam.*
Erythrina orientalis (L.) Merr.
Erythrina parcellii W. Bull
Erythrina variegata var. *orientalis* (L.) Merr.
Tetradapa javanorum Osbeck
科名　Leguminosae（マメ科）
英名　Indian coraltree / coraltree / tiger's claw
Part of use　bark
Note 1　—
Note 2　—
注　—

名　称　カクコウ

他名等　Incarvillea sinensis
部位等　全草
備　考　—

他名（参考）　—
漢字表記・生薬名等　角蒿（カクコウ）
Name (Romaji)　KAKUKÔ
Other name (s) (Romaji)　—
学名　*Incarvillea sinensis* Lam.
科名　Bignoniaceae（ノウゼンカズラ科）
英名　trumpet flower
Part of use　whole plant
Note 1　—
Note 2　—
注　—

名　称　カゴソウ

他名等　ウツボグサ
部位等　全草
備　考　—

他名（参考）　—
漢字表記・生薬名等　夏枯草（カゴソウ）、靭草（ウツボグサ）
Name (Romaji)　KAGOSÔ
Other name (s) (Romaji)　UTSUBOGUSA
学名　*Prunella vulgaris* L. var. *lilacina* Nakai
Prunella vulgaris L. ssp. *asiatica* (Nakai) Hara
科名　Labiatae（シソ科）
英名　heal all / self heal / selfheal
Part of use　whole plant
Note 1　—
Note 2　—
注　—

名　称　**カシ***

他名等　ミロバラン
部位等　果実
備　考　—

他名(参考)　—
漢字表記･生薬名等　訶子（カシ）
Name(Romaji)　KASHI*
Other name(s) (Romaji)　MIROBARAN
学名　*Terminalia chebula* Retz.*
科名　Combretaceae（シクンシ科）
英名　chebulic myrobalan / black myrobalan / true myrobalan
Part of use　fruit
Note 1　—
Note 2　—
注　—

名　称　**カシュウ***

他名等　ツルドクダミ
部位等　塊根
備　考　茎・葉は「非医」

他名(参考)　—
漢字表記･生薬名等　何首烏（カシュウ）、蔓戟・蔓毒痛（ツルドクダミ）
Name(Romaji)　KASHÛ*
Other name(s) (Romaji)　TSURUDOKUDAMI
学名　*Polygonum multiflorum* Thunb.*
Fallopia multiflora (Thunb.) Haraldson
Fagopyrum multiflorum (Thunb.) I. Grint.
Reynoutria multiflora (Thunb.) Moldenko
Pleuropterus cordatus Turcz.
科名　Palygonaceae（タデ科）
英名　fo ti / fleeceflower / Chinese knotweed
Part of use　tuber
Note 1　stem, leaf：non-drug category
Note 2　—
注　—

名　称　**カスカラサグラダ***

他名等　—
部位等　樹皮
備　考　—

他名(参考)　—
漢字表記･生薬名等　カスカラサグラダ
Name(Romaji)　KASUKARASAGURADA*
Other name(s) (Romaji)　—
学名　*Rhamnus purshiana* DC.*
Frangula purshiana (DC.) J.G. Cooper*
科名　Rhamnaceae（クロウメモドキ科）
英名　cascara sagrada / bearberry / cascara / chittem bark / sacred bark / chittam bark / western buckthorn
Part of use　bark
Note 1　—
Note 2　—
注　—

名　称　**カッコウ***

他名等　パチョリ
部位等　地上部
備　考　—

他名(参考)　—
漢字表記･生薬名等　藿香（カッコウ）、川緑（カワミドリ）
Name(Romaji)　KAKKÔ*
Other name(s) (Romaji)　PACHORI
学名　*Agastache rugosa* (Fisch. et C.A. Mey.) Kuntze*（カワミドリ）
Lophanthus rugosus Fisch. et C.A. Mey.（カワミドリ）
Pogostemon cablin (Blanco) Benth.*（パチョリ）
Pogostemon patchouly Pellet.*（パチョリ）
科名　Labiatae（シソ科）
英名　*A. rugosa, L. rugosus*：Chinese giant hyssop / Korean mint
P. cablin, P. patchouly：patchouli plant / patchouly
Part of use　aerial part
Note 1　—
Note 2　KAKKÔ is identical with KAWAMIDORI. KAWAMIDORI is also listed in the item of "Name".
注　カッコウは別項のカワミドリと同一。

名　称　**カッコン***

他名等　クズ
部位等　根
備　考　種子・葉・花・クズ澱粉は「非医」

他名(参考)　—
漢字表記･生薬名等　葛根（カッコン）、葛（クズ）
Name(Romaji)　KAKKON*

Other name(s) (Romaji)　KUZU
学名　*Pueraria lobata* (Willd.) Ohwi*
Pueraria montana (Lour.) Merr. var. *lobata* (Willd.) Maesen et S.M. Almeida ex Sanjappa et Predeep*
科名　Leguminosae (マメ科)
英名　kudzu
Part of use　root
Note 1　seed, leaf, flower, starch：non-drug category
Note 2　—
注　—

名　称　**カッシア・アウリキュラータ***

他名等　**ミミセンナ／Cassia　auriculata**
部位等　樹皮
備　考　—

他名(参考)　—
漢字表記・生薬名等　—
Name(Romaji)　KASSHIA・AURIKYURÂTA*
Other name(s) (Romaji)　MIMISENNA
学名　*Cassia auriculata* L.*
Senna auriculata (L.) Roxb.*
科名　Leguminosae (マメ科)
英名　tanner's cassia / matara tea
Part of use　bark
Note 1　—
Note 2　—
注　—

名　称　**カバ***

他名等　**カバカバ／シャカオ**
部位等　全草
備　考　kawakawaは「医」

他名(参考)　—
漢字表記・生薬名等　カバカバ
Name(Romaji)　KABA*
Other name(s) (Romaji)　KABAKABA／SHAKAO
学名　*Piper methysticum* G. Forst.*
科名　Piperaceae (コショウ科)
英名　kava / awa / kava kava / kava pepper / yangona / yaqona
Part of use　whole plant
Note 1　kawakawa：drug category
Note 2　—
注　—

名　称　**カラバル豆**

他名等　—
部位等　豆
備　考　—

他名(参考)　—
漢字表記・生薬名等　カラバル豆
Name(Romaji)　KARABARUMAME
Other name(s) (Romaji)　—
学名　*Physostigma venenosum* Balf.
科名　Leguminosae (マメ科)
英名　calabar bean / ordeal bean
Part of use　bean
Note 1　—
Note 2　—
注　—

名　称　**カロコン***

他名等　**オオカラスウリ／キカラスウリ／シナカラスウリ**
部位等　根
備　考　果実・種子は「非医」

他名(参考)　トウカラスウリ (唐烏瓜)、チョウセンカラスウリ (朝鮮烏瓜)
漢字表記・生薬名等　栝楼根 (カロコン)、大烏瓜 (オオカラスウリ)、黄烏瓜 (キカラスウリ)、支那烏瓜 (シナカラスウリ)
Name(Romaji)　KAROKON*
Other name(s) (Romaji)　ÔKARASUURI／KIKARASUURI／SHINAKARASUURI
学名　*Trichosanthes bracteata* Voigt (オオカラスウリ)
Trichosanthes kirilowii Maxim.* (トウカラスウリ、シナカラスウリ、チョウセンカラスウリ)
Trichosanthes kirilowii Maxim. var. *japonica* (Miq.) Kitam. (キカラスウリ)
科名　Cucurbitaceae (ウリ科)
英名　tricosanthes / Chinese cucumber / Mongolian snake gourd / Chinese snake gourd
Part of use　root
Note 1　fruit, seed：non-drug category
Note 2　—
注　—

名　称　カロライナジャスミン*

他名等　—
部位等　全草
備　考　—

他名（参考）　—
漢字表記・生薬名等　—
Name（Romaji）　KARORAINAJASUMIN*
Other name(s) (Romaji)　—
学名　*Gelsemium sempervirens*（L.）J. St.-Hil.*
科名　Loganiaceae（マチン科）
英名　Carolina jasmine / gelsemium / yellow jasmine / evening trumpet flower / woodbine / yellow jessamine
Part of use　whole plant
Note 1　—
Note 2　—
注　—

名　称　kawakawa

他名等　Macropiper excelsum
部位等　全草
備　考　カバは「医」

他名（参考）　—
漢字表記・生薬名等　—
Name（Romaji）　KAWAKAWA
Other name(s) (Romaji)　—
学名　*Macropiper excelsum*（G. Forst.）Miq.
科名　Piperaceae（コショウ科）
英名　New Zealand pepper tree / pepper tree / kawa / taakawa / Maori bush basil / Maori kava
Part of use　whole plant
Note 1　kava：drug category
Note 2　—
注　—

名　称　カワミドリ*

他名等　—
部位等　地上部
備　考　—

他名（参考）　カッコウ（藿香）、パチョリ
漢字表記・生薬名等　川緑（カワミドリ）
Name（Romaji）　KAWAMIDORI*
Other name(s) (Romaji)　—
学名　*Agastache rugosa*（Fisch. et C.A. Mey.）Kuntze*
Lophanthus rugosus Fisch. et C.A. Mey.
科名　Labiatae（シソ科）
英名　Chinese giant hyssop / Korean mint
Part of use　aerial part
Note 1　—
Note 2　KAWAMIDORI is identical with KAKKÔ. KAKKÔ is also listed in the item of “Name”.
注　カワミドリは別項のカッコウと同一。

名　称　カワラタケ*

他名等　—
部位等　菌糸体
備　考　子実体は「非医」

他名（参考）　—
漢字表記・生薬名等　瓦茸（カワラタケ）
Name（Romaji）　KAWARATAKE*
Other name(s) (Romaji)　—
学名　*Coriolus versicolor*（L.）Quél.*
Trametes versicolor（L.）Lloyd*
科名　Polyporaceae（サルノコシカケ科）
英名　Turkey tails
Part of use　mycelium
Note 1　fruit body：non-drug category
Note 2　—
注　—

名　称　カンショウコウ*

他名等　—
部位等　根
備　考　—

他名（参考）　カンショウ（甘松）、カンヨウカンショウ（寛葉甘松）
漢字表記・生薬名等　甘松香（カンショウコウ）
Name（Romaji）　KANSHÔKÔ*
Other name(s) (Romaji)　—
学名　*Nardostachys jatamansi*（Jones ex Roxb.）DC.*
Valeriana jatamansi Jones ex Roxb.*
Nardostachys chinensis Batalin*
科名　Valerianaceae（オミナエシ科）
英名　jatamansi / Indian nard / Indian spikenard / nard / spoon-leaf nardostachys / Chinese spikenard / Chinese nardostachys
Part of use　root
Note 1　—
Note 2　—
注　—

名　称　**カントウカ***

他名等　フキタンポポ
部位等　花蕾
備　考　葉・幼若花茎は「非医」

他名(参考)　—
漢字表記・生薬名等　款冬花（カントウカ）、蕗蒲公英（フキタンポポ）
Name(Romaji)　KANTÔKA*
Other name(s)(Romaji)　FUKITANPOPO
学名　*Tussilago farfara* L.*
科名　Compositae（キク科）
英名　coltsfoot
Part of use　bud
Note 1　leaf, young scape：non-drug category
Note 2　—
注　—

名　称　**キササゲ**

他名等　シジツ／トウキササゲ
部位等　果実
備　考　—

他名(参考)　シナキササゲ（支那楸）
漢字表記・生薬名等　木大角豆（キササゲ）、梓実（シジツ）、唐楸（トウキササゲ）
Name(Romaji)　KISASAGE
Other name(s)(Romaji)　SHIJITSU／TÔKISASAGE
学名　*Catalpa ovata* G. Don（キササゲ）
Catalpa bungei C.A. Mey.（トウキササゲ）
科名　Bignoniaceae（ノウゼンカズラ科）
英名　*C. ovata*：Chinese catalpa / yellow catalpa / Japanese catalpa
C. bungei：Manchurian catalpa / Chinese catalpa / Chinese catawba
Part of use　fruit
Note 1　—
Note 2　—
注　—

名　称　**キナ***

他名等　アカキナノキ
部位等　根皮・樹皮
備　考　—

他名(参考)　—
漢字表記・生薬名等　キナ、赤機那樹・赤規那樹（アカキナノキ）
Name(Romaji)　KINA*
Other name(s)(Romaji)　AKAKINANOKI
学名　*Cinchona succirubra* Pav. et Klotzsch（アカキナノキ）
Cinchona pubescens Vahl*（アカキナノキ）
Cinchona ledgeriana Moens ex Trimen*（ボリビアキナノキ）
Cinchona officinalis L.*（キナノキ）
Cinchona calisaya Wedd.*
科名　Rubiaceae（アカネ科）
英名　red cinchona / Jesuit's bark / Peruvian bark / red quinine / fever bark tree / ledgerbark cinchona
Part of use　root bark, bark
Note 1　—
Note 2　—
注　—

名　称　**キョウカツ***

他名等　—
部位等　根・根茎
備　考　—

他名(参考)　—
漢字表記・生薬名等　羌活（キョウカツ）
Name(Romaji)　KYÔKATSU*
Other name(s)(Romaji)　—
学名　*Notopterygium incisum* K.C. Ting ex H.T. Chang*
Notopterygium forbesii H. Boissieu*
Hansenia weberbaueriana (Fedde ex H. Wolff) Pimenov et Kljuykov
Hansenia forbessi (H. Boissieu) Pimenov et Kljuykov
科名　Umbelliferae（セリ科）
英名　notopterygium
Part of use　root, rhizome
Note 1　—
Note 2　—
注　—

名　称　**キョウニン***

他名等　アンズ／クキョウニン／ホンアンズ
部位等　種子
備　考　カンキョウニンは「非医」

他名(参考)　—
漢字表記・生薬名等　杏仁（キョウニン）、杏（アンズ）、苦杏仁（クキョウニン）、本杏（ホンアンズ）

Name (Romaji)　KYÔNIN*
Other name (s) (Romaji)　ANZU／KUKYÔNIN／HON' ANZU
学名　*Prunus armeniaca* L.*（ホンアンズ）
Prunus armeniaca L. var. *ansu* Maxim.（アンズ）
Prunus sibirica L.（モウコアンズ）
Armeniaca vulgaris Lam.*（アンズ）
科名　Rosaceae（バラ科）
英名　apricot / Siberian apricot / ansu apricot
Part of use　seed
Note 1　Kankyonin, seed containing amygdalin less than 2%：non-drug category
Note 2　—
注　—

名　称　**キンリュウカ属**

他名等　ストロファンツス／Strophanthus属
部位等　種子・木部
備　考　—

他名(参考)　—
漢字表記･生薬名等　ストロファンツス子
Name (Romaji)　KINRYÛKA-ZOKU
Other name (s) (Romaji)　SUTOROFANTSUSU
学名　*Strophanthus caudatus* Kurz
Strophanthus kombe Oliv.
Strophanthus hispidus DC.
Strophanthus gratus (Wall. et Hook. ex Benth) Baill.（ストロファンツス）
Strophanthus divaricatus (Lour.) Hook. et Arn.
科名　Apocynaceae（キョウチクトウ科）
英名　goat horns
Part of use　seed, xylem
Note 1　—
Note 2　—
注　—

名　称　**グアシャトンガ***

他名等　—
部位等　葉
備　考　—

他名(参考)　—
漢字表記･生薬名等　—
Name (Romaji)　GUASHATONGA*
Other name (s) (Romaji)　—
学名　*Casearia sylvestris* Sw.*
Samyda parviflora L.
Casearia parviflora L.
Anavinga samyda Gaertn. f.
科名　Flacourtiaceae（イイギリ科）
英名　wild coffee / cafeillo / guayabillo / papelite / casearia / crack open / guassatonga
Part of use　leaf
Note 1　—
Note 2　—
注　—

名　称　**クジン***

他名等　クララ
部位等　根
備　考　—

他名(参考)　—
漢字表記･生薬名等　苦参（クジン）
Name (Romaji)　KUJIN*
Other name (s) (Romaji)　KURARA
学名　*Sophora flavescens* Aiton*
科名　Leguminosae（マメ科）
英名　shrubby sophora / light-yellow sophora
Part of use　root
Note 1　—
Note 2　—
注　—

名　称　**クスノハガシワ***

他名等　—
部位等　樹皮
備　考　—

他名(参考)　カマラ、ルソンシュウモウ（呂宋楸毛）
漢字表記･生薬名等　カマラ
Name (Romaji)　KUSUNOHAGASHIWA*
Other name (s) (Romaji)　—
学名　*Mallotus philippensis* (Lam.) Müll. Arg.*
Rottlera tinctoria Roxb.*
科名　Euphorbiaceae（トウダイグサ科）
英名　kamala tree / orange kamala / red kamala / monkey face tree
Part of use　bark
Note 1　—
Note 2　—
注　—

名　称　グラビオラ*

他名等　サーサップ／トゲバンレイシ／オランダドリアン
部位等　種子
備　考　果実は「非医」

他名(参考)　—
漢字表記･生薬名等　刺蕃荔枝（トゲバンレイシ）
Name(Romaji)　GURABIORA*
Other name(s) (Romaji)　SÂSAPPU／TOGEBANREISHI／ORANDADORIAN
学名　*Annona muricata* L.*
Annona macrocarpa auct.
科名　Annonaceae（バンレイシ科）
英名　guanabana / graviola / soursop / prickly custard apple
Part of use　seed
Note 1　fruit：non-drug category
Note 2　—
注　—

名　称　グリフォニア・シンプリシフォリア

他名等　—
部位等　種子
備　考　—

他名(参考)　—
漢字表記･生薬名等　—
Name(Romaji)　GURIFONIA・SHINPURISHIFORIA
Other name(s) (Romaji)　—
学名　*Griffonia simplicifolia* (Vahl ex DC.) Baill.
Bandeiraea simplicifolia (Vahl ex DC.) Benth.
Schotia simplicifolia Vahl ex DC.
科名　Leguminosae（マメ科）
英名　griffonia
Part of use　seed
Note 1　—
Note 2　—
注　—

名　称　クロウメモドキ属

他名等　ソリシ／Rhamnus属
部位等　果実
備　考　—

他名(参考)　—
漢字表記･生薬名等　黒梅擬（クロウメモドキ）、鼠李子（ソリシ）
Name(Romaji)　KUROUMEMODOKI-ZOKU
Other name(s) (Romaji)　SORISHI
学名　*Rhamnus* L.
科名　Rhamunaceae（クロウメモドキ科）
英名　buckthorn
Part of use　fruit
Note 1　—
Note 2　—
注　—

名　称　ケイガイ*

他名等　—
部位等　全草
備　考　—

他名(参考)　アリタソウ（有田草）
漢字表記･生薬名等　荊芥（ケイガイ）
Name(Romaji)　KEIGAI*
Other name(s) (Romaji)　—
学名　*Schizonepeta tenuifolia* (Benth.) Briq.*
Nepeta tenuifolia Benth.*
科名　Labiatae（シソ科）
英名　schizonepeta
Part of use　whole plant
Note 1　—
Note 2　—
注　—

名　称　ケシ*

他名等　—
部位等　全草（発芽防止処理された種子・種子油は除く）
備　考　発芽防止処理された種子・種子油は「非医」

他名(参考)　—
漢字表記･生薬名等　芥子（ケシ）、阿片（アヘン）
Name(Romaji)　KESHI*
Other name(s) (Romaji)　—
学名　*Papaver somniferum* L.*
科名　Papaveraceae（ケシ科）
英名　opium poppy / poppy / opium / oilseed poppy / small opium poppy / wild poppy
Part of use　whole plant (except seed treated with prevention of germination and seed oil)
Note 1　seed treated with prevention of germination and seed oil：non-drug category
Note 2　—
注　—

名　称　**ケファエリス属***

他名等　トコン／Cephaelis属
部位等　根
備　考　—

他名（参考）　—
漢字表記・生薬名等　吐根（トコン）
Name（Romaji）　KEFAERISU-ZOKU*
Other name(s)（Romaji）　TOKON
学名　*Cephaelis* Sw.
Cephaelis ipecacuanha (Brot.) A. Rich*
Cephaelis acuminata H. Karst.*
科名　Rubiaceae（アカネ科）
英名　ipecac / ipecacuanha / Brazilian ipecac / Rio ipecac
Part of use　root
Note 1　—
Note 2　—
注　—

名　称　**ケンゴシ***

他名等　アサガオ
部位等　種子
備　考　葉・花は「非医」

他名（参考）　—
漢字表記・生薬名等　牽牛子（ケンゴシ）、朝顔（アサガオ）
Name（Romaji）　KENGOSHI*
Other name(s)（Romaji）　ASAGAO
学名　*Pharbitis nil* (L.) Choisy*
Ipomoea nil (L.) Roth*
科名　Convolvulaceae（ヒルガオ科）
英名　white-edge morning glory / Japanese morning glory
Part of use　seed
Note 1　leaf, flower : non-drug category
Note 2　—
注　—

名　称　**ゲンジン***

他名等　ゴマノハグサ
部位等　根
備　考　—

他名（参考）　—
漢字表記・生薬名等　玄参（ゲンジン）、胡麻葉草（ゴマノハグサ）
Name（Romaji）　GENJIN*
Other name(s)（Romaji）　GOMANOHAGUSA
学名　*Scrophularia ningpoensis* Hemsl.*
科名　Scrophulariaceae（ゴマノハグサ科）
英名　scrophularia
Part of use　root
Note 1　—
Note 2　—
注　—

名　称　**ゲンチアナ***

他名等　—
部位等　根・根茎
備　考　花は「非医」

他名（参考）　—
漢字表記・生薬名等　ゲンチアナ
Name（Romaji）　GENCHIANA*
Other name(s)（Romaji）　—
学名　*Gentiana lutea* L.*
科名　Gentianaceae（リンドウ科）
英名　gentian / yellow gentian / great yellow gentian
Part of use　root, rhizome
Note 1　flower : non-drug category
Note 2　—
注　—

名　称　**ゲンノショウコ**

他名等　—
部位等　地上部
備　考　—

他名（参考）　ゲンソウ（玄草）
漢字表記・生薬名等　現之証拠（ゲンノショウコ）
Name（Romaji）　GENNOSHÔKO
Other name(s)（Romaji）　—
学名　*Geranium thunbergii* Sieb. ex Lindl. et Paxton
Geranium nepalense var. *thunbergii* (Sieb. ex Lindl. et Paxton) Kudo
科名　Geraniaceae（フウロウソウ科）
英名　geranium herb
Part of use　aerial part
Note 1　—
Note 2　—
注　—

名　称　**コウブシ***

他名等　**サソウ／ハマスゲ**
部位等　根茎
備　考　―

他名(参考)　シャソウ（沙草）
漢字表記・生薬名等　香附子（コウブシ）、沙草（サソウ）、浜菅（ハマスゲ）
Name (Romaji)　KÔBUSHI*
Other name(s) (Romaji)　SASÔ／HAMASUGE
学名　*Cyperus rotundus* L.*
科名　Cyperaceae（カヤツリグサ科）
英名　cyperus / nut grass / nut sedge / galine gale
Part of use　rhizome
Note 1　―
Note 2　―
注　―

名　称　**コウフン**

他名等　**コマントウ**
部位等　全草
備　考　―

他名(参考)　ダンチョウグサ（断腸草）
漢字表記・生薬名等　鉤吻（コウフン）、胡蔓藤（コマントウ）、治葛（カマツ）
Name (Romaji)　KÔFUN
Other name(s) (Romaji)　KOMANTÔ
学名　*Gelsemium elegans* (Gardener et Champ.) Benth.
科名　Loganiaceae（マチン科）
英名　Chinese gelsemium
Part of use　whole plant
Note 1　―
Note 2　―
注　―

名　称　**コウボク***

他名等　**ホウノキ**
部位等　樹皮
備　考　―

他名(参考)　―
漢字表記・生薬名等　厚朴（コウボク）、朴木（ホウノキ）
Name (Romaji)　KÔBOKU*
Other name(s) (Romaji)　HÔNOKI
学名　*Magnolia obovata* Thunb.*（ホウノキ）
Magnolia hypoleuca Sieb. et Zucc.*（ホウノキ）
Magnolia officinalis Rehd. et E.H. Wils.*（コウボク）
Magnolia officinalis Rehd. et E.H. Wils. var. *biloba* Rehd. et E.H. Wils.*（凹葉厚朴）
科名　Magnoliaceae（モクレン科）
英名　Japanese white bark magnolia / magnolia / magnolia bark / Japanese big-leaf magnolia / two-lobe magnolia
Part of use　bark
Note 1　―
Note 2　―
注　―

名　称　**コウホン***

他名等　**―**
部位等　根・根茎
備　考　―

他名(参考)　―
漢字表記・生薬名等　藁本（コウホン）、遼藁本（リョウコウホン）
Name (Romaji)　KÔHON*
Other name(s) (Romaji)　―
学名　*Ligusticum sinense* Oliv.*（コウホン）
Ligusticum jeholense (Nakai et Kitag.) Nakai et Kitag.*（リョウコウホン、ムレイセンキュウ）
科名　Umbelliferae（セリ科）
英名　Chinese lovage / Sichuan lovage
Part of use　root, rhizome
Note 1　―
Note 2　―
注　―

名　称　**ゴールデンシール***

他名等　**カナダヒドラスチス**
部位等　根茎
備　考　―

他名(参考)　―
漢字表記・生薬名等　ヒドラスチス根
Name (Romaji)　GÔRUDENSHÎRU*
Other name(s) (Romaji)　KANADAHIDORASUCHISU
学名　*Hydrastis canadensis* L.*
科名　Ranunculaceae（キンポウゲ科）
英名　goldenseal / yellow puccoon / yellow root / orange root
Part of use　rhizome
Note 1　―
Note 2　―

注　—

名　称　**コケモモヨウ***

他名等　コケモモ
部位等　葉
備　考　果実は「非医」

他名（参考）　—
漢字表記・生薬名等　苔桃葉（コケモモヨウ）
Name（Romaji）　KOKEMOMOYÔ*
Other name(s)（Romaji）　KOKEMOMO
学名　*Vaccinium vitis-idaea* L.*
科名　Ericaceae（ツツジ科）
英名　lingonberry / lingenberry / cowberry / foxberry / northern mountain cranberry / alpine cranberry / mountain cranberry / partridge berry / rock cranberry
Part of use　leaf
Note 1　fruit：non-drug category
Note 2　—
注　—

名　称　**ゴシツ***

他名等　イノコヅチ／ヒナタイノコヅチ
部位等　根
備　考　—

他名（参考）　—
漢字表記・生薬名等　牛膝（ゴシツ）、イノコヅチ（豕槌）、ヒナタイノコヅチ（日向猪小槌）
Name（Romaji）　GOSHITSU*
Other name(s)（Romaji）　INOKOZUCHI／HINATAINO-KOZUCHI
学名　*Achyranthes fauriei* H. Lév. et Vaniot
Achyranthes bidentata Blume*
科名　Amaranthaceae（ヒユ科）
英名　achyranthes / pig's knee / ox knee
Part of use　root
Note 1　—
Note 2　—
注　—

名　称　**ゴシュユ***

他名等　ホンゴシュユ
部位等　果実
備　考　—

他名（参考）　—
漢字表記・生薬名等　呉茱萸（ゴシュユ）、本呉茱萸（ホンゴシュユ）
Name（Romaji）　GOSHUYU*
Other name(s)（Romaji）　HONGOSHUYU
学名　*Euodia ruticarpa*（A. Juss）Hook. f. et Thomson*（ゴシュユ）
Evodia rutaecarpa Benth.（ゴシュユ）
Euodia officinalis Dode（ホンゴシュユ）
Evodia officinalis Dode（ホンゴシュユ）
Euodia bodinieri Dode（ゴシュユ）
Evodia bodinieri Dode（ゴシュユ）
科名　Rutaceae（ミカン科）
英名　evodia / evodia fruit
Part of use　fruit
Note 1　—
Note 2　—
注　—

名　称　**コジョウコン***

他名等　イタドリ
部位等　根茎
備　考　若芽は「非医」

他名（参考）　—
漢字表記・生薬名等　虎杖根（コジョウコン）、虎杖（イタドリ）
Name（Romaji）　KOJÔKON*
Other name(s)（Romaji）　ITADORI
学名　*Polygonum cuspidatum* Sieb. et Zucc.*
Reynoutria japonica Houtt.
科名　Polygonaceae（タデ科）
英名　Japanese knotweed / Japanese fleeceflower / giant knotweed
Part of use　rhizome
Note 1　young sprout：non-drug category
Note 2　—
注　—

名　称　**ゴボウシ***

他名等　ゴボウ
部位等　果実
備　考　根・葉は「非医」

他名(参考)　—
漢字表記・生薬名等　牛蒡子（ゴボウシ）、牛蒡（ゴボウ）
Name (Romaji)　GOBÔSHI*
Other name (s) (Romaji)　GOBÔ
学名　*Arctium lappa* L.*
Arctium edule Beger
Lappa major Gaertn.
Lappa officinalis All.
科名　Compositae（キク科）
英名　burdock / harlock / gobo / begger's buttons / edible burdock / great burdock / greater burdock / lappa
Part of use　fruit
Note 1　root, leaf : non-drug category
Note 2　—
注　—

名　称　**ゴミシ***

他名等　チョウセンゴミシ
部位等　果実
備　考　—

他名(参考)　—
漢字表記・生薬名等　五味子（ゴミシ）、朝鮮五味子（チョウセンゴミシ）
Name (Romaji)　GOMISHI*
Other name (s) (Romaji)　CHÔSENGOMISHI
学名　*Schisandra chinensis* (Turcz.) Baill.*
科名　Schisandraceae（マツブサ科）
英名　schisandra / schizandra / northern schisandra / Chinese magnolia vine / five flavor fruit / magnolia vine
Part of use　fruit
Note 1　—
Note 2　—
注　—

名　称　**コロシントウリ***

他名等　—
部位等　果実
備　考　—

他名(参考)　—
漢字表記・生薬名等　コロシント、コロシント瓜（コロシントウリ）
Name (Romaji)　KOROSHINTO-URI*
Other name (s) (Romaji)　—
学名　*Citrullus colocynthis* (L.) Schrad.*
Colocynthis vulgaris Schrad.
科名　Cucurbitadeae（ウリ科）
英名　colocynth / bitter apple / bitter gourd / bitter cucumber / wild gourd / vine of Sodem
Part of use　fruit
Note 1　—
Note 2　—
注　—

名　称　**コロンボ***

他名等　—
部位等　根
備　考　—

他名(参考)　—
漢字表記・生薬名等　コロンボ
Name (Romaji)　KORONBO*
Other name (s) (Romaji)　—
学名　*Jateorhiza columba* Miers*
科名　Menispermaceae（ツヅラフジ科）
英名　calumba / colombo
Part of use　root
Note 1　—
Note 2　—
注　—

名　称　**コンズランゴ***

他名等　—
部位等　樹皮
備　考　—

他名(参考)　—
漢字表記・生薬名等　コンズランゴ
Name (Romaji)　KONZURANGO*
Other name (s) (Romaji)　—
学名　*Marsdenia cundurango* Rchb. f.*

科名　Asclepiadaceae（ガガイモ科）
英名　condurango / condor vine
Part of use　bark
Note 1　—
Note 2　—
注　—

名　称　**コンドデンドロン属**

他名等　**コンドデロデンドロン属／バリエラ／パレイラ根**
部位等　樹皮・根
備　考　—

他名(参考)　—
漢字表記・生薬名等　パレイラ根（パレイラコン）
Name (Romaji)　KONDODENDORON-ZOKU
Other name (s) (Romaji)　KONDODERODENDORON-ZOKU／BARIERA／PAREIRAKON
学名　*Chondrodendron* Ruiz et Pav. *corr.* Miers（バリエラ属）
Chondrodendron tomentosum Ruiz et Pav.
科名　Menispermaceae（ツヅラフジ科）
英名　wild grape / Peruvian's wild grape / pareira / pareira root / pareira brava
Part of use　bark, root
Note 1　—
Note 2　KONDODENDORON-ZOKU and KONDODERODENDORON-ZOKU in the items of "Name" and "Other names" respectively are incorrect. The correct name is KONDORODENDORON-ZOKU.
注　「名称」に記載されているコンドデンドロン属および「他名等」に記載されているコンドデロデンドロン属は、正しくはコンドロデンドロン属である。

名　称　**コンミフォラ属**

他名等　**アラビアモツヤク／モツヤク／モツヤクジュ／ミルラ／Commiphora属**
部位等　全木（ガムググルの樹脂を除く）
備　考　ガムググル（Commiphora mukul）の樹脂は「非医」

他名(参考)　—
漢字表記・生薬名等　没薬（モツヤク）、没薬樹（モツヤクジュ）
Name (Romaji)　KONMIFORA-ZOKU
Other name (s) (Romaji)　ARABIAMOTSUYAKU／MOTSUYAKU／MOTSUYAKUJU／MIRURA
学名　*Commiphora* Jacq.
科名　Burseraceae（カンラン科）
英名　myrrh tree
Part of use　whole tree (except resin of *Commiphora mukul*)
Note 1　resin of *Commiphora mukul*：non-drug category
Note 2　—
注　—

サ行

名　称　**サイコ**

他名等　**ミシマサイコ**
部位等　根
備　考　葉は「非医」

他名(参考)　—
漢字表記・生薬名等　柴胡（サイコ）、三島柴胡（ミシマサイコ）
Name (Romaji)　SAIKO
Other name (s) (Romaji)　MISHIMASAIKO
学名　*Bupleurum falcatum* L.
科名　Umbelliferae（セリ科）
英名　bupleurum / Chinese throughwax / Sickle hare's ear / Sickle-leaf hare's ear
Part of use　root
Note 1　leaf：non-drug category
Note 2　—
注　—

名　称　**サイシン***

他名等　**ウスバサイシン／ケイリンサイシン**
部位等　全草
備　考　—

他名(参考)　ウスゲサイシン（薄毛細辛）
漢字表記・生薬名等　細辛（サイシン）、薄葉細辛（ウスバサイシン）、鶏林細辛（ケイリンサイシン）
Name (Romaji)　SAISHIN*
Other name (s) (Romaji)　USUBASAISHIN／KEIRINSAISHIN
学名　*Asarum sieboldii* (Miq.) F. Maek.*（ウスバサイシン）
Asarum sieboldii (Miq.) var. *seoulense* Nakai（ウスゲサイシン）
Asarum heterotropoides (F. Schmidt) F. Maek. var. *mandschuricum* (Maxim.) F. Maek.*（ケイリンサ

イシン）
Asarum heterotropoides F. Schmidt var. *mandshuricum* (Maxim.) Kitag.* （ケイリンサイシン）
科名 Aristrochiaceae（ウマノスズクサ科）
英名 Chinese wild ginger / Manchurian wild ginger / Siebold's wild ginger
Part of use whole plant
Note 1 —
Note 2 —
注 —

名　称 **サビナ**

他名等 —
部位等 枝葉・球果
備　考 —

他名（参考） サビナビャクシン（サビナ柏槇）
漢字表記・生薬名等 —
Name (Romaji) SABINA
Other name (s) (Romaji) —
学名 *Juniperus sabina* L.
科名 Cupressaceae（ヒノキ科）
英名 savin / savin juniper / savina / hoarfrost juniper / tamarix juniper / Spanish savin juniper / tam
Part of use branch and leaf, cone
Note 1 —
Note 2 —
注 —

名　称 **サルカケミカン**

他名等 —
部位等 茎
備　考 —

他名（参考） サラカキ
漢字表記・生薬名等 猿掛蜜柑（サルカケミカン）
Name (Romaji) SARUKAKEMIKAN
Other name (s) (Romaji) —
学名 *Toddalia asiatica* (L.) Lam.
科名 Rutaceae（ミカン科）
英名 wild orange tree / orange tree / forest paper
Part of use stem
Note 1 —
Note 2 —
注 —

名　称 **サワギキョウ**

他名等 —
部位等 全草
備　考 —

他名（参考） ミゾカクシ（溝隠）、磯桔梗（イソギキョウ）、インディアン・タバコ
漢字表記・生薬名等 沢桔梗（サワギキョウ）、山梗菜（サンコウサイ）
Name (Romaji) SAWAGIKYÔ
Other name (s) (Romaji) —
学名 *Lobelia sessilifolia* Lamb.
科名 Campanulaceae（キキョウ科）
英名 —
Part of use whole plant
Note 1 —
Note 2 —
注 —

名　称 **サンキライ***

他名等 ケナシサルトリイバラ／Smilax glabra
部位等 塊茎・根茎
備　考 葉は「非医」、サンキライ以外のシオデ属の葉・根は「非医」

他名（参考） ドブクリョウ（土茯苓）、ワサンキライ（和山帰来）
漢字表記・生薬名等 山帰来（サンキライ）、ケナシ猿捕茨（ケナシサルトリイバラ）、菝葜（バッカツ）
Name (Romaji) SANKIRAI*
Other name (s) (Romaji) KENASHISARUTORIIBARA
学名 *Smilax glabra* Roxb.* （ケナシサルトリイバラ）
Smilax china L.* （サルトリイバラ）
科名 Liliaceae（ユリ科）
英名 Chinese smilax / glabrous greenbrier / greenbrier / catbrier / China root
Part of use tuber, rhizome
Note 1 leaf：non-drug category
leaf and root of *Smilax* L. except *Smilax glabra* and *Smilax china*：non-drug category
Note 2 —
注 —

名　称　**サンズコン***

他名等　―
部位等　根・根茎
備　考　―

他名(参考)　コウズコン（広豆根）
漢字表記・生薬名等　山豆根（サンズコン）
Name(Romaji)　SANZUKON*
Other name(s) (Romaji)　―
学名　*Sophora subprostrata* Chun et T.C. Chen*
Sophora tonkinensis Gagnep.*
科名　Leguminosae（マメ科）
英名　Vietnamese sophora
Part of use　root, rhizome
Note 1　―
Note 2　―
注　―

名　称　**ジオウ***

他名等　アカヤジオウ／カイケイジオウ
部位等　茎・根
備　考　―

他名(参考)　ジュクジオウ（熟地黄）
漢字表記・生薬名等　地黄（ジオウ）、赤矢地黄（アカヤジオウ）、懐慶地黄（カイケイジオウ）
Name(Romaji)　JIÔ*
Other name(s) (Romaji)　AKAYAJIÔ／KAIKEIJIÔ
学名　*Rehmannia glutinosa* Libosch. var. *purprea* Makino（アカヤジオウ）
Rehmannia glutinosa（Gaertn.）Libosch. ex Fisch. et C.A. Mey.*（カイケイジオウ）
Rehmannia glutinosa var. *huechingensis* Chao et Shih（カイケイジオウ）
科名　Scrophulariaceae（ゴマノハグサ科）
英名　rehmannia
Part of use　stem, root
Note 1　―
Note 2　―
注　―

名　称　**シオン***

他名等　―
部位等　根・根茎
備　考　―

他名(参考)　―
漢字表記・生薬名等　紫苑（シオン）
Name(Romaji)　SHION*
Other name(s) (Romaji)　―
学名　*Aster tataricus* L. f.*
科名　Compositae（キク科）
英名　Tatarian aster / Tatar aster / Tarter aster / Chinese aster
Part of use　root, rhizome
Note 1　―
Note 2　―
注　―

名　称　**ジギタリス属***

他名等　Digitalis属
部位等　葉
備　考　―

他名(参考)　―
漢字表記・生薬名等　ジギタリス
Name(Romaji)　JIGITARISU-ZOKU*
Other name(s) (Romaji)　―
学名　*Digitalis* L.
Digitalis purpurea L.*
科名　Scrophulariaceae（ゴマノハグサ科）
英名　digitalis / fox glove / purple fox glove / common fox glove
Part of use　leaf
Note 1　―
Note 2　―
注　―

名　称　**シキミ**

他名等　ハナノキ
部位等　実
備　考　―

他名(参考)　シキビ（樒、樒、梻）、ハナシバ（花柴）
漢字表記・生薬名等　樒（シキミ）、花の木（ハナノキ）
Name(Romaji)　SHIKIMI
Other name(s) (Romaji)　HANANOKI
学名　*Illicium anisatum* L.
Illicium religiosum Sieb. et Zucc.
Illicium japonicum Sieb. et Masam.
科名　Illiciaceae（シキミ科）
英名　Japanese anise tree / Japanese star anise
Part of use　fruit
Note 1　―
Note 2　―

注　—

名　称　**ジコッピ***

他名等　クコ
部位等　根皮
備　考　果実・葉は「非医」

他名（参考）　—
漢字表記・生薬名等　地骨皮（ジコッピ）、拘杞（クコ）
Name（Romaji）　JIKOPPI*
Other name(s)（Romaji）　KUKO
学名　*Lycium chinense* Mill.*
　　Lycium barbarum L.*
科名　Solaneceae（ナス科）
英名　*L. chinense*：lycium / Chinese boxthorn / Chinese wolfberry
　　L. barbarm：lycium / barbary wolf berry / matrimony vine
Part of use　root bark
Note 1　fruit, leaf：non-drug category
Note 2　—
注　—

名　称　**シコン***

他名等　ムラサキ
部位等　根
備　考　—

他名（参考）　—
漢字表記・生薬名等　紫根（シコン）、紫草（ムラサキ）
Name（Romaji）　SHIKON*
Other name(s)（Romaji）　MURASAKI
学名　*Lithospermum erythrorhizon* Sieb. et Zucc.*
科名　Boraginaceae（ムラサキ科）
英名　red-root / lithospermum / red-root gromwell
Part of use　root
Note 1　—
Note 2　—
注　—

名　称　**シッサス・クアドラングラリス***

他名等　ヒスイカク
部位等　全草
備　考　—

他名（参考）　—
漢字表記・生薬名等　翡翠閣（ヒスイカク）
Name（Romaji）　SHISSASU・KUADORANGURARISU*
Other name(s)（Romaji）　HISUIKAKU
学名　*Cissus quadrangularis* L.*
　　Vitis quadrangularis（L.）Wall. ex Wight et Arn.*
科名　Vitaceae（ブドウ科）
英名　winged treebine / veldt grape / bonesetter / edible stemed vine / devil's backbone
Part of use　whole plant
Note 1　—
Note 2　—
注　—

名　称　**シツリシ***

他名等　ハマビシ
部位等　果実
備　考　—

他名（参考）　—
漢字表記・生薬名等　蒺藜子（シツリシ）、浜菱（ハマビシ）
Name（Romaji）　SHITSURISHI*
Other name(s)（Romaji）　HAMABISHI
学名　*Tribulus terrestris* L.*
科名　Zygophyllaceae（ハマビシ科）
英名　puncture vine / puncturevine caltrop / small caltrops
Part of use　fruit
Note 1　—
Note 2　—
注　—

名　称　**シマハスノハカズラ***

他名等　フンボウイ／Stephania tetranda
部位等　茎・茎根
備　考　—

他名（参考）　—
漢字表記・生薬名等　粉防已（フンボウイ）、漢防已（カンボウイ）
Name（Romaji）　SHIMAHASUNOHAKAZURA*
Other name(s)（Romaji）　FUNBÔI
学名　*Stephania tetrandra* S. Moore*
科名　Menispermaceae（ツヅラフジ科）
英名　stephania
Part of use　stem, rhizome
Note 1　—
Note 2　—
注　—

名　称　**シャクヤク***

他名等　—
部位等　根
備　考　花は「非医」

他名（参考）　セキシャク（赤芍）、ビャクシャク（白芍）
漢字表記・生薬名等　芍薬（シャクヤク）、白芍（ビャクシャク）、赤芍（セキシャク）
Name（Romaji）　SHAKUYAKU*
Other name（s）（Romaji）　—
学名　*Paeonia lactiflora* Pall.*（シャクヤク）
Paeonia albiflora Pall.*（ビャクシャク）
Paeonia veitchii Lynch*（セキシャク）
科名　Paeoniaceae（ボタン科）
英名　peony / Chinese peony / common garden peony / red peony root / white peony root
Part of use　root
Note 1　flower：non-drug category
Note 2　—
注　—

名　称　**ジャショウ***

他名等　オカゼリ
部位等　果実・茎・葉
備　考　果実はジャショウシともいう

他名（参考）　オヤブジラミ（雄藪虱）
漢字表記・生薬名等　蛇床子（ジャショウシ）、岡芹（オカゼリ）
Name（Romaji）　JASHÔ*
Other name（s）（Romaji）　OKAZERI
学名　*Cnidium monnieri*（L.）Cusson*（オカゼリ）
Selinum monnieri L.（オカゼリ）
Torilis scabra（Thunb.）DC.（オヤブジラミ）
Torilis japonica（Houtt.）DC.（ヤブジラミ）
科名　Umbelliferae（セリ科）
英名　cnidium / Monnier's snowparsely
Part of use　fruit, stem, leaf
Note 1　fruit is called "JASHÔSHI".
Note 2　—
注　—

名　称　**シュクシャ***

他名等　シャジン＜砂仁＞／シュクシャミツ
部位等　種子の塊・成熟果実
備　考　シャジン＜沙参＞の根は「非医」

他名（参考）　—
漢字表記・生薬名等　縮砂（シュクシャ）、砂仁（シャジン）、縮砂蔤（シュクシャミツ）
Name（Romaji）　SHUKUSHA*
Other name（s）（Romaji）　SHAJIN／SHUKUSHAMITSU
学名　*Amomum xanthioides* Wall. ex Baker
Amomum villosum Lour. var. *xanthioides*（Wall. ex Baker）T.L. Wu et S.J. Chen*
科名　Zingiberaceae（ショウガ科）
英名　Chinese amomum / bastard cardamom / wild siamese cardamom
Part of use　a lump of seeds, riped fruit
Note 1　root of *Adenophora tetraphylla, Adenophora stricta, Adenophora hunanensis* or *Adenophora triphylla*：non-drug category
Note 2　—
注　—

名　称　**ショウブコン***

他名等　カラムスコン／ショウブ
部位等　根茎
備　考　—

他名（参考）　—
漢字表記・生薬名等　菖蒲根（ショウブコン）、カラムス根、菖蒲（ショウブ）
Name（Romaji）　SHÔBUKON*
Other name（s）（Romaji）　KARAMUSUKON／SHÔBU
学名　*Acorus calamus* L.*
科名　Araceae（サトイモ科）
英名　calamus / acorus / sweet calamus
Part of use　rhizome
Note 1　—
Note 2　—
注　—

名　称　**ショウボクヒ**

他名等　クヌギ／ボクソク
部位等　樹皮
備　考　—

他名（参考）　コナラ（小楢）、ミズナラ（水楢）、アベマキ

（阿部槙）
漢字表記･生薬名等　橡木皮（ショウボクヒ）、櫟（クヌギ）、樸樕（ボクソク）
Name(Romaji)　SHÔBOKUHI
Other name(s)(Romaji)　KUNUGI／BOKUSOKU
学名　*Quercus acutissima* Carruth.（クヌギ）
Quercus serrata Murray（コナラ）
Quercus mongolica Fisch. ex Ledeb.（ミズナラ）
Quercus variabilis Blume（アベマキ）
科名　Fegaceae（ブナ科）
英名　Japanese chestnut oak / konara oak / sawtooth oak / Chinese cork oak / Mongolian oak
Part of use　bark
Note 1　—
Note 2　—
注　—

名　称　ショウマ*

他名等　サラシナショウマ
部位等　根茎
備　考　アカショウマの根は「非医」

他名(参考)　—
漢字表記･生薬名等　升麻（ショウマ）、晒菜升麻（サラシナショウマ）
Name(Romaji)　SHÔMA*
Other name(s)(Romaji)　SARASHINASHÔMA
学名　*Cimicifuga simplex* (DC.) Turcz.（サラシナショウマ）
Cimicifuga dahurica (Turcz.) Maxim.*（ショウマ）
Cimicifuga heracleifolia Kom.*（ショウマ）
Cimicifuga foetida L.*（ショウマ）
科名　Ranunculaceae（キンポウゲ科）
英名　Chinese cimicifuga / Dahurian bugbane / large-leaf bugbane
Part of use　rhizome
Note 1　root of *Astilbe thunbergii*：non-drug category
Note 2　—
注　—

名　称　ショウリク*

他名等　ヤマゴボウ／Phytolacca esculenta
部位等　根
備　考　ヤマゴボウ（*Cirsium dipsacolepis*）の根は「非医」

他名(参考)　—
漢字表記･生薬名等　商陸（ショウリク）、山牛蒡（ヤマゴボウ）
Name(Romaji)　SHÔRIKU*
Other name(s)(Romaji)　YAMAGOBÔ
学名　*Phytolacca esculenta* Van Houtte*
Phytolacca acinosa Roxb.*
科名　Phytolaccaceae（ヤマゴボウ科）
英名　Indian poke / Indian pokeweed / Chinese poke / sweet belladonna / food pokeberry
Part of use　root
Note 1　root of *Cirsium dipsacolepis*：non-drug category
Note 2　—
注　—

名　称　シンイ*

他名等　コブシ／タムシバ
部位等　花蕾
備　考　—

他名(参考)　—
漢字表記･生薬名等　辛夷（シンイ）、拳・辛夷（コブシ）、田虫葉（タムシバ）
Name(Romaji)　SHIN'I*
Other name(s)(Romaji)　KOBUSHI／TAMUSHIBA
学名　*Magnolia salicifolia* (Sieb. et Zucc.) Maxim.（タムシバ）
Magnolia kobus DC.（コブシ）
Magnolia biondii Pamp.*（コブシ）
Magnolia sprengeri Pamp.*（コブシ）
Magnolia heptapeta (Buc'hoz) Dandy（ハクモクレン）
Magnolia denudata Desr.（ハクモクレン）
科名　Magnoliaceae（モクレン科）
英名　*M. salicifolia*：anise magnolia / Japanese willow-leaf magnolia
M. kobus：kobus magnolia
M. biondii, M. sprengeri：magnolia
M. heptapeta（=*M. denudata*）：lilytree / yu lan / yu lan magnolia
Part of use　bud
Note 1　—
Note 2　—
注　—

名　称　ジンコウ*

他名等　—
部位等　材・樹脂
備　考　—

他名(参考)　—

漢字表記・生薬名等　沈香（ジンコウ）
Name (Romaji)　JINKÔ*
Other name (s) (Romaji)　—
学名　*Aquilaria agallocha* Roxb.*
Aquilaria malaccensis Lam.*
Aquilaria crassna Pierre ex Lecomte
Aquilaria sinensis (Lour.) Gilg.*
Aquilaria filaria (Oken) Merr.
科名　Thymelaeaceae（ジンチョウゲ科）
英名　*A. agallocha*, *A. malaccensis*：agar wood / aloes wood
A. sinensis：Chinese agarwood
Part of use　wood, resin
Note 1　—
Note 2　—
注　—

名　称　**スイサイ***

他名等　ミツガシワ
部位等　葉
備　考　—

他名（参考）　—
漢字表記・生薬名等　睡菜（スイサイ）、睡菜葉（スイサイヨウ）、三槲・三柏（ミツガシワ）
Name (Romaji)　SUISAI*
Other name (s) (Romaji)　MITSUGASHIWA
学名　*Menyanthes trifoliata* L.*
科名　Menyanthaceae（ミツガシワ科）
英名　bog bean / bog myrtle / buck bean / marsh trefoil / marsh clover
Part of use　leaf
Note 1　—
Note 2　—
注　—

名　称　**スカルキャップ***

他名等　—
部位等　根
備　考　根以外は「非医」

他名（参考）　タツナミソウ（立浪草）
漢字表記・生薬名等　—
Name (Romaji)　SUKARUKYAPPU*
Other name (s) (Romaji)　—
学名　*Scutellaria lateriflora* L.*
科名　Labiatae（シソ科）
英名　skullcap / blue skullcap / scullcap / mad dog scullcap
Part of use　root
Note 1　whole plant except root：non-drug category
Note 2　—
注　—

名　称　**スズラン***

他名等　—
部位等　全草
備　考　—

他名（参考）　—
漢字表記・生薬名等　鈴蘭（スズラン）
Name (Romaji)　SUZURAN*
Other name (s) (Romaji)　—
学名　*Convallaria majalis* L.*
Convallaria majalis L. var. *keiskei* (Miq.) Makino
Convallaria majalis L. var. *majalis*
科名　Liliaceae（ユリ科）
英名　lily of the valley / European lily of the valley
Part of use　whole plant
Note 1　—
Note 2　—
注　—

名　称　**セイコウ***

他名等　カワラニンジン
部位等　帯果・帯花枝葉
備　考　—

他名（参考）　—
漢字表記・生薬名等　青蒿（セイコウ）、河原人参（カワラニンジン）
Name (Romaji)　SEIKÔ*
Other name (s) (Romaji)　KAWARANINJIN
学名　*Artemisia apiacea* Hance*
Artemisia carvifolia var. *apiacea* (Hance) Pamp.
Artemisia caruifolia Buch.-Ham. ex Roxb.
科名　Compositae（キク科）
英名　Chinese wormwood
Part of use　aerial part with flower or fruit
Note 1　—
Note 2　—
注　—

名　称　セイヨウトチノキ*

他名等　—
部位等　種子
備　考　樹皮・葉・花・芽は「非医」、トチノキの種子は「非医」

他名(参考)　ウマグリ（馬栗）、ヨウシュトチノキ（洋種栃の木）、マロニエ
漢字表記･生薬名等　西洋栃の木（セイヨウトチノキ）
Name (Romaji)　SEIYÔTOCHINOKI*
Other name (s) (Romaji)　—
学名　*Aesculus hippocastanum* L.*
Aesculus hippocastanum f. *memmingeri* (K. Koch) Schelle
科名　Hippocastanaceae（トチノキ科）
英名　horse chestnut / common horse chestnut / European horse chestnut / conker tree / marronier
Part of use　seed
Note 1　bark, leaf, flower, sprout：non-drug category
seed of *Aesculus turbinata*：non-drug category
Note 2　—
注　—

名　称　セイヨウヤドリギ*

他名等　ソウキセイ／ヤドリギ
部位等　枝葉梢・茎・葉
備　考　—

他名(参考)　—
漢字表記･生薬名等　西洋宿木・西洋寄生木（セイヨウヤドリギ）、桑寄生（ソウキセイ）、宿木（ヤドリギ）
Name (Romaji)　SEIYÔYADORIGI*
Other name (s) (Romaji)　SÔKISEI／YADORIGI
学名　*Viscum album* L.*（セイヨウヤドリギ）
Viscum album L. var. *coloratum* (Komar.) Ohwi（ヤドリギ）
科名　Loranthaceae（ヤドリギ科）
英名　European mistletoe / common mistletoe / mistletoe
Part of use　foliage, stem, leaf
Note 1　—
Note 2　—
注　—

名　称　セキサン

他名等　ヒガンバナ／マンジュシャゲ
部位等　鱗茎
備　考　—

他名(参考)　ジゴクバナ（地獄花）
漢字表記･生薬名等　石蒜（セキサン）、彼岸花（ヒガンバナ）、曼珠沙華（マンジュシャゲ）、石蒜根（セキサンコン）
Name (Romaji)　SEKISAN
Other name (s) (Romaji)　HIGANBANA／MANJUSHAGE
学名　*Lycoris radiata* (L'Hér.) Herb.
科名　Amaryllidaceae（ヒガンバナ科）
英名　red spider lily / spider lily / higanbana
Part of use　bulb
Note 1　—
Note 2　—
注　—

名　称　セキショウコン*

他名等　セキショウ
部位等　根茎
備　考　茎は「非医」

他名(参考)　—
漢字表記･生薬名等　石菖根（セキショウコン）、石菖（セキショウ）
Name (Romaji)　SEKISHÔKON*
Other name (s) (Romaji)　SEKISHÔ
学名　*Acorus gramineus* Sol. ex Aiton*
Acorus tatarinowii Schott.*
科名　Araceae（サトイモ科）
英名　grass-leaf sweet flag / grass-leaf calamus / slender sweet flag
Part of use　rhizome
Note 1　stem：non-drug category
Note 2　—
注　—

名　称　セキナンヨウ

他名等　オオカナメモチ／シャクナゲ
部位等　葉
備　考　—

他名(参考)　—
漢字表記･生薬名等　石楠葉（セキナンヨウ）、大要黐（オ

オカナメモチ）、石南花（シャクナゲ）
Name(Romaji)　SEKINAN'YÔ
Other name(s) (Romaji)　ÔKANAMEMOCHI／SHAKUNAGE
学名　*Photinia serrulata* Lindl.（オオカナメモチ）
Rhododendron degronianum Carr.（シャクナゲ）
科名　Rosaceae（バラ科）
Ericaceae（ツツジ科）
英名　*P. serrulata*：low photinia / Chinese hawthorn / Taiwanese photinia
R. degronianum：Yakushima rhododendron
Part of use　leaf
Note 1　—
Note 2　ÔKANAMEMOCHI（*P. serrulata*）：Rosaceae
SHAKUNAGE（*R. degronianum*）：Ericaceae
注　オオカナメモチ（*P. serrulata*）はバラ科、シャクナゲ（*R. degronianum*）はツツジ科。

名　称　セネガ*

他名等　ヒロハセネガ
部位等　根
備　考　—

他名(参考)　—
漢字表記・生薬名等　セネガ、広葉セネガ（ヒロハセネガ）
Name(Romaji)　SENEGA*
Other name(s) (Romaji)　HIROHASENEGA
学名　*Polygala senega* L. var. *latifolia* Torrey et Gray（ヒロハセネガ）
Polygala senega L.*（セネガ）
科名　Polygalaceae（ヒメハギ科）
英名　seneca snakeroot / senega snakeroot / senega root
Part of use　root
Note 1　—
Note 2　—
注　—

名　称　センキュウ*

他名等　—
部位等　根茎
備　考　葉は「非医」

他名(参考)　ブキュウ（撫芎）
漢字表記・生薬名等　川芎・川窮・芎窮（センキュウ）
Name(Romaji)　SENKYÛ*
Other name(s) (Romaji)　—
学名　*Cnidium officinale* Makino*
Ligusticum ibukiense Yabe*
Ligusticum chuanxiong Hort.*
科名　Umbelliferae（セリ科）
英名　senkyu
Part of use　rhizome
Note 1　leaf：non-drug category
Note 2　—
注　—

名　称　ゼンコ*

他名等　—
部位等　根
備　考　—

他名(参考)　ノダケ（野竹）
漢字表記・生薬名等　前胡（ゼンコ）
Name(Romaji)　ZENKO*
Other name(s) (Romaji)　—
学名　*Peucedanum praeruptorum* Dunn*
Peucedanum decursivum（Miq.）Maxim.*
Angelica decrursiva（Miq.）Franch. et Sav.
科名　Umbelliferae（セリ科）
英名　peucedanum / hog fennel
Part of use　root
Note 1　—
Note 2　—
注　—

名　称　センコツ

他名等　コウホネ
部位等　根茎
備　考　茎は「非医」

他名(参考)　—
漢字表記・生薬名等　川骨（センコツ）、河骨（コウホネ）
Name(Romaji)　SENKOTSU
Other name(s) (Romaji)　KÔHONE
学名　*Nuphar japonicum* DC.
科名　Nymphaeaceae（スイレン科）
英名　ko-hone
Part of use　rhizome
Note 1　stem：non-drug category
Note 2　—
注　—

名　称　**センソウ<茜草>***

他名等　**アカネ／アカミノアカネ／セイソウ**
部位等　根
備　考　センソウ<仙草>の全草は「非医」

他名(参考)　—
漢字表記･生薬名等　茜草（センソウ、セイソウ、アカミノアカネ)、赤根（アカネ)、茜草根（センソウコン、セイソウコン）
Name(Romaji)　SENSÔ*
Other name(s) (Romaji)　AKANE／AKAMINOAKANE／SEISÔ
学名　*Rubia akane* Nakai
Rubia cordifolia L.*
科名　Rubiaceae（アカネ科）
英名　Indian madder / Bengal madder
Part of use　root
Note 1　whole plant of *Mesona chinensis* or *Mesona procumbens*：non-drug category
Note 2　—
注　—

名　称　**センナ***

他名等　**アレキサンドリア・センナ／チンネベリ・センナ**
部位等　果実・小葉・葉柄・葉軸
備　考　茎は「非医」

他名(参考)　—
漢字表記･生薬名等　センナ実（センナジツ)、番瀉葉（バンシャヨウ、チンネベリ・センナ）
Name(Romaji)　SENNA*
Other name(s) (Romaji)　AREKISANDORIA・SENNA／CHINNEBERI・SENNA
学名　*Cassia acutifolia* Delile*
Cassia angustifolia Vahl*
Senna alexandrina Mill. *
科名　Leguminosae（マメ科）
英名　senna / Alexandrian senna / Tinnevelly senna / true senna / Indian senna
Part of use　fruit, leaf, petiole, lamina
Note 1　stem：non-drug category
Note 2　—
注　—

名　称　**センダン***

他名等　**クレンシ／クレンピ／トキワセンダン／Melia azedarach**
部位等　果実・樹皮
備　考　葉は「非医」、トウセンダン（Melia toosendan）の果実・樹皮は「医」

他名(参考)　—
漢字表記･生薬名等　楝檀（センダン)、苦楝子（クレンシ)、苦楝皮（クレンピ)、常盤楝檀（トキワセンダン）
Name(Romaji)　SENDAN*
Other name(s) (Romaji)　KURENSHI／KURENPI／TOKIWASENDAN
学名　*Melia azedarach* L.*
Melia toosendan Sieb. et Zucc.*
科名　Meliaceae（センダン科）
英名　Indian lilac / melia / Persian lilac / Chinaberry / China tree / pagoda tree
Part of use　fruit, bark
Note 1　leaf：non-drug category
fruit and bark of *Melia toosendan*：drug category
Note 2　—
注　—

名　称　**センプクカ***

他名等　**オグルマ**
部位等　花
備　考　—

他名(参考)　—
漢字表記･生薬名等　旋覆花（センプクカ)、小車（オグルマ）
Name(Romaji)　SENPUKUKA*
Other name(s) (Romaji)　OGURUMA
学名　*Inula britannica* L. ssp. *japonica*（Thunb.）Kitam.
Inula britannica var. *japonica*（Thunb.）Franch. et Sav.*
科名　Compositae（キク科）
英名　British elecampane / Japanese elecampane / British inula
Part of use　flower
Note 1　—
Note 2　—
注　—

名　称　**センブリ**

他名等　トウヤク
部位等　全草
備　考　—

他名(参考)　—
漢字表記・生薬名等　千振（センブリ）、当薬（トウヤク）
Name(Romaji)　SENBURI
Other name(s)(Romaji)　TÔYAKU
学名　*Swertia japonica* Makino
Swertia japonica (Schult.) Makino
Ophelia japonica (Schult.) Griseb.
科名　Gentianaeceae（リンドウ科）
英名　senburi
Part of use　whole plant
Note 1　—
Note 2　—
注　—

名　称　**ソウカ***

他名等　—
部位等　果実
備　考　—

他名(参考)　—
漢字表記・生薬名等　草菓（ソウカ）
Name(Romaji)　SÔKA*
Other name(s)(Romaji)　—
学名　*Amomum tsao-ko* Crevost et Lemarié*
科名　Zingiberaceae（ショウガ科）
英名　tsaoko amomum / tsao ko / cao guo
Part of use　fruit
Note 1　—
Note 2　—
注　—

名　称　**ソウシシ***

他名等　トウアズキ
部位等　種子
備　考　—

他名(参考)　—
漢字表記・生薬名等　相思子（ソウシシ）、唐小豆（トウアズキ）
Name(Romaji)　SÔSHISHI*
Other name(s)(Romaji)　TÔAZUKI
学名　*Abrus precatorius* L.*
Glycine abrus L.
科名　Leguminosae（マメ科）
英名　precatory / jequirity / Indian licorice / rosary pea / crab's eye
Part of use　seed
Note 1　—
Note 2　—
注　—

名　称　**ソウジシ**

他名等　オナモミ
部位等　果実
備　考　—

他名(参考)　—
漢字表記・生薬名等　蒼耳子（ソウジシ）、菜耳（オナモミ）
Name(Romaji)　SÔJISHI
Other name(s)(Romaji)　ONAMOMI
学名　*Xanthium strumarium* L.
科名　Compositae（キク科）
英名　California bur / Canada cocklebur / Siberian cocklebur / cocklebur
Part of use　fruit
Note 1　—
Note 2　—
注　—

名　称　**ソウジュツ***

他名等　ホソバオケラ
部位等　根茎
備　考　—

他名(参考)　—
漢字表記・生薬名等　蒼朮（ソウジュツ）、細葉朮（ホソバオケラ）
Name(Romaji)　SÔJUTSU*
Other name(s)(Romaji)　HOSOBAOKERA
学名　*Atractylodes lancea* (Thunb.) DC.*
Atractylodes chinensis (Bunge) Koidz.*
科名　Compositae（キク科）
英名　cang-zhu atractylodes / southern tsangshu
Part of use　rhizome
Note 1　—
Note 2　—
注　—

名　称　**ソウハクヒ***

他名等　**クワ／マグワ**
部位等　根皮
備　考　葉・花・実（集合果）は「非医」

他名(参考)　—
漢字表記・生薬名等　桑白皮（ソウハクヒ）、桑（クワ）、真桑（マグワ）、桑根白皮（ソウコンハクヒ）
Name (Romaji)　SÔHAKUHI*
Other name (s) (Romaji)　KUWA／MAGUWA
学名　*Morus alba* L.*
科名　Moraceae（クワ科）
英名　white mulberry
Part of use　root bark
Note 1　leaf, flower, fruit (aggregate fruit) : non-drug category
Note 2　—
注　—

名　称　**ソテツ**

他名等　—
部位等　種子
備　考　—

他名(参考)　—
漢字表記・生薬名等　蘇鉄（ソテツ）、蘇鉄子（ソテツシ）、蘇鉄実（ソテツジツ）
Name (Romaji)　SOTETSU
Other name (s) (Romaji)　—
学名　*Cycas revoluta* Thunb.
科名　Cycadaceae（ソテツ科）
英名　Japanese sago palm / Japanese fern palm / sago cycas / sotetsu nut
Part of use　seed
Note 1　—
Note 2　—
注　—

名　称　**ソボク***

他名等　**スオウ**
部位等　心材
備　考　—

他名(参考)　—
漢字表記・生薬名等　蘇木（ソボク）、蘇芳（スオウ）
Name (Romaji)　SOBOKU*
Other name (s) (Romaji)　SUÔ
学名　*Caesalpinia sappan* L.*
科名　Leguminosae（マメ科）
英名　sappan wood / sappan lignum / Brazil wood / Indian red wood / Japan wood
Part of use　heart wood
Note 1　—
Note 2　—
注　—

タ行

名　称　**ダイオウ***

他名等　**ヤクヨウダイオウ**
部位等　根茎
備　考　葉は「非医」

他名(参考)　—
漢字表記・生薬名等　大黄（ダイオウ）、薬用大黄（ヤクヨウダイオウ）
Name (Romaji)　DAIÔ*
Other name (s) (Romaji)　YAKUYÔDAIÔ
学名　*Rheum palmatum* L.*
Rheum tanguticum Maxim. ex Balf.*
Rheum officinale Baill.*
Rheum coreanum Nakai
科名　Polygonaceae（タデ科）
英名　Chinese rhubarb / Tibetan rhubarb / Turkey rhubarb / ornamental rhubarb
Part of use　rhizome
Note 1　leaf : non-drug category
Note 2　—
注　—

名　称　**ダイフクヒ***

他名等　**ビンロウ**
部位等　果皮
備　考　種子は「非医」

他名(参考)　—
漢字表記・生薬名等　大腹皮（ダイフクヒ）、檳榔（ビンロウ）、檳榔皮（ビンロウヒ）
Name (Romaji)　DAIFUKUHI*
Other name (s) (Romaji)　BINRÔ
学名　*Areca catechu* L.*
科名　Palmae（ヤシ科）
英名　catechu / betel palm / betelnut palm / areca nut

Part of use　pericarp
Note 1　seed：non-drug category
Note 2　—
注　—

名　称　**タクシャ***

他名等　サジオモダカ
部位等　塊茎
備　考　—

他名(参考)　—
漢字表記・生薬名等　澤瀉（タクシャ）、匙面高（サジオモダカ）
Name(Romaji)　TAKUSHA*
Other name(s) (Romaji)　SAJIOMODAKA
学名　*Alisma orientale* (Sam.) Juz.*
　　Alisma plantago-aquatica L. var. *orientale* Sam.*
科名　Alismataceae（オモダカ科）
英名　Asian water plantain
Part of use　tuber
Note 1　—
Note 2　—
注　—

名　称　**ダミアナ***

他名等　—
部位等　葉
備　考　—

他名(参考)　—
漢字表記・生薬名等　ダミアナ
Name(Romaji)　DAMIANA*
Other name(s) (Romaji)　—
学名　*Turnera diffusa* Willd. ex Schult.*
　　Turnera microphylla Ham.
科名　Turneraceae（トルネア科）
英名　damiana / Mexican holly
Part of use　leaf
Note 1　—
Note 2　—
注　—

名　称　**タユヤ***

他名等　—
部位等　根
備　考　—

他名(参考)　—
漢字表記・生薬名等　—
Name(Romaji)　TAYUYA*
Other name(s) (Romaji)　—
学名　*Cayaponia tayuya* (Vell.) Cogn.*
　　Trianosperma tayuya (Vell.) Mart.*
　　Bryonia tayuya Vell.
科名　Cucurbitaceae（ウリ科）
英名　tayuya
Part of use　root
Note 1　—
Note 2　—
注　—

名　称　**タンジン***

他名等　—
部位等　根
備　考　葉は「非医」

他名(参考)　—
漢字表記・生薬名等　丹参（タンジン）、木乳羊（モクニュウヨウ）
Name(Romaji)　TANJIN*
Other name(s) (Romaji)　—
学名　*Salvia miltiorrhiza* Bunge*
科名　Labiatae（シソ科）
英名　Chinese salvia / Chinese sage / red-root sage / dan shen
Part of use　root
Note 1　leaf：non-drug category
Note 2　—
注　—

名　称　**チクジョ**

他名等　—
部位等　稈の内層
備　考　—

他名(参考)　ハチク（葉竹）、マダケ（真竹）
漢字表記・生薬名等　竹茹（チクジョ）
Name(Romaji)　CHIKUJO
Other name(s) (Romaji)　—

学名　*Bambusa tuldoides* Munro
Phyllostachys nigra Munro var. *henonis* Stapf ex Rendl.
Phyllostachys bambusoides Sieb. et Zucc.
Bambusa spp.
Dendrocalamus spp.
科名　Gramineae（イネ科）
英名　bamboo / henon bamboo / black bamboo
Part of use　caulis
Note 1　—
Note 2　—
注　—

名　称　**チクセツニンジン***

他名等　トチバニンジン
部位等　根茎
備　考　—

他名（参考）　—
漢字表記・生薬名等　竹節人参（チクセツニンジン）、栃葉人参（トチバニンジン）
Name (Romaji)　CHIKUSETSUNINJIN*
Other name (s) (Romaji)　TOCHIBANINJIN
学名　*Panax japonicus* (T. Nees) C.A. Mey.*
Panax pseudoginseng Wall. var. *japonicus* (C.A. Mey.) G. Hoo et C.J. Tseng*
科名　Araliaceae（ウコギ科）
英名　Japanese ginseng / bamboo ginseng
Part of use　rhizome
Note 1　—
Note 2　—
注　—

名　称　**チノスポラ・コルディフォリア***

他名等　Tinospora cordifolia
部位等　全草
備　考　—

他名（参考）　イボツヅラフジ（疣葛藤）
漢字表記・生薬名等　—
Name (Romaji)　CHINOSUPORA・KORUDIFORIA*
Other name (s) (Romaji)　—
学名　*Tinospora cordifolia* (Willd.) Miers ex Hook. f. et Thoms.*
科名　Menispermaceae（ツヅラフジ科）
英名　Indian tinospora / guduchi
Part of use　whole plant
Note 1　—
Note 2　—
注　—

名　称　**チモ***

他名等　ハナスゲ
部位等　根茎
備　考　—

他名（参考）　—
漢字表記・生薬名等　知母（チモ）、花菅（ハナスゲ）
Name (Romaji)　CHIMO*
Other name (s) (Romaji)　HANASUGE
学名　*Anemarrhena asphodeloides* Bunge*
科名　Liliaceae（ユリ科）
英名　anemarrhena
Part of use　rhizome
Note 1　—
Note 2　—
注　—

名　称　**チョウセンアサガオ属***

他名等　チョウセンアサガオ
部位等　種子・葉・花
備　考　—

他名（参考）　—
漢字表記・生薬名等　朝鮮朝顔（チョウセンアサガオ）、曼陀羅花（マンダラゲ）、曼陀羅葉（マンダラヨウ）、曼陀羅子（マンダラシ）、洋金花（ヨウキンカ）、ダツラ葉（ダツラヨウ）
Name (Romaji)　CHÔSEN'ASAGAO-ZOKU*
Other name (s) (Romaji)　CHÔSEN'ASAGAO
学名　*Datura* L.
Datura metel L.*
Datura stramonium L.*
科名　Solanaceae（ナス科）
英名　horn-of-plenty / jimson weed / stramonium / thorn apple / angel's trumpet / devil's trumpet / metel
Part of use　seed, leaf, flower
Note 1　—
Note 2　—
注　—

名　称　**チョウトウコウ***

他名等　カギカズラ／トウカギカズラ
部位等　とげ
備　考　葉は「非医」

他名(参考)　—
漢字表記・生薬名等　釣藤鈎（チョウトウコウ）、鈎葛（カギカズラ）、唐鈎葛（トウカギカズラ）
Name(Romaji)　CHÔTÔKÔ*
Other name(s)(Romaji)　KAGIKAZURA／TÔKAGI-KAZURA
学名　*Uncaria rhynchophylla* (Miq.) Jacks.*
Uncaria sinensis (Oliv.) Havil
Uncaria macrophylla Wall.
科名　Rubiaceae（アカネ科）
英名　uncaria rhynchohylla / gambir
Part of use　thorn
Note 1　leaf：non-drug category
Note 2　—
注　—

名　称　**チョレイ***

他名等　チョレイマイタケ
部位等　菌核
備　考　—

他名(参考)　—
漢字表記・生薬名等　猪苓（チョレイ）、猪苓舞茸（チョレイマイタケ）
Name(Romaji)　CHOREI*
Other name(s)(Romaji)　CHOREIMAITAKE
学名　*Polyporus umbellatus* (Pers.) Fr.*
Grifola umbellata (Pers.：Fr.) Pilát*
科名　Polyporaceae（サルノコシカケ科）
英名　zhu ling
Part of use　sclerotium
Note 1　—
Note 2　—
注　—

名　称　**デンドロビウム属***

他名等　セッコク／ホンセッコク／Dendrobium属
部位等　茎
備　考　—

他名(参考)　—
漢字表記・生薬名等　石斛（セッコク）
Name(Romaji)　DENDOROBIUMU-ZOKU*
Other name(s)(Romaji)　SEKKOKU／HONSEKKOKU
学名　*Dendrobium* Sw.
Dendrobium officinale K. Kimura et Migo*（ホンセッコク）
科名　Orchidaceae（ラン科）
英名　dendrobium / Chinese orchid
Part of use　stem
Note 1　—
Note 2　—
注　—

名　称　**テンナンショウ***

他名等　—
部位等　塊茎
備　考　—

他名(参考)　マイヅルテンナンショウ（異葉天南星、舞鶴天南星）
漢字表記・生薬名等　天南星（テンナンショウ）
Name(Romaji)　TENNANSHÔ*
Other name(s)(Romaji)　—
学名　*Arisaema heterophyllum* Blume*
Arisaema erubescens (Wall.) Schott.*
Arisaema amurense Maxim.*
Arisaema serratum (Thunb.) Schott.*
科名　Araceae（サトイモ科）
英名　Chinese arisaema / Japanese arisaema
Part of use　tuber
Note 1　—
Note 2　—
注　—

名　称　**テンマ***

他名等　オニノヤガラ
部位等　塊茎
備　考　—

他名(参考)　—
漢字表記・生薬名等　天麻（テンマ）、鬼矢柄（オニノヤガラ）
Name(Romaji)　TENMA*
Other name(s)(Romaji)　ONINOYAGARA
学名　*Gastrodia elata* Blume*
科名　Orchidaceae（ラン科）
英名　gastrodia
Part of use　tuber
Note 1　—

Note 2 —
注 —

名 称 **テンモンドウ***

他名等 クサスギカズラ
部位等 根
備 考 種子・葉・花は「非医」

他名(参考) —
漢字表記・生薬名等 天門冬（テンモンドウ）、草杉葛（クサスギカズラ）
Name (Romaji) TENMONDÔ*
Other name (s) (Romaji) KUSASUGIKAZURA
学名 *Asparagus cochinchinensis* (Lour.) Merr.*
科名 Liliaceae（ユリ科）
英名 Chinese asparagus
Part of use root
Note 1 seed, leaf, flower：non-drug category
Note 2 —
注 —

名 称 **トウガシ***

他名等 トウガ
部位等 種子
備 考 果実は「非医」

他名(参考) トウカニン（冬瓜仁）、ハクカシ（白瓜子）、カモウリ（氈瓜）、チョウセンウリ（朝鮮瓜）
漢字表記・生薬名等 冬瓜子（トウガシ）、冬瓜（トウガ）、冬瓜仁（トウカニン）
Name (Romaji) TÔGASHI*
Other name (s) (Romaji) TÔGA
学名 *Benincasa hispida* (Thunb.) Cogn.*
Benincasa cerifera Savi.*
Benincasa cerifera Savi. f. *emarginata* K. Kimura et Sugiyama
Cucurbita hispida Thunb.
科名 Cucurbitaceae（ウリ科）
英名 winter melon / wax gourd / white pumpkin / white gourd
Part of use seed
Note 1 fruit：non-drug category
Note 2 —
注 —

名 称 **トウキ***

他名等 オニノダケ／カラトウキ
部位等 根
備 考 葉は「非医」

他名(参考) —
漢字表記・生薬名等 当帰（トウキ）、鬼土当帰（オニノダケ）、唐当帰（カラトウキ）
Name (Romaji) TÔKI*
Other name (s) (Romaji) ONINODAKE／KARATÔKI
学名 *Angelica acutiloba* (Sieb. et Zucc.) Kitag.（トウキ）
Angelica acutiloba (Sieb. et Zucc.) Kitag. var. *sugiyamae* Hikino（ホッカイトウキ）
Angelica sinensis (Oliv.) Diels*（カラトウキ）
Angelica gigas Nakai（オニノダケ）
科名 Umbelliferae（セリ科）
英名 dong quai / Chinese angelica
Part of use root
Note 1 leaf：non-drug category
Note 2 —
注 —

名 称 **トウジン***

他名等 ヒカゲノツルニンジン
部位等 根
備 考 —

他名(参考) —
漢字表記・生薬名等 党参（トウジン）、日陰蔓人参（ヒカゲノツルニンジン）
Name (Romaji) TÔJIN*
Other name (s) (Romaji) HIKAGENOTSURUNINJIN
学名 *Codonopsis pilosula* (Franch.) Nannf.*（ヒカゲノツルニンジン）
Codonopsis silvestris Kom.*（ヒカゲノツルニンジン）
Codonopsis pilosula Nannf. var. *modesta* (Nannf.) L.T. Shen（トウジン）
Codonopsis tangshen Oliv.*（トウジン）
科名 Campanulaceae（キキョウ科）
英名 codonopsis / bellflower / Sichuan dang shen
Part of use root
Note 1 —
Note 2 —
注 —

名　称　**トウシンソウ***

他名等　**イ／イグサ／Juncus effusus**
部位等　全草
備　考　地上部の熱水抽出（100℃ 8 分以上又は同等以上の方法）後の残渣は「非医」

他名(参考)　—
漢字表記･生薬名等　灯心草・燈芯草（トウシンソウ）、藺（イ）、藺草（イグサ）
Name(Romaji)　TÔSHINSÔ*
Other name(s) (Romaji)　I／IGUSA
学名　*Juncus effusus* L.*
Juncus effusus L. var. *decipiens* Buchenau
Juncus decipiens (Buchenau) Nakai
科名　Juncaceae（イグサ科）
英名　soft rush / bulrush / lamp rush
Part of use　whole plant
Note 1　residue of boiled water extraction of aerial part (longer than 8minutes at 100℃ or equivalent methods)：non-drug category
Note 2　—
注　—

名　称　**トウセンダン***

他名等　**クレンシ／クレンピ／センレンシ／Melia toosendan**
部位等　果実・樹皮
備　考　センダン(Melia azedarach)の果実・樹皮は「医」、センダン(Melia azedarach)の葉は「非医」

他名(参考)　—
漢字表記･生薬名等　唐栴檀（トウセンダン）、苦楝子（クレンシ）、苦楝皮（クレンピ）、川楝子（センレンシ）
Name(Romaji)　TÔSENDAN*
Other name(s) (Romaji)　KURENSHI／KURENPI／SENRENSHI
学名　*Melia toosendan* Sieb. et Zucc.*（トウセンダン）
Melia azedarach L.*（センダン）
科名　Meliaceae（センダン科）
英名　melia / China berry / China tree / pagoda tree / Persian lilac / pride-of-India / pride-of-China
Part of use　fruit, bark
Note 1　fruit and bark of *Melia azedarach*：drug category
leaf of *Melia azedarach*：non-drug category
Note 2　—
注　—

名　称　**トウニン***

他名等　—
部位等　種子
備　考　葉・花は「非医」

他名(参考)　—
漢字表記･生薬名等　桃仁（トウニン）
Name(Romaji)　TÔNIN*
Other name(s) (Romaji)　—
学名　*Prunus persica* (L.) Batsch*（モモ）
Amygdalus persica L.*（モモ）
Prunus persica (L.) Batsch var. *davidiana* (Carrière) Maxim.（ノモモ）
Prunus davidiana (Carrière) Franch.（ノモモ）
Prunus vulgaris Mill.*（モモ）
科名　Rosaceae（バラ科）
英名　peach
Part of use　seed
Note 1　leaf, flower：non-drug category
Note 2　—
注　—

名　称　**トウリョウソウ**

他名等　—
部位等　全草
備　考　—

他名(参考)　—
漢字表記･生薬名等　冬凌草（トウリョウソウ）
Name(Romaji)　TÔRYÔSÔ
Other name(s) (Romaji)　—
学名　*Rabdosia rubescens* (Hemsl.) Hara
Isodon rubescens (Hemsl.) Hara
科名　Labiatae（シソ科）
英名　blushred rabdosia / isodon rubescens
Part of use　whole plant
Note 1　—
Note 2　—
注　—

名　称　**ドクカツ***

他名等　ウド／ドッカツ／Aralia cordata
部位等　根茎
備　考　軟化茎は「非医」、シシウド（Angelica pubescens／Angelica bisserata）の根茎・軟化茎は「非医」

他名(参考)　シシウド（猪独活）、トウドクカツ（唐独活）
漢字表記･生薬名等　独活（ドクカツ、ウド、ドッカツ）
Name (Romaji)　DOKUKATSU*
Other name (s) (Romaji)　UDO／DOKKATSU
学名　*Aralia cordata* Thunb.（ウド、和独活、韓独活）
Angelica pubescens Maxim.*（シシウド、香独活）
Angelica laxiflora Diels（川独活）
Angelica megaphylla Diels（川独活）
科名　Araliaceae（ウコギ科）
Umbelliferae（セリ科）
英名　*Aralia cordata*：Japanese asparagus / Japanese spikenard / spikenard / udo
Angelica pubescens：pubescent angelica
Part of use　rhizome
Note 1　soft stem：non-drug category
rhizome and soft stem of *Angelica pubescens*（= *Angelica bisserata*）：non-drug category
Note 2　UDO（*Aralia cordata*）：Araliaceae
SHISHIUDO（*Angelica pubescens*）：Umbelliferae.
注　ウド（*Aralia cordata*）はウコギ科、シシウド（*Angelica pubescens*）はセリ科。

名　称　**トシシ***

他名等　ネナシカズラ／マメダオシ
部位等　種子
備　考　—

他名(参考)　—
漢字表記･生薬名等　菟絲子（トシシ）、根無葛（ネナシカズラ）、豆倒し（マメダオシ）
Name (Romaji)　TOSHISHI*
Other name (s) (Romaji)　NENASHIKAZURA／MAMEDAOSHI
学名　*Cuscuta japonica* Chois.*（ネナシカズラ）
Cuscuta epilinum Weihe（ネナシカズラ）
Cuscuta chinensis Lam.*（ハマネナシカズラ）
Cuscuta australis R. Br.*（マメダオシ）
科名　Convolvulaceae（ヒルガオ科）
英名　*C. japonica*：Japanese dodder / Japanese cuscuta
C. chinensis：Chinese dodder / Chinese cuscuta / Japanese cuscuta
Part of use　seed
Note 1　—
Note 2　—
注　—

名　称　**トチュウ***

他名等　—
部位等　樹皮
備　考　果実・葉・葉柄・木部は「非医」

他名(参考)　—
漢字表記･生薬名等　杜仲（トチュウ）
Name (Romaji)　TOCHÛ*
Other name (s) (Romaji)　—
学名　*Eucommia ulmoides* Oliv.*
科名　Eucommiaceae（トチュウ科）
英名　eucommia / Chinese gutta percha / Chinese rubber tree / hardy rubber tree
Part of use　bark
Note 1　fruit, leaf, petiole, xylem：non-drug category
Note 2　—
注　—

名　称　**ドモッコウ***

他名等　オオグルマ
部位等　根
備　考　—

他名(参考)　—
漢字表記･生薬名等　土木香（ドモッコウ）、大車（オオグルマ）
Name (Romaji)　DOMOKKÔ*
Other name (s) (Romaji)　ÔGURUMA
学名　*Inula helenium* L.*
科名　Compositae（キク科）
英名　elecampane / velvet dock / scabwort
Part of use　root
Note 1　—
Note 2　—
注　—

名　称　**トリカブト属**

他名等　トリカブト／ブシ／ヤマトリカブト
部位等　塊根
備　考　—

他名(参考)　—

漢字表記・生薬名等　鳥兜（トリカブト）、附子（ブシ）、山鳥兜（ヤマトリカブト）
Name (Romaji)　TORIKABUTO-ZOKU
Other name (s) (Romaji)　TORIKABUTO／BUSHI／YAMATORIKABUTO
学名　*Aconitum* L.
科名　Ranunculaceae（キンポウゲ科）
英名　aconite / monkshood / wolfbane
Part of use　root tuber
Note 1　—
Note 2　—
注　—

ナ行

名　称　ナンテンジツ*

他名等　シロミナンテン／ナンテン
部位等　果実
備　考　—

他名（参考）　—
漢字表記・生薬名等　南天実（ナンテンジツ）、白実南天（シロミナンテン）、南天（ナンテン）
Name (Romaji)　NANTENJITSU*
Other name (s) (Romaji)　SHIROMINANTEN／NANTEN
学名　*Nandina domestica* Thunb.*（ナンテン）
Nandina domestica Thunb. f. *leucocarpa* Makino（シロミナンテン、シロナンテン）
科名　Berberidaceae（メギ科）
英名　nandina / Chinese bamboo / heavenly bamboo / sacred bamboo / southern heaven bamboo
Part of use　fruit
Note 1　—
Note 2　—
注　—

名　称　ニガキ

他名等　—
部位等　木部（樹皮除く）
備　考　—

他名（参考）　—
漢字表記・生薬名等　苦木（ニガキ）
Name (Romaji)　NIGAKI
Other name (s) (Romaji)　—
学名　*Picrasma quassioides* (D. Don) Benn.
Picrasma ailanthoides (Bunge) Planch.
科名　Simaroubaceae（ニガキ科）
英名　nigaki / shurni
Part of use　xylem (except bark)
Note 1　—
Note 2　—
注　—

名　称　ニチニチソウ*

他名等　—
部位等　全草
備　考　—

他名（参考）　—
漢字表記・生薬名等　日々草（ニチニチソウ）
Name (Romaji)　NICHINICHISÔ*
Other name (s) (Romaji)　—
学名　*Vinca rosea* L.*
Catharanthus roseus (L.) G. Don*
科名　Apocynaceae（キョウチクトウ科）
英名　Madagascar periwinkle / old maid / rose periwinkle / rosy periwinkle / bright eyes
Part of use　whole plant
Note 1　—
Note 2　—
注　—

ハ行

名　称　バイケイソウ属

他名等　コバイケイソウ／シュロソウ／バイケイソウ
部位等　全草
備　考　—

他名（参考）　—
漢字表記・生薬名等　梅蕙草（バイケイソウ）、小梅蕙草（コバイケイソウ）、棕櫚草（シュロソウ）、藜芦根（リロコン）
Name (Romaji)　BAIKEISÔ-ZOKU
Other name (s) (Romaji)　KOBAIKEISÔ／SHUROSÔ／BAIKEISÔ
学名　*Veratrum* L.
Veratrum album L. ssp. *oxysepalum* (Turcz.) Hult.（バイケイソウ）
Veratrum stamineum Maxim.（コバイケイソウ）

Veratrum maackii Regel var. *japonicum* (Baker) T. Shimizu（シュロソウ）
科名 Liliaceae（ユリ科）
英名 hellebore
Part of use whole plant
Note 1 —
Note 2 —
注 —

名　称　バイモ*

他名等 アミガサユリ
部位等 鱗茎
備　考 —

他名(参考) —
漢字表記・生薬名等 貝母（バイモ）、網笠百合（アミガサユリ）
Name(Romaji) BAIMO*
Other name(s) (Romaji) AMIGASAYURI
学名 *Fritillaria verticillata* Willd. var. *thunbergii* (Miq.) Baker
Fritillaria thunbergii Miq.*
科名 Liliaceae（ユリ科）
英名 Zhejiang fritillary
Part of use bulb
Note 1 —
Note 2 —
注 —

名　称　ハクシジン*

他名等 —
部位等 種子
備　考 —

他名(参考) ハクシニン(白子仁)、コノテガシワ(児手柏)、ソクハクヨウ（側柏葉）
漢字表記・生薬名等 柏子仁（ハクシニン、ハクシジン）
Name(Romaji) HAKUSHIJIN*
Other name(s) (Romaji) —
学名 *Thuja orientalis* L.*
Biota orientalis (L.) Endl.*
Platycladus orientalis (L.) Franco*
科名 Cupressaceae（ヒノキ科）
英名 oriental arborvitae
Part of use seed
Note 1 —
Note 2 HAKUSHIJIN is the seed of SOKUHAKUYÔ (*Thuja orientalis* L.). Branch and leaf of SOKUHAKUYÔ are listed in the "non-drug" category. HAKUSHININ but not HAKUSHIJIN is common.
注 ハクシジンはソクハクヨウの種子。ソクハクヨウの枝及び葉は「非医」リストに掲載されている。ハクシジンではなくハクシニンのほうが一般的。

名　称　ハクセンピ*

他名等 —
部位等 根皮
備　考 —

他名(参考) —
漢字表記・生薬名等 白蘚皮（ハクセンピ）
Name(Romaji) HAKUSENPI*
Other name(s) (Romaji) —
学名 *Dictamnus dasycarpus* Turcz.*
科名 Rutaceae（ミカン科）
英名 dense-fruit dittany
Part of use root bark
Note 1 —
Note 2 —
注 —

名　称　ハクトウオウ*

他名等 —
部位等 茎・葉
備　考 —

他名(参考) オキナグサ（翁草）、ヒロハオキナグサ（広葉翁草）
漢字表記・生薬名等 白頭翁（ハクトウオウ）
Name(Romaji) HAKUTÔÔ*
Other name(s) (Romaji) —
学名 *Pulsatilla chinensis* (Bunge) Regel*
科名 Ranunculaceae（キンポウゲ科）
英名 Chinese pulsatilla
Part of use stem, leaf
Note 1 —
Note 2 —
注 —

名　称　ハクトウスギ

他名等　**ウンナンコウトウスギ**
部位等　樹皮・葉
備　考　心材は「非医」

他名(参考)　―
漢字表記・生薬名等　白豆杉（ハクトウスギ）、雲南紅豆杉（ウンナンコウトウスギ）
Name(Romaji)　HAKUTÔSUGI
Other name(s)(Romaji)　UNNANKÔTÔSUGI
学名　*Pseudotaxus chienii*（W.C. Cheng）W.C. Cheng（ハクトウスギ）
Taxus yunnanensis W.C. Cheng et L.K. Fu（ウンナンコウトウスギ）
Taxus wallichiana Zucc. var. *wallichiana*（ウンナンコウトウスギ）
科名　Taxaceae（イチイ科）
英名　*P. chienii*：white berry yew
T. yunnanensis：Himalayan yew
Part of use　bark, leaf
Note 1　heart wood：non-drug category
Note 2　―
注　―

名　称　バクモンドウ*

他名等　**コヤブラン／ジャノヒゲ／ヤブラン／リュウノヒゲ**
部位等　根の膨大部
備　考　―

他名(参考)　カツヨウバクトウ（闊葉麦冬）
漢字表記・生薬名等　麦門冬（バクモンドウ）、小藪蘭（コヤブラン）、蛇の髭（ジャノヒゲ）、藪蘭（ヤブラン）、龍の髭（リュウノヒゲ）
Name(Romaji)　BAKUMONDÔ*
Other name(s)(Romaji)　KOYABURAN／JANOHIGE／YABURAN／RYÛNOHIGE
学名　*Liriope spicata* Lour.（コヤブラン）
Liriope muscari Bailey（ヤブラン）
Ophiopogon japonicus（L. f.）Ker Gawl.*（ジャノヒゲ）
Ophiopogon ohwii Okuyama（ナガバノジャノヒゲ）
科名　Liliaceae（ユリ科）
英名　creeping lilyturf / ophiopogon / snake's beard / dwarf lilyturf / mond grass
Part of use　root tuber
Note 1　―
Note 2　―
注　―

名　称　ハゲキテン*

他名等　**―**
部位等　根
備　考　―

他名(参考)　―
漢字表記・生薬名等　巴戟天（ハゲキテン）
Name(Romaji)　HAGEKITEN*
Other name(s)(Romaji)　―
学名　*Morinda officinalis* F.C. How*
科名　Rubiaceae（アカネ科）
英名　morinda
Part of use　root
Note 1　―
Note 2　―
注　―

名　称　ハシリドコロ属*

他名等　**ハシリドコロ／ロート根**
部位等　根
備　考　―

他名(参考)　ロート（莨菪）
漢字表記・生薬名等　走野老（ハシリドコロ）、莨菪根（ロートコン）
Name(Romaji)　HASHIRIDOKORO-ZOKU*
Other name(s)(Romaji)　HASHIRIDOKORO／RÔTOKON
学名　*Scopolia* Jacq.
Scopolia japonica Maxim.（ロート根）
Scopolia carniolica Jacq.*（ロート根）
Scopolia parviflora（Dunn）Nakai（ロート根）
科名　Solanaceae（ナス科）
英名　scopolia / Russian belladonna
Part of use　root
Note 1　―
Note 2　―
注　―

名　称　ハズ*

他名等　**―**
部位等　種子
備　考　―

他名(参考)　―
漢字表記・生薬名等　巴豆（ハズ）
Name(Romaji)　HAZU*

Other name(s) (Romaji)　—
学名　*Croton tiglium* L.*
科名　Euphorbiaceae（トウダイグサ科）
英名　purging croton / croton oil plant
Part of use　seed
Note 1　—
Note 2　—
注　—

名　称　**ハルマラ***

他名等　—
部位等　全草・種子
備　考　—

他名（参考）　—
漢字表記・生薬名等　ハルマラ
Name (Romaji)　HARUMARA*
Other name(s) (Romaji)　—
学名　*Peganum harmala* L.*
科名　Zygophyllaceae（ハマビシ科）
英名　hermal / Syrian rue / African rue / wild rue / foreign henna
Part of use　whole plant, seed
Note 1　—
Note 2　—
注　—

名　称　**ハンゲ***

他名等　カラスビシャク
部位等　塊茎
備　考　—

他名（参考）　—
漢字表記・生薬名等　半夏（ハンゲ）、烏柄杓（カラスビシャク）
Name (Romaji)　HANGE*
Other name(s) (Romaji)　KARASUBISHAKU
学名　*Pinellia ternata* (Thunb.) Makino ex Breitenb.*
科名　Araceae（サトイモ科）
英名　pinellia / pinellia root
Part of use　tuber
Note 1　—
Note 2　—
注　—

名　称　**ヒマシ油***

他名等　トウゴマ／ヒマ
部位等　種子油
備　考　—

他名（参考）　—
漢字表記・生薬名等　蓖麻子油（ヒマシユ）、唐胡麻（トウゴマ）、蓖麻（ヒマ）
Name (Romaji)　HIMASHI-YU*
Other name(s) (Romaji)　TÔGOMA／HIMA
学名　*Ricinus communis* L.*
科名　Euphorbiaceae（トウダイグサ科）
英名　castor bean / castor oil plant / palma christi
Part of use　seed oil
Note 1　—
Note 2　—
注　—

名　称　**ビャクシ***

他名等　ヨロイグサ
部位等　根
備　考　—

他名（参考）　—
漢字表記・生薬名等　白芷（ビャクシ）、鎧草（ヨロイグサ）
Name (Romaji)　BYAKUSHI*
Other name(s) (Romaji)　YOROIGUSA
学名　*Angelica dahurica* (Hoffm.) Benth. et Hook. f. ex Franch. et Sav.*
科名　Umbelliferae（セリ科）
英名　fragrant angelica / Dahurian angelica
Part of use　root
Note 1　—
Note 2　—
注　—

名　称　**ビャクジュツ***

他名等　オオバナオケラ／オケラ
部位等　根茎
備　考　—

他名（参考）　—
漢字表記・生薬名等　白朮（ビャクジュツ）、大花朮（オオバナオケラ）、朮（オケラ）
Name (Romaji)　BYAKUJUTSU*
Other name(s) (Romaji)　ÔBANAOKERA／OKERA
学名　*Atractylodes ovata* (Thunb.) DC.*（オオバナオケ

ラ）
Atractylodes macrocephala Koidz.*（オオバナオケラ）
Atractylodes japonica Koidz. ex Kitam.（オケラ）
科名 Compositae（キク科）
英名 Cang'zhu atractylodes / bai-zhu atractylodes
Part of use rhizome
Note 1 —
Note 2 —
注 —

名　称 **ビャクダン***

他名等 —
部位等 心材・油
備　考 —

他名（参考） —
漢字表記・生薬名等 白壇（ビャクダン）、壇香（ダンコウ）、沈香（ジンコウ）
Name（Romaji） BYAKUDAN*
Other name（s）（Romaji） —
学名 *Santalum album* L.*
科名 Santalaceae（ビャクダン科）
英名 sandalwood / white sandalwood / yellow sandalwood / East Indian sandalwood / white saunders / yellow saunders
Part of use heart wood, oil
Note 1 —
Note 2 —
注 —

名　称 **ビャクブ***

他名等 —
部位等 肥大根
備　考 —

他名（参考） —
漢字表記・生薬名等 百部（ビャクブ）
Name（Romaji） BYAKUBU*
Other name（s）（Romaji） —
学名 *Stemona japonica*（Blume）Miq.*（タチビャクブ）
Stemona sessilifolia（Miq.）Franch. et Sav.*（ツルビャクブ）
Stemona tuberosa Lour.*（タマビャクブ）
科名 Stemonaeceae（ビャクブ科）
英名 stemona / Japanese stemona / sessile stemona / tuberous stemona
Part of use succulent root
Note 1 —
Note 2 —
注 —

名　称 **ヒュウガトウキ**

他名等 Angelica furcijuga
部位等 根
備　考 —

他名（参考） ニホンヤマニンジン（日本山人参）、ウズ
漢字表記・生薬名等 日向当帰（ヒュウガトウキ）
Name（Romaji） HYÛGATÔKI
Other name（s）（Romaji） —
学名 *Angelica furcijuga* Kitag.
Angelica tenuisecta（Makino）Makino var. *furucijuga*（Kitag.）H. Ohba
科名 Umbelliferae（セリ科）
英名 Angelica furcijuga
Part of use root
Note 1 —
Note 2 —
注 —

名　称 **ヒヨス属***

他名等 ヒヨス
部位等 種子・葉
備　考 —

他名（参考） —
漢字表記・生薬名等 ヒヨス
Name（Romaji） HIYOSU-ZOKU*
Other name（s）（Romaji） HIYOSU
学名 *Hyoscyamus* L.
Hyoscyamus niger L.*
科名 Solanaceae（ナス科）
英名 henbane
Part of use seed, leaf
Note 1 —
Note 2 —
注 —

名　称　フクジュソウ属

他名等　ガンジツソウ／Adonis属
部位等　全草
備　考　—

他名(参考)　マンサク（万作）
漢字表記・生薬名等　福寿草（フクジュソウ)、元日草（ガンジツソウ）
Name(Romaji)　FUKUJUSÔ-ZOKU
Other name(s) (Romaji)　GANJITSUSÔ
学名　*Adonis* L.
Adonis amurensis Regel et Radde
科名　Ranunculaceae（キンポウゲ科）
英名　Amur adonis / far east Amur adonis
Part of use　whole plant
Note 1　—
Note 2　—
注　—

名　称　ブクシンボク*

他名等　—
部位等　菌核に含まれる根
備　考　—

他名(参考)　マツホド（松塊）
漢字表記・生薬名等　茯神木（ブクシンボク）
Name(Romaji)　BUKUSHINBOKU*
Other name(s) (Romaji)　—
学名　Pine root of stump on which *Wolfiporia cocos* (F.A. Wolf) Ryvarden et Gilb.* (=*Poria cocos* (Fr.) Wolf*) is radicicolous.
科名　Polyporaceae（サルノコシカケ科）
英名　poria cocos / hoelen / Indian bread / polyporus
Part of use　root surrounded with sclerotium
Note 1　—
Note 2　See BUKURYÔ on this list.
注　ブクリョウの項を参照のこと。

名　称　フクボンシ*

他名等　ゴショイチゴ
部位等　未成熟集果
備　考　—

他名(参考)　—
漢字表記・生薬名等　覆盆子（フクボンシ)、御所苺（ゴショイチゴ）
Name(Romaji)　FUKUBONSHI*
Other name(s) (Romaji)　GOSHOICHIGO
学名　*Rubus chingii* Hu*
Rubus officinalis Koidz.*
科名　Rosaceae（バラ科）
英名　palm-leaf raspberry
Part of use　unriped aggregate fruit
Note 1　—
Note 2　—
注　—

名　称　ブクリョウ*

他名等　マツホド
部位等　菌核
備　考　—

他名(参考)　—
漢字表記・生薬名等　茯苓（ブクリョウ)、松塊（マツホド）
Name(Romaji)　BUKURYÔ*
Other name(s) (Romaji)　MATSUHODO
学名　*Wolfiporia cocos* (F.A. Wolf) Ryvarden et Gilb.*
Poria cocos (Fr.) Wolf*
Pachyma hoelen Rumph.
科名　Polyporaceae（サルノコシカケ科）
英名　poria / hoelen / Indian bread / polyporus
Part of use　sclerotium
Note 1　—
Note 2　See BUKUSHINBOKU on this list.
注　ブクシンボクの項を参照のこと。

名　称　フジコブ

他名等　フジ
部位等　フジコブ菌が寄生し生じた瘤
備　考　茎（フジコブ菌が寄生し生じた瘤以外）は「非医」

他名(参考)　—
漢字表記・生薬名等　藤瘤（フジコブ)、藤（フジ）
Name(Romaji)　FUJIKOBU
Other name(s) (Romaji)　FUJI
学名　*Wisteria floribunda* (Willd.) DC.（フジ、ノダフジ）
Wisteria brachybotrys Sieb. et Zucc.（ヤマフジ）
科名　Legminosae（マメ科）
英名　Japanese wisteria
Part of use　knob being parasitic with *Erwinia herbicola* pv. *milletiae*
Note 1　stem except knob being parasitic with *Erwinia herbicola* pv. *milletiae*：non-drug category
Note 2　—
注　—

名　称　**フタバアオイ**

他名等　—
部位等　全草
備　考　—

他名(参考)　ドサイシン（土細辛）
漢字表記・生薬名等　双葉葵（フタバアオイ）
Name(Romaji)　FUTABAAOI
Other name(s) (Romaji)　—
学名　*Asarum caulescens* Maxim.
Japonasarum caulescens (Maxim.) Nakai
科名　Aristrochiaceae（ウマノスズクサ科）
英名　flowering plants
Part of use　whole plant
Note 1　—
Note 2　—
注　—

名　称　**フラングラ皮***

他名等　セイヨウイソノキ
部位等　樹皮
備　考　—

他名(参考)　—
漢字表記・生薬名等　フラングラ皮（フラングラヒ）、西洋磯木（セイヨウイソノキ）
Name(Romaji)　FURANGURAHI*
Other name(s) (Romaji)　SEIYÔISONOKI
学名　*Rhamnus frangula* L.*
Frangula alnus Mill.*
科名　Rhamnaceae（クロウメモドキ科）
英名　frangula / alder buckthorn / glossy buckthorn
Part of use　bark
Note 1　—
Note 2　—
注　—

名　称　**ヘパティカ・ノビリス***

他名等　ミスミソウ／ユキワリソウ／Hepatica nobilis
部位等　全草
備　考　—

他名(参考)　—
漢字表記・生薬名等　三角草（ミスミソウ）、雪割草（ユキワリソウ）
Name(Romaji)　HEPATIKA・NOBIRISU*
Other name(s) (Romaji)　MISUMISÔ／YUKIWARISÔ
学名　*Hepatica nobilis* Schreb.*
Anemone hepatica L.*
Hepatica nobilis Schreb. var. *japonica* Nakai
科名　Ranunculaceae（キンポウゲ科）
英名　kidneywort / liver wort / hepatica
Part of use　whole plant
Note 1　—
Note 2　—
注　—

名　称　**ヘラオモダカ**

他名等　—
部位等　塊茎
備　考　—

他名(参考)　—
漢字表記・生薬名等　箆面高（ヘラオモダカ）
Name(Romaji)　HERAOMODAKA
Other name(s) (Romaji)　—
学名　*Alisma canaliculatum* A. Braun et C.D. Bouché
科名　Alismataceae（オモダカ科）
英名　—
Part of use　tuber
Note 1　—
Note 2　—
注　—

名　称　**ベラドンナ属***

他名等　ベラドンナ
部位等　根
備　考　—

他名(参考)　オオカミナスビ（狼茄子）、オオハシリドコロ（大走野老）、セイヨウハシリドコロ（西洋走野老）
漢字表記・生薬名等　ベラドンナ根（ベラドンナコン）
Name(Romaji)　BERADONNA-ZOKU*
Other name(s) (Romaji)　BERADONNA
学名　*Atropa* L.
Atropa belladonna L.*
科名　Solanaceae（ナス科）
英名　belladonna / deadly nightshade
Part of use　root
Note 1　—
Note 2　—
注　—

名　称　ボウイ

他名等　オオツヅラフジ
部位等　根茎・つる性の茎
備　考　—

他名(参考)　—
漢字表記・生薬名等　防已（ボウイ）、大葛藤（オオツヅラフジ）
Name(Romaji)　BÔI
Other name(s) (Romaji)　ÔTSUZURAFUJI
学名　*Sinomenium acutum*（Thunb.）Rehder et E.H. Wilson
科名　Menispermaceae（ツヅラフジ科）
英名　—
Part of use　rhizome, lianous stem
Note 1　—
Note 2　—
注　—

名　称　ボウコン*

他名等　チガヤ／ビャクボウコン
部位等　根茎
備　考　—

他名(参考)　—
漢字表記・生薬名等　茅根（ボウコン）、茅（チガヤ）、白茅根（ビャクボウコン）
Name(Romaji)　BÔKON*
Other name(s) (Romaji)　CHIGAYA／BYAKUBÔKON
学名　*Imperata cylindrica*（L.）P. Beauv.（チガヤ）
Imperata cylindrica（L.）P. Beauv. var. *major*（Nees）C.E. Hubb.*
Imperata cylindrica（L.）P. Beauv. var. *koenigii*（Retz.）Durand et Schinz
科名　Gramineae（イネ科）
英名　imperata / alang-alang / blady grass / cogon / Japanese blood grass / woolly grass
Part of use　rhizome
Note 1　—
Note 2　—
注　—

名　称　ホウセンカ*

他名等　—
部位等　種子
備　考　種子以外は「非医」

他名(参考)　トウコツソウ（透骨草）
漢字表記・生薬名等　鳳仙花（ホウセンカ）、鳳仙子（ホウセンシ）、急性子（キュウセイシ）
Name(Romaji)　HÔSENKA*
Other name(s) (Romaji)　—
学名　*Impatiens balsamina* L.*
科名　Balsaminaceae（ツリフネソウ科）
英名　garden balsam / rose balsam / impatiens / jewelweed / alegria / belen
Part of use　seed
Note 1　whole plant except seed：non-drug category
Note 2　—
注　—

名　称　ホウビソウ

他名等　イノモトソウ
部位等　全草
備　考　—

他名(参考)　—
漢字表記・生薬名等　鳳尾草（ホウビソウ）、井の許草（イノモトソウ）
Name(Romaji)　HÔBISÔ
Other name(s) (Romaji)　INOMOTOSÔ
学名　*Pteris multifida* Poir.
科名　Pteridaceae（イノモトソウ科）
英名　Chinese brake / spider brake / spider fern
Part of use　whole plant
Note 1　—
Note 2　—
注　—

名　称　ボウフウ*

他名等　—
部位等　根・根茎
備　考　—

他名(参考)　トウスケボウフウ（藤助防風）、ハマオオネ（浜大根）
漢字表記・生薬名等　防風（ボウフウ）
Name(Romaji)　BÔFÛ*
Other name(s) (Romaji)　—

学名　*Saposhnikovia divaricata* (Turcz.) Schischk.*
Ledebouriella seseloides auct. non (Hoffm.) H. Wolf
科名　Umbelliferae（セリ科）
英名　siler
Part of use　root, rhizome
Note 1　—
Note 2　—
注　—

名　称　**ホオウ***

他名等　ガマ／ヒメガマ
部位等　花粉
備　考　花粉以外は「非医」、ガマ・ヒメガマ以外の花粉は「非医」

他名（参考）　—
漢字表記・生薬名等　蒲黄（ホオウ）、蒲（ガマ）、姫蒲（ヒメガマ）
Name (Romaji)　HOÔ*
Other name (s) (Romaji)　GAMA／HIMEGAMA
学名　*Typha latifolia* L.*（ガマ）
Typha angustifolia L.*（ヒメガマ）
Typha angustata Bory et Chaub.*（ヒメガマ）
科名　Typhaceae（ガマ科）
英名　cat-tail / bulrush / common cattail / Cossack asparagus
Part of use　pollen
Note 1　whole plant except pollen：non-drug category
Pollen other than *Typha latifolia, Typha angustifolia* and *Typha angustata*：non-drug category
Note 2　—
注　—

名　称　**ホオズキ属**

他名等　サンショウコン／Physalis属
部位等　根
備　考　食用ホオズキの果実は「非医」

他名（参考）　—
漢字表記・生薬名等　酸漿・鬼灯（ホオズキ）、酸漿根（サンショウコン）
Name (Romaji)　HÔZUKI-ZOKU
Other name (s) (Romaji)　SANSHÔKON
学名　*Physalis* L.
科名　Solanaceae（ナス科）
英名　Chinese lantern plant
Part of use　root
Note 1　fruit of strawberry tomato (*Physalis pruinosa*)：non-drug category
Note 2　—
注　—

名　称　**ボスウェリア属**

他名等　ニュウコウ／Boswellia属
部位等　全木（ボスウェリア・セラータの樹脂を除く）
備　考　ボスウェリア・セラータ（Boswellia serrata）の樹脂は「非医」

他名（参考）　—
漢字表記・生薬名等　乳香（ニュウコウ）
Name (Romaji)　BOSUWERIA-ZOKU
Other name (s) (Romaji)　NYÛKÔ
学名　*Boswellia* Roxb.
科名　Burseraceae（カンラン科）
英名　frankincense
Part of use　whole tree (except resin of *Boswellia serrata*)
Note 1　resin of *Boswellia serrata*：non-drug category
Note 2　—
注　—

名　称　**ボタンピ***

他名等　ボタン
部位等　根皮
備　考　葉・花は「非医」

他名（参考）　—
漢字表記・生薬名等　牡丹皮（ボタンピ）、牡丹（ボタン）
Name (Romaji)　BOTANPI*
Other name (s) (Romaji)　BOTAN
学名　*Paeonia suffruticosa* Andr.*
Paeonia moutan Sims*
科名　Paeoniaceae（ボタン科）
英名　tree peony / mountain peony
Part of use　root bark
Note 1　leaf, flower：non-drug category
Note 2　—
注　—

名　称　**ポテンティラ・アンセリナ***

他名等　**トウツルキンバイ／ケツマ／Potentilla anserina**
部位等　全草
備　考　—

他名（参考）　—
漢字表記・生薬名等　蕨麻（ケツマ）、鵝絨委陵菜（トウツルキンバイ）
Name (Romaji)　POTENTIRA・ANSERINA*
Other name(s) (Romaji)　TÔTSURUKINBAI／KETSUMA
学名　*Potentilla anserina* L.*
　　Argentina anserina (L.) Rydb.*
科名　Rosaceae（バラ科）
英名　silverweed
Part of use　whole plant
Note 1　—
Note 2　—
注　—

名　称　**ポドフィルム属***

他名等　**ヒマラヤハッカクレン／Podophyllum属**
部位等　根・根茎
備　考　—

他名（参考）　アメリカハッカクレン（アメリカ八角蓮）
漢字表記・生薬名等　ポドフィルム、ヒマラヤ八角蓮（ヒマラヤハッカクレン）
Name (Romaji)　PODOFIRUMU-ZOKU*
Other name(s) (Romaji)　HIMARAYAHAKKAKUREN
学名　*Podophyllum* L.
　　Podophyllum hexandrum Royle*（ヒマラヤハッカクレン）
　　Podophyllum peltatum L.*（アメリカハッカクレン）
科名　Berberidaceae（メギ科）
英名　*P. hexandrum*：mayapple / Himalayan mayapple
　　P. peltatum：mayapple / American mandrake / wild mandrake / wild lemon / raccoon berry / wild jalap
Part of use　root, rhizome
Note 1　—
Note 2　—
注　—

マ行

名　称　**マオウ***

他名等　—
部位等　地上茎
備　考　—

他名（参考）　—
漢字表記・生薬名等　麻黄（マオウ）
Name (Romaji)　MAÔ*
Other name(s) (Romaji)　—
学名　*Ephedra sinica* Staph*
　　Ephedra intermedia Schrenk et C.A. Mey.*
　　Ephedra equisetina Bunge*
科名　Ephedraceae（マオウ科）
英名　ma-huang / ephedra / Chinese ephedra / Chinese jointfir
Part of use　terrestrial stem
Note 1　—
Note 2　—
注　—

名　称　**マクリ**

他名等　—
部位等　全藻
備　考　—

他名（参考）　マクリモ（万久利母）
漢字表記・生薬名等　海人草（マクリ、カイニンソウ、カイジンソウ）
Name (Romaji)　MAKURI
Other name(s) (Romaji)　—
学名　*Digenea simplex* (Wulfen) C. Agardh
科名　Rhodomelaceae（フジマツモ科）
英名　makuri / kaijinso
Part of use　whole algae
Note 1　—
Note 2　—
注　—

名　称　マシニン*

他名等　アサ
部位等　発芽防止処理されていない種子
備　考　発芽防止処理されている種子は「非医」

他名(参考)　—
漢字表記・生薬名等　麻子仁（マシニン）、火麻仁（カマニン）、麻（アサ）
Name (Romaji)　MASHININ*
Other name (s) (Romaji)　ASA
学名　*Cannabis sativa* L.*
科名　Moraceae（クワ科）
英名　hemp / Indian hemp / marijuana / marihuana
Part of use　seed without treatment for prevention of germination
Note 1　seed treated for prevention of germination : non-drug category
Note 2　—
注　—

名　称　マチン属*

他名等　ホミカ／マチンシ
部位等　種子
備　考　—

他名(参考)　—
漢字表記・生薬名等　ホミカ、馬銭子（マチンシ）
Name (Romaji)　MACHIN-ZOKU*
Other name (s) (Romaji)　HOMIKA／MACHINSHI
学名　*Strychnos* L.
Strychnos nux-vomica L.*（ホミカ）
科名　Loganiaceae（マチン科）
英名　nux-vomica / nux-vomica tree / poison-nut tree / strychnine tree
Part of use　seed
Note 1　—
Note 2　—
注　—

名　称　マルバタバコ*

他名等　アステカタバコ
部位等　葉
備　考　—

他名(参考)　—
漢字表記・生薬名等　丸葉煙草（マルバタバコ）、アステカ煙草（アステカタバコ）
Name (Romaji)　MARUBATABAKO*
Other name (s) (Romaji)　ASUTEKATABAKO
学名　*Nicotiana rustica* L.*
科名　Solanaceae（ナス科）
英名　Aztec tobacco / Indian tobacco / native tobacco / wild tobacco / small tobacco
Part of use　leaf
Note 1　—
Note 2　—
注　—

名　称　マンケイシ*

他名等　ハマゴウ
部位等　果実
備　考　—

他名(参考)　—
漢字表記・生薬名等　蔓荊子（マンケイシ）、浜栲（ハマゴウ）
Name (Romaji)　MANKEISHI*
Other name (s) (Romaji)　HAMAGÔ
学名　*Vitex rotundifolia* L. f.*（ハマゴウ）
Vitex trifolia L.*（ミツバハマゴウ）
科名　Verbenaceae（クマツヅラ科）
英名　*V. rotundifolia* : round-leaf chaste tree
V. trifolia : simple leaf tree / hand of Mary / Indian privet
Part of use　fruit
Note 1　—
Note 2　—
注　—

名　称　マンドラゴラ属*

他名等　マンドラゴラ
部位等　根
備　考　—

他名(参考)　—
漢字表記・生薬名等　マンドラゴラ
Name (Romaji)　MANDORAGORA-ZOKU*
Other name (s) (Romaji)　MANDORAGORA
学名　*Mandragora* L.
Mandragora officinarum L.*
科名　Solanaceae（ナス科）
英名　mandrake
Part of use　root
Note 1　—
Note 2　—

注　—

名　称　**ミゾカクシ**

他名等　—
部位等　全草
備　考　—

他名(参考)　—
漢字表記･生薬名等　溝隠（ミゾカクシ）、半辺蓮（ハンペンレン）
Name (Romaji)　MIZOKAKUSHI
Other name (s) (Romaji)　—
学名　*Lobelia chinensis* Lour.
科名　Campanulaceae（キキョウ科）
英名　Chinese lobelia / creeping lobelia
Part of use　whole plant
Note 1　—
Note 2　—
注　—

名　称　**ミツモウカ***

他名等　—
部位等　花
備　考　—

他名(参考)　ワタフジウツギ（綿藤空木）
漢字表記･生薬名等　密蒙花（ミツモウカ）
Name (Romaji)　MITSUMÔKA*
Other name (s) (Romaji)　—
学名　*Buddleja officinalis* Maxim.*
科名　Buddlejaceae（フジウツギ科）
英名　buddleia / buddleja / butterfly bush
Part of use　flower
Note 1　—
Note 2　—
注　—

名　称　**ムイラプアマ***

他名等　—
部位等　根
備　考　根以外は「非医」

他名(参考)　—
漢字表記･生薬名等　ムイラプアマ
Name (Romaji)　MUIRAPUAMA*
Other name (s) (Romaji)　—
学名　*Ptychopetalum olacoides* Benth.*
Ptychopetalum uncinatum Anselmino*
科名　Olacaceae（ボロボロノキ科）
英名　muira puama / marapuama
Part of use　root
Note 1　whole plant except root : non-drug category
Note 2　—
注　—

名　称　**モウオウレン***

他名等　—
部位等　ひげ根
備　考　—

他名(参考)　オウレン（黄蓮）
漢字表記･生薬名等　毛黄蓮（モウオウレン）
Name (Romaji)　MÔÔREN*
Other name (s) (Romaji)　—
学名　*Coptis japonica* (Thunb.) Makino*（オウレン）
Coptis chinensis Franch.*（オウレン）
Coptis deltoidea C.Y. Cheng et Hsiao*（オウレン）
Coptis teeta Wall.*（オウレン）
Coptis japonica (Thunb.) Makino var. *japonica*（キクバオウレン）
Coptis japonica (Thunb.) Makino var. *major* (Miq.) Satake（コセリバオウレン）
科名　Ranunculaceae（キンポウゲ科）
英名　coptis / Japanese goldthread / Chinese goldthread / Indian goldthread / Tibetan goldthread
Part of use　fibrous root
Note 1　—
Note 2　MÔÔREN is identical with ÔREN, but their parts of use are different each other. ÔREN is also listed in the item of “Name” and its leaf is classified in the “non-drug” category.
注　モウオウレンは別項のオウレンと同一。但し､「部位等」の記載が異なっている。オウレンの葉は「非医」とされている。

名　称　**モクゾク***

他名等　トクサ
部位等　全草
備　考　—

他名(参考)　—
漢字表記･生薬名等　木賊（モクゾク）、砥草（トクサ）
Name (Romaji)　MOKUZOKU*
Other name (s) (Romaji)　TOKUSA

学名 *Equisetum hyemale* L.*
科名 Equisetaceae（トクサ科）
英名 scouring rush / shave grass / rough horsetail
Part of use whole plant
Note 1 —
Note 2 —
注 —

名 称 **モクツウ***

他名等 アケビ／ツウソウ
部位等 つる性の茎
備 考 実は「非医」

他名（参考） —
漢字表記・生薬名等 木通（モクツウ、アケビ）、通草（ツウソウ）
Name（Romaji） MOKUTSÛ*
Other name（s）（Romaji） AKEBI／TSÛSÔ
学名 *Akebia quinata*（Thunb. ex Houtt.）Decne.*
Akebia trifoliata（Thunb.）Koidz.*（ミツバアケビ）
科名 Lardizabalaceae（アケビ科）
英名 akebia / five leaf akebia / chocolate vine
Part of use lianous stem
Note 1 fruit：non-drug category
Note 2 —
注 —

名 称 **モクベッシ**

他名等 ナンバンキカラスウリ／モクベツシ
部位等 種子
備 考 —

他名（参考） —
漢字表記・生薬名等 木鼈子（モクベッシ、モクベツシ）、南蛮木烏瓜（ナンバンキカラスウリ）
Name（Romaji） MOKUBESSHI
Other name（s）（Romaji） NANBANKIKARASUURI／MOKUBETSUSHI
学名 *Momordica cochinchinensis*（Lour.）K. Spreng.
科名 Cucurbitaceae（ウリ科）
英名 spiny bitter gourd / spiny bitter cucumber / balsam pear / Chinese cucumber / sweet gourd
Part of use seed
Note 1 —
Note 2 —
注 —

名 称 **モッコウ***

他名等 —
部位等 根
備 考 —

他名（参考） —
漢字表記・生薬名等 木香（モッコウ）
Name（Romaji） MOKKÔ*
Other name（s）（Romaji） —
学名 *Saussurea lappa*（Decne.）C.B. Clarke*
Saussurea costus（Falc.）Lipsh.*
Aucklandia lappa Decne.*
科名 Compositae（キク科）
英名 costus / aucklandia
Part of use root
Note 1 —
Note 2 —
注 —

ヤ行

名 称 **ヤクチ***

他名等 —
部位等 果実
備 考 —

他名（参考） —
漢字表記・生薬名等 益智（ヤクチ）
Name（Romaji） YAKUCHI*
Other name（s）（Romaji） —
学名 *Alpinia oxyphylla* Miq.*
科名 Zingiberaceae（ショウガ科）
英名 sharp-leaf galangal / black cardamom / bitter cardamon
Part of use fruit
Note 1 —
Note 2 —
注 —

名 称 **ヤクモソウ***

他名等 メハジキ
部位等 全草
備 考 —

他名（参考） —

漢字表記・生薬名等　益母草（ヤクモソウ）、目弾（メハジキ）
Name(Romaji)　YAKUMOSÔ*
Other name(s) (Romaji)　MEHAJIKI
学名　*Leonurus japonicus* Houtt.*（メハジキ）
Leonurus sibiricus L.*（ホソバメハジキ）
科名　Labiatae（シソ科）
英名　*L. japonicus*：Chinese motherwort
L. sibiricus：Siberian motherwort
Part of use　whole plant
Note 1　—
Note 2　MEHAJIKI (*Lenuras japonicus* Houtt.) in the item of "Other names" on this list is identical with REONURUSUSÔ which is listed in the "non-drug" category.
注　本項の「他名等」に記載されているメハジキと「非医」植物リストのレオヌルスソウは同一。

名　称　ヤボランジ*

他名等　—
部位等　葉
備　考　—

他名(参考)　—
漢字表記・生薬名等　ヤボランジ
Name(Romaji)　YABORANJI*
Other name(s) (Romaji)　—
学名　*Pilocarpus pennatifolius* Lem.*
Pilocarpus jaborandi Holmes*
Pilocarpus microphyllus Staph ex Wardleworth*
科名　Rutaceae（ミカン科）
英名　*P. pennatifolius*：jaborandi / Paraguay jaborandi
P. jaborandi：jaborandi / Pernam buco jaborandi
P. microphyllus：jaborandi / Maranhao jaborandi
Part of use　leaf
Note 1　—
Note 2　—
注　—

名　称　ヤラッパ*

他名等　—
部位等　脂・根
備　考　—

他名(参考)　—
漢字表記・生薬名等　ヤラッパ根（ヤラッパコン）、ヤラッパ脂（ヤラッパシ）
Name(Romaji)　YARAPPA*
Other name(s) (Romaji)　—
学名　*Ipomoea purga* (Wender.) Hayne*
科名　Convolvulaceae（ヒルガオ科）
英名　jalap / Veracruz jalap
Part of use　resin, root
Note 1　—
Note 2　—
注　—

名　称　ユキノハナ属

他名等　**オオユキノハナ／ユキノハナ**
部位等　鱗茎
備　考　—

他名(参考)　マツユキソウ（待雪草）
漢字表記・生薬名等　大雪の花（オオユキノハナ）、雪の花（ユキノハナ）
Name(Romaji)　YUKINOHANA-ZOKU
Other name(s) (Romaji)　ÔYUKINOHANA／YUKINOHANA
学名　*Galanthus* L.
Galanthus elwesii Hook. f.（オオユキノハナ）
Galanthus nivalis L.（ユキノハナ、マツユキソウ）
科名　Amaryllidaceae（ヒガンバナ科）
英名　*G. elwesii*：snowdrop / giant snowdrop / greater snowdrop
G. nivalis：snowdrop / common snowdrop / fair maids of February
Part of use　bulb
Note 1　—
Note 2　—
注　—

名　称　ヨヒンベ*

他名等　—
部位等　樹皮
備　考　—

他名(参考)　—
漢字表記・生薬名等　ヨヒンベ皮（ヨヒンベヒ）
Name(Romaji)　YOHINBE*
Other name(s) (Romaji)　—
学名　*Pausinystalia johimbe* (K. Schum.) Pierre ex Beille*
Corynanthe yohimbe K. Schum.*
科名　Rubiaceae（アカネ科）
英名　yohimbe / johimbe
Part of use　bark
Note 1　—

Note 2 —
注 —

ラ行

名 称 ラタニア*

他名等 —
部位等 根
備 考 —

他名(参考) —
漢字表記・生薬名等 ラタニア根（ラタニアコン）
Name (Romaji) RATANIA*
Other name (s) (Romaji) —
学名 *Krameria lappacea* (Dombey) Burdet et B.B. Simpson*
Krameria triandra Ruiz et Pav.*
科名 Krameriaceae（クラメリア科）
英名 rhatany / rhatania / Peruvian krameria / Peruvian rhatany
Part of use root
Note 1 —
Note 2 —
注 —

名 称 ランソウ*

他名等 フジバカマ
部位等 全草
備 考 —

他名(参考) ハイラン（佩蘭）
漢字表記・生薬名等 蘭草（ランソウ）、藤袴（フジバカマ）
Name (Romaji) RANSÔ*
Other name (s) (Romaji) FUJIBAKAMA
学名 *Eupatorium fortunei* Turcz.*
Eupatorium japonicum Thunb.
科名 Compositae（キク科）
英名 Chinese eupatorium / fortune's thoroughwort
Part of use whole plant
Note 1 —
Note 2 —
注 —

名 称 リュウタン*

他名等 トウリンドウ／リンドウ
部位等 根・根茎
備 考 —

他名(参考) —
漢字表記・生薬名等 竜胆（リュウタン）、唐竜胆（トウリンドウ）、竜胆（リンドウ）
Name (Romaji) RYÛTAN*
Other name (s) (Romaji) TÔRINDÔ／RINDÔ
学名 *Gentiana scabra* Bunge*（トウリンドウ）
Gentiana scabra Bunge var. *buergeri* (Miq.) Maxim. ex Franch. et Sav.（リンドウ）
Gentiana manshurica Kitag.*（マンシュウリンドウ）
Gentiana triflora Pall.*（エゾリンドウ）
Gentiana triflora Pall. var. *japonica* (Kusn.) H. Hara（エゾリンドウ）
科名 Gentianaceae（リンドウ科）
英名 *G. scabra* : scabrous gentian / Japanese gentian
G. triflora : three flower gentian
G. manshurica : Manshurian gentian
Part of use root, rhizome
Note 1 —
Note 2 —
注 —

名 称 リョウキョウ*

他名等 —
部位等 根茎
備 考 —

他名(参考) コウリョウキョウ（高良姜）
漢字表記・生薬名等 良姜（リョウキョウ）
Name (Romaji) RYÔKYÔ*
Other name (s) (Romaji) —
学名 *Alpinia officinarum* Hance*
科名 Zingiberaceae（ショウガ科）
英名 lesser galangal / Chinese galangal / Chinese ginger
Part of use rhizome
Note 1 —
Note 2 —
注 —

名　称　**レンギョウ***

他名等　**連翹**
部位等　果実
備　考　葉は「非医」

他名(参考)　—
漢字表記・生薬名等　連翹（レンギョウ）
Name (Romaji)　RENGYÔ*
Other name (s) (Romaji)　RENGYÔ
学名　*Forsythia suspensa* (Thunb.) Vahl*（レンギョウ）
Forsythia viridissima Lindl.（シナレンギョウ）
科名　Oleaceae（モクセイ科）
英名　forsythia / goldenbells
Part of use　fruit
Note 1　leaf : non-drug category
Note 2　—
注　—

名　称　**ロウハクカ***

他名等　—
部位等　樹皮・花
備　考　—

他名(参考)　ヨウテイコウ（羊蹄甲）
漢字表記・生薬名等　老白花（ロウハクカ）
Name (Romaji)　RÔHAKUKA*
Other name (s) (Romaji)　—
学名　*Bauhinia variegata* L.*
科名　Leguminosae（マメ科）
英名　mountain ebony / orchid tree
Part of use　bark, flower
Note 1　—
Note 2　—
注　—

名　称　**ロコン***

他名等　ヨシ
部位等　根茎
備　考　根茎以外は「非医」

他名(参考)　—
漢字表記・生薬名等　芦根（ロコン）、葦（ヨシ）
Name (Romaji)　ROKON*
Other name (s) (Romaji)　YOSHI
学名　*Phragmites communis* Trin.*
Phragmites australis (Cav.) Trin. ex Steud.*
科名　Gramineae（イネ科）
英名　phragmites / common reed
Part of use　rhizome
Note 1　whole plant except rhizome : non-drug category
Note 2　—
注　—

名　称　**ロベリアソウ***

他名等　—
部位等　全草
備　考　—

他名(参考)　—
漢字表記・生薬名等　ロベリア草（ロベリアソウ）
Name (Romaji)　ROBERIASÔ*
Other name (s) (Romaji)　—
学名　*Lobelia inflata* L.*
科名　Campanulaceae（キキョウ科）
英名　lobelia / Indian tobacco / puke weed
Part of use　whole plant
Note 1　—
Note 2　—
注　—

2．動物由来物等

2. Substances originated in animals

網掛け部分：網掛け部分には「名称」、「他名等」、「部位等」、「備考」の４項目が含まれる。これらの項目は食薬区分リストの表記に準拠し、そのまま一切の変更を加えずに記載した。

注１）「名称」及び「他名等」の欄については、生薬名、一般名及び起源動物名、該当する部位等を記載している。

注２）リストに掲載されている成分本質（原材料）のうち、該当する部位について、「部位等」の欄に記載している。

注３）他の部位が別のリストに掲載されている場合等、その取扱いが紛らわしいものについては、備考欄にその旨記載している。

注４）備考欄の「非医」は「医薬品的効能効果を標ぼうしない限り医薬品と判断しない成分本質（原材料）リスト」に掲載されていることを示す。

Shaded section：The shaded section consists of four items：Name, Other name(s), Part of use, and Remarks. These items are shown exactly as recorded in the food and drug classification lists without any changes having been made whatsoever.

1) The "Name" and "Other name(s)" entries include the crude drug name, common name, and source animal name, and the relevant part of use.
2) Of the ingredients (raw materials) included in the list, the relevant part used is included in the "Part of use" entry.
3) Where other parts are included in other lists, notes are entered in the "Remarks" column if there could be any confusion over the handling.
4) Where the "Remarks" column shows "non-drug (非医)", the substance is included in the "List of ingredients (raw materials) not deemed drugs unless claiming medicinal efficacy".

動物由来等の原材料の見方
(Notation of a substance originated in animal(s).)

名　称 他名等 部位等 備　考	**Name** **Other name(s)** **Part of Use** **Remarks** 食薬区分リストの記載事項とその内容。 The shaded section consists of the following four items which are exactly shown as recorded in the food and drug classification lists without any changes.
他名(参考)	食薬区分リストには載っていないが、実際に使用されている名称。 **Other name(s) (for reference)**：Names in actual use but not recorded in the food and drug classification list.
漢字表記・生薬名等	「名称」「他名等」の漢字表記と読み。それらの生薬、漢方等における名称の漢字表記と読み。 **Kanji notation and crude drug name**：The kanji notations of "Name" and "Other name(s)" along with the names (kanji) used in crude drug and/or Kampo medicine (traditional Japanese medicine), etc.
Name(Romaji)	「名称」のローマ字表記。 Roman alphabet (romaji) of the "Name" in the food and drug classification list.
Other name(s) (Romaji)	「他名等」のローマ字表記。 Roman alphabet (romaji) of the "Other name(s)" in the food and drug classification list.
学名 **科名** **英名**	**Scientific name(s)** **Family name** **English name(s)** 「名称」または「他名等」の学名、科名、英名。 Scientific name(s), Family name and English name(s) of the "Name" or "Other name(s)".
Part of use	「部位等」の英訳。 English translation of the "Part of use" in the food and drug classification list.
Note 1	「備考」の英訳。 English translation of the content of "Remarks" in the food and drug classification list.
Note 2	下記「注」の英訳。 English translation of "Note (注)" in the last item.
注	食薬区分リストの記載事項についての補足情報等。 **Note**：Comments or supplementary information on the content of the food and drug classification records are given.

カ行

名 称 カイクジン

他名等 オットセイ／ゴマフアザラシ
部位等 陰茎・睾丸
備 考 骨格筋抽出物は「非医」

他名(参考) —
漢字表記・生薬名等 海狗腎（カイクジン）、海豹（ゴマフアザラシ）、海狗・膃肭臍（オットセイ）
Name(Romaji) KAIKUJIN
Other name(s) (Romaji) OTTOSEI／GOMAFUAZARASHI
学名 *Phoca vitulina* L.（ゴマフアザラシ、アザラシ科）
Callorhinus ursinus L.（オットセイ、アシカ科）
Otoes ursinus L.（オットセイ、アシカ科）
Otaria ursinus Gray（オットセイ、アシカ科）
科名 Phocidae（アザラシ科）
Otariidae（アシカ科）
英名 —
Part of use penis, testis
Note 1 scheletal muscle extract：non-drug catgory
Note 2 Male genital organs (penis, testis) of other Phocidae species may be used as KAIKUJIN.
注 その他のアザラシ科動物の雄の生殖器もカイクジンとして使用されている可能性がある。

名 称 ケツエキ

他名等 —
部位等 ヒト血液
備 考 ウシ・シカ・ブタの血液・血漿は「非医」

他名(参考) —
漢字表記・生薬名等 血液（ケツエキ）
Name(Romaji) KETSUEKI
Other name(s) (Romaji) —
学名 *Homo sapiens* L.
科名 Hominidae（ヒト科）
英名 human blood
Part of use human blood
Note 1 blood of bovine, deer or swine：non-drug category
Note 2 —
注 —

名 称 コウクベン

他名等 イヌ／クインラン／ボクインキョウ／ボクインケイ
部位等 陰茎・睾丸
備 考 —

他名(参考) コウクジン（広狗腎）、オウクジン（黄狗腎）
漢字表記・生薬名等 広狗鞭（コウクベン）、牝狗陰茎（ボクインキョウ、ボクインケイ）
Name(Romaji) KÔKUBEN
Other name(s) (Romaji) INU／KUINRAN／BOKUINKYÔ／BOKUINKEI
学名 *Canis lupus familiaris* L.
科名 Canidae（イヌ科）
英名 dog / domestic dog
Part of use penis, testis
Note 1 —
Note 2 —
注 —

名 称 ゴオウ

他名等 ウシ
部位等 胆嚢中の結石
備 考 —

他名(参考) ドセイ（土精）、チュウゲン（丑玄）、チュウホウ（丑宝）
漢字表記・生薬名等 犀黄（ゴオウ）、牛黄（ゴオウ）
Name(Romaji) GOÔ
Other name(s) (Romaji) USHI
学名 *Bos taurus* L. var. *domesticus* Gmelin（ウシ）
Bubalus arnee Kerr（スイギュウ、アジアスイギュウ）
科名 Bovidae（ウシ科）
英名 oriental bezoar
Part of use bovine gallstone
Note 1 —
Note 2 GOÔ is the calculus formed in gallbladder, bile duct or hepatic duct of bovine or buffalo.
注 ゴオウは黄牛(和名：ウシ)、水牛(和名：スイギュウ)の胆嚢、胆管または肝管中の結石。

名　称　**ココツ**

他名等　**トラ**
部位等　骨格
備　考　ワシントン条約で輸入が禁止されている

他名(参考)　コケイコツ（虎脛骨）
漢字表記・生薬名等　虎骨（ココツ）
Name(Romaji)　KOKOTSU
Other name(s) (Romaji)　TORA
学名　*Panthera tigris* L.
Felis tigris Pock
Leo tigris Elite
科名　Felidae（ネコ科）
英名　tiger bone
Part of use　schelton
Note 1　Tiger bone is on the CITES list.
Note 2　—
注　—

名　称　**コツズイ**

他名等　**—**
部位等　ヒト骨髄
備　考　ウシ骨髄は「非医」

他名(参考)　—
漢字表記・生薬名等　骨髄（コツズイ）
Name(Romaji)　KOTSUZUI
Other name(s) (Romaji)　—
学名　*Homo sapiens* L.
科名　Hominidae（ヒト科）
英名　human bone marrow
Part of use　human bone marrow
Note 1　bovine bone marrow：non-drug category
Note 2　—
注　—

名　称　**ゴレイシ**

他名等　**—**
部位等　モモンガ亜科動物の糞
備　考　—

他名(参考)　—
漢字表記・生薬名等　五霊脂（ゴレイシ）
Name(Romaji)　GOREISHI
Other name(s) (Romaji)　—
学名　*Trogopterus xanthipes* Milne-Edwards
科名　Ptauristidae（ムササビ科）
英名　feces of Pteromyinae spp.
Part of use　feces of Pteromyinae spp.
Note 1　—
Note 2　—
注　—

サ行

名　称　**シベット**

他名等　**ジャコウネコ／レイビョウコウ**
部位等　香嚢腺から得た分泌液
備　考　—

他名(参考)　—
漢字表記・生薬名等　霊猫香（レイビョウコウ）、麝香猫（ジャコウネコ）
Name(Romaji)　SHIBETTO
Other name(s) (Romaji)　JAKÔNEKO／REIBYÔKÔ
学名　*Viverra zibetha* L.（インドジャコウネコ）
Viverricula indica É. Geoffroy Saint-Hilaire（コジャコウネコ）
科名　Viverridae（ジャコウネコ科）
英名　secretion from large Indian civet / small Indian civet
Part of use　secretion from anal gland
Note 1　—
Note 2　—
注　—

名　称　**ジャコウ**

他名等　**ジャコウジカ**
部位等　雄の麝香腺から出た分泌物
備　考　ワシントン条約で輸入が禁止されている

他名(参考)　—
漢字表記・生薬名等　麝香（ジャコウ）、麝香鹿（ジャコウジカ）
Name(Romaji)　JAKÔ
Other name(s) (Romaji)　JAKÔJIKA
学名　*Moschus moschiferus* L.
科名　Cervidae（シカ科）
英名　musk
Part of use　secretion from musk gland
Note 1　Musk is on the CITES list.
Note 2　—
注　—

名　称　ジャドク

他名等　ヘビ
部位等　蛇毒
備　考　ヘビ全体は「非医」

他名(参考)　—
漢字表記・生薬名等　蛇毒（ジャドク）
Name(Romaji)　JADOKU
Other name(s) (Romaji)　HEBI
学名　—（snake venom）
科名　主に以下に属するもの（Mainly belonging to the followings）:
Elapidae（コブラ科）
Viperidae（クサリヘビ科）
Colubridae（ナミヘビ科）
英名　snake venom
Part of use　snake venom
Note 1　whole snake：non-drug category
Note 2　—
注　—

名　称　ジリュウ

他名等　カッショクツリミミズ
部位等　全形
備　考　—

他名(参考)　キュウイン（蚯蚓）、ジリュウカン（地竜干）、カンジリュウ（乾地竜）、ジリュウニク（地竜肉）、コウジリュウ（広地竜）、ドジリュウ（土地竜）
漢字表記・生薬名等　地竜・地龍（ジリュウ）
Name(Romaji)　JIRYÛ
Other name(s) (Romaji)　KASSHOKUTSURIMIMIZU
学名　*Pheretima asiatica* Michaelsen（広地竜、フトミミズ科）
Pheretima aspergillum E. Perrier（広地竜、フトミミズ科）
Allolobophora caliginosa Ant. Druges（土地竜、ツリミミズ科）
Aporrectodea trapezoides Dugès（土地竜、ツリミミズ科）
科名　Megascolecidae（フトミミズ科）
Lumbricidae（ツリミミズ科）
英名　earthworm / ground dragon / night crawlers / oligochaetes
Part of use　whole body
Note 1　—
Note 2　—
注　—

名　称　センソ

他名等　シナヒキガエル
部位等　毒腺分泌物
備　考　—

他名(参考)　—
漢字表記・生薬名等　蟾酥（センソ）、支那蟇・支那蟾蜍（シナヒキガエル）
Name(Romaji)　SENSO
Other name(s) (Romaji)　SHINAHIKIGAERU
学名　*Bufo bufo gargarizans* Cantor（シナヒキガエル）
Bufo melanosticus Schneider（ヘリグロヒキガエル）
科名　Bufonidae（ヒキガエル科）
英名　toad venom
Part of use　secretion from venom gland
Note 1　—
Note 2　—
注　—

名　称　センタイ

他名等　アブラゼミ／クマゼミ
部位等　蛻殻
備　考　—

他名(参考)　ゼンタイ・センタイ（蝉退）、センゼイ（蝉蛻）、センカク（蝉殻）、センイ（蝉衣）
漢字表記・生薬名等　蝉退（センタイ）、油蝉・鳴蜩（アブラゼミ）、熊蝉（クマゼミ）
Name(Romaji)　SENTAI
Other name(s) (Romaji)　ABURAZEMI／KUMAZEMI
学名　*Cryptotympana atrata* Fabr.（スジアカクマゼミ）
Graptopsaltria nigrofuscata Motshulsky（アブラゼミ）
科名　Cicadidae（セミ科）
英名　cicada slough
Part of use　cicada slough
Note 1　—
Note 2　—
注　—

タ行

名　称　胎盤

他名等　シカシャ
部位等　ヒト胎盤
備　考　ウシ・ヒツジ・ブタの胎盤は「非医」

他名(参考)　ジンポウ（人胞）、ホウイ（胞衣）、タイイ（胎衣）、コントンイ（混沌衣）、ブッケサ（佛袈裟）、コンゲンイ（混元衣）、プラセンタ
漢字表記・生薬名等　胎盤（タイバン）、紫河車・只河車（シカシャ）、坎気（ケンキ）
Name (Romaji)　TAIBAN
Other name (s) (Romaji)　SHIKASHA
学名　*Homo sapiens* L.
科名　Hominidae（ヒト科）
英名　human placenta
Part of use　human placenta
Note 1　placenta of bovine, sheep or swine：non-drug category
Note 2　—
注　—

名　称　胆汁・胆嚢

他名等　ウシ／クマ／ブタ
部位等　ウシ・クマ・ブタの胆汁・胆嚢
備　考　コイ・ヘビの胆嚢は「非医」

他名(参考)　ユウタン（熊胆）、クマノイ（熊の胆）、ユウシ（熊脂）、ギュウタン（牛胆）、ボクタン（牡狗胆）、トンタン（豚胆）
漢字表記・生薬名等　胆汁（タンジュウ）、胆嚢（タンノウ）
Name (Romaji)　TANJÛ／TANNÔ
Other name (s) (Romaji)　USHI／KUMA／BUTA
学名　*Bos taurus* L. var. *domesticus* Gmelin（ウシ、ウシ科）
Selenarctos thibetanus Cuvier（ツキノワグマ、クマ科）
Ursus arctos L.（ヒグマ、クマ科）、その他近縁種
Sus scrofa domesticus Gray（ブタ、イノシシ科）
科名　Bovidae（ウシ科）
Ursidae（クマ科）
Suidae（イノシシ科）
英名　bile / gallbladder
Part of use　bile and gallbladder of bovine, bear or swine
Note 1　gallbladder of carp or snake：non-drug category
Note 2　—
注　—

ハ行

名　称　バホウ

他名等　ウマ
部位等　胃腸結石
備　考　—

他名(参考)　サクトウ（鮓荅）、バフンセキ（馬糞石）、ウマノタマ（馬の玉）、ヘイサラバサラ、ベゾアール
漢字表記・生薬名等　馬宝（バホウ）
Name (Romaji)　BAHÔ
Other name (s) (Romaji)　UMA
学名　*Equus caballus* L.
科名　Equidae（ウマ科）
英名　gastrointestinal calculous / bezoar
Part of use　gastrointestinal calculous
Note 1　—
Note 2　—
注　—

名　称　ボウチュウ

他名等　アブ
部位等　全虫
備　考　—

他名(参考)　ウシアブ（牛虻）、サンカクウシアブ（三角牛虻）、タイワンシロアブ（台湾白虻）、ヒメシロアブ（姫白虻）
漢字表記・生薬名等　虻虫（ボウチュウ）、虻（アブ）
Name (Romaji)　BÔCHÛ
Other name (s) (Romaji)　ABU
学名　*Tabanus trigonus* Coquillett（ウシアブ、三角牛虻）
Tabanus amaenus Walker（タイワンシロフアブ）
Tabanus cordiger Meigen（ヒメシロフアブ）
科名　Tabanidae（アブ科）
英名　gadfly / horsefly
Part of use　whole body
Note 1　—
Note 2　BÔCHÛ is the dried imaginal whole body of female gadfly. Tabanus species other than those written here are also used as BÔCHÛ.

注　ボウチュウはアブの雌の成虫の全乾燥体である。ここに記載した以外の種もある。

ラ行

名　称　リュウコツ

他名等　—
部位等　古代哺乳動物の骨の化石
備　考　—

他名(参考)　カリュウコツ（花竜骨）、ドリュウコツ（土竜骨）
漢字表記・生薬名等　竜骨・龍骨（リュウコツ）
Name(Romaji)　RYÛKOTSU
Other name(s) (Romaji)　—
学名　大型哺乳動物の化石（Fossil bone of large mammals：e.g. *Stegodon orientalis* Owen（東方剣歯象）、*Rhinoceros sinensis* Owen（中国犀））
科名　(Proboscida（チョウビ目）
Perrisodactyla（キテイ目), etc.)
英名　fossil dragon / longgu
Part of use　fossil bone of ancient mammals
Note 1　—
Note 2　There are other species besides the examples written in the item of “scientific name”.
注　ここに記載した以外の種もある。

名　称　レイヨウカク

他名等　サイカレイヨウ
部位等　角
備　考　—

他名(参考)　サイガレイヨウ（賽加羚羊）
漢字表記・生薬名等　羚羊角（レイヨウカク）、賽加羚羊（サイカレイヨウ、サイガレイヨウ）
Name(Romaji)　REIYÔKAKU
Other name(s) (Romaji)　SAIKAREIYÔ
学名　*Saiga tatarica* L.（サイカレイヨウ、サイガレイヨウ）
科名　Bovidae（ウシ科）
英名　saiga tatarica horn
Part of use　horn
Note 1　—
Note 2　—
注　—

名　称　ロクジョウ

他名等　シベリアジカ／マンシュウアカジカ／マンシュウジカ／ワピチ
部位等　雄の幼角
備　考　—

他名(参考)　バロクジョウ（馬鹿茸）、カロクジョウ（花鹿茸）、カンジョウ（砍茸）、キョジョウ（鋸茸）
漢字表記・生薬名等　鹿茸（ロクジョウ）
Name(Romaji)　ROKUJÔ
Other name(s) (Romaji)　SHIBERIAJIKA／MANSHÛAKAJIKA／MANSHÛJIKA／WAPICHI
学名　*Cervus* (*Cervus*) *elaphus* L. var. *xanthopygus* Milne-Edwards（マンシュウアカジカ）
Cervus (*Shika*) *nippon* Temminck var. *mantchuricus* Swinhoe（マンシュウジカ）
Cervus canadensis Erxleben（アメリカアカシカ、ワピチ）
科名　Cervidae（シカ科）
英名　hairy deer horn / hairy antler
Part of use　male juvenile horn
Note 1　—
Note 2　—
注　—

名　称　ロクベン

他名等　ロクジン
部位等　シカの陰茎・睾丸
備　考　—

他名(参考)　ロクインケイ（鹿陰茎）
漢字表記・生薬名等　鹿鞭（ロクベン）、鹿腎（ロクジン）
Name(Romaji)　ROKUBEN
Other name(s) (Romaji)　ROKUJIN
学名　*Cervus* (*Cervus*) *elaphus* L. var. *xanthopygus* Milne-Edwards（マンシュウアカジカ）
Cervus (*Shika*) *nippon* Temminck var. *mantchuricus* Swinhoe（マンシュウジカ）
科名　Cervidae（シカ科）
英名　penis or testis of deer
Part of use　penis or testis of deer
Note 1　—
Note 2　—
注　—

3．その他（化学物質等）

3. Other substances (chemicals, vitamins and minerals, etc.)

網掛け部分：網掛け部分には「名称」、「他名等」、「部位等」、「備考」の４項目が含まれる。これらの項目は食薬区分リストの表記に準拠し、そのまま一切の変更を加えずに記載した。

注１）他の部位が別のリストに掲載されている場合等、その取扱いが紛らわしいものについては、備考欄にその旨記載している。

注２）備考欄の「非医」は「医薬品的効能効果を標ぼうしない限り医薬品と判断しない成分本質（原材料）リスト」に掲載されていることを示す。

注３）消化酵素の名称については、同様の機能を持つものとしての総称として使用されているものを含む。

Shaded section：The shaded section consists of four items：Name, Other name(s), Part of use, and Remarks. These items are shown exactly as recorded in the food and drug classification lists without any changes having been made whatsoever.

1) Where other parts are included in other lists, notes are entered in the "Remarks" column if there could be any confusion over the handling.

2) Where the "Remarks" column shows "non-drug (非医)", the substance is included in the "List of ingredients (raw materials) not deemed drugs unless claiming medicinal efficacy".

3) The names for digestive enzymes include general terms used for substances with the same function.

その他（化学物質等）の原材料の見方
(Notation of a substance (chemical(s), vitamin(s) and mineral(s), etc.)

名　称 **他名等** **部位等** **備　考**	**Name** **Other name(s)** **Part of Use** **Remarks**	食薬区分リストの記載事項とその内容。 The shaded section consists of the following four items which are exactly shown as recorded in the food and drug classification lists without any changes.
Name	成分の英名 English name of the ingredient.	
Other name(s)	「他名等」の英名 The English translation of "Other name(s)".	
IUPAC Name		
CAS No.		
Synonyms		
分子式	**Molecular formula**	
特性・カテゴリー	**Properties and category**	
Note 1	「部位等」及び「備考」の英訳 English translation of "Part of use" and the content of "Remarks" in the food and drug classification list.	
Note 2	下記「注」の英訳。 English translation of "Note (注)" in the last item.	
注「医」	その他補足情報等 **Note** : Comments or supplementary information on the content of the food and drug classification records are given.	
構造式	**The structural formula**	

ア行

名　称　アスピリン

他名等　アセチルサリチル酸
部位等　—
備　考　—

Name　Aspirin
Other name(s)　Acetylsalicylic acid
IUPAC Name　2-acetyloxybenzoic acid
CAS No.　50-78-2
Synonyms　*o*-(Acetyloxy)benzoic acid / Acylpyrin / Ecotrin / Polopiryna / Colfarit
分子式　$C_9H_8O_4$
特性・カテゴリー　鎮痛剤(プロトタイプ：軽・中等度の痛み)／The prototypical analgesic used in the treatment of mild to moderate pain.
Note 1　—
Note 2　Anti-inflammatory and antipyretic properties and act as an inhibitor of cyclooxygenase which results in the inhibition of the biosynthesis of prostaglandins. Inhibit platelet aggregation and used in the prevention of arterial and venous thrombosis.
注　オキシゲナーゼ阻害剤として作用（プロスタグランジン生成抑制）、解熱消炎剤。血小板凝集抑制、血栓予防。

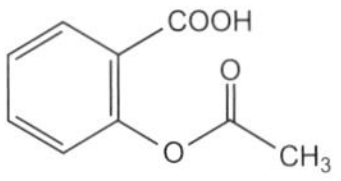

名　称　アセチルアシッド

他名等　Acetil acid／4-ethoxy-3-(1-methyl-7-oxo-3-propyl-6,7-dihydro-1*H*-pyrazolo[4,3-*d*]pyrimidin-5-yl)benzoic acid
部位等　—
備　考　—

Name　Acetil Acid
Other name(s)　Acetil acid / 4-ethoxy-3-(1-methyl-7-oxo-3-propyl-6,7-dihydro-1*H*-pyrazolo[4,3-*d*]pyrimidin-5-yl)benzoic acid
IUPAC Name　—
CAS No.　—
Descarbonsildenafil (Similar compound of acetyl acid)：104393-45-5
Synonyms　—
Descarbonsildenafil (Similar compound of acetyl acid)：N-[2-Dimethylamino)ethyl]-4-ethoxy-3-(1-methyl-7-oxo-3-propyl-6,7-dihydro-1*H*-pyrazolo[4,3-*d*]pyrimidin-5-yl)benzenesulfonamide
分子式　$C_{18}H_{20}N_4O_4$
Descarbonsildenafil (Similar compound of acetyl acid)：$C_{17}H_{22}N_6O_3S$
特性・カテゴリー　シルデナフィル類似物質／Sildenafil analogue
Note 1　—
Note 2　Descarbonsildenafil (Similar compound of acetyl acid)：Sildenafil analogue was detected in a functional coffee sample labelled to have male sexual performance enhancement effects. (A case in overseas)
注　Descarbonsildenafil（シルデナフィル類似物質）：シルナデフィル類似の作用を持つ。強精作用を謳ったコーヒーに含まれていた。（海外の事例）

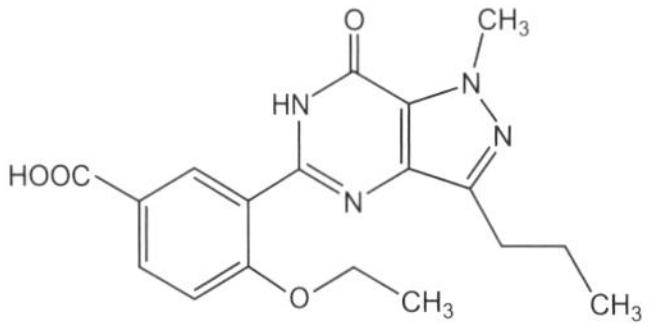

Acetil acid

名　称　アミノタダラフィル

他名等　Aminotadalafil
部位等　—
備　考　—

Name　Aminotadalafil
Other name(s)　Aminotadalafil
IUPAC Name　—
CAS No.　385769-84-6
Synonyms　Amino tadalafil / ((6R,12aR)-2-amino-6-(1,3-benzodioxol-5-yl)-2,3,6,7,12,12a-hexahydropyrazino(1',2':1,6)pyrido(3,4-*b*)indole-1,4-dione
分子式　$C_{21}H_{18}N_4O_4$
特性・カテゴリー　タダラフィル（Cialis®、勃起障害経口治療剤）の誘導体／Derivative of Tadarafil (Cialis®, an oral drug for erectile dysfunction)
Note 1　—
Note 2　—
注　—

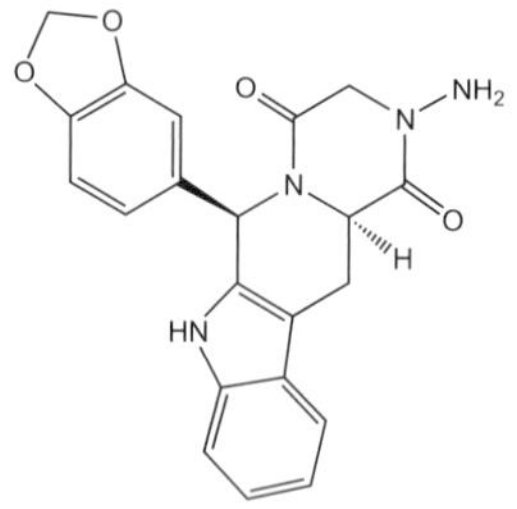

called 5-ureidohydantoin.

Note 1 —

Note 2 A urea hydantoin that is found in urine and plants and is used in dermatological preparations.

注 尿中及び植物に存在し、化粧品等外用剤に用いられる。

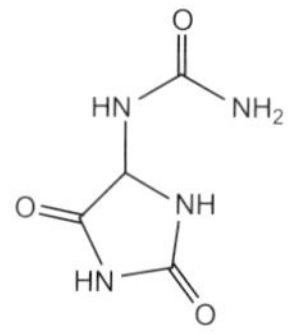

名 称 アミラーゼ

他名等 ジアスターゼ

部位等 —

備 考 —

Name Amylase

Other name(s) Diastase

IUPAC Name 4-alpha-D-glucan glucanohydrolase (IUBMB Enzyme Nomenclature)

CAS No. Amylase：9000-92-4
alpha-Amylase (EC 3.2.1.1)：9000-90-2

Synonyms alpha-Amylase / Glycogenase / Endoamylase / Taka-amylase / (alpha-D-Glucopyranosyl-(1-4))$_n$-alpha-D-glucopyranose / 1,4-alpha-D-Glucan glucanohydrolase

分子式 —

特性・カテゴリー 澱粉分解酵素／Catalyzing the hydrolysis of alpha 1→4 glucosidic likages of polysaccharides such as glycogen and satarch.

Note 1 —

Note 2 —

注 —

名 称 アラントイン

他名等 —

部位等 —

備 考 —

Name Allantoin

Other name(s) —

IUPAC Name (2,5-dioxoimidazolidin-4-yl)urea

CAS No. 97-59-6

Synonyms 5-Ureidoimidazolidine-2,4-dione / 5-(Carbamoylamino)hydantoin

分子式 $C_4H_6N_4O_3$

特性・カテゴリー グリオキシル酸のジウレイド。別名5-ウレイドヒダントイン。尿酸の中間代謝物（ヒトの場合）。／Diureido of glyoxylic acid in human. An intermediate metabolite of uric acid and it is also

名 称 アロイン

他名等 バルバロイン

部位等 —

備 考 アロエの成分

Name Alloin, Aloin

Other name(s) Barbaloin

IUPAC Name (10S)-1,8-dihydroxy-3-(hydroxymethyl)-10-[(2S,3R,4R,5S,6R)-3,4,5-trihydroxy-6-(hydroxymethyl)oxan-2-yl]-10*H*-anthracen-9-one

CAS No. 1415-73-2

Synonyms Barbaloin / Aloin A / (10S)-1,8-Dihydroxy-3-(hydroxymethyl)-10beta-beta-D-glucopyranosyl-9,10-dihydroanthracene-9-one

分子式 $C_{21}H_{22}O_9$

特性・カテゴリー 植物成分。緩下薬として用いる。／Botanical constituent. Laxative.

Note 1 Component of Aloe spp.

Note 2 —

注 —

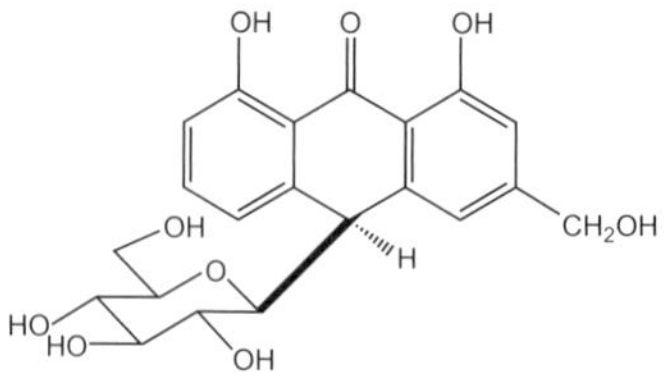

名 称 アンジオテンシン

他名等 —
部位等 —
備 考 —

Name Angiotensin
Other name(s) —
IUPAC Name Angiotensin II：(3S)-3-amino-4-[[(2S)-1-[[(2S)-1-[[(2S)-1-[[(2S,3S)-1-[[(2S)-1-[(2S)-2-[[(1S)-1-carboxy-2-phenylethyl]carbamoyl]pyrrolidin-1-yl]-3-(1*H*-imidazol-5-yl)-1-oxopropan-2-yl]amino]-3-methyl-1-oxopentan-2-yl]amino]-3-(4-hydroxyphenyl)-1-oxopropan-2-yl]amino]-3-methyl-1-oxobutan-2-yl]amino]-5-(diaminomethylideneamino)-1-oxopentan-2-yl]amino]-4-oxobutanoic acid
CAS No. Angiotensin II：4474-91-3
Synonyms Angiotensin II：Angiotensin / Ang II / Human angiotensin II / Asp-Arg-Val-Tyr-Ile-His-Pro-Phe (human)
分子式 Angiotensin II：$C_{50}H_{71}N_{13}O_{12}$
特性・カテゴリー アミノ酸8残基よりなるペプチドホルモン。血管収縮による血圧上昇をもたらす。／The octapeptide amide that causes vasoconstriction and a subsequent increase in blood pressure.
Note 1 —
Note 2 Produced from angiotensin I by angiotensin converting enzyme. (Angiotensin II is described as a representative substance of Angiotensin.)
注 アンジオテンシン変換酵素によって、アンジオテンシンIから生成される。(Angiotensin IIで代表させた)

Asp - Arg - Val - Tyr - Ile - His - Pro - Phe - OH (angiotensinII)

名 称 アンドロステンジオン

他名等 —
部位等 —
備 考 —

Name Androstenedione
Other name(s) —
IUPAC Name (8R,9S,10R,13S,14S)-10,13-dimethyl-2,6,7,8,9,11,12,14,15,16-decahydro-1*H*-cyclopenta[a]phenanthrene-3,17-dione
CAS No. 63-05-8
Synonyms Androst-4-ene-3,17-dione / 4-Androstene-3,17-dione / 4-Androstenedione / Androtex / 3,17-Dioxoandrost-4-ene
分子式 $C_{19}H_{26}O_2$
特性・カテゴリー テストステロン、エストロン、エストラジオールの前駆体。／Precursor to testosterone as well as estrone and estradiol.
Note 1 —
Note 2 A delta-4 C19 steroid that is produced not only in the testis, but also in the ovary and the adrenal cortex.
注 delta-4 C19ステロイド。精巣、卵巣、副腎皮質で生成。

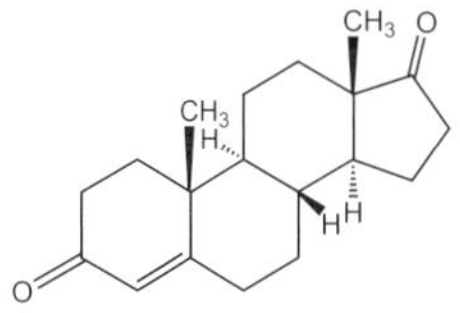

名 称 イミダゾサガトリアジノン

他名等 Imidazosagatriadinone
部位等 —
備 考 —

Name Imidazosagatriadinone
Other name(s) Imidazosagatriadinone
IUPAC Name —
CAS No. —
Synonyms —
分子式 —
特性・カテゴリー バルデナフィルの誘導体／Derivative of vardenafil
Note 1 —
Note 2 There is no chemical information on imidazosagatriadinone.
注 イミダゾサガトリアジノンに関する化学情報はない。

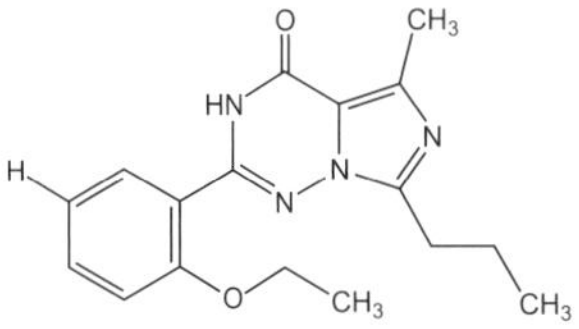

名 称 **インベルターゼ**

他名等 インベルチン／サッカラーゼ／β-フルクトフラノシダーゼ
部位等 —
備 考 —

Name Invertase
Other name(s) Invertin / Saccharase / beta-Fructofuranosidase
IUPAC Name beta-D-fructofuranoside fructohydrolase (IUBMB Enzyme Nomenclature)
CAS No. beta-Fructofuranosidase (EC 3.2.1.26) : 9001-57-4
Invertase (as a whole) (EC 3.2.1.26) : 9001-57-4
Synonyms —
分子式 —
特性・カテゴリー ショ糖を果糖とブドウ糖に加水分解する酵素／Catalyze the hydrolysis of sucrose into fructose and glucose.
Note 1 —
Note 2 Inveltase has the enzymatic function of beta-Fructofuranosidase. CAS No. of beta-Fructofranosidase is based on BRENDA, and that of Invertase (as a whole) is based on Merk Index.
注 インベルターゼはβ-フルクトフラノシダーゼの酵素機能を持つ。
β-フルクトフラノシダーゼのCAS No.はBRENDAによる。インベルターゼ（全体として）のCAS No.はMerk Indexによる。

名 称 **ウデナフィル**

他名等 Udenafil
部位等 —
備 考 —

Name Udenafil
Other name(s) Udenafil
IUPAC Name 3-(1-methyl-7-oxo-3-propyl-4*H*-pyrazolo[4,3-*d*]pyrimidin-5-yl)-N-[2-(1-methylpyrrolidin-2-yl)ethyl]-4-propoxybenzenesulfonamide
CAS No. 268203-93-6
Synonyms Zydena
分子式 $C_{25}H_{36}N_6O_4S$
特性・カテゴリー シルデナフィル（Viagra®、勃起障害経口治療剤）の誘導体／Derivative of Sildenafil (Viagra®, an oral drug for erectile dysfunction)
Note 1 —
Note 2 —
注 —

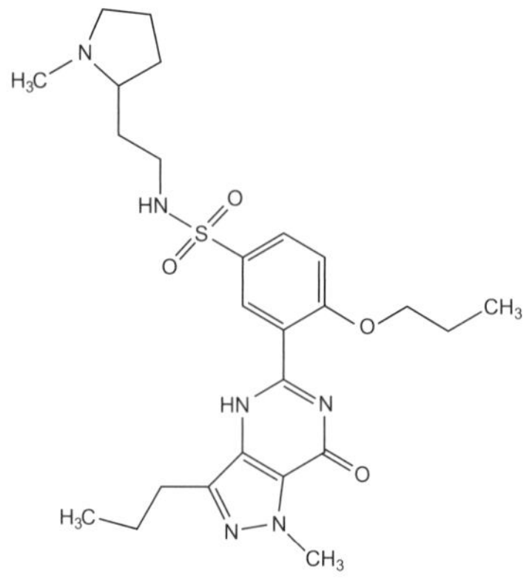

名 称 **S-アデノシル-L-メチオニン**

他名等 SAMe
部位等 —
備 考 —

Name S-adenosyl-L-methionine
Other name(s) SAMe
IUPAC Name (2S)-2-amino-4-[[(2S,3S,4R,5R)-5-(6-aminopurin-9-yl)-3,4-dihydroxyoxolan-2-yl]methyl-methylsulfonio]butanoate
CAS No. 29908-03-0
Synonyms SAM-e / Methioninyladenylate / S-Adenosylmethionine
分子式 $C_{15}H_{22}N_6O_5S$
特性・カテゴリー 抗炎症作用を有する。慢性肝疾患の治療に用いられてきた。／Possesses anti-inflammatory activity and has been used in treatment of chronic liver disease.
Note 1 —
Note 2 Physiologic methyl radical donor involved in enzymatic transmethylation reactions and present in all living organisms.
注 メチル基転移酵素反応にメチルラジカルとしての生理作用を持つ。すべての生物に存在する。

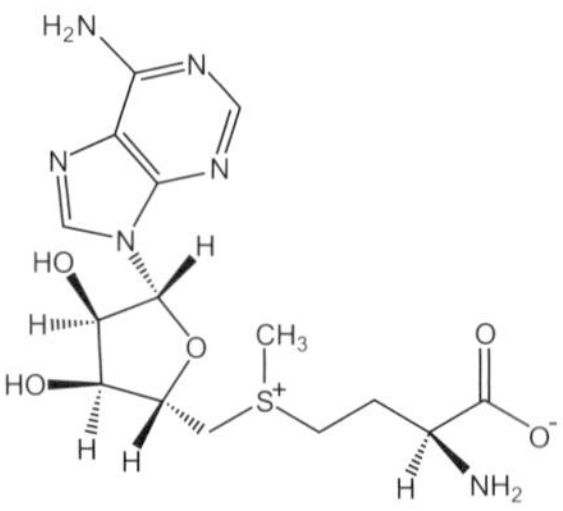

名　称　**N-オクチルノルタダラフィル**

他名等　N-octylnortadalafil
部位等　—
備　考　—

Name　N-octylnortadalafil
Other name(s)　N-octylnortadalafil
IUPAC Name　—
CAS No.　1173706-35-8
Synonyms　(6R,12aR)-6-(1,3-Benzodioxole-5-yl)-2,3,6,7,12,12a-hexahydro-2-octylpyrazino[1',2':1,6]pyrido[3,4-b]indole-1,4-dione / (6R)-2-Octyl-6alpha-(1,3-benzodioxole-5-yl)-2,3,6,7,12,12a beta-hexahydropyrazino[1',2':1,6]pyrido[3,4-b]indole-1,4-dione
分子式　$C_{29}H_{33}N_3O_4$
特性・カテゴリー　タダラフィル（Cialis®、勃起障害経口治療剤）の誘導体／Derivative of Tadarafil (Cialis®, an oral drug for erectile dysfunction)
Note 1　—
Note 2　—
注　—

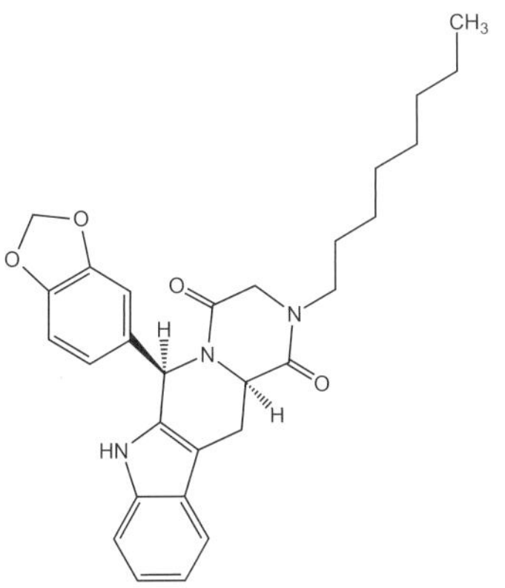

名　称　**N-ニトロソフェンフルラミン**

他名等　—
部位等　—
備　考　—

Name　N-nitroso-fenfluramine
Other name(s)　—
IUPAC Name　—
CAS No.　19023-40-6
Synonyms　N-Nitrosofenfluramine / N-Nitroso-fenfluramin / N-Ethyl-N-nitroso-α-methyl-3-(trifluoromethyl)benzeneethanamine / N-Nitroso-bis-(2-hydroxy-propyl)amine
分子式　$C_{12}H_{15}F_3N_2O$
特性・カテゴリー　フェンフルラミンのニトロソ誘導体で、セロトニンの取り込みを抑制する作用物質／Nitroso compound of fenfluramine and blocks serotonin uptake and provokes transport-mediated serotonin release.
Note 1　—
Note 2　Fenfluramine is an adrenergic drug, serotonin agonist and beta-adrenergic drug, and used as an appetite depressant.
注　フェンフルラミンはアドレナリン作動薬、セロトニン作動薬、βアドレナリン作動薬で、食欲抑制薬として用いられていた。

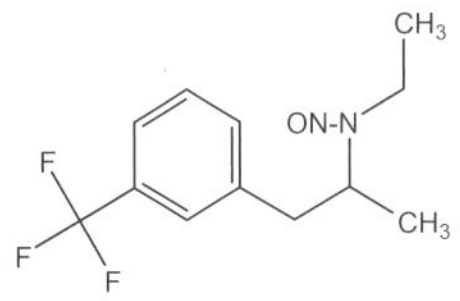

名　称　**エフェドリン**

他名等　—
部位等　—
備　考　—

Name　Ephedrine
Other name(s)　—
IUPAC Name　(1R,2S)-2-(methylamino)-1-phenylpropan-1-ol
CAS No.　299-42-3
Synonyms　Senedrine / Mandrin / [R,(-)]-α-[(S)-1-(Methylamino)ethyl]benzyl alcohol / (1R,2S)-2-(Methylamino)-1-phenyl-1-propanol / (1R,2S)-2-Methylamino-1-phenylpropane-1-ol
分子式　$C_{10}H_{15}NO$
特性・カテゴリー　アドレナリン作動物質として喘息、心不全、鼻炎、尿失禁に用いられ、中枢神経刺激剤としてナルコレプシーやうつ病に用いられてきた。／Adrenergic agent used for asthma, heart failure, rhinitis, and urinary incontinence, and for its central nervous system stimulatory effects in the treatment of narcolepsy and depression.
Note 1　—
Note 2　A phenethylamine found in *Ephedra sinica*. Pseudoephedrine is an isomer.
注　麻黄に含まれるフェネチルアミン。Pseudoephedrineの異性体。

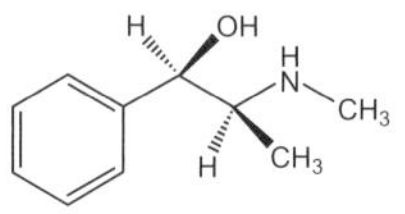

カ行

名　称　カオリン

他名等　—
部位等　—
備　考　—

Name　Kaolin
Other name(s)　—
IUPAC Name　oxo-oxoalumanyloxy-[oxo(oxoalumanyloxy)silyl]oxysilane;dihydrate
CAS No.　1332-58-7
Synonyms　Donnagel / Alphagloss / Aluminum silicate / Aluminium silicate hydroxide / Surround
分子式　$H_2Al_2Si_2O_8 \cdot H_2O$
特性・カテゴリー　含水ケイ酸アルミニウム。止瀉剤（吸着剤）として利用されてきた。／A hydrous Alminum silicate. Used as an antidiarrheal (absorbent).
Note 1　—
Note 2　Kaolin is named after Kao-ling (Chinese : “high ridge”) and contains mainly the clay mineral kaolinite.
注　カオリンは中国名「高嶺」に由来し、カオリナイト（カオリン石）を主成分鉱物として含む粘土。

名　称　カタラーゼ

他名等　—
部位等　—
備　考　—

Name　Catalase
Other name(s)　—
IUPAC Name　—
CAS No.　Catalase (EC 1.11.1.6) : 9001-05-2
Synonyms　Caperase / Equilase / Optidase / Catalase-peroxidase
分子式　—
特性・カテゴリー　酵素：過酸化水素を分解して水と酸素を生じる反応を促進。／Enzyme : Promoting reactions involving the decomposition of hydrogen peroxide to water and oxygen.
Note 1　—
Note 2　—
注　—

名　称　カルボデナフィル

他名等　Carbodenafil
部位等　—
備　考　—

Name　Carbodenafil
Other name(s)　Carbodenafil
IUPAC Name　—
CAS No.　—
Synonyms　—
分子式　$C_{24}H_{32}N_6O_3$
特性・カテゴリー　シルデナフィル（Viagra®、勃起障害経口治療剤）の誘導体／Derivative of Sildenafil (Viagra®, an oral drug for erectile dysfunction)
Note 1　—
Note 2　There is almost no data.
注　殆どデータ無し。

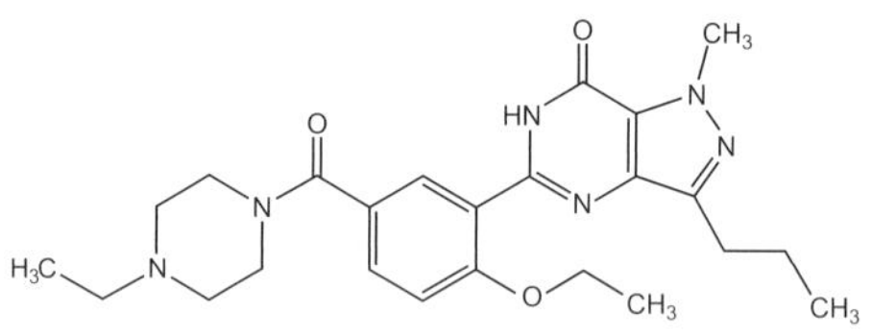

名　称　キサントアントラフィル

他名等　Xanthoanthrafil
部位等　—
備　考　—

Name　Xanthoanthrafil
Other name(s)　Xanthoanthrafil
IUPAC Name　N-[(3,4-dimethoxyphenyl)methyl]-2-(1-hydroxypropan-2-ylamino)-5-nitrobenzamide
CAS No.　Xanthoanthrafil : 1020251-53-9
(R)-Xanthoanthrafil : 247568-68-9
Synonyms　Benzamidenafil / N-(3,4-dimethoxybenzyl)-2-((2-hydroxy-1-methylethyl)amino)-5-nitrobenzamide
分子式　$C_{19}H_{23}N_3O_6$
特性・カテゴリー　シルデナフィル（Viagra®、勃起障害経口治療剤）の誘導体／Derivative of Sildenafil (Viagra®, an oral drug for erectile dysfunction)
Note 1　—

Note 2 —
注 —

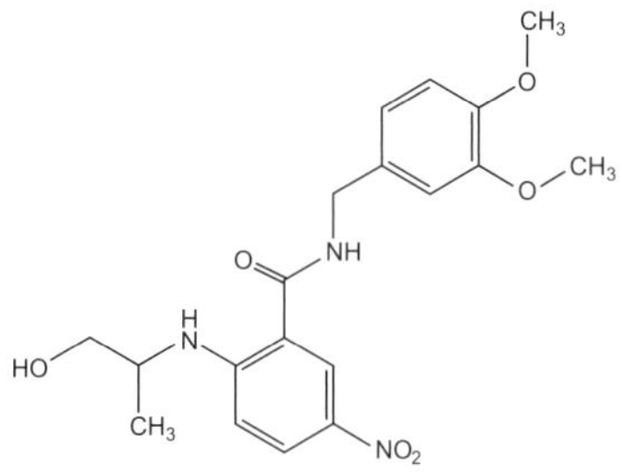

名 称 γ-オリザノール

他名等 —
部位等 —
備 考 —

Name gamma-Oryzanol
Other name(s) —
IUPAC Name —
CAS No. 11042-64-1
Synonyms Caclate / Gamma-OZ / γ-Oryzanol
分子式 $C_{40}H_{58}O_4$
特性・カテゴリー 穀類、米糠油に含まれる。閉経期症候群の治療、血中コレステロール及び中性脂肪の低下作用。/Found in grains and isolated from rice bran oil : used to treat menopausal symptoms and to lower blood cholesterol and triglyceride levels.
Note 1 —
Note 2 —
注 —

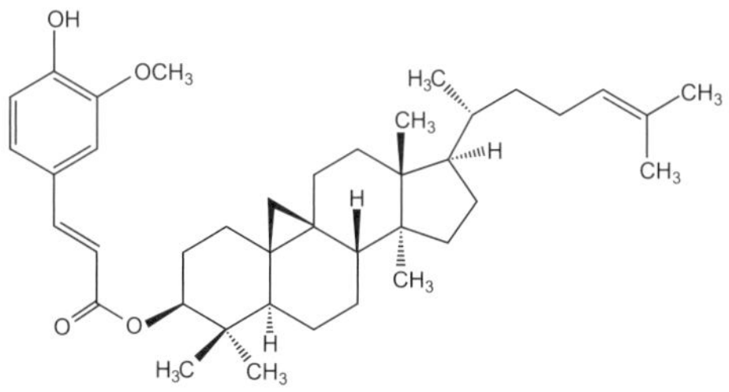

名 称 グアイフェネジン

他名等 —
部位等 —
備 考 —

Name Guaifenesin
Other name(s) —
IUPAC Name 3-(2-methoxyphenoxy)propane-1,2-diol
CAS No. 93-14-1
Synonyms Guaiacol glyceryl ether / Guaiphenesin / Glycerol guaiacolate
分子式 $C_{10}H_{14}O_4$
特性・カテゴリー 去痰薬。筋弛緩作用があり、多くの鎮咳剤に用いられる。/An expectorant that also has some muscle relaxing action. It is used in many cough preparations.
Note 1 —
Note 2 The Japanese name "GUAIFENEJIN" should be "GUAIFENESHIN".
注 名称のグアイフェネジンはグアイフェネシンとした方が良い。

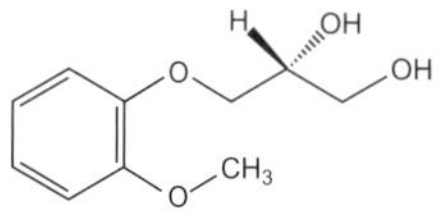

名 称 グルタチオン

他名等 —
部位等 —
備 考 —

Name Glutathione
Other name(s) —
IUPAC Name (2S)-2-amino-5-[[(2R)-1-(carboxymethylamino)-1-oxo-3-sulfanylpropan-2-yl]amino]-5-oxopentanoic acid
CAS No. 70-18-8
Synonyms N-[N-(L-γ-Glutamyl)-L-cysteinyl]glycine / GSH
分子式 $C_{10}H_{17}N_3O_6S$
特性・カテゴリー 細胞内で様々な機能を有するトリペプチド。多くの薬物に抱合して、可溶化し排泄を促す。幾つかの酵素の補酵素となり、タンパク質のジスルフィド結合の再形成に関与し、また、過酸化物を減少させる作用を有する。/A tripeptide with many roles in cells. It conjugates to drugs to make them more soluble for excretion, is a cofactor for some enzymes, is involved in protein disulfide bond rearrangement and reduces peroxides.
Note 1 —
Note 2 —
注 —

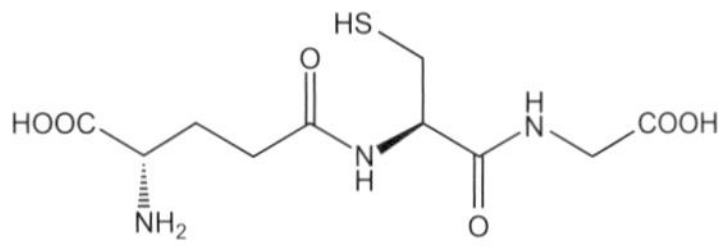

名　称　クロロプレタダラフィル

他名等　Chloropretadalafil
部位等　—
備　考　—

Name　Chloropretadalafil
Other name(s)　Chloropretadalafil
IUPAC Name　methyl(1R,3R)-1-(1,3-benzodioxol-5-yl)-2-(2-chloroacetyl)-1,3,4,9-tetrahydropyrido[3,4-*b*]indole-3-carboxylate
CAS No.　171489-59-1
Synonyms　(1R,3R)-Methyl 1-(benzo[d][1,3]dioxol-5-yl)-2-(2-chloroacetyl)-2,3,4,9-tetrahydro-1*H*-pyrido[3,4-*b*]indole-3-carboxylate / (1R,3R)-Methyl-1,2,3,4-tetrahydro-2-chloroacetyl-1-(3,4-methylenedioxyphenyl)-9*H*-pyrido[3,4-*b*]indole-3-carboxylate
分子式　$C_{22}H_{19}ClN_2O_5$
特性・カテゴリー　タダラフィル（Cialis®、勃起障害経口治療剤）の誘導体／Derivative of Tadarafil (Cialis®, an oral drug for erectile dysfunction)
Note 1　—
Note 2　—
注　—

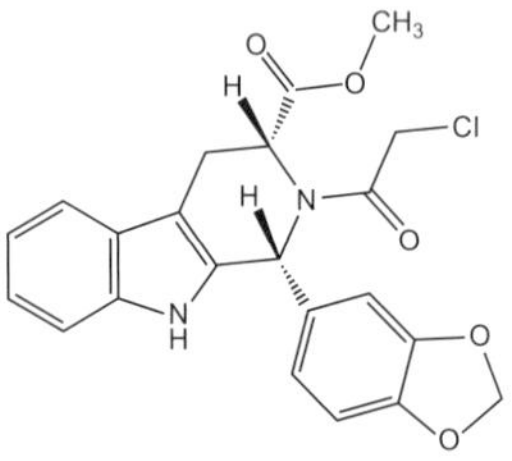

名　称　ゲンデナフィル

他名等　Gendenafil
部位等　—
備　考　—

Name　Gendenafil
Other name(s)　Gendenafil
IUPAC Name　5-(5-acetyl-2-ethoxyphenyl)-1-methyl-3-propyl-4*H*-pyrazolo[4,3-*d*]pyrimidin-7-one
CAS No.　147676-66-2
Synonyms　5-(5-Acetyl-2-ethoxyphenyl)-1,6-dihydro-1-methyl-3-propyl-7*H*-pyrazolo(4,3-*d*)pyrimidin-7-one
分子式　$C_{19}H_{22}N_4O_3$
特性・カテゴリー　シルデナフィル（Viagra®、勃起障害経口治療剤）の誘導体／Derivative of Sildenafil (Viagra®, an oral drug for erectile dysfunction)
Note 1　—
Note 2　—
注　—

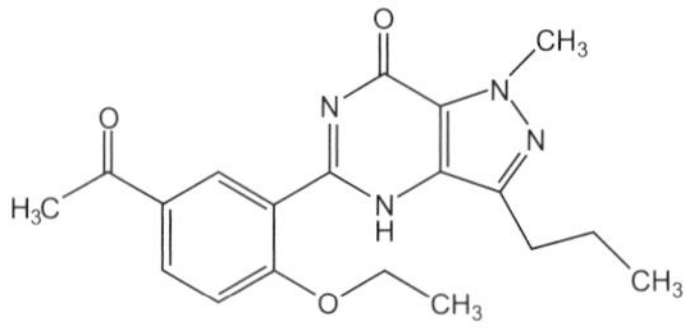

サ行

名　称　GBL

他名等　ガンマブチロラクトン
部位等　—
備　考　—

Name　GBL
Other name(s)　gamma-Butyrolactone
IUPAC Name　dihydrofuran-2(3*H*)-one
CAS No.　96-48-0
Synonyms　4-Butyrolactone / 1,4-Butanolide / Dihydro-2(3*H*)-furanone
分子式　$C_4H_6O_2$
特性・カテゴリー　γ-アミノ酪酸から生体内で生成し、γ-ヒドロキシ酪酸の前駆体になる。／An endogenous compound made from gamma-aminobutyrate and is the precursor of gamma-hydroxybutyrate.
Note 1　—
Note 2　—
注　—

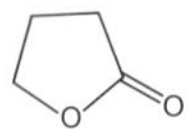

名　称　**シクロフェニール**

他名等　—
部位等　—
備　考　—

Name　Cyclofenil
Other name(s)　—
IUPAC Name　[4-[(4-acetyloxyphenyl)-cyclohexylidenemethyl]phenyl]acetate
CAS No.　2624-43-3
Synonyms　Ondogyne / Cyclofenyl / bis(*p*-Acetoxyphenyl)cyclohexylidenemethane
分子式　$C_{23}H_{24}O_4$
特性・カテゴリー　性腺刺激、排卵誘発因子。不妊、無月経の治療に用いる。クロミフェンより弱い。／A gonadal stimulant and inducer of ovulation. It is used in the treatment of infertility and amenorrhea, but is thought to be less effective than clomiphene.
Note 1　—
Note 2　—
注　—

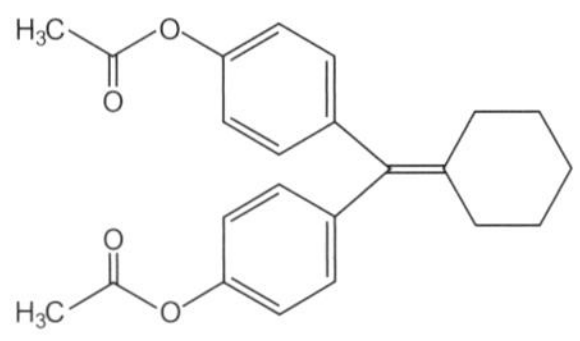

名　称　**シクロペンチナフィル**

他名等　Cyclopentynafil
部位等　—
備　考　—

Name　Cyclopentynafil
Other name(s)　Cyclopentynafil
IUPAC Name　—
CAS No.　—
Synonyms　(4-Cyclopentylpiperazine-1-yl)[3-(1-methyl-3-propyl-6,7-dihydro-7-oxo-1H-pyrazolo[4,3-d]pyrimidine-5-yl)-4-(ethoxy)phenyl]sulfone / 1-Methyl-3-propyl-5-[2-ethoxy-5-(4-cyclopentylpiperazinosulfonyl)phenyl]-6,7-dihydro-1*H*-pyrazolo[4,3-*d*]pyrimidine-7-one
分子式　$C_{26}H_{36}N_6O_4S$
特性・カテゴリー　シルデナフィル（Viagra®、勃起障害経口治療剤）の誘導体／Derivative of Sildenafil (Viagra®, an oral drug for erectile dysfunction)
Note 1　—
Note 2　—
注　—

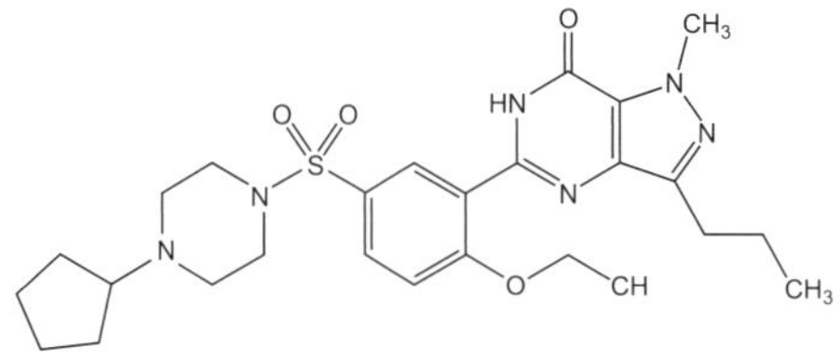

名　称　**臭化水素酸デキストロメトルファン**

他名等　Dextromethorphan Hydrobromide
部位等　—
備　考　—

Name　Dextromethorphan hydrobromide
Other name(s)　Dextromethorphan hydrobromide
IUPAC Name　—
CAS No.　125-69-9
Synonyms　(9S,13S,14S)-3-Methoxy-17-methylmorphinan monohydrobromide monohydrate / Racemethrophan / Astomari / Dextophan / Medicon
分子式　$C_{18}H_{26}BrNO$
特性・カテゴリー　鎮咳薬。NMDA（N-methyl D-spartate）レセプターの拮抗薬。非拮抗チャネルブロッカーとして作用。／Antitussive. This compound is an NMDA (N-methyl D-aspartate) receptor antagonist and acts as a non-competitive channel blocker.
Note 1　—
Note 2　See Dextromethorphan in this list.
注　別項のデキストロメトルファンを参照

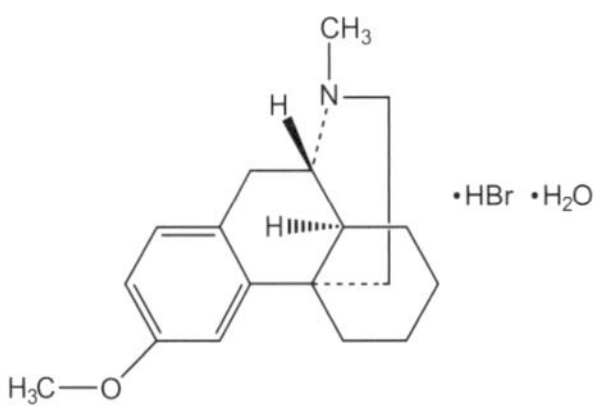

名　称　シルデナフィル

他名等　Sildenafil
部位等　—
備　考　—

Name　Sildenafil
Other name (s)　Sildenafil
IUPAC Name　5-[2-ethoxy-5-(4-methylpiperazin-1-yl)sulfonylphenyl]-1-methyl-3-propyl-4*H*-pyrazolo[4,3-*d*]pyrimidin-7-one
CAS No.　139755-83-2
Synonyms　Revatio® / Viagra® (Sildenafil citrate)
分子式　$C_{22}H_{30}N_6O_4S$
特性・カテゴリー　血管作動性薬剤として勃起障害の治療及び肺動脈性高血圧（PAH）の症状改善に用いる。５型ホスホジエステラーゼ（PDE-5）の酵素活性阻害作用により、cGMPのレベルを上昇させ、効力を発揮する。／Sildenfail is a vasoactive agent used to treat erectile dysfunction and reduce symptoms in patients with pulmonary arterial hypertension (PAH). Sildenafil elevates levels of the second messenger, cGMP, by inhibiting its breakdown via phosphodiesterase type 5 (PDE-5).
Note 1　—
Note 2　Viagra® is sildenafil citrate. See Homosildenafil in this list.
注　Viagra®はシルデナフィルのクエン酸塩
別項のホモシルデナフィルを参照

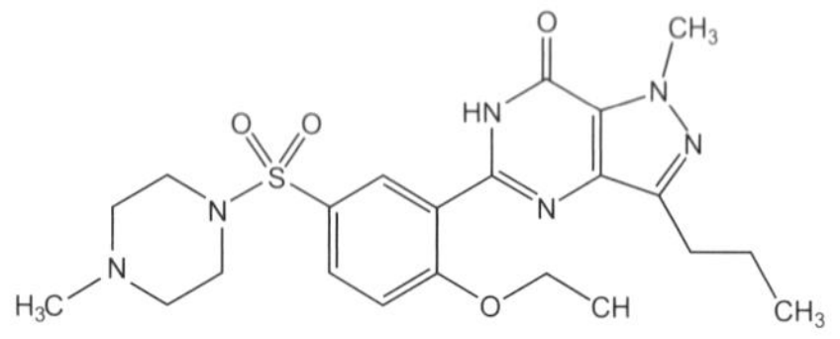

名　称　スルフォンアミド

他名等　—
部位等　—
備　考　—

Name　Sulphonamide
Other name (s)　—
IUPAC Name　—
CAS No.　—
Synonyms　—
分子式　—
特性・カテゴリー　—
Note 1　—
Note 2　Not possible to identify a compound because sulphoneamide means sulphoneamide bond.
注　スルフォンアミド結合を意味するので、対象が絞れない。スルフォンアミドとしての単独の存在はない。

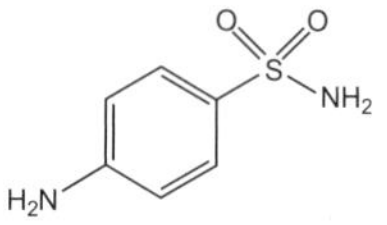

Sulfanilamide

※スルフォンアミドの１例としてスルファニルアミドの構造式を示す。

名　称　セキテッコウ

他名等　赤鉄鉱／タイシャセキ
部位等　—
備　考　鉱石

Name　Hematite
Other name (s)　Hematite
IUPAC Name　iron(3+);oxygen(2-)
CAS No.　1309-37-1
Synonyms　Ferric oxide / Raphisiderite / Specularite / Haematite / Red iron ore
分子式　Fe_2O_3
特性・カテゴリー　ミネラル／Mineral
Note 1　Mineral ore
Note 2　—
注　—

タ行

名　称　タウリン

他名等　—
部位等　—
備　考　—

Name　Taurine
Other name (s)　—
IUPAC Name　2-aminoethanesulfonic acid
CAS No.　107-35-7
Synonyms　2-Aminoethanesulfonic acid / L-Taurine / 2-Aminoethylsulfonic acid / Ethanesulfonic acid
分子式　$C_2H_7NO_3S$
特性・カテゴリー　哺乳類の発達の過程で重要な必須栄養

素。牛胆汁から得られ、胆汁酸に強力な抱合剤である。／Esential nutrient, important during mammalian development. It is isolated mostly from ox bile and strongly conjugates bile acids.

Note 1 —

Note 2 —

注 —

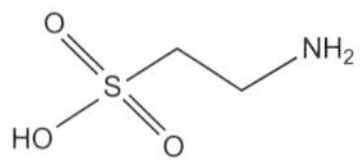

名　称　**タダラフィル**

他名等　**Tadalafil**

部位等　—

備　考　—

Name　Tadalafil

Other name(s)　Tadalafil

IUPAC Name　(2R,8R)-2-(2H-1,3-benzodioxol-5-yl)-6-methyl-3,6,17-triazatetracyclo[8.7.0.0^{3,8}.0^{11,16}]heptadeca-1(10),11,13,15-tetraene-4,7-dione

CAS No.　171596-29-5

Synonyms　Cialis® / (6R,12aR)-6-(1,3-Benzodioxole-5-yl)-2,3,6,7,12,12a-hexahydro-2-methylpyrazino[1',2':1,6]pyrido[3,4-b]indole-1,4-dione

分子式　$C_{22}H_{19}N_3O_4$

特性・カテゴリー　勃起障害経口治療剤／Oral drug for erectile dysfunction

Note 1 —

Note 2 —

注 —

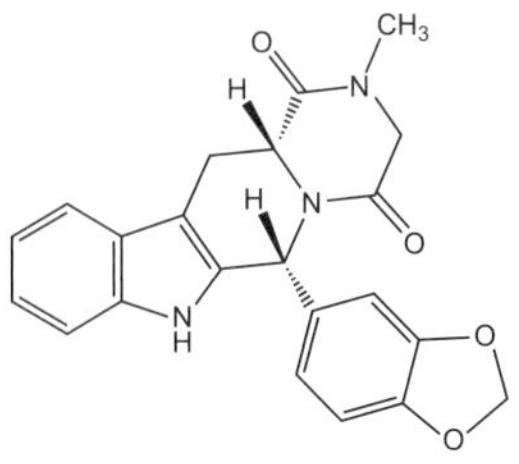

名　称　**脱*N,N*-ジメチルシブトラミン**

他名等　**Des-*N,N*-dimethyl-sibutramine**

部位等　—

備　考　—

Name　Des-N,N-dimethyl-sibutramine

Other name(s)　Des-N,N-dimethyl-sibutramine

IUPAC Name　—

CAS No.　84467-54-9

Synonyms　Cyclobutanemethanamine / N-Didesmethylsibutramine / 1-[1-(4-Chlorophenyl)cyclobutyl]-3-methylbutylamine / 1-(4-Chlorophenyl)-α-(2-methylpropyl)cyclobutanemethanamine

分子式　$C_{15}H_{22}ClN$

特性・カテゴリー　シブトラミン（経口肥満症治療薬）の誘導体／Derivative of sibutramine (an oral drug for obesity)

Note 1 —

Note 2 —

注 —

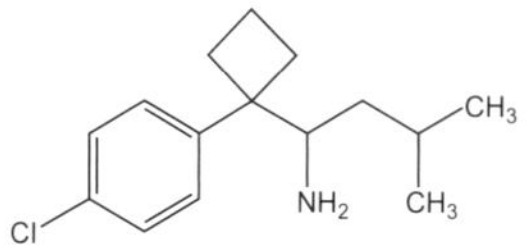

名　称　**脱*N*-メチルシブトラミン**

他名等　**Des-*N*-methyl-sibutramine**

部位等　—

備　考　—

Name　Des-N-methyl-sibutramine / N-(Desmethylsibutramine hydrochloride)

Other name(s)　Des-N-methyl-sibutramine / N-(Desmethylsibutramine hydrochloride)

IUPAC Name　N-Desmethylsibutramine hydrochloride：1-[1-(4-chlorophenyl)cyclobutyl]-N,3-dimethylbutan-1-amine；hydrochloride

CAS No.　N-Desmethylsibutramine hydrochloride：84467-94-7

Synonyms　N-Desmethylsibutramine hydrochloride：1-(4-Chlorophenyl)-N-methyl-α-(2-methylpropyl)-cyclobutanemethanamine Hydrochloride

分子式　N-Desmethylsibutramine hydrochloride：$C_{16}H_{25}Cl_2N$

特性・カテゴリー　シブトラミン（経口肥満症治療薬）の誘導体／Derivative of sibutramine (an oral drug for obesity)

Note 1 —

Note 2 —

注 —

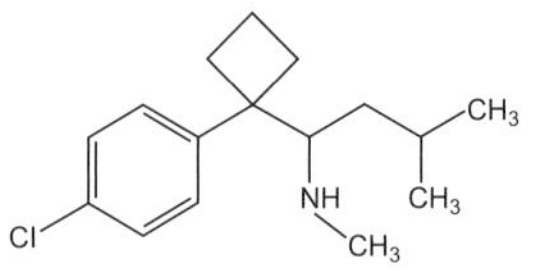

名　称　**チオアイルデナフィル**

他名等　**Thioaildenafil**
部位等　—
備　考　—

Name　Thioaildenafil
Other name(s)　Thioaildenafil
IUPAC Name　5-[5-[(3S,5R)-3,5-dimethylpiperazin-1-yl]sulfonyl-2-ethoxyphenyl]-1-methyl-3-propyl-4*H*-pyrazolo[4,3-*d*]pyrimidine-7-thione
CAS No.　856190-47-1
Synonyms　Sulfoaildenafil / Thiomethisosildenafil / (3R,5S)-rel-1-[[3-(4,7-Dihydro-1-methyl-3-propyl-7-thioxo-1*H*-pyrazolo[4,3-*d*]pyrimidin-5-yl)-4-ethoxyphenyl]sulfonyl]-3,5-dimethyl-piperazine
分子式　$C_{23}H_{32}N_6O_3S_2$
特性・カテゴリー　シルデナフィル（Viagra®、勃起障害経口治療剤）の誘導体／Derivative of Sildenafil (Viagra®, an oral drug for erectile dysfunction)
Note 1　—
Note 2　—
注　—

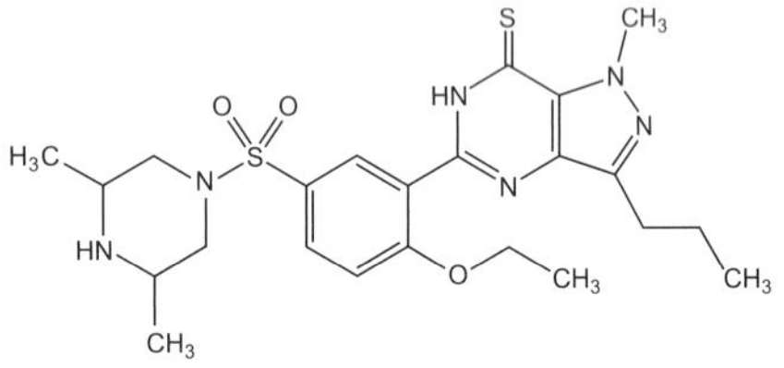

名　称　**チオキナピペリフィル**

他名等　**Thioquinapiperifil**
部位等　—
備　考　—

Name　Thioquinapiperifil
Other name(s)　Thioquinapiperifil
IUPAC Name　—
CAS No.　—
Synonyms　3-Ethyl-8-[2-[4-(hydroxymethyl)piperidino]benzylamino]-2,3-dihydro-1*H*-imidazo[4,5-*g*]quinazoline-2-thione / 8-[[2-[4-(Hydroxymethyl)piperidine-1-yl]benzyl]amino]-3-ethyl-3*H*-imidazo[4,5-*g*]quinazoline-2(1*H*)-thione
分子式　$C_{24}H_{28}N_6OS$
特性・カテゴリー　シルデナフィル（Viagra®、勃起障害経口治療剤）の誘導体／Derivative of Sildenafil (Viagra®, an oral drug for erectile dysfunction)
Note 1　—
Note 2　—
注　—

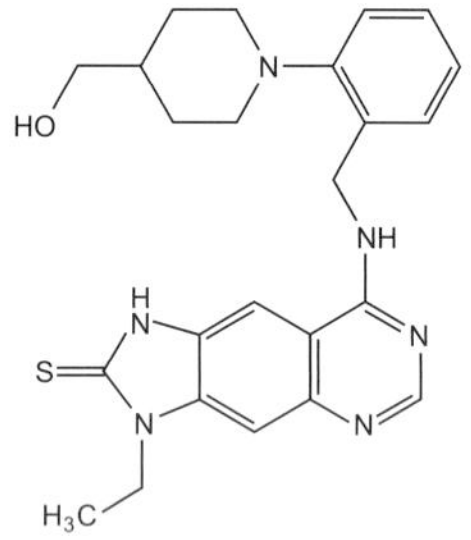

名　称　**チオデナフィル**

他名等　**Thiodenafil**
部位等　—
備　考　—

Name　Thiodenafil
Other name(s)　Thiodenafil
IUPAC Name　—
CAS No.　—
Synonyms　Thiosildenafil / 1-Methyl-3-propyl-5-[2-ethoxy-5-(4-methylpiperazinosulfonyl)phenyl]-1*H*-pyrazolo[4,3-*d*]pyrimidine-7(6*H*)-thione / 1-Methyl-3-propyl-5-[2-ethoxy-5-(4-methylpiperazinosulfonyl)phenyl]-6,7-dihydro-1*H*-pyrazolo[4,3-*d*]pyrimidine-7-thione
分子式　$C_{22}H_{30}N_6O_3S_2$
特性・カテゴリー　シルデナフィル（Viagra®、勃起障害経口治療剤）の誘導体／Derivative of Sildenafil (Viagra®, an oral drug for erectile dysfunction)
Note 1　—
Note 2　—
注　—

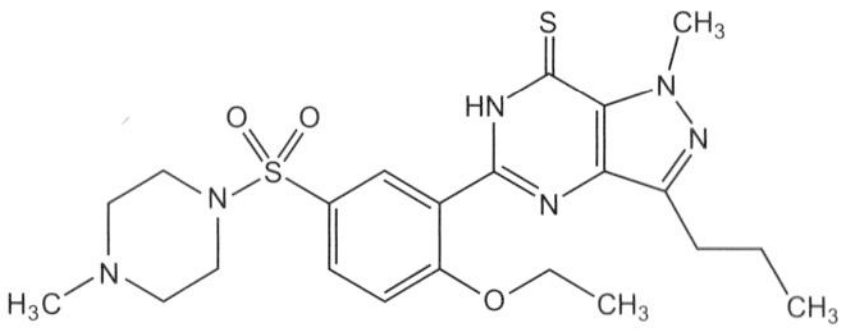

名　称　DHEA

他名等　デヒドロエピアンドロステロン
部位等　—
備　考　—

Name　DHEA
Other name(s)　Dehydroepiandrosterone
IUPAC Name　(3S,8R,9S,10R,13S,14S)-3-hydroxy-10,13-dimethyl-1,2,3,4,7,8,9,11,12,14,15,16-dodecahydrocyclopenta[a]phenanthren-17-one
CAS No.　53-43-0
Synonyms　Androstenolone / Dehydroisoandrosterone / 3beta-Hydroxy-5-androsten-17-one
分子式　$C_{19}H_{28}O_2$
特性・カテゴリー　副腎や性腺で生産されるステロイドホルモン／A major C19 steroid produced by the adrenal glands and gonads
Note 1　—
Note 2　—
注　—

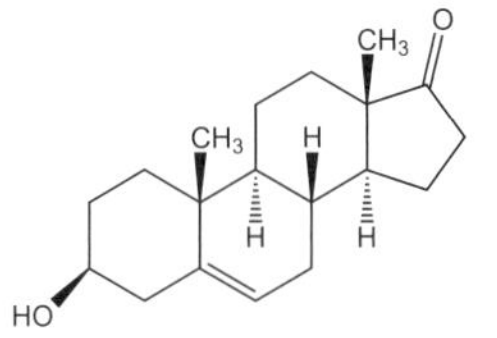

名　称　1-デオキシノジリマイシン

他名等　DNJ
部位等　—
備　考　—

Name　1-Deoxynojirimycin
Other name(s)　DNJ
IUPAC Name　(2R,3R,4R,5S)-2-(hydroxymethyl)piperidine-3,4,5-triol
CAS No.　19130-96-2
Synonyms　1,5-Deoxy-1,5-imino-D-mannitol / 1-Deoxymannojirimycin / Moranoline
分子式　$C_6H_{13}NO_4$
特性・カテゴリー　α-グルコシダーゼ阻害剤。抗ウィルス作用を有す。／An alpha-glucosidase inhibitor with antiviral action.
Note 1　—
Note 2　—
注　—

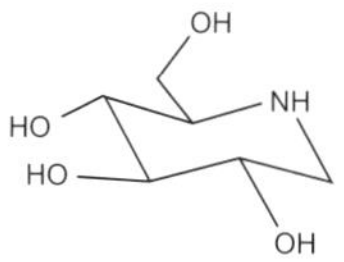

名　称　デキストロメトルファン

他名等　Dextromethorphan
部位等　—
備　考　—

Name　Dextromethorphan
Other name(s)　Dextromethorphan
IUPAC Name　—
CAS No.　125-71-3
Synonyms　d-Methorphan / Levomethorphan / (+)-3-Methoxy-N-methylmorphinon / (+)-3-Methoxy-17-methylmorphinan / [9α,13α,14α,(+)]-3-Methoxy-17-methylmorphinan
分子式　$C_{18}H_{25}NO$
特性・カテゴリー　中枢性非麻薬性鎮咳薬／An antitussive drug (Central non-narcotic antitussive drug)
Note 1　—
Note 2　See Dextromethorphan hydrobromide in this list.
注　別項の臭化水素デキストロメトルファンを参照

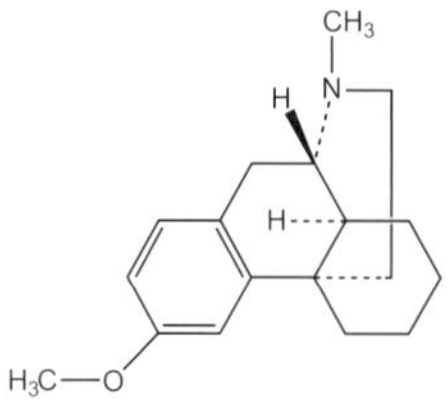

ナ行

名　称　ニコチン

他名等　—
部位等　—
備　考　—

Name　Nicotine
Other name(s)　—
IUPAC Name　3-[(2S)-1-methylpyrrolidin-2-yl]pyridine
CAS No.　54-11-5

Synonyms (S)-3-(1-methylpyrrolidin-2-yl)pyridine
分子式 $C_{10}H_{14}N_2$
特性・カテゴリー ニコチン性コリン作動性受容体のアゴニスト。強くニューロンを刺激し、最終的にシナプス伝達をブロックする。／Prototypical agonist at nicotinic cholinergic receptors where it dramatically stimulates neurons and ultimately blocks synaptic transmission.
Note 1 —
Note 2 Nicotine is highly toxic alkaloid.
注 毒性の強いアルカロイド。

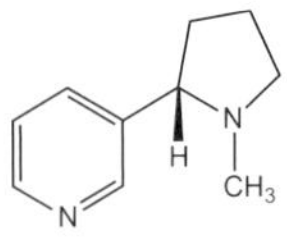

名 称 ニトロデナフィル

他名等 Nitrodenafil
部位等 —
備 考 —

Name Nitrodenafil
Other name(s) Nitrodenafil
IUPAC Name 5-(2-ethoxy-5-nitrophenyl)-1-methyl-3-propyl-4*H*-pyrazolo[4,3-*d*]pyrimidin-7-one
CAS No. 147676-99-1
Synonyms 5-(2-Ethoxy-5-nitrophenyl)-1-methyl-3-propyl-1*H*-pyrazolo[4,3-*d*]pyrimidine-7(6*H*)-one
分子式 $C_{17}H_{19}N_5O_4$
特性・カテゴリー シルデナフィル（Viagra®、勃起障害経口治療剤）の誘導体／Derivative of Sildenafil (Viagra®, an oral drug for erectile dysfunction)
Note 1 —
Note 2 —
注 —

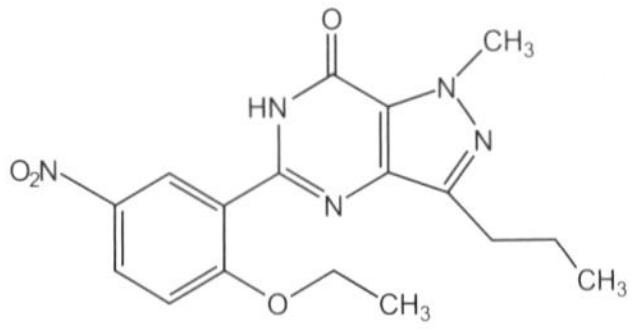

名 称 ノルネオシルデナフィル

他名等 Norneosildenafil
部位等 —
備 考 —

Name Norneosildenafil
Other name(s) Norneosildenafil
IUPAC Name 5-(2-ethoxy-5-piperidin-1-ylsulfonylphenyl)-1-methyl-3-propyl-4*H*-pyrazolo[4,3-*d*]pyrimidin-7-one
CAS No. 371959-09-0
Synonyms Norneo sildenafil / 5-[2-Ethoxy-5-(1-piperidinylsulfonyl)phenyl]-1,6-dihydro-1-methyl-3-propyl-7*H*-pyrazolo[4,3-*d*]pyrimidin-7-one / 1-[[3-(4,7-Dihydro-1-methyl-7-oxo-3-propyl-1*H*-pyrazolo[4,3-*d*]pyrimidin-5-yl)-4-ethoxyphenyl]sulfonyl]piperidine
分子式 $C_{22}H_{29}N_5O_4S$
特性・カテゴリー シルデナフィル（Viagra®、勃起障害経口治療剤）の誘導体／Derivative of Sildenafil (Viagra®, an oral drug for erectile dysfunction)
Note 1 —
Note 2 —
注 —

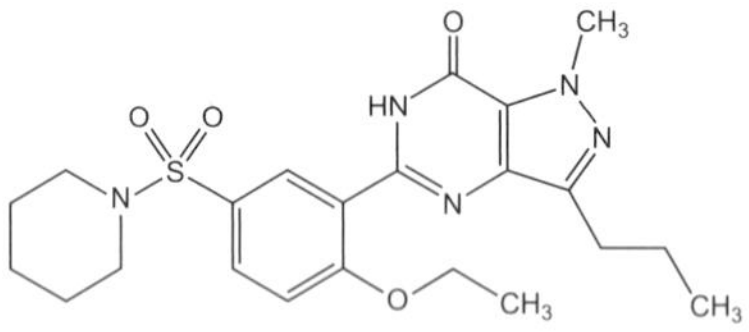

名 称 ノルホンデナフィル

他名等 Norhongdenafil
部位等 —
備 考 —

Name Norhongdenafil
Other name(s) Norhongdenafil
IUPAC Name —
CAS No. —
Synonyms 1-Methyl-3-propyl-5-[2-ethoxy-5-(4-methylpiperazinoacetyl)phenyl]-6,7-dihydro-1*H*-pyrazolo[4,3-*d*]pyrimidine-7-one
分子式 $C_{24}H_{32}N_6O_3$
特性・カテゴリー シルデナフィル（Viagra®、勃起障害経口治療剤）の誘導体／Derivative of Sildenafil (Viagra®, an oral drug for erectile dysfunction)
Note 1 —

Note 2 —
注 —

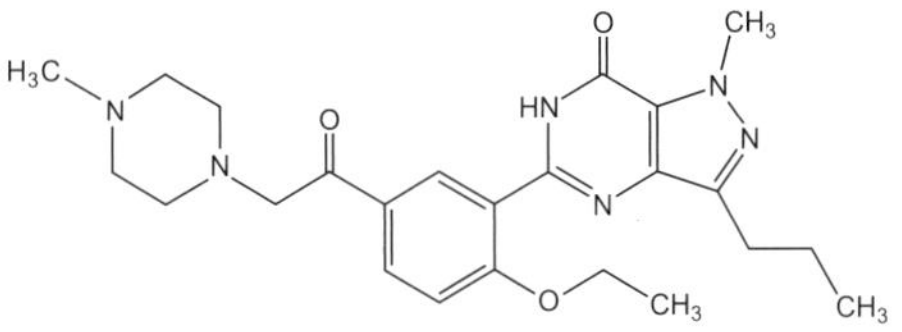

ハ行

名　称　パパイン

他名等 —
部位等 —
備　考 パパイア、パイナップル加工品は「非医」

Name Papain
Other name(s) —
IUPAC Name —
CAS No. Papain (EC 3.4.22.2) (transferred from EC 3.4.4.10) : 9001-73-4
Synonyms Papayotin / Summetrin / Veraldon / Papaine
分子式 —
特性・カテゴリー タンパク質分解酵素（遊離のSH基が必要）／Proteolytic enzymes that needs a free sulfhydryl groups for activity
Note 1 products obtained by processing papaya and pineapple : non-drug category
Note 2 —
注 —

名　称　バルデナフィル

他名等 Vardenafil
部位等 —
備　考 —

Name Vardenafil
Other name(s) Vardenafil
IUPAC Name 2-[2-ethoxy-5-(4-ethylpiperazin-1-yl) sulfonylphenyl]-5-methyl-7-propyl-1*H*-imidazo[5,1-*f*][1,2,4]triazin-4-one
CAS No. 224785-90-4
Synonyms Levitra® / Vivanza® / 2-[2-Ethoxy-5-(4-ethylpiperazinosulfonyl)phenyl]-5-methyl-7-propyl-3,4-dihydroimidazo[5,1-*f*][1,2,4]triazine-4-one
分子式 $C_{23}H_{32}N_6O_4S$
特性・カテゴリー 勃起障害経口治療剤／Oral drug for erectile dysfunction
Note 1 —
Note 2 —
注 —

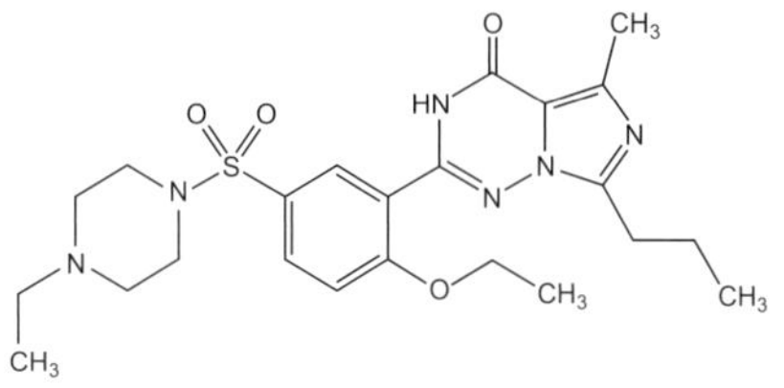

名　称　ハルマリン

他名等 Harmaline
部位等 —
備　考 —

Name Harmaline
Other name(s) Harmaline
IUPAC Name 7-methoxy-1-methyl-3,4-dihydro-2*H*-pyrido[3,4-*b*]indole
CAS No. 304-21-2
Synonyms Dihydroharmine / Harmidine / 3,4-Dihydroharmine / O-Methylharmalol
分子式 $C_{13}H_{14}N_2O$
特性・カテゴリー 中枢神経刺激剤。可逆的MAO阻害剤（RIMA）。／Central nervous system stimulant. Riversible inhibitor of monoamine oxidase type-A (RIMA).
Note 1 —
Note 2 A dihydro compound of Harmine
注 ハルミンのジヒドロ化合物

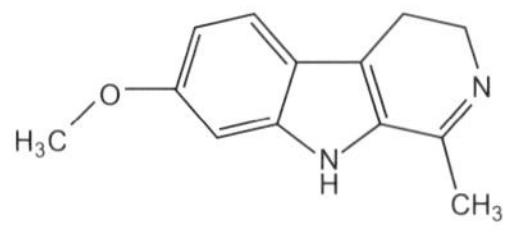

名　称　ハルミン

他名等 Harmine
部位等 —
備　考 —

Name Harmine
Other name(s) Harmine

IUPAC Name 7-methoxy-1-methyl-9*H*-pyrido[3,4-*b*]indole
CAS No. 442-51-3
Synonyms Banisterine / Leucoharmine / 7-Methoxy-1-methyl-9*H*-pyrido[3,4-*b*]indole
分子式 $C_{13}H_{12}N_2O$
特性・カテゴリー ハルマラ（ハマビシ科）の種子等より得られるアルカロイド。アマゾン領域で使用される幻覚飲料の成分の1つ。／Alkaloid isolated from seeds of *Peganum harmala* L.(Zygophyllaceae), etc. One of the active ingredients of hallucinogenic drinks made in the western Amazon region.
Note 1 —
Note 2 —
注 —

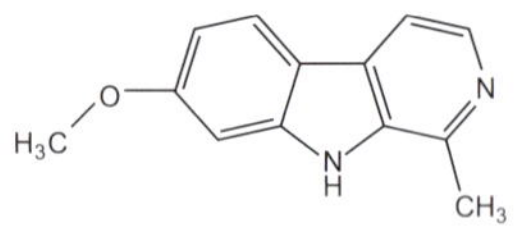

名　称　パンクレアチン

他名等 —
部位等 —
備　考 —

Name Pancreatin
Other name(s) —
IUPAC Name —
CAS No. 8049-47-6
Synonyms Pancreatic extracts
分子式 —
特性・カテゴリー リパーゼ、アミラーゼ及びプロテアーゼを含む酵素濃縮物。パンクレアチンは膵外分泌細胞で産生される消化酵素の混合物。／Enzyme concentrates containing lipase, amylase, and protease. Pancreatin is a mixture of several digestive enzymes produced by the exocrine cells of the pancreas.
Note 1 —
Note 2 —
注 —

名　称　BD

他名等 1,4-ブタンジオール
部位等 —
備　考 —

Name BD
Other name(s) 1,4-Butanediol
IUPAC Name butane-1,4-diol
CAS No. 110-63-4
Synonyms 1,4-Butylene glycol / Tetramethylene glycol
分子式 $C_4H_{10}O_2$
特性・カテゴリー 鎮静作用物質／Sedative
Note 1 —
Note 2 1,3-Butanediol and 2,3-Butanediol are not included in this item. It is limited to 1,4-Butandiol.
注 1,3-Butanediolと2,3-Butanediolも存在するが、ここでは1,4-Butandiolに限定される。

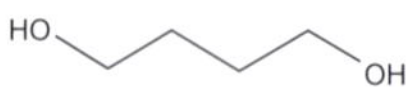

名　称　BDD

他名等 ジメチル-4,4'-ジメトキシ-5,6,5',6'-ジメチレンジオキシビフェニル-2,2'-ジカルボキシレート
部位等 —
備　考 —

Name BDD
Other name(s) Dimethyl-4,4'-dimethoxy-5,6,5',6'-dimethylenedioxybiphenyl-2,2'-dicarboxylate
IUPAC Name methyl 7-methoxy-4-(7-methoxy-5-methoxycarbonyl-1,3-benzodioxol-4-yl)-1,3-benzodioxole-5-carboxylate
CAS No. 73536-69-3
Synonyms Bifendate / Bifendatatum / Dimethyl 7,7'-dimethoxy-4,4'-bi-1,3-benzodioxole-5,5'-dicarboxylate / 7,7'-dimethoxy-(4,4'-bis-1,3-benzodioxole)-5,5'-dicarboxylic acid dimethyl ester
分子式 $C_{20}H_{18}O_{10}$
特性・カテゴリー 免疫反応促進剤。酵素-基質結合を阻害する物質として知られている。／Immune enhancer. Substance which inhibits normal substrate-enzyme combination.
Note 1 —
Note 2 —
注 —

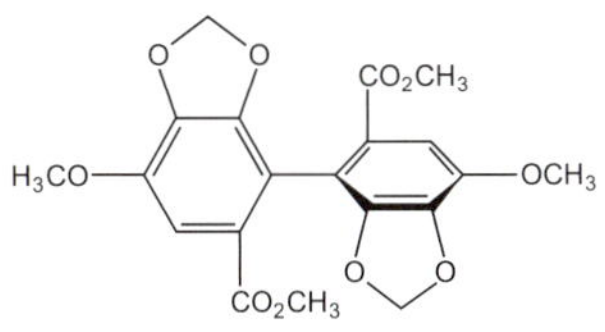

名　称　ヒドロキシチオホモシルデナフィル

他名等　Hydroxythiohomosildenafil
部位等　—
備　考　—

Name　Hydroxythiohomosildenafil
Other name(s)　Hydroxythiohomosildenafil
IUPAC Name　5-[2-ethoxy-5-[4-(2-hydroxyethyl)piperazin-1-yl]sulfonylphenyl]-1-methyl-3-propyl-4*H*-pyrazolo[4,3-*d*]pyrimidine-7-thione
CAS No.　479073-82-0
Synonyms　Thiohydroxyhomosildenafil / Sulfohydroxyhomosildenafil / Hydroxythiohomo sildenafil / Night bullet
分子式　$C_{23}H_{32}N_6O_4S_2$
特性・カテゴリー　シルデナフィル（Viagra®、勃起障害経口治療剤）の誘導体／Derivative of Sildenafil (Viagra®, an oral drug for erectile dysfunction)
Note 1　—
Note 2　—
注　—

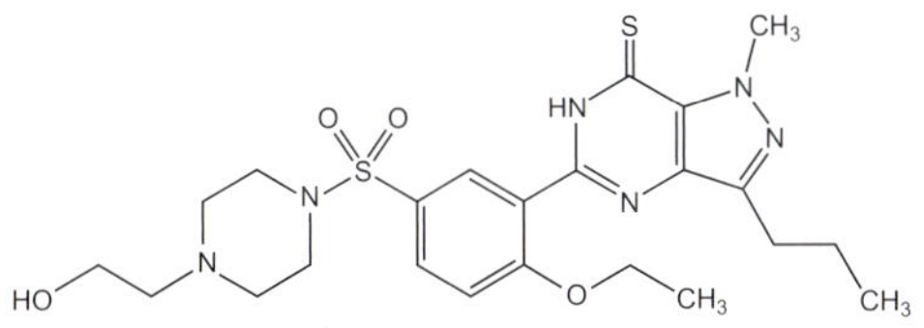

名　称　5-HTP（ヒドロキシトリプトファン）

他名等　L-5-Hydroxy-tryptophan
部位等　—
備　考　—

Name　5-HTP (5-Hydroxy-tryptophan)
Other name(s)　L-5-Hydroxy-tryptophan
IUPAC Name　2-amino-3-(5-hydroxy-1*H*-indol-3-yl) propanoic acid
CAS No.　5-Hydroxytryptophan：56-69-9
5-Hydroxy-L-tryptophan：4350-09-8
Synonyms　5-Hydroxy-DL-tryptophan / DL-5-Hydroxytryptophan / (+-)-5-Hydroxytryptophan / DL-Hydroxytryptophan / 5-Hydroxy-L-tryptophan
分子式　$C_{11}H_{12}N_2O_3$
特性・カテゴリー　抗鬱薬。セロトニンの再吸収抑制によりセロトニン作動系に作用。／Antidepressant. Act on serotonergic systems, especially by inhibiting serotonin reuptake.
Note 1　—
Note 2　The immediate precursor in the biosynthesis of serotonin from tryptophan. It is used as an antiepileptic and antidepressant.
注　トリプトファンからセロトニンへの体内合成の直前の前駆物質。抗てんかん薬及び抗鬱薬として使用される。

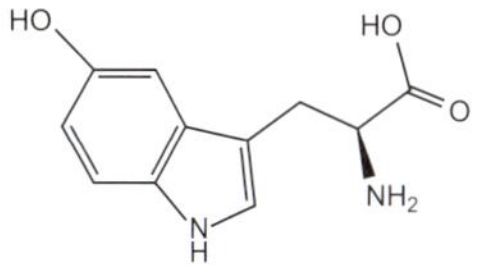

名　称　ヒドロキシホモシルデナフィル

他名等　Hydroxyhomosildenafil
部位等　—
備　考　—

Name　Hydroxyhomosildenafil
Other name(s)　Hydroxyhomosildenafil
IUPAC Name　5-[2-ethoxy-5-[4-(2-hydroxyethyl)piperazin-1-yl]sulfonylphenyl]-1-methyl-3-propyl-4*H*-pyrazolo[4,3-*d*]pyrimidine-7-thione
CAS No.　139755-85-4
Synonyms　Hydroxyhomo sildenafil
分子式　$C_{23}H_{32}N_6O_5S$
特性・カテゴリー　シルデナフィル（Viagra®、勃起障害経口治療剤）の誘導体／Derivative of Sildenafil (Viagra®, an oral drug for erectile dysfunction)
Note 1　—
Note 2　—
注　—

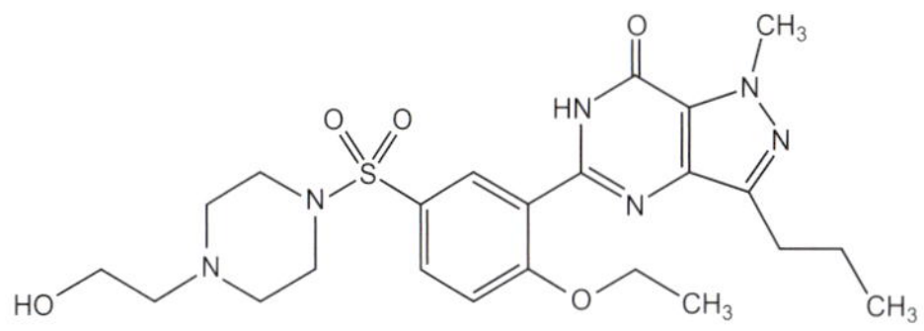

名　称　ヒドロキシホンデナフィル

他名等　Hydroxyhongdenafil
部位等　—
備　考　—

Name　Hydroxyhongdenafil
Other name(s)　Hydroxyhongdenafil
IUPAC Name　5-[2-ethoxy-5-[2-[4-(2-hydroxyethyl)piperazin-1-yl]acetyl]phenyl]-1-methyl-3-propyl-4*H*-pyrazolo[4,3-*d*]pyrimidin-7-one
CAS No.　147676-56-0
Synonyms　Hydroxyacetildenafil / Hydroxy acetildenafil
分子式　$C_{25}H_{34}N_6O_4$
特性・カテゴリー　シルデナフィル（Viagra®、勃起障害経口治療剤）の誘導体／Derivative of Sildenafil (Viagra®, an oral drug for erectile dysfunction)
Note 1　—
Note 2　—
注　—

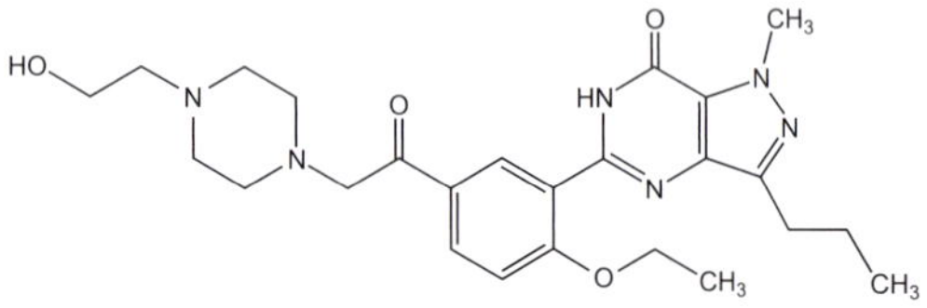

名　称　ビンカミン

他名等　—
部位等　—
備　考　—

Name　Vincamine
Other name(s)　—
IUPAC Name　(3alpha, 14beta, 16alpha)-14,15-dihydro-14-hydroxyeburnamenine-14-carboxylic acid methyl ester
CAS No.　1617-90-9
Synonyms　methyl(3alpha,14beta,16alpha)-14-hydroxy-14,15-dihydroeburnamenine-14-carboxylate
分子式　$C_{21}H_{26}N_2O_3$
特性・カテゴリー　末梢血管拡張薬。ヒメツルニチニチソウの主要アルカロイド／Peripheral vasodilator. A major alkaloid of *Vinca minor* L.
Note 1　—
Note 2　—
注　—

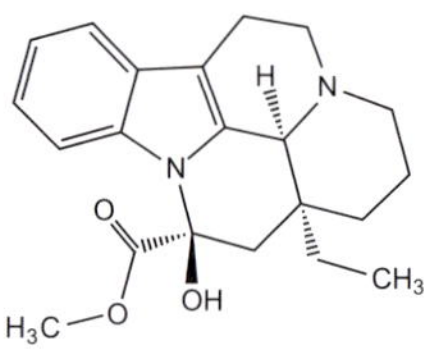

名　称　プソイドバルデナフィル

他名等　ピペリデナフィル／Pseudovardenafil／Piperidenafil
部位等　—
備　考　—

Name　Pseudovardenafil
Other name(s)　PIPERIDENAFIRU (in KATAKANA) / Pseudovardenafil / Piperidenafil
IUPAC Name　2-(2-ethoxy-5-piperidin-1-ylsulfonylphenyl)-5-methyl-7-propyl-1*H*-imidazo[5,1-*f*][1,2,4]triazin-4-one
CAS No.　224788-34-5
Synonyms　Pseudo vardenafil / Piperadino vardenafil / Piperidino-vardenafil
分子式　$C_{22}H_{29}N_5O_4S$
特性・カテゴリー　シルデナフィル（Viagra®、勃起障害経口治療剤）の誘導体／Derivative of Sildenafil (Viagra®, an oral drug for erectile dysfunction)
Note 1　—
Note 2　—
注　—

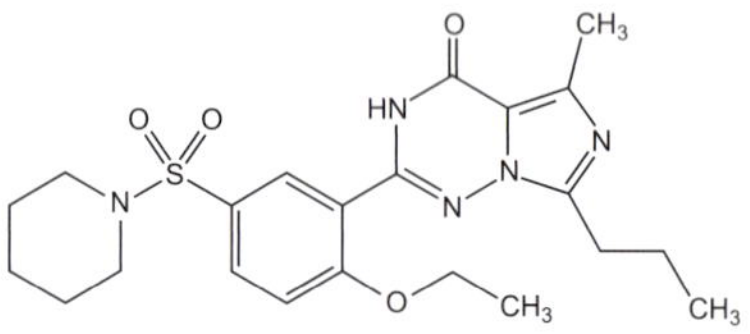

名　称　ブフォテニン

他名等　Bufotenine
部位等　—
備　考　—

Name　Bufotenine
Other name(s)　Bufotenine
IUPAC Name　3-[2-(dimethylamino)ethyl]-1*H*-indol-5-ol
CAS No.　487-93-4
Synonyms　Bufotenin / Cinobufotenine / N,N-Dimethyl-

serotonin / N,N-Dimethyl-5-hydroxytryptamine
分子式 $C_{12}H_{16}N_2O$
特性・カテゴリー 幻覚発現性セロトニン類似物質。ヒキガエル科シナヒキガエル等の耳腺分泌物に含まれる強心ステロイド。生薬名は蟾酥（センソ）。／Hallucinogenic serotonin analogue. A cardiotonic steroid found in the secretion from parotoid gland of *Bufo bufo gargarizans* Cantor, etc. belonging to Bufonidae. Its name as a Kampo medicine, the traditional Japanese medicine, is SENSO.
Note 1 —
Note 2 —
注 —

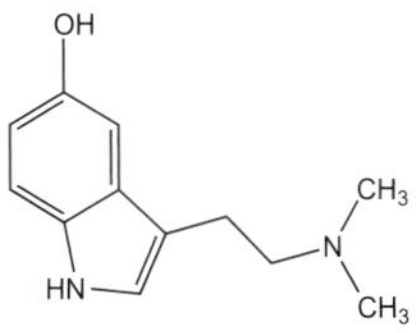

名　称　プロスタグランジン

他名等 —
部位等 —
備　考 —

Name Prostaglandin
Other name(s) —
IUPAC Name —
CAS No. —
Synonyms —
分子式 —
特性・カテゴリー プロスタン酸骨格をもつ一群の生理活性物質。アラキドン酸からシクロオキシゲナーゼの作用によって生合成されるエイコサノイドの1つで、様々な強い生理活性を有す。／A group of bioactive compounds derived from unsaturated 20-carbon fatty acids, prostanoic acid, primarily arachidonic acid, via the cyclooxygenase pathway. They are extremely potent mediators of a diverse group of physiological processes.
Note 1 —
Note 2 —
注 —

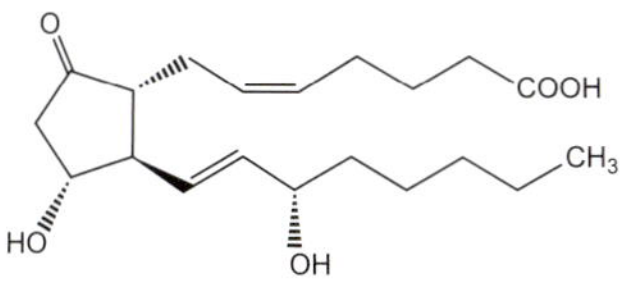

Prostaglandin E_2

名　称　プロテアーゼ

他名等 —
部位等 —
備　考 —

Name Protease
Other name(s) —
IUPAC Name —
CAS No. —
Synonyms —
分子式 —
特性・カテゴリー タンパク質・ペプチド加水分解酵素の総称で、非常に多くの酵素が存在するので、単一の酵素に特定できない。／Protease refers to a group of enzymes which catalytic function is to hydrolyze proteins.
Note 1 —
Note 2 —
注 —

名　称　ブロメライン

他名等 —
部位等 —
備　考 —

Name Bromelain
Other name(s) —
IUPAC Name —
CAS No. Fruit bromelain（EC 3.4.22.33）：9001-00-7
Stem bromelain（EC 3.4.22.32）：37189-34-7
Synonyms Edemase / Bromelains / Ananas / Stem bromelain / Juice bromelain / Fruit bromelain
分子式 —
特性・カテゴリー パイナップル果実ジュース及び茎より得られるタンパク質分解酵素及び凝乳酵素／Protein-digesting and milk-clotting enzymes found in pineapple fruit juice and stem tissues.
Note 1 —
Note 2 —
注 —

名　称　ペプシン

他名等　—
部位等　—
備　考　—

Name　Pepsin
Other name (s)　—
IUPAC Name　—
CAS No.　Pepsin A（EC 3.4.23.1）：9001-75-6
　Pepsin B（EC 3.4.23.2）：9025-48-3
Synonyms　Pepsin A / Pepsin B
分子式　—
特性・カテゴリー　胃液中の主要消化酵素：タンパク質のプロテオース及びペプトンへの分解をコントロールする。／Principle digestive enzym of gastric juice：controls the degradation of proteins to proteoses and peptones.
Note 1　—
Note 2　—
注　—

名　称　ホモシルデナフィル

他名等　Homosildenafil
部位等　—
備　考　—

Name　Homosildenafil
Other name (s)　—
IUPAC Name　5-[2-ethoxy-5-(4-ethylpiperazin-1-yl) sulfonylphenyl]-1-methyl-3-propyl-4*H*-pyrazolo[4,3-*d*]pyrimidin-7-one
CAS No.　642928-07-2
Synonyms　—
分子式　$C_{23}H_{32}N_6O_4S$
特性・カテゴリー　シルデナフィル（Viagra®、勃起障害経口治療剤）の誘導体／Derivative of Sildenafil（Viagra®, an oral drug for erectile dysfunction）
Note 1　—
Note 2　See Sildenafil in this list.
注　別項のシルデナフィルを参照。

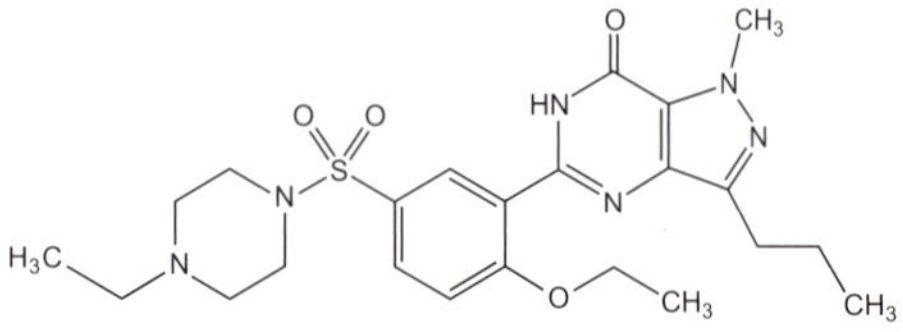

名　称　ホモチオデナフィル

他名等　Homothiodenafil
部位等　—
備　考　—

Name　Homothiodenafil
Other name (s)　Homothiodenafil
IUPAC Name　Thiohomosildenafil：5-[2-ethoxy-5-(4-ethylpiperazin-1-yl) sulfonylphenyl]-1-methyl-3-propyl-4*H*-pyrazolo[4,3-*d*]pyrimidine-7-thione
CAS No.　479073-80-8
Synonyms　Thiohomosildenafil：Sulfohomosildenafil / Thiohomo sildenafil / Homosildenafil thione
分子式　$C_{23}H_{32}N_6O_3S_2$
特性・カテゴリー　シルデナフィル（Viagra®、勃起障害経口治療剤）の誘導体／Derivative of Sildenafil（Viagra®, an oral drug for erectile dysfunction）
Note 1　—
Note 2　—
注　—

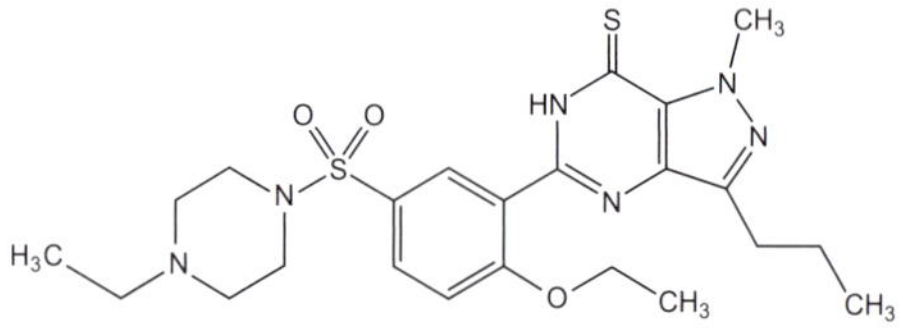

名　称　ホンデナフィル

他名等　アセチルデナフィル／Hongdenafil／Acetildenafil
部位等　—
備　考　—

Name　Hongdenafil
Other name (s)　ASECHIRUDENAFIRU（in KATAKANA）/ Hongdenafil / Acetildenafil
IUPAC Name　5-[2-ethoxy-5-[2-(4-ethylpiperazin-1-yl) acetyl]phenyl]-1-methyl-3-propyl-4*H*-pyrazolo[4,3-*d*]pyrimidin-7-one
CAS No.　831217-01-7
Synonyms　Sildenafil / 5-[2-Ethoxy-5-[2-[4-ethylpiperazine-1-yl]acetyl]phenyl]-1-methyl-3-propyl-1*H*-pyrazolo[4,3-*d*]pyrimidine-7(6*H*)-one / 5-[2-Ethoxy-5-[2-(4-ethylpiperazin-1-yl) acetyl]phenyl]-1-methyl-3-propyl-4*H*-pyrazolo[4,3-*d*]pyrimidin-7-one
分子式　$C_{25}H_{34}N_6O_3$
特性・カテゴリー　シルデナフィル（Viagra®、勃起障害経口治療剤）の誘導体／Derivative of Sildenafil（Viagra®, an oral drug for erectile dysfunction）

Note 1　—

Note 2　—

注　—

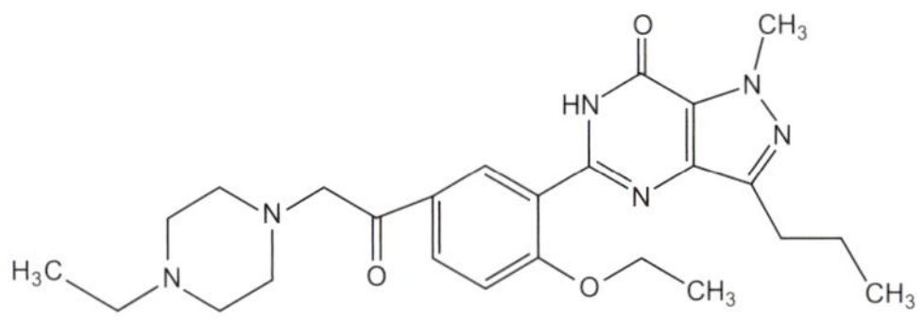

マ行

名　称　マグノフロリン

他名等　Magnoflorine

部位等　—

備　考　—

Name　Magnoflorine

Other name(s)　Magnoflorine

IUPAC Name　(6aS)-2,10-dimethoxy-6,6-dimethyl-5,6,6a,7-tetrahydro-4*H*-dibenzo[de,g]quinoline-6-ium-1,11-diol

CAS No.　Magnoflorine：2141-09-5
Thalictrin：75026-31-2

Synonyms　Thalictrin / Escholin / Thalictrine / (s)-5,6,6a,7-tetrahydro-1,11-dihydroxy-2,10-dimethoxy-6,6-dimethyl-4h-dibenzo[de,g]quinolinium

分子式　$C_{20}H_{24}NO_4^+$

特性・カテゴリー　植物成分。イカリソウ、メギ、オウレン、ホウノキ等に含まれるアポルフィン型イソキノリンアルカロイド。LDLリポタンパクの酸化に対して抗酸化活性を有す。／Botanical constituent. Aporphine-type of isoquinoline alkaloid containd in *Epimedium* spp., *Berberis* spp., *Coptis* spp. or *Magnolia* spp.. Anti-oxidant activity against the oxidation of low density lipoprotein (LDL).

Note 1　—

Note 2　—

注　—

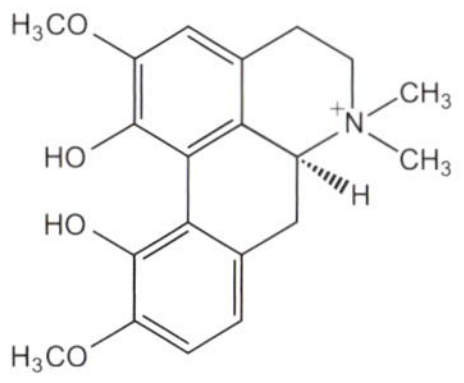

名　称　マルターゼ

他名等　α-グルコシダーゼ

部位等　—

備　考　—

Name　Maltase

Other name(s)　alpha-Glucosidase

IUPAC Name　—

CAS No.　alpha-Glucosidase（EC 3.2.1.20）：9001-42-7

Synonyms　Glucoinvertase / Glucosidosucrase / alpha-D-Glucoside glucohydrolase / alpha-Glucoside hydrolase / alpha-1,4-Glucosidase

分子式　—

特性・カテゴリー　マルトース加水分解酵素／Catalyzes the hydrolysis of maltose to the simple sugar glucose

Note 1　—

Note 2　—

注　—

名　称　ムタプロデナフィル

他名等　Mutaprodenafil

部位等　—

備　考　—

Name　Mutaprodenafil

Other name(s)　Mutaprodenafil

IUPAC Name　Nitrosoprodenafil：N-[2-[5-[5-(2,6-dimethylpiperidin-4-yl)sulfonyl-2-ethoxyphenyl]-1-methyl-3-propylpyrazolo[4,3-*d*]pyrimidin-7-yl]oxy-1,3-thiazol-5-yl]-N-methylnitrous amide

CAS No.　Mutaprodenafil：138577-30-1

Synonyms　Nitrosoprodenafil / Nitroprodenafil

分子式　Mutaprodenafil：$C_{27}H_{35}N_9O_5S_2$
Nitrosoprodenafil：$C_{28}H_{36}N_8O_5S_2$

特性・カテゴリー　シルデナフィル（Viagra®、勃起障害経口治療剤）の誘導体／Derivative of Sildenafil（Viagra®, an oral drug for erectile dysfunction）

Note 1　—

Note 2　—

注　—

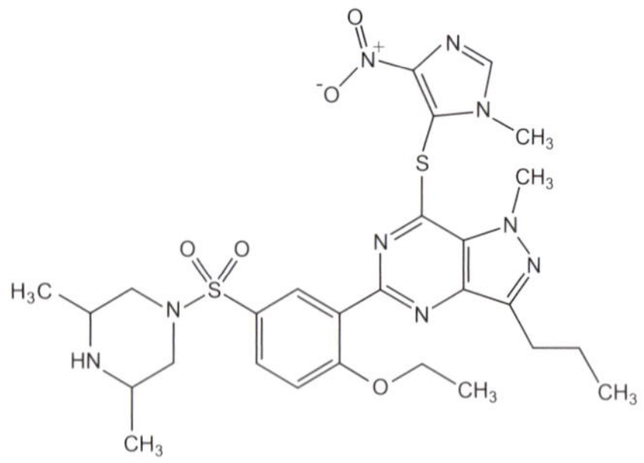

名　称　**メチソシルデナフィル**

他名等　Methisosildenafil
部位等　—
備　考　—

Name　Methisosildenafil
Other name(s)　Methisosildenafil
IUPAC Name　5-[5-[(3S,5R)-3,5-dimethylpiperazin-1-yl]sulfonyl-2-ethoxyphenyl]-1-methyl-3-propyl-4*H*-pyrazolo[4,3-*d*]pyrimidin-7-one
CAS No.　496835-35-9
Synonyms　Aildenafil / Dimethylsildenafil / Dimethyl sildenafil
分子式　$C_{23}H_{32}N_6O_4S$
特性・カテゴリー　シルデナフィル（Viagra®、勃起障害経口治療剤）の誘導体／Derivative of Sildenafil (Viagra®, an oral drug for erectile dysfunction)
Note 1　—
Note 2　—
注　—

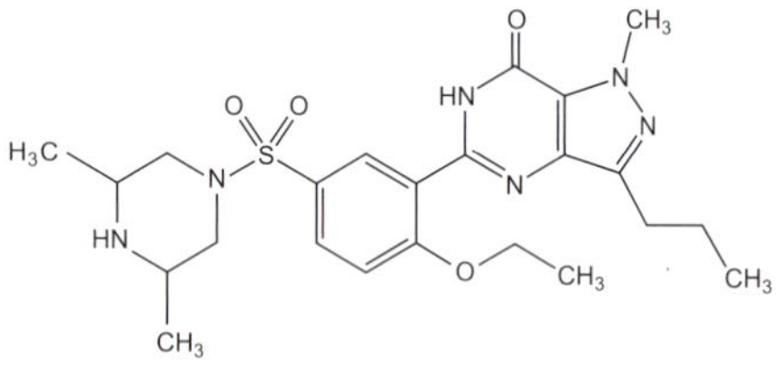

名　称　**メラトニン**

他名等　松果体ホルモン
部位等　—
備　考　—

Name　Melatonin
Other name(s)　Pineal gland hormone
IUPAC Name　N-[2-(5-methoxy-1*H*-indol-3-yl)ethyl]acetamide
CAS No.　73-31-4
Synonyms　N-Acetyl-5-methoxytryptamine / 5-Methoxy-N-acetyltryptamine / Melovine® / Melatonex® / Vivitas®
分子式　$C_{13}H_{16}N_2O_2$
特性・カテゴリー　生体アミン。動物、植物、微生物に含まれる。哺乳類では松果体で生産される。ヒトではメラトニン受容体を活性化させる。／Biogenic amine. Melatonin is found in animals, plants and microbes. In mammals, it is produced by the pineal gland. In human, Melatonin activates its receptors.
Note 1　—
Note 2　—
注　—

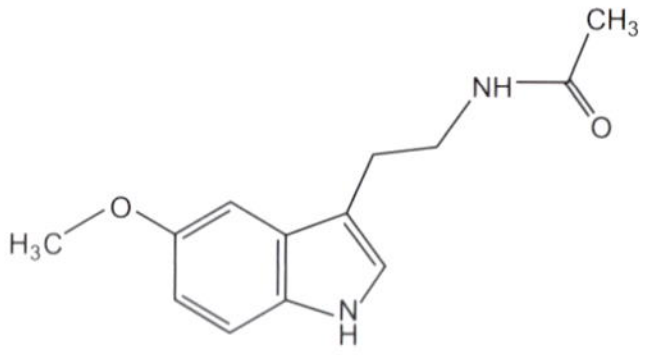

ヤ行

名　称　**ヨウキセキ**

他名等　—
部位等　—
備　考　鉱石

Name　Actinolite
Other name(s)　—
IUPAC Name　—
CAS No.　77536-66-4
Synonyms　—
化学組成（Chemical composition）　$Ca_2(Mg,Fe)_5Si_8O_{22}(OH)_2$ (Mg / (Mg+Fe) = 0.5–0.9)
特性・カテゴリー　鉱石／mineral (Ore)
Note 1　Mineral (Ore)
Note 2　Component of asbestos. YÔKI-SEKI which English name is actinolite is also known as RYOKUSEN-SEKI or TÔRYOKUSEN-SEKI.
注　アスベスト（石綿）の成分。
ヨウキセキ（陽起石）は、リョクセンセキ（緑閃石）、トウリョクセンセキ（透緑閃石）ともいう。

ラ行

名　称　ラクターゼ

他名等　β-ガラクトシダーゼ
部位等　—
備　考　—

Name　Lactase
Other name(s)　beta-Galactosidase
IUPAC Name　—
CAS No.　beta-Galactosidase (EC 3.2.1.23)：9031-11-2
Synonyms　Lactase-phlorizin hydrolase / lactose galactohydrolase
分子式　—
特性・カテゴリー　乳糖加水分解酵素／Hydrolase enzyme that catalyzes the hydrolysis of beta-galactosides into monosaccharides.
Note 1　—
Note 2　—
注　—

名　称　リパーゼ

他名等　—
部位等　—
備　考　—

Name　Lipase
Other name(s)　—
IUPAC Name　—
CAS No.　Triacylglycerol lipase (EC 3.1.1.3)：9001-62-1
Synonyms　Triacylglycerol lipase / Triacylglycerol acylhydrolase
分子式　—
特性・カテゴリー　脂質加水分解酵素（エステラーゼ）、特にトリグリセライド（グリセロールの脂肪酸エステル）を脂肪酸とグリセロールに分解する。／Esterase, Hydrolyzing fat (present in ester form, such as glycerides) yielding fatty acids and glycerol.
Note 1　—
Note 2　—
注　—

名　称　ルンブルキナーゼ

他名等　—
部位等　—
備　考　—

Name　Lumbrokinase
Other name(s)　—
IUPAC Name　—
CAS No.　556743-18-1
Synonyms　—
分子式　—
特性・カテゴリー　タンパク質分解酵素。線維素溶解活性、血小板凝集能を増し、血液粘度を上げる。／Protease, promote healthy fibrinolytic activity, platelet coagulation functions and blood viscosity.
Note 1　—
Note 2　Fibrinolytic enzyme present in the earthworm *Lumbricus rubellus* (Syn. *L. bimatus*). It has been investigated as an experimental antithrombotic agent.
注　食用アカミミズ（*Lumbricus rubellus*, 異名：*L. bimatus*）に含まれる線維素溶解酵素。実験的抗血栓剤として研究されている。

第 3 部　添付資料

Part 3　Appendix

1．既存添加物名簿収載品目リスト
List of existing food additives

2．天然香料基原物質リスト
List of plant or animal sources of natural flavorings

3．一般に食品として飲食に供されている物であって添加物として使用される品目リスト
List of substances which are generally provided for eating or drinking as foods and which are also used as food additives

4．無承認無許可医薬品の指導取締りについて（昭和46年６月１日薬発第476号）
Regulatory control of unapproved/unpermitted drugs (1 June 1971, PAB Notification No. 476)

5．無承認無許可医薬品の監視指導について（昭和62年９月22日薬監第88号）
Inspection and guidance of unapproved/unpermitted drugs (22 September 1987, PAB Notification No. 88)

6．「「医薬品的効能効果を標ぼうしない限り医薬品と判断しない成分本質（原材料）」の食品衛生法上の取り扱いの改正について」の一部改正について（平成26年３月14日食安基発0314第１号）
Partial amendments to the 'Amending the handling of "List of ingredients (raw materials) not deemed drugs unless claiming medicinal efficacy" under the Food Sanitation Act' (14 March 2014, Department of Food Safety, Standards and Evaluation Division Notification No. 0314-1)

7．欧州医薬品庁(EMA) ハーブ医薬品委員会によるハーブ素材評価リスト（2014年７月８日現在）
List of herbal substances designated for assessment by the European Medicines Agency's Committee on Herbal Medicinal Products (HMPC) (as of July 8, 2014)

8．第36改正 米国薬局方及び第31改正 国民医薬品集におけるダイエタリーサプリメント，オフィシャルモノグラフ（2013）
Lists of USP 36-NF 31 (2013) Dietary Supplements , Official Monographs

9．日本薬局方（第16改正）収載生薬の学名表記について
On the scientific names of crude drugs listed in the Japanese Pharmacopoeia (The 16th Edition)

〈1．～3．〉平成22年10月20日消食表第377号通知「食品衛生法に基づく添加物の表示等について」の別添１、２、3

〈1．～3．〉Labeling of additives based on the Food Sanitation Act (Food Labeling Division, Consumer Affairs Agency Notification No. 377) Attachment table 1, 2 and 3

添付資料 1
既存添加物名簿収載品目リスト

Appendix 1
List of existing food additives

既存添加物名簿収載品目リスト

番号	品名 名称	品名 別名	簡略名又は類別名	基原・製法・本質	用途	備考
1	アウレオバシジウム培養液 （アウレオバシジウム培養液から得られた、β-1,3-1,6-グルカンを主成分とするものをいう。）			黒酵母（Aureobasidium pullulans）の培養液より、分離して得られたものである。主成分はβ-1,3-1,6-グルカンである。	増粘安定剤	Aureobasidium cultured solution
2	アガラーゼ			担子菌（Coliolus）又は細菌（Bacillus, Pseudomonas）の培養液より、水で抽出して得られたものである。	酵素	Agarase
3	アクチニジン			マタタビ科キウイ（Actinidia chinensis PLANCH）の果肉より、搾汁して得られたもの、又はこれを、冷時～室温時水で抽出して得られたもの、若しくは膜で濃縮して得られたものである。	酵素	Actinidine
4	アグロバクテリウムスクシノグリカン （アグロバクテリウムの培養液から得られた、クスシノグリカンを主成分とするものをいう。）		スクシノグリカン	細菌（Agrobacterium tumefaciences）の培養液より、分離して得られた多糖類である。主成分はスクシノグリカンである。	増粘安定剤	Agrobacterium succinoglycan
5	アシラーゼ			糸状菌（Aspergillus ochraceus, Aspergillus melleus）の培養液より、水で抽出して得られたもの、冷時～室温時除菌したもの、又はこれより、冷時エタノールで処理して得られたものである。	酵素	Acylase
6	アスコルビン酸オキシダーゼ	アスコルベートオキシダーゼ ビタンミンCオキシダーゼ	オキシダーゼ V.Cオキシダーゼ	ウリ、カボチャ、キャベツ、キュウリ若しくはホウレンソウより、搾汁して得られたもの、冷時～室温時水で抽出して得られたもの、冷時アセトンで処理して得られたもの、又は糸状菌（Trichoderma lignorum）若しくは放線菌（Eupenicillium brefeldianum）の培養液より、除菌後、濃縮して得られたものである。	酵素	Ascorbate oxidase
7	L-アスパラギン		アスパラギン	植物性タンパク質を、加水分解し、分離して得られたものである。成分はL-アスパラギンである。	調味料 強化剤	L-Asparagine
8	L-アスパラギン酸		アスパラギン酸	発酵又は酵素法により得られたものを、分離して得られたものである。成分はL-アスパラギン酸である。	調味料	L-Aspartic acid
9	アスペルギルステレウス糖たん白質 （アスペルギルステレウスの培養液から得られた、糖タンパク質を主成分とするものをいう。）	ムタステイン		糸状菌（Aspergillus terreus）によるブドウ糖、殿粉及び大豆ミールの発酵培養液を除菌し、硫酸アンモニウムにより分画した後、脱塩して得られたものである。主成分は糖タンパク質である。	製造用剤	Aspergillus terreus glycoprotein
10	α-アセトラクタートデカルボキシラーゼ	α-アセトラクテートデカルボキシラーゼ	リアーゼ	細菌（Bacillus subtilis, Serratia）の培養液より、室温時水で抽出して得られたものである。	酵素	α-Acetolactate decarboxylase
11	5'-アデニル酸	アデノシン5'-一リン酸	5'-AMP	酵母（Candida utilis）の菌体より、水で抽出した核酸を酵素で加水分解した後、分離して得られたものである。成分は5'-アデニル酸である。	強化剤	5'-Adenylic acid
12	アナトー色素 （ベニノキの種子の被覆物から得られた、ノルビキシン及びビキシンを主成分とするものをいう。）		アナトー カロチノイド カロチノイド色素 カロテノイド カロテノイド色素	ベニノキ科ベニノキ（Bixa orellane LINNE）の種子の被覆物より、熱時油脂若しくはプロピレングリコールで抽出して得られたもの、室温時ヘキサン若しくはアセトンで抽出し、溶媒を除去して得られたもの、又は熱時アルカル性水溶液で抽出し、加水分解し、中和し	着色料	Annatto extract

番号	品名 名称	品名 別名	簡略名又は類別名	基原・製法・本質	用途	備考
				て得られたものである。主色素はビキシン及びノルビキシンである。黄色～橙色を呈する。		
13	アマシードガム（アマの種子から得られた、多糖類を主成分とするものをいう。）		アマシード	アマ科アマ（Linum usitatissimum LINNE）の種子の胚乳部分より、室温時～温時水又は含水アルコールで抽出して得られたものである。主成分は多糖類である。	増粘安定剤	Linseed gum Linseed extract
14	アミノペプチダーゼ			細菌（Aeromonas caviae, Lactobacillus casei, Lactococcus lactis）の培養液より、分離して得られたものである。	酵素	Aminopeptidase
15	α-アミラーゼ	液化アミラーゼ G3分解酵素	アミラーゼ カルボヒドラーゼ	糸状菌（Aspergillus aureus, Aspergillus niger, Aspergillus oryzae）、細菌（Alcaligenes latus, Arthrobacter, Bacillus amyloliquefaciens, Bacillus licheniformis, Bacillus stearothermophilus, Bacillus subtilis, Sulfolobus solfataricus）若しくは放線菌（Thermomonospora viridis）の培養液より、又は麦芽より、冷時～室温時水で抽出して得られたもの、除菌したもの若しくは濃縮したもの、冷時エタノール、含水エタノール若しくはアセトンで処理して得られたもの、又は硫酸アンモニウム等で分画した後、脱塩処理して得られたものである。	酵素	α-Amylase
16	β-アミラーゼ		アミラーゼ カルボヒドラーゼ	糸状菌（Aspergillus oryzae）、放線菌（Streptomyces）若しくは細菌（Bacillus amyloliquefaciens, Bacillus polymyxa, Bacillus subtilis）の培養液より、又は麦芽若しくは穀類の種子より、冷時～室温時水で抽出して得られたもの若しくは濃縮して得られたもの、又は冷時エタノールで処理して得られたものである。	酵素	β-Amylase
17	L-アラニン		アラニン	タンパク質原料の加水分解又は発酵若しくは酵素法により得られたものを、分離して得られたものである。成分はL-アラニンである。	調味料 強化剤	L-Alanine
18	アラビアガム（アカシアの分泌液から得られた、多糖類を主成分とするものをいう。）	アカシアガム	アカシア	アカシア属植物（Acacia senegal Willdenow又はAcacia seyal Delile）の分泌液を、乾燥して得られた、又はこれを脱塩して得られた多糖類を主成分とするものである。	増粘安定剤	Gum Arabic Arabic gum Acacia gum
19	アラビノガラクタン			マツ科セイヨウカラマツ（Larix occidentalis NUTT.）又はその他同属植物の根又は幹より、室温時水で抽出して得られたものである。成分は多糖類（構成糖はガラクトース、アラビノース等）である。	増粘安定剤	Arabino galactan
20	L-アラビノース		アラビノース	アラビアガム、ガディガム、コーンファイバー又はテンサイのパルプ（シュガービートパルプ）の多糖類（アラビナン等）を、加水分解し、分離して得られたものである。成分はL-アラビノースである。	甘味料	L-Arabinose
21	L-アルギニン		アルギニン	タンパク質原料の加水分解により又は糖類を原料とした発酵により得られたものを、分離して得られたものである。成分はL-アルギニンである。	調味料 強化剤	L-Arginine
22	アルギン酸	昆布類粘質物		褐藻類（Phaeophyceae）より、温時～熱時水又はアルカリ性水溶液で抽出し、精製して得られたものである。成分はアルギン酸である。	増粘安定剤	Alginic acid

番号	品名		簡略名又は類別名	基原・製法・本質	用途	備考
	名称	別名				
23	アルギン酸リアーゼ			細菌（Alteromonas macleodii, Flavobacterium maltivolum, Pseudomonas, Xanthomonas）の培養液より、室温時水で抽出して得られたものである。	酵素	Alginate lyase
24	アルミニウム	アルミ末		^{27}Al	着色料	Aluminium
25	アントシアナーゼ			糸状菌（Aspergillus oryzae, Aspergillus niger, Penicillium decumbens）の培養液より、又は麦芽若しくは穀類の種子より、冷時～室温時水で抽出して得られたもの又はこれを冷時エタノール又は含水エタノールで処理して得られたものである。	酵素	Anthocyanase
26	イソアミラーゼ	枝切り酵素		細菌（Bacillus, Flavobacterium odoratum, Pseudomonas amyloderamosa）の培養液より、冷時～室温時除菌後、冷時～室温時濃縮して得られたものである。	酵素	Isoamylase
27	イソアルファー苦味酸 （ホップの花から得られた、イソフムロン類を主成分とするものをいう。）	イソアルファー酸	ホップ	クワ科ホップ（Humulus lupulus LINNE）の雌花より、水、二酸化炭素又は有機溶剤で抽出し、熱処理して得られたものである。主成分はイソフムロン類である。	苦味料等	Iso-α-bitter acid
28	イソマルトデキストラナーゼ			細菌（Arthrobacter）の培養液より、水で抽出して得られたものである。	酵素	Isomaltodextranase
29	イタコン酸	メチレンコハク酸		麹菌（Aspergillus terreus）による澱粉又は粗糖発酵培養液より、分離して得られたものである。成分はイタコン酸である。	酸味料	Itaconic acid
30	イナワラ灰抽出物 （イネの茎又は葉の灰化物から抽出して得られたものをいう。）	ワラ灰抽出物	植物灰抽出物	イネ科イネ（Oryza sativa LINNE）の茎又は葉を灰化したものより、室温時水で抽出して得られたものであって、アルカリ金属及びアルカリ土類金属を含む。	製造用剤	Rice straw ash extract
31	イヌリナーゼ	イヌラーゼ		糸状菌（Aspergillus aculeatus, Aspergillus niger, Aspergillus phoenicis, Penicillium purpurogenum, Trichoderma）の培養液より、室温時水で抽出して得られたものである。	酵素	Inulinase
32	イノシトール	イノシット		「フィチン酸」を分解したものより、又はアカザ科サトウダイコン（Beta vulgaris LINNE var.rapa DUMORTIER）の糖液又は糖蜜より、分離して得られたものである。成分はイノシトールである。	強化剤	Inositol
33	インベルターゼ	サッカラーゼ シュークラーゼ スクラーゼ		糸状菌（Aspergillus aculeatus, Aspergillus awamori, Aspergillus niger）、細菌（Arthrobacter, Bacillus）又は酵母（Kluyveromyces lactis, Saccharomyces cerevisiae）の培養液より、冷時～室温時菌体を回収して得られたもの、冷時～室温時水若しくはアルカリ性水溶液で抽出して得られたもの、冷時～室温時濃縮して得られたもの、又はアセトン若しくはアルコールで処理し、イオン交換処理後、アセトン若しくはアルコールで処理及び透析除去したものである。	酵素	Invertase
34	ウェランガム （アルカリゲネスの培養液から得られた、多糖類を主成分とするものをいう。）	ウェラン多糖類		グラム陰性細菌（Alcaligenes）の培養液より、分離して得られた多糖類である。	増粘安定剤	Welan gum
35	ウコン色素 （ウコンの根茎から得られた、クルクミンを主成分とするもの	クルクミン ターメリック色素	ウコン	ウコン（Curcuma longa Linne）の根茎から得られた、クルクミンを主成分とするものである。食用油脂を含むことがある。	着色料	Turmeric oleoresin Curcumin

番号	品名 名称	品名 別名	簡略名又は類別名	基原・製法・本質	用途	備考
	をいう。)					
36	ウルシロウ (ウルシの果実から得られた、グリセリンパルミタートを主成分とするものをいう。)			ウルシ科ウルシ (Rhus verniciflua LINNE) の果実より、融解、さらして得られたものである。主成分はグリセリンパルミタートである。	ガムベース 光沢剤	Urushi Wax
37	ウレアーゼ		アミダーゼ	乳酸菌 (Lactobacillus fermentum) 又は細菌 (Arthrobacter) の培養液を、室温時水で抽出し、冷時エタノールで処理して得られたもの、又は濃縮し、微温時エタノールで処理して得られたものである。	酵素	Urease
38	エキソマルトテトラオヒドロラーゼ	G4生成酵素	アミラーゼ カルボヒドラーゼ	細菌 (Pseudomonas stutzeri) の培養液より、室温時除菌し、膜で濃縮して得られたもの、又はこれをエタノールで処理して得られたものである。	酵素	Exomaltotetraohydrolase
39	エステラーゼ			動物の肝臓、魚類、糸状菌 (Aspergillus)、細菌 (Pseudomonas) 若しくは酵母 (Candida, Torulopsis) の培養液より、冷時～室温時水で抽出して得られたもの、除菌したもの若しくは濃縮したもの、又は冷時～室温時エタノール若しくは含水エタノールで処理して得られたものである。	酵素	Esterase
40	エレミ樹脂 (エレミの分泌液から得られた、β-アミリンを主成分とするものをいう。)			カンラン科エレミ (Canarium luzonicum A.GRAY.) の分泌液を、乾燥して得られたものである。主成分はβ-アミリンである。	増粘安定剤 ガムベース	Elemi resin
41	塩水湖水低塩化ナトリウム液 (塩水湖水から塩化ナトリウムを析出分離して得られた、アルカリ金属塩類及びアルカリ土類金属塩類を主成分とするものをいう。)		塩水湖水ミネラル液	塩水湖の塩水を、天日蒸散により濃縮し、塩化ナトリウムを析出分離し、残りの液体をろ過したものである。主成分はアルカリ金属塩類及びアルカリ土類金属塩類である。	調味料	Sodium chloride-decreased brine (saline lake)
42	オゾケライト	セレシン		ワックスシュールの鉱脈に含まれるロウを精製したものである。主成分はC_{29}～C_{53}の炭化水素である。	ガムベース	Ozokerite
43	オゾン			O_3	製造用剤	Ozone
44	オリゴガラクチュロン酸			「ペクチン」をペクチナーゼで酵素分解し、限外ろ過して得られたものであって、ガラクチュロン酸の1～9量体の混合物からなる。	製造用剤	Oligogalacturonic acid
45	γ-オリザノール (米ぬか又は胚芽油から得られた、ステロールとフェルラ酸及びトリテルペンアルコールとフェルラ酸のエステルを主成分とするものをいう。)		オリザノール	イネ科イネ (Oryza sativa LINNE) の種子より得られる米ぬか又は胚芽油より、室温時含水エタノール及びn-ヘキサン又はアセトンで分配した後、含水エタノール画分から得られたものである。主成分はステロールとフェルラ酸及びトリテルペンアルコールとフェルラ酸のエステルである。	酸化防止剤	γ-Oryzanol
46	オレガノ抽出物 (オレガノの葉から得られた、カルバクロール及びチモールを主成分とするものをいう。)			シソ科オレガノ (Origanum vulgare LINNE) の葉より、室温時～温時エタノール、含水エタノール又はヘキサンで抽出して得られたものである。成分としてチモール及びカルバクロールを含む。	製造用剤	Oregano extract
47	オレンジ色素 (アマダイダイの果実又は果皮から得られた、カロテン及びキサントフィルを主成分とするものをいう。)		カロチノイド カロチノイド色素 カロテノイド カロテノイド色素 果実色素	ミカン科アマダイダイ (Citrus sinensis OSBECK) の果実又は果皮より、搾汁したもの、又は熱時エタノール、ヘキサン若しくはアセトンで抽出し、溶媒を除去して得られたものである。主色素はβ-クリプトキサンチンの	着色料	Orange colour

番号	品名 名称	品名 別名	簡略名又は類別名	基原・製法・本質	用途	備考
				脂肪酸エステルである。黄色を呈する。		
48	海藻灰抽出物 (褐藻類の灰化物から得られた、ヨウ化カリウムを主成分とするものをいう。)			褐藻類を焼成灰化したものより、水で抽出して得られたものである。主成分はヨウ化カリウムである。	製造用剤	Seaweed ash extract
49	カオリン	白陶土	不溶性鉱物性物質	天然の含水ケイ酸アルミニウムを精製したものである。	製造用剤	Kaolin
50	カカオ色素 (カカオの種子から得られた、アントシアニンの重合物を主成分とするものをいう。)	ココア色素	カカオ フラボノイド フラボノイド色素	アオギリ科カカオ(Theobroma cacao LINNE)の種子(カカオ豆)を発酵後、焙焼したものより、温時弱アルカリ性水溶液で抽出し、中和して得られたものである。主色素はアントシアニンが熱により重合したものである。褐色を呈する。	着色料	Cacao colour
51	カキ色素 (カキの果実から得られた、フラボノイドを主成分とするものをいう。)		果実色素 フラボノイド フラボノイド色素	カキノキ科カキ(Diospyros kaki THUNB.)の果実を発酵後、焙焼したものより、温時含水エタノールで抽出して得られたもの、又は温時弱アルカリ性水溶液で抽出し、中和して得られたものである。主色素はフラボノイドである。赤褐色を呈する。	着色料	Japanese persimmon colour
52	花こう斑岩		麦飯石 不溶性鉱物性物質	花こう斑岩を洗浄、粉砕したものを、乾燥後、滅菌して得られたものである。	製造用剤	Granite porphyry
53	カシアガム (エビスグサモドキの種子を粉砕して得られた、多糖類を主成分とするものをいう。)	カッシャガム		マメ科エビスグサモドキ(Cassia tora LINNE)の種子の胚乳部を、粉砕して得られたものである。主成分は多糖類である。	増粘安定剤	Cassia gum
54	カタラーゼ		オキシダーゼ	ブタの肝臓より、水で抽出して得られたもの、又は糸状菌(Aspergillus aculeatus, Aspergillus awamori, Aspergillus foetidus, Aspergillus niger, Aspergillus phoenicis, Penicillium amagasakiense) 細菌(Micrococcus lyzodeikticus)若しくは酵母(Saccharomyces)の培養液より、冷時～室温時水で抽出して得られたもの、温時溶菌後、除菌し、冷時～室温時濃縮して得られたもの、又はこれを冷時エタノールで処理して得られたものである。	酵素	Catalase
55	活性炭 (含炭素物質を炭化し、賦活化して得られたものをいう。)			鋸屑、木片、ヤシ殻の植物性繊維質、亜炭又は石油等の含炭素物質を炭化後、賦活化を行って得られたものである。	製造用剤	Active carbon
56	活性白土		不溶性鉱物性物質	酸性白土を硫酸処理して得られたものである。主成分は含水ケイ酸アルミニウムである。	製造用剤	Activated acid clay
57	ガティガム (ガティノキの分泌液から得られた、多糖類を主成分とするものをいう。)		ガティ	ガティノキ(Anogeissus latifolia Wallich)の分泌液から得られた、多糖類を主成分とするものである。	増粘安定剤	Gum ghatti
58	カテキン			ツバキ科チャ(Camellia sinensis O.KZE.)の茎若しくは葉、マメ科ペグアセンヤク(Acacia catechu WILLD.)の幹枝又はアカネ科ガンビール(Uncaria gambir ROXBURGH)の幹枝若しくは葉より、乾留した後、水又はエタノールで抽出し、精製して得られたもの、又は熱時水で抽出した後、メタノール若しくは酢酸エチルで分配して得られたものである。成分はカテキン類である。	酸化防止剤	Catechin

番号	品名 名称	品名 別名	簡略名又は類別名	基原・製法・本質	用途	備考
59	カードラン (アグロバクテリウム又はアルカリゲネスの培養液から得られた、β-1,3-グルカンを主成分とするものをいう。)		ブドウ糖多糖	アグロバクテリウム属菌 (Agrobacterium biovar 1) 又はリゾビウム属菌 (Rhizobium radiobacter) の培養液から得られた、β-1,3-グルカンを主成分とするものである。	増粘安定剤 製造用剤	Curdlan
60	カフェイン (抽出物) (コーヒーの種子又はチャの葉から得られた、カフェインを主成分とするものをいう。)		カフェイン	アカネ科コーヒー (Coffea arabica LINNE) の種子 (コーヒー豆) 又はツバキ科チャ (Camellia sinensis O.KZE.) の葉より、水又は二酸化炭素で抽出し、分離、精製して得られたものである。主成分はカフェインである。	苦味料等	Caffeine (extract)
61	カラギナン (イバラノリ、キリンサイ、ギンナンソウ、スギノリ又はツノマタの全藻から得られた、ι-カラギナン、κ-カラギナン及びλ-カラギナンを主成分とするものをいう。)	カラギーナン カラゲナン カラゲーナン カラゲニン			増粘安定剤	Carrageenan
	加工ユーケマ藻類		ユーケマ	カラギナン (イバラノリ属 (Hypnea)、キリンサイ属 (Eucheuma)、ギンナンソウ属 (Iridaea)、スギノリ属 (Gigartina) 又はツノマタ属 (Chondrus) の藻類の全藻から得られた、ι-カラギナン、κ-カラギナン及びλ-カラギナンを主成分とするものをいう。) の一つである。		Semirefined carrageenan Processed eucheuma algae Processed red algae
	精製カラギナン		紅藻抽出物	カラギナン (イバラノリ属 (Hypnea)、キリンサイ属 (Eucheuma)、ギンナンソウ属 (Iridaea)、スギノリ属 (Gigartina) 又はツノマタ属 (Chondrus) の全藻から得られた、ι-カラギナン、κ-カラギナン及びλ-カラギナンを主成分とするものをいう。) の一つである。ショ糖、ブドウ糖、マルトース、乳糖又はデキストリンを含むことがある。		Purified carrageenan Refined carrageenan
	ユーケマ藻末		ユーケマ	ミリン科キリンサイ属 (Eucheuma) の全藻を、乾燥、粉砕して得られたものである。		Powdered red algae
62	α-ガラクトシダーゼ	メリビアーゼ	カルボヒドラーゼ	糸状菌 (Aspergillus aculeatus, Aspergillus awamori, Aspergillus niger, Aspergillus phoenicis, Mortierella) 又は細菌 (Bacillus stearothermophilus) の培養液より、室温時～微温時水、酸性水溶液若しくはアルカリ性水溶液で抽出して得られたもの、冷時含水エタノールで処理したもの、又は除菌後、濃縮して得られたものである。	酵素	α-Galactosidase
63	β-ガラクトシダーゼ	ラクターゼ	カルボヒドラーゼ	動物の臓器より、冷時～微温時水で抽出して得られたもの、又は糸状菌 (Aspergillus oryzae, Penicillium multicolor, Rhizopus oryzae)、細菌 (Bacillus circulans, Streptococcus) 若しくは酵母 (Kluyveromyces fragillus, Kluyveromyces lactis, Saccharomyces) の培養液より、冷時～室温時水で抽出して得られたもの、室温時自己消化処理して得られたもの、冷時～室温時濃縮したもの、冷時エタノール、含水エタノール若しくはアセトンで処理して得られたもの、又は硫酸アンモニウム等で分画した後、脱塩処理して得られたものである。	酵素	β-Galactosidase (Lactase)

番号	品名 名称	品名 別名	簡略名又は類別名	基原・製法・本質	用途	備考
64	カラシ抽出物 (カラシナの種子から得られた、イソチオシアン酸アリルを主成分とするものをいう。)	マスタード抽出物		アブラナ科カラシナ (Brassica juncea LINNE) の種子の脂肪油を除いた圧搾粕より、水蒸気蒸留により得られたものである。主成分はイソチオシアン酸アリルである。	製造用剤	Mustard extract
65	カラメルⅠ (でん粉加水分解物、糖蜜又は糖類の食用炭水化物を熱処理して得られたものをいう。ただし、「カラメルⅡ」、「カラメルⅢ」及び「カラメルⅣ」を除く。)	カラメル	カラメル色素	でん粉加水分解物、糖蜜又は糖類の食用炭水化物を、熱処理して得られたもの、又は酸若しくはアルカリを加えて熱処理して得られたもので、亜硫酸化合物及びアンモニウム化合物を使用していないものである。	着色料 製造用剤	Caramel Ⅰ (plain)
66	カラメルⅡ (でん粉加水分解物、糖蜜又は糖類の食用炭水化物に亜硫酸化合物を加えて熱処理して得られたものをいう。ただし、「カラメルⅣ」を除く。)	カラメル	カラメル色素	でん粉加水分解物、糖蜜又は糖類の食用炭水化物に、亜硫酸化合物を加えて、又はこれに酸若しくはアルカリを加えて熱処理して得られたもので、アンモニウム化合物を使用していないものである。	着色料 製造用剤	Caramel Ⅱ (caustic sulfite process)
67	カラメルⅢ (でん粉加水分解物、糖蜜又は糖類の食用炭水化物にアンモニウム化合物を加えて熱処理して得られたものをいう。ただし、「カラメルⅣ」を除く。)	カラメル	カラメル色素	でん粉加水分解物、糖蜜又は糖類の食用炭水化物に、アンモニウム化合物を加えて、又はこれに酸若しくはアルカリを加えて熱処理して得られたもので、亜硫酸化合物を使用していないものである。	着色料 製造用剤	Caramel Ⅲ (ammonia process)
68	カラメルⅣ (でん粉加水分解物、糖蜜又は糖類の食用炭水化物に亜硫酸化合物及びアンモニウム化合物を加えて熱処理して得られたものをいう。	カラメル	カラメル色素	でん粉加水分解物、糖蜜又は糖類の食用炭水化物に、亜硫酸化合物及びアンモニウム化合物を加えて、又はこれに酸若しくはアルカリを加えて熱処理して得られたものである。	着色料 製造用剤	Caramel Ⅳ (sulfite ammonia process)
69	カラヤガム (カラヤ又はキバナワタモドキの分泌液から得られた、多糖類を主成分とするものをいう。)		カラヤ	カラヤ (Sterculia urens Roxburgh) 又はキバナワタモドキ (Cochlospermum gossypium de Candolle) の分泌液から得られた、多糖類を主成分とするものである。	増粘安定剤	Karaya gum
70	カルナウバロウ (ブラジルロウヤシの葉から得られた、ヒドロキシセロチン酸セリルを主成分とするものをいう。)	カルナウバワックス ブラジルワックス	植物ワックス	ブラジルロウヤシ (Copernicia prunifera H.E.Moore (Copernicia cerifera Martius)) の葉から得られた、ヒドロキシセロチン酸セリルを主成分とするものである。	ガムベース 光沢剤	Carnauba wax Brazil wax
71	カルボキシペプチダーゼ			イネ科コムギ (Triticum aestivum LINNE) の種皮及び果皮 (ふすま) より、酢酸水溶液で抽出したもの、又は糸状菌 (Aspergillus) 若しくは酵母 (Saccharomyces cerevisiae) の培養液より、冷時～室温時水で抽出して得られたもの若しくは冷時～室温時濃縮し、冷エタノールで処理して得られたものである。	酵素	Carboxypeptidase
72	カロブ色素 (イナゴマメの種子の胚芽を粉砕して得られたものをいう。)	カロブジャーム	カロブ フラボノイド フラボノイド色素	マメ科イナゴマメ (Ceratonia siliqua LINNE) の種子の胚芽を、粉砕して得られたものである。淡黄色を呈する。	着色料 製造用剤	Carob germ colour
73	カロブビーンガム (イナゴマメの種子の胚乳を粉砕し、又は溶解し、沈殿して得られたものをいう。)	ローカストビーンガム	ローカスト	イナゴマメ (Ceratonia siliqua Linne) の種子の胚乳を粉砕し，又は溶解し，沈殿して得られたものである。ショ糖，ブドウ糖，乳糖，デキストリン又はマルトースを含むことがある。	増粘安定剤	Carob bean gum Locust bean gum
74	カワラヨモギ抽出物 (カワラヨモギの全草から得られた、カピリンを主成分とするものをいう。)		カラワヨモギ	キク科カワラヨモギ (Artemisia capillaris THUNB.) の全草より、室温時エタノール若しくは含水エタノールで抽出して得られたもの、又は水蒸気蒸留して得られたものである。	保存料	Rumput roman extract

番号	品名		簡略名又は類別名	基原・製法・本質	用途	備考
	名称	別名				
				有効成分はカピリン等である。		
75	カンゾウ抽出物 （ウラルカンゾウ、チョウカカンゾウ又はヨウカンゾウの根又は根茎から得られた、グリチルリチン酸を主成分とするものをいう。）	カンゾウエキス グリチルリチン リコリス抽出物	カンゾウ カンゾウ甘味料 リコリス	ウラルカンゾウ（Glycyrrhiza uralensis Fischer），チョウカカンゾウ（Glycyrrhiza inflata Batalin），ヨウカンゾウ（Glycyrrhiza glabra Linne），又はそれらの近縁植物の根若しくは根茎から得られた，グリチルリチン酸を主成分とするものである。本品には，粗製物と精製物がある。	甘味料	Licorice extract
76	カンゾウ油性抽出物 （ウラルカンゾウ、チョウカカンゾウ又はヨウカンゾウの根又は根茎から得られた、フラボノイドを主成分とするものをいう。）		油性カンゾウ	マメ科ウラルカンゾウ（Glycyrrhiza uralensis FISCHER）、マメ科チョウカカンゾウ（Glycyrrhiza inflata BATALIN）又はマメ科ヨウカンゾウ（Glycyrrhiza glabra LINNE）の根又は根茎を水で洗浄した残渣より、室温時～温時エタノール、アセトン又はヘキサンで抽出して得られたものである。主成分はフラボノイドである。	酸化防止剤	Licorice oil extract
77	カンデリラロウ （カンデリラの茎から得られた、ヘントリアコンタンを主成分とするものをいう。）	カンデリラワックス キャンデリラロウ キャンデリラワックス	植物ワックス	カンデリラ（Euphorbia antisyphilitica Zuccarini又はEuphorbia cerifera Alcocer）の茎から得られた、ヘントリアコンタンを主成分とするものである。	ガムベース 光沢剤	Candelilla wax
78	キサンタンガム （キサントモナスの培養液から得られた、多糖類を主成分とするものをいう。）	キサンタン多糖類 ザンサンガム	キサンタン	キサントモナス属菌（Xanthomonas campestris）の培養液から得られた、多糖類を主成分とするものである。ブドウ糖、乳糖、デキストリン又はマルトースを含むことがある。	増粘安定剤	Xanthan gum
79	キシラナーゼ			糸状菌（Aspergillus aculeatus, Aspergillus niger, Trichoderma koningii, Trichoderma longibrachiatum reesei, Trichoderma viride）の培養液より、分離して得られたものである。	酵素	Xylanase
80	D-キシロース		キシロース	木材又はアオイ科ワタ（Gossypium arboretum LINNE）、イネ科イネ（Oryza sativa LINNE）、イネ科サトウキビ（Saccharum officinarum LINNE）若しくはイネ科トウモロコシ（Zea Mays LINNE）又はその他同属植物の茎、実又は殻より、熱時酸性水溶液で加水分解し、分離して得られたものである。成分はD-キシロースである。	甘味料	D-Xylose
81	キチナーゼ			糸状菌（Trichoderma harzianum, Trichoderma reesei）、放線菌（Amycolatopsis orientalis, Streptomyces）又は細菌（Aeromonas）の培養液より、冷時～室温時除菌後、濃縮し、硫酸アンモニウムで分画したもの、若しくはエタノールで処理したものから得られたものである。	酵素	Chitinase
82	キチン			エビ、カニ等甲殻類の甲殻又はイカの甲を、室温時～温時酸性水溶液で炭酸カルシウムを除去した後、温時～熱時弱アルカル性水溶液でタンパク質を除去したもので、N-アセチル-D-グルコサミンの多量体からなる。	増粘安定剤	Chitin
83	キトサナーゼ			細菌（Aeromonas, Bacillus）又は糸状菌（Aspergillus niger, Trichoderma reesei, Trichoderma viride, Verticillium）の培養液より、除菌後、冷時～微温時濃縮したもの又	酵素	Chitosanase

番号	品名 名称	品名 別名	簡略名又は類別名	基原・製法・本質	用途	備考
				はエタノール若しくはアセトンで処理して得られたものである。		
84	キトサン			「キチン」を、温時～熱時水酸化ナトリウム水溶液で脱アセチル化したもので、D-グルコサミンの多量体からなる。	増粘安定剤 製造用剤	Chitosan
85	キナ抽出物 （アカキナの樹皮から得られた、キニジン、キニーネ及びシンコニンを主成分とするものをいう。）			アカネ科アカキナ（Cinchona succirubra PAVON）の樹皮より、水又はエタノール等で抽出して得られたものである。有効成分はキニーネ、キニジン及びシンコニンである。	苦味料等	Redbark cinchona extract
86	キハダ抽出物 （キハダの樹皮から得られた、ベルベリンを主成分とするものをいう。）		キハダ	ミカン科キハダ（Phellodendron amurense RUPR.）の樹皮より、水又はエタノールで抽出して得られたものである。主成分はベルベリンである。	苦味料等	Phellodendron bark extract
87	魚鱗箔 （魚類の上皮部から抽出して得られたものをいう。）			イワシ科マイワシ（Sardinops melanosticta TEMMINCK et SCHLEGEL）、タチウオ科タチウオ（Trichiurus lepturus LINNE）又はニシン科ニシン（Clupea pallasi CUVIER et VALENCIENNES）の魚体の上皮部を採り、室温時水又は弱アルカリ性水溶液で洗浄後、室温時エタノールで抽出して得られたものである。主色素は不明であるが、グアニンを含む。白色～淡黄灰色を呈する。	着色料	Fish scale foil
88	キラヤ抽出物 （キラヤの樹皮から得られた、サポニンを主成分とするものをいう。）	キラヤサポニン	サポニン	キラヤ（Quillaja saponaria Molina）の樹皮から得られた、サポニンを主成分とするものである。	乳化剤	Quillaia extract Quillaja extract
89	金	金箔		^{197}Au	着色料 製造用剤	Gold
90	銀	銀箔		^{107}Ag, ^{109}Ag	着色料	Silver
91	グァーガム （グァーの種子から得られた、多糖類を主成分とするものをいう。ただし、「グァーガム酵素分解物」を除く。）	グァーフラワー グァルガム	グァー	グァー（Cyamopsis tetragonolobus Taubert）の種子から得られた、多糖類を主成分とするものである。ショ糖、ブドウ糖、乳糖又はデキストリンを含むことがある。	増粘安定剤	Guar gum
92	グァーガム酵素分解物 （グァーの種子を粉砕し、分解して得られた、多糖類を主成分とするものをいう。）	グァーフラワー酵素分解物 グァルガム酵素分解物	グァー分解物	「グァーガム」を、酵素（α-ガラクトシダーゼ、ヘミセルラーゼ）で分解して得られたものである。主成分は多糖類である。	増粘安定剤	Enzymatically hydrolyzed guar gum
93	グアヤク脂 （ユソウボクの幹枝から得られた、グアヤコン酸、グアヤレチック酸及びβ-レジンを主成分とするものをいう。）			ハマビシ科ユソウボク（Guajacum officinale LINNE）の幹枝を、加熱して得られたものである。有効成分は、グアヤコン酸、グアヤレチック酸及びβ-レジンである。	酸化防止剤	Guaiac resin Guajac resin
94	グアヤク樹脂 （ユソウボクの分泌液から得られた、α-グアヤコン酸及びβ-グアヤコン酸を主成分とするものをいう。）			ハマビシ科ユソウボク（Guaiacum officinale LINNE）の分泌液を、室温時エタノールで抽出し、ろ液からエタノールを留去して得られたものである。主構成成分はα-、β-グアヤコン酸である。	ガムベース	Guajac resin (extract)
95	クエルセチン	ケルセチン	ルチン分解物	「ルチン（抽出物）」を、酵素又は酸性水溶液で加水分解して得られたものである。成分はクエルセチンである。	酸化防止剤	Quercetin
96	クチナシ青色素 （クチナシの果実から得られたイリドイド配糖体とタンパク質		クチナシ クチナシ色素	クチナシ（Gardenia augusta Merrill又はGardenia jasminoides Ellis）の果実から得られたイリドイド配糖体とタンパク質分解物の	着色料	Gardenia blue

番号	品名 名称	品名 別名	簡略名又は類別名	基原・製法・本質	用途	備考
	分解物の混合物にβ-グルコシダーゼを添加して得られたものをいう。)			混合物に、β-グルコシダーゼを添加して得られたものである。デキストリン又は乳糖を含むことがある。		
97	クチナシ赤色素 (クチナシの果実から得られたイリドイド配糖体のエステル加水分解物とタンパク質分解物の混合物にβ-グルコシダーゼを添加して得られたものをいう。)		クチナシ クチナシ色素	クチナシ(Gardenia augusta Merrill又はGardenia jasminoides Ellis)の果実から得られたイリドイド配糖体のエステル加水分解物とタンパク質分解物の混合物に、β-グルコシダーゼを添加して得られたものである。デキストリン又は乳糖を含むことがある。	着色料	Gardenia red
98	クチナシ黄色素 (クチナシの果実から得られた、クロシン及びクロセチンを主成分とするものをいう。)		カロチノイド カロチノイド色素 カロテノイド カロテノイド色素 クチナシ クチナシ色素 クロシン	クチナシ(Gardenia augusta Merrill又はGardenia jasminoides Ellis)の果実から得られた、クロシン及びクロセチンを主成分とするものである。デキストリン又は乳糖を含むことがある。	着色料	Gardenia yellow
99	グッタハンカン (グッタハンカンの分泌液から得られた、アミリンアセタート及びポリイソプレンを主成分とするものをいう。)			アカテツ科グッタハンカン(Palaquium leiocarpum BOERL.)の幹枝より得られたラテックスを、熱時水で洗浄し、水溶成分を除去したものより得られたものである。主成分はトランスポリイソプレン及びアミリンアセタートである。	ガムベース	Gutta hang kang
100	グッタペルカ (グッタペルカの分泌液から得られた、ポリイソプレンを主成分とするものをいう。)			アカテツ科グッタペルカ(Palaquium gutta BURCK.)の幹枝より得られたラテックスを、熱時水で洗浄し、水溶成分を除去したものより得られたものである。主成分はトランスポリイソプレンである。	ガムベース	Gutta percha
101	クリストバル石		不溶性鉱物性物質	鉱床より採掘したクリストバル石を、粉砕乾燥、800〜1200℃で焼成、又は塩酸処理して焼成したものである。	製造用剤	Cristobalite
102	グルカナーゼ		カルボヒドラーゼ ヘミセルラーゼ	糸状菌(Aspergillus aculeatus, Aspergillus niger, Humicola insolens, Rhizopus delemar, Trichoderma harzianum, Trichoderma longibrachiatum, Trichoderma viride)、担子菌(Pycnoporus coccineus)、細菌(Arthrobacter, Bacillus subtilis, Pseudomonas paucimobilis)若しくは酵母(Saccharomyces)の培養液より、冷時〜微温時水若しくは酸性水溶液で抽出して得られたもの、除菌後、冷時〜室温時濃縮したもの、冷時エタノール、含水エタノール若しくはアセトンで処理して得られたもの、又は除菌後、硫酸アンモニウム等で分画した後、脱塩処理して得られたものである。	酵素	Glucanase
103	グルコアミラーゼ	糖化アミラーゼ	アミラーゼ カルボヒドラーゼ	糸状菌(Acremonium, Aspergillus, Humicola grisea, Rhizopus delemar, Rhizopus niveus)、担子菌(Corticium rolfsii)、細菌(Bacillus, Pseudomonas)又は酵母(Saccharomyces)の培養液より、冷時〜室温時水で抽出して得られたもの、冷時〜室温時除菌後、濃縮したもの、冷時〜室温時濃縮後、エタノール、含水エタノール若しくはアセトンで処理して得られたもの、又は硫酸アンモニウム等で分画した後、脱塩処理して得られたものである。	酵素	Glucoamylase
104	グルコサミン			「キチン」を、塩酸で加水分解し、分離して	増粘安定剤	Glucosamine

番号	品名 名称	品名 別名	簡略名又は類別名	基原・製法・本質	用途	備考
				得られたものである。成分はグルコサミンである。	製造用剤	
105	α-グルコシダーゼ	マルターゼ		糸状菌（Absidia, Acremonium, Aspergillus）、細菌（Bacillus, Pseudomonas）若しくは酵母（Saccharomyces）の培養液より、冷時～室温時水で抽出して得られたもの、又は冷時～室温時濃縮後、冷時エタノールで処理して得られたものである。	酵素	α-Glucosidase
106	β-グルコシダーゼ	ゲンチオビアーゼ セロビアーゼ		ソテツ科ソテツ（Cycas revoluta THUNB.）より、冷時～微温時水で抽出して得られたもの、又は糸状菌（Aspergillus aculeatus, Aspergillus niger, Aspergillus pulverulentus, Penicillium decumbens, Trichoderma harzianum, Trichoderma longibrachiatum, Trichoderma reesei）若しくは細菌（Bacillus）の培養液より、冷時～微温時水で抽出して得られたもの、冷時～室温時濃縮したもの、又は冷時エタノール若しくは含水エタノールで処理して得られたものである。	酵素	β-Glucosidase
107	α-グルコシルトランスフェラーゼ	4-α-グルカノトランスフェラーゼ 6-α-グルカノトランスフェラーゼ		細菌（Agrobacterium radiobacter, Arthrobacter, Bacillus, Erwinia, Pimelobacter, Protaminobacter, Pseudomonas, Serratia, Thermus）の培養液又はバレイショ（Solanum tuberosum LINNE）の塊茎より、冷時～室温時除菌したもの、冷時水で抽出して得られたもの、又は冷時～室温時濃縮して得られたものである。なお、基質特異性により、4-α-グルカノトランスフェラーゼ、6-α-グルカノトランスフェラーゼと呼ばれるものがある。	酵素	α-Glucosyltransferase 4-α-Glucanotransferase 6-α-Glucanotransferase
108	α-グルコシルトランスフェラーゼ処理ステビア （「ステビア抽出物」から得られた、α-グルコシルステビオシドを主成分とするものをいう。）	酵素処理ステビア	ステビア ステビア甘味料 糖転移ステビア	『ステビア抽出物』に、α-グルコシルトランスフェラーゼを用いてD-グルコースを付加して得られたものである。α-グルコシルステビオシドを主成分とする。	甘味料	α-Glucosyltransferase treated stevia
109	グルコースイソメラーゼ			糸状菌（Aspergillus）、放線菌（Actinoplanes missouriensis, Streptomyces griseofuscus, Streptomyces murinus, Streptomyces phaeochromogenes, Streptomyces rubiginosus）又は細菌（Bacillus coagulans）の培養液より、室温時水で抽出して得られたものである。	酵素	Glucose isomerase
110	グルコースオキシダーゼ			糸状菌（Aspergillus aculeatus, Aspergillus niger, Penicillium）の培養液より、冷時～室温時水で抽出して得られたもの、又は冷時～微温時溶菌後、除菌したもの、又は冷時～室温時濃縮後、冷時エタノールで処理して得られたものである。	酵素	Glucose oxidase
111	グルタミナーゼ		アミダーゼ	枯草菌（Bacillus subtilis）、糸状菌（Aspergillus）又は酵母（Candida）の培養液より、冷時～室温時水で抽出して得られたもの、冷時～室温時濃縮したもの、冷時エタノール、含水エタノール若しくはアセトンで処理して得られたもの、又は硫酸アンモニウム等で分画した後、脱塩処理して得られたものである。	酵素	Glutaminase
112	L-グルタミン		グルタミン	糖類を原料とした発酵により得られたものから分離して得られたものである。成分はL-	調味料 強化剤	L-Glutamine

番号	品名 名称	品名 別名	簡略名又は類別名	基原・製法・本質	用途	備考
				グルタミンである。		
113	グレープフルーツ種子抽出物 (グレープフルーツの種子から得られた、脂肪酸及びフラボノイドを主成分とするものをいう。)		グレープフルーツ種子	ミカン科グレープフルーツ(Citrus paradisi MACF.)の種子より、水又はエタノールで抽出して得られたものである。主成分は脂肪酸及びフラボノイドである。	製造用剤	Grapefruit seed extract
114	クーロー色素 (ソメモノイモの根から抽出して得られたものをいう。)	ソメモノイモ色素	フラボノイド フラボノイド色素	ヤマノイモ科ソメモノイモ(Dioscorea matsudai HAYATA)の根より、熱時水、弱アルカリ性水溶液若しくはプロピレングリコールで抽出したもの、又は室温時含水エタノールで抽出して得られたものである。赤褐色を呈する。	着色料	Kooroo colour Matsudai colour
115	クローブ抽出物 (チョウジのつぼみ、葉又は花から得られた、オイゲノールを主成分とするものをいう。)	チョウジ抽出物	チョウジ油	フトモモ科チョウジ(Syzygium aromaticum MERRILL et PERRY)のつぼみ、葉又は花より、エタノール又はアセトンで抽出して得られたもの、又は水蒸気蒸留により得られたものである。主成分はオイゲノール等である。	酸化防止剤	Clove extract
116	クロロフィリン		葉緑素	「クロロフィル」を、温時アルカリ性エタノール水溶液で加水分解し、希塩酸で中和した後、含水エタノールで抽出して得られたものである。主成分はマグネシウムクロロフィリンである。緑色を呈する。	着色料	Chlorophylline
117	クロロフィル		葉緑素	緑色植物より得られた、クロロフィル類を主成分とするものである。食用油脂を含むことがある。	着色料	Chlorophyll
118	くん液 (サトウキビ、竹材、トウモロコシ又は木材を燃焼して発生したガス成分を捕集し、又は乾溜して得られたものをいう。)	スモークフレーバー			製造用剤	Smoke flavourings
	木酢液			サトウキビ、竹材、トウモロコシ又は木材を、乾留して得られたものである。		Wood vinegar Pyroligneous acid
	リキッドスモーク			サトウキビ、竹材、トウモロコシ又は木材を、限定された空気の存在下で、燃焼して発生したガス成分を捕集して得られたものである。		Liquid smoke
119	ケイソウ土		不溶性鉱物性物質	ケイソウに由来する二酸化ケイ素で、乾燥品、焼成品及び融剤焼成品があり、それぞれをケイソウ土(乾燥品)、ケイソウ土(焼成品)及びケイソウ土(融剤焼成品)と称する。焼成品は、800~1,200℃で焼成したものであり、融剤焼成品は、少量の炭酸のアルカリ塩を添加して800~1,200℃で焼成したものである。融剤焼成品のうち酸洗い品については、焼成品の規定(性状を除く)を準用する。	製造用剤	Diatomaceous earth
120	ゲンチアナ抽出物 (ゲンチアナの根又は根茎から得られた、アマロゲンチン及びゲンチオピクロシドを主成分とするものをいう。)			リンドウ科ゲンチアナ(Gentiana lutea LINNE)の根又は根茎より、水又はエタノールで抽出して得られたものである。有効成分はゲンチオピクロシド(ゲンチオピクリン)及びアマロゲンチンである。	苦味料等	Gentian root extract
121	高級脂肪酸(動植物性油脂又は動植物性硬化油脂を加水分解して得られたものをいう。)		脂肪酸	動植物性油脂又は動植物性硬化油脂より、加水分解したものより得られたものである。	製造用剤	Higher fatty acid
122	香辛料抽出物 (アサノミ、アサフェチダ、ア	スパイス抽出物	香辛料 スパイス	アサノミ、アサフェチダ、アジョワン、アニス、アンゼリカ、ウイキョウ、ウコン、オレ	苦味料等	Spice extracts

番号	品名 名称	品名 別名	簡略名又は類別名	基原・製法・本質	用途	備考
	ジョワン、アニス、アンゼリカ、ウイキョウ、ウコン、オールスパイス、オレガノ、オレンジピール、カショウ、カッシア、カモミール、カラシナ、カルダモン、カレーリーフ、カンゾウ、キャラウェー、クチナシ、クミン、クレソン、クローブ、ケシノミ、ケーパー、コショウ、ゴマ、コリアンダー、サッサフラス、サフラン、サボリー、サルビア、サンショウ、シソ、シナモン、シャロット、ジュニパーベリー、ショウガ、スターアニス、スペアミント、セイヨウワサビ、セロリー、ソーレル、タイム、タマネギ、タマリンド、タラゴン、チャイブ、チャービル、ディル、トウガラシ、ナツメグ、ニガヨモギ、ニジェラ、ニンジン、ニンニク、バジル、パセリ、ハッカ、バニラ、パプリカ、ヒソップ、フェネグリーク、ペパーミント、ホースミント、マジョラム、ミョウガ、ラベンダー、リンデン、レモングラス、レモンバーム、ローズ、ローズマリー、ローレル又はワサビから抽出し、又はこれを水蒸気蒸留して得られたものをいう。ただし、「ウコン色素」、「オレガノ抽出物」、「オレンジ色素」、「カラシ抽出物」、「カンゾウ抽出物」、「カンゾウ油性抽出物」、「クチナシ黄色素」、「クローブ抽出物」、「ゴマ油不けん化物」、「シソ抽出物」、「ショウガ抽出物」「精油除去ウイキョウ抽出物」、「セイヨウワサビ抽出物」、「セージ抽出物」、「タマネギ色素」、「タマリンド色素」、「タマリンドシードガム」、「タンニン（抽出物)」、「トウガラシ色素」、「トウガラシ水性抽出物」、「ニガヨモギ抽出物」、「ニンジンカロテン」及び「ローズマリー抽出物」を除く。)			ガノ、オールスパイス、オレンジピール、カショウ、カッシア、カモミール、カラシナ、カルダモン、カレーリーフ、カンゾウ、キャラウェー、クチナシ、クミン、クレソン、クローブ、ケシノミ、ケーパー、コショウ、ゴマ、コリアンダー、サッサフラス、サフラン、サボリー、サルビア、サンショウ、シソ、シナモン、シャロット、ジュニパーベリー、ショウガ、スターアニス、スペアミント、セイヨウワサビ、セロリー、ソーレル、タイム、タマネギ、タマリンド、タラゴン、チャイブ、チャービル、ディル、トウガラシ、ナツメグ、ニガヨモギ、ニジェラ、ニンジン、ニンニク、バジル、パセリ、ハッカ、バニラ、パプリカ、ヒソップ、フェネグリーク、ペパーミント、ホースミント、マジョラム、ミョウガ、ラベンダー、リンデン、レモングラス、レモンバーム、ローズ、ローズマリー、ローレル又はワサビより水、エタノール、二酸化炭素若しくは有機溶剤で抽出して得られたもの、又は水蒸気蒸留により得られたものである。		
123	酵素処理イソクエルシトリン（「ルチン酵素分解物」から得られた、α-グルコシルイソクエルシトリンを主成分とするものをいう。)	糖転移イソクエルシトリン	酵素処理ルチン 糖転移ルチン	『ルチン酵素分解物』とでん粉又はデキストリンの混合物に、シクロデキストリングルコシルトランスフェラーゼを用いてD-グルコースを付加して得られたものである。主成分はα-グルコシルイソクエルシトリンである。	酸化防止剤	Enzymatically modified isoquercitrin
124	酵素処理ナリンジン（「ナリンジン」から得られた、α-グルコシルナリンジンを主成分とするものをいう。)	糖転移ナリンジン	ナリンジン	「ナリンジン」とデキストリンの混合物に、シクロデキストリングルコシルトランスフェラーゼを用いてグルコースを付加させたものである。有効成分はα-グルコシルナリンジンである。	苦味料等	Enzymatically modified naringin

番号	品名 名称	品名 別名	簡略名又は類別名	基原・製法・本質	用途	備考
125	酵素処理ヘスペリジン（「ヘスペリジン」にシクロデキストリングルコシルトランスフェラーゼを用いてグルコースを付加して得られたものをいう。）	糖転移ヘスペリジン 糖転移ビタミンP	ヘスペリジン	柑橘類の果皮、果汁、又は種子より、アルカリ性水溶液で抽出して得られるヘスペリジンに、シクロデキストリングルコシルトランスフェラーゼを用いてD-グルコースを付加して得られたものである。	強化剤	Enzymatically modified hesperidin
126	酵素処理ルチン（抽出物）（「ルチン（抽出物）」から得られた、α-グルコシルルチンを主成分とするものをいう。）	糖転移ルチン（抽出物）	酵素処理ルチン 糖転移ルチン	「ルチン（抽出物）」とでん粉又はデキストリンの混合物に、シクロデキストリングルコシルトランスフェラーゼを用いてグルコースをα-1,4付加して得られたものである。主成分はα-グルコシルルチンである。	酸化防止剤 強化剤 着色料	Enzymatically modified rutin(extract)
127	酵素処理レシチン（「植物レシチン」又は「卵黄レシチン」から得られた、ホスファチジルグリセロールを主成分とするものをいう。）		レシチン	「植物レシチン」又は「卵黄レシチン」とグリセリンの混合物に、ホスホリパーゼDを用いて得られたものである。主成分はホスファチジルグリセロールである。	乳化剤	Enzymatically modified lecithin
128	酵素分解カンゾウ（「カンゾウ抽出物」を酵素分解して得られた、グリチルレチン酸-3-グルクロニドを主成分とするものをいう。）		カンゾウ	「カンゾウ抽出物」を、酵素分解して得られたものである。主甘味成分はグリチルレチン酸-3-グルクロニドである。	甘味料	Enzymatically hydrolyzed licorice extract
129	酵素分解リンゴ抽出物（リンゴの果実を酵素分解して得られた、カテキン類及びクロロゲン酸を主成分とするものをいう。）		リンゴ抽出物 リンゴエキス	バラ科リンゴ（<u>Malus</u> <u>pumila</u> MILLER）の果実を搾汁し、パルプを分離した後、得られた上清を酵素処理し、精製して得られたものである。有効成分はクロロゲン酸及びカテキン類である。	酸化防止剤	Enzymatically decomposed apple extract
130	酵素分解レシチン（「植物レシチン」又は「卵黄レシチン」から得られた、フォスファチジン酸及びリゾレシチンを主成分とするものをいう。）		レシチン	アブラナ（<u>Brassica</u> <u>rapa</u> Linne又は<u>Brassica</u> *napus* Linne）若しくはダイズ（<u>Glycine</u> <u>max</u> Merrill）の種子から得られた植物レシチン又は卵黄から得られた卵黄レシチンから得られた、ホスファチジン酸及びリゾレシチンを主成分とするものである。酵素分解植物レシチンと酵素分解卵黄レシチンがある。	乳化剤	Enzymatically decomposed lecithin
131	酵母細胞壁（サッカロミセスの細胞壁から得られた、多糖類を主成分とするものをいう。）	酵母細胞膜		サッカロミセス属菌（<u>Saccharomyces</u> <u>cerevisiae</u>）の細胞壁から得られた、多糖類を主成分とするものである。	増粘安定剤 製造用剤	Yeast cell wall
132	コウリャン色素（コウリャンの種子から得られた、アピゲニニジン及びルテオリニジンを主成分とするものをいう。）	キビ色素	フラボノイド フラボノイド色素	イネ科コウリャン（<u>Sorghum</u> <u>nervosum</u> BESS.）の実及び殻より、温時～熱時水、含水エタノール若しくは酸性含水エタノールで抽出して得られたもの、又は室温時～温時アルカリ性水溶液で抽出し、中和して得られたものである。主色素はアピゲニニジン及びルテオリニジンである。赤褐色を呈する。	着色料	Kaoliang colour
133	コチニール色素（エンジムシから得られた、カルミン酸を主成分とするものをいう。）	カルミン酸色素	カルミン酸 コチニール	エンジムシ（<u>Dactylopius</u> <u>coccus</u> Costa(<u>Coccus</u> <u>cacti</u> Linnaeus)）から得られた，カルミン酸を主成分とするものである。	着色料	Cochineal extract Carminic acid
134	骨炭（ウシの骨から得られた、炭末及びリン酸カルシウムを主成分とするものをいう。）			ウシ（<u>Bos</u> <u>taurus</u> Linne）の骨を、炭化し、粉砕して得られたものである。主成分はリン酸カルシウム及び炭末である。	製造用剤	Bone charcoal
135	骨炭色素（骨を炭化して得られた、炭素を主成分とするものをいう。）	炭末色素	炭末	ウシ科ウシ（<u>Bos</u> <u>taurus</u> LINNE var.<u>domesticus</u> GEMEL.）等の骨を、炭化した物である。主色素は炭素である。黒色を呈する。	着色料	Bone carbon black

番号	品名		簡略名又は類別名	基原・製法・本質	用途	備考
	名称	別名				
136	ゴマ油不けん化物 (ゴマの種子から得られた、セサモリンを主成分とするものをいう。)		ゴマ油抽出物	ゴマ科ゴマ (Sesamum indicum LINNE) の種子又は種子の搾油糟より、エタノールで抽出して得られたものである。主成分はセサモリンである。	酸化防止剤	Sesame seed oil unsaponified matter
137	ゴマ柄灰抽出物 (ゴマの茎又は葉の灰化物から抽出して得られたものをいう。)			ゴマ (Sesamum indicum LINNE) の茎又は葉を灰化し、室温時水で抽出し、上澄み液をろ過して得られたものである。	製造用剤	Sesame straw ash extract
138	ゴム (パラゴムの分泌液から得られた、ポリイソプレンを主成分とするものをいう。ただし、「低分子ゴム」を除く。)	カウチョック		トウダイグサ科パラゴム (Hevea brasiliensis MUELL.-ARG.) の幹枝より得られるラテックスを酸性水溶液で凝固させ、水洗、脱水したものより得られたものである。主成分はシスポリイソプレンである。	ガムベース	Rubber
139	ゴム分解樹脂 (「ゴム」から得られた、ジテルペン、トリテルペン及びテトラテルペンを主成分とするものをいう。)			トウダイグサ科パラゴム (Hevea brasiliensis MUELL.-ARG.) の幹枝より得られるラテックスを、加熱分解したもの、又は酵素分解して得られた低分子の樹脂状物質である。主成分はC_{20}～C_{40}のテルペノイドである。	ガムベース	Resin of depolymerized natural rubber
140	コメヌカ油抽出物 (米ぬか油から得られた、フェルラ酸を主成分とするものをいう。)	コメヌカ油不けん化物		イネ科イネ (Oryza sativa LINNE) の種子より得られる米ぬか油の不けん化物より、エタノールで抽出して得られたものである。有効成分はフェルラ酸である。	酸化防止剤	Rice bran oil extract
141	コメヌカ酵素分解物 (脱脂米ぬかから得られた、フィチン酸及びペプチドを主成分とするものをいう。)			イネ科イネ (Oryza sativa LINNE) の種子より得られる脱脂米ぬかを酵素分解したものより、水で抽出して得られたものである。主成分はペプチド及びフィチン酸である。	酸化防止剤	Enzymatically decomposed rice bran
142	コメヌカロウ (米ぬか油から得られた、リグノセリン酸ミリシルを主成分とするものをいう。)	コメヌカワックス ライスワックス	植物ワックス	イネ科イネ (Oryza sativa LINNE) の種子より得られる米ぬか油より、分離して得られたものである。主成分はリグノセリン酸ミリシルである。	ガムベース 光沢剤	Rice bran wax
143	サイリウムシードガム (ブロンドサイリウムの種皮から得られた、多糖類を主成分とするものをいう。)	サイリウムハスク	サイリウム	ブロンドサイリウム (Plantago ovata Forsskal) の種皮から得られた，多糖類を主成分とするものをいう。ショ糖，ブドウ糖，乳糖，デキストリン又はマルトースを含むことがある。	増粘安定剤	Psyllium seed gum
144	サトウキビロウ (サトウキビの茎から得られた、パルミチン酸ミリシルを主成分とするものをいう。)	カーンワックス ケーンワックス	植物ワックス	イネ科サトウキビ (Saccharum officinarum LINNE) の茎の搾汁残渣より、分離、精製して得られたものである。主成分はパルミチン酸ミリシルである。	ガムベース 光沢剤	Cane wax
145	サバクヨモギシードガム (サバクヨモギの種皮から得られた、多糖類を主成分とするものをいう。)	アルテミシアシードガム サバクヨモギ種子多糖類		キク科サバクヨモギ (Artemisia halodendron TURCZ. ex BESS., Artemisia ordosica KRASCHEN., Artemisias sphaerocephala KRASCH) の種子の外皮を、脱脂、乾燥して得られたものである。主成分は、α-セルロースを基本骨格に持つ、中性多糖類及び酸性多糖類である。	製造用剤 増粘安定剤	Artemisia sphaerocephala seed gum Artemisia seed gum
146	酸性白土		不溶性鉱物性物質	モンモリロナイト系粘土鉱物を精製して得られたものである。主成分は含水ケイ酸アルミニウムである。	製造用剤	Acid clay
147	酸性ホスファターゼ	ホスホモノエステラーゼ		糸状菌 (Aspergillus niger, Aspergillus oryzae) の培養液より、冷時～温時水で抽出し、除菌した後、冷時～室温時濃縮し、冷時エタノール若しくは含水エタノールで処理して得られたものである。	酵素	Acid phosphatase
148	酸素			O_2	製造用剤	Oxygen
149	シアナット色素		シアナット	アカテツ科シアノキ (Butyrospermum	着色料	Shea nut colour

番号	品名 名称	品名 別名	簡略名又は類別名	基原・製法・本質	用途	備考
	（シアノキの果実又は種皮から抽出して得られたものをいう。）		フラボノイド フラボノイド色素	parkii KOTSCHY.）の果実又は種皮より、室温時弱アルカリ性水溶液で抽出し、中和して得られたものである。褐色を呈する。		
150	シアノコバラミン	ビタミンB_{12}	V.B_{12}	放線菌（Streptomyces）又は細菌（Agrobacterium, Bacillus, Flavobacterium, Propionibacterium又はRhizobium）の培養液より、分離して得られたものである。成分はシアノコバラミンである。	強化剤	Cyanocobalamin Vitamin B_{12}
151	シェラック （ラックカイガラムシの分泌液から得られた、アレウリチン酸とシェロール酸又はアレウリチン酸とジャラール酸のエステルを主成分とするものをいう。）	セラック		ラックカイガラムシ（Laccifer spp.）の分泌液から得られた、アレウリチン酸とシェロール酸又はアレウリチン酸とジャラール酸のエステルを主成分とするものである。白シェラック及び精製シェラックがあり、ロウ分を除去していない含ロウ品及びロウ分を除去した脱ロウ品がある。	ガムベース 光沢剤	Shellac
	白シェラック	白セラック 白ラック		カイガラムシ科ラックカイガラムシ（Laccifer lacca KERR）の分泌する樹脂状物質を、温時アルカリ性水溶液で抽出し、漂白したものより得られたものである。主成分はアレウリチン酸とジャラール酸又はアレウリチン酸とシェロール酸のエステル等である。		White shellac
	精製シェラック	精製セラック		カイガラムシ科ラックカイガラムシ（Laccifer lacca KERR）の分泌する樹脂状物質を、室温時エタノールで抽出又は温時アルカリ性水溶液で抽出し、精製して得られたものである。主成分はアレウリチン酸とジャラール酸又はアレウリチン酸とシェロール酸のエステル等である。		Purified shellac
152	シェラックロウ （ラックカイガラムシの分泌液から得られた、ろう分を主成分とするものをいう。）	セラックロウ		カイガラムシ科ラックカイガラムシ（Laccifer lacca KERR）の分泌する樹脂状物質を、室温時エタノール又は温時アルカリ性水溶液に溶解し、ろ液からロウ分を分離して得られたものである。主成分は樹脂酸エステルである。	ガムベース 光沢剤	Shellac wax
153	ジェランガム （シュードモナスの培養液から得られた、多糖類を主成分とするものをいう。）	ジェラン多糖類	ジェラン	スフィンゴモナス属菌（Sphingomonas elodea）の培養液から得られた、多糖類を主成分とするものである。	増粘安定剤	Gellan gum
154	ジェルトン （ジェルトンの分泌液から得られた、アミリンアセタート及びポリイソプレンを主成分とするものをいう。）	ポンチアナック		キョウチクトウ科ジェルトン（Dyera costulata HOOK F., Dyera lowii HOOK F.）の幹枝から得られたラテックスを、熱時水で洗浄し、水溶成分を除去して得られたものである。主成分はアミリンアセタート及びシスポリイソプレンである。	ガムベース	Jelutong
155	シクロデキストリン	サイクロデキスト 分岐サイクロデキストリン 分岐シクロデキストリン	環状オリゴ糖	デンプンを、酵素処理し、非還元性環状デキストリンとして得られたものである。成分はシクロデキストリンである。	製造用剤	Cyclodextrin
156	シクロデキストリングルカノトランスフェラーゼ	シクロデキストリングルコシルトランスフェラーゼ	トランスフェラーゼ	細菌（Bacillus, Brevibacterium, Corynebacterium）の培養液より、冷時～室温時水で抽出して得られたもの、又は除菌後、冷時～室温時濃縮したもの、又はこれを、含水エタノールで処理して得られたものである。	酵素	Cyclodextrin glucanotransferase
157	L-シスチン		シスチン	動物性タンパク質（特に動物毛、羽毛）を、	調味料	L-Cystine

番号	品名 名称	品名 別名	簡略名又は類別名	基原・製法・本質	用途	備考
				加水分解し、分離して得られたものである。成分はL-シスチンである。	強化剤	
158	シソ抽出物 （シソの種子又は葉から得られた、テルペノイドを主成分とするものをいう。）	シソエキス		シソ科シソ（Perilla crispa TANAKA）の種子又は葉より、酸性水溶液又は温時含水エタノールで抽出したものから得られたものである。主成分はテルペノイドである。	製造用剤	Perilla extract
159	シタン色素 （シタンの幹枝から得られた、サンタリンを主成分とするものをいう。）	サンダルウッド色素	サンダルウッド フラボノイド フラボノイド色素	マメ科シタン（Pterocarpus santalinus LINNE）の幹枝より、水、熱時プロピレングルコール又は温時エタノールで抽出して得られたものである。主色素はサンタリンである。紫赤色を呈する。	着色料	Sandalwood red
160	5'-シチジル酸		5'-CMP	酵母（Candida utilis）の菌体より、食塩存在下、水で抽出した核酸を酵素で加水分解した後、分離して得られたものである。成分は5'-シチジル酸である。	強化剤	5'-Cytidylic acid
161	ジャマイカカッシア抽出物 （ジャマイカカッシアの幹枝又は樹皮から得られた、クアシン及びネオクアシンを主成分とするものをいう。）	カッシアエキス	カッシア	ニガキ科ジャマイカカッシア（Quassia excelsa SW.）の幹枝又は樹皮より、水で抽出して得られたものである。有効成分はクアシン及びネオクアシンである。	苦味料等	Jamaica quassia extract
162	ショウガ抽出物 （ショウガの根茎から得られた、ショウガオール及びジンゲロールを主成分とするものをいう。）	ジンジャー抽出物		ショウガ科ショウガ（Zingiber officinale ROSC.）の根茎より、室温時エタノール、アセトン又はヘキサンで抽出して得られたものである。主成分はジンゲロール類及びショウガオール類である。	製造用剤	Ginger extract
163	焼成カルシウム （うに殻、貝殻、造礁サンゴ、ホエイ、骨又は卵殻を焼成して得られた、カルシウム化合物を主成分とするものをいう。）		焼成Ca		強化剤 製造用剤	Calcinated calcium
	うに殻焼成カルシウム		うに殻カルシウム うに殻Ca	うに殻を、焼成して得られたものである。主成分は酸化カルシウムである。		Calcinated sea urchin shell calcium
	貝殻焼成カルシウム		貝カルシウム 貝Ca	貝殻を焼成して得られたものである。成分は酸化カルシウムである。		Calcinated shell calcium
	骨焼成カルシウム		骨カルシウム 骨Ca	獣骨又は魚骨を、焼成して得られたものである。成分はリン酸カルシウムである。		Calcinated bone calcium
	造礁サンゴ焼成カルシウム		コーラルカルシウム コーラルCa サンゴカルシウム サンゴCa	イシサンゴ目の（Scleractinia）の造礁サンゴを、焼成して得られたものである。主成分は酸化カルシウムである。		Calcinated coral calcium
	乳清焼成カルシウム	乳清第三リン酸カルシウム ホエイ第三リン酸カルシウム ホエイリン酸三カルシウム	乳清リン酸カルシウム 乳清リン酸Ca ホエイリン酸カルシウム ホエイリン酸Ca	乳清（酸カゼインホエイ）より乳清タンパクと乳糖を分離、除去したものを、精製し焼成して得られたものである。主成分はリン酸三カルシウムである。		Tricalcium phosphate
	卵殻焼成カルシウム		卵殻カルシウム 卵殻Ca	卵殻を焼成して得られたものである。主成分は酸化カルシウムである。		Calcinated eggshell calcium
164	植物性ステロール （油糧種子から得られた、フィトステロールを主成分とするものをいう。）	フィトステロール	ステロール	油糧種子を粉砕し、抽出して得られた植物性油脂より、室温時～温時メタノール、エタノール、イソプロパノール、酢酸エチル、アセトン、又はヘキサンで抽出したものより得られたものである。主成分はフィトステロールである。	乳化剤	Vegetable sterol

番号	品名 名称	品名 別名	簡略名又は類別名	基原・製法・本質	用途	備考
165	植物炭末色素 (植物を炭化して得られた、炭素を主成分とするものをいう。)	炭末色素	炭末	植物を、水蒸気賦活法で高温に加熱し炭化したものである。主色素は炭素である。黒色を呈する。	着色料	Vegetable carbon black
166	植物レシチン (アブラナ又はダイズの種子から得られた、レシチンを主成分とするものをいう。)	レシチン		アブラナ科アブラナ (Brassica campestris LINNE)、マメ科ダイズ (Glycine max MERRILL) の種子より得られた油脂より、分離して得られたものである。主成分はレシチンである。	乳化剤	Vegetable lecithin
167	しらこたん白抽出物 (魚類の精巣から得られた、塩基性タンパク質を主成分とするものをいう。)	しらこたん白 しらこ分解物 プロタミン	核たん白 しらこ	アイナメ (Hexagrammos otakii Jordan et Starks)、カラフトマス (Oncorhynchus gorbuscha(Walbaum))、シロザケ (Oncorhynchus keta(Walbaum))、ベニサケ (Oncorhynchus nerka(Walbaum))、カツオ (Katsuwonus pelamis(Linnaeus)) 又はニシン (Clupea pallasii Valenciennes) の精巣から得られた、塩基性タンパク質を主成分とするものである。	保存料	Milt protein
168	水素			H_2	製造用剤	Hydrogen
169	ステビア抽出物 (ステビアの葉から抽出して得られた、ステビオール配糖体を主成分とするものをいう。)	ステビアエキス ステビオサイド ステビオシド レバウジオシド レバウディオサイド	ステビア ステビア甘味料	ステビア (Stevia rebaudiana Bertoni) の葉から抽出して得られた、ステビオール配糖体を主成分とするものである。	甘味料	Stevia extract
170	ステビア末 (ステビアの葉を粉砕して得られた、ステビオール配糖体を主成分とするものをいう。)		ステビア	キク科ステビア (Stevia rebaudiana BERTONI) の葉を、粉末としたものである。主甘味成分はステビオール配糖体 (ステビオシド及びレバウジオシド) である。	甘味料	Powdered stevia
171	スピルリナ色素 (スピルリナの全藻から得られた、フィコシアニンを主成分とするものをいう。)	スピルリナ青色素	スピルリナ青	スピルリナ (Spirulina platensis Geitler) の全藻から得られた、フィコシアニンを主成分とするものである。デキストリン又は乳糖を含むことがある。	着色料	Spirulina colour
172	スフィンゴ脂質 (米ぬかから得られた、スフィンゴシン誘導体を主成分とするものをいう。)			イネ科イネ (Oryza sativa LINNE) の種子又は小麦 (Triticum aestivum LINNE) の胚芽から得られた米ぬかより、室温時～温時エタノール、含水エタノール、イソプロピルアルコール、アセトン、ヘキサン又は酢酸エチルで抽出したものより得られたものである。主成分はスフィンゴシン誘導体である。	乳化剤	Sphingolipid
173	生石灰			石灰石を、焼成して得られたものである。主成分は酸化カルシウムである。	製造用剤	Quicklime
174	精油除去ウイキョウ抽出物 (ウイキョウの種子から得られた、グルコシルシナピルアルコールを主成分とするものをいう。)	精油除去フェンネル抽出物		セリ科ウイキョウ (Foeniculum vulgare LINNE) の種子を水蒸気蒸留した残渣より、熱時水で抽出し、濃縮して得られたものである。主成分は4-O-α-D-グルコシルシナピルアルコールである。	酸化防止剤	Essential oil-removed fennel extract
175	セイヨウワサビ抽出物 (セイヨウワサビの根から得られた、イソチオシアナートを主成分とするものをいう。)	ホースラディッシュ抽出物		アブラナ科セイヨウワサビ (Armoracia rusticana P.GAERTN., B.MEYER et SCHERB.) の根を、粉砕後、水蒸気蒸留で抽出して得られたものである。主成分はイソチオシアナートである。	酸化防止剤 製造用剤	Horseradish extract
176	ゼイン (トウモロコシの種子から得られた、植物性タンパク質を主成分とするものをいう。)	トウモロコシたん白		イネ科トウモロコシ (Zea mays LINNE) の種子を粉末化したものより、エタノール又はアセトンで抽出し、精製して得られたものである。主成分はプロラミンに属する植物性タ	製造用剤	Zein

番号	品名 名称	品名 別名	簡略名又は類別名	基原・製法・本質	用途	備考
				ンパク質である。		
177	ゼオライト		不溶性鉱物性物質	鉱床より採掘したゼオライトを精製して得られたものである。主成分は結晶性アルミノケイ酸塩である。	製造用剤	Zeolite
178	セージ抽出物 （サルビアの葉から得られた、カルノシン酸及びフェノール性ジテルペンを主成分とするものをいう。）			シソ科サルビア（Salvia officinalis LINNE）の葉より、水、エタノール又はヘキサンで抽出して得られたものである。有効成分はフェノール性ジテルペノイド（ジテルペン）及びカルノシン酸である。	酸化防止剤	Sage extract
179	セピオライト			鉱石セピオライトを、粉砕して得られたものである。主成分はイノケイ酸のマグネシウム塩である。	製造用剤	Sepiolite
180	L-セリン		セリン	タンパク質原料の加水分解により、又は糖類を原料とした発酵により得られたものを、分離して得られたものである。成分はL-セリンである。	調味料 強化剤	L-Serine
181	セルラーゼ	繊維素分解酵素	カルボヒドラーゼ	糸状菌（Acremonium cellulolyticus, Aspergillus aculeatus, Aspergillus awamori, Aspergillus niger, Humicola insolens, Trichoderma harzianum, Trichoderma insolens, Trichoderma koningii, Trichoderma longibrachiatum, Trichoderma reesei, Trichoderma viride）、担子菌（Corticium, Irpex, Pycnoporus coccineus）、放線菌（Actinomyces, Streptomyces）若しくは細菌（Bacillus circulans, Bacillus subtillis）の培養液より、冷時～微温時水で抽出して得られたもの、又は冷時～室温時濃縮後、冷時エタノール若しくは含水エタノールで処理して得られたものである。	酵素	Cellulase
182	粗製海水塩化カリウム （海水から塩化ナトリウムを析出分離して得られた、塩化カリウムを主成分とするものをいう。）			海水を、濃縮し、塩化ナトリウムを析出分離させた後、そのろ液を、室温まで冷却し、析出分離させたものである。主成分は塩化カリウムである。	調味料	Crude potassium chloride(sea water)
183	粗製海水塩化マグネシウム （海水から塩化カリウム及び塩化ナトリウムを析出分離して得られた、塩化マグネシウムを主成分とするものをいう。）	塩化マグネシウム含有物		海水より、塩化ナトリウムを析出分離し、その母液を冷却して析出する塩化カリウム等を分離した残りのものである。主成分は塩化マグネシウムである。	製造用剤	Crude magnesium chloride(sea water)
184	ソバ柄灰抽出物 （ソバの茎又は葉の灰化物から抽出して得られたものをいう。）		植物灰抽出物	タデ科ソバ（Fagopyrum esculentum MOENCH.）の茎又は葉を灰化したものより、熱時水で抽出して得られたものであって、アルカリ金属及びアルカリ土類金属を含む。	製造用剤	Buckwheat ash extract
185	ソルバ （ソルバの分泌液から得られた、アミリンアセタート及びポリイソプレンを主成分とするものをいう。）	ペリージョ ペンダーレ レッチェカスピ		キョウチクトウ科ソルバ（Couma macrocarpa BARB. RODR.）の幹枝から得られたラテックスを、熱時水で洗浄し、水溶成分を除去して得られたものである。主成分はアミリンアセタート及びシスポリイソプレンである。	ガムベース	Sorva Leche caspi
186	ソルビンハ （ソルビンハの分泌液から得られた、アミリンアセタート及びポリイソプレンを主成分とするものをいう。）	ソルバペケーニャ		キョウチクトウ科ソルビンハ（Couma utilis MUELL.）の幹枝より得られたラテックスを、熱時水で洗浄し、水溶成分を除去して得られたものである。主成分はアミリンアセタート及びシスポリイソプレンである。	ガムベース	Sorvinha

番号	品名 名称	品名 別名	簡略名又は類別名	基原・製法・本質	用途	備考
187	ダイズサポニン (ダイズの種子から得られた、サポニンを主成分とするものをいう。)		サポニン	マメ科ダイズ (Glycine max MERRILL) の種子を粉砕し、水又はエタノールで抽出し、精製して得られたものである。主成分はサポニン (ソヤサポニン等) である。	乳化剤	Soybean saponin
188	タウマチン (タウマトコッカスダニエリの種子から得られた、タウマチンを主成分とするものをいう。)	ソーマチン		タウマトコッカス・ダニエリ (Thaumatococcus daniellii Bentham) の種子から得られた、タウマチンを主成分とするものである。	甘味料	Thaumatin
189	タウリン (抽出物) (魚類又はほ乳類の臓器又は肉から得られた、タウリンを主成分とするものをいう。)		タウリン	魚介類又は哺乳動物の臓器又は肉から得られた、タウリンを主成分とするものである。	調味料	Taurine(extract)
190	タマネギ色素 (タマネギのりん茎から得られた、クエルセチンを主成分とするものをいう。)		フラボノイド フラボノイド色素 野菜色素	ユリ科タマネギ (Allium cepa LINNE) のりん茎より、温時～熱時水若しくは含水エタノールで抽出して得られたもの、又は温時～熱時弱アルカリ性水溶液で抽出し、中和して得られたものである。主色素はクエルセチンである。黄色を呈する。	着色料	Onion colour
191	タマリンド色素 (タマリンドの種子から得られた、フラボノイドを主成分とするものをいう。)		フラボノイド フラボノイド色素	マメ科タマリンド (Tamarindus indica LINNE) の種子を焙焼したものより、温時弱アルカリ性水溶液で抽出し、中和して得られたものである。主色素はフラボノイドである。赤褐色を呈する。	着色料	Tamarind colour
192	タマリンドシードガム (タマリンドの種子から得られた、多糖類を主成分とするものをいう。)	タマリンドガム タマリンド種子多糖類	タマリンド	タマリンド (Tamarindus indica Linne) の種子から得られた、多糖類を主成分とするものである。ショ糖、ブドウ糖、乳糖、デキストリン又はマルトースを含むことがある。	増粘安定剤	Tamarind seed gum
193	タラガム (タラの種子から得られた、多糖類を主成分とするものをいう。)			タラ (Caesalpinia spinosa Kuntze) の種子から得られた、多糖類を主成分とするものである。ショ糖、ブドウ糖、乳糖、デキストリン又はマルトースを含むことがある。	増粘安定剤	Tara gum
194	タルク		不溶性鉱物性物質	天然の含水ケイ酸マグネシウムを精選したもので、ときに少量のケイ酸アルミニウムを含む。	ガムベース 製造用剤	Talc
195	胆汁末 (胆汁から得られた、コール酸及びデソキシコール酸を主成分とするものをいう。)	コール酸 デソキシコール酸		動物の胆汁を、粉末化して得られたものである。主成分はコール酸及びデソキシコール酸である。	乳化剤	Powdered bile
196	単糖・アミノ酸複合物 (アミノ酸と単糖類の混合物を加熱して得られたものをいう。)		糖・アミノ酸複合物	アミノ酸と単糖類の混合液を、常圧下で加熱して得られたものである。	酸化防止剤	Amino acid-sugar reaction product
197	タンナーゼ			糸状菌 (Aspergillus oryzae) の培養液より、冷時～室温時水で抽出して得られたもの、又は濃縮後、冷時～室温時エタノール若しくは含水エタノールで処理して得られたものである。	酵素	Tannase
198	タンニン (抽出物) (カキの果実、五倍子、タラ末、没食子又はミモザの樹皮から得られた、タンニン及びタンニン酸を主成分とするものをいう。)	タンニン酸 (抽出物)	タンニン タンニン酸		製造用剤	Tannin(extract)
	柿タンニン	柿渋 柿抽出物		カキ科カキ (Diospyros kaki THUNB.) の実より、搾汁したもの、又は水若しくはエタノールで抽出して得られたものである。主成		Tannin of persimmon

番号	品名 名称	品名 別名	簡略名又は類別名	基原・製法・本質	用途	備考
				分はタンニン及びタンニン酸である。		
	植物タンニン			五倍子、タラ末又は没食子から得られた、タンニン及びタンニン酸を主成分とするものである。		Vegetable tannin
	ミモザタンニン			マメ科ミモザ（Acacia dealbata LINNE）の樹皮より、水又はエタノールで抽出して得られたものである。主成分はタンニン及びタンニン酸である。		Tannin of silver wattle
199	チクル（サポジラの分泌液から得られた、アミリンアセタート及びポリイソプレンを主成分とするものをいう。）	クラウンガム チクブル ニスペロ		アカテツ科サポジラ（Achras zapota LINNE）の幹枝より得られたラテックスを、脱水したものより得られたものである。主成分はアミリンアセタート及びポリイソプレンである。	ガムベース	Chicle Chiquibul Crown gum Nispero
200	窒素			N_2	製造用剤	Nitrogen
201	チャ乾留物（チャの葉を乾留して得られたものをいう。）			ツバキ科チャ（Camellia sinensis O.KZE.）の葉より製した茶を、乾留して得られたものである。有効成分は特定できないが、アミノ酸、カフェイン、タンニン、カテキン類を含む。	製造用剤	Tea dry distillate
202	チャ抽出物（チャの葉から得られた、カテキン類を主成分とするものをいう。）	ウーロンチャ抽出物 緑茶抽出物		ツバキ科チャ（Camellia sinensis O.KZE.）の葉より製した茶より、室温時、温時又は熱時、水、酸性水溶液、含水エタノール、エタノール、含水メタノール、メタノール、アセトン、酢酸エチル又はグリセリン水溶液で抽出したものより得られたものである。成分としてカテキン類を含む。なお、チャの葉の処理方法によりウーロンチャ抽出物と呼ばれるものがある。	酸化防止剤 製造用剤	Tea extract
203	チルテ（チルテの分泌液から得られた、アミリンアセタート及びポリイソプレンを主成分とするものをいう。）			トウダイグサ科チルテ（Cnidoscolus elasticus LUNDELL.）の幹枝より得られたラテックスを、熱時水で洗浄し、水溶成分を除去して得られたものである。主成分はアミリンアセタート及びポリイソプレンである。	ガムベース	Chilte
204	L-チロシン	L-チロジン	チロシン チロジン	動物性若しくは植物性タンパク質の加水分解により、又は糖類を原料とした発酵により得られたものを、分離して得られたものである。成分はL-チロシンである。	調味料 強化剤	L-Tyrosine
205	ツヌー（ツヌーの分泌液から得られた、アミリンアセタート及びポリイソプレンを主成分とするものをいう。）			クワ科ツヌー（Castilla fallax COOK）の幹枝より得られたラテックスを、脱水したものより得られたものである。主成分はアミリンアセタート及びポリイソプレンである。	ガムベース	Tunu
206	ツヤプリシン（抽出物）（ヒバの幹枝又は根から得られた、ツヤプリシン類を主成分とするものをいう。）	ヒノキチオール（抽出物）	ヒノキチオール	アスナロ（ヒバ）（Thujopsis dolabrata Siebold et Zuccarini）の幹枝又は根から得られた、ツヤプリシン類を主成分とするものである。	保存料	Thujaplicin (extract) Hinokitiol (extract)
207	5′-デアミナーゼ			糸状菌（Aspergillus melleus, Aspergillus oryzae）の培養液より、冷時～室温時水で抽出して得られたもの、又は冷時～室温時濃縮後、冷時エタノールで処理して得られたものである。	酵素	5′-Deaminase
208	低分子ゴム（パラゴムの分泌液を分解して得られた、ポリイソプレンを主成分とするものをいう。）			トウダイグサ科パラゴム（Hevea brasiliensis MUELL.-ARG.）の幹枝より得られるラテックスを、加熱分解して得られたもの、又は酵素分解して得られたものである。主成分	ガムベース	Depolymerized natural rubber

番号	品名 名称	品名 別名	簡略名又は類別名	基原・製法・本質	用途	備考
				はシスポリイソプレンである。		
209	テオブロミン			アオギリ科カカオ（Theobroma cacao LINNE）の種子、アオギリ科コーラ（Cola acuminata SCHOTT et ENDL.）の種子又はツバキ科チャ（Camellia sinensis O. KZE.）の葉より、水又はエタノールで抽出し、分離して得られたものである。成分はテオブロミンである。	苦味料等	Theobromine
210	デキストラナーゼ			糸状菌（Chaetomium erraticum, Chaetomium gracile, Penicillium lilacinum）の培養液より、冷時～室温時水若しくは酸性水溶液で抽出して得られたもの、除菌後、冷時～室温時濃縮したもの、又は冷時エタノールで処理して得られたものである。	酵素	Dextranase
211	デキストラン		ブドウ糖多糖	グラム陽性細菌（Leuconostoc mesenteroides又はStreptococcus equinus）の培養液より、分離して得られたものである。成分はデキストランである。	増粘安定剤	Dextran
212	鉄			^{54}Fe, ^{56}Fe, ^{57}Fe, ^{58}Fe	強化剤 製造用剤	Iron
213	デュナリエラカロテン （デュナリエラの全藻から得られた、β-カロテンを主成分とするものをいう。）	藻類カロチン 藻類カロテン デュナリエラカロチン ドナリエラカロチン ドナリエラカロテン 抽出カロチン 抽出カロテン	カロチノイド カロチノイド色素 カロチン カロチン色素 カロテノイド カロテノイド色素 カロテン カロテン色素	デュナリエラ（Dunaliella bardawil又はDunaliella salina）の全藻から得られた、β-カロテンを主成分とするものである。食用油脂を含むことがある。	強化剤 着色料	Dunaliella carotene
214	銅			^{63}Cu, ^{65}Cu	製造用剤	Copper
215	トウガラシ色素 （トウガラシの果実から得られた、カプサンチン類を主成分とするものをいう。）	カプシカム色素 パプリカ色素	カロチノイド カロチノイド色素 カロテノイド カロテノイド色素	トウガラシ（Capsicum annuum Linne）の果実から得られた、カプサンチン類を主成分とするものである。食用油脂を含むことがある。	着色料	Paprika colour Paprika oleoresin
216	トウガラシ水性抽出物 （トウガラシの果実から抽出して得られた、水溶性物質を主成分とするものをいう。）	カプシカム水性抽出物 パプリカ水性抽出物	カプシカム抽出物 トウガラシ抽出物 パプリカ抽出物	ナス科トウガラシ（Capsicum annuum LINNE）の果実より、室温時含水エタノールで抽出したもので、タンパク質、ペプチド、ビタミンCを含む。	製造用剤	Capsicum water-soluble extract
217	動物性ステロール （魚油又は「ラノリン」から得られた、コレステロールを主成分とするものをいう。）	コレステロール	ステロール	魚油の不けん化物又は「ラノリン」より、加水分解したもの、又は有機溶剤で抽出したものより得られたものである。主成分はコレステロールである。	乳化剤	Cholesterol
218	トコトリエノール			イネ（Oryza sativa Linne）の米ぬか油、アブラヤシ（Elaeis guineensis Jacquin）のパーム油等より分別精製して得られたものである。主成分はトコトリエノールである。食用油脂を含むことがある。	酸化防止剤	Tocotrienol
219	d-α-トコフェロール	α-ビタミンE 抽出トコフェロール 抽出ビタミンE	抽出V.E トコフェロール α-トコフェロール ビタミンE V.E	油糧種子から得られた植物油脂又はミックストコフェロール（植物油脂から得られたd-α-トコフェロール、d-β-トコフェロール、d-γ-トコフェロール及びd-δ-トコフェロールを主成分とするものをいう。）より分離して得られた、d-α-トコフェロールを主成分とするものである。食用油脂を含むこと	酸化防止剤 強化剤	d-α-Tocopherol

番号	品名 名称	品名 別名	簡略名又は類別名	基原・製法・本質	用途	備考
				がある。		
220	d-γ-トコフェロール	γ-ビタミンE 抽出トコフェロール 抽出ビタミンE	抽出V.E トコフェロール γ-トコフェロール ビタミンE V.E	油糧種子から得られた植物油脂又はミックストコフェロール（植物油脂から得られたd-α-トコフェロール、d-β-トコフェロール、d-γ-トコフェロール及びd-δ-トコフェロールを主成分とするものをいう。）より分離して得られた、d-γ-トコフェロールを主成分とするものである。食用油脂を含むことがある。	酸化防止剤 強化剤	d-γ-Tocopherol
221	d-δ-トコフェロール	δ-ビタミンE 抽出トコフェロール 抽出ビタミンE	抽出V.E トコフェロール δ-トコフェロール ビタミンE V.E	油糧種子から得られた植物油脂又はミックストコフェロール（植物油脂から得られたd-α-トコフェロール、d-β-トコフェロール、d-γ-トコフェロール及びd-δ-トコフェロールを主成分とするものをいう。）より分離して得られた、d-δ-トコフェロールを主成分とするものである。食用油脂を含むことがある。	酸化防止剤 強化剤	d-δ-Tocopherol
222	トマト色素 （トマトの果実から得られた、リコピンを主成分とするものをいう。）	トマトリコピン	カロチノイド カロチノイド色素 カロテノイド カロテノイド色素 野菜色素	トマト（Lycopersicon esculentum Miller）の果実から得られた、リコピンを主成分とするものである。食用油脂を含むことがある。	着色料	Tomato colour Tomato lycopene
223	トラガントガム （トラガントの分泌液から得られた、多糖類を主成分とするものをいう。）		トラガント	トラガント（Astragalus gummifer Labillardiere）の分泌液から得られた、多糖類を主成分とするものである。	増粘安定剤	Tragacanth gum
224	トランスグルコシダーゼ			糸状菌（Aspergillus niger, Aspergillus usamii）、細菌（Sulfolobus solfataricus）の培養液より、冷時～室温時除菌したもの、冷時～室温時濃縮したもの、又は冷時エタノールで処理して得られたものである。	酵素	Transglucosidase
225	トランスグルタミナーゼ			動物の肝臓より、又は放線菌（Streptomyces, Streptoverticillium mobaraense）若しくは細菌（Bacillus）の培養液より、室温時水で抽出後、冷時エタノールで処理して得られたものである。	酵素	Transglutaminase
226	トリプシン			動物の膵臓又は魚類若しくは甲殻類の臓器から得られた、たん白質分解酵素である。乳糖又はデキストリンを含むことがある。	酵素	Trypsin
227	トレハロース			担子菌（Aguricus等）、細菌（Arthrobacter, Brevibacterium, Pimelobacter, Pseudomonas, Thermus等）又は酵母（Saccharomyces等）の培養ろ液又は菌体より、水若しくはアルコールで抽出して得られたもの、これを酵素によるでん粉の糖化液より分離して得られたもの、又はマルトースを酵素処理して得られたものである。成分はトレハロースである。	製造用剤	Trehalose
228	トレハロースホスホリラーゼ			細菌（Plesiomonas）の培養液の菌体を酵素（リゾチーム）処理した後、冷時～室温時水で抽出して得られたものである。	酵素	Trehalose phosphorylase
229	トロロアオイ （トロロアオイの根から得られた、多糖類を主成分とするものをいう。）			アオイ科トロロアオイ（Abelmoschus manihot MED.）の根を、乾燥、粉砕して得られたものである。主成分は多糖類である。	増粘安定剤	Tororoaoi

番号	品名		簡略名又は類別名	基原・製法・本質	用途	備考
	名称	別名				
230	納豆菌ガム (納豆菌の培養液から得られた、ポリグルタミン酸を主成分とするものをいう。)	納豆菌粘質物	ポリグルタミン酸	納豆菌 (Bacillus subtilis) の培養液から得られた、ポリグルタミン酸を主成分とするものである。	増粘安定剤 製造用剤	Bacillus natto gum
231	ナフサ	石油ナフサ		石油蒸留物を、精製して得られたものである。成分はパラフィン系及びナフタレン系炭化水素である。	製造用剤	Petroleum naphtha
232	生コーヒー豆抽出物 (コーヒーの種子から得られた、クロロゲン酸及びポリフェノールを主成分とするものをいう。)			アカネ科コーヒー (Coffea arabica LINNE) の種子より、温時アスコルビン酸又はクエン酸酸性水溶液で抽出して得られたものである。有効成分は、クロロゲン酸及びポリフェノールである。	酸化防止剤	Coffee bean extract
233	ナリンジナーゼ	ナリンギナーゼ		糸状菌 (Aspergillus usamii, Penicillium decumbens) の培養液より、冷時〜室温時水で抽出し、冷時〜室温時濃縮後、冷時エタノールで処理して得られたものである。	酵素	Naringinase
234	ナリンジン	ナリンギン		グレープフルーツ (Citrus × paradisi Macfadyen) の果皮、果汁又は種子より、水又はエタノール若しくはメタノールで抽出し、分離して得られたものである。成分はナリンジンである。	苦味料等	Naringin
235	ニガーグッタ (ニガーグッタの分泌液から得られた、アミリンアセタート及びポリイソプレンを主成分とするものをいう。)			クワ科ニガーグッタ (Ficus platyphylla DELILE.) の幹枝より得られたラテックスを、熱時水で洗浄し、水溶成分を除去して得られたものである。主成分はアミリンアセタート及びポリイソプレンである。	ガムベース	Niger gutta
236	ニガヨモギ抽出物 (ニガヨモギの全草から得られた、セスキテルペンを主成分とするものをいう。)		ニガヨモギ	キク科ニガヨモギ (Artemisia absinthium LINNE) の全草より、水又は室温時エタノールで抽出して得られたものである。主成分はセスキテルペン (アブシンチン等) である。	苦味料等	Absinth extract
237	ニッケル			^{58}Ni, ^{60}Ni, ^{61}Ni, ^{62}Ni, ^{64}Ni	製造用剤	Nickel
238	ニンジンカロテン (ニンジンの根から得られた、カロテンを主成分とするものをいう。)	キャロットカロチン キャロットカロテン ニンジンカロチン 抽出カロチン 抽出カロテン	カロチノイド カロチノイド色素 カロチン カロチン色素 カロテノイド カロテノイド色素 カロテン カロテン色素	ニンジン (Daucus carota Linne) の根から得られた、カロテンを主成分とするものである。食用油脂を含むことがある。	強化剤 着色料	Carrot carotene
239	ばい煎コメヌカ抽出物 (米ぬかから得られた、マルトールを主成分とするものをいう。)			イネ科イネ (Oryza sativa LINNE) の米ぬかを脱脂し、ばい煎したものを、熱時水で抽出後、温時エタノールでタンパク質を除去したものである。成分としてマルトールを含む。	製造用剤	Roasted rice bran extract
240	ばい煎ダイズ抽出物 (ダイズの種子から得られた、マルトールを主成分とするものをいう。)			マメ科ダイズ (Glycine max MERRILL) の種子を脱脂し、ばい煎したものより、熱時水で抽出後、温時エタノールでタンパク質を除去して得られたものである。成分としてマルトールを含む。	製造用剤	Roasted soybean extract
241	パーオキシダーゼ	ペルオキシダーゼ		アブラナ科セイヨウワサビ (Armoracia rusticana)、アブラナ科ダイコン (Rahpauns acanthiformis) 若しくはキュウリ科キュウリ (Cucumis sativus) より搾汁したもの、又は糸状菌 (Alternaria, Aspergillus oryzae, Coprinus cinereus, Oidiodendron) 若しくは	酵素	Peroxidase

番号	品名 名称	品名 別名	簡略名又は類別名	基原・製法・本質	用途	備考
				細菌（Bacillus）の培養液より、冷時～室温時水で抽出して得られたもの、若しくは冷時～室温時濃縮後、エタノールで処理して得られたものである。		
242	白金			^{192}Pt, ^{194}Pt, ^{195}Pt, ^{196}Pt, ^{198}Pt	製造用剤	Platinum
243	パパイン			パパイヤ（Carica papaya Linne）の果実より得られた、たん白質分解酵素である。乳糖又はデキストリンを含むことがある。	酵素	Papain
244	パーム油カロテン（アブラヤシの果実から得られた、カロテンを主成分とするものをいう。）	パーム油カロチン 抽出カロチン 抽出カロテン	カロチノイド カロチノイド色素 カロチン カロチン色素 カロテノイド カロテノイド色素 カロテン カロテン色素	アブラヤシ（Elaeis guineensis Jacquin）の果実から得られた、カロテンを主成分とするものである。食用油脂を含むことがある。	強化剤 着色料	Palm oil carotene
245	パーライト		不溶性鉱物性物質	鉱物性二酸化ケイ素を800～1,200℃で焼成したものである。	製造用剤	Perlite
246	パラジウム			^{102}Pd, ^{104}Pd, ^{105}Pd, ^{106}Pd, ^{108}Pd, ^{110}Pd	製造用剤	Palladium
247	パラフィンワックス	パラフィン		石油の常圧及び減圧蒸留留出油から得た固形の炭化水素の混合物で、主として直鎖状の飽和炭化水素からなる。	ガムベース 光沢剤	Paraffin wax
248	パンクレアチン			動物のすい臓より、室温時水で抽出し、冷時～室温時アセトンで処理して得られたものである。	酵素	Pancreatin
249	ヒアルロン酸		ムコ多糖	鶏冠より、微温時～温時水、アルカリ性水溶液若しくは酸性水溶液で抽出し、エタノール若しくは含水エタノールで処理、若しくは酵素処理した後エタノール若しくは含水エタノールで処理し、精製して得られたもの、又は細菌（Streptcoccus zooepidemicus）の培養液を、冷時～温時、除菌し、エタノール若しくは含水エタノールで処理し、精製して得られたものである。成分はヒアルロン酸である。	製造用剤	Hyaluronic acid
250	微結晶セルロース（パルプから得られた、結晶セルロースを主成分とするものをいう。）	結晶セルロース	セルロース	パルプから得られた、結晶セルロースを主成分とするものである。乾燥物及び含水物がある。	製造用剤	Microcryrstalline cellulose
251	微小繊維状セルロース（パルプ又は綿を微小繊維状にして得られた、セルロースを主成分とするものをいう。）		セルロース	パルプ又は綿を微小繊維状にして得られた、セルロースを主成分とするものである。	増粘安定剤 製造用剤	Microfibrillated cellulose
252	L-ヒスチジン		ヒスチジン	タンパク質原料の加水分解により、又は糖類を原料とした発酵により得られたものを、分離して得られたものである。成分はL-ヒスチジンである。	調味料 強化剤	L-Histidine
253	ビートレッド（ビートの根から得られた、イソベタニン及びベタニンを主成分とするものをいう。）	アカビート色素	アカビート 野菜色素	ビート（Beta vulgaris Linne）の根から得られた、イソベタニン及びベタニンを主成分とするものである。デキストリン又は乳糖を含むことがある。	着色料	Beet red
254	L-ヒドロキシプロリン	L-オキシプロリン	オキシプロリン ヒドロキシプロリン	ゼラチン等を、加水分解し、分離して得られたものである。主成分はL-ヒドロキシプロリンである。	調味料 強化剤	L-Hydroxyproline

番号	品名 名称	品名 別名	簡略名又は類別名	基原・製法・本質	用途	備考
255	ヒマワリ種子抽出物 (ヒマワリの種子から得られた、イソクロロゲン酸及びクロロゲン酸を主成分とするものをいう。)	ヒマワリエキス ヒマワリ種子エキス ヒマワリ抽出物	ヒマワリ種子	キク科ヒマワリ(Helianthus annuus LINNE)の種子又は種子の搾油粕より、熱時水又は含水エタノールで抽出して得られたものである。有効成分はイソクロロゲン酸及びクロロゲン酸である。	酸化防止剤	Sunflower seed extract
256	ひる石		不溶性鉱物性物質	鉱床より採掘したひる石を、1000℃で焼成し、洗浄した後、乾燥して得られたものである。主成分はケイ酸塩である。	製造用剤	Vermiculite
257	ファーセレラン (フルセラリアの全藻から得られた、多糖類を主成分とするものをいう。)			ススカケベニ科フルセラリア(Furcellaria fastigiata HUD.)の全藻より、熱時水又はアルカリ性水溶液で抽出して得られたものである。主成分は多糖類である。	増粘安定剤	Furcellaran
258	ファフィア色素 (ファフィアの培養液から得られた、アスタキサンチンを主成分とするものをいう。)		カロチノイド カロチノイド色素 カロテノイド カロテノイド色素	酵母(Phaffia rhodozyma MILLER)の培養液より、室温時アセトン、エタノール、含水エタノール、ヘキサン又はこれらの混合液で抽出し、溶媒を除去して得られたものである。主色素はアスタキサンチンである。橙~赤色を呈する。	着色料	Phaffia colour
259	フィシン	ファイシン		クワ科イチジク(Ficus carica LINNE)又はクワ科ヒゴ(Ficus glabrata H.B. et K.)の樹液を、乾燥したもの、又はこれより、冷時~室温時水で抽出して得られたものである。成分はフィシンである。	酵素	Ficin
260	フィターゼ		ホスホヒドロラーゼ	糸状菌(Aspergillus niger)の培養液より水で抽出し、濃縮して得られたものである。	酵素	Phytase
261	フィチン酸 (米ぬか又はトウモロコシの種子から得られた、イノシトールヘキサリン酸を主成分とするものをいう。)			イネ科イネ(Oryza sativa LINNE)の種子より得られた米ぬか又はイネ科トウモロコシ(Zea mays LINNE)の種子より、室温時水又は酸性水溶液で抽出し、精製して得られたものである。主成分はイノシトールヘキサリン酸である。	酸味料 製造用剤	Phytic acid
262	フィチン(抽出物) (米ぬか又はトウモロコシの種子から得られた、イノシトールヘキサリン酸マグネシウムを主成分とするものをいう。)		フィチン	イネ科イネ(Oryza sativa LINNE)の種子より得られた米ぬか又はイネ科トウモロコシ(Zea mays LINNE)の種子より、室温時水で抽出して得られたものである。主成分はイノシトールヘキサリン酸マグネシウムである。	製造用剤	Phytin(extract)
263	フェリチン		鉄たん白 鉄たん白質	ウシ科ウシ(Bos taurus LINNE)の脾臓より、熱時水で抽出し、塩析法で分画し、膜ろ過により得られたものである。成分はフェリチンである。	強化剤	Ferritin
264	フェルラ酸			イネ科イネ(Oryza sativa LINNE)の糠より得られた米糠油を、室温時弱アルカル性下で含水エタノール及びヘキサンで分配した後、含水エタノール画分に得られたγ-オリザノールを、加圧下熱時硫酸で加水分解し、精製して得られたもの、又は細菌(Pseudomonas)を、フトモモ科チョウジノキ(Syzygium aromaticum MERRILL et PERRY)のつぼみ及び葉より水蒸気蒸留で得られた丁子油、又は丁子油から精製して得られたオイゲノールを含む培養液で培養し、その培養液を、分離、精製して得られたものである。成分はフェルラ酸である。	酸化防止剤	Ferulic acid
265	フクロノリ抽出物 (フクロノリの全藻から得られ	フクロノリ多糖類		フクロフノリ(Gloiopeltis furcata J.Agardh)の全藻から得られた、多糖類を主成分とする	増粘安定剤	Fukuronori extract

番号	品名		簡略名又は類別名	基原・製法・本質	用途	備考
	名称	別名				
	た、多糖類を主成分とするものをいう。)	フクロフノリ多糖類 フクロフノリ抽出物		ものである。ショ糖、ブドウ糖、乳糖、デキストリン又はマルトースを含むことがある。		
266	ブタン			石油若しくは天然ガス成分中、n-ブタンの沸点付近の留分である。	製造用剤	Butane
267	ブドウ果皮色素 (アメリカブドウ又はブドウの果皮から得られた、アントシアニンを主成分とするものをいう。)	エノシアニン	アントシアニン アントシアニン色素 ブドウ色素	アメリカブドウ(Vitis labrusca Linne)又はブドウ(Vitis vinifera Linne)の果皮から得られた、アントシアニンを主成分とするものである。デキストリン又は乳糖を含むことがある。	着色料	Grape skin colour Grape skin extract
268	ブドウ果皮抽出物 (アメリカブドウ又はブドウの果皮から得られた、ポリフェノールを主成分とするものをいう。)			ブドウ科アメリカブドウ(Vitis labrusca LINNE)又はブドウ科ブドウ(Vitis vinifera LINNE)のうち、生食用又は醸造用ブドウの甲州、シャルドネ若しくはリースリング種の果皮搾粕より、室温時~微温時エタノールで抽出して得られたものである。主成分はポリフェノールである。	製造用剤	Grape skin-derived substance
269	ブドウ種子抽出物 (アメリカブドウ又はブドウの種子から得られた、プロアントシアニジンを主成分とするものをいう。)		プロアントシアニジン	ブドウ科アメリカブドウ(Vitis labrusca LINNE)又はブドウ科ブドウ(Vitis vinifera LINNE)の種子より、熱時水、温時エタノール若しくは室温時アセトンで抽出したものより得られたもの、又はこの抽出物を、酵母を用いて発酵処理したものより得られたもの、若しくはタンナーゼにより加水分解処理したものより得られたものである。主成分はプロアントシアニジンである。	酸化防止剤 製造用剤	Grape seed extract
270	ブラジルカンゾウ抽出物 (ブラジルカンゾウの根から得られた、ペリアンドリンを主成分とするものをいう。)	ペリアンドリン	ブラジルカンゾウ	マメ科ブラジルカンゾウ(Periandra dulcis MART.)の根より、水で抽出したものより得られたものである。甘味成分はペリアンドリンである。	甘味料	Brazilian licorice extract
271	フルクトシルトランスフェラーゼ			糸状菌(Aspergillus, Penicillium roqueforti)又は細菌(Arthrobacter, Bacillus)の培養液より、冷時~室温時水で抽出して得られたもの、又は除菌後、冷時~室温時濃縮して得られたものである。	酵素	Fructosyl transferase
272	プルラナーゼ		アミラーゼ カルボヒドラーゼ	細菌(Bacillus, Klebsiella, Sulfolobus solfataricus)の培養液より、冷時~室温時水で抽出して得られたもので、除菌したもの、冷時~室温時濃縮したもの、冷時エタノール、含水エタノール若しくはアセトンで処理して得られたもの、又は硫酸アンモニウム等で分画した後、脱塩処理して得られたものである。	酵素	Pullulanase
273	プルラン			糸状菌(Aureobasidium pullulans)の培養液より、分離して得られた多糖類である。成分はプルランである。	増粘安定剤 製造用剤	Pullulan
274	プロテアーゼ	たん白分解酵素		動物、魚類若しくは甲殻類の筋肉若しくは臓器より、冷時~温時水で抽出して得られたもの、又は糸状菌(Aspergillus melleus, Aspergillus niger, Aspergillus oryzae, Aspergillus saitoi, Aspergillus, sojae, Monascus pilosus, Monascus purpureus, Mucor circinelloides, Mucor javanicus, Mucor miehei, Mucor rouxii, Penicillium citrinum, Peni-	酵素	Protease

番号	品名 名称	品名 別名	簡略名又は類別名	基原・製法・本質	用途	備考
				cillium duponti, Rhizomucor miehei, Rhizopus chinensis, Rhizopus delemar, Rhizopus niveus, Rhizopus oryzae)、担子菌（Pycnoporus coccineus)、放線菌（Streptomyces)、細菌（Bacillus amyloliquefaciens, Bacillus coagulans J4, Bacillus lentus, Bacillus licheniformis, Bacillus polymixa, Bacillus stearothermophilus, Bacillus subtilis, Bacillus thermoproteolyticus, Pseudomonas paucimobilis）若しくは酵母（Saccharomyces）の培養より、冷時～室温時水で抽出して得られたもの、除菌したもの、冷時～室温時濃縮したもの、冷時～室温時樹脂精製して得られたもの、若しくはこれより、冷時エタノール、含水エタノール若しくはアセトンで処理して得られたもの若しくは硫酸アンモニウム等で分画した後、脱塩処理して得られたものである。		
275	プロパン			石油若しくは天然ガス成分中、n-プロパンの沸点付近の留分である。	製造用剤	Propane
276	プロポリス抽出物 （ミツバチの巣から得られた、フラボノイドを主成分とするものをいう。）			ミツバチ科ミツバチ（Apis mellifera LINNE, Apis indica RODOSZKOWSKI）の巣より、エタノールで抽出して得られたものである。主成分はフラボノイドである。	酸化防止剤	Propolis extract
277	ブロメライン	ブロメリン		パイナップル（Ananas comosus Merrill）の果実又は根茎より得られた、たん白質分解酵素である。乳糖又はデキストリンを含むことがある。	酵素	Bromelain
278	L-プロリン		プロリン	タンパク質原料の加水分解により、又は糖類を原料とした発酵により得られたものを、分離して得られたものである。成分はL-プロリンである。	調味料 強化剤	L-Proline
279	分別レシチン （「植物レシチン」又は「卵黄レシチン」から得られた、スフィンゴミエリン、フォスファチジルイノシトール、フォスファチジルエタノールアミン及びフォスファチジルコリンを主成分とするものをいう。）	レシチン分別物 レシチン		「植物レシチン」又は「卵黄レシチン」より、室温時～温時メタノール、エタノール、含水エタノール、イソプロピルアルコール、アセトン、ヘキサン又は酢酸エチルで抽出して得られたものである。主成分は、フォスファチジルコリン、フォスファチジルエタノールアミン、フォスファチジルイノシトール、スフィンゴミエリンである。	乳化剤	Fractionated lecithin Cephalin Lipoinositol
280	粉末セルロース （パルプを分解して得られた、セルロースを主成分とするものをいう。ただし、「微結晶セルロース」を除く。）		セルロース	パルプを分解して得られた、セルロースを主成分とするものである。	製造用剤	Powdered cellulose
281	粉末モミガラ （イネのもみ殻から得られた、セルロースを主成分とするものをいう。）			イネ科イネ（Oryza sativa LINNE）のもみ殻を、微粉砕して得られたものである。主成分はセルロースである。	ガムベース	Powdered rice hulls
282	ペカンナッツ色素 （ピーカンの果皮又は渋皮から得られた、フラボノイドを主成分とするものをいう。）	ピーカンナッツ色素	フラボノイド フラボノイド色素	クルミ科ピーカン（Carya pecan ENGL. et GRAEBN.）の果皮又は渋皮より、熱時水若しくは含水エタノールで抽出して得られたもの又は熱時酸性水溶液で抽出し、中和して得られたものである。主色素はフラボノイドである。褐色を呈する。	着色料	Pecan nut colour
283	ヘキサン			主として n-ヘキサン（C_6H_{14}）を含む。	製造用剤	Hexane
284	ペクチナーゼ		カルボヒドラーゼ	糸状菌（Aspergillus aculeatus, Aspergillus	酵素	Pectinase

番号	品名 名称	品名 別名	簡略名又は類別名	基原・製法・本質	用途	備考
				alliaceus, Aspergillus awamori, Aspergillus japonicus, Aspergillus niger, Aspergillus pulverulentus, Aspergillus usamii, Rhizopus oryzae, Trichoderma)、細菌（Bacillus subtilis)、担子菌（Corticium）若しくは酵母（Trichosporon）の培養液より、冷時～微温時水で抽出して得られたもの、除菌したもの、冷時～室温時濃縮したもの、又は冷時エタノール若しくは含水エタノールで処理して得られたものである。		
285	ペクチン			かんきつ類、リンゴ等から得られた、部分的にメチルエステル化されたポリガラクチュロン酸などの水溶性多糖類を成分とするものである。ショ糖、ブドウ糖、乳糖又はデキストリンを含むことがある。	増粘安定剤	Pectin
286	ペクチン分解物 (「ペクチン」から得られた、ガラクチュロン酸を主成分とするものをいう。)		分解ペクチン	「ペクチン」を、酵素で分解して得られたものである。主成分はガラクチュロン酸である。	保存料	Pectin digests
287	ヘゴ・イチョウ抽出物 (イチョウ及びヘゴの葉から抽出して得られたものをいう。)			ヘゴ科ヘゴ（Cyathea fauriei COPEL.）及びイチョウ科イチョウ（Ginkgo biloba LINNE）の葉を9：1の比率で混合し、熱時水で抽出して得られたものである。	酸化防止剤	Hego-Ginkgo leaf extract
288	ヘスペリジナーゼ			糸状菌（Aspergillus, Penicillium decumbens）の培養液より、冷時～室温時水で抽出し、冷時～室温時濃縮後、冷時エタノールで処理して得られたものである。	酵素	Hesperidinase
289	ヘスペリジン	ビタミンP		柑橘類の果皮、果汁又は種子より、室温時アルカリ性水溶液で抽出して得られたものである。成分はヘスペリジンである。	強化剤	Hesperidin Vitamin P
290	ベタイン			テンサイ（Beta vulgaris Linne）の糖蜜より、分離して得られたものである。成分はベタインである。	調味料	Betaine
291	ベニコウジ黄色素 (ベニコウジカビの培養液から得られた、キサントモナシン類を主成分とするものをいう。)	モナスカス黄色素	紅麹 紅麹色素 モナスカス モナスカス色素	子のう菌類ベニコウジカビ（Monascus purpureus WENT.）の培養液を乾燥し、粉砕したものより、微温時弱塩酸酸性エタノールで抽出し、中和して得られたものである。主色素はキサントモナシン類である。黄色を呈する。	着色料	Monascus yellow
292	ベニコウジ色素 (ベニコウジカビの培養液から得られた、アンカフラビン及びモナスコルブリンを主成分とするものをいう。)	モナスカス色素	紅麹 モナスカス	ベニコウジカビ（Monascus pilosus又はMonascus purpureus）の培養液から得られた、アンカフラビン類及びモナスコルブリン類を主成分とするものである。	着色料	Monascus colour
293	ベニバナ赤色素 (ベニバナの花から得られた、カルタミンを主成分とするものをいう。)	カーサマス赤色素	フラボノイド フラボノイド色素 紅花赤 紅花色素	ベニバナ（Carthamus tinctorius Linne）の花から得られた、カルタミンを主成分とするものである。デキストリン又は乳糖を含むことがある。	着色料	Carthamus red
294	ベニバナ黄色素 (ベニバナの花から得られた、サフラーイエロー類を主成分とするものをいう。)	カーサマス黄色素	フラボノイド フラボノイド色素 紅花黄 紅花色素	ベニバナ（Carthamus tinctorius Linne）の花から得られた、サフラーイエロー類を主成分とするものである。デキストリン又は乳糖を含むことがある。	着色料	Carthamus yellow
295	ベネズエラチクル (ベネズエラチクルの分泌液から得られた、アミリンアセター	カプーレ		アカテツ科ベネズエラチクル（Manilkara williamsii STANDL.）の幹枝より得られるラテックスを、脱水したものより得られたもの	ガムベース	Venezuelan chicle

番号	品名 名称	品名 別名	簡略名又は類別名	基原・製法・本質	用途	備考
	ト及びポリイソプレンを主成分とするものをいう。)			である。主成分はアミリンアセタート及びポリイソプレンである。		
296	ペプシン			動物又は魚類から得られた、たん白質分解酵素である。乳糖又はデキストリンを含むことがある。	酵素	Pepsin
297	ヘプタン			石油成分中、n-ヘプタンの沸点付近の留分である。	製造用剤	Heptane
298	ペプチダーゼ			糸状菌（Aspergillus niger, Aspergillus oryzae, Aspergillus sojae, Rhizopus oryzae）若しくは細菌（Bacillus, Lactococcus lactis）の培養液より、冷時～室温時水で抽出して得られたもの、除菌したもの、若しくはこれより、冷時エタノールで処理して得られたもの、又は培養液を固液分離、濃縮、ろ過して得られたものである。	酵素	Peptidase
299	ヘマトコッカス藻色素 (ヘマトコッカスの全藻から得られた、アスタキサンチンを主成分とするものをいう。)		カロチノイド カロチノイド色素 カロテノイド カロテノイド色素	ヘマトコッカス（Haematococcus spp.）の全藻から得られた、アスタキサンチン類を主成分とするものである。食用油脂を含むことがある。	着色料	Haematococcus algae colour
300	ヘミセルラーゼ	ペントサナーゼ	カルボヒドラーゼ	枯草菌（Bacillus subtilis）、糸状菌（Aspergillus aculeatus, Aspergillus awamori, Aspergillus niger, Aspergillus oryzae, Aspergillus usamii, Humicola insolens, Trichoderma harzianum, Trichoderma koningii, Trichoderma longibrachiatum, Trichoderma viride）若しくは担子菌（Corticium, Pycnoporus coccineus）の培養液より、冷時～微温時水で抽出して得られたもの、除菌したもの、冷時～室温時濃縮したもの、冷時エタノール若しくは含水エタノールで処理して得られたもの、又は培養液を固液分離、濃縮、ろ過して得られたものである。	酵素	Hemicellulase
301	ヘム鉄			ヘモグロビンをタンパク分解酵素で処理したものより、分離して得られたものである。主成分はヘム鉄である。	強化剤	Heme iron
302	ヘリウム			^{2}He	製造用剤	Helium
303	ベントナイト		不溶性鉱物性物質	鉱床より採掘して得られたベントナイトを乾燥して得られたものである。主成分は含水ケイ酸アルミニウムである。	製造用剤	Bentonite
304	ホスホジエステラーゼ			糸状菌（Aspergillus niger, Penicillium citrinum）の培養液より、冷時～室温時水で抽出し、冷時エタノールで処理して得られたものである。	酵素	Phosphodiesterase
305	ホスホリパーゼ	ホスファチダーゼ レシチナーゼ		動物のすい臓若しくはアブラナ科キャベツ（Brassica oleracea LINNE）より、冷時～室温時水で抽出して得られたもの、又は糸状菌（Aspergillus oryzae, Aspergillus niger）、担子菌（Corticium）、放線菌（Actinomadura, Nocardiopsis）若しくは細菌（Bacillus）の培養液より、冷時～室温時水で抽出して得られたもの、除菌したもの、冷時～室温時濃縮したもの、又はこれより含水エタノール若しくは含水アセトンで処理して得られたもの、樹脂精製後、アルカリ性水溶液で処理したものである	酵素	Phospholipase

番号	品名		簡略名又は類別名	基原・製法・本質	用途	備考
	名称	別名				
306	没食子酸			ウルシ科ヌルデ（Rhus javanica LINNE）に発生する五倍子、ブナ科（Quercus infectoria OlIV.）に発生する没食子より、水、エタノール又は有機溶剤で抽出したタンニン、又はマメ科タラ（Caesalpinia spinosa(MOLINA)KUNTZE）の実の莢より、温時水で抽出したタンニンを、アルカリ又は酵素（タンナーゼ）により加水分解して得られたものである。成分は没食子酸である。	酸化防止剤	Gallic acid
307	ホホバロウ （ホホバの果実から得られた、イコセン酸イコセニルを主成分とするものをいう。）	ホホバワックス		ツゲ科ホホバ（Simmondsia californica NUTT.）の果実より採油したホホバ脂より、分離して得られた高融点ロウ物質である。主成分はイコセン酸イコセニルである。	ガムベース	Jojoba wax
308	ポリフェノールオキシダーゼ	フェノラーゼ		糸状菌（Alternaria, Aspergillus niger, Coriolus）若しくは担子菌（Cyathus, Polyporus cinereus, Pycnoporus coccineus, Polyporus versicolor, Trametes）の培養液より、冷時～室温時水で抽出して得られたもの、冷時～室温時濃縮したもの、冷時エタノール、含水エタノール若しくはアセトンで処理して得られたもの、除菌後、冷時含水エタノールで処理して得られたもの、又は硫酸アンモニウム等で分画した後、脱塩処理して得られたものである	酵素	Polyphenol oxidase
309	ε-ポリリシン	ε-ポリリジン	ポリリジン	放線菌（Streptomyces albulus）の培養液より、イオン交換樹脂を用いて吸着、分離して得られたものである。成分はε-ポリリシンである。デキストリンを含むことがある。	保存料	ε-Polylysine
310	マイクロクリスタリンワックス	ミクロクリスタリンワックス		石油の減圧蒸留の残渣油又は重質留出油から得られた固形の炭化水素の混合物で、主として分枝状及び直鎖状の飽和炭化水素からなる。	ガムベース 光沢剤	Microcrystalline wax
311	マクロホモプシスガム （マクロホモプシスの培養液から得られた、多糖類を主成分とするものをいう。）	マクロホモプシス多糖類		マクロホモプシス属菌（Macrophomopsis (Fisicoccum)）の培養液から得られた、多糖類を主成分とするものである。ショ糖、ブドウ糖、乳糖、デキストリン又はマルトースを含むことがある。。	増粘安定剤	Macrophomopsis gum
312	マスチック （ヨウニュウコウの分泌液から得られた、マスチカジエノン酸を主成分とするものをいう。）			ウルシ科ヨウニュウコウ（Pistacia lentiscus LINNE）の分泌液より、低沸点部を蒸留により除去し、熱時エタノールで抽出し、エタノールを留去して得られたものである。主構成成分はマスチカジエノン酸である。	ガムベース	Mastic gum
313	マッサランドバチョコレート （マッサランドバチョコレートの分泌液から得られた、アミリンアセタート及びポリイソプレンを主成分とするものをいう。）			アカテツ科マッサランドバチョコレート（Manilkara solimoesensis GILLY.）の幹枝より得られたラテックスを、熱時水で洗浄し、水溶成分を除去して得られたものである。主成分はアミリンアセタート及びポリイソプレンである。	ガムベース	Massaranduba chocolate
314	マッサランドババラタ （マッサランドババラタの分泌液から得られた、アミリンアセタート及びポリイソプレンを主成分とするものをいう。）			アカテツ科マッサランドババラタ（Manilkara huberi(DUCKE)CHEVAL.）の幹枝より得られたラテックスを、熱時水で洗浄し、水溶成分を除去して得られたものである。主成分はアミリンアセタート及びポリイソプレンである。	ガムベース	Massaranduba balata
315	マリーゴールド色素 （マリーゴールドの花から得ら		カロチノイド カロチノイド色素	マリーゴールド（Tagetes patula Linne若しくはTagetes erecta Linne又はそれらの種間	着色料	Marigold colour

番号	品名 名称	品名 別名	簡略名又は類別名	基原・製法・本質	用途	備考
	れた、キサントフィルを主成分とするものをいう。)		カロテノイド カロテノイド色素 マリーゴールド	雑種)の花から得られた、キサントフィルを主成分とするものである。		
316	マルトースホスホリラーゼ			細菌(Plesiomonas)の培養液の菌体を酵素(リゾチーム)処理した後、冷時～室温時水で抽出して得られたものである	酵素	Maltose phosphorylase
317	マルトトリオヒドロラーゼ	G3生成酵素	アミラーゼ カルボヒドラーゼ	糸状菌(Penicillium)又は細菌(Bacillus subtilis, Microbacterium)の培養液より、冷時～室温時除菌した後、濃縮して得られたものである。	酵素	Maltotriohydrolase
318	未焼成カルシウム (貝殻、真珠の真珠層、造礁サンゴ、骨又は卵殻を乾燥して得られた、カルシウム塩を主成分とするものをいう。)		未焼成Ca		強化剤	Non-calcinated calcium
	貝殻未焼成カルシウム		貝カルシウム 貝Ca	貝殻を、殺菌、乾燥し、粉末にして得られたものである。主成分は炭酸カルシウムである。		Non-calcinated shell calcium
	骨未焼成カルシウム		骨カルシウム 骨Ca	獣骨又は魚骨を、殺菌、乾燥し、粉末にして得られたものである。主成分はリン酸カルシウムである。		Non-calcinated bone calcium
	サンゴ未焼成カルシウム		コーラルカルシウム コーラルCa サンゴカルシウム サンゴCa	イシサンゴ目(Scleractinia)の造礁サンゴを、殺菌、乾燥し、粉末にして得られたものである。主成分は炭酸カルシウムである。		Non-calcinated coral calcium
	真珠層未焼成カルシウム		真珠層カルシウム 真珠層Ca	ウグイスガイ科アコヤガイ(Pinctada fucata)から得られる真珠の核を除いた真珠層を、殺菌、乾燥し、粉末にして得られたものである。主成分は炭酸カルシウムである。		Non-calcinated mother-of-pearl layer calcium
	卵殻未焼成カルシウム		卵殻カルシウム 卵殻Ca	卵殻を、殺菌、乾燥し、粉末にして得られたものである。主成分は炭酸カルシウムである。		Non-calcinated eggshell calcium
319	ミックストコフェロール (植物性油脂から得られた、d-α-トコフェロール、d-β-トコフェロール、d-γ-トコフェロール及びd-δ-トコフェロールを主成分とするものをいう。)	ミックスビタミンE 抽出トコフェロール 抽出ビタミンE	抽出V.E トコフェロール ビタミンE V.E ミックスV.E	植物性油脂から得られた、d-α-トコフェロール、d-β-トコフェロール、d-γ-トコフェロール及びd-δ-トコフェロールを主成分とするものである。食用油脂を含むことがある。	酸化防止剤 強化剤	Mixed tocopherols
320	ミツロウ (ミツバチの巣から得られた、パルミチン酸ミリシルを主成分とするものをいう。)	オウロウ ビースワックス ベースワックス		ミツバチ(Apis spp.)の巣から得られた、パルミチン酸ミリシルを主成分とするものである。	ガムベース 光沢剤	Bees wax
321	ミルラ (ボツヤクの分泌液から抽出して得られたものをいう。)	ミル		カンラン科ボツヤク(Commiphora mukul ENGL.)の分泌液より、低沸点部を蒸留により除去し、室温時エタノールで抽出し、エタノールを留去して得られたものである。成分としてコミホールを含む。	ガムベース	Myrrh
322	ムラサキイモ色素 (サツマイモの塊根から得られた、シアニジンアシルグルコシド及びペオニジンアシルグルコシドを主成分とするものをいう。)		アントシアニン アントシアニン色素 野菜色素	サツマイモ(Ipomoea batatas Poiret)の塊根から得られた、シアニジンアシルグルコシド及びペオニジンアシルグルコシドを主成分とするものである。デキストリン又は乳糖を含むことがある。	着色料	Purple sweet potato colour

番号	品名 名称	品名 別名	簡略名又は類別名	基原・製法・本質	用途	備考
323	ムラサキトウモロコシ色素（トウモロコシの種子から得られた、シアニジン-三-グルコシドを主成分とするものをいう。）	ムラサキコーン色素	アントシアニン アントシアニン色素	トウモロコシ（Zea mays Linne）の種子から得られた、シアニジン3-グルコシドを主成分とするものである。デキストリン又は乳糖を含むことがある。	着色料	Purple corn colour
324	ムラサキヤマイモ色素（ヤマイモの塊根から得られた、シアニジンアシルグルコシドを主成分とするものをいう。）		アントシアニン アントシアニン色素 ムラサキヤマイモ 野菜色素	ヤマノイモ科ヤマイモ（Dioscorea alata LINNE）の紫色の塊根より、室温時水又は弱酸性水溶液で抽出して得られたものである。主色素はシアニジンアシルグルコシドである。紫赤色を呈する。	着色料	Purple yam colour
325	ムラミダーゼ			放線菌（Actinomyces, Streptomyces）又は細菌（Bacillus）の培養液より、冷時～室温時除菌後、冷時～室温時濃縮し、冷時含水エタノールで抽出して得られたものである。	酵素	Muramidase
326	メナキノン（抽出物）（アルトロバクターの培養液から得られた、メナキノン-四を主成分とするものをいう。）	ビタミンK_2(抽出物)	ビタミンK_2 ビタミンK V.K_2 V.K メナキノン	アルトロバクター属菌（Arthrobacter nicotianae）の培養液から得られた、メナキノン-4を主成分とするものである。	強化剤	Menaquinone (extract) Vitamin K_2(extract)
327	メバロン酸			酵母（Saccharomycopsis fibuligera）によるコーンスチープリカー又はカゼイン由来のペプトンを主原料とする発酵培養液より、有機溶剤で抽出して得られたものである。成分はメバロン酸である。	製造用剤	Mevalonic acid
328	メラロイカ精油（メラロイカの葉から得られた、精油を主成分とするものをいう。）			フトモモ科メラロイカ（Melaleuca alternifolia CHEEL）の葉より、水蒸気蒸留により得られたものである。成分は精油（α-テルピネン及びγ-テルピネン等）である。	酸化防止剤	Melaleuca oil
329	モウソウチク乾留物（モウソウチクの茎を乾留して得られたものをいう。）		竹乾留物	イネ科モウソウチク（Phyllostachys heterocycla MITF.）の茎をチップ状にしたものを、減圧加熱下で乾留したものより得られたものである。	製造用剤	Mousouchiku dry distillate
330	モウソウチク抽出物（モウソウチクの茎の表皮から得られた、2,6-ジメトキシ-1,4-ベンゾキノンを主成分とするものをいう。）			イネ科モウソウチク（Phyllostachys heterocycla MITF.）の茎の表皮を、粉砕したものより、微温時エタノールで抽出して得られたものである。成分として2,6-ジメトキシ-1,4-ベンゾキノンを含む。	製造用剤	Mousouchiku extract
331	木材チップ（ハシバミ又はブナの幹枝を粉砕して得られたものをいう。）	シュペーネ		カバノキ科ハシバミ（Corylus heterophylla FISCHER var.thunberglii BLUME）又はブナ科ブナ（Fagus crenata BLUME）の幹枝を熱水殺菌したものを、粉砕して得られたものである。	製造用剤	Wood chip
332	木炭（竹材又は木材を炭化して得られたものをいう。）			イネ科マダケ（Phyllostachys bambusoides SIEB. et ZUCC.）若しくはイネ科モウソウチク（Phyllostachys heterocycla MITF.）の茎又はカバノキ科シラカバ（Betula platyphylla SUKAT. var. japonica HARA）、チョウセンマツ（Pinus koraiensis SIEB. et ZUCC.）、ブナ科ウバメガシ（Quercus phylliraeoides）等の幹枝又は種子を、炭化して得られたものである。	製造用剤	Charcoal
333	モクロウ（ハゼノキの果実から得られた、グリセリンパルミタートを主成分とするものをいう。）	日本ロウ ハゼ脂	植物ワックス	キクウルシ科ハゼノキ（Rhus succedanea LINNE）の果実より、融解、さらしたものより得られたものである。主成分はグリセリンパルミタートである。	カムベース	Japan wax
334	木灰			ブナ科ブナ（Fagus crenata BLUME）等の	製造用剤	Timber ash

番号	品名		簡略名又は類別名	基原・製法・本質	用途	備考
	名称	別名				
	(竹材又は木材を灰化して得られたものをいう。)			幹枝を、灰化して得られたものである。		
335	木灰抽出物 (「木灰」から抽出して得られたものをいう。)			ブナ科ブナ (Fagus crenata BLUME)、クスノキ科クスノキ (Cinnamomum Camphora SIEB.) 等の幹枝を灰化して得られた灰化物を、精製して得られたものである。	製造用剤	Timber ash extract
336	モモ樹脂 (モモの分泌液から得られた、多糖類を主成分とするものをいう。)		ピーチガム	バラ科モモ (Prunus persica BATSCH) の幹枝の樹脂成分を、分離して得られたものである。主成分は多糖類である。	増粘安定剤	Peach gum
337	ヤマモモ抽出物 (ヤマモモの果実、樹皮又は葉から抽出して得られたものをいう。)			ヤマモモ (Myrica rubra Siebold et Zuccarini) の果実、樹皮又は葉から抽出して得られたものである。主成分はミリシトリンである。	酸化防止剤	Chinese bayberry extract
338	ユッカフォーム抽出物 (ユッカアラボレセンス又はユッカシジゲラの全草から得られた、サポニンを主成分とするものをいう。)	ユッカ抽出物	ユッカフォーム ユッカ・フォーム	ユッカ・ブレビフォリア (Yucca brevifolia Engelmann) 又はユッカ・シジゲラ (Yucca schidigera Roezl ex Ortgies) の全草から得られた、サポニンを主成分とするものである。	乳化剤 製造用剤	Yucca foam extract Yucca joshua tree
339	ラカンカ抽出物 (ラカンカの果実から得られた、モグロシド類を主成分とするものをいう。)	ラカンカエキス	ラカンカ	ラカンカ (Siraitia grosevenorii C. Jeffrey ex A. M. Lu & Zhi Y. Zhang (Momordica grosvenori Swingle)) の果実から得られた、モグロシド類を主成分とするものである。	甘味料	Rakanka extract
340	ラクトパーオキシダーゼ			脱脂生乳又は乳清より、イオン交換樹脂で分離して得られたものである。	酵素	Lactoperoxidase
341	ラクトフェリン濃縮物 (ほ乳類の乳から得られた、ラクトフェリンを主成分とするものをいう。)		ラクトフェリン	ほ乳類の乳を脱脂分離したもの又は乳清より、精製し、濃縮して得られたものである。主成分は、ラクトフェリンである。	製造用剤	Lactoferrin concentrates
342	ラック色素 (ラックカイガラムシの分泌液から得られた、ラッカイン酸類を主成分とするものをいう。)	ラッカイン酸	ラック	ラックカイガラムシ (Laccifer spp.) の分泌液から得られた、ラッカイン酸類を主成分とするものである。	着色料	Lac colour
343	ラノリン (ヒツジの毛に付着するろう様物質から得られた、高級アルコールと α-ヒドロキシ酸のエステルを主成分とするものをいう。)	羊毛ロウ		ヒツジの毛に付着するろう様物質から得られた、高級アルコールと α-ヒドロキシ酸のエステルを主成分とするものである。	ガムベース 光沢剤	Lanolin
344	ラムザンガム (アルカリゲネスの培養液から得られた、多糖類を主成分とするものをいう。)	ラムザン多糖類	ラムザン	スフィンゴモナス属菌 (Sphingomonas sp.) の培養液から得られた、多糖類を主成分とするものである。ショ糖、ブドウ糖、乳糖、デキストリン又はマルトースを含むことがある。	増粘安定剤	Rhamsan gum
345	L-ラムノース		ラムノース	「ルチン (抽出物)」又はミカン科アマダイダイ (Citrus sinensis OSBECK) 若しくはミカン科ウンシュウミカン (Citrus unshiu MARCOV.) の果皮、樹皮若しくは花に含まれる配糖体、又は大豆油、菜種油若しくはコーン油を発酵、濃縮分離して得られたものを、加水分解し、分離して得られたものである。成分はL-ラムノースである。	甘味料	L-Rhamnose
346	卵黄レシチン (卵黄から得られた、レシチンを主成分とするものをいう。)	レシチン		卵黄より得られた卵黄油より、分離して得られたものである。主成分はレシチンである。	乳化剤	Yolk lecithin

番号	品名 名称	品名 別名	簡略名又は類別名	基原・製法・本質	用途	備考
347	L-リシン	L-リジン	リシン リジン	糖類を原料とした発酵により得られたものを、分離して得られたものである。成分はL-リシンである。	調味料 強化剤	L-Lysine
348	リゾチーム	卵白リゾチーム		卵白より、アルカリ性水溶液及び食塩水で処理し、樹脂精製して得られたもの、又は樹脂処理若しくは加塩処理した後、カラム精製若しくは再結晶により得られたもので、細菌の細胞壁物質を溶解する酵素である。	酵素	Lysozyme
349	リパーゼ	脂肪分解酵素	エステラーゼ	動物若しくは魚類の臓器、又は動物の舌下部より、冷時～微温時水で抽出して得られたもの又は糸状菌（Aspergillus awamori, Aspergillus niger, Aspergillus oryzae, Aspergillus phoenicis, Aspergillus usamii, Geotrichum candidum, Humicola, Mucor javanicus, Mucor miehei, Penicillium camembertii, Penicillium chrysogenum, Penicillum roquefortii, Rhizomucor miehei, Rhizopus delemar, Rhizopus japonicus, Rhizopus miehei, Rhizopus niveus, Rhizopus oryzae）、放線菌（Streptomyces）、細菌（Alcaligenes, Arthrobactor, Chromobacterium viscosum, Pseudomonas, Serratia marcescens）又は酵母（Candida）の培養液より、冷時～微温時水で抽出して得られたもの、除菌したもの、冷時～室温時濃縮したもの、又はエタノール、、含水エタノール若しくはアセトンで処理して得られたものである。	酵素	Lipase
350	リポキシゲナーゼ	リポキシダーゼ		植物油粕より、又は糸状菌（Rhizopus）の培養液より、水で抽出して得られたものである。	酵素	Lipoxygenase
351	D-リボース		リボース	グラム陽性細菌（Bacillus pumilus又はBacillus subtilis）によるD-グルコースの発酵培養液より、分離して得られたものである。成分はD-リボースである。	甘味料	D-Ribose
352	流動パラフィン	ミネラルオイルホワイト	パラフィン	石油から得た炭化水素類の混合物である。	製造用剤	Liquid paraffin
353	リンターセルロース （ワタの単毛から得られた、セルロースを主成分とするものをいう。）		セルロース	アオイ科ワタ（Gossypium hirsutum LINNE）の実の単毛を、精製して得られたものである。主成分はセルロースである。	製造用剤	Linter cellulose
354	ルチン酵素分解物 （「ルチン（抽出物）」から得られた、イソクエルシトリンを主成分とするものをいう。）		イソクエルシトリン	ルチン（抽出物）（アズキ（Vigna angularis Ohwi et H. Ohashi）の全草、エンジュ（Sophora japonica Linne）のつぼみ若しくは花又はソバ（Fagopyrum esculentum Moench）の全草から得られた、ルチンを主成分とするものをいう。）を酵素処理した後、精製して得られたものである。主成分はイソクエルシトリンである。	酸化防止剤	Enzymatically decomposed rutin
355	ルチン（抽出物） （アズキの全草、エンジュのつぼみ若しくは花又はソバの全草から得られた、ルチンを主成分とするものをいう。）		フラボノイド ルチン		酸化防止剤 着色料	Rutin(extract)
	エンジュ抽出物			ルチン（抽出物）のうちエンジュ（Sophora japonica Linne）のつぼみ又は花より、水、エタノール又はメタノールで抽出し、溶媒を		Enju extract Japanese pagoda tree extract

番号	品名 名称	別名	簡略名又は類別名	基原・製法・本質	用途	備考
				除去して得られたものである。主成分はルチンである。		
	アズキ全草抽出物			マメ科アズキ（Azukia angularis OHWI）の全草より、水又はエタノールで抽出して得られたものである。主成分はルチンである。		Azuki extract
	ソバ全草抽出物			タデ科ソバ（Fagopyrum esculentum MOENCH）の全草より、水又はエタノールで抽出して得られたものである。主成分はルチンである。		Buckwheat extract
356	ルテニウム			^{96}Ru, ^{98}Ru, ^{99}Ru, ^{100}Ru, ^{101}Ru, ^{102}Ru, ^{104}Ru	製造用剤	Ruthenium
357	レイシ抽出物（マンネンタケの菌糸体若しくは子実体又はその培養液から抽出して得られたものをいう。）	マンネンタケ抽出物	レイシ	サルノコシカケ目マンネンタケ（Ganoderma lucidum KARST.）の菌糸体若しくは子実体、又はその培養液より、水、エタノール又は二酸化炭素で抽出して得られたものである。	苦味料等	Mannentake extract
358	レッチュデバカ（レッチュデバカの分泌液から得られた、アミリンエステルを主成分とするものをいう。）			クワ科レッチュデバカ（Brosimum utile (H.B.K)PITT.）の幹枝から得られたラテックスを、熱時水で洗浄し、水溶成分を除去して得られたものである。主成分はアミリンエステルである。	ガムベース	Leche de vaca
359	レバン（枯草菌の培養液から得られた、多糖類を主成分とするものをいう。）	フラクタン		枯草菌（Bacillus subtilis(EHR.)COHN）によるショ糖又はラフィノースの発酵培養液より、分離して得られたものである。主成分は多糖類である。	増粘安定剤	Levan
360	レンネット	キモシン レンニン		反すう動物の第四胃より、室温時～微温時水若しくは酸性水溶液で抽出して得られたもの、又は酵母菌（Kluyveromyces lactis）、糸状菌（Mucor miehei, Mucor pusillus LINDT, Mucor spp., Rhizomucor miehei）、担子菌（Irpex lacteus）若しくは細菌（Bacillus cereus, Crypnohectria parasitica, Escherichia coli K-12等）の培養液より、室温時～微温時水若しくは酸性水溶液で抽出して得られたもの、室温時濃縮したもの、又は、冷時エタノール若しくは含水エタノールで処理して得られたものである。	酵素	Rennet
361	L-ロイシン		ロイシン	動物性若しくは植物性タンパク質の加水分解により、又は糖類を原料とした発酵法により得られたものより、分離して得られたものである。成分はL-ロイシンである。	調味料 強化剤	L-Leucine
362	ログウッド色素（ログウッドの心材から得られた、ヘマトキシリンを主成分とするものをいう。）			マメ科ログウッド（Haematoxylon campechianum）の心材より、熱時水で抽出して得られたものである。主色素はヘマトキシリンである。黒褐色を呈する。	着色料	Logwood colour
363	ロシディンハ（ロシディンハの分泌液から得られた、アミリンアセタート及びポリイソプレンを主成分とするものをいう。）	ロジディンハ		アカテツ科シデロキシロン属（Sideroxylon）の幹枝より得られたラテックスを、脱水したものより得られたものである。主成分はアミリンアセタート及びポリイソプレンである。	ガムベース	Rosidinha
364	ロシン（マツの分泌液から得られた、アビエチン酸を主成分とするものをいう。）	ロジン		マツ科マツ（Pinus palustris MILL.）の樹皮の分泌液より、低沸点部を蒸留により除去して得られたものである。主構成成分はアビエチン酸である。	ガムベース	Rosin
365	ローズマリー抽出物（マンネンロウの葉又は花から得られた、カルノシン酸、カル	マンネンロウ抽出物		シソ科マンネンロウ（Rosmarinus officinalis LINNE）の葉又は花より、二酸化炭素、温時～熱時含水エタノール若しくはエタノール	酸化防止剤	Rosemary extract

番号	品名 名称	品名 別名	簡略名又は類別名	基原・製法・本質	用途	備考
	ノソール及びロスマノールを主成分とするものをいう。)			で抽出して得られたもの、又は温時～熱時ヘキサン、メタノール若しくは含水メタノールで抽出し、溶媒を除去して得られたものである。有効成分は、フェノール性ジテルペノイド（ロスマノール、カルノソール及びカルノシン酸等）である。		

添付資料 2
天然香料基原物質リスト

Appendix 2
List of plant or animal sources of natural flavorings

天然香料基原物質リスト

基原物質名	別　名	備　考
アイスランドモス	アイスランド苔	Iceland moss
アカヤジオウ		Akayajio
アケビ		Akebia
アサ	麻	Hemp
アサフェチダ		Asafetida
アジアンタム		Maidenhair fern
アジョワン		Ajowan
アズキ	小豆	Red beans
アスパラサスリネアリス	ルイボス、ロオイボス	Rooibos
アップルミント		Apple mint
アーティチョーク	チョウセンアザミ	Artichoke
アニス		Anise
アボカド		Avocado
アマ		Flax
アマチャ	甘茶	Amacha
アマチャヅル		Amachazuru
アミガサユリ		Amigasayuri
アミリス		Amyris
アーモンド		Almond
アリタソウ		Aritaso
アルカンナ		Alkanet
アルテミシア		Artemisia
アルニカ		Arnica
アルファルファ		Alfalfa
アロエ		Aloe
アロニア		Chokeberry
アンゴスツラ		Angostura
アンゴラウィード		Angola weed
アンズ	アプリコット	Apricot
アンズタケ		Anzutake, Chanterelle
アンゼリカ	アンゲリカ	Angelica
アンバー		Amber
アンバーグリス	竜涎香	Ambergris
アンブレット		Ambrette
イカ		Squid
イカリソウ		Ikariso
イグサ		Rush
イースト	酵母	Yeasts
イタドリ		Itadori

基原物質名	別　名	備　考
イチゴ	ストロベリー	Strawberry
イチゴノキ	ストロベリーツリー	Strawberry tree
イチジク	フィグ	Fig
イチョウ		Ginkgo, Gingko
イヌゴマ	ベトニー	Betony
イノコヅチ		Inokozuchi
イランイラン		Ylang-ylang
イワオウギ		Iwaohgi
インペラトリア		Imperatoria
インモルテル		Immortelle, Everlasting flower
ウィンターグリーン		Wintergreen
ウォータークレス	オランダガラシ	Water cress
ウコギ		Ukogi
ウコン	ターメリック	Turmeric
ウスバサイシン		Usubasaishin
ウッドラフ	クルマバソウ	Woodruff
ウニ		Sea urchin
ウメ		Ume, Japanese apricot
ウーロンチャ		Oolong tea
エゴマ		Egoma
エノキダケ		Enokidake
エビ		Lobster, Prawn, Shrimp
エビスグサ		Ebisugusa
エリゲロン		Erigeron
エルダー	セイヨウニワトコ	Elder
エレウテロコック		Eleutherococcus
エレカンペン		Elecampane
エレミ		Elemi
エンゴサク		Engosaku
エンジュ		Enju, Japanese-pagoda-tree
エンダイブ	キクヂシャ	Endive
欧州アザミ		Blessed thistle
オウレン		Goldthread
オオアザミ		Milk thistle
オオバコ	プランテン	Plantain
オカゼリ		Cnidium fruit
オキアミ		Krill
オーク		Oak
オークモス		Oak moss

基原物質名	別　名	備　考
オケラ		Okera
オスマンサス	モクセイ	Osmanthus
オポポナックス		Opoponax
オミナエシ		Ominaeshi
オモダカ		Sagiomodaka
オランダセンニチ		Para cress
オリガナム		Origanum
オリス		Orris
オリバナム	乳香	Olibanum
オリーブ		Olive
オールスパイン		Allspice
オレンジ		Orange
オレンジフラワー		Orange flower
カイ	貝	Shellfish
海藻	シーウィード	Seaweed
カイニンソウ		Kaininso
カカオ	ココア	Cacao
カキ	柿	Japanese persimmon
カサイ	果菜	Fruit vegetables
カシューナッツ		Cashew nut
カスカラ		Cascara
カスカリラ		Cascarilla
カストリウム	海狸香	Castoreum
カタクリ		Katakuri
カツオブシ		Dried bonito
カッシー		Cassie
カッシャフィスチュラ		Purging cassia
カテキュ		Catechu
カニ		Crab
カーネーション		Carnation
カノコソウ		Valerian
カモミル		Camomile
カヤプテ		Cajeput, Cajuput
カラクサケマン		Fumitory
カラシ	マスタード	Mustard
カラスウリ		Karasuuri
カラスビシャク		Karasubishaku, Dragon root
カラバッシュナツメグ		Calabash nutmeg
ガラナ		Guarana

基原物質名	別　名	備　考
カラマンシー	シキキツ	Calamondin
カラミント		Calamint
カラムス		Calamus
ガランガ		Galanga
カーラント		Currant
カリッサ		Carissa, Karanda
カリン		Chinese quince
カルダモン	ショウズク	Cardamon
ガルバナム		Galbanum
カレー		Curry powder
カレーリーフ	カリーリーフ	Curry leaf
カワミドリ		Kawamidori
カンゾウ	リコリス	Licorice
ガンビア		Gambir
カンラン		Chinese olive
キウィーフルーツ		Kiwifruit
キカイガラタケ		Kikaigaratake
キキョウ		Kikyo, Baloon flower
キク		Chrysanthemum
キクラゲ		Kikurage, Jew's-ear
キササゲ		Kisasage
ギシギシ		Gishigishi, Dock
キダチアロエ		Kidachi aloe
キナ		Cinchona
キハダ		Kihada
キバナオウギ		Kibanaohgi
ギボウシ		Giboshi
ギムネマシルベスタ		Gymnema sylvestre
キャットニップ	イヌハッカ	Catnip
キャラウェイ	ヒメウイキョウ	Caraway
キャロブ	イナゴマメ、カロブ	Carob, Locust bean
キュウリ	キューカンバー	Cucumber
キラヤ		Quillaja, Quillaia
キンミズヒキ		Agrimony
グァバ		Guava
グァヤク		Guaiacum
クコ		Kuko
クサスギカズラ		Kusasugikazura
クサボケ	シドミ	Kusaboke, Dwarf Japanese quince

基原物質名	別　名	備　考
クズ		Kuzu, Thunberg kudzu vine
クスノキ		Camphor tree
クスノハガシワ		Kamala
グーズベリー		Gooseberry
クチナシ	ガーデニア	Gardenia
クベバ		Cubeb
クマコケモモ		Bearberry
グミ		Gumi, Oleaster
クミン		Cumin
グラウンドアイビー	カキドウシ	Ground ivy
クララ	クサエンジュ	Kurara
クラリセージ		Clary sage
クランベリー		Cranberry
クリ	チェスナッツ	Chestnut
クルミ	ウォルナッツ	Walnut
クリーム		Cream
グレインオブパラダイス		Grains of paradise
クレタディタニー		Dittany of Crete
グレープフルーツ		Grapefruit
クローバー		Clover
クローブ		Clove
クロモジ		Kuromoji
クロレラ		Chlorella
クワ	マルベリー	Mulberry
クワッシャ	ニガキ	Quassia
ケイパー	ケーパー	Caper
ゲットウ	月桃	Getto
ケード		Cade
ケブラコ		Quebracho
ゲルマンダー		Germander
ケンチュール		Kencur
ケンポナシ		Kenponashi, Japanese raisin tree
ゲンノショウコ	フウロソウ	Gennoshoko
コウジ		Koji
コウタケ		Koutake
コウチャ	紅茶	Black tea
コウホネ		Kohone
コカ		Coca
コガネバナ		Koganebana

基原物質名	別　名	備　考
コクトウ	黒糖	Brown sugar
コクルイ	穀類	Cereals
ココナッツ	ココヤシ	Coconut
ココメグサ	アイブライト	Eyebright
ゴシュユ		Goshuyu
コショウ	ペパー	Pepper
コスタス		Costus
コストマリー		Costmary
コパイバ		Copaiba
コーヒー		Coffee
コブシ	ヤマモクレン	Kobushi
ゴボウ		Burdock
ゴマ	セサミ	Sesame
コーラ		Cola
コリアンダー	コエンドロ	Coriander
コルツフート	フキタンポポ	Coltsfoot
ゴールデンロッド		Golden rod
コロンボ		Colombo
コンサイ	根菜	Root and tuber vegetables
コンズランゴ		Kondurango
コンブ		Kombu kelp
コンフリー		Comfrey
サイプレス	イトスギ、シプレス	Cypress
魚	フィッシュ	Fish
サクラ		Cherry tree
サクランボ	チェリー	Cherry
ザクロ	グレナディン	Common pomegranate
サケカス	酒粕	Pressed sake cake
ササ		Sasa, Bamboo grass
ササクサ		Sasakusa
サーチ		Sea buckthorn
サッサフラス		Sassafras
サフラン		Saffron
サポジラ		Sapodilla
サボテン		Cactus
サラシナショウマ		Sarashinashoma
サルサパリラ		Sarsaparilla
サルシファイ	セイヨウゴボウ	Salsify
サルノコシカケ		Sarunokoshikake

基原物質名	別　名	備　考
サンザシ	ホウソーン	Hawthorn
サンシュユ		Sanshuyu
サンショウ		Japanese pepper
サンタハーブ		Santa herb
サンダラック		Sandarac
サンダルウッド	ビャクダン	Sandalwood
サンダルレッド	シタン	Red sandalwood
シイタケ		Shiitake
ジェネ	エニシダ	Genet
シソ		Perilla
シダー	セダー	Cedar
シトラス	カンキツ	Citrus
シトロネラ		Citronella
シヌス		Schinus molle
シベット	霊猫香	Civet
シマルーバ		Simarouba
シメジ		Shimeji
シャクヤク		Shakuyaku, Chinese peony
ジャスミン		Jasmin
ジャノヒゲ		Janohige
ジャボランジ	ヤボランジ	Jaborandi
シャロット		Shallot
シュクシャ		Shukusha
ジュウニヒトエ	ビューグル	Bugle
ジュニパーベリー	ネズ	Juniper berry
ショウガ	ジンジャー	Ginger
ショウユ		Soy sauce
ショウユカス		Pressed soy sauce cake
ジョウリュウシュ	蒸留酒	Spirits
ショウロ		Shoro
シルバーウィード		Silver weed
シロタモギタケ	ブナシメジ	Elm-mushroom
ジンセン	高麗ニンジン	Ginseng
シンナモン		Cinnamon
酢	ビネガー	Vinegar
スイカ	ウォーターメロン	Watermelon
スイセン	ナルシス	Narcissus
スギ		Sugi, Peacock pine
スターアニス	ダイウイキョウ	Star anise

基原物質名	別　名	備　考
スターフルーツ	キャランボラ	Starfruit, Carambora
スチラックス		Styrax
スッポン		Suppon, Snapping turtle
スッポンタケ		Suppontake
ズドラベッツ		Zdravetz
スネークルート		Snakeroot, Serpentary
スパイクナード		Spikenard
スピンネル		Spignel
スプルース	ヘムロック	Spruce
スペアミント	ミドリハッカ	Spearmint
スベリヒユ		Suberihiyu, Pigweed
スローベリー		Sloe berry
セイボリー	キダチハッカ	Savory
セイヨウダイコンソウ		Avens, Herb bennet
セイヨウナナカマド		Rowan tree, European mountain ash
セキショウ		Sekisho
セージ		Sage
ゼドアリー		Zedoary
セネガ		Senega
ゼラニウム		Geranium
セロリー		Celery
センキュウ		Senkyu
センタウリア		Centaury
センダン		Sendan
セントジョーンズウォルト	セイヨウオトギリソウ	St.John's wort
センナ		Senna
ソース		Sauces
ダイオウ	ルバーブ	Rhubarb
ダイズ	大豆	Soybeans
タイム	タチジャコウソウ	Thyme
タケノコ		Bamboo shoot
タコ		Octopus
タデ		Tade, Water pepper
ダバナ		Davana
タマゴ	エッグ	Egg
タマゴタケ		Royal agaric
タマネギ	オニオン	Onion
タマリンド		Tamarind
ダミアナ		Damiana

基原物質名	別　名	備　考
タモギタケ	ヒメヒラタケ	Tamogitake
タラゴン	エストラゴン	Tarragon
タラノキ		Tara, Angelica tree
タンジー	ヨモギギク	Tansy
タンジェリン	マンダリン	Tangerine, Mandarin
タンポポ	ダンデリオン	Dandelion
チェリモラ	チェリモヤ	Cherimoya
チェリーローレル		Cherry laurel
チェリーワイルド		Wild cherry
チガヤ		Chigaya
チコリ		Chicory
チーズ		Cheese
チチタケ		Chichitake
チャイブ		Chive
チャービル		Chervil
チャンパカ		Champac
チュベローズ	月下香	Tuberose
チョウセンゴミシ		Chosengomishi
チラータ		Chirata
ツクシ		Tsukushi, Fern-ally
ツケモノ	漬物	Pickled products
ツタ		Ivy
ツバキ	カメリア	Camellia
ツユクサ		Tsuyukusa
ツリガネニンジン		Tsuriganeninjin
ツルドクダミ		Tsurudokudami
ディアタング	リアトリス	Deertongue
ティスル	キバナアザミ	Thistle
ディタニー		Dittany
ディル	イノンド	Dill
デーツ	ナツメヤシ	Date palm
テンダイウヤク		Lindera root
テンマ		Tenma
テンリョウチャ		Tenryocha
トウガラシ	カプシカム	Capsicum
トウキ		Toki
ドウショクブツタンパクシツ	動植物蛋白質	Proteins
ドウショクブツユシ	動植物油脂	Oil and fats
トウミツ	糖蜜、モラセス	Molasses

基原物質名	別　名	備　考
トウモロコシ	コーン	Maize
ドクダミ		Dokudami
トチュウ		Tochu
ドッググラス		Dog grass, Couch grass
トマト		Tomato
ドラゴンブラッド		Doragon's blood
ドリアン		Durian
トリュフ		Truffle
トルーバルサム		Tolu balsam
トンカ	トンコ	Tonka beans
ナギナタコウジュ		Naginatakoju
ナシ	ペア	Pear
ナスターシャム		Common nasturtium
ナッツ		Nut
ナットウ	納豆	Natto
ナツメ		Jujube
ナツメグ	ニクヅク、メース	Nutmeg, Mace
ナデシコ		Nadeshiko
ナメコ		Nameko
ナラタケ		Naratake
ナンテン		Nanten
ニアウリ		Ti-tree
ニュウサンキンバイヨウエキ	乳酸菌培養液	Cultured lactic acid bacteria solution
ニレ	エルム	Elm
ニンジン	キャロット	Carrot
ニンニク	ガーリック	Garlic
ネズミモチ		Nezumimochi
ネットル	イラクサ	Nettle
ネムノキ		Nemunoki, Silk tree
ノットグラス	ニワヤナギ	Knotgrass
ノリ	海苔	Nori, Laver
バイオレット	スミレ	Violet
パイナップル		Pineapple
ハイビスカス	ローゼル	Hibiscus. Roselle
麦芽	モルト	Malt
ハコベ		Hakobe, Common chickweed
バシクルモン		Basikurumon
バジル	メボウキ	Basil
ハス		Lotus

基原物質名	別　名	備　考
ハスカップ		Hasukappu
パースニップ	アメリカボウフウ	Parsnip
パセリ	オランダゼリ	Parsley
バター		Butter
バターオイル		Butter oil
バターミルク		Butter milk
バーチ	カバノキ	Birch
ハチミツ	ハネー	Honey
パチュリー	パチョリ	Patchouli
ハッカ		Corn-mint, Japanese mint
バックビーン		Buckbeans
ハッコウシュ	発酵酒	Fermented alcoholic beverages
ハッコウニュウ	発酵乳	Fermented milk
ハッコウミエキ	発酵味液	Fermented seasoning solution
パッションフルーツ	クダモノトケイソウ	Passion fruit
ハツタケ		Hatsutake
バッファローベリー		Buffaloberry
ハトムギ		Job's tears
ハナスゲ		Hanasuge
バナナ		Banana
バニラ	ワニラ	Vanilla
ハネーサックル	スイカズラ	Honeysuckle
パパイヤ		Papaya
バーベリー	メギ	Barberry
ハマゴウ		Hamago
ハマスゲ		Hamasuge
ハマナス		Hamanasu, Rugosa rose
ハマボウフウ		Hamabofu
ハマメリス		Winter bloom
バラ	ローズ	Rose
パルマローザ		Palmarosa
パンダナ		Pandanus
バンレイシ	シャカトウ	Sugar apple, Sweet sop
ヒキオコシ		Hikiokoshi
ヒシ		Hishi, Water chestnut
ピスタチオ		Pistachio
ヒソップ	ヤナギハッカ	Hyssop
ヒッコリー		Hickory
ピーナッツ	ラッカセイ	Peanut

基原物質名	別　名	備　考
ヒノキ		Hinoki
ヒバ		Hiba
ピプシシワ		Common popsissewa
ヒマワリ		Sunflower
ヒメハギ		Himehagi
ヒヤシンス		Hyacinth
ヒヨドリバナ		Eupatorium
ヒラタケ		Hiratake
ビワ		Biwa, Loquat
ピンピネラ		Burnet
ビンロウ		Areca nut, Betel nut
フェイジョア		Feijoa, Pineapple guava
フェネグリーク	コロハ	Fenugreek
フェンネル	ショウウイキョウ	Fennel
フジバカマ		Fujibakama
フジモドキ		Fujimodoki
フスマ		Bran
フーゼル油		Fusel oil
プチグレイン		Petitgrain
ブチュ	ブッコ	Buchu
ブドウ	グレープ	Grape
ブドウサケカス	ブドウ酒粕	Wine lees
フトモモ		Rose apple
ブナ		Beech
ブナハリタケ		Bunaharitake
ブラックキャラウェイ	ニジェラ	Black caraway, Nigella
ブラックベリー		Blackberry
プラム	スモモ	Plum
ブリオニア		Bryonia
プリックリーアッシュ	アメリカサンショウ	Prickly ash
プリムローズ	サクラソウ	Primrose
プルネラ	ウツボグサ	Prunella, Self-heal
ブルーベリー		Blueberry
ブレッドフルーツ	パンノキ	Breadfruit
ヘイ		Hay
ベイ		Bay
ヘーゼルナッツ	ハシバミ	Hazelnut
ヘザー	ヒース	Heather
ベチバー	ベチベルソウ	Vetiver

基原物質名	別　名	備　考
ベーテル	キンマ	Betel
ベニノキ		Annatto
ベニバナ	サフラワー	Safflower
ペニーロイヤル	メグサハッカ	Pennyroyal
ペパーミント	セイヨウハッカ	Peppermint
ヘビ		Snake
ペピーノ		Pepino
ペプトン		Peptone
ペリトリー		Pellitory
ベルガモット		Bergamot
ベルガモットミント		Bergamot mint
ペルーバルサム		Peru balsam
ベルベナ	バーベナ、ベルベイン	Verbena, Vervain
ベロニカ		Veronica
ベンゾイン	安息香	Benzoin
ヘンナ		Henna
ボアドローズ	ローズウッド	Rosewood
ホアハウンド	ニガハッカ	Hoarhound
ホウ		Haw
ホウキタケ		Houkitake
ホウショウ	芳樟	Houshou
ボウフウ		Saposhinikovia root
ホエイ		Whey
ホオノキ		Honoki
ホースミント	ヤグルマハッカ	Horsemint
ホースラディッシュ	セイヨウワサビ、ワサビダイコン	Horseradish
ボタン		Moutan bark
ホップ		Hop
ポピー		Poppy
ポプラ		Poplar
ポポー		Papaw
ホホバ		Jojoba
ホヤ		Sea squirt
ボルドー		Boldo
ボロニア		Boronia
マイタケ		Maitake
マグウォルト		Mugwort
マシュマロー	ウスベニタチアオイ	Marshmallow
マジョラム	マヨラナ	Marjoram

基原物質名	別　名	備　考
マスティック		Mastic
マソイ		Massoi
マタタビ		Matatabi, Silver vine
マチコ		Matico
マツ	パイン	Pine
マツオウジ		Matsuoji
マッシュルーム		Mushroom
マツタケ		Matsutake
マツブサ		Matusbusa
マツホド		Matsuhodo
マテチャ	マテ	Mate tea
マメ		Beans
マリーゴールド		Marigold
マルバダイオウ	食用ダイオウ	Garden rhubarb, Edible rhubarb
マルメロ	クインス	Quince
マレイン		Mullein
マロー	ゼニアオイ	Mallow
マンゴー		Mango
マンゴスチン		Mangosteen
マンナノキ		Manna ash
ミカン		Mikan
ミシマサイコ		Mishimasaiko
ミソ	味噌	Miso, Soybean paste
ミツマタ		Mitsumata
ミツロウ	オウロウ、ビースワックス、ベースワックス	Bees wax
ミート	肉	Meat
ミモザ		Mimosa
ミョウガ		Myoga
ミルク		Milk
ミルテ		Myrtle
ミルフォイル	セイヨウノコギリソウ	Milfoil
ミルラ	没薬	Myrrh
ミロバラン		Myrobalan
ムカゴニンジン	スキレット	Skirret
ムギチャ	ムギ茶	Roasted barley
ムスク		Musk
ムラサキ		Murasaki, Gromwell
メスキート		Mesquite
メドウスィート	シモツケソウ	Meadowsweet

基原物質名	別　名	備　考
メハジキ		Mehajiki
メープル	サトウカエデ	Maple
メリッサ	バーム	Melissa, Balm
メリロット		Melilot
メロン		Melon
モウセンゴケ		Sundew
モニリアバイヨウエキ	モニリア培養液	Cultured Moniliaceae solution
モミノキ	ファー	Fir
モモ	ピーチ	Peach
モロヘイヤ		Jew's mallow
ヤクチ		Yakuchi
ヤドリギ		Mistletoe
ヤマブシタケ		Yamabushi take
ヤマモモ		Chinese bayberry
ユーカリ		Eucalyptus
ユキノシタ		Yukinoshita
ユズ		Yuzu
ユッカ		Yucca
ユリ	リリー	Lily
ヨウサイ	葉菜	Leaf vegetables
ヨロイザク		Yoroigusa
ライオンズフート		Lion's foot
ライチ		Litchi
ライフエバーラスティングフラワー		Life-everlasting flower
ライム		Lime
ライラック	リラ	Lilac
ラカンカ		Rakanka, Lo han kuo
ラカンショウ		Long-leaved podocarp
ラズベリ		Raspberry
ラタニア		Rhatany
ラディッシュ	ハツカダイコン	Radish
ラブダナム	システ	Labdanum, Ciste
ラベンダー		Lavender
ラングウォルト		Lungwort
ラングモス		Lungmoss
ランブータン		Ramboutan
リキュール		Liqueur
リーク		Leek
リツェア	タイワンヤマクロモジ	Litsea

基原物質名	別　名	備　考
リナロエ		Linaloe
リュウガン		Longan
リュウゼツラン		Century plant
リョウフンソウ		Ryofunso
リョクチャ	緑茶	Green tea
リンゴ	アップル	Apple
リンデン	ボダイジュ	Linden
リンドウ		Gentian
ルー	ヘンルーダ	Rue
ルリジサ		Borage
レセダ	モクセイソウ	Reseda
レモン		Lemon
レモングラス		Lemongrass
レンギョウ		Rengyo
レンゲ		Renge
レンブ		Wax jambu, Mankil
ローズマリー	マンネンロウ	Rosemary
ロベージ		Lovage
ローレル	ゲッケイジュ	Laurel
ロンゴザ		Longose
ワサビ		Wasabi
ワスレナグサ		Forger me not, Mouse ears
ワタフジウツギ		Watafujiutsugi
ワームウッド	ニガヨモギ	Wormwood
ワームシード		Wormseed
ワラビ		Warabi, Eagle fern
ワレモコウ		Waremoko, Garden burnet

添付資料 3
一般に食品として飲食に供されている物であって添加物として使用される品目リスト

Appendix 3
List of substances which are generally provided for eating or drinking as foods and which are also used as food additives

一般に食品として飲食に供されている物であって添加物として使用される品目リスト

品名		簡略名又は類別名	基原・製法・本質	用途	備考
名称	別名				
アカキャベツ色素	ムラサキキャベツ色素	アカキャベツ アントシアニン アントシアニン色素 野菜色素	アブラナ科キャベツ（Brassica oleracea LINNE var.capitata DC.）の赤い葉（赤キャベツ、紫キャベツ）より、室温時弱酸性水溶液で抽出して得られたものである。主色素はシアニジンアシルグリコシドである。赤色～紫赤色を呈する。	着色料	Red cabbage colour
アカゴメ色素		アカゴメ アントシアニン アントシアニン色素	イネ科イネ（Oryza sativa LINNE）の赤い種子（赤米）より、温時水、弱酸性水溶液又は含水エタノールで抽出して得られたものである。主色素はシアニジン-3-グルコシド等である。赤色を呈する。	着色料	Red rice colour
アカダイコン色素		アカダイコン アントシアニン アントシアニン色素 野菜色素	アブラナ科ダイコン（Raphanus sativus LINNE）の赤紫の根（赤ダイコン）より、室温時水、弱酸性水溶液又は含水エタノールで抽出して得られたものである。主色素はペラルゴニジンアシルグリコシドである。	着色料	Red radish colour
アズキ色素		アズキ	マメ科アズキ（Azukia angularis OHWI）の種子より水で抽出して得られたもの、又はこれを乾燥したものである。赤色を呈する。	着色料	Azuki colour
アマチャ抽出物	アマチャエキス	アマチャ	ユキノシタ科アマチャ（Hydrangea macrophylla SER. var.thungbergii MAKINO）の葉より、水で抽出して得られたものである。甘味成分はフィロズルシンである。	甘味料	Amacha extract Hydrangea leaves extract
イカスミ色素		イカ墨	コウイカ科モンゴウイカ（Sepia officinalis LINNAEUS）等の墨袋の内容物を水洗いしたものより、弱酸性含水エタノール及び含水エタノールで洗浄し、乾燥したものである。主色素はユーメラニンである。黒色を呈する。	着色料	Sepia colour
ウグイスカグラ色素		アントシアニン アントシアニン色素 果実色素 ベリー色素	スイカズラ科クロミノウグイスカグラ（Lonicera caerulea LINNE var.emphyllocalyx NAKAI）の果実より、搾汁したもの、又は水で抽出して得られたものである。主色素はアントシアニンである。赤色～青色を呈する。	着色料	Uguisukagura colour
ウコン	ターメリック			着色料	Turmeric
エタノール	エチルアルコール	アルコール 酒精	デンプン、糖蜜を原料とし、糖化、発酵後、蒸留して得られたものである。成分は専売法による発酵アルコールである。	製造用剤	Ethanol
エルダーベリー色素		アントシアニン アントシアニン色素 果実色素 ベリー色素	スイカズラ科エルダーベリー（Sambucus caerulea RAFIN., Sambucus canadensis LINNE, Sambucus nigra LINNE）の果実より、搾汁したもの、又は室温時～微温時水若しくは酸性水溶液で抽出して得られたものである。主色素は、シアニジングリコシド、デルフィニジングリコシドである。赤色～青色を呈する。	着色料	Elderberry colour
オクラ抽出物			アオイ科オクラ（Abelmoschus escaulentus MOENCH）のさやより、水で抽出して得られた粘質物である。	増粘安定剤	Okra extract
オリーブ茶			モクセイ科オリーブ（Olea europaea LINNE）の葉より、茶と同様の製法により製したものである。	着色料 苦味料等	Olive tea
海藻セルロース		セルロース	海藻を、乾燥、粉砕して得られたセルロースである。	増粘安定剤	Seaweed cellulose
カウベリー色素		アントシアニン アントシアニン色素 果実色素	ツツジ科コケモモ（Vaccinium Vitis-Idaea LINNE）の果実より、搾汁したもの、又は水で抽出して得られたものである。主色素はシアニ	着色料	Cowberry colour

品名		簡略名又は類別名	基原・製法・本質	用途	備考
名称	別名				
		ベリー色素	ジングリコシド及びデルフィニジングリコシドである。赤色～青色を呈する。		
果汁 ウグイスカグラ果汁	フルーツジュース ウグイスカグラジュース			着色料	Fruit juice Uguisukagura juice
エルダーベリー果汁	エルダーベリージュース				Elderberry juice
オレンジ果汁	オレンジジュース				Orange juice
カウベリー果汁	カウベリージュース				Cowberry juice
グースベリー果汁	グースベリージュース				Gooseberry juice
クランベリー果汁	クランベリージュース				Cranberry juice
サーモンベリー果汁	サーモンベリージュース				Salmonberry juice
ストロベリー果汁	ストロベリージュース				Strawberry juice
ダークスィートチェリー果汁	ダークスィートチェリージュース				Dark sweet cherry juice
チェリー果汁	チェリージュース				Cherry juice
チンブルベリー果汁	スィムブルベリージュース				Thimbleberry juice
デュベリー果汁	デュベリージュース				Dewberry juice
パイナップル果汁	パイナップルジュース				Pineapple juice
ハクルベリー果汁	ハクルベリージュース				Huckleberry juice
ブドウ果汁	ブドウジュース、グレープ果汁、グレープジュース				Grape juice
ブラックカーラント果汁	ブラックカーラントジュース				Black currant juice
ブラックベリー果汁	ブラックベリージュース				Blackberry juice
プラム果汁	プラムジュース				Plum juice
ブルーベリー果汁	ブルーベリージュース				Blueberry juice
ベリー果汁	ベリージュース				Berry juice
ボイセンベリー果汁	ボイセンベリージュース				Boysenberry juice
ホワートルベリー果汁	ホワートルベリージュース				Whortleberry juice
マルベリー果汁	マルベリージュース				Mulberry juice
モレロチェリー果汁	モレロチェリージュース				Morello cherry juice
ラズベリー果汁	ラズベリージュース				Raspberry juice
レッドカーラント果汁	レッドカーラントジュース				Red currant juice
レモン果汁	レモンジュース				Lemon juice
ローガンベリー果汁	ローガンベリージュース				Loganberry juice
カゼイン	酸カゼイン	乳たん白	牛乳又は脱脂乳より、酸処理による沈殿によって得られたタンパク質である。	製造用剤	Casein
褐藻抽出物	褐藻粘質物		アラメ、オキナワモズク、コンブ又はワカメより、水で抽出して得られたものである。成分はポリウロン酸及び硫酸多糖である。	増粘安定剤	Kelp extract

品名		簡略名又は類別名	基原・製法・本質	用途	備考
名称	別名				
カンゾウ末		カンゾウ	マメ科ウラルカンゾウ（Glycyrrhiza uralensis FISCHER）、マメ科チョウカカンゾウ（Glycyrrhiza inflata BATALIN）又は、マメ科ヨウカンゾウ（Glycyrrhiza glabra LINNE）の根茎を粉砕したものである。甘味成分はグリチルリチン酸である。	甘味料	Powdered licorice
寒天				製造用剤	Agar
グーズベリー色素		アントシアニン アントシアニン色素 果実色素 ベリー色素	ユキノシタ科グースベリー（Ribes grossularia LINNE）の果実より、搾汁したもの、又は水で抽出して得られたものである。主色素はアントシアニンである。赤色～青色を呈する。	着色料	Gooseberry colour
クランベリー色素		アントシアニン アントシアニン色素 果実色素 ベリー色素	ツツジ科クランベリー（Oxycoccus macrocarpus PERS.）の果実より、搾汁したもの、又は水で抽出して得られたものである。主色素はシアニジングリコシド、ペラルゴニジングリコシドである。赤色～青色を呈する。	着色料	Cranberry colour
グルテン				増粘安定剤	Gluten
グルテン分解物				増粘安定剤	Gluten decomposites
クロレラ抽出液		クロレラエキス	緑藻類クロレラ（Chlorella）を、熱時水で抽出後、濃縮、精製して得られたものである。	調味料 製造用剤	Chlorella extract
クロレラ末			緑藻類クロレラ（Chlorella）を、乾燥し、粉末化したものである。	着色料	Powdered chlorella
ココア	ココアパウダー			着色料	Cocoa
小麦粉				製造用剤	Wheat flour
コムギ抽出物			イネ科コムギ（Triticum aestivum LINNE）の種子（玄麦）を、ばい煎後、熱時水で抽出して得られたものである。	製造用剤	Wheat extract
コラーゲン				製造用剤	Collagen
コンニャクイモ抽出物	グルコマンナン		サトイモ科コンニャク（Amorphophallus konjac）の根茎を、乾燥、粉砕後、含水エタノールで洗浄して得られたもの、又はこれを冷時～温時水で抽出して得られたもので、グルコースとマンノースで構成される多糖類からなる。	増粘安定剤 製造用剤	Konjac extract
サツマイモセルロース		セルロース	ヒルガオ科サツマイモ（Ipomoea batatas POIR.）の塊根より得られたものである。主成分はセルロースである。	製造用剤 増粘安定剤	Sweetpotato cellulose
サフラン				着色料	Saffron
サフラン色素		カロチノイド カロチノイド色素 カロテノイド カロテノイド色素 クロシン サフラン	アヤメ科サフラン（Crocus sativus LINNE）の雌芯頭より、エタノールで抽出して得られたものである。主色素は、カロテノイド系のクロシン、クロセチンである。黄色を呈する。	着色料	Saffron colour
サーモンベリー色素		アントシアニン アントシアニン色素 果実色素 ベリー色素	バラ科サーモンベリー（Rubus spectabilis PURSH.）の果実より、搾汁したもの、又は水で抽出して得られたものである。主色素はアントシアニンである。赤色～青色を呈する。	着色料	Salmonberry colour
シソ色素		アントシアニン アントシアニン色素 野菜色素	シソ科シソ（Perilla frutescens BRITT. var. acuta KUDO）の葉より、室温時水、弱酸性水溶液又は含水エタノールで抽出して得られたものである。主色素は、シソニン、マロニルシソニンである。赤色～赤紫色を呈する。	着色料	Beefsteak plant colour Perilla colour
ストロベリー色素		アントシアニン アントシアニン色素	バラ科オランダイチゴ（Fragaria ananassa DUCHESNE）の果実より、搾汁したもの、又	着色料	Strawberry colour

品名 名称	品名 別名	簡略名又は類別名	基原・製法・本質	用途	備考
		果実色素 ベリー色素	は水で抽出して得られたものである。主色素は、シアニジングリコシド、ペラルゴニジングリコシドである。赤色～青色を呈する。		
ゼラチン				製造用剤	Gelatin
ダイズ多糖類	ダイズヘミセルロース		マメ科ダイズ（Glycine max MERRILL）の種子から得られた多糖類である。主成分はヘミセルロースである。	製造用剤 増粘安定剤	Soybean polysaccharides
ダイダイ抽出物			ミカン科ダイダイ（Citrus aurantium LINNE）の果皮より、エタノールで抽出して得られたものである。主成分はリモニンである。	苦味料等	Daidai extract
ダークスィートチェリー色素		アントシアニン アントシアニン色素 果実色素 チェリー色素	バラ科セイヨウミザクラ（Prunus avium LINNE）の果実より、搾汁したもの、又は室温時～温時水若しくは弱酸性水溶液で抽出して得られたものである。主色素はアントシアニンである。赤色～赤紫色を呈する。	着色料	Dark sweet cherry colour
チェリー色素		アントシアニン アントシアニン色素 果実色素	バラ科カラミザクラ（Prunus pauciflora BUNGE）の果実より、搾汁したもの、又は室温時～温時水若しくは弱酸性水溶液で抽出して得られたものである。主色素はシアニジングリコシドである。赤色～赤紫色を呈する。	着色料	Cherry colour
チコリ色素		チコリ 野菜色素	キク科キクニガナ（Cichorium intybus LINNE）の根をばい煎したものより、温時水で抽出して得られたものである。黄褐色を呈する。	着色料	Chicory colour
茶		抹茶		着色料	Tea
チンブルベリー色素	スィムブルベリー色素	アントシアニン アントシアニン色素 果実色素 ベリー色素	バラ科クロミキイチゴ（Robus occidentalis LINNE）の果実より、搾汁したもの、又は水で抽出して得られたものである。主色素はアントシアニンである。赤色～青色を呈する。	着色料	Thimbleberry colour
デュベリー色素		アントシアニン アントシアニン色素 果実色素 ベリー色素	バラ科オオナワシロイチゴ（Rubus caesius LINNE）の果実より、搾汁したもの、又は水で抽出して得られたものである。主色素はアントシアニンである。赤色～青色を呈する。	着色料	European dewberry colour
トウモロコシセルロース	コーンセルロース	セルロース	イネ科トウモロコシ（Zea mays LINNE）の種皮から得られたものである。主成分はセルロース、ヘミセルロース及びリグニンである。	製造用剤	Corn cellulose
ナタデココ	醸造セルロース 発酵セルロース	セルロース		増粘安定剤 製造用剤	Fermentation-derived cellulose
乳酸菌濃縮物		乳酸菌	乳酸菌を培養した後、集菌、濃縮し、凍結又は乾燥したものである。	酵素	Lactic acid bacteria concentrates
ノリ色素	海苔色素		ウシケノリ科アマノリ（Porphyra tenera KJELLM.）の葉より、温時水又は弱酸性水溶液で抽出して得られたものである。主色素はフィコエリトリンである。桃色～赤色を呈する。	着色料	Laver colour
ハイビスカス色素	ローゼル色素	アントシアニン アントシアニン色素 ローゼル	アオイ科ローゼル（Hibiscus sabdariffa LINNE）の花弁及び萼部より、室温時水で抽出して得られたものである。主色素はデルフィニジン-3-サンブビオシド等である。赤色～紫赤色を呈する。	着色料	Hibiscus colour
麦芽抽出物	麦芽エキス	モルトエキス	イネ科オオムギ（Hordeum vulgare LINNE）の麦芽又はこれを焙煎したものを室温時～温時水で抽出して得られたものである。	着色料	Malt extract
ハクルベリー色素		アントシアニン アントシアニン色素 果実色素	ツツジ科ブラックハクルベリー（Gaylussacia baccata C.KOCH.）の果実より、搾汁したもの、又は水で抽出して得られたものである。主色素	着色料	Black huckleberry colour

品名		簡略名又は類別名	基原・製法・本質	用途	備考
名称	別名				
		ベリー色素	はアントシアニンである。赤色～青色を呈する。		
パプリカ粉末				着色料	Paprika
ブドウ果汁色素		アントシアニン アントシアニン色素 果実色素 ブドウ色素	ブドウ科アメリカブドウ（Vitis Labrusca LINNE）又はブドウ科ブドウ（Vitis vinifera LINNE）の果実より、搾汁し、沈殿を除去して得られたものである。主色素はマルビジン-3-グルコシド等である。赤色～赤紫色を呈する。	着色料	Grape juice colour
ブラックカーラント色素		アントシアニン アントシアニン色素 果実色素 ベリー色素	ユキノシタ科クロフサスグリ（Ribes nigrum LINNE）の果実より、搾汁したもの、又は室温時～微温時水若しくは弱酸性水溶液で抽出して得られたものである。主色素はデルフイニジン-3-ルチノシド等である。赤色～青色を呈する。	着色料	Black currant colour
ブラツクベリー色素		アントシアニン アントシアニン色素 果実色素 ベリー色素	バラ科ヨーロッパブラックベリー（Rubus fruticosus LINNE）の果実より、搾汁したもの、又は水で抽出して得られたものである。主色素はシアニジングリコシドである。赤色～青色を呈する。	着色料	Black berry colour
プラム色素		アントシアニン アントシアニン色素 果実色素	バラ科プラム（Prunus domestica LINNE）の果実より、エタノールで抽出して得られたものである。主色素はシアニジングルコシド等である。赤色～赤紫色を呈する。	着色料	Plum colour
ブルーベリー色素		アントシアニン アントシアニン色素 果実色素 ベリー色素	ツツジ科ハイブッシュブルーベリー（Vaccinium corymbosum LINNE）又はツツジ科ロースィートブルーベリー（Vaccinium angustifolium AIT.）の果実より、搾汁したもの、又は室温時～微温時水若しくは弱酸性水溶液で抽出して得られたものである。主色素はアントシアニンである。赤色～青色を呈する。	着色料	Blueberry colour
ボイセンベリー色素		アントシアニン アントシアニン色素 果実色素 ベリー色素	バラ科エゾイチゴ（Rubus strigosus MICHX.）の果実より、搾汁したもの、又は室温時～微温時水若しくは弱酸性水溶液で抽出して得られたものである。主色素はシアニジン-3-グルコシド等である。赤色～青色を呈する。	着色料	American red raspberry colour Boysenberry colour
ホエイソルト	乳清ミネラル ホエイミネラル		乳清（チーズホエイ）より、乳清タンパクと乳糖を分離除去し、精製して得られたものである。成分は、カリウム、カルシウム、ナトリウム等の塩類である。	調味料	Whey salt Whey mineral
ホップ抽出物	ホップエキス	ホップ		苦味料等	Hop extract
ホワートルベリー色素		アントシアニン アントシアニン色素 果実色素 ベリー色素 ビルベリー色素	ツツジ科ホワートルベリー（Vaccinium myrtillus LINNE）の果実より、搾汁したもの、水若しくはエタノールで抽出して得られたもの、又は室温時メタノールで抽出し、溶媒を除去したものである。主色素はマルビジングルコシド等である。赤色～青色を呈する。	着色料	Whortleberry colour
マルベリー色素		アントシアニン アントシアニン色素 果実色素 ベリー色素	クワ科ブラックマルベリー（Morus nigra LINNE）又はクワ科ホワイトマルベリー（Morus alba LINNE）の果実より、搾汁したもの、又は水で抽出して得られたものである。主色素はシアニジングルコシド等である。赤色～青色を呈する。	着色料	Mulberry colour
マンナン				増粘安定剤	Mannan
モレロチェリー色素		アントシアニン アントシアニン色素 果実色素 チェリー色素	バラ科モレロチェリー（Prunus cerasus LINNE var.austera LINNE）の果実より、室温時～温時エタノールで抽出して得られたものである。主色素はシアニジングリコシルルチノシ	着色料	Morello cherry colour

品名		簡略名又は類別名	基原・製法・本質	用途	備考
名称	別名				
			ド等である。赤色～赤紫色を呈す。		
野菜ジュース アカキャベツジュース アカビートジュース シソジュース タマネギジュース トマトジュース ニンジンジュース	ベジタブルジュース			着色料	Vegetable juice Red cabbage juice Beet red juice Beefsteak plant juice Onion juice Tomato juice Carrot juice
ヨモギ抽出物			キク科ヨモギ（Artemisia princeps PAMPAN.）の茎又は葉より、水又はエタノールで抽出して得られたものである。主成分はカフェタンニン及び精油類である。	苦味料等	Mugwort extract
ラズベリー色素		アントシアニン アントシアニン色素 果実色素 ベリー色素	バラ科セイヨウキイチゴ（Rubus Idaeus LINNE）の果実より、搾汁したもの、又は室温時～微温時水若しくは弱酸性水溶液で抽出して得られたものである。主色素はシアニジングリコシドである。赤色～青色を呈する。	着色料	Raspberry colour
卵白				製造用剤	Egg white
レッドカーラント色素		アントシアニン アントシアニン色素 果実色素 ベリー色素	ユキノシタ科アカスグリ（Ribes sativum SYME.）の果実より、搾汁したもの、又は水で抽出して得られたものである。主色素は、ペラルゴニジンガラクトシド、ペチュニジンガラクトシド等である。赤色～青色を呈する。	着色料	Red currant colour
レンネットカゼイン		カゼイン 乳たん白		増粘安定剤	Rennet casein
ローガンベリー色素		アントシアニン アントシアニン色素 果実色素 ベリー色素	バラ科ローガンベリー（Rubus loganobaccus BAILEY）の果実より、搾汁したもの、又は水で抽出して得られたものである。主色素はシアニジングリコシドである。赤色～青色を呈する。	着色料	Loganberry colour

添付資料 4
無承認無許可医薬品の指導取締りについて

（昭和46年 6 月 1 日薬発第476号）

Appendix 4
Regulatory control of unapproved/unpermitted drugs

(1 June 1971, PAB Notification No. 476)

無承認無許可医薬品の指導取締りについて

昭和46年6月1日　薬発第476号
各都道府県知事あて厚生省薬務局長通知

［改正　昭和58年4月1日　薬発第273号
昭和62年9月22日　薬発第827号
平成2年11月22日　薬発第1179号
平成10年3月31日　医薬発第344号
平成12年4月5日　医薬発第392号
平成13年3月27日　医薬発第243号
平成14年11月15日　医薬発第1115003号
平成16年3月31日　薬食発第0331009号
平成19年4月17日　薬食発第0417001号
平成21年2月20日　薬食発第0220001号
平成23年1月20日　薬食発0120第1号
平成24年1月23日　薬食発0123第3号
平成25年7月10日　薬食発0710第2号］

昨今、その本質、形状、表示された効能効果、用法用量等から判断して医薬品とみなされるべき物が、食品の名目のもとに製造（輸入を含む。以下同じ。）販売されている事例が少なからずみうけられている。

かかる製品は、薬事法上医薬品として、その製造、販売、品質、表示、広告等について必要な規制を受けるべきものであるにもかかわらず、食品の名目で製造販売されているため、

⑴　万病に、あるいは、特定疾病に効果があるかのごとく表示広告されることにより、これを信じて服用する一般消費者に、正しい医療を受ける機会を失わせ、疾病を悪化させるなど、保健衛生上の危害を生じさせる、
⑵　不良品及び偽薬品が製造販売される、
⑶　一般人の間に存在する医薬品及び食品に対する概念を崩壊させ、医薬品の正しい使用が損われ、ひいては、医薬品に対する不信感を生じさせる、
⑷　高貴な成分を配合しているかのごとく、あるいは特殊な方法により製造したかのごとく表示広告して、高価な価格を設定し、一般消費者に不当な経済的負担を負わせる、

等の弊害をもたらすおそれのある事例がみられている。

このため、従来より各都道府県の協力をえて、薬事法等の規定に基づく厳重な指導取締りを行なってきたところであるが、業者間に認識があさく、現在、なお医薬品の範囲に属する物であるにもかかわらず、食品として製造販売されているものがみられることは極めて遺憾なことである。

ついては、今般、今まで報告されてきた事例等を参考として、人が経口的に服用する物のうち「医薬品の範囲に関する基準」（以下「基準」という。）を別紙のとおり定めたので、今後は、下記の点に留意のうえ、貴管下関係業者に対して、遺憾のないように指導取締りを行なわれたい。

（仮訳：Provisional Translation）

Regulatory control of unapproved/unpermitted drugs

(1 June 1971, PAB Notification No. 476)
Notification by the Director of Pharmaceutical Affairs Bureau (PAB), Ministry of Health and Welfare (MHW) to the Prefectural Governors

Amended	1 April 1983	PAB Notification No. 273
	22 September 1987	PAB Notification No. 827
	22 November 1990	PAB Notification No. 1179
	31 March 1998	PMSB Notification No. 344
	5 April 2000	PMSB Notification No. 392
	27 March 2001	PMSB Notification No. 243
	15 November 2002	PMSB Notification No. 1115003
	31 March 2004	PFSB Notification No. 0331009
	17 April 2007	PFSB Notification No. 0417001
	20 February 2009	PFSB Notification No. 0220001
	20 January 2011	PFSB Notification 0120 No. 1
	23 January 2012	PFSB Notification 0123 No. 3
	10 July 2013	PFSB Notification 0710 No. 2

In recent years, there have been more than a few cases of substances manufactured (or imported ; same below) and marketed under the name of foods that should have been deemed drugs, from an assessment of their nature, form, efficacy labeling, dosage and administration methods, and other factors.

Such products are manufactured and marketed as foods, even though the manufacture, marketing, quality, labeling, and advertising of these products should be regulated as a drug under the Pharmaceutical Affairs Act (PAA). This could result in harmful situations, such as:

(1) General consumers may believe the marketing claims that they can treat certain or all diseases and decide to take the product ; this may result in general consumers not seeking out appropriate healthcare such that their condition worsens, which could cause harm from the perspective of health and hygiene.
(2) Faulty or fake products could be manufactured and marketed.
(3) Laypeople may become confused over the concept of what is a drug and what is a food, stop using drugs correctly, and even start to distrust drugs.
(4) General consumers could experience unfair economic losses if the product is advertised as containing the very best ingredients or manufactured using special process and is therefore expensively priced.

Strict regulatory control based on the PAA and other acts and ordinances has been attempted with the cooperation of the prefectures, but the situation has become highly unsatisfactory, with little understanding between businesses and products that should be classified within the scope of drugs being manufactured and marketed as foods.

“Standards for the Scope of Drugs” (hereinafter“Standards”) have been defined (see attachment) for oral substances for human use, with reference to previous examples reported, so we now wish to draw the attention of those businesses involved to the points listed below and provide guidance to resolve this unsatisfactory situation.

記

1．医薬品の該当性については、薬事法第２条における定義に照らし合わせて判断されるべきものであり、本基準は、当該判断に資するよう、過去の判断を例示しているものであることから、医薬品の該当性は、その目的、成分本質（原材料）等を総合的に検討の上、判断すること。

2．基準により医薬品の範囲に属する物は、薬事法の規制を受けるべきものであるので、この旨関係業者に周知徹底し、同法の規定に基づく承認及び許可を受けたものでなければ、製造販売しないよう強力に指導されたいこと。なお、その表示事項、形状等の改善により、食品として製造販売する物にあっては、表示事項については直ちに、また、形状等については、昭和46年11月までに所要の改善措置を講じさせること。

3．これらの指導にもかかわらず、基準により医薬品の範囲に属する物を食品として製造販売する業者に対しては、薬事法及びその他の関連法令に基づき、告発等の厳重な措置を講じられたいこと。

4．ドリンク剤及びドリンク剤類似清涼飲料水の取扱いについては、今後とも、基準準中専ら医薬品として使用される物として例示したような成分本質の物についても、清涼飲料水に配合しないよう指導されたいこと。

(別紙)

医薬品の範囲に関する基準

人が経口的に服用する物が、薬事法（昭和35年法律第145号）第２条第１項第２号又は第３号に規定する医薬品に該当するか否かは、医薬品としての目的を有しているか、又は通常人が医薬品としての目的を有するものであると認識するかどうかにより判断することとなる。通常人が同項第２号又は第３号に掲げる目的を有するものであると認識するかどうかは、その物の成分本質（原材料）、形状（剤型、容器、包装、意匠等をいう。）及びその物に表示された使用目的・効能効果・用法用量並びに販売方法、販売の際の演述等を総合的に判断すべきものである。

したがって、医薬品に該当するか否かは、個々の製品について、上記の要素を総合的に検討のうえ判定すべきものであり、その判定の方法は、Ⅰの「医薬品の判定における各要素の解釈」に基づいて、その物の成分本質（原材料）を分類し、効能効果、形状及び用法用量が医薬品的であるかどうかを検討のうえ、Ⅱの「判定方法」により行うものとする。

ただし、次の物は、原則として、通常人が医薬品としての目的を有するものであると認識しないものと判断して差し支えない。

1　野菜、果物、調理品等その外観、形状等から明らかに食品と認識される物

2　健康増進法（平成14年法律第103号）第26条の規定に基づき許可を受けた表示内容を表示する特別用途食品

Notes:

1. The definitions in Article 2 of the PAA should be referred to when evaluating a substance to determine whether it is a drug. These standards are resources for the relevant assessments and also provide examples of previous decisions, so they can be used for evaluating whether a substance is a drug in combination with consideration of its purpose, ingredients (raw materials), and other factors.

2. A substance that is deemed a drug according to the standards should be regulated under the PAA. We stress that businesses involved with such a substance should be fully aware of this and not manufacture and market the substance if they have not obtained the approvals and permissions based on this Act. For substances to be manufactured and marketed as a food after improvements are made to the product labeling, form, or other factors, the required steps for improvement must be taken immediately for labeling and before November 1971 for the form and other factors.

3. Businesses manufacturing and marketing as foods those substances that are categorized as drugs based on the standards, regardless of these instructions, will be prosecuted and have other severe measures imposed, based on the PAA and other relevant acts and ordinances.

4. For tonic drinks and soft drinks similar to tonic drinks, the regulations indicate that soft drinks should not be combined with ingredients previously demonstrated as being substances used exclusively for drugs according to standards currently under development.

[Attachment]

Standards for the Scope of Drugs

Whether an oral substance for human use is deemed a drug and regulated under the PAA (Act No. 145 of 1960) Articles 2-1-2 and 2-1-3 is determined according to whether the substance has the purpose of a drug and whether laypeople recognize that the substance has the purpose of a drug. Whether lay people recognize that the substance has the purpose of a drug as described in Articles 2-1-2 and 2-1-3 is determined through a comprehensive review of the substance's ingredients (raw materials); form (dosage form, container, packaging, design, and so on); the substance labeling in terms of intended use, efficacy, and dosage and administration methods; marketing methods; and the sales pitch at the time of sale.

Accordingly, whether a substance is deemed a drug should be determined following a comprehensive investigation of the above factors for each individual product. This decision can be made by categorizing the substance's ingredients (raw materials) and investigating whether the efficacy, form, and dosage and administration methods are like those for a drug, in accordance with"I. Interpreting various factors when determining whether a substance is a drug", and using the methods in"II. Determination methods".
However, in principle it may be decided that lay people would not recognize the following substances as having the purpose of a drug:

1. Vegetables, fruit, food preparation products, and other substances that are clearly recognized as foods from their external appearance and form
2. Foods with special dietary use (FOSDU) labeled with information that has received permission based on Article 26 of the Health Promotion Act (Act No. 103 of 2002)

Ⅰ　医薬品の判定における各要素の解釈

1　物の成分本質（原材料）からみた分類

物の成分本質（原材料）が、専ら医薬品として使用される成分本質（原材料）であるか否かについて、別添1「食薬区分における成分本質（原材料）の取扱いについて」（以下「判断基準」という。）により判断することとする。

なお、その物がどのような成分本質（原材料）の物であるかは、その物の成分、本質、起源、製法等についての表示、販売時の説明、広告等の内容に基づいて判断して差し支えない。

判断基準の1．に該当すると判断された成分本質（原材料）については、別添2「専ら医薬品として使用される成分本質（原材料）リスト」にその例示として掲げることとする。

なお、別添2に掲げる成分本質（原材料）であっても、医薬部外品として承認を受けた場合には、当該成分本質（原材料）が医薬部外品の成分として使用される場合がある。

また、判断基準の1．に該当しないと判断された成分本質（原材料）については、関係者の利便を考え、参考として別添3「医薬品的効能効果を標ぼうしない限り医薬品と判断しない成分本質（原材料）リスト」にその例示として掲げることとする。

なお、当該リストは医薬品の該当性を判断する際に参考とするために作成するものであり、食品としての安全性等の評価がなされたもののリストではないことに留意されたい。

2　医薬品的な効能効果の解釈

その物の容器、包装、添付文書並びにチラシ、パンフレット、刊行物、インターネット等の広告宣伝物あるいは演述によって、次のような効能効果が表示説明されている場合は、医薬品的な効能効果を標ぼうしているものとみなす。また、名称、含有成分、製法、起源等の記載説明においてこれと同様な効能効果を標ぼうし又は暗示するものも同様とする。

なお、食品衛生法施行規則（昭和23年厚生省令第23号）第21条第1項第1号シの規定に基づき、厚生労働大臣が定める基準に従い、栄養成分の機能の表示等をする栄養機能食品（以下「栄養機能食品」という。）にあっては、その表示等を医薬品的な効能効果と判断しないこととして差し支えない。

㈠　疾病の治療又は予防を目的とする効能効果

（例）　糖尿病、高血圧、動脈硬化の人に、胃・十二指腸潰瘍の予防、肝障害・腎障害をなおす、ガンがよくなる、眼病の人のために、便秘がなおる等

㈡　身体の組織機能の一般的増強、増進を主たる目的とする効能効果

ただし、栄養補給、健康維持等に関する表現はこの限りでない。

（例）　疲労回復、強精（強性）強壮、体力増強、食欲増進、老化防止、勉学能力を高める、回春、若返り、精力をつける、新陳代謝を盛んにする、内分泌機能を盛んにする、解毒機能を高める、心臓の働きを高める、血液を浄化する、病気に対する自然治癒能力が増す、胃腸の消化吸収を増す、健胃整腸、病中・病後に、成長促進等

I. Interpreting various factors when determining whether a substance is a drug

1. Categories for a substance's ingredients (raw materials)

Appendix 1"Handling the ingredients (raw materials) on the food and drug classification lists" (hereinafter "evaluation criteria") should be used to determine whether or not the ingredient (raw material) is an ingredient (raw material) used exclusively for drugs.

Assessment of what type of ingredients (raw materials) are found in a substance can be based on the labeling showing the ingredients, characteristics, source, and manufacturing methods ; the explanation at the time of sale ; and the content of advertising and other materials.

Examples of ingredients (raw materials) deemed consistent with evaluation criterion 1 can be found in the "List of ingredients (raw materials) used exclusively for drugs".

Ingredients (raw materials) listed in Appendix 2 may sometimes be used as ingredients for quasi-drugs if they have been approved as a quasi-drug.

For reference purposes, examples of ingredients (raw materials) not deemed consistent with evaluation criterion 1 can be found in Appendix 3:"List of ingredients (raw materials) not deemed drugs unless claiming medicinal efficacy"for the convenience of interested parties.

This List has been produced for reference purposes when determining whether an ingredient is a drug. Note that it is not a list of ingredients evaluated for safety etc. when used as a food.

2. Interpreting medicinal efficacy

An item is considered to be claiming medicinal efficacy if the sales pitch or advertising material, including the substance's container, packaging, package insert or product leaflet, pamphlets, publications, or web-based advertising, displays information on efficacy as described below. The same approach is taken if information displayed, including the name, constituent ingredients, manufacturing methods, and source, claim similar efficacy or suggest as much.

Note that for foods with nutrient function claims (FNFCs) that display the function of the nutrient ingredients in accordance with the standards defined by the Health, Labour and Welfare Minister, based on the regulations outlined in Article 21-1-1(L) of the Ministerial Ordinance for Enforcement of the Food Sanitation Act (MHW Ordinance No. 23, 1948), this labeling can be evaluated as not claiming medicinal efficacy.

(1) Efficacy to treat or prevent a disease
Examples: For people with diabetes, high blood pressure, or arteriosclerosis ; to prevent stomach and duodenal peptic ulcers ; cures liver and kidney dysfunction ; improves cancer ; for people with eye disease ; cures constipation ; etc.

(2) Efficacy mainly to promote or generally augment the structure and function of the body. This definition does not apply to expressions related to nutritional support and maintaining health.
Examples: Recovery from fatigue, tonic, boosts stamina, promotes appetite, prevents aging, increases ability to study, rejuvenation, feel young again, greater vitality, boosts metabolism, boosts endocrine function, increases ability to detoxify, increases cardiac function, cleanses the blood, improves natural healing powers against disease, increases digestion and absorption in the gut, regulates gastrointestinal function, during and after illness, promotes growth, etc.

㈢　医薬品的な効能効果の暗示

(a)　名称又はキャッチフレーズよりみて暗示するもの

（例）　延命○○、○○の精（不死源）、○○の精（不老源）、薬○○、不老長寿、百寿の精、漢方秘法、皇漢処方、和漢伝方等

(b)　含有成分の表示及び説明よりみて暗示するもの

（例）　体質改善、健胃整腸で知られる○○○○を原料とし、これに有用成分を添加、相乗効果をもつ等

(c)　製法の説明よりみて暗示するもの

（例）　本邦の深山高原に自生する植物○○○○を主剤に、△△△、×××等の薬草を独特の製造法（製法特許出願）によって調製したものである。等

(d)　起源、由来等の説明よりみて暗示するもの

（例）　○○○という古い自然科学書をみると胃を開き、鬱（うつ）を散じ、消化を助け、虫を殺し、痰なども無くなるとある。こうした経験が昔から伝えられたが故に食膳に必ず備えられたものである。等

(e)　新聞、雑誌等の記事、医師、学者等の談話、学説、経験談などを引用又は掲載することにより暗示するもの

（例）　医学博士○○○○の談

「昔から赤飯に○○○をかけて食べると癌にかからぬといわれている。………癌細胞の脂質代謝異常ひいては糖質、蛋白代謝異常と○○○が結びつきはしないかと考えられる。」等

3　医薬品的な形状の解釈

錠剤、丸剤、カプセル剤及びアンプル剤のような剤型は、一般に医薬品に用いられる剤型として認識されてきており、これらの剤型とする必要のあるものは、医薬品的性格を有するものが多く、また、その物の剤型のほかに、その容器又は被包の意匠及び形態が市販されている医薬品と同じ印象を与える場合も、通常人が当該製品を医薬品と認識する大きな要因となっていることから、原則として、医薬品的形状であった場合は、医薬品に該当するとの判断が行われてきた。

しかし、現在、成分によって、品質管理等の必要性が認められる場合には、医薬品的形状の錠剤、丸剤又はカプセル剤であっても、直ちに、医薬品に該当するとの判断が行われておらず、実態として、従来、医薬品的形状とされてきた形状の食品が消費されるようになってきていることから、「食品」である旨が明示されている場合、原則として、形状のみによって医薬品に該当するか否かの判断は行わないこととする。ただし、アンプル形状など通常の食品としては流通しない形状を用いることなどにより、消費者に医薬品と誤認させることを目的としていると考えられる場合は、医薬品と判断する必要がある。

4　医薬品的な用法用量の解釈

医薬品は、適応疾病に対し治療又は予防効果を発揮し、かつ、安全性を確保するために、服用時期、服用間隔、服用量等の詳細な用法用量を定めることが必要不可欠である。したがって、ある物の使用方法として服用時期、服用間隔、服用量等の記載がある場合には、原則として医薬品的な用法用量とみなすものとし、次のような事例は、これに該当するものとする。ただし、調理の目的のために、使用方法、使用量等を定めているものについてはこの限りでない。

(3) Suggestions of medicinal efficacy

(a) Suggestions from the name or strapline
Examples: Long life XX, XX vigor (source of immortality), XX vigor (source of eternal youth), drug XX, perpetual youth and longevity, live to 100, secret Kampo medicine (traditional Japanese medicine)/ traditional Chinese medicine formula, royal traditional medicine, traditional Japanese/ Chinese medicine, etc.

(b) Suggestions from the labeling of constituent ingredients and their explanations
Examples: Improves physical condition, ingredients include XXXX known to regulate gastrointestinal function, with added effective ingredients, produces synergistic effects, etc.

(c) Suggestions from explanations of the manufacturing methods
Example: The plant XXXX native to the deep mountain tablelands of Japan is the main agent, combined with YYY, ZZZ, and other medicinal plants using a special manufacturing method (patent pending), etc.

(d) Suggestions from explanations of the source and origin
Example: According to XXX, an ancient book on the natural sciences, this stimulates appetite, eliminates depression, aids digestion, cures bad moods, and improves maladies. This experience has been handed down through the ages and is something that should be added to all food.

(e) Suggestions from publications or extracts from discussions by doctors and academics, theories, or real-life experiences, or articles in newspapers or journals, etc.
Example:
Conversation with XXXX M.D.
"Long ago, it was said that if you ate sekihan festive red rice sprinkled with YYY, you would not get cancer … It is possible that abnormalities in the lipid metabolism or sugar/protein metabolism in cancer cells could be linked to ZZZ."

3. Interpreting medicinal form

Dosage forms such as tablets, pills, capsules, and ampoules are generally recognized as being the dosage forms used for pharmaceuticals. In many cases, these dosage forms are needed because of the medicinal properties of the product. As well as the dosage form, products marketed in containers, packaging designs, or shapes that give the same impression as a pharmaceutical could be recognized by the layperson as a drug. Therefore, in the past, if a product has a medicinal form, in principle it has been deemed a drug.

However, today, not all products with medicinal forms (tablets, pills, or capsules) are immediately deemed a drug if there is a recognized need for that form depending on the ingredient (for example for quality management purposes). In practice, because foods are now consumed in forms previously considered to be medicinal, if the product clearly states that it is a"food", in principle the product will not be deemed a drug purely because of its form. However, if the product is supplied as an ampoule or another form that is not usual for a normal food and the design is considered to be for the purpose of misleading the consumer into thinking it is a drug, then the product must be deemed a drug.

4. Interpreting medicinal dosage and administration methods

Pharmaceuticals treat or prevent an indicated disease and detailed dosage and administration methods must be defined (including timing of administration, intervals between administration, and dose to be administered) in order to ensure safety. Therefore, if information is provided on the timing of administration, intervals between administration, and dose to be administered etc. for a substance, in principle, these are considered to be medicinal dosage and administration methods. The examples given below meet this definition. However, this definition does not apply to usage methods and usage amounts etc. defined for the purpose of food preparation.

一方、食品であっても、過剰摂取や連用による健康被害が起きる危険性、その他合理的な理由があるものについては、むしろ積極的に摂取の時期、間隔、量等の摂取の際の目安を表示すべき場合がある。

これらの実態等を考慮し、栄養機能食品にあっては、時期、間隔、量等摂取の方法を記載することについて、医薬品的用法用量には該当しないこととして差し支えない。

ただし、この場合においても、「食前」「食後」「食間」など、通常の食品の摂取時期等とは考えられない表現を用いるなど医薬品と誤認させることを目的としていると考えられる場合においては、引き続き医薬品的用法用量の表示とみなすものとする。

（例）　１日２～３回、１回２～３粒
　　　　１日２個
　　　　毎食後、添付のサジで２杯づつ
　　　　成人１日３～６錠
　　　　食前、食後に１～２個づつ
　　　　お休み前に１～２粒

Ⅱ　判定方法

人が経口的に服用する物について、Ｉの「医薬品の判定における各要素の解釈」に基づいて、その成分本質（原材料）を分類し、その効能効果、形状及び用法用量について医薬品的であるかどうかを検討のうえ、以下に示す医薬品とみなす範囲に該当するものは、原則として医薬品とみなすものとする。なお、２種以上の成分が配合されている物については、各成分のうちいずれかが医薬品と判定される場合は、当該製品は医薬品とみなすものとする。

ただし、当該成分が薬理作用の期待できない程度の量で着色、着香等の目的のために使用されているものと認められ、かつ、当該成分を含有する旨標ぼうしない場合又は当該成分を含有する旨標ぼうするが、その使用目的を併記する場合等総合的に判断して医薬品と認識されるおそれのないことが明らかな場合には、この限りでない。

医薬品とみなす範囲は次のとおりとする。

㈠　効能効果、形状及び用法用量の如何にかかわらず、判断基準の１．に該当する成分本質（原材料）が配合又は含有されている場合は、原則として医薬品の範囲とする。

㈡　判断基準の１．に該当しない成分本質（原材料）が配合又は含有されている場合であって、以下の①から③に示すいずれかに該当するものにあっては、原則として医薬品とみなすものとする。
　①　医薬品的な効能効果を標ぼうするもの
　②　アンプル形状など専ら医薬品的形状であるもの
　③　用法用量が医薬品的であるもの

However, when a substance is a food but there is a risk of harm to health from over consumption or continuous use or there is some other rational explanation, the product should claim suggested standards for when the product should be used, at what intervals, and in what amounts.

Given the above, FNFCs may be deemed as not having medicinal dosage and administration methods if they provide information on when the product should be used, at what intervals, and in what amounts etc.

However, even in this case, a product will be deemed as claiming medicinal dosage and administration methods if it uses expressions not normally associated with eating normal food (for example, before meal, after meal, or between meals) with the intent of misleading the consumer into thinking the product is a drug.

Examples:
A dose of two or three pieces taken two or three times daily
Two pieces per day
Two spoonfuls (using the attached spoon) after every meal
3-6 tablets a day for adults
One or two pieces before and after meal
One or two pieces before bed

II. Determination methods

Whether an orally taken substance for human use is considered to be a drug is determined by first categorizing the substance's ingredients (raw materials) and investigating whether the efficacy, form, and dosage and administration methods are like those for a drug, in accordance with"I. Interpreting various factors when determining whether a substance is a drug". Substances that fall within the scope of substances considered to be drugs shown below are, in principle, considered to be drugs. For substances that comprise a combination of two or more ingredients, if any of the ingredients are determined as drugs, then the product is considered to be a drug.

However, this definition does not apply when there is clearly no chance of the substance being recognized as a drug, based on a comprehensive assessment of whether an ingredient is confirmed as being used in amounts not expected to produce a pharmacological effect for the purpose of coloring, flavoring, etc. and when the product does not claim to contain the relevant ingredient or when the product does claim to contain the relevant ingredient but information on the intended use is also provided.
The scope of substances considered to be drugs is as follows.

(1) A substance is, in principle, considered to fall within the scope of drugs if it contains ingredients (raw materials), alone or in combination, that comply with evaluation criterion 1, regardless of its efficacy, form, and dosage and administration methods.
(2) A substance is, in principle, considered to fall within the scope of drugs if it complies with any of points (1) through (3) below, even if it contains ingredients (raw materials), alone or in combination, that do not comply with evaluation criterion 1.
1) Items that claim to have medicinal efficacy
2) Items in an exclusively medicinal form, such as an ampoule
3) Items with medicinal dosage and administration methods

(別添1) 食薬区分における成分本質（原材料）の取扱いについて

1.「専ら医薬品として使用される成分本質（原材料）リスト」の考え方

(1)　専ら医薬品としての使用実態のある物
　解熱鎮痛消炎剤、ホルモン、抗生物質、消化酵素等専ら医薬品として使用される物

(2)　(1)以外の動植物由来物（抽出物を含む。)、化学的合成品等であって、次のいずれかに該当する物。ただし、一般に食品として飲食に供されている物を除く。
①　毒性の強いアルカロイド、毒性タンパク等、その他毒劇薬指定成分（別紙参照）に相当する成分を含む物（ただし、食品衛生法で規制される食品等に起因して中毒を起こす植物性自然毒、動物性自然毒等を除く）
②　麻薬、向精神薬及び覚せい剤様作用がある物（当該成分及びその構造類似物（当該成分と同様の作用が合理的に予測される物に限る）並びにこれらの原料植物）
③　処方せん医薬品に相当する成分を含む物であって、保健衛生上の観点から医薬品として規制する必要性がある物

注1）ビタミン、ミネラル類及びアミノ酸（別紙参照）を除く。ただし、ビタミン誘導体については、食品衛生法の規定に基づき使用される食品添加物である物を除き、「専ら医薬品として使用される成分本質（原材料）リスト」に収載される物とみなす。
注2）当該成分本質（原材料）が薬理作用の期待できない程度の量で着色、着香等の目的のために使用されているものと認められ、かつ、当該成分本質（原材料）を含有する旨標ぼうしない場合又は当該成分本質（原材料）を含有する旨標ぼうするが、その使用目的を併記する場合等総合的に判断して医薬品と認識されるおそれがないことが明らかな場合には、「専ら医薬品として使用される成分本質（原材料）リスト」に収載されていても、医薬品とみなさない。
注3）「医薬品的効能効果を標ぼうしない限り医薬品と判断しない成分本質（原材料）リスト」に収載されている原材料であっても、水、エタノール以外の溶媒による抽出を行った場合には、当該抽出成分について、上記の考え方に基づいて再度検討を行い、「専ら医薬品として使用される成分本質（原材料）リスト」に収載すべきかどうか評価する。

2. 新規成分本質（原材料）の判断及び判断する際の手続き

(1)「専ら医薬品として使用される成分本質（原材料）リスト」にも、「医薬品的効能効果を標ぼうしない限り医薬品と判断しない成分本質（原材料）リスト」にも収載されていない成分本質（原材料）を含む製品を輸入販売又は製造する事業者は、あらかじめ、当該成分本質（原材料）の学名、使用部位、薬理作用又は生理作用、毒性、麻薬・覚せい剤様作用、国内外での医薬品としての承認前例の有無、食習慣等の資料を都道府県薬務担当課（室）を通じて、厚生労働省医薬食品局監視指導・麻薬対策課あて提出し、その判断を求めることができる。

[Attachment 1] Handling of ingredients (raw materials) in the Food and Drug Classification in Japan

1. Basic approach to"List of ingredients (raw materials) used exclusively for drugs"

(1) Substances actually used exclusively as a drug
Substances used exclusively as a drug, including antipyretic analgesic anti-inflammatories, hormones, antibiotics, and digestive enzymes

(2) Substances not included in (1) of plant or animal origin (including extracts) or chemically synthesized products, etc. that comply with any of the following definitions. However, this excludes substances generally supplied for eating or drinking as a food.

① Substances that include ingredients that are highly toxic alkaloids, toxic proteins, etc. or other ingredients designated as poisonous or deleterious drugs (see attachment). (However, this excludes natural plant toxins and natural animal toxins that cause food poisoning from foods etc. regulated under the Food Sanitation Act.)

② Substances that act like narcotic drugs, psychotropic drugs, and stimulants [the relevant ingredients and structurally similar substances (limited to substances that could be logically expected to have a similar action as the relevant ingredient) and the raw material plants].

③ Substances that include ingredients equivalent to prescribed pharmaceuticals that need to be regulated as drugs from the perspective of health and hygiene.

Note 1) Excludes vitamins, minerals, and amino acids (see attachment). However, vitamin derivatives are substances included in the"List of ingredients (raw materials) used exclusively for drugs"with the exception of food additives used in accordance with the Food Sanitation Act.

Note 2) A substance is not deemed a pharmaceutical, even if it is included in the"List of ingredients (raw materials) used exclusively for drugs", if there is clearly no chance of the substance being recognized as a drug, based on a comprehensive assessment of whether an ingredient is confirmed as being used in amounts not expected to produce a pharmacological effect for the purpose of coloring, flavoring, etc. and when the product does not claim to contain the relevant ingredient or when the product does claim to contain the relevant ingredient but information on the intended use is also provided.

Note 3) Even for raw materials listed on the"List of ingredients (raw materials) not deemed drugs unless claiming medicinal efficacy", if they have been extracted using a solvent other than water and/or ethanol, the extract must be re-investigated based on the approach above and evaluated as to whether they should be listed on the"List of ingredients (raw materials) used exclusively for drugs".

2. Procedures for assessing and evaluating new ingredients (raw materials)

(1) Businesses manufacturing or importing products including ingredients that are not included in the"List of ingredients (raw materials) used exclusively for drugs"and the"List of ingredients (raw materials) not deemed drugs unless claiming medicinal efficacy"should, in advance, seek assessment by submitting to the Compliance and Narcotics Division (CND), Pharmaceutical and Food Safety Bureau (PFSB), Ministry of Health, Labour and Welfare (MHLW), via the Division of Pharmaceutical Affairs, Prefectural Health Department (Bureau), materials on the scientific names of the relevant ingredients (raw materials), part of use, pharmacological action and physiological action, toxicity, narcotic- and stimulant-like effects, previous examples of approval as a drug in Japan and overseas, and dietary habits.

(2)　監視指導・麻薬対策課は、提出された資料により、上記1の考え方に基づき学識経験者と協議を行い、専ら医薬品として使用される成分本質（原材料）への該当性を判断する。この場合、事業者に対し追加資料の要求をする場合がある。

(3)　監視指導・麻薬対策課は、「専ら医薬品として使用される成分本質（原材料）リスト」に該当せず、効能効果の標ぼう等からみて食品としての製造（輸入）、販売等が行われる場合には、食品安全部関係各課（室）に情報提供を行う。

また、当該リストは定期的に公表するものとする。

3．その他

「医薬品的効能効果を標ぼうしない限り医薬品と判断しない成分本質（原材料）リスト」及び「専ら医薬品として使用される成分本質（原材料）リスト」は、今後、新たな安全性に関する知見等により、必要に応じて変更することがある。

(参考)

ハーブについては、次の文献等を参考にする。

・Jeffrey B.Harborne FRS,Herbert Baxter：Dictionary of Plant Toxins, Willey
・The Complete German Commission E Monographs Therapeutic Guide to Herbal Medicines（The American Botanical Council）
・Botanical Safety Handbook（American Herbal Products Association）
・Richard Evans Schultes, Albert Hofmann：The Botany and Chemistry of Hallucinogens, Charles C. Thomas Publisher
・Poisonous Plants：Lucia Woodward
・WHO monographs on selected medicinal plants
・John H. Wiersema, Blanca Leon：World Economic Plants
・中薬大辞典：小学館
・和漢薬：医歯薬出版株式会社

(別紙)

○毒薬・劇薬指定基準（注略）

(1)　急性毒性（概略の致死量：mg／kg）が次のいずれかに該当するもの。
1）経口投与の場合、毒薬が30mg/kg、劇薬が300mg/kg以下の値を示すもの。
2）皮下投与の場合、毒薬が20mg/kg、劇薬が200mg/kg以下の値を示すもの。
3）静脈内（腹腔内）投与の場合、毒薬が10mg/kg、劇薬が100mg/kg以下の値を示すもの。

(2)　次のいずれかに該当するもの。なお、毒薬又は劇薬のいずれに指定するかは、その程度により判断する。
1）原則として、動物に薬用量の10倍以下の長期連続投与で、機能又は組織に障害を認めるもの
2）通例、同一投与法による致死量と有効量の比又は毒性勾配から、安全域が狭いと認められるもの
3）臨床上中毒量と薬用量が極めて接近しているもの
4）臨床上薬用量において副作用の発現率が高いもの又はその程度が重篤なもの
5）臨床上蓄積作用が強いもの

(2) The CND will consult with science experts on the materials submitted, using the basic approach outlined above in 1, and decide whether the ingredients (raw materials) will be deemed as used exclusively for drugs. The business may sometimes be asked to submitted additional information.

(3) If the CND decides that the ingredient (raw material) should not be on the"List of ingredients (raw materials) used exclusively for drugs"and that it is manufactured (imported) and marketed as a food based on the efficacy claims, etc., the information will be supplied to the relevant divisions (bureaus) belonging to the Department of Food Safety.
The relevant lists are published regularly.

3. Other

The"List of ingredients (raw materials) not deemed drugs unless claiming medicinal efficacy"and the"List of ingredients (raw materials) used exclusively for drugs"will be revised as needed according to new findings on safety etc.

(Reference)

The following references are used for herbs.
- Jeffrey B. Harborne FRS, Herbert Baxter: Dictionary of Plant Toxins, Wiley
- The Complete German Commission E Monographs Therapeutic Guide to Herbal Medicines (The American Botanical Council)
- Botanical Safety Handbook (American Herbal Products Association)
- Richard Evans Schultes, Albert Hofmann: The Botany and Chemistry of Hallucinogens, Charles C. Thomas Publisher
- Poisonous Plants: Lucia Woodward
- WHO monographs on selected medicinal plants
- John H. Wiersema, Blanca Leon: World Economic Plants
- Chuyaku Daijiten (The Dictionary of Chinese Medicines): Shogakukan
- Wakan-yaku (Japanese and Chinese Medicine): Ishiyaku Pub., Inc.

[Attachment]

○ Standards for designation as poisonous or deleterious (abbreviated)

(1) Acute toxicity defined as one of the following (lethal dose in overview: mg/kg).
  1) Values with oral administration are up to 30mg/kg for a poisonous drug and 300mg/kg for a deleterious drug.
  2) Values with subcutaneous administration are up to 20mg/kg for a poisonous drug and 200mg/kg for a deleterious drug.
  3) Values with intravenous (peritoneal) administration are up to 10mg/kg for a poisonous drug and 100mg/kg for a deleterious drug.

(2) Substance that complies with one of the following. Note that whether a drug is designated as poisonous or deleterious is determined according to degree.
  1) In principle, long-term continuous administration to animals at less than 10x the therapeutic dose disrupts functions or tissues.
  2) In general, the safety margin is narrow, based on the toxicity gradient or the ratio of the lethal dose and effective dose using the same administration method
  3) In the clinical setting, the toxic dose and the therapeutic dose are extremely close
  4) In the clinical setting, there is a high incidence of side effects at the therapeutic dose or side effects are severe
  5) In the clinical setting, the drug has a strong cumulative effect

6）臨床上薬用量において薬理作用が激しいもの

○注１に規定するアミノ酸は、以下のとおりとする。

・アスパラギン、アスパラギン酸、アラニン、アルギニン、イソロイシン、グリシン、グルタミン、グルタミン酸、シスチン、システイン、セリン、チロシン、トリプトファン、トレオニン、バリン、ヒスチジン、4-ヒドロキシプロリン、ヒドロキシリジン、フェニルアラニン、プロリン、メチオニン、リジン、ロイシン

※　別添２（専ら医薬品として使用される成分本質（原材料）リスト）および別添３（医薬品的効能効果を標ぼうしない限り医薬品として判断しない成分本質（原材料）リスト）は、本書の第１部および第２部に相当するため、添付を割愛する。

6) In the clinical setting, the drug produces an extreme pharmacological action at the therapeutic dose

○Amino acids specified in Note 1 are as follows.

・Asparagine, aspartic acid, alanine, arginine, isoleucine, glycine, glutamine, glutamic acid, cystine, cysteine, serine, tyrosine, tryptophan, threonine, valine, histidine, 4-hydroxyproline, hydroxylysine, phenylalanine, proline, methionine, lysine, leucine

※Attachments 2 and 3 are equivalent to Sections 1 and 2 of this publication, so are not attached here.

添付資料 5
無承認無許可医薬品の監視指導について

（昭和62年 9 月22日薬監第88号）

Appendix 5
Inspection and guidance of unapproved/unpermitted drugs

(22 September 1987, PAB Notification No. 88)

無承認無許可医薬品の監視指導について

（昭和62年９月22日　薬監第88号）
（各都道府県衛生主管部（局）長宛　厚生省薬務局監視指導課長通知）

〔改正　平成２年11月22日　薬監第65号
平成10年３月31日　医薬監第62号
平成12年４月５日　医薬監第31号
平成13年３月27日　医薬監麻発第333号
平成14年11月15日　医薬監麻発第1115016号
平成16年３月31日　薬食監麻発第0331004号
平成19年４月17日　薬食監麻発第0417001号〕

標記については、昭和46年６月１日薬発第476号厚生省薬務局長通知「無承認無許可医薬品の指導取締りについて」により行つてきたところであるが、今般、同通知の別紙「医薬品の範囲に関する基準」の一部が昭和62年９月22日薬発第827号薬務局長通知をもつて改正されたことに合わせ、監視指導の一層の徹底を図るため、別添のとおり、「無承認無許可医薬品監視指導マニュアル」を定めたので、今後とも監視指導に遺漏のないようよろしく御配意願いたい。

〔別添〕

無承認無許可医薬品監視指導マニュアル

目次

Ⅰ　無承認無許可医薬品の指導取締りについて
　1　薬事法の目的
　2　医薬品と食品
　3　無承認無許可医薬品の指導取締りの必要性
　4　医薬品の範囲に関する基準と本マニュアルについて
Ⅱ　基本的考え方と判定方法による判定について
　1　基本的な考え方
　2　「判定方法」の意義
　3　具体的な判断方法
　4　「明らかに食品と認識される物」の解釈
　5　特別用途食品の取扱い
　6　「判定方法」についての解説
Ⅲ　物の成分本質（原材料）からみた分類について
　1　基本的な考え方
　2　例示成分本質（原材料）の分類の変更等
　3　表示、販売時の説明、広告等の内容による判断
　4　着色、着香等の目的で使用される場合の取扱い
　5　抽出成分等の取扱い
　6　植物等の部位による取扱いの違い
　7　生薬名の使用
Ⅳ　医薬品的な効能効果について

（仮訳：Provisional Translation）

Inspection and guidance of unapproved/unpermitted drugs

(22 September 1987, PAB Notification No. 88)
Notification by the Director of Compliance and Narcotics Division (CND), Pharmaceutical Affairs Bureau (PAB), Ministry of Health and Welfare (MHW) to the Heads of the Prefectural Health Management Divisions

Amended	22 November 1990	PAB Notification No. 65
	31 March 1998	PMSB Notification No. 62
	5 April 2000	PMSB Notification No. 31
	27 March 2001	PMSB/CND Notification No. 333
	15 November 2002	PMSB/CND Notification No. 1115016
	31 March 2004	PMSB/CND Notification No. 0331004
	17 April 2007	PMSB/CND Notification No. 0417001

The title was previously"Regulatory control of unapproved/unpermitted drugs", Notification by the Director of the PAB, MHW (1 June 1971, PAB Notification No. 476). However, part of the Appendix"Standards on the Scope of Drugs"in this Notification were amended according to the Notification by the Director of the PAB (22 September 1987, PAB Notification No. 827) and the"Manual for regulatory control of unapproved/unpermitted drugs"was defined, as an Appendix, in order to make regulatory control more consistent. Please ensure that these are taken into consideration for regulatory control in the future.

[Appendix]

Contents of the"Manual for regulatory control of unapproved/unpermitted drugs"

Ⅰ. Regulatory control of unapproved/unpermitted drugs
1. Objective of the PAA
2. Drugs and foods
3. Need for regulatory control of unapproved/unpermitted drugs
4. Standards on scope of drugs and this Manual
Ⅱ. Basic approach and assessment using determination methods
1. Basic approach
2. Significance of"determination methods"
3. Specific evaluation methods
4. Interpreting"Substances that are clearly recognized as foods"
5. Dealing with food for special dietary use (FOSDU)
6. Interpreting"determination methods"
Ⅲ. Categories for a substance's ingredients (raw materials)
1. Basic approach
2. Examples of changes to the categories for ingredients (raw materials)
3. Evaluation based on the labeling, sales pitch at the time of sale, and advertising
4. Treatment of items used as colorings, flavorings, etc.
5. Handling of extracts etc.
6. Differences in handling according to plant or animal part used
7. Use of crude drug names
Ⅳ. Medicinal efficacy

1　基本的な考え方
2　医薬品的な効能効果の標ぼうの方法
3　栄養補給に関する表現
4　「健康維持」、「健康増進」等の表現
5　医薬品的な効能効果の暗示
V　医薬品的な形状について
VI　医薬品的な用法用量について
1　基本的な考え方
2　医薬品的な用法用量の範囲
3　摂取方法、調理法等の表現
4　栄養補給のための摂取量の表現
5　過食を避けるため摂取の上限量を示す表現

I　無承認無許可医薬品の指導取締りについて

現在の国民の最大の関心事の一つは、自ら、あるいは家族の健康であるといわれており、国民の健康に対する志向は近年非常な高まりを見せている。このような状況を反映して、健康食品と称するものが流通するようになってきたが、いわゆる健康食品の中には医薬品的な効能効果を標ぼうするなど、医薬品に該当するにもかかわらず食品として流通し、消費者の健康に好ましからざる影響を及ぼすものもあるのが実情である。昭和58年度に経済企画庁が中心となって行った「『健康食品』の販売等に関する総合実態調査」においても、「医薬品的な効能効果や用法用量が表示されている場合もあり、これを信じて摂取する消費者に正しい医療を受ける機会を失わせ、疾病を悪化させるなどの保健衛生上の危害を生じさせるおそれがある。」との指摘がなされている。

本マニュアルは、薬事法第2条第1項第2号又は第3号の医薬品に該当する物が食品と称して販売されることのないよう、医薬品の範囲についての具体的な判断のポイントを示すことにより、医薬品の範囲をより明確化し、無承認無許可医薬品の流通防止を図ることを目的として作成したものである。

1　薬事法の目的

医薬品は、人の生命、健康に直接かかわるものであり、その品質、有効性及び安全性を確保することが重要である。効果のないもの、有害であるものが誤って医薬品として使用された場合には、人の生命を失わせる危険さえある。また、専門的な医学・薬学の知識を持たない通常人には、その物が何であり、どのような疾病に、どのように使用したら効果があるかを判断することは不可能である。したがって、医薬品については、その特殊性にかんがみ、その品質、有効性及び安全性が適正なもののみが供給されることが必要であり、医薬品の製造、輸入、販売等を規制し、その品質、有効性及び安全性の確保を図ることが重要である。

薬事法は、医薬品の使用によってもたらされる国民の健康への積極的、消極的被害を未然に防止するため、医薬品に関する事項を規制し、その品質、有効性及び安全性を確保することを目的としている。医薬品を製造又は輸入しようとする者は、その医薬品について承認を受ける必要があり（その物の有効性及び安全性を確認するために必要である。）、その有効性及び安全性が確認された医薬品を製造又は輸入しようとする者は、製造所又は営業所ごとに許可を受ける必要がある（承認された物を承認されたとおりに製造・輸入できるような人的物的要件を確認するために必要である。）。また、医薬品を販売しようとする者は、販売業の許可を受ける必要がある。これら必要な承認・許可を取得していない医薬品は、無承認無許可医薬品として取り締まらなければならない。

1. Basic approach
2. Methods of claiming medicinal efficacy
3. Expressions related to nutritional support
4. Expressions on"maintaining health"or"promoting health"
5. Suggestions of medicinal efficacy
V. Medicinal form
VI. Medicinal dosage and administration methods
1. Basic approach
2. Scope of medicinal dosage and administration methods
3. Expressions on how to eat or prepare
4. Expressions on amounts to take for nutritional support
5. Expressions describing maximum amounts to eat to avoid overconsumption

I. Regulatory control of unapproved/unpermitted drugs

Personal health and the health of one's family is a key issue for the general public today. The population has becoming increasingly interested in public health in recent years, as can be seen in the spread of so-called health foods. These products are distributed as foods, even though they could be classified as drugs because of the medicinal effects some health foods have, and they sometimes have undesirable effects on consumer health. A comprehensive survey on the sale of health foods, conducted by the Economic Planning Agency in 1983, suggested that some products displayed medicinal effects and dosage and administration guides, and consumers could believe the claims made and use health foods for particular conditions, thereby missing out on the opportunity to receive the appropriate healthcare and resulting in the worsening of a disease, which could damage health overall.

This Manual was produced with the objective of preventing the distribution of unapproved/unpermitted drugs, by clarifying the scope of drugs and providing specific points for assessing the scope of drugs, to ensure that substances that are classified as drugs under the Pharmaceutical Affairs Act(PAA) Articles 2-1-2 and 2-1-3 are not sold as foods.

1. Objective of the PAA

Drugs have a direct impact on people's lives and health, so it is important to ensure they are of appropriate quality, efficacy, and safety. People can die if ineffective or harmful substances are mistakenly used as drugs. It is also not possible for a layperson with no specialist medical or pharmacological knowledge to decide what a substance is, how it should be used for what disease, and what effects it will produce. Accordingly, it is important to consider the particular characteristics of drugs ; ensure only drugs of an appropriate quality, efficacy, and safety are supplied ; regulate drug manufacture, import, and sale ; and ensure drug quality, efficacy, and safety.

The PAA is aimed at ensuring drug quality, efficacy, and safety, and regulating various drug-related matters to prevent active and passive harm to public health through the use of drugs. Parties intending to manufacture or import drugs need to obtain approval for that drug(needed to confirm the drug's efficacy and safety), while parties intending to manufacture or import drugs of confirmed efficacy and safety need to obtain permission for each manufacturing and sales site(needed to confirm the human and physical requirements are in place for the manufacture and import of the approved drug in line with that approval). Parties intending to sell drugs need to obtain permission for the sales business. Drugs for which these required approvals and permissions have not been obtained must be controlled as unapproved/unpermitted drugs.

2　医薬品と食品

では、どのような物が薬事法により医薬品として規制を受けるのか。薬事法においては、医薬品として規制を受けるべき物を、次のように定義している。

〔薬事法第２条第１項〕
一　日本薬局方に収められている物
二　人又は動物の疾病の診断、治療又は予防に使用されることが目的とされている物であって、機械器具、歯科材料、医療用品及び衛生用品でないもの（医薬部外品を除く。）
三　人又は動物の身体の構造又は機能に影響を及ぼすことが目的とされている物であって、機械器具等でないもの（医薬部外品及び化粧品を除く。）

薬事法の立法趣旨が、前述のとおり医薬品の使用によってもたらされる国民の健康への積極的、消極的被害を未然に防止しようとする点にあるとすると、薬事法第２条第１項第２号又は第３号に規定する医薬品には、同法第14条又は第19条の２に基づいて承認を受けた医薬品のみならず、その物の成分本質（原材料）、形状、効能効果、用法用量等を総合的に判断して、その物が「人又は動物の疾病の診断、治療又は予防に使用されることが目的とされている」又は「人又は動物の身体の構造又は機能に影響を及ぼすことが目的とされている」と通常人が認識する物も含まれる。すなわち、口から摂取される物が医薬品に該当するか否かは、その物が薬事法第２条第１項第２号又は第３号に掲げる目的を持つものと認識されるか否かによって判断されることとなる。この場合、その薬理作用の有無は問題とはならないと解される。このような現行薬事法における医薬品の範囲についての考え方は、旧薬事法におけるものと変わるものではない。

一方、食品衛生法において食品とは次のように定義されている。

〔食品衛生法第４条第１項〕
この法律で食品とは、すべての飲食物をいう。但し、薬事法に規定する医薬品及び医薬部外品は、これを含まない。

医薬品の定義及び食品の定義により明らかなように、口から摂取される物は、医薬品等と食品のどちらかに該当することになり、口から摂取される物のうち、医薬品等に該当しないもののみが食品とされることになる。

3　無承認無許可医薬品の指導取締りの必要性

無承認無許可医薬品には模造に係る医薬品や医薬品と称しているが承認・許可を取得していない物、それに食品と称しているが医薬品とみなされるべき物とがあるが、判断が困難なのは最後の範疇に属するものであり、多くはいわゆる健康食品と呼ばれるものである。

いわゆる健康食品について薬事法との関係で問題になる点は、医薬品として承認を受けるべき物が食品の名目のもとに製造・販売されるという点である。

医薬品に該当する物が、薬事法に基づく承認・許可を取得せずに食品として製造・販売されるとなると、

①　一般消費者の間にある、医薬品と食品に対する概念を混乱させ、ひいては医薬品に対する不信感を生じさせるおそれがある、

2. Drugs and foods

What substances are regulated as drugs under the PAA ? The PAA includes the following definition for substances that must be regulated as drugs.

[PAA Article 2-1]

1) Substances included in the Japanese Pharmacopeia
2) Substances used for the purpose of diagnosing, treating, or preventing disease in humans or animals and that are not machinery and appliances, dental materials, or medical or sanitary items(hereinafter termed machinery and appliances) (excluding quasi-drugs)
3) Substances used for the purpose of affecting the physical structure or function of humans or animals and that are not machinery and appliances(excluding quasi-drugs and cosmetics)

The legislative intent of the PAA is to prevent active or passive harm to public health brought about by the use of drugs as described above. Accordingly, drugs regulated under PAA Articles 2-1-2 and 2-1-3 include drugs that have been approved in line with PAA Articles 14 and 19-2, as well as substances recognized by the layperson as being"used for the purpose of diagnosing, treating, or preventing disease in humans or animals"and"used for the purpose of affecting the physical structure or function of humans or animals"through comprehensive consideration of the ingredients(raw materials), form, efficacy, and dosage and administration methods. In other words, whether an oral substance is a drug or not can be determined by recognizing whether or not the intended use of that substance is as outlined in the PAA Articles 2-1-2 and 2-1-3. In this case, the existence of a pharmacological action is not considered problematic. The views on the scope of drugs in the current PAA do not differ from those in the previous PAA.

The Food Sanitation Act defines foods as follows.

[Food Sanitation Act Article 4-1]

Under this Act, foods are defined as all substances eaten or drunk. However, the definition does not include drugs regulated under the PAA and quasi-drugs.

As is clear from the definitions of drugs and food, oral substances can be considered either drugs or foods and only those oral substances not deemed drugs etc. are defined as foods.

3. Need for regulatory control of unapproved/unpermitted drugs

Unapproved/unpermitted drugs include counterfeit drugs, substances termed drugs for which approval/permission has not been obtained, and substances that are termed foods but should be deemed drugs. This last category is the most difficult to determine and many of the substances that fall into this category are so-called health foods.

Defining the relationship between the PAA and so-called health foods is problematic because substances that should be approved as drugs are being manufactured and marketed under the name of foods.

If substances deemed drugs are manufactured and marketed as foods without obtaining the approvals/permissions required in the PAA, the following issues arise:

1) General consumers may become confused over the concept of what is a drug and what is a food, and start to distrust drugs.

② 有効性が確認されていないにもかかわらず、疾病の治療等が行えるかのような認識を与えて販売されることから、これを信じて摂取する一般消費者に、正しい医療を受ける機会を失わせ、疾病を悪化させるなど保健衛生上の危害を生じさせるおそれがある、

等の問題がある。

国民の健康への積極的、消極的被害を未然に防止するため、このような無承認無許可医薬品は、厳正に取り締まらなければならない。

成分本質（原材料）、形状、効能効果等から見て医薬品に該当する物が、承認・許可を得なくても製造・販売することができるとすると、何故に薬事法があり、何故に承認・許可制度があるのかという疑問を惹起させることになり、医薬品の品質、有効性及び安全性を担保している承認・許可制度その他の各種の規制を実質的に無意味化することになる。それはとりもなおさず、前述した薬事法の立法趣旨、目的を否定することにつながり、国民の保健衛生にとって由々しき問題を投げかける。無承認無許可医薬品の製造・販売を認めることは、国民の健康への積極的、消極的被害を未然に防止する観点からは許されるものではない。

4　医薬品の範囲に関する基準と本マニュアルについて

薬事法第2条第1項第2号又は第3号に規定する医薬品に該当するか否かについては、昭和46年6月1日薬発第476号厚生省薬務局長通知「無承認無許可医薬品の指導取締りについて」（以下「通知」という。）の中で「医薬品の範囲に関する基準」（以下「基準」という。）として、例示を含めて、具体的な判断のための基準が示されているところであるが、さらに、本マニュアルは、この基準について、過去の指導事例等をもとに解説を加えたものである。また、ここに記載のない事項についても薬事法の立法趣旨に照らして判断されなければならない。

なお、本マニュアルは食品の範囲にある物の是非等を論ずるものではないことは言うまでもなく、本マニュアルにおいて、医薬品に該当するとは断定できないとされた物については、食品衛生法、健康増進法、不当景品類及び不当表示防止法等他法令に抵触することのないよう、栄養・食品担当部局及び景表法担当部局等関係部局に照会するよう指導されたい。

Ⅱ　基本的考え方と判定方法による判定について

〈通知本文抜粋〉

人が経口的に服用する物が、薬事法（昭和35年法律第145号）第2条第1項第2号又は第3号に規定する医薬品に該当するか否かは、医薬品としての目的を有しているか、又は通常人が医薬品としての目的を有するものであると認識するかどうかにより判断することとなる。通常人が同項第2号又は第3号に掲げる目的を有するものであると認識するかどうかは、その物の成分本質（原材料）、形状（剤型、容器、包装、意匠等をいう。）及びその物に表示された使用目的・効能効果・用法用量並びに販売方法、販売の際の演述等を総合的に判断すべきものである。

したがって、医薬品に該当するか否かは、個々の製品について、上記の要素を総合的に検討のうえ判定すべきものであり、その判定の方法は、Ⅰの「医薬品の判定における各要素の解釈」に基づいて、その物の成分本質（原材料）を分類し、効能効果、形状及び用法用量が医薬品的であるかどうかを検討のうえ、Ⅱの「判定方法」により行うものとする。

2) Even though these substances have not been confirmed as efficacious, general consumers may use them in the belief that the marketing claims for treating certain diseases are true ; this may result in general consumers not seeking out appropriate healthcare such that their condition worsens, which could cause harm from the perspective of health and hygiene.

Unapproved/unpermitted drugs must be strictly controlled in order to prevent active and passive harm to public health.

If the manufacture and marketing of substances deemed drugs, based on their ingredients (raw materials), form, efficacy, and so on, are allowed without obtaining approval/permission, it brings into question the existence of the PAA and of approval/permission systems and actually renders meaningless the various other approval/permission systems that ensure drug quality, efficacy, and safety. In other words, this would negate the legislative intent and purpose of the PAA, as described above, and could raise serious health and hygiene issues for the general public. Allowing the manufacture and marketing of unapproved/unpermitted drugs cannot be permitted from the perspective of preventing active and passive harm to public health.

4. Standards on scope of drugs and this Manual

A Notification by the Director of the PAB, MHW (1 June 1971, PAB Notification No. 476) entitled "Regulatory control of unapproved/unpermitted drugs" (hereinafter "the Notification") contains a section entitled "Standards for scope of drugs" (hereinafter "Standards") that provides specific standards, as well as examples, to determine whether a substance is classified as a drug and regulated according to the PAA Articles 2-1-2 and 2-1-3. This Manual provides additional explanations, based on previous regulatory examples. Where there are situations not described in this Manual, a decision should be made with reference to the legislative intent of the PAA.

Obviously, this Manual does not discuss issues surrounding substances that fall within the scope of foods. For items where it cannot be determined whether a substance should be deemed a drug, enquiries should be made with departments responsible for nutrition/food and the Act against Unjustifiable Premiums and Misleading Representations to prevent any conflict with the Food Sanitation Act, the Health Promotion Act, the Act against Unjustifiable Premiums and Misleading Representations, and other acts and ordinances.

Ⅱ. Basic approach and assessment using determination methods

<Extract from the Notification text>

Whether an oral substance for human use is deemed a drug and regulated under the PAA (Act No. 145 of 1960) Articles 2-1-2 and 2-1-3 is determined according to whether the substance has the purpose of a drug and whether laypeople recognize that the substance has the purpose of a drug. Whether laypeople recognize that the substance has the purpose of a drug as described in Articles 2-1-2 and 2-1-3 is determined through a comprehensive review of the substance's ingredients (raw materials) ; form (dosage form, container, packaging, design, and so on) ; the substance labeling in terms of intended use, efficacy, and dosage and administration methods ; marketing methods ; and the sales pitch at the time of sale.

Accordingly, whether a substance is deemed a drug should be determined following a comprehensive investigation of the above factors for each individual product. This decision can be made by categorizing the substance's ingredients (raw materials) and investigating whether the efficacy, form, and dosage and administration methods are like those for a drug, in accordance with "I. Interpreting various factors when determining whether a substance is a drug", and using the methods in "II. Determination methods".

ただし、次の物は、原則として、通常人が医薬品としての目的を有するものであると認識しないものと判断して差し支えない。

1　野菜、果物、調理品等その外観、形状等から明らかに食品と認識される物

2　健康増進法（平成14年法律第103号）第26条の規定に基づき許可を受けた表示内容を表示する特別用途食品

〈通知本文抜粋〉

Ⅱ　判定方法

人が経口的に服用する物について、Ⅰの「医薬品の判定における各要素の解釈」に基づいて、その成分本質（原材料）を分類し、その効能効果、形状及び用法用量について医薬品的であるかどうかを検討のうえ、以下に示す医薬品とみなす範囲に該当するものは、原則として医薬品とみなすものとする。なお、２種以上の成分が配合されている物については、各成分のうちいずれかが医薬品と判定される場合は、当該製品は医薬品とみなすものとする。

ただし、当該成分が薬理作用の期待できない程度の量で着色、着香等の目的のために使用されているものと認められ、かつ、当該成分を含有する旨標ぼうしない場合又は当該成分を含有する旨標ぼうするが、その使用目的を併記する場合等総合的に判断して医薬品と認識されるおそれのないことが明らかな場合には、この限りでない。

医薬品とみなす範囲は次のとおりとする。

㈠　効能効果、形状及び用法用量の如何にかかわらず、判断基準の１．に該当する成分本質（原材料）が配合又は含有されている場合は、原則として医薬品の範囲とする。

㈡　判断基準の１．に該当しない成分本質（原材料）が配合又は含有されている場合であって、以下の①から③に示すいずれかに該当するものにあっては、原則として医薬品とみなすものとする。
①　医薬品的な効能効果を標ぼうするもの
②　アンプル形状など専ら医薬品的形状であるもの
③　用法用量が医薬品的であるもの

1　基本的な考え方

「人が経口的に服用する物が、薬事法第２条第１項第２号又は第３号に規定する医薬品に該当するか否かは、医薬品としての目的を有しているか、又は通常人が医薬品としての目的を有するものであると認識するかどうかにより判断することとなる。通常人が同項第２号又は第３号に掲げる目的を有するものであると認識をするかどうかは、その物の成分本質（原材料）、形状（剤型、容器、包装、意匠等をいう。）及びその物に表示された使用目的・効能効果・用法用量並びに販売方法、販売の際の演述等を総合的に判断すべきものである。」とする本文は、医薬品の範囲に関する基本的な考え方を示したものである。

However, in principle it may be decided that laypeople would not recognize the following substances as having the purpose of a drug:

1．Vegetables, fruit, food preparation products, and other substances that are clearly recognized as foods from their external appearance and form

2．Foods with special dietary use(FOSDU)labeled with information that has received permission based on Article 26 of the Health Promotion Act(Act No. 103 of 2002)

<Extract from the Notification text>

II. Determination methods

Whether an oral substance for human use is considered to be a drug is determined by first categorizing the substance's ingredients(raw materials)and investigating whether the efficacy, form, and dosage and administration methods are like those for a drug, in accordance with"I. Interpreting various factors when determining whether a substance is a drug". Substances that fall within the scope of substances considered to be drugs shown below are, in principle, considered to be drugs. For substances that comprise a combination of two or more ingredients, if any of the ingredients are determined as drugs, then the product is considered to be a drug.

However, this definition does not apply when there is clearly no chance of the substance being recognized as a drug, based on a comprehensive assessment of whether an ingredient is confirmed as being used in amounts not expected to produce a pharmacological effect for the purpose of coloring, flavoring, etc. and when the product does not claim to contain the relevant ingredient or when the product does claim to contain the relevant ingredient but information on the intended use is also provided.

The scope of substances considered to be drugs is as follows.

(1) A substance is, in principle, considered to fall within the scope of drugs if it contains ingredients(raw materials), alone or in combination, that comply with evaluation criterion 1, regardless of its efficacy, form, and dosage and administration methods.

(2) A substance is, in principle, considered to fall within the scope of drugs if it complies with any of points ① through ③ below, even if it contains ingredients(raw materials), alone or in combination, that do not comply with evaluation criterion 1.
① Items that claim to have medicinal efficacy
② Items in an exclusively medicinal form, such as an ampoule
③ Items with medicinal dosage and administration methods

1．Basic approach

The following text defines the basic approach on the scope of drugs.
"Whether an oral substance for human use is deemed a drug and regulated under the PAA Articles 2-1-2 and 2-1-3 is determined according to whether the substance has the purpose of a drug and whether laypeople recognize that the substance has the purpose of a drug. Whether laypeople recognize that the substance has the purpose of a drug as described in Articles 2-1-2 and 2-1-3 is determined through a comprehensive review of the substance's ingredients(raw materials) ; form(dosage form, container, packaging, design, and so on) ; the substance labeling in terms of intended use, efficacy, and dosage and administration methods ; marketing methods ; and the sales pitch at the time of sale."

その物が医薬品に該当するか否かの判断は、具体的には、個々の製品について、その物の成分本質（原材料）を分類し、効能効果、形状及び用法用量が医薬品的であるかどうかを検討のうえ行うものであるが、通知本文にあるとおり、あくまでも総合的に判断して通常人がその物を医薬品の目的を有するものと認識するか否かに基づくべきとの基本的な考え方を忘れてはならない。

なお、「医薬品ではありません。」等医薬品でない旨標ぼうしたとしても、そのことをもって医薬品に該当しないということにはならない。

2　「判定方法」の意義

⑴　経口的に摂取される物が医薬品に該当する場合には、薬事法に基づき、所要の承認・許可を取得しない限り、製造、輸入、販売することが禁じられることとなるため、医薬品に該当するか否かの総合判断の判断基準は一律でなければならない。このため、総合判断の具体的な判定のための方法として「判定方法」が示されている。

⑵　その物が医薬品に該当するか否かの判断は、原則としてこの「判定方法」により行うものとし、「医薬品とみなす範囲」に該当する物は、当該成分本質（原材料）が着色、着香等の目的のために使用される場合等、総合的に判断して医薬品と認識されるおそれのないことが明らかな場合を除いて、原則として医薬品に該当するものである。

3　具体的な判断方法

その物が医薬品に該当するか否かの判断に当たっては、第一に医薬品としての目的を有しているか否かを確認する必要があること。また、医薬品の目的を有するものと認識するか否かの判断については、原則として次のような方法により行うものとする。

①　その物の原材料を確認し、その原材料について「Ⅲ　物の成分本質（原材料）からみた分類について」に基づき、どの分類に該当するかを判定する。

当該原材料が例示成分本質（原材料）として掲げられていない場合には、当課あて照会すること。

なお、その際には、学名、使用部位、薬理作用又は生理作用、毒性、麻薬・覚せい剤様作用、国内外での医薬品としての承認前例の有無、食習慣等の資料について、当該成分本質（原材料）を配合又は含有する製品を製造又は輸入しようとする者より徴求する等し、添付したうえで、照会すること。

②　その物の剤型を確認し、その剤型が「Ⅴ　医薬品的な形状について」に基づき、専ら医薬品的な剤型に該当するか否かの判定を行い、さらにその物の容器又は被包の意匠及び形態を検討して、その物の形状が総合的にみて医薬品的であるか否かを判断する。

③　「Ⅳ　医薬品的な効能効果について」及び「Ⅵ　医薬品的な用法用量について」に基づき、その物の容器、被包等の表示、添付文書、パンフレット、チラシ等に医薬品的な効能効果、用法用量が標ぼうされているか否かを判断する。

④　①で確認した成分本質（原材料）の分類に対応する「判定方法」中の「医薬品とみなす範囲」に従って、②で判断した形状及び③で判断した効能効果、用法用量を組み合わせて総合的に判断する。

Whether a substance falls within the scope of drugs should be determined by categorizing the substance's ingredients (raw materials) and investigating whether the efficacy, form, and dosage and administration methods are like those for a drug. However, as shown in the Notification text, it is important to remember the basic approach that the decision should be a comprehensive one and based on whether laypeople recognize that the substance has the purpose of a drug.

Even if an item claims that it is not a drug, for example by stating "This is not a drug", this should not be used as the basis for deciding that the item is not a drug.

2. Significance of "determination methods"

(1) The PAA bans the manufacture, import, and sale of orally ingested substances that fall under the scope of drugs, unless the necessary approvals and permissions have been obtained, so the criteria used to make a comprehensive decision on whether a substance is deemed a drug must be consistent. The "determination methods" therefore show methods for specific assessments in the comprehensive decision.

(2) The decision on whether a substance is deemed a drug should, in principle, be made using the "determination methods" and substances that fall within the scope of substances deemed drugs are, in principle, considered to be drugs, with the exception of cases where there is clearly no possibility that a substance is recognized as a drug following a comprehensive assessment, for example where the ingredients (raw materials) in question are used for the purpose of coloring, flavoring, etc.

3. Specific evaluation methods

The first step in making a decision on whether a substance is deemed a drug should involve determining whether the substance has the purpose of a drug. The following methods should, in principle, be used to determine whether the substance has the purpose of a drug.

① Confirm the raw materials in the substance and determine which category the raw materials fall into based on "III. Categories for a substance's ingredients (raw materials)."
If a particular raw material is not listed as an example ingredient (raw material), enquiries should be made with the relevant departments.
In this case, enquiries should attach the following information obtained from the party intending to manufacture or import the product containing the relevant ingredients (raw materials), in combination or alone: scientific name, part of use, pharmacological or physiological action, toxicity, narcotic- or stimulant-like action, whether there are previous examples of approval as a drug in Japan or overseas, and eating habits.

② Confirm the substance's dosage form, determine whether it is an exclusively medicinal dosage form based on "V. Medicinal forms" and investigate the design and shape of the container or packaging to decide whether the form is like a drug from an overall perspective.

③ Determine whether claims are made for medicinal efficacy and dosage and administration methods in the item labeling on the container or packaging, in the package insert, or in pamphlets and leaflets, based on "IV. Medicinal efficacy" and "VI. Medicinal dosage and administration methods".

④ Make a comprehensive evaluation combining assessment of the form, as evaluated in ②, and the efficacy and dosage and administration methods, as evaluated in ③, in line with the "scope of substances considered to be drugs" in the "determination methods" for the corresponding category of ingredients (raw materials) confirmed in ①.

このために、後述する各要素についての医薬品的であるか否かの範囲を十分理解することが必要である。

4 「明らかに食品と認識される物」の解釈

(1) 通常の食生活において、その物の食品としての本質を経験的に十分認識していて、その外観、形状等より容易に食品であることがわかるものは、その物の食品としての本質に誤認を与えることはないため、通常人がその物を医薬品と誤認するおそれはない。

したがって、医薬品の目的を有するものであるという認識を与えるおそれのないこのような物は、医薬品に該当しないことは明らかであり、その成分本質（原材料）、形状、効能効果、用法用量について個々に検討し、後述する「判定方法」に従って判定するまでもない。通知本文中のただし書はこの旨を明記したものである。

(2) その物がここでいう「明らかに食品と認識される物」に該当するか否かは、食生活の実態を十分勘案し、外観、形状及び成分本質（原材料）からみて社会通念上容易に食品と認識されるか否かにより判断するものである。

通常人が社会通念上容易に通常の食生活における食品と認識するものとは、例えば次のような物が考えられる。ただし、特定の成分を添加したもの、遺伝子組み換え技術を用いたものなど、医薬品としての目的を持つことが疑われるものについては、個別に判断する必要がある。

① 野菜、果物、卵、食肉、海藻、魚介等の生鮮食料品及びその乾燥品（ただし、乾燥品のうち医薬品としても使用される物を除く。）

（例）トマト、キャベツ、リンゴ、牛肉、豚肉、鰯、秋刀魚、鮪　等

② 加工食品

（例）豆腐、納豆、味噌、ヨーグルト、牛乳、チーズ、バター、パン、うどん、そば、緑茶、紅茶、ジャスミン茶、インスタントコーヒー、ハム、かまぼこ、コンニャク、清酒、ビール、まんじゅう、ケーキ　等

③ ①、②の調理品

（例）飲食店等で提供される料理、弁当、惣菜及びこれらの冷凍食品・レトルト食品　等

④ 調味料

（例）醤油、ソース　等

(3) なお、「明らかに食品と認識される物」について行われる標ぼうにあっては、虚偽誇大な表現については不当景品類及び不当表示防止法第４条第１項第１号に、また、場合によっては健康増進法第32条の２等他法令に抵触するおそれがあるので、栄養・食品担当部局等関係部局に照会するよう指導すること。

5 特別用途食品の取扱い

(1) 健康増進法第26条の規定に基づき厚生労働大臣の許可を受けた特別用途食品の表示内容については、栄養・食品担当部局の指導が行われるものである。

A full understanding of the various factors described below is needed to determine the scope of whether a substance is a drug or not.

4. Interpreting"Substances that are clearly recognized as foods"

(1) Laypeople would not mistake the substance as a drug because, during the course of normal dietary habits, they have sufficient experience to recognize that the substance is actually a food and they do not make mistakes over substances that can be easily identified as food from their external appearance or form.
Accordingly, substances that are unlikely to be recognized as having the purpose of a drug are clearly not deemed drugs and they do not need to have their ingredients(raw materials), form, efficacy, and dosage and administration methods investigated separately for a decision to be made using the "determination methods". This is clearly stated in the provisos in the text of the Notification.

(2) Whether the substance is clearly recognized as a food or not should be determined by taking into full account actual dietary habits and determining whether the commonly held view is that it could easily be recognized as a food from the perspective of the external appearance, form, and ingredients(raw materials).
The following are examples of substances that would be recognized as a food by laypeople based on commonly held views on normal dietary habits. However, individual decisions need to be made for substances suspected as having the purpose of a drug, such as those with special added ingredients or where genetic recombination technologies have been used.

① Vegetables, fruits, egg, meat, seaweed, seafood, and other fresh foods or dried products of the same foods(however, the dried products excludes substances also used for drugs).
Examples: tomato, cabbage, apple, beef, pork, sardine, Pacific saury, tuna, etc.

② Processed foods
Examples: tofu, natto, miso, yoghurt, milk, cheese, butter, bread, udon noodles, soba noodles, green tea, black tea, jasmine tea, instant coffee, ham, kamaboko fish sausage, konnyaku, refined sake, beer, steamed bun, cake, etc.

③ Prepared products that use ① and ②
Examples: food, lunch boxes, and side dishes supplied by restaurants and other outlets, and chilled foods or packaged and sterilized foods, etc.

④ Seasonings
Examples: soy sauce, sauce, etc.

(3) For claims made on"substances that are clearly recognized as food", Article 4-1-1 of the Act, the Act against Unjustifiable Premiums and Misleading Representations states that enquires should be made with the relevant departments responsible for nutrition/food if false and exaggerated language is used, as in some cases this may be in violation of Article 32-2 of the Health Promotion Act and other acts and ordinances.

5. Dealing with food for special dietary use(FOSDU)

(1) FOSDU that has received the permission of the Health, Labour and Welfare Minister, in accordance with Article 26 of the Health Promotion Act, should be labeled in line with the instructions from the departments responsible for nutrition/food.

(2)　容器包装、説明書、広告、パンフレット等に許可を受けた表示内容を超えて医薬品的な効能効果の標ぼうが行われた場合にも、その標ぼう内容について、まず栄養・食品担当部局に照会するよう指導すること。

6 「判定方法」についての解説

「判定方法」による判定によることなく、当然に、医薬品に該当しないとされた物（前記4「『明らかに食品と認識される物』の解釈」及び前記5「特別用途食品の取扱い」に示されたもの）以外の物については、その成分本質（原材料）に応じて、原則として「判定方法」により医薬品に該当するか否かを判断するものである。

以下、各成分本質（原材料）の分類ごとの判定について解説する。

(1)　専ら医薬品として使用される成分本質（原材料）について

ア 「専ら医薬品として使用される成分本質（原材料）」（基準の別添1（以下「判断基準」という。）の1．に該当する物）に該当する成分本質（原材料）の物は、専ら医薬品として使用され、薬事法第2条第1項第2号又は第3号の目的を有することが明らかであるため、その物又はこれを配合若しくは含有する物は、効能効果、形状、用法用量の如何にかかわらず原則として医薬品と判断する。

イ　次のような場合には、専ら医薬品として使用される成分本質（原材料）が含有されている場合であっても直ちに医薬品には該当しない。

(ア)　着色、着香等の目的のために使用されているものと認められる場合には、専ら医薬品として使用される成分本質（原材料）が含有されていても、当該成分を含有する旨を標ぼうしない場合又は当該成分を含有する旨を標ぼうするが、その使用目的を併記する場合には、当該成分が含有されていないものとみなして差し支えない。

(イ)　(ア)に準ずる場合であって、総合的に判断して医薬品と認識されるおそれのないことが明らかなときには、医薬品には該当しないと解して差し支えない。

なお、医薬品に該当しない場合にあっても、食品に専ら医薬品として使用される成分本質（原材料）を配合又は含有させることの適否については、栄養・食品担当部局に照会するほか、虚偽誇大な表現については不当景品類及び不当表示防止法第4条第1号に、また、場合によっては健康増進法等他法令に抵触するおそれがあるので、栄養・食品担当部局等関係部局に照会するよう指導すること。

(2)　医薬品的効能効果を標ぼうしない限り医薬品と判断しない成分本質（原材料）について

ア 「医薬品的効能効果を標ぼうしない限り医薬品と判断しない成分本質（原材料）」（判断基準の1．に該当しない物）に該当する成分本質（原材料）の物は、通知の「医薬品とみなす範囲」に示されたとおり、医薬品的な効能効果を標ぼうする場合は原則として医薬品に該当するほか、アンプル形状など専ら医薬品的形状である場合又は用法用量が医薬品的であるものは原則として医薬品に該当する。

ここでいう「専ら医薬品的形状である場合」とは、「V　医薬品的な形状について」において、専ら医薬品的な剤型に該当すると判断された剤型の場合及び剤型、容器又は被包の意匠及び形態等のすべてを総合的に判断し、通常人に医薬品と誤認させることを目的としていると考えられる場合をいう。

(2) If claims for medicinal efficacy are made above and beyond the permitted label contents on the container/packaging, product leaflet, advertising, or pamphlets etc., the details of these claims should be initially referred to the departments responsible for nutrition/food.

6. Interpreting"determination methods"

The decision on whether a substance is deemed a drug should be made, in principle, by using the"determination methods"according to the substance's ingredients(raw materials), apart from substances that are clearly not deemed drugs and do not need to be evaluated using the"determination methods" [as shown above in 4. Interpreting"Substances that are clearly recognized as foods"and 5. Dealing with food for special dietary use (FOSDU)].
Below, we interpret the determination for each category of ingredient(raw materials).

(1) Ingredients(raw materials)used exclusively for drugs

a) An ingredient(raw material)that falls under the scope of"Ingredients(raw materials)used exclusively for drugs" [entities consistent with point 1 in attachment 1 on standards(hereinafter"assessment criteria")]are used exclusively for drugs and therefore clearly have the purpose described in the PAA Articles 2-1-2 and 2-1-3, so such substances or items containing such substances, alone or in combination, should, in principle, be deemed drugs regardless of their efficacy, form, and dosage and administration methods.

b) For the cases outlined below, substances are not immediately deemed drugs even if they contain ingredients(raw materials)used exclusively for drugs.

i) Where the substance is recognized as being used for the purpose of coloring or flavoring, even if that substance contains an ingredient(raw material)that is exclusively used for drugs, the substance can be considered to not contain that ingredient if its intended use is written on the labeling and the substance does not claim to contain the relevant ingredient or when the substance does claim to contain the relevant ingredient but information on the intended use is also provided.

ii) For a substance consistent with point i)and where comprehensive consideration has determined that there is clearly no chance of the substance being recognized as a drug, the substance can be determined as not falling under the scope of drugs.
Even if an entity is not deemed a drug, the departments responsible for nutrition/food should be contacted over whether it is appropriate for a food to contain or include a combination of an ingredients(raw materials)used exclusively for drugs, or the departments responsible for nutrition/food and other matters should be contacted if false and exaggerated claims may conflict with Article 4-1-1 of the Act against Unjustifiable Premiums and Misleading Representations or, in some cases, the Health Promotion Act and other acts and ordinances.

(2) Ingredients(raw materials)not deemed drugs unless claiming medicinal efficacy

a) Ingredients(raw materials)consistent with"Ingredients(raw materials)not deemed drugs unless claiming medicinal efficacy" (substances not consistent with determination methods point 1)are, in principle, deemed drugs if claims are made about medicinal efficacy, as shown in"Scope of substances considered to be drugs"in the Notification, or are, in principle, deemed drugs if they are in an exclusively medicinal form such as an ampoule or have medicinal dosage and administration methods.
Here"if they are in an exclusively medicinal form"is relevant if the dosage form is considered to be an exclusively medicinal form and if, following a comprehensive assessment of the dosage form and the design and shape of the container or packaging, the purpose of the design may be to cause laypeople to mistake the substance for a drug.

イ　医薬品的効能効果を標ぼうしない限り医薬品と判断しない成分本質（原材料）が含有されている物で、通知の「医薬品とみなす範囲」に該当する場合であっても、直ちに医薬品には該当しない場合もあるが、これについては「(1)専ら医薬品として使用される成分本質（原材料）について」のイと同様に取り扱うものとする。

Ⅲ　物の成分本質（原材料）からみた分類について

〈通知本文抜粋〉

物の成分本質（原材料）が、専ら医薬品として使用される成分本質（原材料）であるか否かについて、別添1「食薬区分における成分本質（原材料）の取扱いについて」（以下「判断基準」という。）により判断することとする。

なお、その物がどのような成分本質（原材料）の物であるかは、その物の成分、本質、起源、製法等についての表示、販売時の説明、広告等の内容に基づいて判断して差し支えない。

判断基準の1．に該当すると判断された成分本質（原材料）については、別添2「専ら医薬品として使用される成分本質（原材料）リスト」にその例示として掲げることとする。

なお、別添2に掲げる成分本質（原材料）であっても、医薬部外品として承認を受けた場合には、当該成分本質（原材料）が医薬部外品の成分として使用される場合がある。

また、判断基準の1．に該当しないと判断された成分本質（原材料）については、関係者の利便を考え、参考として別添3「医薬品的効能効果を標ぼうしない限り医薬品と判断しない成分本質（原材料）リスト」にその例示として掲げることとする。

なお、当該リストは医薬品の該当性を判断する際に参考とするために作成するものであり、食品としての安全性等の評価がなされたもののリストではないことに留意されたい。

〈通知本文抜粋〉

Ⅱ　判定方法

人が経口的に服用する物について、Ⅰの「医薬品の判定における各要素の解釈」に基づいて、その成分本質（原材料）を分類し、その効能効果、形状及び用法用量について医薬品的であるかどうかを検討のうえ、以下に示す医薬品とみなす範囲に該当するものは、原則として医薬品とみなすものとする。なお、2種以上の成分が配合されている物については、各成分のうちいずれかが医薬品と判定される場合は、当該製品は医薬品とみなすものとする。

ただし、当該成分が薬理作用の期待できない程度の量で着色、着香等の目的のために使用されているものと認められ、かつ、当該成分を含有する旨標ぼうしない場合又は当該成分を含有する旨標ぼうするが、その使用目的を併記する場合等総合的に判断して医薬品と認識されるおそれのないことが明らかな場合には、この限りでない。

1　基本的な考え方

(1)　その物が医薬品に該当するか否かは、その物の成分本質（原材料）を分類し、その効能効果、形状及び用法用量について医薬品的であるかどうかを検討し、総合的に判断するものである。

成分本質（原材料）の分類に当たっては、医薬品としての使用実態及び食品としての認識の程度を踏まえ、判断基準により判断することとする。

b) Even if substances containing ingredients (raw materials) not deemed drugs unless claiming medicinal efficacy do fall under the "Scope of substances considered to be drugs" in the Notification, in some cases they may be immediately classified as not drugs, in which case they are handled in the same way as point b) of "(1) Ingredients (raw materials) used exclusively for drugs".

Ⅲ. Categories for a substance's ingredients (raw materials)

<Extract from the Notification text>

Appendix 1 "Handling the ingredients (raw materials) on the food and drug classification lists" (hereinafter "evaluation criteria") should be used to determine whether or not the ingredient (raw material) is an ingredient (raw material) used exclusively for drugs.
Assessment of what type of ingredients (raw materials) are found in a substance can be based on the labeling showing the ingredients, characteristics, source, and manufacturing methods; the explanation at the time of sale; and the content of advertising and other materials.
Examples of ingredients (raw materials) deemed consistent with evaluation criterion 1 can be found in the "List of ingredients (raw materials) used exclusively for drugs" in Appendix 2.
Ingredients (raw materials) listed in Appendix 2 may sometimes be used as ingredients for quasi-drugs if they have been approved as a quasi-drug.
For reference purposes, examples of ingredients (raw materials) not deemed consistent with evaluation criterion 1 can be found in Appendix 3: "List of ingredients (raw materials) not deemed drugs unless claiming medicinal efficacy" for the convenience of interested parties.
This List has been produced for reference purposes when determining whether an ingredient is a drug. Note that it is not a list of ingredients evaluated for safety etc. when used as a food.

<Extract from the Notification text>

Ⅱ. Determination methods

Whether an oral substance for human use is considered to be a drug is determined by first categorizing the substance's ingredients (raw materials) and investigating whether the efficacy, form, and dosage and administration methods are like those for a drug, in accordance with "I. Interpreting various factors when determining whether a substance is a drug". Substances that fall within the scope of substances considered to be drugs shown below are, in principle, considered to be drugs. For substances that comprise a combination of two or more ingredients, if any of the ingredients are determined as drugs, then the product is considered to be a drug.
However, this definition does not apply when there is clearly no chance of the substance being recognized as a drug, based on a comprehensive assessment of whether an ingredient is confirmed as being used in amounts not expected to produce a pharmacological effect for the purpose of coloring, flavoring, etc. and when the product does not claim to contain the relevant ingredient or when the product does claim to contain the relevant ingredient but information on the intended use is also provided.

1. Basic approach

(1) Whether a substance is deemed a drug or not is determined by categorizing that substance's ingredients (raw materials) and comprehensively investigating whether it has medicinal efficacy, shape, and dosage and administration methods.
The category for the ingredient (raw material) should be decided based on the evaluation criteria, reflecting the actual use as a drug and the degree of recognition as a food.

医薬品としての使用実態がある場合とは、原則として、厚生労働大臣が医薬品として承認・許可を与えている場合をいうが、必要な場合には、外国での医薬品としての使用実態をも参考とするものとする。例えば、ある成分本質（原材料）が我が国では医薬品として承認・許可を受けたことはないが、外国において医薬品としての有効性が科学的に認められている場合には、これを勘案して当該成分本質（原材料）を「専ら医薬品として使用されている物」と判断する場合もある。

また、食品としての認識についても外国の実態を参考とする。例えば、日本では食品としての認識がない場合又は不明な場合にあっても、外国で広く食品として使用されているときには、これも参考とする。

なお、例えば、伝承的に疾病時にのみその治療又は症状の緩和の目的で使用されているものは、食品としての認識があるものとはみなさない。

(2)　上記の「基本的な考え方」に従って、判断基準により専ら医薬品として使用される成分本質（原材料）及び医薬品的効能効果を標ぼうしない限り食品と認められる成分本質（原材料）に分類する。

2　例示成分本質（原材料）の分類の変更等

(1)　通知に示された各成分本質（原材料）の分類は、国内外、特に国内における今後の食生活の変化、新たな安全性等の知見等により将来変更となる可能性がある。また、現在医薬品として使用されていない物であっても、将来医薬品として承認・許可を取得した場合には、分類が変更となる可能性がある。

その物を医薬品として開発しながら、一方で承認・許可の取得に時間と費用がかかるということで食品と称して医薬品まがいに製造・販売することは認められない。

(2)　例示された成分の末尾に「等」とされているとおり、通知に示された各成分本質（原材料）は一例であり、例示されていないことをもって各分類に該当しないということではない。

(3)　医薬品的効能効果を標ぼうしない限り医薬品と判断しない成分本質（原材料）リストに掲載されているものであっても、食品衛生法等の規制により食品又は食品添加物として使用できない場合もあることに留意すること。

3　表示、販売時の説明、広告等の内容による判断

その物の成分本質（原材料）が何であるかの判断は、通知本文にあるとおり、表示、販売時の説明、広告等の内容に基づいて行うものとする。これは、通常人には、その物の成分本質（原材料）を分析して確認することは不可能であり、その物の成分本質（原材料）が何であるかを認識するのは、その物の表示等によるほかはないためである。

したがって、実際に配合又は含有されていない成分本質（原材料）であっても、配合又は含有されている旨を標ぼうする場合には、その成分本質（原材料）が配合又は含有されているものとみなして判断する。

なお、専ら医薬品として使用される成分本質（原材料）については、当該成分本質（原材料）が配合又は含有されていることが判明した場合には、これに従って判断する。

4　着色、着香等の目的で使用される場合の取扱い

次に示すように、当該成分が医薬品の目的をもって使用されたものではない場合であって、通常人に医薬品的な認識を与えるおそれがないときには、当該成分は含有されていないものとみなして差し支えない。

If the ingredient is actually used as a drug, then in principle the Health, Labour and Welfare Minister may need to give approval/permission as a drug ; if this is needed, the actual use as a drug overseas should be referred to. For example, an ingredient(raw material)has not been given approval/permission as a drug in Japan, but if its effectiveness as a drug is scientifically proven overseas, this could be taken into account and the ingredient(raw material)could be deemed an ingredient used exclusively for drugs.

The situation overseas can also be taken into account for recognition as a food. For example, if an ingredient is not recognized as a food in Japan or the situation is unclear, the widespread use overseas of that ingredient as a food could be taken into account.

In another example, substances that traditionally are only used to alleviate symptoms or for therapy during times of sickness would not be deemed as being recognized as a food.

(2) Ingredients(raw materials)are categorized in line with the above"basic approach", based on the assessment criteria, as either ingredients(raw materials)used exclusively for drugs or as ingredients (raw materials)not deemed drugs unless claiming medicinal efficacy.

2. Examples of changes to the categories for ingredients(raw materials)

(1) The category for each ingredient(raw material)shown in the Notification could change in the future, because of changing dietary habits in Japan and overseas(particularly in Japan)or new findings on safety and other issues. Furthermore, substances not currently used as drugs could be approved/permitted as drugs in the future, in which case the categories may change.

Parties are not allowed to manufacture and market pseudo-drugs as foods while developing the substance as a drug and investing time and money into obtaining the necessary approvals/permissions.

(2) Ingredients given as an example have"etc."included after their name to indicate that the ingredients (raw materials)shown in the Notification are only examples. If a substance is not included in the examples, it does not mean that it does not belong in one of the categories.

(3) Note that even items that are included in the"List of ingredients(raw materials)not deemed drugs unless claiming medicinal efficacy"cannot in some cases be used as foods or food additives according to regulations including the Food Sanitation Act.

3. Evaluation based on the labeling, sales pitch at the time of sale, and advertising

Evaluation of what ingredients(raw materials)a substance contains is made based on the contents of labeling, sales pitch at the time of sale, advertising, and other factors, as described in the Notification text. This method is used because a layperson cannot use analysis to confirm the ingredients(raw materials)in a substance and can only rely on the labeling and other information about the substance to see what the ingredients(raw materials)are.

Accordingly, if a substance does not actually contain a particular ingredient(raw material), alone or in combination, but the item claims to contain that ingredient(raw material), alone or in combination, then the item is evaluated as though it did contain that ingredient(raw material), alone or in combination.

Note that for ingredients(raw materials)used exclusively for drugs, if it is established that the relevant ingredient(raw material)is present, alone or in combination, the item will be evaluated on this basis.

4. Treatment of items used as colorings, flavorings, etc.

As shown below, if a particular ingredient is not used for a medicinal purpose, that ingredient can be handled as though it were not present in the item if there is no chance that the ingredient will be recognized as medicinal by a layperson.

なお、この場合にあっても、食品添加物等としての使用の適否については、食品担当部局に照会するほか、表示の方法によっては、食品衛生法、不当景品類及び不当表示防止法等他法令に抵触するおそれがあるので、食品担当部局等関係部局に照会するよう指導すること。

(1)　含有されている成分が、着色、着香等の目的のために使用されているものと認められ、かつ、当該成分を含有する旨を標ぼうしない場合又は当該成分を含有する旨を標ぼうするが、その使用目的を併記する場合には、当該成分が含有されていないものとみなして差し支えない。この場合、医薬品的な効能効果、用法用量を標ぼうしないことはもちろんである。

（例）

成分本質（原材料）	用　　途
γ-オリザノール	酸化防止剤
キナ	苦味料等
ゲンチアナ	苦味料等
シコン	着色料
ニガキ	苦味料等

(2)　また、食品の製造過程において使用されたものの、最終の食品中には含有されない場合又は最終の食品中に含有される場合であっても失活している場合についても、(1)と同様、当該成分を使用した旨若しくは含有する旨を標ぼうしない場合又は当該成分を使用した旨若しくは含有する旨を標ぼうするが、その使用目的を併記する場合には、当該成分が使用又は含有されていないものとみなして差し支えない。この場合、医薬品的な効能効果、用法用量を標ぼうしないことはもちろんである。

(3)　なお、食品の製造過程において使用される物又は食品の加工保存のために使用される物が単独で流通する場合がある（例えば、調理用としての炊飯用のアミラーゼや肉軟化用のパパイン等）が、これらは医薬品の目的を有するものではないので、食品調理用である旨等その目的を明確に標ぼうする場合には、医薬品には該当しない。

（例）

成分本質（原材料）	用　　途
アミラーゼ	でんぷん質の糖化
パパイン	ビール等の清澄剤 肉軟化剤

5　抽出成分等の取扱い

「医薬品的効能効果を標ぼうしない限り医薬品と判断しない成分本質（原材料）リスト」に収載されている成分本質（原材料）であっても、水、エタノール以外の溶媒による抽出を行った場合には、当該抽出成分について、判断基準の考え方に基づいて再度検討を行い、「専ら医薬品として使用される成分本質（原材料）リスト」に収載すべきかどうか評価することとする。

例えば、玄米胚芽（米糠）等の食品中には、元来γ-オリザノール等の成分が含有されているが、このような成分をその食品から抽出精製した場合には、当該抽出成分自体の分類は、原材料となった食品の分類とは別に、当該抽出成分の医薬品又は食品としての認識の程度を勘案して判断するものとする。

Even in this case, whether a substance is suitable for use as a food additive etc. should be referred to the departments responsible for food, while enquiries about labeling methods should be referred to the relevant departments responsible for food and other matters, as there may be a conflict with the Food Sanitation Act, the Act against Unjustifiable Premiums and Misleading Representations, and other acts and ordinances.

(1) A substance can be considered to not contain a particular ingredient if the ingredient in the substance is recognized as being used for coloring, flavoring, etc. and where the product does not claim to contain the relevant ingredient or the product does claim to contain the relevant ingredient, but the labeling also includes its intended use. In this case, the substance obviously does not make any claims about medicinal efficacy and dosage and administration methods.
Example:

Ingredient(raw material)	Use
Gamma-oryzanol	Antioxidant
Cinchona	Bitter flavoring, etc.
Gentian	Bitter flavoring, etc.
Lithospermum root	Coloring
Quassia amara	Bitter flavoring, etc.

(2) Where a substance is used in the food manufacturing process but is not contained in the final food product or where it may be contained in the final food product but could be inactive, the substance can be considered to not contain the relevant ingredient, as in point(1), if the product does not claim to contain or use the relevant ingredient or the product does claim to contain or use the relevant ingredient, but the labeling also includes its intended use. In this case, the substance obviously does not make any claims about medicinal efficacy and dosage and administration methods.

(3) Substances used during food manufacturing process and substances used to preserve processed foods can be distributed separately(for example, amylase as a food preparation ingredient for rice cooking or papain to tenderize meat), but these do not have the purpose of a drug, so they are not deemed drugs if they claim to be for food preparation and clearly specify their purpose.
Example:

Ingredient(raw material)	Use
Amylase	Break down complex sugars(starch)
Papain	Clarifying agent for beer etc. Meat tenderizer

5. Handling of extracts etc.

Even ingredients(raw materials) listed on the"List of ingredients(raw materials) not deemed drugs unless claiming medicinal efficacy", if they have been extracted using a solvent other than water and/or ethanol, the extract must be re-investigated using the evaluation criteria approach and evaluated as to whether they should be listed on the"List of ingredients(raw materials) used exclusively for drugs".

For example, foods like unpolished rice germ(rice bran), etc. naturally contain gamma-oryzanol and other constituents, but if such constituents are extracted and purified from the food, the category for the relevant extract is different from the category for the food where the extract originated. The extract is evaluated with reference to the degree of recognition as a drug or a food.

玄米胚芽（米糠）は通常の食生活において食品と認識されているものであり、医薬品的効能効果を標ぼうしない限り食品と認められる成分本質（原材料）に該当するが、γ-オリザノールは、医薬品として使用されている成分であり、専ら医薬品として使用される成分本質（原材料）に該当し、玄米胚芽（米糠）とγ-オリザノールとはその取扱いが異なっている。

その物の成分本質（原材料）を例えば玄米胚芽（米糠）とみなすか又はγ-オリザノールとみなすかについては、原則としてその物の名称、原材料等の表示、説明等に基づいてその物の成分本質（原材料）がどのように認識されるかにより判断するものとし、次のすべての条件を満たす場合には、その物の成分本質（原材料）は玄米胚芽（米糠）であると判断して差し支えないものとする。

なお、この場合、その物が原材料となった食品の本質を失っていないものであることは当然である。

① 「食品」の文字を容器、被包前面及び内袋にわかりやすく記載する等食品である旨が明示されていること
② 原材料となった食品又はその加工品である旨が明示されていること
③ その物の成分本質（原材料）に誤解を与えるような特定成分の強調がなされていないこと

下表右欄に掲げる食品は、それぞれ左欄に掲げる成分を含有しているが、これらの食品を原材料とした物については、上記のすべての条件を満たす場合にあっては、その成分本質（原材料）はそれぞれ右欄に掲げる食品とみなされ、同表右欄に示す分類となる。また、上記の条件を満たさない場合であって、左欄に掲げる成分を成分本質（原材料）とする物と認識されるときには、当該品の成分本質（原材料）はそれぞれ左欄に掲げる成分とみなされ、同表左欄に示す分類となる。

成分例（専ら医薬品として使用される成分本質（原材料）に分類される物）	食品例（医薬品的効能効果を標ぼうしない限り医薬品と判断しない成分本質（原材料）に分類される物）
グルタチオン	酵母
タウリン	たこ、いわし等の魚介類加工品
γ-オリザノール	玄米胚芽（米糠）
パパイン	パパイヤ加工品
ブロメライン	パイナップル加工品

6　植物等の部位による取扱いの違い

「判定方法」の専ら医薬品として使用される成分本質（原材料）に分類される成分本質（原材料）のうち、動植物に由来する成分については、必ずしもその基源植物等の全体を指すものではなく、医薬品として使用されている部位（薬用部位）のみを指すものである。

例えば、クコについては、根皮（ジコッピ）は薬用部位に該当し、これが専ら医薬品として使用される成分本質（原材料）に分類されるが、果実及び葉は医薬品的効能効果を標ぼうしない限り食品と認められる成分本質（原材料）に分類される。

Unpolished rice germ (rice bran) is recognized as a food in normal dietary habits and is considered an ingredient (raw material) not deemed as a drug unless making claims of medicinal efficacy. However, gamma-oryzanol is an ingredient used as a drug and so is considered an ingredient (raw material) used exclusively for drugs. In this example, unpolished rice germ (rice bran) and gamma-oryzanol are therefore handled differently.

Whether a substance's ingredient (raw material) is considered, for example, unpolished rice germ (rice bran) or gamma-oryzanol is in principle determined by how the substance's name, labeling of raw materials, etc., and explanations etc. of the ingredients (raw materials) are recognized. If all the conditions given below are met, the ingredient (raw material) could be considered as unpolished rice germ (rice bran).
Note that, in this case, the properties of the food used as the raw material in this substance are not lost.

① The product is shown to be a food with the word "food" clearly written on the container, front of the outer packaging, and inner packaging.
② The product is shown to be a food raw material or a processed product of that food
③ The ingredients (raw materials) for the substance do not stress specific ingredients in a way that may cause a misunderstanding

Foods listed in the right column of the table below contain the ingredients given on the relevant line in the left column. If substances that use these foods as raw materials meet all the conditions above, their ingredients (raw materials) are considered to be the foods shown in the right column and they are categorized as shown in the right column of the table. If the substances do not meet all the conditions outlined above and they are recognized as substances with ingredients (raw materials) in the left column, the relevant ingredients (raw materials) are considered to be the ingredients shown in the left column and they are categorized as shown in the left column of the table.

Example ingredient [Substances categorized as ingredients (raw materials) used exclusively for drugs]	Example food [Substances categorized as ingredients (raw materials) not deemed drugs unless claiming medicinal efficacy]
Glutathione	Yeast
Taurine	Processed seafood products, such as octopus, sardines, etc.
Gamma-oryzanol	Unpolished rice germ (rice bran)
Papain	Processed papaya products
Bromelain	Processed pineapple products

6. Differences in handling according to plant or animal part used

Of the ingredients (raw materials) categorized using the determination methods as ingredients (raw materials) used exclusively for drugs, ingredients of animal and plant origin must not simply be described as the overall source plant or animal, but must only be described in terms of the part used as a drug (medicinal part).

For example, with the Chinese wolfberry *Lycium chinense*, the root bark (Lycium bark) is deemed a medicinal part and is categorized as an ingredient (raw material) used exclusively for drugs, but the fruit and leaves are categorized as ingredients (raw materials) not deemed drugs unless claiming medicinal efficacy.

上記のとおり医薬品として使用されている植物等には、薬用部位でなく食品として使用される部位があるが、薬用部位を使用していない場合であっても、当該生薬名又は当該基源植物名のみを標ぼうし、その使用部位を明示していないときには、薬用部位が使用されているものとみなして判断する。

7　生薬名の使用

「判定方法」の医薬品的効能効果を標ぼうしない限り医薬品と判断しない成分本質（原材料）に該当する成分本質（原材料）の中には、医薬品としても使用される物もあるため、当該成分本質（原材料）を食品として使用する場合には、食品として認識されやすいように、その成分本質（原材料）の標ぼうに当たっては、原則として基源植物名等を使用し、生薬名は使用しないこととする。これは、生薬名を使用した場合には、食品と認識されにくく、医薬品的な認識を与えるおそれがあるためである。

（例）

生　薬　名	基源植物名等
サンヤク（山薬）	ヤマノイモ、ナガイモ
ショウキョウ（生薑）	ショウガ
タイソウ（大棗）	ナツメ
ボレイ	カキ殻
ヨクイニン	ハトムギ

Ⅳ　医薬品的な効能効果について

〈通知本文抜粋〉

その物の容器、包装、添付文書並びにチラシ、パンフレット、刊行物、インターネット等の広告宣伝物あるいは演述によって、次のような効能効果が表示説明されている場合は、医薬品的な効能効果を標ぼうしているものとみなす。また、名称、含有成分、製法、起源等の記載説明においてこれと同様な効能効果を標ぼうし又は暗示するものも同様とする。

なお、食品衛生法施行規則（昭和23年厚生省令第23号）第21条第１項第１号シの規定に基づき、厚生労働大臣が定める基準に従い、栄養成分の機能の表示等をする栄養機能食品（以下「栄養機能食品」という。）にあっては、その表示等を医薬品的な効能効果と判断しないこととして差し支えない。

㈠　疾病の治療又は予防を目的とする効能効果

㈡　身体の組織機能の一般的増強、増進を主たる目的とする効能効果
　　ただし、栄養補給、健康維持等に関する表現はこの限りでない。

㈢　医薬品的な効能効果の暗示

(a)　名称又はキャッチフレーズよりみて暗示するもの

(b)　含有成分の表示及び説明よりみて暗示するもの

(c)　製法の説明よりみて暗示するもの

(d)　起源、由来等の説明よりみて暗示するもの

(e)　新聞、雑誌等の記事、医師、学者等の談話、学説、経験談などを引用又は掲載することにより暗示するもの

As shown above, plants and other substances used as drugs can have non-medicinal parts that are used as food, but even when the non-medicinal part is used, if the part used is not clearly described and the product only claims the relevant crude drug name or name of the relevant plant source, the substance is evaluated as though the medicinal part were used.

7. Use of crude drug names

Of the ingredients (raw materials) categorized using the determination methods as ingredients (raw materials) not deemed drugs unless claiming medicinal efficacy, some substances are also used as drugs, so if the relevant ingredient (raw material) is used as a food, the claims for that ingredient (raw material) should, in principle, use the name of the source plant, etc. and not the crude drug name, in order to make it more easily recognizable as a food. If the crude drug name is used, the product is difficult to recognize as a food and it could result in the product being considered a drug.

Example:

Crude drug name	Name of source plant, etc.
Sanyaku (Dioscorea Rhizoma)	Japanese yam, Chinese yam
Shokyo (Zingiberis Rhizoma)	Ginger
Taiso (Jujubae Fructus)	Jujube fruit
Borei (Ostreae Concha)	Oyster shell
Yokuinin (Coicis Semen)	Job's tears

Ⅳ. Medicinal efficacy

<Extract from the Notification text>

An item is considered to be claiming medicinal efficacy if the sales pitch or advertising material, including the substance's container, packaging, package insert or product leaflet, pamphlets, publications, or web-based advertising, displays information on efficacy as described below. The same approach is taken if information displayed, including the name, constituent ingredients, manufacturing methods, and source, claim similar efficacy or suggest as much.

Note that for foods with nutrient function claims (FNFCs) that display the function of the nutrient ingredients in accordance with the standards defined by the Health, Labour and Welfare Minister, based on the regulations outlined in Article 21-1-1 (L) of the Ministerial Ordinance for Enforcement of the Food Sanitation Act (MHW Ordinance No. 23, 1948), this labeling can be evaluated as not claiming medicinal efficacy.

(1) Efficacy to treat or prevent a disease

(2) Efficacy mainly to promote or generally augment the structure and function of the body ; this definition does not apply to expressions related to nutritional support and maintaining health.

(3) Suggestions of medicinal efficacy

 (a) Suggestions from the name or strapline

 (b) Suggestions from the display of constituent ingredients and their explanations

 (c) Suggestions from explanations of the manufacturing methods

 (d) Suggestions from explanations of the source and origin

 (e) Suggestions from publications or extracts from discussions by doctors and academics, theories, or real-life experiences, or articles in newspapers or journals, etc.

1　基本的な考え方

疾病の治療又は予防を目的とする効能効果及び身体の組織機能の一般的増強、増進を主たる目的とする効能効果の標ぼうは、医薬品的な効能効果の標ぼうに該当する。

この場合、明示的であると暗示的であるとを問わない。

また、外国語で標ぼうされた場合であっても同様に取り扱う。

2　医薬品的な効能効果の標ぼうの方法

(1)　本基準で標ぼうとは、その物の販売に関連して次により行われるすべての表示説明をいう。

①　その物の容器、包装、添付文書等の表示物

②　その物のチラシ、パンフレット等

③　テレビ、ラジオ、新聞、雑誌、インターネット等によるその物の広告

④　「驚異の○○」、「○○のすべて」等と題する小冊子、書籍

⑤　「○○の友」等の会員誌又は「○○ニュース」、「○○特報」等の情報紙

⑥　新聞、雑誌等の記事の切り抜き、書籍、学術論文等の抜粋

⑦　代理店、販売店に教育用と称して配布される商品説明（関連）資料

⑧　使用経験者の感謝文、体験談集

⑨　店内及び車内等における吊り広告

⑩　店頭、訪問先、説明会、相談会、キャッチセールス等においてスライド、ビデオ等又は口頭で行われる演述等

⑪　その他特定商品の販売に関連して利用される前記に準ずるもの

(2)　(1)の④ないし⑩により行われる標ぼうについては、特定商品名を示していない場合であっても、特定商品の説明を求める者に提供したり、特定商品を説明するものとして商品と同一売場に置いたり、特定商品の購入申込書とともに送付する等により特定商品の説明を行っているときは、当該特定商品について医薬品的な効能効果を標ぼうしているものとみなす。

すなわち、その物の容器、包装、添付文書等には医薬品的な効能効果の標ぼうは行われていないが、特定商品名を明示しない書籍、小冊子、情報紙等に医薬品的な効能効果を標ぼうし、これらを販売活動の中で特定商品に結び付けて利用している場合には、すべて当該製品についての医薬品的な効能効果の標ぼうとみなす。

3　栄養補給に関する表現

(1)　「栄養補給」の表現について

ア　「栄養補給」という表現自体は、医薬品的な効能効果には該当しないが、次のような、疾病等による栄養成分の欠乏時等を特定した表現は、医薬品的な効能効果に該当する。

（例）・病中病後の体力低下時（の栄養補給）に

・胃腸障害時（の栄養補給）に

なお、医薬品的な効能効果に該当しない表現であっても、虚偽誇大な表現については不当景品類及び不当表示防止法第4条第1号に、また、場合によっては健康増進法第32条の2等他法令に抵触するおそれがあるので、食品としての表現の適否については、栄養・食品担当部局等関係部局に照会するよう指導すること。

1. Basic approach

Claims of efficacy to treat or prevent a disease or to promote or generally augment the structure and function of the body are considered as claims for medicinal efficacy.
In this case, no distinction is made between explicitly stated or suggested claims.
Furthermore, the substance is handled the same way even if the claims were made in a foreign language.

2. Methods of claiming medicinal efficacy

(1) Claims according to these criteria are all explanations for an item for sale displayed in the following ways.

① Items displayed on the substance's container, packaging, or package insert, etc.
② Flyers, leaflets, etc. on the substance
③ Advertising for the substance via TV, radio, newspapers, journals, or the internet, etc.
④ Pamphlets and books with titles like "Miracle XXX" or "All XXX", etc.
⑤ Member-only magazines such as "Friends of XXX" or publications such as "XXX News" or "XX Special Edition"
⑥ Clippings of articles from newspapers or journals, etc. and extracts from books or scientific papers, etc.
⑦ Product information (related) materials distributed in the name of education at agents and sales outlets
⑧ Expressions of thanks by product users and compilations of testimonies
⑨ Hanging advertising in stores or vehicles
⑩ Presentations etc. conducted using slides, by video, or orally in stores, during visits, at briefing meetings, at roundtable discussions, or unscrupulous sales practices
⑪ Other practices that comply with the above used for the sale of specific products

(2) For claims made as described in points (1)-④ through (1)-⑩ above, even if the specific product name is not stated, the conclusion is that claims for medicinal efficacy for that specific product are being made if information on a specific product is given by way of supply to an individual requesting information on that product, placement of specific product information in the same sales space as the product, or dispatch along with a purchasing form for that specific product.

Therefore, claims for medicinal efficacy are being made for all products where claims for medicinal efficacy are made in books, pamphlets, or information sheets that do not mention the specific product's name and where these items are linked to the specific product during sales activities, even if no claims for medicinal efficacy are made on the product's container, packaging, or package insert, etc.

3. Expressions related to nutritional support

(1) Expressions used for nutritional support

a) The actual phrase "nutritional supplement" is not considered as medicinal efficacy, but specific expressions on nutritional deficiencies caused by diseases etc., as shown below, are considered to be medicinal efficacy.

Example: · (Nutritional support) for when the body is weak during and after a disease
· (Nutritional support) for gastrointestinal dysfunction

Even with expressions not considered to be medicinal efficacy, there can be conflicts with Article 4-1-1 of the Act against Unjustifiable Premiums and Misleading Representations or in some cases Article 32-2 of the Health Promotion Act and other acts and ordinances if any false and exaggerated language is used. Departments responsible for nutrition/food and other relevant departments should be contacted for guidance on the suitability of expressions for food.

イ　特定時期の栄養補給については、正常状態でありながら通常の生理現象として特に栄養成分の需要が増大することが医学的、栄養学的に確認されている発育期、妊娠授乳期等において、その栄養成分の補給ができる旨の表現は、直ちに医薬品的な効能効果には該当しない。

なお、この場合にあっても、虚偽誇大な表現については不当景品類及び不当表示防止法第４条第１号に、また、場合によっては健康増進法第32条の２等他法令に抵触するおそれがあるので、食品としての表現の適否については、栄養・食品担当部局等関係部局に照会するよう指導すること。

ウ　栄養補給と標ぼうしながら、頭髪、目、皮膚等の特定部位への栄養補給ができる旨を標ぼうし、当該部位の改善、増強等ができる旨暗示する表現は、医薬品的な効能効果に該当する。

(2)　栄養成分に関する表現について

ア　栄養成分の体内における作用を示す表現は、医薬品的な効能効果に該当する。ただし、栄養機能食品において、栄養成分の機能として認められた表示の範囲を除く。

(例)・○○は体内でホルモンのバランスを調整しています。

なお、特定商品に関連しない栄養に関する一般的な知識の普及については、この限りでない。

イ　具体的な作用を標ぼうせずに単に健康維持に重要であることを示す表現又はタンパク質、カルシウム等生体を構成する栄養成分について構成成分であることを示す表現は、直ちに医薬品的な効能効果には該当しない。

なお、この場合にあっても、虚偽誇大な表現については不当景品類及び不当表示防止法第４条第１号に、また、場合によっては健康増進法第32条の２等他法令に抵触するおそれがあるので、食品としての表現の適否については、栄養・食品担当部局等関係部局に照会するよう指導すること。

４「健康維持」、「健康増進」等の表現

(1)「健康維持」、「美容」の表現は、医薬品的な効能効果に該当しない。

なお、虚偽誇大な表現については不当景品類及び不当表示防止法第４条第１号に、また、場合によっては健康増進法第32条の２等他法令に抵触するおそれがあるので、食品としての表現の適否については、栄養・食品担当部局等関係部局に照会するよう指導すること。

(2)「健康増進」の表現は、身体諸機能の向上を暗示するものであるが、「食品」の文字を容器、被包前面及び内袋にわかりやすく記載する等食品である旨が明示されている場合であって、総合的に判断して医薬品と認識されるおそれのないことが明らかなときには、「健康増進」の標ぼうのみをもって医薬品に該当するとは断定できないものの、虚偽誇大な表現については不当景品類及び不当表示防止法第４条第１号に、また、場合によっては健康増進法第32条の２等他法令に抵触するおそれがあるので、食品としての表現の適否については、栄養・食品担当部局等関係部局に照会するよう指導すること。

b) Expressions on providing nutritional support are not immediately considered as medicinal efficacy if they are for nutritional support at specific times, for example during periods of growth, pregnancy, or lactation where the individual is in a normal condition but there are increased nutritional demands as part of the normal physiology, confirmed medically and nutritionally.
Even under these circumstances, there can be conflicts with Article 4-1-1 of the Act against Unjustifiable Premiums and Misleading Representations or in some cases Article 32-2 of the Health Promotion Act and other acts and ordinances if any false and exaggerated language is used. Departments responsible for nutrition/food and other relevant departments should be contacted for guidance on the suitability of expressions for food.

c) Expressions are considered to be medicinal efficacy if claims are made for nutritional support and the language claims that it is possible to provide nutritional support for specific areas, such as the hair, eyes, or skin, or the language suggests it is possible to improve or strengthen a particular area.

(2) Expressions relating to nutrients

a) Expressions on the actions of nutrients within the body are considered to be medicinal efficacy. However, this excludes the approved range of expressions on nutrient functions for FNFCs.
Example: ・XX adjusts the hormone balance within the body
Note that this definition does not apply to the use of general knowledge on nutrition not related to a specific product.

b) Expressions indicating an important role in simply maintaining health without claims for a specific action or expressions indicating a nutrient plays a structural role in the body, such as proteins or calcium, are not immediately considered to be medicinal efficacy.
Even in this case, there can be conflicts with Article 4-1-1 of the Act against Unjustifiable Premiums and Misleading Representations or in some cases Article 32-2 of the Health Promotion Act and other acts and ordinances if any false and exaggerated language is used. Departments responsible for nutrition/food and other relevant departments should be contacted for guidance on the suitability of expressions for food.

4. Expressions on"maintaining health"or"promoting health"

(1) Expressions on"maintaining health"or"beauty"are not considered to be claiming medicinal efficacy.
Note that there can be conflicts with Article 4-1-1 of the Act against Unjustifiable Premiums and Misleading Representations or in some cases Article 32-2 of the Health Promotion Act and other acts and ordinances if any false and exaggerated language is used. Departments responsible for nutrition/food and other relevant departments should be contacted for guidance on the suitability of expressions for food.

(2) Expressions on"promoting health"suggest improved bodily functions. However, the claim can be decided as only for"promoting health"and the product not considered a drug if a comprehensive evaluation has determined that there is clearly no possibility of the product being recognized as a drug, for example if a product is clearly labeled as a food with the word"Food"clearly written on the container, front of the outer packaging, or inner packaging. Note that there can be conflicts with Article 4-1-1 of the Act against Unjustifiable Premiums and Misleading Representations or in some cases Article 32-2 of the Health Promotion Act and other acts and ordinances if any false and exaggerated language is used. Departments responsible for nutrition/food and other relevant departments should be contacted for guidance on the suitability of expressions for food.

5　医薬品的な効能効果の暗示

次に掲げるような方法による医薬品的な効能効果の暗示は、いずれも医薬品的な効能効果を標ぼうするものに該当する。

これらに該当するもののうち文学的、詩歌的表現については、成分本質（原材料）、形状等を勘案し、総合的に判断して当該品が直ちに医薬品に該当しない場合もあるが、原則としては医薬品的な効能効果の標ぼうに該当する。

(1)　名称又はキャッチフレーズよりみて暗示するもの

(例)・薬○○
・漢方秘法

(2)　含有成分の表示及び説明よりみて暗示するもの

(例)・体質改善、健胃整腸で知られる○○○○を原料とし、これに有用成分を添加、相乗効果をもつ。

(3)　製法の説明よりみて暗示するもの

(例)・本邦の深山高原に自生する植物○○○○を主剤に、△△△、×××等の薬草を独特の製造法（製法特許出願）によって調整したものである。

(4)　起源、由来等の説明よりみて暗示するもの

「神農本草経」や「本草綱目」などの古書の薬効に関する記載の引用等により古来より薬効が認められていることを示す表現もこれに該当する。

(例)・○○○という古い自然科学書をみると胃を開き、鬱（うつ）を散じ、消化を助け、虫を殺し、痰なども無くなるとある。こうした経験が昔から伝えられたが故に食膳に必ず備えられたものである。

(5)　新聞、雑誌等の記事、医師、学者等の談話、学説、経験談などを引用又は掲載することにより暗示するもの

(例)・医学博士○○○○の談
「昔から赤飯に○○○をかけて食べると癌にかからぬといわれている。……癌細胞の脂質代謝異常ひいては糖質、蛋白代謝異常と○○○が結びつき　はしないかと考えられる。」

(6)　高麗人参と同等又はそれ以上の薬効を有する旨の表現により暗示するもの

(例)・高麗人参にも勝るという薬効が認められています。

(7)「健康チェック」等として、身体の具合、症状等をチェックさせ、それぞれの症状等に応じて摂取を勧めることにより暗示するもの

(8)「○○○の方に」等の表現により暗示するもの

「○○○の方にお勧めします。」等の摂取を勧める対象を示す表現は、次に示すように対象者の表現如何によっては医薬品的な効能効果に該当する。

5. Suggestions of medicinal efficacy

Suggestions of medicinal efficacy using one of the methods listed below are all considered claims for medicinal efficacy.

The use of literary or poetic expressions may, in principle, be considered as claims of medicinal efficacy, although a product may not immediately be deemed a drug following a comprehensive assessment taking into account the ingredients (raw materials) and shape, etc.

(1) Suggestions from the name or strapline

Examples: ・Drug XX

・Secret Kampo medicine (traditional Japanese medicine)/traditional Chinese medicine formula

(2) Suggestions from the display of ingredients and their explanations

Example: ・XXXX, known to improve the constitution and regulate gastrointestinal function, is used as a raw material, providing additional synergistic effects with these useful ingredients.

(3) Suggestions from explanations of the manufacturing methods

Example: ・The plant XXXX native to the deep mountain tablelands of Japan is the main agent, combined with YYY, ZZZ, and other medicinal plants using a special manufacturing method (patent pending)

(4) Suggestions from explanations of the source and origin

This refers to expressions that suggest drug efficacy was recognized in ancient times, based on quotations on drug efficacy in ancient tomes such as Shennong Bencao Jing (Shennong's Herb-Root Classic) and Bencao Gangmu (Compendium of Materia Medica).

Example: ・According to XXX, an ancient book on the natural sciences, this stimulates appetite, eliminates depression, aids digestion, cures bad moods, and improves maladies. This experience has been handed down through the ages and is something that should be added to all food.

(5) Suggestions from publications or extracts from discussions by doctors and academics, theories, or real-life experiences, or articles in newspapers or journals, etc.

Example: ・Conversation with XXXX M.D.

"Long ago, it was said that if you ate sekihan festive red rice sprinkled with YYY, you would not get cancer … It is possible that abnormalities in the lipid metabolism or sugar/protein metabolism in cancer cells could be linked to ZZZ."

(6) Suggestions from expressions on drug efficacy equivalent or superior to Asian ginseng (*Panax ginseng*)

Example: ・Known to be more efficacious than Asian ginseng

(7) Suggestions that recommend ingestion in line with each individual symptom, through a health check-up that assesses physical health, symptoms, and other factors

(8) Suggestions using expressions like "For those with XXX"

Expressions that recommend particular individuals ingest the food, such as "Recommended for those with XXX", are considered to be claiming medicinal efficacy depending on the type of expressions used for the target audience, as shown below.

なお、医薬品的な効能効果に該当しない場合にあっても、虚偽誇大な表現については不当景品類及び不当表示防止法第４条第１号に、また、場合によっては健康増進法第32条の２等他法令に抵触するおそれがあるので、食品としての表現の適否については、栄養・食品担当部局等関係部局に照会するよう指導すること。

ア　疾病を有する者、疾病の予防を期待する者、好ましくない身体状態にある者を対象とする旨の表現は、医薬品的な効能効果に該当する。

（例）・便秘ぎみの方に
　　　・○○病が気になる方に
　　　・身体がだるく、疲れのとれない方に

イ　「健康維持」、「美容」を目的とする趣旨の表現は、直ちに医薬品的な効能効果には該当しない。

（例）・健康を保ちたい方に

ウ　「栄養補給」を目的とする趣旨の表現は、直ちに医薬品的な効能効果には該当しない。

（例）・偏食がちな方に
　　　・野菜の足りない方に

⑼　「好転反応」に関する表現により暗示するもの

「摂取すると、一時的に下痢、吹出物などの反応がでるが、体内浄化、体質改善等の効果の現れである初期症状であり、そのまま摂取を続けることが必要である」等として不快症状が出ても、それを「好転反応」、「めんけん（瞑眩）反応」等と称して効果の証であると説明しているものがあるが、このような標ぼうは、医薬品的な効能効果の標ぼうに該当する。

なお、このような表現は、危害の発見を遅らせ、適正な医療の機会を失わせる等の保健衛生上の危害が発生するおそれが強い。

⑽　「効用」、「効果」、「ききめ」等の表現により暗示するもの

疾病名等の具体的な表現はしないが、特定製品の摂取により、「効果」、「効用」、「ききめ」又は「効能効果」等がある旨を標ぼうすることは、成分本質（原材料）、形状等の如何によっては医薬品的な認識を与えることとなるので、医薬品的な効能効果の標ぼうに該当するおそれがある。

（例）・１か月以上飲み続けないと効果はありません。
　　　・大学病院でもその効用が認められています。
　　　・医薬品のように速効性はありませんが、２～３か月飲み続ければ、その効果は必ずお分かりいただけます。

⑾　「薬」の文字により暗示するもの

（例）・生薬、妙薬、民間薬、薬草、漢方薬
　　　・薬用されている、薬効が認められる健康茶であるため薬効は表示できませんが、詳しくは「神農本草経」、「本草綱目」、「広辞苑」などでお調べ下さい。

Note that even if the product is not considered to be claiming medicinal efficacy, there can be conflicts with Article 4-1-1 of the Act against Unjustifiable Premiums and Misleading Representations or in some cases Article 32-2 of the Health Promotion Act and other acts and ordinances if any false and exaggerated language is used. Departments responsible for nutrition/food and other relevant departments should be contacted for guidance on the suitability of expressions for food.

a) A product is considered to be claiming medicinal efficacy if it uses expressions targeting individuals with a disease, individuals hoping to prevent a disease, or individuals in poor physical condition.

Example:

・For those prone to constipation
・For those concerned about XX disease
・For those who feel sluggish or constantly tired

b) Expressions on"maintaining health"or"beauty"are not immediately considered to be claiming medicinal efficacy.

Example:

・For those who want to stay healthy

c) Expressions on"nutritional support"are not immediately considered to be claiming medicinal efficacy.

Example:

・For those who tend to have an unbalanced diet
・For those who don't eat enough vegetables

(9) Suggestions from expressions on"detoxification reactions"

A product is considered to be claiming medicinal efficacy if unpleasant symptoms are described as"detoxification reactions"or"a healing crisis"and are explained as proving the product is taking effect, for example claims that"when the product is taken, you may experience a temporary reaction such as diarrhea or acne, but this is just the first signs of the body cleansing itself and your health improving ; it is important to keep taking the product".

Note that such expressions could cause harm from a health and hygiene perspective if there is a delay in discovering the problem or the individual misses out on the opportunity to seek appropriate healthcare.

(10) Suggestions from expressions such as"benefit","useful", or"effective"

Products could be considered to be claiming medicinal efficacy if they do not specify the disease name, but they do claim"benefit","useful","effective", or"efficacy"because there is a recognized medicinal impact depending on the ingredients(raw materials)or form, etc.

Examples:

・Only effective when taken continuously for one month or more
・This product is even recognized by university hospitals as useful.
・Will not produce a rapid effect like a pharmaceutical, but you will definitely see benefits when taken continuously for two or three months.

(11) Suggestions from the words"drug"or"medicine"

Examples:

・Crude drug, wonder drug, folk medicine, medicinal plant, Kampo medicine(traditional Japanese medicine)/traditional Chinese medicine
・This is a health tea for medicinal use recognized for its efficacy ; details of the efficacy cannot be displayed here ; for more information please refer to the Shennong Bencao Jing(Shennong's Herb-Root Classic), Bencao Gangmu(Compendium of Materia Medica), or Kojien Japanese Dictionary.

Ⅴ　医薬品的な形状について

〈通知本文抜粋〉

錠剤、丸剤、カプセル剤及びアンプル剤のような剤型は、一般に医薬品に用いられる剤型として認識されてきており、これらの剤型とする必要のあるものは、医薬品的性格を有するものが多く、また、その物の剤型のほかに、その容器又は被包の意匠及び形態が市販されている医薬品と同じ印象を与える場合も、通常人が当該製品を医薬品と認識する大きな要因となっていることから、原則として、医薬品的形状であった場合は、医薬品に該当するとの判断が行われてきた。

しかし、現在、成分によって、品質管理等の必要性が認められる場合には、医薬品的形状の錠剤、丸剤又はカプセル剤であっても、直ちに、医薬品に該当するとの判断が行われておらず、実態として、従来、医薬品的形状とされてきた形状の食品が消費されるようになってきていることから、「食品」である旨が明示されている場合、原則として、形状のみによって医薬品に該当するか否かの判断は行わないこととする。ただし、アンプル形状など通常の食品としては流通しない形状を用いることなどにより、消費者に医薬品と誤認させることを目的としていると考えられる場合は、医薬品と判断する必要がある。

(1)　その物の形状とは、剤型（アンプル剤、ハードカプセル剤、ソフトカプセル剤、錠剤、丸剤、粉末状・顆粒状及びこれらの分包、液状等）のほか、ガラスビン、紙箱、ビニール袋等のその物の容器又は被包の形態や、その容器又は被包に書かれている図案、写真、図面及び表示されている文字の字体、デザイン等のすべてを含んだものをいう。その物の形状が医薬品的であるか否かの判断は、その物の剤型のほか、その容器又は被包の意匠及び形態を総合的に勘案し、通常人に医薬品的な形状であるとの認識を与えるか否かによりなされるものである。

(2)　専ら医薬品的な剤型である物を除き、その容器等に「食品」である旨を明示している場合は、原則、形状のみによって医薬品に該当するか否かの判断は行わないこととする。ただし、剤型、その物の容器又は被包の形態等のすべてを総合的に判断し、通常人に医薬品と誤認させることを目的としていると考えられる場合は、専ら医薬品的な形状に該当する。

(3)　専ら医薬品的な剤型である物は、その容器又は被包の意匠及び形態の如何にかかわらず、専ら医薬品的形状に該当する。

(4)　専ら医薬品的な剤型には、アンプル剤のほか、用法を考慮して、舌下錠や液状のもののうち舌下に滴下するもの等粘膜からの吸収を目的とするもの、液状のもののうちスプレー管に充填して口腔内に噴霧して口腔内に作用させることを目的とするもの等がある。

V. Medicinal form

<Extract from the Notification text>

Dosage forms such as tablets, pills, capsules, and ampoules are generally recognized as being the dosage forms used for pharmaceuticals. In many cases, these dosage forms are needed because of the medicinal properties of the product. As well as the dosage form, products marketed in containers, packaging designs, or shapes that give the same impression as a pharmaceutical could be recognized by the layperson as a drug. Therefore, in the past, if a product has a medicinal form, in principle it has been deemed a drug.

However, today, not all products with medicinal forms(tablets, pills, or capsules)are immediately deemed a drug if there is a recognized need for that form depending on the ingredient(for example for quality management purposes). In practice, because foods are now consumed in forms previously considered to be medicinal, if the product clearly states that it is a"food", in principle the product will not be deemed a drug purely because of its form. However, if the product is supplied as an ampoule or another form that is not usual for a normal food and the design is considered to be for the purpose of misleading the consumer into thinking it is a drug, then the product must be deemed a drug.

(1) A substance's form includes the dosage form(ampoule, hard capsule, soft capsule, tablet, pill, powder/granules and powder/granules in individual sachet doses or liquid forms)as well as the form of the container or packaging for that substance(glass bottle, paper box, or plastic bag)and the design(diagrams, photographs, words on the container or packaging). Whether a substance is in a medicinal form is determined according to whether a layperson would recognize it as a medicinal form, taking into full account the dosage form and the shape and design of the container or packaging.

(2) Apart from substances that have a dosage form used exclusively for pharmaceuticals, if the container etc. clearly states that it is a"food", in principle the product will not be deemed a drug purely because of its form. However, if a comprehensive assessment has been made of the dosage form, shape of the container or packaging, etc. and the design is considered to be for the purpose of misleading the consumer into thinking it is a drug, then the product is deemed a drug.

(3) Substances that have a dosage form used exclusively for pharmaceuticals will be deemed as having a form used exclusively for pharmaceuticals regardless of the shape and design of the container or packaging.

(4) Dosage forms used exclusively for pharmaceuticals include ampoules, as well as substances that are intended for absorption via mucous membranes(for example, sublingual tablets or liquid forms that are dropped under the tongue), and substances that are intended to act within the mouth cavity (whereby a spray can is filled with the substance in a liquid form for spraying in the mouth).

Ⅵ　医薬品的な用法用量について

〈通知本文抜粋〉

医薬品は、適応疾病に対し治療又は予防効果を発揮し、かつ、安全性を確保するために、服用時期、服用間隔、服用量等の詳細な用法用量を定めることが必要不可欠である。したがって、ある物の使用方法として服用時期、服用間隔、服用量等の記載がある場合には、原則として医薬品的な用法用量とみなすものとし、次のような事例は、これに該当するものとする。ただし、調理の目的のために、使用方法、使用量等を定めているものについてはこの限りでない。

一方、食品であっても、過剰摂取や連用による健康被害が起きる危険性、その他合理的な理由があるものについては、むしろ積極的に摂取の時期、間隔、量等の摂取の際の目安を表示すべき場合がある。

これらの実態等を考慮し、栄養機能食品にあっては、時期、間隔、量等摂取の方法を記載することについて、医薬品的用法用量には該当しないこととして差し支えない。

ただし、この場合においても、「食前」「食後」「食間」など、通常の食品の摂取時期等とは考えられない表現を用いるなど医薬品と誤認させることを目的としていると考えられる場合においては、引き続き医薬品的用法用量の表示とみなすものとする。

（例）１日２～３回、１回２～３粒
　　　１日２個
　　　毎食後、添付のサジで２杯づつ
　　　成人１日３～６錠
　　　食前、食後に１～２個づつ
　　　お休み前に１～２粒

1　基本的な考え方

(1)　医薬品は、疾病の治療、予防等の使用目的を有し、そのために服用されるものであるから、その目的を達成するためには一定量を服用する必要がある一方、過量に服用した場合にはその薬理作用のためかえって有害作用を及ぼすおそれもあり、有効性、安全性を確保するためには、その服用に関する詳細な指示が必要である。このため、医薬品には、その有効性、安全性の確保という観点から、用法用量として服用時期、服用間隔、服用量が定められている。

(2)　その物の用法用量、特に服用時期及び服用間隔は、その物に一定の効果を期待して初めて設定できる性格の強いものであり、これを定めることは、一定の効果を期待して用法用量が記載されている医薬品と認識されやすい。

したがって、その物の使用方法として、服用時期、服用間隔、服用量等の標ぼうのある場合には、原則として医薬品的な用法用量とみなすものとする。

(3)　一方、食品であっても、過剰摂取や連用による健康被害が起きる危険性、その他合理的な理由があるものについては、むしろ積極的に摂取の時期、間隔、量等の摂取の際の目安を表示すべき場合がある。

これらの実態等を考慮し、栄養機能食品にあっては、時期、間隔、量等摂取の方法を記載することについて、医薬品的用法用量には該当しないこととして差し支えない。

Ⅵ. Medicinal dosage and administration methods

<Extract from the Notification text>

Pharmaceuticals treat or prevent the indicated disease and detailed dosage and administration methods must be defined (including timing of administration, intervals between administration, and dose to be administered) in order to ensure safety. Therefore, if information is provided on the timing of administration, intervals between administration, and dose to be administered etc. for a substance, in principle, these are considered to be medicinal dosage and administration methods. The examples given below meet this definition. However, this definition does not apply to usage methods and usage amounts etc. defined for the purpose of food preparation.

When a substance is a food but there is a risk of harm to health from over consumption or continuous use or there is some other rational explanation, the product should claim suggested standards for when the product should be used, at what intervals, and in what amounts.

Given the above, FNFCs may be deemed as not having medicinal dosage and administration methods if they provide information on when the product should be used, at what intervals, and in what amounts.

However, even in this case, a product will be deemed as claiming medicinal dosage and administration methods if it uses expressions not normally associated with eating normal food (for example, before eating, after eating, or between meals) with the intent of misleading the consumer into thinking the product is a drug.

Examples: A dose of two or three pieces taken two or three times daily
Two pieces per day
Two spoonfuls (using the attached spoon) after every meal
3–6 tablets a day for adults
One or two pieces before or after meal
One or two pieces before bed

1. Basic approach

(1) Pharmaceuticals are used to treat or prevent disease, etc. and are taken for this purpose, so they need to be taken in specific amounts if they are to achieve their purpose. However, if taken in excessive amounts, the pharmacological action can have a harmful effect. Therefore, in order to ensure both efficacy and safety, detailed instructions are needed on how they should be taken. Therefore, dosage and administration methods define when the drug should be taken, at what intervals, and in what dose in order to ensure the drug is both effective and safe.

(2) The dosage and administration methods for a substance, particularly the timing and intervals, are first set according to the expected effects of the substance. The use of defined dosage and administration methods means that a product could be recognized as a drug with dosage and administration methods that are expected to produce a certain effect.
Therefore, if the usage methods for a substance include when to take the substance, at what interval, and in what amount, in principle that substance will be deemed as having medicinal dosage and administration methods.

(3) However, when a substance is a food but there is a risk of harm to health from overconsumption or continuous use or there is some other rational explanation, the product should claim suggested standards for when the product should be used, at what intervals, and in what amounts.
In light of the above, FNFCs may be deemed as not having medicinal dosage and administration methods if they provide information on when the product should be used, at what intervals, and in what amounts.

(4)　ただし、この場合においても、「食前」「食後」「食間」など、通常の食品の摂取時期等とは考えられない表現を用いるなど医薬品と誤認させることを目的としていると考えられる場合においては、引き続き医薬品的用法用量の表示とみなすものとする。

2　医薬品的な用法用量の範囲

医薬品的な用法用量の範囲は、次のとおりである。

(1)　服用時期、服用間隔、服用量等を定めるものは、医薬品的な用法用量に該当する。

（例）・1日3回毎食後、1回2粒が適当です。

・1日1回添付の小サジで、大人は3杯、小児は1杯半、幼児は1杯です。この使用量をよく守ることが大切です。サジですくって、直接嘗めとって下さい。湯や水に溶かして飲むのは良法ではありません。

・本製品は、1日2～3回、1回につき2～3粒程度お飲み下さい。なお、○○を飲用後、体調がよくなった場合は、1日3回から2回、2回から1回と、徐々に回数を減らし、その後も1日1回、2～3粒程度お飲み下さい。

(2)　症状に応じた用法用量を定めるものは、医薬品的な用法用量に該当する。

（例）・高血圧の方は、1日に10粒
便秘の方は、1日に3粒
適宜、体調にあわせてお召し上がり下さい。

・便秘の特にひどい方（便秘薬の常用の方）は、夜の空腹時に便秘薬を飲み、朝の空腹時に○○○を飲んで下さい。便秘がよくなれば便秘薬より○○○だけを飲んで下さい。

・心臓が弱い方や病気中の方は、一週間程度は通常量の倍ぐらいの量にし、様子を見て下さい。

(3)　一日量を定めるものは、服用時期、服用間隔を示さない場合であっても、医薬品的な認識を与えるおそれがあるので、原則として医薬品的な用法用量に該当するが、「食品」の文字を容器、被包前面及び内袋にわかりやすく記載する等食品である旨を明記する場合であって次に該当するときは、直ちに医薬品的な用法用量には該当しない。

なお、この場合であっても、食品についての表現の適否については、栄養・食品担当部局等関係部局に照会するよう指導すること。

ア　原材料となった食品との相関を示し、原材料となった食品の通常の食生活における摂取量等を勘案して、適当量を一応の目安として定めるもの

（例）・本品○粒は100gのマイワシ○匹分に相当するビタミンが含まれていますので、日常の食事の内容に応じて適宜お召し上がり頂いて結構です。

イ　「栄養補給の食品として」等食品としての目安量であることを明示して、適当量を一応の目安として定めるもの

(4) However, even in this case, a product will be deemed as claiming medicinal dosage and administration methods if it uses expressions not normally associated with eating normal food (for example, before meal, after meal, or between meals) with the intent of misleading the consumer into thinking the product is a drug.

2. Scope of medicinal dosage and administration methods

The scope of medicinal dosage and administration methods is as follows.

(1) The definition of when the product should be taken, at what intervals, and in what dose etc. is deemed as a medicinal dosage and administration method.

Examples:
- Two pieces taken three times daily after meals
- Once daily dosing with 3 spoonfuls for adults, 1.5 spoonfuls for children, and 1 spoonful for infants. It is important to use the exact amounts. Measure using the spoon and take immediately. Dissolving in hot or cold water is not recommended.
- Around two or three pieces of this product should be taken two or three times daily. If the condition improves after taking XX, gradually reduce the dose from three times to two times daily, then from twice to once daily. Thereafter, take two or three pieces once daily.

(2) Dosage and administration methods defined according to symptoms are deemed to be medicinal dosage and administration methods.

Examples:
- Ten pieces daily for those with high blood pressure
  Three pieces daily for those with constipation
  Please take in appropriate amounts according to your physical condition
- Individuals with particularly bad constipation (who are constantly taking laxatives) should take a laxative on an empty stomach at night and take XXX on an empty stomach in the morning. Once the constipation improves, only take XXX instead of a laxative.
- Individuals with a weak heart or who are sick should take double the usual amount for around 1 week and see how they progress.

(3) Defining a daily dose could be recognized as medicinal, even if when to take the product and at what intervals is not specified, so in principle a product with a defined daily dose is deemed as having a medicinal dosage and administration method. However, a product may not immediately be deemed as having a medicinal dosage and administration method if it is clearly marked as a food (for example with the word "food" clearly marked on the container, front of the outer packaging, and inner packaging) and it complies with the definitions listed below.

Note that even in this case enquiries should be made with the departments responsible for nutrition/food and other relevant departments as to whether the expressions used are appropriate for a food.

a) Items that have a correlation with food used as a raw material and where general standards are defined for appropriate amounts to take with consideration to the amounts of raw material food that is ingested with normal dietary habits.

Example:
- X pieces of this product contain same amount of vitamins as found in 100g sardines, so this product can be enjoyed in appropriate amounts as part of your daily diet.

b) "Foods for nutritional support" and other products that display suggested standards for the food amounts and define general standards for appropriate amounts

(例)・栄養補給の食品として1日10粒ぐらい（○～○個、○個以内）を目安としてお召し上がりになるのが適当です。

(4)　1か月、3か月等一定期間の服用量を目安として定めるものは、1日の服用量を容易に換算できることから、1日量を定めるものと同様と考えられるが、「食品」の文字を容器、被包前面及び内袋にわかりやすく記載する等食品である旨を明記する場合には、直ちに医薬品的な用法用量には該当しない。

なお、この場合であっても、食品についての表現の適否については、栄養・食品担当部局等関係部局に照会するよう指導すること。

(例)・1か月に約3瓶を目安として適宜お召し上がり下さい。

(5)　服用時期を定めるものは、「食後のデザートに」、「ティータイムに」、「食事とともに」等医薬品の服用時期の表現とはみなされない場合のほかは、原則として医薬品的な用法用量に該当するが、当該食品のより効率的な摂取を図るために摂取時期を定める必要があると客観的に認められる場合にあっては、「食品」の文字を容器、被包前面及び内袋にわかりやすく記載する等食品である旨を明記して摂取時期を定めることは、直ちに医薬品的な用法用量には該当しない。

なお、この場合であっても、食品についての表現の適否については、栄養・食品担当部局等関係部局に照会するよう指導すること。

3　摂取方法、調理法等の表現

(1)　医薬品に特有な服用方法と同様の表現は、医薬品的な認識を与えるおそれがある。

(例)・オブラートに包んでお飲み下さい。

(2)　次のような食品としての摂取方法、調理法等を示すものは、医薬品的な用法用量には該当しない。

なお、この場合であっても、食品についての表現の適否については、栄養・食品担当部局等関係部局に照会するよう指導すること。

ア　水、ミルク、ジュース等の飲料に溶いて摂取するものなどその使用方法、使用量等を定めているもの

(例)・そのまま飲まれても結構ですが、ジュース、ミルクに溶かして飲まれると美味です。

・1パックに水500cc程を注いで、4～5分してからお飲み下さい。

・本品は、添付のカップ1杯を5倍にうすめてお飲み下さい。

・噛んでおいしくお召し上がり下さい。

イ　調理の目的のために使用するもので、その使用方法、使用量等を定めているもの

(例)・炊飯時に1合のお米に対して、1粒入れて炊きますとおいしく炊き上がります。

・スープ、みそ汁、煮物等お料理にお使い下さい。

Example:
・Around ten pieces(X-Y pieces, no more than Z pieces)can be taken daily as a food for nutritional support

(4) Products that define standards for the amount to be taken over a particular period, such as one month or three months, can be easily converted to daily amounts to be taken, so are considered to be the same as products defining daily amounts. However, a product may not immediately be deemed as having a medicinal dosage and administration method if it is clearly marked as a food(for example with the word"food"clearly marked on the container, front of the outer packaging, and inner packaging).
Note that even in this case enquiries should be made with the departments responsible for nutrition/food and other relevant departments as to whether the expressions used are appropriate for a food.
Example: Enjoy in appropriate amounts, such as around three bottles over a one-month period.

(5) Products that define when they should be taken, even if they use expressions not deemed as medicinal, such as"for dessert after your meal","for a tea break", and"with your meal", are considered in principle to have medicinal dosage and administration methods. However, a product may not immediately be deemed as having a medicinal dosage and administration method if it is subjectively recognized as requiring definitions for when to ingest in order to make eating this food more effective and the product is clearly marked as a food(for example with the word"food"clearly marked on the container, front of the outer packaging, and inner packaging).
Note that even in this case enquiries should be made with the departments responsible for nutrition/food and other relevant departments as to whether the expressions used are appropriate for a food.

3. Expressions on how to eat or prepare

(1) Expressions similar to special administration methods for pharmaceuticals may result in the product being recognized as a drug.
Example: ・Wrap in oblate(thin film of edible starch)before taking

(2) Products with the following methods for food ingestion and preparation are not considered to have medicinal dosage and administration methods.
Note that even in this case enquiries should be made with the departments responsible for nutrition/food and other relevant departments as to whether the expressions used are appropriate for a food.

a) Defined usage methods and amounts that include dissolving in water, milk, juice, or another drink before taking
Example: ・Can be taken as is, but also tastes great when dissolved in juice or milk first.
・Pour one pack into around 500mL of water and leave for four or five minutes before drinking.
・Dilute one cup(attached)of this product five times before drinking.
・Tasty when chewed.

b) Usage methods and amounts defined for use in food preparation
Example: ・Add one piece for every cup of rice being cooked for a better taste
・Use in soups, miso soup, and stews

(3)　医薬品的な用法用量に該当しない摂取方法、調理法等を標ぼうする場合であっても、「用法用量」といった医薬品的な標題を付さず、「召し上がり方」等の食品的な標題とし、医薬品的な認識を与えないようにする必要がある。

4　栄養補給のための摂取量の表現

不必要な摂取を抑え又は過量摂取による危害を防ぐため、摂取量を示す次の例のような表現は、直ちに医薬品的な用法用量には該当しないが、必要量を超えて通常の食品では摂取できないほど多量で、薬理作用が期待できる程度の量を勧める摂取量の表現は、栄養補給に必要な量を示す表現とは認められず、医薬品的な用法用量に該当するおそれがある。

なお、医薬品的な用法用量に該当しない場合であっても、健康増進法第32条の２等他法令に抵触するおそれがあるので、食品についての表現の適否については、栄養・食品担当部局等関係部局に照会するよう指導すること。

(例)・通常１日１粒で必要な栄養成分の補給ができます。液状の温かいお料理には人数分の量を入れてよくかき混ぜてお召し上がり下さい。

5　過食を避けるため摂取の上限量を示す表現

過量に摂取した場合に生じる危害を防止するため摂取の上限量を一日量として示す表現は、直ちに医薬品的な用法用量には該当しないが、食品についての表現の適否については、栄養・食品担当部局等関係部局に照会するよう指導すること。

(3) Even when a product does not use medicinal dosage and administration methods in instructions on how to eat or prepare the food, such instructions should not be presented in a way that may result in it being recognized as a drug. For example, food terminology should be used, such as"How best to enjoy/suggested dose"instead of a medicinal title like"Dosage and administration".

4. Expressions on amounts to take for nutritional support

Expressions on amounts to take, like those listed below, to prevent harm from overconsumption or curb unnecessary intake are not immediately deemed as medicinal dosage and administration methods. However, expressions on amounts to take that recommend large amounts(more than necessary and more than could be eaten for a normal food)or amounts expected to produce a pharmacological effect may not be recognized as describing the necessary amounts for nutritional support and could be deemed as medicinal dosage and administration methods.

Note that even if the product is not deemed as having medicinal dosage and administration methods, there could be conflict with Article 32-2 of the Health Promotion Act and other acts and ordinances, so enquiries should be made with the departments responsible for nutrition/food and other relevant departments as to whether the expressions used are appropriate for a food.

Example: ・Normally one piece daily can provide the necessary nutrients. Mix through warm, liquid food in the appropriate amount for the number of people and enjoy.

5. Expressions describing maximum amounts to eat to avoid overconsumption

Expressions describing maximum daily amounts to eat to prevent harm if the food was consumed to excess are not immediately deemed medicinal dosage and administration methods, but enquiries should be made with the departments responsible for nutrition/food and other relevant departments as to whether the expressions used are appropriate for a food.

添付資料 6
「「医薬品的効能効果を標ぼうしない限り医薬品と判断しない成分本質（原材料）」の食品衛生法上の取り扱いの改正について」の一部改正について

（平成26年 3 月14日食安基発0314第 1 号）

Appendix 6
Partial amendments to the 'Amending the handling of "Ingredients (raw materials) not deemed drugs unless claiming medicinal efficacy" under the Food Sanitation Act'

(14 March 2014, Department of Food Safety, Standards and Evaluation Division Notification No. 0314-1)

「「医薬品的効能効果を標ぼうしない限り医薬品と判断しない成分本質（原材料）」の食品衛生法上の取扱いの改正について」の一部改正について

平成26年３月14日　食安基発0314第１号
各都道府県、保健所設置市、特別区衛生主管部（局）長あて
厚生労働省医薬食品局食品安全部基準審査課長通知

「無承認無許可医薬品の指導取締りについて」（昭和46年６月１日付け薬発第476号）の別紙「医薬品の範囲に関する基準」の別添３「医薬品的効能効果を標ぼうしない限り医薬品と判断しない成分本質（原材料）リスト」に収載されているものに係る食品衛生法（昭和22年法律第233号）上の取扱いについては、「「医薬品的効能効果を標ぼうしない限り医薬品と判断しない成分本質（原材料）」の食品衛生法上の取扱いの改正について」（平成19年８月17日付け食安基発第0817001号。以下「19年通知」という。）をもって示しているところであるが、今般、「医薬品の範囲に関する基準の一部改正について」（平成24年１月23日付け薬食発0123第３号及び平成25年７月10日付け薬食発0710第2　号）により「医薬品の範囲に関する基準」が改正されたことから、19　年通知の別添を下記のとおり改正することとしたので、貴職におかれては御了知の上、貴管内関係者に対する指導等について遺憾のないよう取り計らわれたい。

記

別添の２の⑸中「N-アセチルグルコサミン」の次に「、５-アミノレブリン酸リン酸塩」、「オクタコサノール」の次に「、オロト酸（フリー体、カリウム塩、マグネシウム塩に限る）」、「コエンザイムA」の次に「、コリン安定化オルトケイ酸」、「ヒドロキシリシン」の次に「、ピロロキノリンキノン二ナトリウム塩」、「リグナン」の次に「及びtrans-レスベラトロール」を加える。

別添の２の⑸中「リグナン」の前の「及び」を削除する。

（参考：改正後全文）

（別添２）

「医薬品的効能効果を標ぼうしない限り医薬品と判断しない成分本質（原材料）」の食品衛生法上の取扱い

1　「医薬品的効能効果を標ぼうしない限り医薬品と判断しない成分本質（原材料）リスト」（以下「同リスト」という。）の基本的な考え方

「医薬品的効能効果を標ぼうしない限り医薬品と判断しない」とは、医薬品的効能効果を標ぼうしない限り薬事法の規制を受けないという趣旨であり、同リストに収載されているものを食品又は食品添加物として使用する場合には、当然に食品衛生法の規制の対象となるものであることに留意されたい。

（仮訳：Provisional Translation）

Partial amendments to the'Amending the handling of "Ingredients(raw materials)not deemed drugs unless claiming medicinal efficacy" under the Food Sanitation Act'

Department of Food Safety, Standards and Evaluation Division Notification No. 0314-1
14 March 2014

For the attention of the Directors of the Hygiene Management Departments (Bureaus)
in the Prefectures, Cities with Public Health Centers, and Special Wards

Director of Department of Food Safety, Standards and Evaluation Division, Pharmaceutical and Food Safety Bureau (PFSB),
Ministry of Health, Labour and Welfare (MHLW)

The"Amendments on the handling under the Food Sanitation Act of ingredients (raw materials) not deemed drugs unless claiming medicinal efficacy" (Department of Food Safety, Standards and Evaluation Division Notification No. 0817001 17 August 2007 ; hereinafter"2007 Notification") describes the handling of substances included in the"List of ingredients (raw materials) not deemed drugs unless claiming medicinal efficacy" [Attachment 3 of"Standards on Scope of Drugs"that is an appendix to the Notification"Regulatory control of unapproved/unpermitted drugs" (PAB Notification No. 476, 1 June 1971)] under the Food Sanitation Act (Act No. 233, 1947). However, the attachment of the 2007 Director's Notification have now been amended, as described below, because the amendments were made to the"Standards on Scope of Drugs"because of the "Partial Amendments to Standards on Scope of Drugs" (PFSB Notification 0123 No. 3, 23 January 2012 and PFSB Notification 0710 No.2, 10 July 2013). Please make the necessary arrangements so that the relevant parties are instructed in these amendments.

Note:

", 5-Aminolevulinic acid・phosphate"after"N-acetyl glucosamine",", orotic acid (limited to free body, potassium salt and magnesium salt)"after"octacosanol",", choline-stabilized orthosilicic acid"after"coenzyme A",", pyrroloquinoline quinone disodium salt"after"hydroxylysine", and", and trans-resveratrol"after"lignans"have been added in Attachment 2 (5).
"And"before"lignans"has been deleted in Attachment 2 (5).

(Reference: Full text after amendments)

(Attachment 2)

Handling under the Food Sanitation Act of"Ingredients (raw materials) not deemed drugs unless claiming medicinal efficacy"

1. Basic approach to the"List of ingredients (raw materials) not deemed drugs unless claiming medicinal efficacy" (hereafter"the List")
   The phrase"not deemed drugs unless claiming medicinal efficacy"means that the substance is not regulated under the Pharmaceutical Affairs Act (PAA) unless claims are made that the substance has medicinal efficacy. Note that substances are regulated under the Food Sanitation Act if they are included on the List and are used as foods or food additives.

2　同リストの取扱いについて

(1)　同リスト中「1．植物由来物等」及び「2．動物由来物等」については、既存添加物に該当するものか、一般に飲食に供されている物かを直ちに判断し難いものも含まれているため、管下関係者への指導に際しては、その点御留意願いたく、疑義がある場合には、あらかじめ、その使用目的、食経験等の資料を厚生労働省医薬食品局食品安全部基準審査課添加物係あて提出し、食品添加物に該当するか否かの判断を受けるよう指導されたい。

(2)　同リスト中「3．その他（化学物質等）」のうち以下に示すものは、食品添加物に該当する。これらについて、食品衛生法施行規則別表第1及び既存添加物名簿（平成8年厚生省告示第120号）に収載されているもの以外のものを使用することは、食品衛生法第10条違反となるので留意されたい。

また、食品衛生法施行規則（昭和23年厚生省令第23号）別表第1及び既存添加物名簿に収載されているものにあっては、食品、添加物等の規格基準（昭和34年厚生省告示第370号）に規定する食品添加物としての規格及び基準を遵守する必要があること。

ア　指定添加物

亜鉛、アスパラギン酸、アラニン、イソロイシン、カリウム、カルシウム、キシリトール、クエン酸、グリシン、グリセリン、グルコン酸亜鉛、グルコン酸鉄、グルタミン酸、ケイ素、システイン、脂肪酸、酒石酸、鉄、鉄クロロフィリンナトリウム、銅、トリプトファン、トレオニン、ナイアシン、バリン、パントテン酸、ビオチン、ヒスチジン、ビタミンA、ビタミンB1、ビタミンB2、ビタミンB6、ビタミンC、ビタミンD、ビタミンE、フェニルアラニン、ベータカロチン、マグネシウム、メチオニン、葉酸及びリジン

イ　既存添加物

アスパラギン、アスタキサンチン注1）、アスパラギン酸、アラニン、イノシトール（D-chiro-イノシトールを含む）注2）、カテキン、カフェイン、カラギーナン、カリウム、カルシウム、カロチン、岩石粉、キチン、キトサン、金、グアガム、クルクミン、グルコサミン塩酸塩、グルタミン、クロロフィル、ケルセチン、サポニン、シスチン、脂肪酸、植物性酵素・果汁酵素、植物性ステロール、セリン、タルク、チロシン、鉄、銅、トコトリエノール、トレハロース、麦飯石、ヒアルロン酸、ヒスチジン、ビタミンB12、ビタミンE、ビタミンK（メナキノン）、4-ヒドロキシプロリン、フィコシアニン、フェリチン鉄、フェルラ酸注3）、プルラン、プロアントシアニジン、プロポリス、プロリン、ヘスペリジン、ヘマトコッカス藻色素、ヘム鉄、マグネシウム、ムコ多糖類、木灰、ラクトフェリン、リジン、流動パラフィン、ルチン、ルテイン、レシチン及びロイシン

注1）当品目は、通常は、既存添加物「ヘマトコッカス藻色素」に包含されるものと思料されるが、食品衛生法第10条に基づく指定がなされていない食品添加物に該当する場合もあることに留意されたい。
注2）当品目は、通常は、既存添加物「イノシトール」に包含されるものと思料されるが、食品衛生法第10条に基づく指定がなされていない食品添加物に該当する場合もあることに留意されたい。
注3）当品目は、通常は、既存添加物「フェルラ酸」に包含されるものと思料されるが、食品衛生法第10条に基づく指定がなされていない食品添加物に該当する場合もあることに留意されたい。

(3)　同リスト「3．その他（化学物質等）」のうち以下に示すものは、現在食品衛生法第10条に基づく指定がなされていないため、食品の製造等に使用する場合には、新たに食品添加物としての指定を受ける必要があること。

2. Handling the List

(1) Sections 1. Substances of plant origin and 2. Substances of animal origin on the List can include existing additives or substances where it is difficult to immediately determine whether it is generally supplied as food or drink. This point should be noted when giving guidance to relevant parties and, if questions arise, information on the substance's intended purpose, eating experiences, and other matters should be submitted in advance to those in charge of additives at the Department of Food Safety, Standards and Evaluation Division of the MHLW's PFSB to obtain guidance on whether the substance should be deemed a food additive.

(2) Listed below are substances deemed food additives under section 3. Other (chemical substances, etc.) of the List. The use of substances other than those listed in Annexed Table 1 of the Ordinance for Enforcement of the Food Sanitation Act and the List of existing food additives (MHW Notice No. 120, 1996) could be in violation of Article 10 of the Food Sanitation Act.
Furthermore, substances listed in Annexed Table 1 of the Ordinance for Enforcement of the Food Sanitation Act (MHW Ordinance No. 23, 1948) and the List of existing food additives must comply with the standards and criteria for food additives as regulated under the Standards for food, additives, etc. (MHW Notice No. 370, 1959).

a) Designated additives
Zinc, aspartic acid, alanine, isoleucine, potassium, calcium, xylitol, citric acid, glycine, glycerin, zinc gluconate, ferrous gluconate, glutamic acid, silicon, cysteine, fatty acid, tartaric acid, iron, sodium iron chlorophyllin, copper, tryptophan, threonine, niacin, valine, pantothenic acid, biotin, histidine, vitamin A, vitamin B1, vitamin B2, vitamin B6, vitamin C, vitamin D, vitamin E, phenylalanine, beta-carotene, magnesium, methionine, folic acid, and lysine.

b) Existing additives
Asparagine, astaxanthin (note 1), aspartic acid, alanine, inositol (including D-chiro-inositol) (note 2), catechin, caffeine, carrageenan, potassium, calcium, carotene, rock powder, chitin, chitosan, gold, guar gum, curcumin, glucosamine HCl, glutamine, chlorophyll, quercetin, saponin, cysteine, fatty acid, plant enzymes/fruit juice enzymes, phytosterol, serine, talc, tyrosine, iron, copper, tocotrienol, trehalose, Maifan stone (bakuhanseki), hyaluronic acid, histidine, vitamin B12, vitamin E, vitamin K (menaquinone), 4-hydroxyproline, phycocyanin, ferritin iron, ferulic acid (note 3), pullulan, proanthocyanidin, propolis, proline, hesperidin, Haematococcus algae colour, heme iron, magnesium, mucopolysaccharide, wood ashes, lactoferrin, lysine, liquid paraffin, rutin, lutein, lecithin, and leucine.

Note 1) While this item is generally considered to be included in the existing additive Haematococcus algae pigment, it can also be defined as a food additive without designation based on Article 10 of the Food Sanitation Act.
Note 2) While this item is generally considered to be included in the existing additive inositol, it can also be defined as a food additive without designation based on Article 10 of the Food Sanitation Act.
Note 3) While this item is generally considered to be included in the existing additive ferulic acid, it can also be defined as a food additive without designation based on Article 10 of the Food Sanitation Act.

(3) Listed below are substances under section 3. Other (chemical substances, etc.) of the List that currently are not specified as additives according to Article 10 of the Food Sanitation Act, so if they are used in the manufacture of food, etc., they need to receive designation as a new food additive.

クロム（Ⅲ）、セレン、ビタミンK（フィトナジオン、メナジオン）、ピコリン酸クロム、フッ素、マンガン、モリブデン、ヨウ素及びリン

(4) 同リスト「３．その他（化学物質等）」のうち以下に示すものは、「一般に食品として飲食に供される物であって添加物として使用されるもの」として取扱うこと。

なお、以下に示すものの製造の過程に用いられる溶媒等については、食品添加物に該当しないが、人の健康を損なうおそれがある不純物の混入等がないよう、製造業者等に対し、製品について規格を設定する等の指導を徹底されたい注１）。また、食品の製造の過程において使用される溶媒等は、食品添加物に該当することに留意されたい。

アルブミン、イオウ（ただし、メチルサリフォニルメタンとして）、イコサペント酸（EPA）、イヌリン、オリゴ糖、オルニチン、果糖、L-カルニチン注２）、L-シトルリン、還元麦芽糖、環状重合乳酸（ただし、乳酸オリゴマーとして）、γ-アミノ酪酸、絹（ただし、絹タンパクとして）、グルコマンナン、クレアチン、ゲルマニウム注３）、コエンザイムQ10、コラーゲン、コンドロイチン硫酸注４）、植物繊維、食物繊維、ゼラチン、チオクト酸注５）、デキストリン、ドコサヘキサエン酸（DHA）、ドロマイト鉱石、乳清、乳糖、フルボ酸、ホスファチジルセリン、リノール酸及びリノレン酸

注１）残留溶媒の規格設定の指導にあっては、「食品、添加物等の規格基準」の第２添加物の　E　製造基準において規定されている溶媒に対する基準や「医薬品の残留溶媒ガイドライン」（平成10年３月30日付け医薬審第307号厚生省医薬安全局審査管理課長通知。以下「残留溶媒ガイドライン」という。）等を参考にされたい。なお、トルエンなど食品衛生法において参考となる基準がなく、残留溶媒ガイドラインを参考とする場合にあっては、医薬品と食品の相違を鑑み、十分配慮することが必要である。

注２）本成分の使用に当たっては、米国では許容一日摂取量（ADI）が20mg/kg/日と評価されていることや、スイスでは1,000mg/日を摂取の条件としていることなどから、過剰摂取しないように配慮するとともに、消費者への情報提供を適切に行うこと。

注３）ゲルマニウムについては、「ゲルマニウムを含有させた食品の取扱いについて（昭和63年10月12日付け衛新第12号生活衛生局長通知）」により、その取扱いについて指導をお願いしているところである。

注４）コンドロイチン硫酸ナトリウムは指定添加物である。

注５）本成分の使用に当たっては、国内において医療用医薬品「チオクト酸」として「通常成人１日１回10～25mgを静脈内、筋肉内又は皮下に注射」の旨の用法・用量が設定されていること等から、食品等事業者においては、自らの責任において食品の安全性を確保するため、過剰摂取しないよう必要な配慮をするとともに、消費者への情報提供を適切に行うこと。

(5) 同リスト「３．その他（化学物質等）」のうち以下に示すものについては、食品添加物に該当する可能性が考えられるため、該当するものを輸入、販売、製造等をしようとする事業者がいる場合には、あらかじめ、その使用目的、食経験等の資料を厚生労働省医薬食品局食品安全部基準審査課添加物係あて提出し、食品添加物に該当するか否かの判断を受けるよう指導されたい。

Chromium (III), selenium, vitamin K (phytonadione, menadione), chromium picolinate, fluorine, manganese, molybdenum, iodine, and phosphorous.

(4) Listed below are substances under section 3. Other (chemical substances, etc.) of the List that are handled as"substances generally supplied as food products to eat or drink and used as additives".
Note that solvents etc. used in the manufacturing of the substances shown below are not defined as food additives but, manufacturers etc. need to follow guidance carefully, including established product standards, to ensure that there is no contamination with impurities that could be harmful to health (Note 1). Take particular note that solvents etc. used during manufacturing processes for food are defined as food additives.

Albumin, sulfur (but as methylsulfonylmethane), eicosapentaenoic acid (EPA), inulin, oligosaccharide, ornithine, fructose, L-carnitine (note 2), L-citrulline, reduced maltose, cyclic polylactate (but as lactic acid oligomer), gamma-aminobutyric acid, silk (but as silk protein), glucomannan, creatine, germanium (note 3), coenzyme Q10, collagen, chondroitin sulfate (note 4), vegetable fiber, dietary fiber, gelatin, thioctic acid (note 5), dextrin, docosahexaenoic acid (DHA), dolomite mineral, whey, lactose, fulvic acid, phosphatidyl serine, linoleic acid and linolenic acid.

Note 1) Please refer to guidance on standards for residual solvent, including standards for solvents regulated in manufacturing standards E, No. 2 additives in"Standards for foods, additives, etc." and"Guidelines on pharmaceutical residual solvents" (Notification from the Director of the Evaluation and Licensing Division, Pharmaceutical and Food Safety Bureau, MHLW, PFSB/ELD Notification No. 307, 30 March 1998 ; hereinafter"residual solvent guidelines"). Note that when referring to the residual solvent guideline for toluene and other substances where there are no reference standards in the Food Sanitation Act, special care should be taken to reflect the differences between pharmaceuticals and foods.

Note 2) With the use of this ingredient, care should be taken to avoid overconsumption, because the acceptable daily intake (ADI) is defined as 20mg/kg/day in the US and Switzerland sets conditions of 1,000mg/day for intake, and the consumer should be informed as appropriate.

Note 3) Guidance on the handling of germanium has been requested from"Handling of foods containing germanium" (Notification from the Director of the Environmental Health Bureau, Eishin No. 12, 12 October 1988).

Note 4) Chondroitin sulfate sodium is a designated additive.

Note 5) With the use of this ingredient, necessary care should be taken to avoid overconsumption, as food business operators have a voluntary responsibility to ensure food safety because in Japan dosage and administration of thioctic acid as an ethical drug is defined as"10-25mg via an intravenous, intramuscular, or subcutaneous injection once daily for a normal adult", and the consumer should be informed as appropriate.

(5) Listed below are substances under section 3. Other (chemical substances, etc.) of the List that may be defined as food additives, so if a business operator intends to import, market, or manufacture, etc. these substances, information on the substances' intended purpose, eating experiences, and other matters should be submitted in advance to those in charge of additives at the Department of Food Safety, Standards and Evaluation Division of the MHLW's PFSB to obtain guidance on whether the substance should be deemed a food additive.

N-アセチルグルコサミン、5-アミノレブリン酸リン酸塩、アリシン、アントシアニジン、イオウ（ただし、メチルサリフォニルメタンを除く）、イソフラキシジン、雲母、オクタコサノール、オロト酸（フリー体、カリウム塩、マグネシウム塩に限る）、環状重合乳酸（ただし、乳酸オリゴマーを除く）、キトサンオリゴ糖、絹（ただし、絹タンパクを除く）、sn-グリセロ(3)ホスホコリン、クレアチン・エチルエステル塩酸塩、コエンザイムA、コリン安定化オルトケイ酸、コンドロムコタンパク、シスタチオン、スクワレン、スーパーオキシドディスムターゼ（SOD）、炭焼の乾留水、石膏、セラミド、ビスベトヒドロキシ-3-メチルブチレートモノハイドレート、ヒドロキシリシン、ピロロキノリンキノン二ナトリウム塩、リグナン及びtrans-レスベラトロール

N-acetyl glucosamine, 5-aminolevulinic acid・phosphate, allicin, anthocyanidin, sulfur (but excluding methylsulfonylmethane), isofraxidine, mica, octacosanol, orotic acid (limited to free body, potassium salt and magnesium salt), cyclic polylactate (but excluding lactic acid oligomer), chitosan oligosaccharide, silk (but excluding silk protein), sn-glycero(3)phosphocholine, creatine ethylester hydrochloride, coenzyme A, choline-stabilized orthosilicic acid, chondromucoprotein, cystathione, squalene, superoxide dismutase (SOD), charcoal dry-distilled water, gypsum (calcium sulfate), ceramide, bis(3hydroxy-3-methylbutyrate)monohydrate, hydroxylysine, pyrroloquinoline quinone disodium salt, lignan, and trans-resveratrol.

添付資料 7
欧州医薬品庁（EMA）ハーブ医薬品委員会による
ハーブ素材評価リスト（2014年7月8日現在）

Appendix 7
List of herbal substances designated for assessment by the European Medicines Agency' s Committee on Herbal Medicinal Products (HMPC) (as of July 8, 2014)

欧州医薬品庁（EMA）ハーブ医薬品委員会によるハーブ素材評価リスト

本リストはDirective 2004/24/EC（欧州（EU）伝統的ハーブ医薬品指令）に基づき、欧州医薬品庁に設置されたハーブ医薬品委員会（Committee on Herbal Medicinal Products, HMPC）が評価対象としたハーブ素材の一覧である。各ハーブ素材の評価段階は、リストの右端の略号（アルファベット）によって示されている。ハーブ素材がHMPCの評価により、ヒトに対する有効性と安全性に関する科学的データの要件および使用年数に関する条件を満たしていると判断された場合、当該ハーブ素材についてのモノグラフが作成され、欧州ハーブモノグラフ（Community herbal monograph）に登録される。当該ハーブ素材のモノグラフがさらに一定の要件を満たていると評価された場合は、最終的に欧州リスト（Community list）に収載される。欧州ハーブモノグラフあるいは欧州リストは、Directive 2004/24/ECに基づき、伝統的ハーブ医薬品の製造承認申請あるいは登録申請手続きを簡略化するための資料として用いられる。

[Status type]

R：Rapporteur assigned（評価者指名済み）
C：ongoing call for scientific data（科学的データを追加要求中）
D：Draft under discussion（評価書作成中）
P：Draft published（評価書公表）
PF：Assessment close to finalisation (pre-final)（最終評価段階）
F：Final opinion adopted（評価終了）

2014.07.08現在

No.	Latin name of the genus	Latin name of herbal substance	Botanical name of plant	English common name of herbal substance	Status
1	Achillea	Millefolii herba	*Achillea millefolium* L.	Yarrow	F
2	Achillea	Millefolii flos	*Achillea millefolium* L.	Yarrow Flower	F
3	Adhatoda	Adhatodae vasicae folium	*Adhatoda vasica* Nees	Malabar-nut leaf	F
4	Aesculus	Hippocastani semen	*Aesculus hippocastanum* L.	Horse-Chestnut Seed	F
5	Aesculus	Hippocastani cortex	*Aesculus hippocastanum* L.	Horse-chestnut bark	F
6	Agropyron	Agropyri repentis rhizoma	*Agropyron repens* (L.) P. Beauv.	Couch grass rhizome	F
7	Allium	Allii cepae bulbus	*Allium cepa* L.	Onion	F
8	Aloe	Aloe bardadensis / Aloe capensis	*Aloe barbadensis* Miller / *Aloe ferox* Miller	Aloes	F
9	Althaea	Althaeae radix	*Althaea officinalis* L.	Marshmallow Root	F
10	Andrographis	Andrographidis paniculatae folium	*Andrographis paniculata* Nees, folium	Kalmegh	F
11	Angelica	Angelicae sinensis radix	*Angelica sinensis* (Oliv.) Diels	Winter Cherry Root	F
12	Arctium	Arctii radix	*Arctium lappa* L.	Burdock Root	F
13	Arctostaphylos	Uvae ursi folium	*Arctostaphylos uva-ursi* (L.) Spreng.	Bearberry Leaf	F
14	Artemisia	Absinthii herba	*Artemisia absinthium* L.	Wormwood	F
15	Avena	Avenae herba	*Avena sativa* L.	Oat Herb	F
16	Avena	Avenae fructus	*Avena sativa* L.	Oat Fruit	F
17	Betula	Betulae folium	*Betula pendula* Roth / *Betula pubescens* Ehrh.	Birch Leaf	F
18	Calendula	Calendulae flos	*Calendula officinalis* L.	Calendula Flower	F
19	Camellia	Camelliae non fermentatum folium	*Camellia sinensis* (L.) Kuntze, non fermentatum folium	Green tea	F
20	Capsella	Bursae pastoris herba	*Capsella bursa-pastoris* (L.) Medikus	Shepherds Purse	F
21	Cassia	Sennae fructus	*Cassia senna* L.; *Cassia angustifolia* Vahl	Senna pods	F
22	Cassia	Sennae folium	*Cassia senna* L.; *Cassia angustifolia* Vahl	Senna leaf	F
23	Centaurium	Centaurii herba	*Centaurium erythraea* Rafn.	Centaury	F
24	Centella	Centellae asiaticae herba	*Centella asiatica* L. Urban	Centella	F
25	Chamaemelum	Chamomillae romanae flos	*Chamaemelum nobile* (L.) All. (*Anthemis nobilis* L.)	Roman Chamomile Flower	F
26	Chelidonium	Chelidonii herba	*Chelidonium majus* L.	Greater Celandine	F
27	Cichorium	Cichorii intybi radix	*Cichorium intybus* L.	Chicory root	F

[Status type]
R：Rapporteur assigned（評価者指名済み）
C：ongoing call for scientific data（科学的データを追加要求中）
D：Draft under discussion（評価書作成中）
P：Draft published（評価書公表）
PF：Assessment close to finalisation（pre-final）（最終評価段階）
F：Final opinion adopted（評価終了）

No.	Latin name of the genus	Latin name of herbal substance	Botanical name of plant	English common name of herbal substance	Status
28	Cimicifuga	Cimicifugae rhizoma	*Cimicifuga racemosa* (L.) Nutt.	Black Cohosh	F
29	Cinnamomum	Cinnamomi cortex	*Cinnamomum veri* J. S. Presl (*Cinnamomum zeylancium* Nees)	Cinnamon	F
30	Cinnamomum	Cinnamomi corticis aetheroleum	*Cinnamomum verum* J. S. Presl (*Cinnamomum zeylanicum* Nees)	Cinnamon Bark Oil	F
31	Citrus	Citri bergamia aetheroleum	*Citrus bergamia* Risso & Poiteau.	Bergamot oil	F
32	Cola	Colae semen	*Cola nitida* (Vent.) Schott et Endl. and its varieties and *Cola acuminata* (P. Beauv.) Schott et Endl.	Cola	F
33	Commiphora	Myrrha, gummi-resina	*Commiphora molmol* Engler	Myrrh	F
34	Cucurbita	Cucurbitae semen	*Cucurbita pepo* L.	Pumpkin seed	F
35	Curcuma	Curcumae longae rhizoma	*Curcuma longa* L.	Turmeric	F
36	Curcuma	Curcumae xanthorrhizae rhizoma	*Curcuma xanthorrhiza* Roxb. (*C. xanthorrhiza* D. Dietrich).	Javanese turmeric	F
37	Cynara	Cynarae folium	*Cynara scolymus* L.	Artichoke Leaf	F
38	Echinacea	Echinaceae angustifoliae radix	*Echinacea angustifolia* DC.	Narrow-leaved coneflower root	F
39	Echinacea	Echinaceae purpureae herba	*Echinacea purpurea* (L.) Moench	Purple Coneflower Herb	F
40	Echinacea	Echinaceae pallidae radix	*Echinacea pallida* (Nutt.) Nutt.	Pale Coneflower Root	F
41	Echinacea	Echinaceae purpureae radix	*Echinacea purpurea* (L.) Moench.	Purple Coneflower Root	F
42	Eleutherococcus	Eleutherococci radix	*Eleutherococcus senticosus* (Rupr. et Maxim.) Maxim.	Eleutherococcus	F
43	Equisetum	Equiseti herba	*Equisetum arvense* L.	Equisetum Stem	F
44	Eucalyptus	Eucalypti aetheroleum	*Eucalyptus globulus* Labill.; *Eucalyptus polybractea* R.T. Baker; *Eucalyptus smithii* R.T. Baker.	Eucalyptus Oil	F
45	Eucalyptus	Eucalypti folium	*Eucalyptus globulus* Labill.	Eucalyptus leaf	F
46	Euphrasia	Euphrasiae herba	*Euphrasia officinalis* L. (mainly subsp. *E. rostkoviana* Hayne)	Eyebright	F
47	Filipendula	Filipendulae ulmariae herba	*Filipendula ulmaria* (L.) Maxim. (= *Spiraea ulmaria* L.).	Meadowsweet	F
48	Filipendula	Filipendulae ulmariae flos	*Filipendula ulmaria* (L.) Maxim. (= *Spiraea ulmaria* L.).	Meadowsweet Flower	F
49	Foeniculum	Foeniculi amari fructus	*Foeniculum vulgare* Miller subsp. *vulgare* var. *vulgare*	Bitter Fennel	F
50	Foeniculum	Foeniculi amari fructus aetheroleum	*Foeniculum vulgare* Miller subsp. *vulgare* var. *vulgare*	Bitter Fennel Fruit Oil	F
51	Foeniculum	Foeniculi dulcis fructus	*Foeniculum vulgare* Miller subsp. *vulgare* var. *dulce* (Miller) Thellung.	Sweet Fennel	F
52	Fraxinus	Fraxini folium	*Fraxinus excelsior* L. and *F. angustifolia* Vahl, folium	Ash Leaf	F
53	Fumaria	Fumariae herba	*Fumaria officinalis* L.,	Fumitory	F
54	Gentiana	Gentianae radix	*Gentiana lutea* L.	Gentian Root	F
55	Glycyrrhiza	Liquiritiae radix	*Glycyrrhiza glabra* L. and/or *Glycyrrhiza inflata* Bat. and/or Glycyrrhiza uralensis Fisch.	Liquorice Root	F
56	Grindelia	Grindeliae herba	Grindelia robusta Nutt., Grindelia squarrosa (Pursh) Dunal, *Grindelia humilis* Hook. et Arn., Grindel	Gumweed herb	F
57	Hamamelis	Hamamelidis cortex	*Hamamelis virginiana* L.	Hamamelis Bark	F
58	Hamamelis	Hamamelidis folium	*Hamamelis virginiana* L.	Hamamelis Leaf	F
59	Hamamelis	Hamamelidis folium et cortex aut ramunculus destillatum	*Hamamelis virginiana* L.	Hamamelis Distillate	F

[Status type]
R：Rapporteur assigned（評価者指名済み）
C：ongoing call for scientific data（科学的データを追加要求中）
D：Draft under discussion（評価書作成中）
P：Draft published（評価書公表）
PF：Assessment close to finalisation (pre-final)（最終評価段階）
F：Final opinion adopted（評価終了）

No.	Latin name of the genus	Latin name of herbal substance	Botanical name of plant	English common name of herbal substance	Status
60	Harpagophytum	Harpagophyti radix	*Harpagophytum procumbens* DC.；*Harpagophytum zeyheri* Decne	Devil's Claw Root	F
61	Hedera	Hederae helicis folium	*Hedera helix* L.	Ivy leaf	F
62	Humulus	Lupuli flos	*Humulus lupulus* L.	Hop Strobile	F
63	Hypericum	Hyperici herba	*Hypericum perforatum* L.	St. John's Wort	F
64	Ilex	Mate folium	*Ilex paraguariensis* St. Hil.	Maté Leaf	F
65	Juglans	Juglandis folium	*Juglans regia* L.	Walnut leaf	F
66	Juniperus	Juniperi pseudo-fructus	*Juniperus communis* L.	Juniper berry	F
67	Juniperus	Juniperi aetheroleum	*Juniperus communis* L.	Juniper Oil	F
68	Lavandula	Lavandulae aetheroleum	*Lavandula angustifolia* Mill. (*L. officinalis* Chaix)	Lavender Oil	F
69	Lavandula	Lavandulae flos	*Lavandula angustifolia* Mill. (*L. officinalis* Chaix)	Lavender	F
70	Leonurus	Leonuri cardiacae herba	*Leonurus cardiaca* L.	Motherwort	F
71	Levisticum	Levistici radix	*Levisticum officinale* Koch.	Lovage root	F
72	Linum	Lini semen	*Linum usitatissimum* L.	Linseed	F
73	Marrubium	Marrubii herba	*Marrubium vulgare* L.	White horehound	F
74	Melilotus	Meliloti herba	*Melilotus officinalis* (L.) Lam.	Melilot	F
75	Melissa	Melissae folium	*Melissa officinalis* L.	Melissa leaf	F
76	Mentha	Menthae piperitae folium	*Mentha x piperita* L.	Peppermint leaf	F
77	Mentha	Menthae piperitae aetheroleum	*Mentha x piperita* L.	Peppermint oil	F
78	Oenothera	Oenotherae biennis oleum	*Oenothera biennis* L.；*Oenothera lamarckiana* L.	Evening Primrose Oil	F
79	Olea	Oleae folium	*Olea europaea* L.	Olive leaf	F
80	Ononis	Ononidis radix	*Ononis spinosa* L. and *Ononis arvensis* L.	Restharrow root	F
81	Origanum	Origani dictamni herba	*Origanum dictamnus* L.	Dittany of Crete herb	F
82	Orthosiphon	Orthosiphonis folium	*Orthosiphon stamineus* Benth.	Java Tea	F
83	Panax	Ginseng radix	*Panax ginseng* C. A. Meyer.	Ginseng	F
84	Passiflora	Passiflorae herba	*Passiflora incarnata* L.	Passion Flower	F
85	Paullinia	Paulliniae semen	*Paullinia cupana* Kunth, semen	Guarana	F
86	Pelargonium	Pelargonii radix	*Pelargonium sidoides* DC；*Pelargonium reniforme* Curt.	Pelargonium root	F
87	Peumus	Boldi folium	*Peumus boldus* Molina	Boldo Leaf	F
88	Phaseolus	Phaseoli fructus (sine semine)	*Phaseolus vulgaris* L.	Green bean pod	F
89	Pimpinella	Anisi aetheroleum	*Pimpinella anisum* L.	Anise Oil	F
90	Pimpinella	Anisi fructus	*Pimpinella anisum* L.	Aniseed	F
91	Plantago	Plantaginis ovatae seminis tegumentum	*Plantago ovata* Forssk.	Ispaghula husk	F
92	Plantago	Psyllii semen	*Plantago afra* L.；*Plantago indica* L.	Psyllium seed	F
93	Plantago	Plantaginis lanceolatae folium	*Plantago lanceolata* L.	Ribwort Plantain	F
94	Plantago	Plantaginis ovatae semen	*Plantago ovata* Forssk.	Ispaghula Seed	F
95	Polypodium	Polypodii rhizoma	*Polypodium vulgare* L.	Polypody Rhizome	F
96	Potentilla	Tormentillae rhizoma	*Potentilla erecta* (L.) Raeusch.	Tormentil	F
97	Primula	Primulae flos	*Primula veris* L.；*Primula elatior* (L.) Hill	Primula flower	F
98	Primula	Primulae radix	*Primula veris* L.；*Primula elatior* (L.) Hill	Primula root	F

[Status type]
R：Rapporteur assigned（評価者指名済み）
C：ongoing call for scientific data（科学的データを追加要求中）
D：Draft under discussion（評価書作成中）
P：Draft published（評価書公表）
PF：Assessment close to finalisation（pre-final）（最終評価段階）
F：Final opinion adopted（評価終了）

No.	Latin name of the genus	Latin name of herbal substance	Botanical name of plant	English common name of herbal substance	Status
99	Quercus	Quercus cortex	*Quercus robur* L.；*Quercus petraea* (Matt.) Liebl.；*Quercus pubescens* Willd.	Oak Bark	F
100	Rhamnus	Frangulae cortex	*Rhamnus frangula* L.	Frangula bark	F
101	Rhamnus	Rhamni purshianae cortex	*Rhamnus purshianus* D.C.	Cascara	F
102	Rheum	Rhei radix	*Rheum palmatum* L.；*Rheum officinale* Baillon	Rhubarb	F
103	Rhodiola	Rhodiolae roseae rhizoma et radix	*Rhodiola rosea* L.	Arctic root	F
104	Ribes	Ribis nigri folium	*Ribes nigrum* L.	Blackcurrant Leaf	F
105	Rosmarinus	Rosmarini aetheroleum	*Rosmarinus officinalis* L.	Rosemary Oil	F
106	Rosmarinus	Rosmarini folium	*Rosmarinus officinalis* L.	Rosemary leaf	F
107	Rubus	Rubi idaei folium	Rubus idaeus L.	Raspberry leaf	F
108	Ruscus	Rusci rhizoma	*Ruscus aculeatus* L.	Butcher's Broom	F
109	Salix	Salicis cortex	*Salix* [various species including *S. purpurea* L.；*S. daphnoides* Vill.；*S. fragilis* L.]	Willow Bark	F
110	Salvia	Salviae officinalis aetheroleum	*Salvia officinalis* L.	Sage Oil	F
111	Salvia	Salviae officinalis folium	*Salvia officinalis* L.	Sage Leaf	F
112	Sambucus	Sambuci fructus	*Sambucus nigra* L.	Elderberry	F
113	Sambucus	Sambuci flos	*Sambucus nigra* L.	Elder Flower	F
114	Solanum	Solani dulcamarae stipites	*Solanum dulcamara* L.	Woody nightshade stem	F
115	Solidago	Solidaginis virgaureae herba	*Solidago virgaurea* L.	European Goldenrod	F
116	Syzygium	Caryophylii flos	*Syzygium aromaticum* (L.) Merill et L. M. Perry	Clove	F
117	Syzygium	Caryophylii floris aetheroleum	*Syzygium aromaticum* (L.) Merill et L. M. Perry	Clove oil	F
118	Tanacetum	Tanaceti parthenii herba	*Tanacetum parthenium* (L.) Schultz Bip.	Feverfew	F
119	Taraxacum	Taraxaci folium	*Taraxacum officinale* Weber ex Wigg.	Dandelion Leaf	F
120	Taraxacum	Taraxaci radix cum herba	*Taraxacum officinale* Weber ex Wigg.	Dandelion Root with Herb	F
121	Thymus	Thymi aetheroleum	*Thymus vulgaris* L.；*Thymus zygis* Loefl. ex L.	Thyme oil	F
122	Thymus	Thymi herba	*Thymus vulgaris* L.；*Thymus zygis* Loefl. ex L.	Thyme	F
123	Thymus / Primula	Thymi herba / Primulae radix	*Thymus vulgaris* L.；*Thymus zygis* Loefl. ex L. / *Primula veris* L.；*Primula elatior* (L.) Hill	Thyme / Primula root	F
124	Tilia	Tiliae tomentosae flos	*Tilia tomentosa* Moench	Silver lime flower	F
125	Tilia	Tiliae flos	*Tilia cordata* Miller, *Tila platyphyllos* Scop., *Tilia x vulgaris* Heyne or their mixtures	Lime flower	F
126	Trigonella	Trigonellae foenugraeci semen	*Trigonella foenum-graecum* L.	Fenugreek	F
127	Urtica	Urticae radix	*Urtica dioica* L.；*Urtica urens* L.	Nettle root	F
128	Urtica	Urticae folium	*Urtica dioica* L.；*Urtica urens* L.	Nettle Leaf	F
129	Urtica	Urticae herba	*Urtica dioica* L.；*Urtica urens* L.	Nettle Herb	F
130	Valeriana	Valerianae radix	*Valeriana officinalis* L.	Valerian Root	F
131	Valeriana/Humulus	Valerianae radix/Lupuli flos	*Valeriana officinalis* L. / *Humulus lupulus* L.	Valerian Root / Hop Strobile	F
132	Verbascum	Verbasci flos	*Verbascum thapsus* L.；*V. densiflorum* Bertol. (*V. thapsiforme* Schrad)；*V. phlomoides* L.	Mullein Flower	F
133	Viola	Violae tricoloris herba cum flore	*Viola tricolor* L.	Wild Pansy	F

[Status type]
R：Rapporteur assigned（評価者指名済み）
C：ongoing call for scientific data（科学的データを追加要求中）
D：Draft under discussion（評価書作成中）
P：Draft published（評価書公表）
PF：Assessment close to finalisation（pre-final）（最終評価段階）
F：Final opinion adopted（評価終了）

No.	Latin name of the genus	Latin name of herbal substance	Botanical name of plant	English common name of herbal substance	Status
134	Viscum	Visci albi herba	*Viscum album* L.	Mistletoe	F
135	Vitex	Agni casti fructus	*Vitex agnus-castus* L.	Agnus Castus Fruit	F
136	Vitis	Vitis viniferae folium	*Vitis vinifera* L.	Grapevine Leaf	F
137	Withania	Withania somnifera radix	*Withania somnifera* (L.) Dunal	Winter-cherry root	F
138	Zingiber	Zingiberis rhizoma	*Zingiber officinale* Roscoe	Ginger	F
139	Symphytum	Symphyti radix	*Symphytum officinale* L.	Comfrey Root	PF
140	Agrimonia	Agrimoniae herba	*Agrimonia eupatoria* L.	Agrimony	P
141	Arnica	Arnicae flos	*Arnica montana* L.	Arnica flower	P
142	Cetraria	Lichen islandicus	*Cetraria islandica* (L.) Acharius s.l.	Iceland moss	P
143	Fucus	Fucus vesiculosus, thallus	*Fucus vesiculosus* L.	Bladderwrack	P
144	Ginkgo	Ginkgo folium	*Ginkgo biloba* L.	Ginkgo Leaf	P
145	Melaleuca	Melaleucae alternifoliae aetheroleum	*Melaleuca alternifolia* (Maiden and Betche) Cheel	Tea-tree oil	P
146	Rosa	Rosae flos	*Rosa centifolia* L.；*Rosa gallica* L.；*Rosa damascena* Mill.	Rose flower	P
147	Sisymbrium	Sisymbrii officinalis herba	*Sisymbrium officinale* (L.) Scop., herba	Hedge mustard	P
148	Allium	Allii sativi bulbus	*Allium sativum* L.	Garlic	D
149	Matricaria	Matricariae flos	*Matricaria recutita* L.	Matricaria Flower	D
150	Matricaria	Matricariae aetheroleum	*Matricaria recutita* L.	Matricaria Oil	D
151	Calendula	Calendulae herba		Marigold	C
152	Centaurea	Cyani flos		Cornflower	C
153	Cistus	Cisti cretici folium/resinum	*Cisti creticus* L.	Pink Rock-Rose	C
154	Epilobium	Epilobii herba		Willow herb	C
155	Glycine	Glycine max, lecithin	*Glycine max* (L.) Merr.	Soyabean	C
156	Helichrysum	Helichrysi flos		Sandy everlasting	C
157	Origanum	Origani majoranae herba	*Origanum majorana* L.	Marjoram	C
158	Paeonia	Paeoniae radix		Peony root	C
159	Pistacia	Pistacia lentiscus, resinum	*Pistacia lentiscus* L.	Mastic tree resin	C
160	Polygonum	Polygoni avicularis herba	Polygonum aviculare L.	Knotweed herb, Common	C
161	Ricinus	Ricini oleum		Castor oil	C
162	Saccharomyces	Saccharomyces cerevisiae/Saccharomyces boulardii		Yeast	C
163	Salvia	Salviae trilobae folium	*Salvia triloba* L.	Sage leaf	C
164	Sideritis	Sideritis herba		Ironwort	C
165	Capsicum	Capsici fructus	*Capsicum annuum* L. var. *minimum* (Miller) Heiser	Capsicum	R
166	Carum	Carvi fructus	*Carum carvi* L.	Caraway fruit	R
167	Carum	Carvi aetheroleum	*Carum carvi* L.	Caraway oil	R
168	Crataegus	Crataegi folium cum flore	*Crataegus* spp, *folium cum* flore	Hawthorn Leaf and Flower	R
169	Crataegus	Crataegi fructus	*Crataegus monogyna* Jacq. (Lindm.)；*Crataegus laevigata* (Poir.) D.C.	Hawthorn Berries	R
170	Eschscholtzia	Eschscholtziae herba cum flore	*Eschscholtzia californi*a Cham.	California poppy	R
171	Fragaria	Fragariae folium	*Fragaria vesca* L.	Wild Strawberry Leaf	R

［Status type］

R：Rapporteur assigned（評価者指名済み）
C：ongoing call for scientific data（科学的データを追加要求中）
D：Draft under discussion（評価書作成中）
P：Draft published（評価書公表）
PF：Assessment close to finalisation（pre-final）（最終評価段階）
F：Final opinion adopted（評価終了）

No.	Latin name of the genus	Latin name of herbal substance	Botanical name of plant	English common name of herbal substance	Status
172	Hieracium	Pilosellae herba cum flore	*Hieracium pilosella* L.	Mouse-ear hawkweed	R
173	Picrorhiza	Picrorhizae kurroae rhizoma et radix	*Picrorhiza kurroa* Royle ex. Benth.	Katula	R
174	Prunus	Prunus africanae cortex	*Prunus africana* (Hook f.) Kalkm.	Pygeum africanum bark	R
175	Serenoa	Sabalis serrulatae fructus	*Serenoa repens* (Bartram) Small (*Sabal serrulata* (Michaux) Nichols	Saw Palmetto Fruit	R
176	Silybum	Silybi mariani fructus	*Silybum marianum* L. Gaertner	Milkthistle Fruit	R
177	Uncaria	Uncariae tomentosae cortex	*Uncariae tomentosae* (Willd.) DC.	Cat's Claw	R
178	Vaccinium	Myrtilli fructus siccus	*Vaccinium myrtillus* L.	Billberry Fruit	R
179	Vaccinium	Myrtilli folium	*Vaccinium myrtillus* L.	Billberry Leaf	R

出典：EUROPEAN MEDICINES AGENCY　SCIENCE MEDICINES HEALTH
http://www.ema.europa.eu/ema/index.jsp?curl=pages/medicines/landing/herbal_search.jsp&mid=WC0b01ac058001fa1d

添付資料 8
第36改正米国薬局方及び第31改正国民医薬品集における
ダイエタリーサプリメント, オフィシャルモノグラフ(2013)

Appendix 8
Lists of USP 36-NF 31 (2013) Dietary Supplements, Official Monographs

第36改正米国薬局方及び第31改正国民医薬品集におけるダイエタリーサプリメント，オフィシャルモノグラフ

米国薬局方（USP）＊1には医薬品の有効成分と製剤の規格（医薬品各条）が掲載されている他、別のセクションにダイエタリーサプリメントの規格（各条）が掲載されている。一方、現在の国民医薬品集（NF）＊2には、医薬品添加物の規格（各条）が掲載されている。

Table 1. はUSP/NFの総論に収載されているダイエタリーサプリメント、**Table 2.** は、USP/NFの公式モノグラフに収載されているダイエタリーサプリメントの基原植物、科名、使用部位を示した表である。

Table 3. は、NF(第31改正)、**Table 4.** は、USP(第36改正）に収載されている医薬品の表である。
尚、USP 36-NF 31の基原植物の命名者名は原書の通りに記載した。

＊1 USP（United States Pharmacopeia）：米国薬局方（原薬、投与形態、および配合製剤）の規格基準書

＊2 NF（the National Formulary）：国民医薬品集（“dietary supplements” ダイエタリーサプリメントと “dietary ingredients” サプリメント成分を含む）の規格基準書

Table 1. General Chapters Information of Dietary Supplements in USP 36 NF 31 (2013)

Dietary Supplement	Original Plants	Family Name	Part of Use
Black Cohosh	*Actaea racemosa* L.	Ranunculaceae	rhizome, root
	Cimicifuga racemosa (L.) Nutt.		
Ginger	*Zingiber officinale* Roscoe	Zingiberaceae	rhizome
Valerian	*Valeriana officinalis* L.	Valerianaceae	subterranean parts
Elm	*Ulmus rubra* Muhl.	Ulmaceae	inner bark
	Ulmus fulva Mich.		

Table 2. Official Monographs of Dietary Supplements in USP 36 NF 31 (2013)

Dietary Supplement	Original Plants	Family Name	Part of Use
American Ginseng	*Panax quinquefolius* L.	Araliaceae	root
Asian Ginseng	*Panax ginseng* C.A. Mey.	Araliaceae	root
Andrographis	*Andrographis paniculata* (Burm.f.) Nees	Acanthaceae	stem, leaf
Ashwagandha	*Withania somnifera* (L.) Dunal	Solanaceae	root
Bacopa	*Bacopa monnieri* (L.) Pennell	Scrophulariaceae	stem, leaf
Powderd Bilberry Extract	*Vaccinium myrtillus* L.	Ericaceae	fruit
Black Cohosh	*Actaea racemosa* L.	Ranunculaceae	rhizome, root
	Cimicifuga racemosa (L.) Nutt.		
Black Pepper	*Piper nigrum* L.	Piperaceae	fruit
Boswellia serrata	*Boswellia serrata* Roxb.	Burseraceae	resin
Cat's Claw	*Uncaria tomentosa* (Willd.) DC.	Rubiaceae	bark

(*Continued*)

Table 2. (*Continued*)

Dietary Supplement	Original Plants	Family Name	Part of Use
Centella asiatica	*Centella asiatica* (L.) Urb.	Apiaceae	aerial parts
	Hydrocotyle asiatica L.		
Chamomile	*Matricaria recutita* L. Rauschert	Asteraceae alt. Compositae	flower
	Matricaria chamomilla L. Rauschert		
	Matricaria chamomilla L var. *courrantiana* Rauschert		
	Chamomilla recutita (L.) Rauschert		
Chaste Tree	*Vitex agnuscastus* L.	Verbenaceae	fruit
Cranberry Liquid Preparation	*Vaccinium macrocarpon* Ait.	Ericaceae	fruit
	Vaccinium oxycoccos L.		
***Crypthecodinium cohnii* Oil**	*Crypthecodinium cohnii*	【algae】	
【Curcuminoids】	*Curcuma longa* L.		rhizome (diarylheptanoids)
Echinacea angustifolia	*Echinacea angustifolia* DC.	Asteraceae	rhizome, root
Echinacea pallida	*Echinacea pallida* (Nutt.) Nutt.	Asteraceae	rhizome, root
***Echinacea purpurea* Aerial Parts**	*Echinacea purpurea* (L.) Moench	Asteraceae	aerial parts
***Echinacea purpurea* Root**	*Echinacea purpurea* (L.) Moench	Asteraceae	rhizome, root
Eleuthero	*Eleutherococcus senticosus* (Rupr. & Maxim.) Maxim.	Araliaceae	rhizome, root
	Acanthopanax senticosus (Rupr. & Maxim.) Harms		
Feverfew	*Tanacetum parthenium* (L.) Sch. Bip.	Asteraceae	leaf
Forskohlii	*Plectranthus barbatus* Andrews	Lamiaceae	root
	Coleus barbatus (Andrews) Benth.		
	Coleus forskohlii Briq.		
Garcinia cambogia	*Garcinia gummi-gutta* (L.) N. Robson	Clusiaceae	pericarp
	Garcinia cambogia (Gaertn.) Desr.		
Powdered Garcinia Hydroxycitrate Extract	*Garcinia cambogia*		
	Garcinia indica		
Garcinia indica	*Garcinia indica* (Thouars) Choisy	Clusiaceae	pericarp
Garlic	*Allium sativum* L.	Liliaceae	bulb
Ginger	*Zingiber officinale* Roscoe	Zingiberaceae	rhizome
Ginkgo	*Ginkgo biloba* L.	Ginkgoaceae	leaf
Goldenseal	*Hydrastis canadensis* L.	Ranunculaceae	root, rhizome

(*Continued*)

Table 2. (*Continued*)

Dietary Supplement	Original Plants	Family Name	Part of Use
Grape Seeds Oligomeric Proanthocyanidins	*Vitis vinifera* L.	Vitaceae	seed
Powdered Decaffeinated Green Tea Extract	*Camellia sinensis* (L.) Kuntze	Theaceae	leaf
	Thea sinensis L.		
Guggul	*Commiphora wightii* (Arnott) Bhandari	Burseraceae	resin
	Commiphora mukul (Hook. ex. Stocks) Engl.		
	Balsamodendrum mukul (Hook.)		
Hawthorn Leaf with Flower	*Crataegus monogyna* Jacq. emend Lindman.	Rosaceae	flower-bearing branches up to 7cm in length
	Crataegus laevigata (Poir.) DC.		
	Crataegus oxycantha Linné		
Horse Chestnut	*Aesculus hippocastanum* L.	Hippocastanaceae	seed
Licorice	*Glycyrrhiza glabra* L.	Fabaceae	root, rhizome, stolon
	Glycyrrhiza uralensis Fish. ex DC.		
Tomato Extract Containing Lycopene	*Lycopersicon esculentum* Mill.	Solanaceae	fruit
Malabar-Nut-Tree, Leaf	*Justicia adhatoda* L.	Acanthaceae	leaf
	Adhatoda vasica Nees		
Maritime Pine	*Pinus pinaster* Aiton	Pinaceae	stem
	Pinus maritima Poir.		
Milk Thistle	*Silybum marianum* (L.) Gaertn.	Asteraceae	fruit
Phyllanthus amarus	*Phyllanthus amarus* Schumach.	Euphorbiaceae	aerial parts
Pygeum	*Prunus africana* (Hook f.) Kalkman	Rosaceae	bark
	Pygeum africanum Hook f.		
Red Clover	*Trifolium pratense* L.	Fabaceae	inflorescence
St. John's Wort	*Hypericum perforatum* L.	Hypericaceae	flower, aerial part
Saw Palmetto	*Serenoa repens* (W.Bartram) Small	Arecaceae	fruit
	Seranoa serrulatum Schult.		
	Sabal serrulata (Michx.) Nutt. ex Schult. & Schult. f.		
【Schizochytrium Oil】	*Schizochytrium*	【algae】	
Powdered Soy Isoflavones Extract	*Glycine max* Merr.	Fabaceae	seed
Stinging Nettle	*Urtica dioica* L. subsp. *dioica*	Urticaceae	root, rhizome

(*Continued*)

Table 2. (*Continued*)

Dietary Supplement	Original Plants	Family Name	Part of Use
Turmeric	*Curcuma longa* L.	Zingiberaceae	rhizome
	C. domestica Val.		
Valerian	*Valeriana officinalis* L.	Valerianaceae	subterranean parts

Table 3. Official Monographs for NF 31 in USP 36 NF 31 (2013)

Crude dug	Original Plants	Family Name	Medicinal part
Acacia	*Acacia senegal* (L.) Wild.	Leguminosae	stem, branche
	other related African species of *Acasia*		
Almond Oil	*Prunus dulcis* (Miller) D.A. Webb	Rosaceae	kernel
	Prunus amygdalus Batsch		
	except for *Prunus dulcis* (Miller) D.A. Webb var. *amara* (De Candolle) Focke		
Anise Oil	*Pimpinella ansium* L.	Apiaceae	fruit
	Illicium verum Hook. f.	Illiciaceae	
Canola Oil	*Brassica napus*	Cruciferae	seed
	Brassica campestris		
Caraway	*Carum carvi* L.	Apiaceae	fruit
Caraway Oil	*Carum carvi* L.	Apiaceae	fruit
Cardamom Oil	*Elettaria cardamomum* (L.) Maton var. *cardamomum*	Zingiberaceae	seed
Cardamom Seed	*Elettaria cardamomum* (L.) Maton var. *cardamomum*	Zingiberaceae	seed
Cherry Juice	*Prunus cerasus* L.	Rosaceae	fruit
Chocolate	*Theobroma cacao* L.	Sterculiaceae	seed
Clove Oil	*Syzygium aromaticum* (L.) Merr. and L. M. Perry	Myrtaceae	flower
Coconut Oil	*Cocos nucifera* L.	Palmae	seed
Coriander Oil	*Coriandrum sativum* L.	Apiaceae	fruit
Corn oil	*Zea mays* Linné	Gramineae	embryo
Cottonseed Oil	*Gossypium hirsutum* Linné	Malvaceae	seed
	other species of *Gossypium*		
Fennel Oil	*Foeniculum vulgare* Mill.	Apiaceae	fruit
Lemon Oil	*Citrus* × *limon* (L.) Osbeck	Rutaceae	fruit

(*Continued*)

Table 3.（*Continued*）

Crude dug	Original Plants	Family Name	Medicinal part
Orange oil	*Citrus sinensis* (L.) Osbeck	Rutaceae	fruit
Sweet Orange Peel Tincture	*Citrus sinensis* (L.) Osbeck	Rutaceae	fruit
Palm Oil	*Elaeis guineensis* Jacq.	Aracaceae	fruit
Peanut Oil	*Arachis hypogaea* Linné	Leguminosae	seed
Peppermint	*Mentha piperita* L.	Labiatae	leaf, flower
Peppermint Oil	*Mentha piperita* Linné	Labiatae	leaf, flower
Fully Hydrogenated Rapeseed Oil	*Brassica napus*	Cruciferae	seed
	Brassica campestris		
Superglycerinated Fully Hydrogenated Rapeseed Oil	*Brassica napus*	Cruciferae	seed
	Brassica campestris		
Rose Oil	*Rosa gallica* L.	Rosaceae	flower
	Rosa damascena Miller		
	Rosa alba L.		
	Rosa centifolia L.		
Sesami Oil	*Sesamum indicum* L.	Pedaliaceae	seed
Hydrogenated Soybean Oil	*Glycine max* Merr.	Fabaceae	seed
Sunflower Oil	*Helianthus annuus* Linnè	Asteraceae alt. Compositae	seed
Vanilla	*Vanilla planifolia* Andrews	Orchidaceae	fruit
	Vanilla tahitensis J. W. Moore		
Zein	*Zea mays* Linné	Gramineae	corn

Table 4. Official Monographs for USP 36 in USP 36 NF 31 (2013)

Crude drug	Original Plants	Family Name	medicinal part
Aloe	*Aloe barbadensis* Mill.	Liliaceae	leaf
	Aloe vera L.		
	Aloe ferox Mill.		
	hybrids of *Aloe ferox* and *Aloe africana* Mill.		
	Aloe spicata Baker		
Belladonna Leaf	*Atropa belladonna* Linné or of its variety *acuminata* Royle ex Lindley	Solanaceae	leaf, flower, fluit

(*Continued*)

Table 4. (*Continued*)

Crude drug	Original Plants	Family Name	medicinal part
Benzoin	*Styrax benzoin* Dryander	Styraceae	balsamic resin
	Styrax paralleloneurus Perkins		
	Styrax tonkinensis (Piérre) Craib ex Hartwich		
	Section *Anthostyrax* of the genus *Styrax*		
Capsicum	*Capsicum frutescens* L.	Solanaceae	fruit
	Capsicum annuum L. var *connoides* Irish		
	Cupsicum annuum var. *longum* Sendt		
Capsicum Oleoresin	*Cupsicum annum* var. *minimum*	Solanaceae	fruit
	C. frutescens		fruit
Cascara sagrada	*Frangula purshiana* (DC.) J. G. Cooper	Rhamnaceae	bark
	Rhamnus purshiana DC		
Castor Oil	*Ricinus communis* L.	Euphorbiaceae	seed
Digitalis	*Digitalis purpurea* Linné	Scrophulariaceae	leaf
Elm	*Ulmus rubra* Muhl.	Ulmaceae	inner bark
	Ulmus fulva Michx.		
Gutta Percha	*Palaquium,*	Sapotaceae	latex
	Payena,		
	Palaquium gutta (Hooker) Baillon		
Ipecac	*Cephaë lis acuminata* Karsten	Rubiaceae	rhizome, root
	Cephaë lis ipecacuanha (Brotero) A. Richard		
Juniper Tar	*Juniperus oxycedrus* L.	Pinaceae	woody portions
Myrrh	*Commiphora molmol* Engler	Burseraceae	resin
	other related species of *Commiphora* other than *Commiphora mukul*		
Plantago Seed	*Plantago psyllium* auct.	Plantaginaceae	seed
	Plantago indica L.		
	Plantago arenaria Waldst. & Kit.		
	Plantago ovata Forssk.		
Psyllium Husk	*Plantago ovata* Forssk.	Plantaginaceae	seed
	Plantago arenaria Waldst. & Kit. *Plantago psyllium* L.		
Rauwolfia Serpentina	*Rauwolfia* (Linne) Bentham ex Kurz	Apocynaceae	root

(*Continued*)

Table 4.（*Continued*）

Crude drug	Original Plants	Family Name	medicinal part
Safflower Oil	*Carthamus tinctorius* L.	Compositae	seed
Senna Leaf	*Senna alexandrina* Mill.	Fabaceae	leaf
	Cassia acutifolia Delile		
	C. angustifolia Vahl		
Sennna Pods	*Senna alexandrina* Mill.	Fabaceae	fruit
	Cassia acutifolia Delile		
	C. angustifolia Vahl		
Sennosides	*Senna alexandrina* Mill.	Fabaceae	leaf, leaf pod（anthraquinines）
	Cassia acutifolia Vahl		
	C. angustifolia Delile		
Soybean Oil	*Glycine max* Merr.	Fabaceae	seed
Tolu Balsam	*Myroxylon balsamum*（L.）Harms	Leguminosae	balsam
Wheat Bran	*Triticum aestivum* L.		fluit
	T. compactum Host		
	T. durum Desf.		

添付資料 9
日本薬局方（第16改正）収載生薬の学名表記について

Appendix 9
On the scientific names of crude drugs listed in the Japanese Pharmacopoeia (The 16th Edition)

日本薬局方収載生薬の学名表記について

日本薬局方収載生薬の基原植物及び基原動物の学名表記法は、論文等で使用される分類学的に用いられる学名表記と若干異なっている。これは、主に局方が学術書ではなく法令であるために生じる問題である。局方での学名の表記と、分類学的に通常使用される学名表記との不一致について、局方利用者の誤解を避ける目的で、本表に、局方で表記した学名と分類学的に通常使用される学名表記との関係を示す。

The notation system of the scientific names for the original plants and animals of crude drugs listed in JP is not necessary the same as the taxonomic system used in the literature. The reason for this is that the JP is not an academic text, but an ordinance. The relationship between the scientific names used in the JP and those generally used taxonomically is indicated in the following table, to avoid misunderstanding by JP users owing to differences in the notation system.

表　日本薬局方の学名表記と分類学的に用いられる学名表記
Table　Scientific names used in the JP and the corresponding taxonomic names

生薬名 Crude Drug	日本薬局方の学名表記＝分類学的に用いられている学名表記（組合わせ明記、命名者簡略標準化） Scientific names used in the JP＝Scientific names being used taxonomically (Combined notation, Standard form for author or authors) 日本薬局方の学名表記とは異なるが分類学的に同一あるいは同一とみなされることがあるもの及び収載種に含まれる代表的な下位分類群。*印のあるものは、日本薬局方で併記されているもの。 Scientific names that are different from those written in JP but identical to them taxonomically or being regarded as identical, and typical subclassified groups belonging to their species. The names marked with"*"are those being written together in JP.	科名 Family
アカメガシワ Mallotus Bark	アカメガシワ *Mallotus japonicus* Mueller Argoviensis ＝*Mallotus japonicus* (Thunb.) Müll. Arg.	Euphorbiaceae トウダイグサ科
アセンヤク Gambir	*Uncaria gambir* Roxburgh ＝*Uncaria gambir* (Hunter) Roxb.	Rubiaceae アカネ科
アマチャ Sweet Hydrangea Leaf	アマチャ *Hydrangea macrophylla* Seringe var. *thunbergii* Makino ＝*Hydrangea macrophylla* (Thunb.) Ser. var. *thunbergii* (Siebold) Makino	Saxifragaceae ユキノシタ科
アラビアゴム Acacia	*Acacia senegal* Willdenow ＝*Acacia senegal* (L.) Willd. その他同属植物	Leguminosae マメ科
アロエ Aloe	*Aloe ferox* Miller ＝*Aloe ferox* Mill. *Aloe ferox* Miller と *Aloe africana* Miller との雑種 ＝*Aloe africana* Mill. *Aloe ferox* Miller と *Aloe spicata* Baker との雑種	Liliaceae ユリ科
アンソッコウ Benzoin	*Styrax benzoin* Dryander ＝*Styrax benzoin* Dryand. その他同属植物	Styracaceae エゴノキ科
イレイセン Clematis Root	サキシマボタンヅル *Clematis chinensis* Osbeck *Clematis mandshurica* Ruprecht ＝*Clematis mandshurica* Rupr. *Clematis hexapetala* Pallas ＝*Clematis hexapetala* Pall.	Ranunculaceae キンポウゲ科
インチンコウ Artemisia Capillaris Flower	カワラヨモギ *Artemisia capillaris* Thunberg ＝*Artemisia capillaris* Thunb.	Compositae キク科

生薬名 Crude Drug	日本薬局方の学名表記＝分類学的に用いられている学名表記（組合わせ明記、命名者簡略標準化） Scientific names used in the JP＝Scientific names being used taxonomically (Combined notation, Standard form for author or authors) 日本薬局方の学名表記とは異なるが分類学的に同一あるいは同一とみなされることがあるもの及び収載種に含まれる代表的な下位分類群。*印のあるものは、日本薬局方で併記されているもの。 Scientific names that are different from those written in JP but identical to them taxonomically or being regarded as identical, and typical subclassified groups belonging to their species. The names marked with"*"are those being written together in JP.	科名 Family
インヨウカク Epimedium Herb	*Epimedium pubescens* Maximowicz ＝*Epimedium pubescens* Maxim.	Berberidaceae メギ科
	Epimedium brevicornu Maximowicz ＝*Epimedium brevicornu* Maxim.	
	Epimedium wushanense T. S. Ying	
	ホザキイカリソウ *Epimedium sagittatum* Maximowicz ＝*Epimedium sagittatum* (Siebold & Zucc.) Maxim.	
	キバナイカリソウ *Epimedium koreanum* Nakai	
	イカリソウ *Epimedium grandiflorum* Morren var. *thunbergianum* Nakai ＝*Epimedium grandiflorum* Morr. var. *thunbergianum* (Miq.) Nakai	
	トキワイカリソウ *Epimedium sempervirens* Nakai	
ウイキョウ Fennel	ウイキョウ *Foeniculum vulgare* Miller ＝*Foeniculum vulgare* Mill.	Umbelliferae セリ科
ウイキョウ油 Fennel Oil	ウイキョウ　*Foeniculum vulgare* Miller ＝*Foeniculum vulgare* Mill.	Umbelliferae セリ科
	Illicium verum Hooker filius ＝*Illicium verum* Hook. f.	Illiciaceae シキミ科
ウコン Turmeric	ウコン *Curcuma longa* Linné ＝*Curcuma longa* L.	Zingiberaceae ショウガ科
ウヤク Lindera Root	テンダイウヤク *Lindera strychnifolia* Fernandez-Villar ＝*Lindera strychnifolia* (Siebold & Zucc.) Fern.-Vill.	Lauraceae クスノキ科
	Lindera aggregata (Sims) Kosterm.	
ウワウルシ Bearberry Leaf	クマコケモモ　*Arctostaphylos uva-ursi* (Linné) Sprengel ＝*Arctostaphylos uva-ursi* (L.) Spreng.	Ericaceae ツツジ科
エイジツ Rose Fruit	ノイバラ　*Rosa multiflora* Thunberg ＝*Rosa multiflora* Thunb.	Rosaceae バラ科
エンゴサク Corydalis Tuber	*Corydalis turtschaninovii* Besser forma *yanhusuo* Y. H. Chou et C. C. Hsu ＝*Corydalis turtschaninovii* Besser f. *yanhusuo* (W. T. Wang) Y. H. Chou & C. C. Hsu	Papaveraceae ケシ科
	Corydalis yanhusuo W. T. Wang	
オウギ Astragalus Root	キバナオウギ *Astragalus membranaceus* Bunge ＝*Astragalus membranaceus* (Fisch.) Bunge	Leguminosae マメ科
	Astragalus mongholicus Bunge	
	Astragalus membranaceus (Fisch.) Bunge var. *mongholicus* (Bunge) Hsiao	
オウゴン Scutellaria Root	コガネバナ *Scutellaria baicalensis* Georgi	Labiatae シソ科
オウセイ Polygonatum Rhizome	ナルコユリ *Polygonatum falcatum* A. Gray	Liliaceae ユリ科
	カギクルマバナルコユリ *Polygonatum sibiricum* Redouté	
	Polygonatum kingianum Collett et Hemsley ＝*Polygonatum kingianum* Collett & Hemsl.	
	Polygonatum cyrtonema Hua	

生薬名 Crude Drug	日本薬局方の学名表記＝分類学的に用いられている学名表記（組合わせ明記、命名者簡略標準化） Scientific names used in the JP＝Scientific names being used taxonomically (Combined notation, Standard form for author or authors) 日本薬局方の学名表記とは異なるが分類学的に同一あるいは同一とみなされることがあるもの及び収載種に含まれる代表的な下位分類群。*印のあるものは、日本薬局方で併記されているもの。 Scientific names that are different from those written in JP but identical to them taxonomically or being regarded as identical, and typical subclassified groups belonging to their species. The names marked with"*"are those being written together in JP.	科名 Family
オウバク Phellodendron Bark	キハダ *Phellodendron amurense* Ruprecht ＝*Phellodendron amurense* Rupr. ヒロハキハダ *Phellodendron amurense* Rupr. var. *sachalinense* F. Schmidt オオバノキハダ *Phellodendron amurense* Rupr. var. *japonicum* (Maxim.) Ohwi ミヤマキハダ *Phellodendron amurense* Rupr. var. *lavallei* (Dode) Sprangue *Phellodendron chinense* Schneider ＝*Phellodendron chinense* C. K. Schneid.	Rutaceae ミカン科
オウレン Coptis Rhizome	オウレン *Coptis japonica* Makino ＝*Coptis japonica* (Thunb.) Makino セリバオウレン *Coptis japonica* (Thunb.) Makino var. *dissecta* (Yatabe) Nakai キクバオウレン *Coptis japonica* (Thunb.) Makino var. *japonica* コセリバオウレン *Coptis japonica* (Thunb.) Makino var. *major* (Miq.) Satake *Coptis chinensis* Franchet ＝*Coptis chinensis* Franch. *Coptis deltoidea* C. Y. Cheng & Hsiao *Coptis teeta* Wallich ＝*Coptis teeta* Wall.	Ranunculaceae キンポウゲ科
オンジ Polygala Root	イトヒメハギ *Polygala tenuifolia* Willdenow ＝*Polygala tenuifolia* Willd.	Polygalaceae ヒメハギ科
ガイヨウ Artemisia Leaf	ヨモギ *Artemisia princeps* Pampanini ＝*Artemisia princeps* Pamp. オオヨモギ *Artemisia montana* Pampanini ＝*Artemisia montana* (Nakai) Pamp.	Compositae キク科
カゴソウ Prunella Spike	ウツボグサ *Prunella vulgaris* Linné var. *lilacina* Nakai ＝*Prunella vulgaris* L. var. *lilacina* Nakai	Labiatae シソ科
カシュウ Polygonum Root	ツルドクダミ *Polygonum multiflorum* Thunberg ＝*Polygonum multiflorum* Thunb.	Polygonaceae タデ科
ガジュツ Zedoary	ガジュツ *Curcuma zedoaria* Roscoe	Zingiberaceae ショウガ科
カッコウ Pogostemon Herb	*Pogostemon cablin* Bentham ＝*Pogostemon cablin* (Blanco) Benth.	Labiatae シソ科
カッコン Pueraria Root	クズ *Pueraria lobata* Ohwi ＝*Pueraria lobata* (Willd.) Ohwi	Leguminosae マメ科
カノコソウ Japanese Valerian	カノコソウ *Valeriana fauriei* Briquet ＝*Valeriana fauriei* Briq. エゾカノコソウ *Valeriana fauriei* Briq. f. *yezoensis* Hara	Valerianaceae オミナエシ科
カロコン Trichosanthes Root	*Trichosanthes kirilowii* Maximowicz ＝*Trichosanthes kirilowii* Maxim. キカラスウリ *Trichosanthes kirilowii* Maximowicz var. *japonicum* Kitamura ＝*Trichosanthes kirilowii* Maxim. var. *japonicum* (Miq.) Kitam. オオカラスウリ *Trichosanthes bracteata* Voigt ＝*Trichosanthes bracteata* (Lam.) Voigt	Cucurbitaceae ウリ科
カンキョウ Processed Ginger	ショウガ *Zingiber officinale* Roscoe	Zingiberaceae ショウガ科

生薬名 Crude Drug	日本薬局方の学名表記＝分類学的に用いられている学名表記（組合わせ明記、命名者簡略標準化） Scientific names used in the JP＝Scientific names being used taxonomically (Combined notation, Standard form for author or authors) 日本薬局方の学名表記とは異なるが分類学的に同一あるいは同一とみなされることがあるもの及び収載種に含まれる代表的な下位分類群。*印のあるものは、日本薬局方で併記されているもの。 Scientific names that are different from those written in JP but identical to them taxonomically or being regarded as identical, and typical subclassified groups belonging to their species. The names marked with"*"are those being written together in JP.	科名 Family
カンゾウ Glycyrrhiza	*Glycyrrhiza uralensis* Fischer ＝*Glycyrrhiza uralensis* Fisch. *Glycyrrhiza glabra* Linné ＝*Glycyrrhiza glabra* L.	Leguminosae マメ科
カンテン Agar	マクサ（テングサ）*Gelidium elegans* Kuetzing その他同属植物 諸種紅そう類	Gelidiaceae テングサ科
キキョウ Platycodon Root	キキョウ *Platycodon grandiflorum* A. De Candolle ＝*Platycodon grandiflorum* (Jacq.) A. DC.	Campanulaceae キキョウ科
キクカ Chrysanthemum Flower	キク *Chrysanthemum morifolium* Ramatuelle ＝*Chrysanthemum morifolium* Ramat. シマカンギク *Chrysanthemum indicum* Linné ＝*Chrysanthemum indicum* L.	Compositae キク科
キササゲ Catalpa Fruit	キササゲ *Catalpa ovata* G. Don *Catalpa bungei* C. A. Meyer ＝*Catalpa bungei* C. A. Mey.	Bignoniaceae ノウゼンカズラ科
キジツ Immature Orange	ダイダイ *Citrus aurantium* Linné var. *daidai* Makino ＝*Citrus aurantium* L. var. *daidai* Makino *Citrus aurantium* L. 'Daidai' ナツミカン *Citrus natsudaidai* Hayata *Citrus aurantium* Linné ＝*Citrus aurantium* L. ハッサク *Citrus aurantium* L. subsp. *hassaku* (Tanaka) Hiroe ＝*Citrus hassaku* hort. ex Tanaka	Rutaceae ミカン科
キョウカツ Notopterygium	*Notopterygium incisum* Ting ex H. T. Chang *Notopterygium forbesii* Boissieu	Umbelliferae セリ科
キョウニン Apricot Kernel	ホンアンズ *Prunus armeniaca* Linné ＝*Prunus armeniaca* L. アンズ *Prunus armeniaca* Linné var. *ansu* Maximowicz ＝*Prunus armeniaca* L. var. *ansu* Maxim. *Prunus sibirica* Linné ＝*Prunus sibirica* L.	Rosaceae バラ科
クコシ Lycium Fruit	クコ *Lycium chinense* Miller ＝*Lycium chinense* Mill. *Lycium barbarum* Linné ＝*Lycium barbarum* L.	Solanaceae ナス科
クジン Sophora Root	クララ *Sophora flavescens* Aiton	Leguminosae マメ科
ケイガイ Schizonepeta Spike	ケイガイ *Schizonepeta tenuifolia* Briquet ＝*Schizonepeta tenuifolia* Briq.	Labiatae シソ科
ケイヒ Cinnamon Bark	*Cinnamomum cassia* Blume	Lauraceae クスノキ科
ケイヒ油 Cinnamon Oil	*Cinnamomum cassia* Blume *Cinnamomum zeylanicum* Nees	Lauraceae クスノキ科

生薬名 Crude Drug	日本薬局方の学名表記＝分類学的に用いられている学名表記（組合わせ明記、命名者簡略標準化） Scientific names used in the JP＝Scientific names being used taxonomically (Combined notation, Standard form for author or authors) 日本薬局方の学名表記とは異なるが分類学的に同一あるいは同一とみなされることがあるもの及び収載種に含まれる代表的な下位分類群。*印のあるものは、日本薬局方で併記されているもの。 Scientific names that are different from those written in JP but identical to them taxonomically or being regarded as identical, and typical subclassified groups belonging to their species. The names marked with"*"are those being written together in JP.	科名 Family
ケツメイシ Cassia Seed	エビスグサ *Cassia obtusifolia* Linné ＝*Cassia obtusifolia* L. *Cassia tora* Linné ＝*Cassia tora* L.	Leguminosae マメ科
ケンゴシ Pharbitis Seed	アサガオ *Pharbitis nil* Choisy ＝*Pharbitis nil* (L.) Choisy	Convolvulaceae ヒルガオ科
ゲンチアナ Gentian	*Gentiana lutea* Linné ＝*Gentiana lutea* L.	Gentianaceae リンドウ科
ゲンノショウコ Geranium Herb	ゲンノショウコ *Geranium thunbergii* Siebold et Zuccarini ＝*Geranium thunbergii* Siebold & Zucc.	Geraniaceae フウロソウ科
コウカ Safflower	ベニバナ *Carthamus tinctorius* Linné ＝*Carthamus tinctorius* L.	Compositae キク科
コウジン Red Ginseng	オタネニンジン *Panax ginseng* C. A. Meyer ＝*Panax ginseng* C. A. Mey. **Panax schinseng* Nees	Araliaceae ウコギ科
コウブシ Cyperus Rhizome	ハマスゲ *Cyperus rotundus* Linné ＝*Cyperus rotundus* L.	Cyperaceae カヤツリグサ科
コウボク Magnolia Bark	ホオノキ *Magnolia obovata* Thunberg ＝*Magnolia obovata* Thunb. **Magnolia hypoleuca* Siebold et Zuccarini ＝*Magnolia hypoleuca* Siebold & Zucc. *Magnolia officinalis* Rehder et Wilson ＝*Magnolia officinalis* Rehder & E. H. Wilson *Magnolia officinalis* Rehder et Wilson var. *biloba* Rehder et Wilson ＝*Magnolia officinalis* Rehder & E. H. Wilson var. *biloba* Rehder & E. H. Wilson	Magnoliaceae モクレン科
ゴオウ Oriental Bezoar	ウシ *Bos taurus* Linné var. *domesticus* Gmelin ＝*Bos taurus* L. var. *domesticus* Gmelin	Bovidae ウシ科
ゴシツ Achyranthes Root	ヒナタイノコズチ *Achyranthes fauriei* Leveille et Vaniot ＝*Achyranthes fauriei* H. Lev. & Vaniot *Achyranthes bidentata* Blume	Amaranthaceae ヒユ科
ゴシュユ Euodia Fruit	ゴシュユ *Euodia ruticarpa* Hooker filius et Thomson ＝*Euodia ruticarpa* (A. Juss.) Hook. f. & Thomson **Evodia rutaecarpa* Bentham ＝*Evodia rutaecarpa* (A. Juss.) Benth. *Tetradium ruticarpum* (A. Juss.) Hartley *Euodia officinalis* Dode **Evodia officinalis* Dode *Evodia rutaecarpa* (A. Juss.) Benth. var. *officinalis* (Dode) Huang *Euodia bodinieri* Dode **Evodia bodinieri* Dode *Evodia rutaecarpa* (A. Juss.) Benth. var. *bodinieri* (Dode) Huang	Rutaceae ミカン科
ゴボウシ Burdock Fruit	ゴボウ *Arctium lappa* Linné ＝*Arctium lappa* L.	Compositae キク科
ゴミシ Schisandra Fruit	チョウセンゴミシ *Schisandra chinensis* Baillon ＝*Schisandra chinensis* (Turcz.) Baill.	Schisandraceae マツブサ科

生薬名 Crude Drug	日本薬局方の学名表記＝分類学的に用いられている学名表記（組合わせ明記、命名者簡略標準化） Scientific names used in the JP＝Scientific names being used taxonomically (Combined notation, Standard form for author or authors) 日本薬局方の学名表記とは異なるが分類学的に同一あるいは同一とみなされることがあるもの及び収載種に含まれる代表的な下位分類群。*印のあるものは、日本薬局方で併記されているもの。 Scientific names that are different from those written in JP but identical to them taxonomically or being regarded as identical, and typical subclassified groups belonging to their species. The names marked with"*"are those being written together in JP.	科名 Family
コロンボ Calumba	*Jateorhiza columba* Miers	Menispermaceae ツヅラフジ科
コンズランゴ Condurango	*Marsdenia cundurango* Reichenbach filius ＝*Marsdenia cundurango* Rchb. f.	Asclepiadaceae ガガイモ科
サイコ Bupleurum Root	ミシマサイコ *Bupleurum falcatum* Linné ＝*Bupleurum falcatum* L. *Bupleurum chinense* DC. *Bupleurum scorzonerifolium* Willd.	Umbelliferae セリ科
サイシン Asiasarum Root	ウスバサイシン *Asiasarum sieboldii* F. Maekawa ＝*Asiasarum sieboldii* (Miq.) F. Maek. *Asarum sieboldii* Miq. ウスゲサイシン *Asarum sieboldii* Miq. var. *seoulense* Nakai ケイリンサイシン *Asiasarum heterotropoides* F. Maekawa var. *mandshuricum* F. Maekawa ＝*Asiasarum heterotropoides* (F. Schmidt) F. Maek. var. *mandshuricum* (Maxim.) F. Maek. *Asarum heterotropoides* F. Schmidt var. *mandshuricum* (Maxim.) Kitag.	Aristolochiaceae ウマノスズクサ科
サフラン Saffron	サフラン *Crocus sativus* Linné ＝*Crocus sativus* L.	Iridaceae アヤメ科
サンキライ Smilax Rhizome	*Smilax glabra* Roxburgh ＝*Smilax glabra* Roxb.	Liliaceae ユリ科
サンザシ Crataegus Fruit	サンザシ *Crataegus cuneata* Siebold et Zuccarini ＝*Crataegus cuneata* Siebold & Zucc. オオミサンザシ *Crataegus pinnatifida* Bunge var. *major* N. E. Brown ＝*Crataegus pinnatifida* Bunge var. *major* N. E. Br.	Rosaceae バラ科
サンシシ Gardenia Fruit	クチナシ *Gardenia jasminoides* Ellis *Gardenia jasminoides* Ellis f. *longicarpa* Z. W. Xie & Okada	Rubiaceae アカネ科
サンシュユ Cornus Fruit	サンシュユ *Cornus officinalis* Siebold et Zuccarini ＝*Cornus officinalis* Siebold & Zucc.	Cornaceae ミズキ科
サンショウ Zanthoxylum Fruit	サンショウ *Zanthoxylum piperitum* De Candolle ＝*Zanthoxylum piperitum* (L.) DC. アサクラザンショウ *Zanthoxylum piperitum* (L.) DC. f. *inerme* Makino	Rutaceae ミカン科
サンソウニン Jujube Seed	サネブトナツメ *Zizyphus jujuba* Miller var. *spinosa* Hu ex H. F. Chou ＝*Zizyphus jujuba* Mill. var. *spinosa* (Bunge) Hu ex H. F. Chou	Rhamnaceae クロウメモドキ科
サンヤク Dioscorea Rhizome	ヤマノイモ *Dioscorea japonica* Thunberg ＝*Dioscorea japonica* Thunb. ナガイモ *Dioscorea batatas* Decaisne ＝*Dioscorea batatas* Decne. *Dioscorea opposita* Thunb.	Dioscoreaceae ヤマノイモ科
ジオウ Rehmannia Root	アカヤジオウ *Rehmannia glutinosa* Liboschitz var. *purpurea* Makino ＝*Rehmannia glutinosa* Libosch. var. *purpurea* Makino *Rehmannia glutinosa* Liboschitz ＝*Rehmannia glutinosa* Libosch.	Scrophulariaceae ゴマノハグサ科
シゴカ Eleutherococcus Senticosus Rhizome	エゾウコギ *Eleutherococcus senticosus* Maximowicz ＝*Eleutherococcus senticosus* (Rupr. & Maxim.) Maxim. **Acanthopanax senticosus* Harms ＝*Acanthopanax senticosus* (Rupr. & Maxim.) Harms	Araliaceae ウコギ科

生薬名 Crude Drug	日本薬局方の学名表記＝分類学的に用いられている学名表記（組合わせ明記、命名者簡略標準化） Scientific names used in the JP＝Scientific names being used taxonomically (Combined notation, Standard form for author or authors) 日本薬局方の学名表記とは異なるが分類学的に同一あるいは同一とみなされることがあるもの及び収載種に含まれる代表的な下位分類群。*印のあるものは、日本薬局方で併記されているもの。 Scientific names that are different from those written in JP but identical to them taxonomically or being regarded as identical, and typical subclassified groups belonging to their species. The names marked with"*"are those being written together in JP.	科名 Family
ジコッピ Lycium Bark	クコ *Lycium chinense* Miller ＝*Lycium chinense* Mill. *Lycium barbarum* Linné ＝*Lycium barbarum* L.	Solanaceae ナス科
シコン Lithospermum Root	ムラサキ *Lithospermum erythrorhizon* Siebold et Zuccarini ＝*Lithospermum erythrorhizon* Siebold & Zucc.	Boraginaceae ムラサキ科
シツリシ Tribulus Fruit	ハマビシ *Tribulus terrestris* Linné ＝*Tribulus terrestris* L.	Zygophyllaceae ハマビシ科
シャクヤク Peony Root	シャクヤク *Paeonia lactiflora* Pallas ＝*Paeonia lactiflora* Pall.	Paeoniaceae ボタン科
ジャショウシ Cnidium Monnieri Fruit	*Cnidium monnieri* Cusson ＝*Cnidium monnieri* (L.) Cusson	Umbelliferae セリ科
シャゼンシ Plantago Seed	オオバコ *Plantago asiatica* Linné ＝*Plantago asiatica* L.	Plantaginaceae オオバコ科
シャゼンソウ Plantago Herb	オオバコ *Plantago asiatica* Linné ＝*Plantago asiatica* L.	Plantaginaceae オオバコ科
ジュウヤク Houttuynia Herb	ドクダミ *Houttuynia cordata* Thunberg ＝*Houttuynia cordata* Thunb.	Saururaceae ドクダミ科
シュクシャ Amomum Seed	*Amomum xanthioides* Wallich ＝*Amomum xanthioides* Wall. *Amomum villosum* Lour. var. *xanthioides* (Wall.) T. L. Wu et Senjen	Zingiberaceae ショウガ科
ショウキョウ Ginger	ショウガ *Zingiber officinale* Roscoe	Zingiberaceae ショウガ科
ショウズク Cardamon	*Elettaria cardamomum* Maton	Zingiberaceae ショウガ科
ショウマ Cimicifuga Rhizome	サラシナショウマ *Cimicifuga simplex* Turczaninow ＝*Cimicifuga simplex* (DC.) Turcz. *Cimicifuga dahurica* Maximowicz ＝*Cimicifuga dahurica* (Turcz.) Maxim. *Cimisifuga heracleifolia* Komarov ＝*Cimisifuga heracleifolia* Kom. *Cimicifuga foetida* Linné ＝*Cimicifuga foetida* L.	Ranunculaceae キンポウゲ科
シンイ Magnolia Flower	タムシバ *Magnolia salicifolia* Maximowicz ＝*Magnolia salicifolia* (Siebold & Zucc.) Maxim. コブシ *Magnolia kobus* De Candolle ＝*Magnolia kobus* DC. *Magnolia biondii* Pampanini ＝*Magnolia biondii* Pamp. *Magnolia sprengeri* Pampanini ＝*Magnolia sprengeri* Pamp. ハクモクレン *Magnolia heptapeta* Dandy ＝*Magnolia heptapeta* (Buchoz) Dandy **Magnolia denudata* Desrousseaux ＝*Magnolia denudata* Desr.	Magnoliaceae モクレン科

生薬名 Crude Drug	日本薬局方の学名表記＝分類学的に用いられている学名表記（組合わせ明記、命名者簡略標準化） Scientific names used in the JP＝Scientific names being used taxonomically (Combined notation, Standard form for author or authors) 日本薬局方の学名表記とは異なるが分類学的に同一あるいは同一とみなされることがあるもの及び収載種に含まれる代表的な下位分類群。*印のあるものは、日本薬局方で併記されているもの。 Scientific names that are different from those written in JP but identical to them taxonomically or being regarded as identical, and typical subclassified groups belonging to their species. The names marked with"*"are those being written together in JP.	科名 Family
セネガ Senega	セネガ *Polygala senega* Linné ＝*Polygala senega* L. ヒロハセネガ *Polygala senega* Linné var. *latifolia* Torrey et Gray ＝*Polygala senega* L. var. *latifolia* Torr. & A.Gray	Polygalaceae ヒメハギ科
センキュウ Cnidium Rhizome	センキュウ *Cnidium officinale* Makino	Umbelliferae セリ科
ゼンコ Peucedanum Root	*Peucedanum praeruptorum* Dunn ノダケ *Angelica decursiva* Franchet et Savatier ＝*Angelica decursiva* (Miq.) Franch. & Sav. **Peucedanum decursivum* Maximowicz ＝*Peucedanum decursivum* (Miq.) Maxim.	Umbelliferae セリ科
センコツ Nuphar Rhizome	コウホネ *Nuphar japonicum* De Candolle ＝*Nuphar japonicum* DC.	Nymphaeaceae スイレン科
センソ Toad Venom	シナヒキガエル *Bufo bufo gargarizans* Cantor *Bufo melanostictus* Schneider	Bufonidae ヒキガエル科
センナ Senna Leaf	*Cassia angustifolia* Vahl *Cassia acutifolia* Delile	Leguminosae マメ科
センブリ Swertia Herb	センブリ *Swertia japonica* Makino ＝*Swertia japonica* (Shult.) Makino	Gentianaceae リンドウ科
ソウジュツ Atractylodes Lancea Rhizome	ホソバオケラ *Atractylodes lancea* De Candolle ＝*Atractylodes lancea* (Thunb.) DC. *Atractylodes chinensis* Koidzumi ＝*Atractylodes chinensis* (DC.) Koidz. 上記種の雑種	Compositae キク科
ソウハクヒ Mulberry Bark	マグワ *Morus alba* Linné ＝*Morus alba* L.	Moraceae クワ科
ソボク Sappan Wood	*Caesalpinia sappan* Linné ＝*Caesalpinia sappan* L.	Leguminosae マメ科
ソヨウ Perilla Herb	シソ *Perilla frutescens* Britton var. *acuta* Kudo ＝*Perilla frutescens* (L.) Britton var. *acuta* (Thunb.) Kudo チリメンジソ *Perilla frutescens* Britton var. *crispa* Decaisne ＝*Perilla frutescens* (L.) Britton var. *crispa*(Thunb.) Decne.	Labiatae シソ科
ダイオウ Rhubarb	*Rheum palmatum* Linné ＝*Rheum palmatum* L. *Rheum tanguticum* Maximowicz ＝*Rheum tanguticum* Maxim. *Rheum officinale* Baillon ＝*Rheum officinale* Baill. *Rheum coreanum* Nakai 上記種の種間雑種	Polygonaceae タデ科
タイソウ Jujube	ナツメ *Zizyphus jujuba* Miller var. *inermis* Rehder ＝*Zizyphus jujuba* Mill. var. *inermis* (Bunge) Rehder	Rhamnaceae クロウメモドキ科
タクシャ Alisma Rhizome	サジオモダカ *Alisma orientale* Juzepczuk ＝*Alisma orientale* (Sam.) Juz. *Alisma plantago-aquatica* L. var. *orientale* Sam.	Alismataceae オモダカ科

生薬名 Crude Drug	日本薬局方の学名表記＝分類学的に用いられている学名表記（組合わせ明記、命名者簡略標準化） Scientific names used in the JP＝Scientific names being used taxonomically (Combined notation, Standard form for author or authors) 日本薬局方の学名表記とは異なるが分類学的に同一あるいは同一とみなされることがあるもの及び収載種に含まれる代表的な下位分類群。*印のあるものは、日本薬局方で併記されているもの。 Scientific names that are different from those written in JP but identical to them taxonomically or being regarded as identical, and typical subclassified groups belonging to their species. The names marked with"*"are those being written together in JP.	科名 Family
チクセツニンジン Panax Japonicus Rhizome	トチバニンジン *Panax japonicus* C. A. Meyer ＝*Panax japonicus* C. A. Mey.	Araliaceae ウコギ科
チモ Anemarrhena Rhizome	ハナスゲ *Anemarrhena asphodeloides* Bunge	Liliaceae ユリ科
チョウジ Clove	チョウジ *Syzygium aromaticum* Merrill et Perry ＝*Syzygium aromaticum* (L.) Merr. & M. L. Perry	Myrtaceae フトモモ科
	**Eugenia caryophyllata* Thunberg ＝*Eugenia caryophyllata* Thunb. *Eugenia caryophyllus* (Spreng.) Bullock & S. G. Harrison	
チョウトウコウ Uncaria Hook	カギカズラ *Uncaria rhynchophylla* Miquel ＝*Uncaria rhynchophylla* (Miq.) Miq.	Rubiaceae アカネ科
	Uncaria sinensis Haviland ＝*Uncaria sinensis* (Oliv.) Havil.	
	Uncaria macrophylla Wallich ＝*Uncaria macrophylla* Wall.	
チョレイ Polyporus Sclerotium	チョレイマイタケ *Polyporus umbellatus* Fries ＝*Polyporus umbellatus* (Pers.) Fries	Polyporaceae サルノコシカケ科
チンピ Citrus Unshiu Peel	ウンシュウミカン *Citrus unshiu* Marcowicz ＝*Citrus unshiu* (Swingle) Marcow.	Rutaceae ミカン科
	Citrus reticulata Blanco 'Unshiu'	
	Citrus reticulata Blanco	
テンマ Gastrodia Tuber	オニノヤガラ *Gastrodia elata* Blume	Orchidaceae ラン科
テンモンドウ Asparagus Tuber	クサスギカズラ *Asparagus cochinchinensis* Merrill ＝*Asparagus cochinchinensis* (Lour.) Merr.	Liliaceae ユリ科
トウガシ Beninacasa Seed	トウガン *Benincasa cerifera* Savi	Cucurbitaceae ウリ科
	Benincasa hispida (Thunb.) Cogn.	
	Benincasa cerifera Savi forma *emarginata* K. Kimura et Sugiyama ＝*Benincasa cerifera* Savi f. *emarginata* K. Kimura & Sugiyama	
トウガラシ Capsicum	トウガラシ *Capsicum annuum* Linné ＝*Capsicum annuum* L.	Solanaceae ナス科
トウキ Japanese Angelica Root	トウキ *Angelica acutiloba* Kitagawa ＝*Angelica acutiloba* (Siebold & Zucc.) Kitag.	Umbelliferae セリ科
	ホッカイトウキ *Angelica acutiloba* Kitagawa var. *sugiyamae* Hikino ＝*Angelica acutiloba* (Siebold & Zucc.) Kitag. var. *sugiyamae* Hikino	
トウニン Peach Kernel	モモ *Prunus persica* Batsch ＝*Prunus persica* (L.) Batsch	Rosaceae バラ科
	Prunus persica Batsch var. *davidiana* Maximowicz ＝*Prunus persica* (L.) Batsch var. *davidiana* (Carrière) Maxim.	
	Prunus davidiana (Carrière) Franch.	

生薬名 Crude Drug	日本薬局方の学名表記＝分類学的に用いられている学名表記（組合わせ明記、命名者簡略標準化） Scientific names used in the JP＝Scientific names being used taxonomically (Combined notation, Standard form for author or authors) 日本薬局方の学名表記とは異なるが分類学的に同一あるいは同一とみなされることがあるもの及び収載種に含まれる代表的な下位分類群。*印のあるものは、日本薬局方で併記されているもの。 Scientific names that are different from those written in JP but identical to them taxonomically or being regarded as identical, and typical subclassified groups belonging to their species. The names marked with"*"are those being written together in JP.	科名 Family
トウヒ Bitter Orange Peel	*Citrus aurantium* Linné ＝*Citrus aurantium* L.	Rutaceae ミカン科
	ダイダイ *Citrus aurantium* Linné var. *daidai* Makino ＝*Citrus aurantium* L. var. *daidai* Makino	
	Citrus aurantium L. 'Daidai'	
トコン Ipecac	*Cephaelis ipecacuanha* (Broterol) A. Richard ＝*Cephaelis ipecacuanha* (Brot.) A. Rich.	Rubiaceae アカネ科
	Cephaelis acuminata Karsten ＝*Cephaelis acuminata* H. Karst.	
トチュウ Eucommia Bark	トチュウ *Eucommia ulmoides* Oliver ＝*Eucommia ulmoides* Oliv.	Eucommiaceae トチュウ科
トラガント Tragacanth	*Astragalus gummifer* Labillardiére ＝*Astragalus gummifer* Labill.	Leguminosae マメ科
ニガキ Picrasma Wood	ニガキ *Picrasma quassioides* Bennet ＝*Picrasma quassioides* (D. Don) Benn.	Simaroubaceae ニガキ科
ニクズク Nutmeg	ニクズク *Myristica fragrans* Houttuyn ＝*Myristica fragrans* Houtt.	Myristicaceae フトモモ科
ニンジン Ginseng	オタネニンジ *Panax ginseng* C. A. Meyer ＝*Panax ginseng* C. A. Mey.	Araliaceae ウコギ科
	**Panax schinseng* Nees	
ニンドウ Lonicera Leaf and Stem	スイカズラ *Lonicera japonica* Thunberg ＝*Lonicera japonica* Thunb.	Caprifoliaceae スイカズラ科
バイモ Fritillaria Bulb	アミガサユリ *Fritillaria verticillata* Willdenow var. *thunbergii* Baker ＝*Fritillaria verticillata* Willd. var. *thunbergii* (Miq.) Baker	Liliaceae ユリ科
	Fritillaria thunbergii Miq.	
バクモンドウ Ophiopogon Tuber	ジャノヒゲ *Ophiopogon japonicus* Ker-Gawler ＝*Ophiopogon japonicus* (L. f.) Ker Gawl.	Liliaceae ユリ科
ハチミツ Honey	ヨーロッパミツバチ *Apis mellifera* Linné ＝*Apis mellifera* L.	Apidae ミツバチ科
	トウヨウミツバチ *Apis cerana* Fabricius	
ハッカ Mentha Herb	ハッカ *Mentha arvensis* Linné var. *piperascens* Malinvaud ＝*Mentha arvensis* L. var. *piperascens* Malinv.	Labiatae シソ科
	ハッカ *Mentha arvensis* L. var. *piperascens* Malinv. を母種とする交配種	
	Mentha haplocalyx Briq.	
ハマボウフウ Glehnia Root and Rhizome	ハマボウフウ *Glehnia littoralis* Fr.Schmidt ex Miquel ＝*Glehnia littoralis* F. Schmidt ex Miq.	Umbelliferae セリ科
ハンゲ Pinellia Tuber	カラスビシャク *Pinellia ternata* Breitenbach ＝*Pinellia ternata* (Thunb.) Breitenb.	Araceae サトイモ科

生薬名 Crude Drug	日本薬局方の学名表記＝分類学的に用いられている学名表記（組合わせ明記、命名者簡略標準化） Scientific names used in the JP＝Scientific names being used taxonomically (Combined notation, Standard form for author or authors) 日本薬局方の学名表記とは異なるが分類学的に同一あるいは同一とみなされることがあるもの及び収載種に含まれる代表的な下位分類群。*印のあるものは、日本薬局方で併記されているもの。 Scientific names that are different from those written in JP but identical to them taxonomically or being regarded as identical, and typical subclassified groups belonging to their species. The names marked with"*"are those being written together in JP.	科名 Family
ビャクゴウ Lilium Bulb	オニユリ *Lilium lancifolium* Thunberg ＝*Lilium lancifolium* Thunb. ハカタユリ *Lilium brownii* F. E. Brown var. *colchesteri* Wilosn ＝*Lilium brownii* F. E. Br. var. *colchesteri*(Van Houtte) E. H. Wilson ex Elwes *Lilium brownii* F. E. Brown var. *viridulum* Baker *Lilium brownii* F. E. Brown ＝*Lilium brownii* F. E. Br. *Lilium pumilum* De Candolle ＝*Lilium pumilum* DC.	Liliaceae ユリ科
ビャクシ Angelica Dahurica Root	ヨロイグサ *Angelica dahurica* Bentham et Hooker filius ex Franchet et Savatier ＝*Angelica dahurica* (Hoffm.) Benth. & Hook. f. ex Franch. & Sav.	Umbelliferae セリ科
ビャクジュツ Atractylodes Rhizome	オケラ *Atractylodes japonica* Koidzumi ex Kitamura ＝*Atractylodes japonica* Koidz. ex Kitam. オオバナオケラ *Atractylodes macrocephala* Koidzumi ＝*Atractylodes macrocephala* Koidz. **Atractylodes ovata* De Candolle ＝*Atractylodes ovata* (Thunb.) DC.	Compositae キク科
ビワヨウ Loquat Leaf	ビワ *Eriobotrya japonica* Lindley ＝*Eriobotrya japonica* (Thunb.) Lindl.	Rosaceae バラ科
ビンロウジ Areca	ビンロウ *Areca catechu* Linné ＝*Areca catechu* L.	Palmae ヤシ科
ブクリョウ Poria Sclerotium	マツホド *Wolfiporia cocos* Ryvarden et Gilbertson ＝*Wolfiporia cocos* (Schw.) Ryv. & Gilbn. **Poria cocos* Wolf ＝*Poria cocos* (Schw.) Wolf	Polyporaceae サルノコシカケ科
ブシ Processed Aconite Root	ハナトリカブト *Aconitum carmichaeli* Debeaux オクトリカブト *Aconitum japonicum* Thunberg ＝*Aconitum japonicum* Thunb.	Ranunculaceae キンポウゲ科
ベラドンナコン Belladonna Root	*Atropa belladonna* Linné ＝*Atropa belladonna* L.	Solanaceae ナス科
ヘンズ Dolichos Seed	フジマメ *Dolichos lablab* Linné ＝*Dolichos lablab* L.	Leguminosae マメ科
ボウイ Sinomenium Stem and Rhizome	オオツヅラフジ *Sinomenium acutum* Rehder et Wilson ＝*Sinomenium acutum* (Thunb.) Rehder & E. H. Wilson	Menispermaceae ツヅラフジ科
ボウコン Imperata Rhizome	チガヤ *Imperata cylindrica* Beauvois ＝*Imperata cylindrica* (L.) P. Beauv. *Imperata cylindrica* (L.) P. Beauv. var. *major* (Nees) C. E. Hubb.	Gramineae イネ科
ボウフウ Saposhnikovia Root and Rhizome	*Saposhnikovia divaricata* Schischkin ＝*Saposhnikovia divaricata* (Turcz.) Schischk.	Umbelliferae セリ科

生薬名 Crude Drug	日本薬局方の学名表記＝分類学的に用いられている学名表記（組合わせ明記、命名者簡略標準化） Scientific names used in the JP＝Scientific names being used taxonomically (Combined notation, Standard form for author or authors) 日本薬局方の学名表記とは異なるが分類学的に同一あるいは同一とみなされることがあるもの及び収載種に含まれる代表的な下位分類群。*印のあるものは、日本薬局方で併記されているもの。 Scientific names that are different from those written in JP but identical to them taxonomically or being regarded as identical, and typical subclassified groups belonging to their species. The names marked with"*"are those being written together in JP.	科名 Family
ボクソク Quercus Bark	クヌギ *Quercus acutissima* Carruthers ＝*Quercus acutissima* Carruth. コナラ *Quercus serrata* Murray ミズナラ *Quercus mongolica* Fischer ex Ledebour var. *crispula* Ohashi ＝*Quercus mongolica* Fisch. ex Ledeb. var. *crispula* (Blume) Ohashi アベマキ *Quercus variabilis* Blume	Fagaceae ブナ科
ボタンピ Moutan Bark	ボタン *Paeonia suffruticosa* Andrews **Paeonia moutan* Sims	Paeoniaceae ボタン科
ホミカ Nux Vomica	*Strychnos nux-vomica* Linné ＝*Strychnos nux-vomica* L.	Loganiaceae マチン科
ボレイ Oyster Shell	カキ *Ostrea gigas* Thunberg ＝*Ostrea gigas* Thunb.	Ostreidae イボタガキ科
マオウ Ephedra Herb	*Ephedra sinica* Stapf *Ephedra intermedia* Schrenk et C. A. Meyer ＝*Ephedra intermedia* Schrenk & C. A. Mey. *Ephedra equisetina* Bunge	Ephedraceae マオウ科
マクリ Digenea	マクリ *Digenea simplex* C. Agardh ＝*Digenea simplex* (Wulfen) C. Agardh	Rhodomelaceae フジマツモ科
マシニン Hemp Fruit	アサ *Cannabis sativa* Linné ＝*Cannabis sativa* L.	Moracea クワ科
モクツウ Akebia Stem	アケビ *Akebia quinata* Decaisne ＝*Akebia quinata* (Thunb. ex Houtt.) Decne. ミツバアケビ *Akebia trifoliata* Koidzumi ＝*Akebia trifoliata* (Thunb.) Koidz.	Lardizabalaceae アケビ科
モッコウ Saussurea Root	*Saussurea lappa* Clarke ＝*Saussurea lappa* (Decne.) C. B. Clarke *Aucklandia lappa* Decne.	Compositae キク科
ヤクチ Bitter Cardamon	*Alpinia oxyphylla* Miquel ＝*Alpinia oxyphylla* Miq.	Zingiberaceae ショウガ科
ヤクモソウ Leonurus Herb	メハジキ *Leonurus japonicus* Houttuyn ＝*Leonurus japonicus* Houtt. *Leonurus sibiricus* Linné ＝*Leonurus sibiricus* L.	Labiatae シソ科
ユウタン Bear Bile	*Ursus arctos* Linné ＝*Ursus arctos* L. その他近縁動物	Ursidae クマ科
ヨクイニン Coix Seed	ハトムギ *Coix lacryma-jobi* Linné var. *mayuen* Stapf ＝*Coix lacryma-jobi* L. var. *mayuen* (Rom. Caill.) Stapf	Gramineae イネ科
リュウガンニク Longan Aril	リュウガン *Euphoria longana* Lamarck ＝*Euphoria longana* Lam. *Dimocarpus longan* Lour.	Sapindaceae ムクロジ科

生薬名 Crude Drug	日本薬局方の学名表記＝分類学的に用いられている学名表記（組合わせ明記、命名者簡略標準化） Scientific names used in the JP＝Scientific names being used taxonomically (Combined notation, Standard form for author or authors) 日本薬局方の学名表記とは異なるが分類学的に同一あるいは同一とみなされることがあるもの及び収載種に含まれる代表的な下位分類群。*印のあるものは、日本薬局方で併記されているもの。 Scientific names that are different from those written in JP but identical to them taxonomically or being regarded as identical, and typical subclassified groups belonging to their species. The names marked with"*"are those being written together in JP.	科名 Family
リュウタン Japanese Gentian	トウリンドウ *Gentiana scabra* Bunge リンドウ *Gentiana scabra* Bunge var. *buergeri* (Miq.) Maxim. *Gentiana manshurica* Kitagawa ＝*Gentiana manshurica* Kitag. *Gentiana triflora* Pallas ＝*Gentiana triflora* Pall. エゾリンドウ *Gentiana triflora* Pall. var. *japonica* Hara	Gentianaceae リンドウ科
リョウキョウ Alpinia Officinarum Rhizome	*Alpinia officinarum* Hance	Zingiberaceae ショウガ科
レンギョウ Forsythia Fruit	レンギョウ *Forsythia suspensa* Vahl ＝*Forsythia suspensa* (Thunb.) Vahl シナレンギョウ *Forsythia viridissima* Lindley ＝*Forsythia viridissima* Lindl.	Oleaceae モクセイ科
レンニク Nelumbo Seed	ハス *Nelumbo nucifera* Gaertner ＝*Nelumbo nucifera* Gaertn.	Nymphacaceae スイレン科
ロジン Rosin	*Pinus*属諸種植物	Pinaceae マツ属
ロートコン Scopolia Rhizome	ハシリドコロ *Scopolia japonica* Maximowicz ＝*Scopolia japonica* Maxim. *Scopolia carniolica* Jacquin ＝*Scopolia carniolica* Jacq. *Scopolia parviflora* Nakai ＝*Scopolia parviflora* (Dunn) Nakai	Solanaceae ナス科
ローヤルゼリー Royal Jelly	ヨーロッパミツバチ *Apis mellifera* Linné ＝*Apis mellifera* L. トウヨウミツバチ *Apis cerana* Fabricius	Apidae ミツバチ科

基原植物に「その他同属植物」などが含まれる場合は、学名の表記はないが本表に記載している。

参考資料
寺林進ら：医薬品医療機器レギュラトリーサイエンス，41(5)，407-418(2010).

出典：第十六改正日本薬局方（平成23年 3月24日　厚生労働省告示第65号）p.2053～2061

参考文献／References

Ⅰ．植物由来物等／Substances originated in plants

1. 学術用語集：植物学編．増訂版．文部省，日本植物学会（編）．丸善，1998
2. 世界有用植物事典．堀田満，他（編）．平凡社，1996
3. 園芸植物大事典．青葉高，他（編），塚本洋太郎（総監修）．小学館，1994
4. 朝日百科　植物の世界．朝日新聞社，1997
5. 中薬大辞典．上海科学技術出版社，小学館（編）．小学館，1998
6. 和漢薬の事典．富山医科薬科大学和漢薬研究所（編），難波恒雄（監）．朝倉書店，2002
7. 生薬の薬効・薬理：モノグラフ．伊田喜光，寺澤捷年（監），鳥居塚和生（編著）．医歯薬出版，2003
8. 漢方のくすりの事典：生薬・ハーブ・民間薬．米田該典（監），鈴木洋（著）．医歯薬出版，1994
9. 天然食品・薬品・香粧品の事典．Albert Y. Leung, Steven Foster（著），小林彰夫，齋藤洋（監訳）．朝倉書店，1999
10. 最新生薬学総覧．新訂第２版．伊沢一男（著）．学文社，1981
11. 図説植物用語事典．清水建美（著）．八坂書房，2001
12. ハーブの写真図鑑：オールカラー世界のハーブ700．レスリー・ブレムネス（著），高橋良孝（監）．日本ヴォーグ社，1995
13. 木の写真図鑑：オールカラー世界の高木500 完璧版．アレン・コーンビス（著），濱谷稔夫（訳・監）．日本ヴォーグ社，1994
14. 野草の写真図鑑：オールカラー英国と北西ヨーロッパのワイルドフラワー500 完璧版．クリストファー・グレイ＝ウィルソン（著），近藤修（訳），高橋良孝（監）．日本ヴォーグ社，1996
15. 植物系統分類の基礎．重版．井上浩，岩槻邦男，柏谷博之，他（著），山岸高旺（編）．北隆館，1997
16. 藻類の多様性と系統．第６版．岩槻邦男，馬渡峻輔（監），千原光雄（編）．裳華房，2007
17. 藻類多様性の生物学．千原光雄（編著）．内田老鶴圃，1997
18. ヤマケイポケットガイド15　きのこ．小宮山勝司（著）．山と溪谷社，2000
19. 山渓カラー名鑑　日本のきのこ．増補改訂新版．保坂健太郎，他（監），今関六也，他（編・解説）．2011
20. 図説熱帯の果樹．岩佐俊吉（著）．養賢堂，2001
21. Herbs of Commerce. 2nd Ed., Michael McGuffin, John T. Kartesz, Albert Y. Leung and Arthur O. Tucker, et al., American Herbal Products Association, 2000
22. Handbook of Phytochemical Constituents of GRAS Herbs and Other Economic Plants, James A. Duke, CRC Press, 2001
23. Dictionary of Economic Plants. 2nd Ed., J. C. Uphof, Lubrecht & Cramer Ltd., 1968
24. Dictionary of Plant Names: Botanical Names and Their Common Name Equivalents. Allen J. Coombes, Timber Press, 1994
25. A Field Guide to Medicinal Plants and Herbs of Eastern and Central North America. 2nd Ed., Steven Foster, James Alan Duke, Houghton Mifflin Harcourt, 2000
26. Simon & Schuster's Guide to Mushrooms. Ed. by Gary H. Lincoff, Simon & Schuster Inc., 1982
27. 500 Popular Tropical Plants. Ed. by Periplus Editions（HK）Ltd., Random House Australia Pty Ltd.,1999
28. The Merck Index: An Encyclopedia of Chemicals, Drugs, and Biologicals. 13th Ed., Merck & Co., Inc., 2001
29. CRC World Dictionary of Plant Names. Umberto Quattrocchi, CRC Press LLC, 2000
30. Tanaka's Cyclopedia of Edible Plants of the World. Ed. by Tyôzaburô Tanaka, Keigaku Pub., 1976
31. The Algae. Chapman V. J., Macmillan & Co Ltd., 1962
32. 米倉浩司・梶田忠（2003-）「BG Plants 和名－学名インデックス」（YList）：http://bean.bio.chiba-u.jp/bgplants/ylist_main.html
33. 跡見群芳譜，嶋田英誠 編：http://www2.mmc.atomi.ac.jp/web01/Flower%20Information%20by%20Vps/Flower%20Albumn/index.htm
34. GKZ植物事典：http://t-webcity.com/~plantdan/index.html

35. KEGG(Kyoto Encyclopedia of Genes and Genomes) DRUG データベース：
http://www.kegg.jp/kegg/drug/drug_ja.html
36. レファレンス協同データベース（国立国会図書館）：http://crd.ndl.go.jp/reference/
37. 伝統医薬データベース（富山大学和漢医薬学総合研究所）：http://dentomed.u-toyama.ac.jp/ja/
38. 民族薬物データベース（富山大学和漢医薬学総合研究所）：
http://ethmed.u-toyama.ac.jp/Search_jp/step1.asp
39. 和漢薬Wikiデータベース（富山大学和漢医薬学総合研究所）：
http://wakandb.u-toyama.ac.jp/wiki/Main_Page
40. 「健康食品」の安全性・有効性情報（独立行政法人国立健康・栄養研究所）：https://hfnet.nih.go.jp/
41. 第十六改正日本薬局方名称データベース（国立医薬品食品衛生研究所）：http://moldb.nihs.go.jp/jp/
42. 野生きのこの世界（公益社団法人 農林水産・食品産業技術振興協会）：
http://www.jataff.jp/kinoko/index.html
43. 外来生物法（環境省自然環境局）：http://www.env.go.jp/nature/intro/index.html
44. フィリピン植物研究会：http://spp2004.web.fc2.com/
45. タイの植物：http://tplant.web.fc2.com/index.html
46. 日本産海藻リスト（「生きもの好きの語る自然誌」）：
http://natural-history.main.jp/Seaweeds_list/Seaweed_list_top.html
47. きのこ図鑑：http://www.kinoco-zukan.net/
48. 薬用植物一覧（公益社団法人日本薬学会HP）：http://www.pharm.or.jp/herb/list.html
49. 写真で見る家畜の有毒植物と中毒（独立行政法人農業・食品産業技術総合研究機構 動物衛生研究所）：
http://www.naro.affrc.go.jp/org/niah/disease_poisoning/plants/index.html
50. 侵入生物データベース（独立行政法人国立環境研究所）：
http://www.nies.go.jp/biodiversity/invasive/index.html
51. くすりの博物館（エーザイ株式会社）：http://www.eisai.co.jp/museum/index.html
52. 植物図鑑DB(日本新薬株式会社)：http://www.nippon-shinyaku.co.jp/herb/db/
53. ナオルコム（丸美屋和漢薬研究所）：http://www.naoru.com/
54. キノコ事典（株式会社タキザワ漢方廠）：http://www.takizawa.asia/encycl_kinoko/
55. キノコの食効、キノコのパワーについて（オートリ薬品）：
http://www.o-tori.jp/kinousyoku/takizawa/manju/kinoko/top.htm
56. 生薬の玉手箱（株式会社ウチダ和漢薬）：
http://www.uchidawakanyaku.co.jp/tamatebako/tamatebako_50.html
57. 家庭の中医学：http://www.sm-sun.com/family/
58. 世界の有用樹種7800種，木の情報発信基地（中川木材産業株式会社）：http://www.woodstar.biz/
59. 松浦薬業株式会社：http://www.matsuura-gp.co.jp/
60. 武田薬品工業株式会社　京都薬用植物園：www.takeda.co.jp/kyoto
61. 『新常用和漢薬集（HP掲載）』(公益社団法人東京生薬協会)：http://www.tokyo-shoyaku.jp/f_wakan/
62. 薬膳情報net：http://www.yakuzenjoho.net/thissite.html
63. イー薬草・ドット・コム：http://www.e-yakusou.com/sou/index.html
64. 木材図鑑（府中家具工業協同組合）：http://www.fuchu.or.jp/~kagu/mokuzai/
65. 北海道水産物検査協会HP：http://h-skk.or.jp/index.php？FrontPage
66. 三河の野草：http://mikawanoyasou.org/
67. 北信州の道草図鑑：http://www.okadanouen.com/zukan/zukan.html
68. 樹の散歩道，木のメモ帳：http://www.geocities.jp/kinomemocho/index.html
69. Metabolomics.jp：http://metabolomics.jp/wiki/Index:PS
70. 沖縄の野草（Okinawa情報局）：http://www.okinawajoho.net/pc/culture/herb/index.html
71. NCBI：http://www.ncbi.nlm.nih.gov/
72. Tropicos：http://www.tropicos.org/Home.aspx
73. World Register of Marine Species：http://www.marinespecies.org/index.php
74. Dr. Duke's Phytochemical and Ethnobotanical Databases：http://www.ars-grin.gov/duke/

75. AlgaeBase：http://www.algaebase.org/
76. The Harvard University Herbaria：http://kiki.huh.harvard.edu/databases/
77. USDA Plants Database：http://plants.usda.gov/java/
78. The International Plant Names Index（IPNI）：http://www.ipni.org/
79. MycoBank：http://www.mycobank.org/
80. Encyclopedia of Life（EOL）-Animals-Plants-Pictures & Information：http://eol.org/
81. NPGS/ GRIN（USDA Agricultural Research Service）：http://www.ars-grin.gov/npgs/
82. The Plant List：http://www.theplantlist.org/
83. Kew Economic Botany Collection：http://www.kew.org/collections/ecbot/index.html
84. eFloras.org：http://www.efloras.org/index.aspx
85. Flora of China：http://flora.huh.harvard.edu/china/
86. Catalogue of Life：2013 Annual Checklist：http://www.catalogueoflife.org/annual-checklist/2013/
87. The Rainforest Plant Database：http://www.rain-tree.com/index.html
88. NewCrop(Purdue University)：http://www.hort.purdue.edu/newcrop/
89. ZipcodeZoo：http://zipcodezoo.com/
90. EFSA：http://www.efsa.europa.eu/
91. Species Fungorum：http://www.speciesfungorum.org/Names/Names.asp
92. Robert W. Freckmann Herbarium：http://wisplants.uwsp.edu/index.html
93. Forest Products Laboratory：http://www.fpl.fs.fed.us/index.php
94. Multilingual Multiscript Plant Name Database（M.M.P.N.D.）：http://www.plantnames.unimelb.edu.au
95. Global Names Index：http://gni.globalnames.org/
96. The U.S. Pharmacopeial Convention：http://www.usp.org/about-usp
97. Australian Tropical Rainforest Plants Edition 6（RFK6）：http://keys.trin.org.au:8080/key-server/data/0e0f0504-0103-430d-8004-060d07080d04/media/Html/index.html
98. Lists of Philippine Herbal Medicinal Plants：http://www.stuartxchange.com/CompleteList.html
99. Ecocrop FAO：http://ecocrop.fao.org/
100. Botanical.com：https://www.botanical.com/index.html
101. Guidechem：http://www.guidechem.com/dictionary/jp/
102. Arctos Multi-Institution, Multi-Collection Museum Database：http://arctos.database.museum/
103. Plants For A Future：http://www.pfaf.org/user/default.aspx
104. Plant Database：http://www.plantdatabase.co.uk/
105. フリー百科事典「ウィキペディア（Wikipedia)」：https://en.wikipedia.org/wiki/Main_Page

Ⅱ．動物由来物等／Substances originated in animals

1. 日本薬局方解説書．第15改正．日本薬局方解説書編集委員会（編），廣川書店，2006
2. 原色和漢薬図鑑．難波恒雄（著）．保育社，1980
3. 中薬大辞典．上海科学技術出版社．小学館（編）．小学館，1990
4. 漢方のくすりの事典－生薬・ハーブ・民間薬－．米田該典（監），鈴木洋（著）．医歯薬出版，1994
5. 和漢薬の事典．難波恒雄（監）．朝倉書店，2002
6. 新・海洋動物の毒―フグからイソギンチャクまで．塩見一雄，長島裕二（著），成山堂書店，2012
7. コイの喫食による特異的食中毒について．浅川学，野口玉雄（著）．FFIジャーナル，217(3)，304，2012
8. 民族薬物データベース（富山大学和漢医薬学総合研究所）：http://ethmed.u-toyama.ac.jp/Search_jp/
9. 伝統薬物データベース（富山大学和漢医薬学総合研究所）：http://dentomed.u-toyama.ac.jp/ja/
10. KEGG（Kyoto Encyclopedia of Genes and Genomes）データベース：http://www.genome.jp/kegg/
11. 侵入生物データベース（独立行政法人国立環境研究所）：http://www.nies.go.jp/biodiversity/invasive/
12. ワシントン条約－貿易管理（経済産業省HP）：

http://www.meti.go.jp/policy/external_economy/trade_control/boekikanri/cites/
13. 生薬の玉手箱（株式会社ウチダ和漢薬）：
http://www.uchidawakanyaku.co.jp/tamatebako/tamatebako_50.html
14. 家庭の中医学：http://www.sm-sun.com/family/index.htm
15. ぼうずコンニャクの市場魚貝類図鑑：http://www.zukan-bouz.com/
16. 薬膳情報.net：http://www.yakuzenjoho.net/index.html
17. 島根の魚（島根県HP）：http://www.pref.shimane.lg.jp/industry/suisan/shinkou/umi_sakana/sakana/
18. 島根大学標本資料類データベース：http://museum-database.shimane-u.ac.jp/specimen/
19. 東京大学総合研究博物館データベース：http://www.um.u-tokyo.ac.jp/web_museum/database.html
20. WoRMS（World Register of Marine Species）：http://www.marinespecies.org/index.php
21. Integrated Taxonomic Information System：http://www.itis.gov/
22. Encyclopedia of Life（EOL）-Animals-Plants-Pictures & Information：http://eol.org/
23. Taxonomy browser（NCBI）：https://www.ncbi.nlm.nih.gov/Taxonomy/Browser/wwwtax.cgi？mode＝Root
24. Wilson & Reeder's Mammal Species of the World Third Edition：
http://www.departments.bucknell.edu/biology/resources/msw3/
25. The Reptile Database：http://www.reptile-database.org/
26. Arctos（Multi-Institution, Multi-Collection Museum Database）：http://arctos.database.museum/
27. AmphibiaWeb：http://amphibiaweb.org/index.html
28. Amphibian Species of the World 6.0, an Online Reference：
http://research.amnh.org/vz/herpetology/amphibia/
29. The Free Dictionary.com：http://encyclopedia.thefreedictionary.com/
30. The IUCN Red List of Threatened Species：http://www.iucnredlist.org/
31. Wikispecies free species directory：http://species.wikimedia.org/wiki/Main_Page
32. AnimalBase：http://www.animalbase.uni-goettingen.de/zooweb/servlet/AnimalBase/AnimalBase/search
33. Digital Taiwan-Culture & Nature：http://culture.teldap.tw/culture/index.php
34. UniProt：http://www.uniprot.org/
35. Femorale - Since 1989：http://www.femorale.com.br
36. Animal Genome Size Database：http://www.genomesize.com/
37. フリー百科事典「ウィキペディア（Wikipedia）」：https://en.wikipedia.org/wiki/Main_Page

Ⅲ．その他（化学物質等）／Other substances（chemicals, vitamins and minerals, etc.）

1. The Merck Index: An Encyclopedia of Chemicals, Drugs, and Biologicals. 14th Ed., Merck & Co., Inc., 2007
2. 健康食品に含有される医薬品成分の分析．守安貴子，他（著）．東京都健康安全研究センター研究年報，62, 25-39, 2011
3. 健康被害情報・無承認無許可医薬品情報（厚生労働省HP）：
http://www.mhlw.go.jp/kinkyu/diet/musyounin.html
4. 日本化学物質辞書Web（独立行政法人科学技術振興機構）：
http://nikkajiweb.jst.go.jp/nikkaji_web/pages/top.html
5. 酵素命名法, 国際生化学分子生物学連合の命名法委員会（NC-IUBMB）：http://www.cudo29.org/enzyme.html
6. 国際化学物質安全性カード（ICSC）-日本語版-（国立医薬品食品衛生研究所）：http://www.nihs.go.jp/ICSC/
7. KEGG（Kyoto Encyclopedia of Genes and Genomes）MEDICUS（Kanehisa Laboratories）：
http://www.kegg.jp/kegg/medicus/
8. DBGET search-ENZYME GenomeNet, Kyoto University Bioinformatics Center.：
http://www.genome.jp/dbget-bin/www_bfind？enzyme
9. 「健康食品」の安全性・有効性情報（独立行政法人国立健康・栄養研究所）：https://hfnet.nih.go.jp/
10. siyaku.com（和光純薬工業株式会社）：http://www.siyaku.com/
11. PubChem Compound, NCBI：http://www.ncbi.nlm.nih.gov/pccompound
12. Chemical Book：http://www.chemicalbook.com/ProductIndex_JP.aspx

13. CAS-NO.org (CAS Registry Number Database)：http://www.cas-no.org/
14. Chemical CAS Database with Global Chemical Suppliers (ChemNet)：http://www.chemnet.com/cas/jp/
15. Common Chemistry Search Chemical Names and CAS Registry Numbers：http://www.commonchemistry.org/
16. DrugBank (Open Data Drug & Drug Target Database), David Wishart, Departments of Computing Science & Biological Sciences, University of Alberta.：http://www.drugbank.ca/
17. National Institutes of Health, Office of Dietary Supplements：http://ods.od.nih.gov/factsheets/list-all/
18. Sidley Chemical Co.,Ltd. HP：http://www.visitchem.com/
19. The database and ontology of Chemical Entities of Biological Interest：http://www.ebi.ac.uk/chebi/
20. Pharmacopeia：http://www.newdruginfo.com/index.asp
21. Guidechem：http://www.guidechem.com/dictionary/jp/
22. MedlinePlus -Health Information from the National Library of Medicine-：http://www.nlm.nih.gov/medlineplus/
23. Minerals Inc. product Data Sheet：http://www.mineralsinc.com/productlist.htm
24. Human Metabolome Database (HMDB)：http://www.hmdb.ca/
25. WebMD：http://www.webmd.com/
26. Encyclopedia Britannica：http://global.britannica.com/
27. Tocris Bioscience：http://www.tocris.com/
28. フリー百科事典「ウィキペディア (Wikipedia)」：https://en.wikipedia.org/wiki/Main_Page

和名索引
Japanese name index

ア

Adonis属 334
アイ 140
藍（アイ） 140
アイギョクシ 37
愛玉子（アイギョクシ） 37
アイスランド苔 37
アイゾーン 82
アイヌネギ（アイヌ葱） 80
アイヌワサビ 219
アイブライト 37, 97
アイリッシュモス 205
亜鉛 241
アオアズキ（青小豆） 214
アオギリ 37
青桐（アオギリ） 37
アオクスリ（青薬） 65
アオダモ 37
アオハダニシキギ（青肌錦木） 158
アオハダニシキギ（青膚錦木） 158
アオバナ（青花） 146
アオマダラウミヘビ 236
青斑海蛇（アオマダラウミヘビ） 236
アカガウクルア 68
アカガエル 229
アカキナノキ 304
赤機那樹（アカキナノキ） 304
赤規那樹（アカキナノキ） 304
アカザ 38
藜（アカザ） 38
アカショウマ 38
赤升麻（アカショウマ） 38
アカダマノキ（赤玉の木） 203
アカツメクサ 38
アカテツ 38
赤鉄（アカテツ） 38
アカナス（赤伽子） 153
アカニレ 39
赤楡（アカニレ） 39
アカネ 320
赤根（アカネ） 320
アカバナムシヨケギク 39
紅花除虫菊（アカバナムシヨケギク） 39
アガーベ 38
アカマムシ（赤蝮） 236
アカミノアカネ 320
茜草（アカミノアカネ） 320
アカミノキ 172
アカメガシワ 39
赤芽柏（アカメガシワ） 39
アカヤジオウ 313
赤矢地黄（アカヤジオウ） 313
アガリクス 39
アガリクス・ブラゼイ 39
アキサンゴ（秋珊瑚） 107
アギタケ 39
阿魏茸（アギタケ） 39
アキニレ（秋楡） 159
アキノキリンソウ 40
秋の麒麟草（アキノキリンソウ） 40
アキョウ 223
阿膠（アキョウ） 223
アクアインカー 163
アグリモニー 124
アグリモニア 124
アケビ 40, 341
通草（アケビ） 40
木通（アケビ） 40, 341
アコヤガイ 233
阿古屋貝（アコヤガイ） 233
アサ 40, 339
麻（アサ） 40, 339
アサガオ 40, 307
朝顔（アサガオ） 40, 307
アサツキ 41
浅葱（アサツキ） 41
アサノミ（麻実） 40
アサマブドウ（浅間葡萄） 90
アザラシ 223
海豹（アザラシ） 223
アシ 41
葦（アシ） 41
蘆（アシ） 41
アジサイ 41
紫陽花（アジサイ） 41
八仙花（アジサイ） 41
アシタグサ 41
明日草（アシタグサ） 41
アシタバ 41
明日葉（アシタバ） 41
アシドフィルス菌 41
アジマメ（味豆） 188
アシュワガンダ 295
アズキ 42
小豆（アズキ） 42
アスコルビン酸 275
アスタキサンチン 241
アステカタバコ 339
アステカ煙草（アステカタバコ） 339
アスナロ 42
翌檜（アスナロ） 42
アスパラギン 241
アスパラギン酸 241
アスピリン 355
アズマニシキガイ 223
吾妻錦貝（アズマニシキガイ） 223
東錦貝（アズマニシキガイ） 223
アセチルアシッド 355
N-アセチルグルコサミン 246
アセチルサリチル酸 355
アセチルデナフィル 374
アセロラ 42
アセンヤク 42
阿仙薬（アセンヤク） 42
アセンヤクノキ（阿仙薬木） 185
アタゴザサ（愛宕笹） 86
アダン 113
厚岸草（アッケシイソウ） 42
アッケシソウ 42
アッサムチャ 142
アップラ 172
アップルミント 43
アーティチョーク 144
S-アデノシル-L-メチオニン 358

穴燕（アナツバメ） 234
アナナス 163
アニス 43
アニール・トレバドール 53
アブ 350
虻（アブ） 350
アファニゾメノン 43
アブラゼミ 349
鳴蜩（アブラゼミ） 349
油蝉（アブラゼミ） 349
アブラナ（油菜） 154
アフリカバオバブ 163
アフリカマンゴノキ 43
アベマキ（阿部槇） 315
阿片（アヘン） 306
アボガド 44
油梨（アボカド） 44
アポン 43
アマ 44
亜麻（アマ） 44
アマガサヘビ 236
雨傘蛇（アマガサヘビ） 236
アマシ 44
亜麻子（アマシ） 44
アマゾンジンセン 121
アマダイダイ（甘橙） 67
アマチャ 44
甘茶（アマチャ） 44
アマチャヅル 44
甘茶蔓（アマチャヅル） 44
アマドコロ 48
甘野老（アマドコロ） 48
アマナ 44
甘菜（アマナ） 44
アマニ油 44
アマニン 44
亜麻仁（アマニン） 44
アマハステビア（甘葉ステビア） 120
アミガサユリ 330
網笠百合（アミガサユリ） 330
アミノタダラフィル 355
γ-アミノ酪酸 251
5-アミノレブリン酸リン酸塩 242
アミラーゼ 356
アムラ（amla） 210
アメリカクガイソウ 184
アメリカ九蓋草（アメリカクガイソウ） 184
アメリカクロミザクラ（アメリカ黒実桜） 219
アメリカサンショウ 45
アメリカ山椒（アメリカサンショウ） 45
アメリカショウマ（アメリカ升麻） 183
アメリカスノキ（アメリカ酢の木） 184
アメリカデイコ 67
亜米利加梯沽（アメリカデイコ） 67
アメリカニンジン 45
アメリカハッカクレン（アメリカ八角蓮） 338
アメリカホドイモ 45
アメリカ塊芋（アメリカホドイモ） 45
アメリカ万作（アメリカマンサク） 171
アメリカ満作（アメリカマンサク） 171
アラガオ 45
アラニン 242
アラビアコーヒー 96
アラビアコーヒーノキ 96
アラビアゴム 45, 185
アラビアゴムノキ 45
アラビアチャノキ 293
アラビアモツヤク 311
アラマンサス・ハイブリダス 122
アラメ 46
阿良米（アラメ） 46
荒布（アラメ） 46
骨海藻（アラメ） 46
アララギ 49, 293
枝杉（アララギ） 293
蘭葱（アララギ） 49
アラントイン 356
アリ 223
アリシン 242
アリタソウ 46, 306
有田草（アリタソウ） 46, 306
アリノコ 223
アルガロバ 50
アルスロスピラ（オルソスピラ）属の藍藻 120
アルテア 46
アルニカ 293
アルピニア 93
アルファバーカ 199
アルファバカ（alfavaca） 199
アルファルファ 46
アルブミン 242
亜茘枝（アレイシ） 213
アレキサンドリア・センナ 320
アロイン 356
アロエ 46, 293
アロマティカ 172
泡立草（アワダチソウ） 40
アワビ 223
鮑（アワビ） 223
アンジオテンシン 357
アンズ 75, 304
杏（アンズ） 75, 304
杏子（アンズ） 75
アンゼリカ 47
安息香（アンソクコウ） 47
アンソクコウノキ 47
アンティリス・ウルネラリア 47
アンティリス・ブルネラリア 47
アンデスポテト 57, 203
アントシアニジン 243
アンドロステンジオン 357
杏仁香（アンニンゴ） 58
アンプラ 172
菴摩羅（アンマラ） 195
アンマロク 210
庵摩勒（アンマロク） 210
按葉（アンヨウ） 208
菴羅（アンラ） 195
アンランジュ（安蘭樹） 201

イ

イ 47, 327
藺（イ） 47, 327
イエハッカ（家薄荷） 167
イオウ 243
イカ 224
イカスミ 224
烏賊墨（イカスミ） 224
イカリソウ 295
碇草（イカリソウ） 295
錨草（イカリソウ） 295
イグサ 47, 327
藺草（イグサ） 47, 327
イクリニン 48
郁李仁（イクリニン） 48
イコサペント酸<EPA> 244
イザヨイバラ 118

十六夜薔薇（イザヨイバラ） 118
イズイ 48
萎蕤（イズイ） 48
磯桔梗（イソギキョウ） 312
イソフラキシジン 244
イソボウキ 112
イソマツ 48
磯松（イソマツ） 48
イソロイシン 244
イタドリ 48, 309
虎杖（イタドリ） 48, 309
イタボガキ（板甫牡蠣） 227
イタリアニンジンボク 127
イチイ 49, 293
一位（イチイ） 49
一位葉（イチイヨウ） 293
イチケンキ（一見喜） 131
イチジク 49
無花果（イチジク） 49
イチネンホウ（一年蓬） 176
イチビ 49
イチビ（苘麻） 150
イチヤクソウ 49
一薬草（イチヤクソウ） 49
イチョウ 50
鴨脚樹（イチョウ） 50
公孫樹（イチョウ） 50
銀杏葉（イチョウヨウ） 50
イトネギ（糸葱） 41
イトヒメハギ 299
糸姫萩（イトヒメハギ） 300
イトマキヒトデ 226
糸巻海星（イトマキヒトデ） 226
糸巻人手（イトマキヒトデ） 226
イナゴマメ 50
蝗豆（イナゴマメ） 50
イヌ 347
イヌキケマン（イヌ黄華蔓） 85
イヌサフラン 293
イヌサンショウ 50
犬山椒（イヌザンショウ） 50
イヌスイバ（犬酸葉） 209
イヌナズナ 50
犬薺（イヌナズナ） 50
イヌノフグリ 50
イヌハッカ 51
犬薄荷（イヌハッカ） 51
イヌホオズキ 51
犬酸漿（イヌホオズキ） 51
イヌリン 244
イネ 51, 94, 100, 101
稲（イネ） 51
イノコヅチ（豕槌） 309
イノシトール 245
D-chiro-イノシトール 266
イノモトソウ 336
井の許草（イノモトソウ） 336
イノンド 176
イバラタツ（茨竜） 226
イバラタツ（刺海馬） 226
イブキジャコウソウ 51, 131
伊吹麝香草（イブキジャコウソウ）
51, 131
イペ 140, 163
イペロッショ 140
イボクサ（疣草） 151
イボツヅラフジ 51, 324
疣葛藤（イボツヅラフジ） 51, 324
イミダゾサガトリアジノン 357
イモノキ（芋の木） 79
イヨウカハンロウ（異葉仮繁縷） 136
刺草（イラクサ） 52
蕁麻（イラクサ） 52
イラクサ属 52
イリス 294
イリス根（イリスコン） 294
遺糧（イリョウ） 106
イレイセン 52, 294
威霊仙（イレイセン） 52, 294
イワオモダカ（岩沢潟） 129
イワオモダカ（岩面高） 129
イワガキ（岩牡蠣） 227
イワシ 224
鰯（イワシ） 224
イワジシャ 52
岩萵苣（イワジシャ） 52
イワタバコ 52
岩煙草（イワタバコ） 52
岩千佐（イワチサ） 52
イワニガナ 52
岩苦菜（イワニガナ） 52
イワベンケイ 52
岩弁慶（イワベンケイ） 52
イワモモ（岩桃） 97
陰茎 224
インゲンマメ 53
隠元豆（インゲンマメ） 53
インスリーナ 53
インチンコウ 294
茵蔯蒿（インチンコウ） 294
インディアン・タバコ 312
インディアンデイト 74
インディアンマルベリー 203
インドアマチャ 53
印度常山（インドアマチャ） 53
インドオオバコ（印度大葉子） 184
インドカラタチ 53, 187
印度枳（インドカラタチ） 53, 187
印度膠樹（インドコウジュ） 100
インドコブラ 230
インドゴムノキ 100
インドサルサ 294
インドシタン 111
インドジャボク 294
印度蛇木（インドジャボク） 295
インドジャボク属 294
インドナガコショウ 54
印度長胡椒（インドナガコショウ）
54
インド乳香 190
インドボダイジュ 54
印度菩提樹（インドボダイジュ） 54
インドヤコウボク 54
印度夜香木（インドヤコウボク） 54
インペティギノサ 54, 140
インペラトリア 54
インベルターゼ 358
インベルチン 358
インヨウカク 295
淫羊藿（インヨウカク） 295

ウ

ウイキョウ 55
茴香（ウイキョウ） 55
茴芹（ウイキン） 43
ウィザニア 295
ウィンベリー 178
ウキヤガラ 55
浮矢柄（ウキヤガラ） 55
ウコギ 55, 96
五加（ウコギ） 55, 96
ウコッケイ 225
烏骨鶏（ウコッケイ） 225
ウコン 55
宇金（ウコン） 55
鬱金（ウコン） 55
ウコンイソマツ 48

鬱金磯松（ウコンイソマツ） 48
ウサギタケ 207
ウシ 223, 224, 228, 229, 232, 233, 347, 350
ウシアブ（牛虻） 350
ウシグサ（牛草） 209
ウシノツメ 166
ウショウ 56
烏樟（ウショウ） 56
ウズ 333
ウスゲサイシン（薄毛細辛） 311
ウスバカマキリ（薄翅蟷螂） 233
ウスバキンゴジカ（薄葉金午時花） 297
ウスバサイシン 311
薄葉細辛（ウスバサイシン） 311
ウスベニアオイ 56, 130
薄紅葵（ウスベニオアイ） 56, 130
ウスベニタチアオイ 46
薄紅立葵（ウスベニタチアオイ） 46
ウゾクコツ 224
烏賊骨（ウゾクコツ） 224
ウチムラサキ（内紫） 185
ウチワサボテン 56
団扇仙人掌（ウチワサボテン） 56
ウチワサボテン属 56
ウチワドコロ 131
団扇野老（ウチワドコロ） 131
ウチワヤシ 56
団扇椰子（ウチワヤシ） 56
ウッドラフ 88
ウツボグサ 300
靭草（ウツボグサ） 300
ウデナフィル 358
ウド 56, 328
独活（ウド） 56, 328
ウドカズラ（独活葛） 150
ウドタラシ 110
ウナギ 225
鰻（ウナギ） 225
ウバイ 57
烏梅（ウバイ） 57
ウベ 57
ウマ 224, 232, 350
ウマグリ（馬栗） 126, 318
ウマゴヤシ 46
ウマスイバ（馬酸葉） 209
馬芹（ウマゼリ） 87
ウマダイコン（馬大根） 219
ウマノアシガタ 57
馬の足形（ウマノアシガタ） 57
ウマノスズクサ属 295
ウマノタマ（馬の玉） 350
ウマビル 235
寛水蛭（ウマビル） 235
長條水蛭（ウマビル） 235
ウマワサビ（馬山葵） 219
ウミガメ 228
海亀（ウミガメ） 228
ウメ 57
梅（ウメ） 57
ウメガサソウ 57
梅笠草（ウメガサソウ） 57
ウヤク 58, 295
烏薬（ウヤク） 58, 295
ウヨウサンシチ（羽葉三七） 176
ウヨウチクセツジン（羽葉竹節参） 176
ウラジロガシ 58
裏白柏（ウラジロガシ） 58
ウルチカソウ 52
ウルメ（潤目） 224
ウルメイワシ（潤鰯） 229
潤目鰯（ウルメイワシ） 224
ウワウルシ 296
ウワミズザクラ 58
上溝桜（ウワミゾザクラ） 58
ウンカロアポ 296
ウンコウ 188
芸香（ウンコウ） 188
ウンシュウミカン 123, 144
温州蜜柑（ウンシュウミカン） 123, 144
ウンナンクテイチャ（雲南苦丁茶） 109
雲南紅豆杉（ウンナンコウトウサン 164
ウンナンコウトウスギ 164, 331
雲南紅豆杉（ウンナンコウトウスギ） 164, 331
雲母 246

エ

エイコサペンタエン酸 244
エイジツ 296
営実（エイジツ） 296
エイボウ（衛矛） 158
依蘭苔（エイランタイ） 37
エキナケア 58
エゴマ 110
荏胡麻（エゴマ） 110
エジプトイボタノキ（エジプト水蝋樹） 109
エジプトイボタノキ（エジプト疣取木） 109
エストラゴン 59
エゾアワビ（蝦夷鮑） 223
エゾウコギ 59, 96
蝦夷五加（エゾウコギ） 59, 96
エゾエンゴサク 296
蝦夷延胡索（エゾエンゴサク） 296
エゾキイチゴ（蝦夷木苺） 124, 212
エゾチチコグサ 59
エゾナナカマド（蝦夷七竈） 156
エゾネギ（蝦夷葱） 41
エゾノチチコグサ 59
蝦夷父子草（エゾノチチコグサ） 59
エゾヘビイチゴ 59
蝦夷蛇苺（エゾヘビイチゴ） 59
エゾムカシヨモギ（蝦夷昔蓬） 141
エゾヨモギ（蝦夷蓬） 210
エゾヨモギギク（蝦夷蓬菊） 210
エーデルワイス 58
エニシダ 60, 296
金雀枝（エニシダ） 60, 296
エノキタケ 60
榎茸（エノキダケ） 60
エビスグサ 60
夷草（エビスグサ） 60
エフェドリン 359
エラブウミヘビ 236
永良部海蛇（エラブウミヘビ） 236
エリカ 81
エリシマム 68
エリスリナ 67, 300
エルカンプーレ 60
エルダー 126
燕窩（エンカ） 234
圓眼（エンガン） 213
エンゴサク 296
延胡索（エンゴサク） 296
エンシショウ 60
燕子掌（エンシショウ） 60, 94
エンジュ 61, 297
槐（エンジュ） 61, 297
エンバク 61
燕麦（エンバク） 61

エンフシ　121
塩麩子（エンフシ）　121
エンベリア　61
エンメイギク　175
延命菊（エンメイギク）　175
エンメイソウ　61
延命草（エンメイソウ）　61

オ

欧茴香（オウウイキョウ）　43
オウカコウ　297
オウカシ　297
黄花仔（オウカシ）　297
オウカボ　297
黄花母（オウカボ）　297
黄花稔（オウカボ）　297
オウギ　62, 298
黄耆（オウギ）　62, 298
オウギヤシ（扇椰子）　56
オウクジン（黄狗腎）　347
オウゴン　62, 298
黄芩（オウゴン）　62, 298
オウゴンカゲツ（黄金花月）　60
オウシュウシラカンバ（欧州白樺）　111
オウシュウトネリコ　126
欧州梣（オウシュウトネリコ）　126
オウシュウハンノキ　62
欧州榛の木（オウシュウハンノキ）　62
黄蜀葵（オウショッキ）　154
オウセイ　62
黄精（オウセイ）　62
オウセキソウ（鴨跖草）　146
オウトウキ（欧当帰）　219
オウニュウ（王乳）　238
オウバク　63, 298
黄柏（オウバク）　63, 298
オウヒ　298
桜皮（オウヒ）　298
オウフルギョウ（王不留行）　63
オウヘンダイリュウシツ（黄辺大龍虱）　237
オウヤクシ　63
黄薬子（オウヤクシ）　63
オウレン　63, 299, 340
黄蓮（オウレン）　63, 299, 340
オオアザミ　161, 194
大薊（オオアザミ）　194
オオアナツバメ　234
オオイタビ　63
大崖爬（オオイタビ）　63
大木蓮子（オオイタビ）　63
オオイナゴマメ　115
オオウミウマ（克氏海馬）　226
オオウメガサソウ　57
大梅笠草（オオウメガサソウ）　57
オオカナメモチ　318
大要黐（オオカナメモチ）　318
オオカマキリ（大刀蜋）　233
オオカマキリ（団螵蛸）　233
オオカミナスビ（狼茄子）　335
オオカラスウリ　74, 302
大烏瓜（オオカラスウリ）　74, 302
オオグルマ　328
大車（オオグルマ）　328
オオクロアリ（大黒蟻）　223
オオサンザシ　106
大山査子（オオサンザシ）　106
オオスグリ（大酸塊）　120
オオスズメバチ（大雀蜂）　235
オオツヅラフジ　336
大葛藤（オオツヅラフジ）　336
オオトカゲ　225
大蜥蜴（オオトカゲ）　225
オオナナカマド（大七竈）　156
オオニンニク　160
大蒜（オオニンニク）　160
オオバコ　63
大葉子（オオバコ）　63
オオハシリドコロ（大走野老）　335
オオバトネリコ（大葉梣）　204
オオバナオケラ　332
大花朮（オオバナオケラ）　332
オオバナサルスベリ　168
大花猿滑（オオバナサルスベリ）　168
大花百日紅（オオバナサルスベリ）　168
オオバニシキギ（大葉錦木）　158
オオバネム（大葉合歓）　178
オオハブソウ　170
オオバボダイジュ（大葉菩提樹）　190
オオハンゴンソウ　64
大反魂草（オオハンゴンソウ）　64
オオビル（大蒜）　160
オオヒレアザミ　64
オオヒレ薊（オオヒレアザミ）　64
オオベニミカン　123
大紅蜜柑（オオベニミカン）　123
オオマツカサノキ　203
オオマツヨイグサ　199
大待宵草（オオマツヨイグサ）　199
オオミサンザシ　106
大実山査子（オオミサンザシ）　106
オオムギ　64
大麦（オオムギ）　64
オオヤモリ　225
大守宮（オオヤモリ）　225
オオユキノハナ　342
大雪の花（オオユキノハナ）　342
オカオグルマ　64
丘小車（オカオグルマ）　64
オカゼリ　315
岡芹（オカゼリ）　315
オカヒジキ　65
岡羊栖菜（オカヒジキ）　65
陸鹿尾菜（オカヒジキ）　65
オカミル（水松）　65
オカミル（陸海松）　65
オキナグサ（翁草）　330
沖縄サンゴ　231
オキナワヤマイモ（沖縄山芋）　57
オギョウ　170
御行（オギョウ）　170
オクタコサノール　247
N-オクチルノルタダラフィル　359
オークモス　145
オグルマ　320
小車（オグルマ）　320
オケラ　332
朮（オケラ）　332
オシダ　299
雄羊歯（オシダ）　299
オシャクシタケ　65
オシャグジタケ　65
オシャクジタケ（鎖陽）　65
オショロソウ（忍路草）　212
オシロイカケ（白粉掛け）　173
オタネニンジン　65
御種人参（オタネニンジン）　65
オットセイ　225, 347
海狗（オットセイ）　347
膃肭臍（オットセイ）　225, 347
オトギリソウ　65
弟切草（オトギリソウ）　65
オートムギ　61
オトメアゼア　65

オドリコソウ　66
踊子草（オドリコソウ）　66
オナジマイマイ（同蝸牛）　227
オナモミ　321
葈耳（オナモミ）　321
オニアザミ　161
オニオオバコ　124
鬼大葉子（オニオオバコ）　124
オニク　157
御肉（オニク）　157
オニサルビア　66
オニノダケ　150, 326
鬼土当帰（オニノダケ）　326
オニノヤガラ　325
鬼矢柄（オニノヤガラ）　325
オニバス　66
鬼蓮（オニバス）　66
オニビシ（鬼菱）　174
オニマツ　184
鬼松（オニマツ）　184
オニユリ　209
鬼百合（オニユリ）　209
オノニス　299
オノニス根（オノニスコン）　299
オノミ（苧実）　40
オペルクリナ・タルペタム　66
オボノ　43
オミナエシ　66
女郎花（オミナエシ）　66
オモト　299
万年青（オモト）　299
オヤブジラミ（雄藪虱）　315
オランダゼリ（和蘭芹）　166
オランダドリアン　87, 306
オランダハッカ　121
オランダビユ　189
和蘭莧（オランダビユ）　189
オランダミツバ　131
オランダ三葉（オランダミツバ）　131
オリゴ糖　247
オリゴ配糖体　247
γ-オリザノール　361
オリーブ　67
オリーブ油　67
オルニチン　248
オレイフ　67
オレゴンブドウ　173
オレンジ　67
オレンジピール　67
オロト酸　248
オンコ　49
オンジ　299
遠志（オンジ）　300

カ

Candida　95
槐（カイ）　297
カイエン　226
海燕（カイエン）　226
カイカ　297
槐花（カイカ）　297
カイカク　297
槐角（カイカク）　297
カイガンショウ　184
海岸松（カイガンショウ）　184
カイガンマツ（海岸松）　184
海金沙（カイキンシャ）　70
海金砂（カイキンシャ）　70
金沙藤（カイキンシャ）　70
カイクジン　347
海狗腎（カイクジン）　347
カイケイジオウ　313
懐慶地黄（カイケイジオウ）　313
カイコ　226
蚕（カイコ）　226
カイコウズ　67
海紅豆（カイコウズ）　67
カイコガ（蚕蛾）　226
槐耳（カイジ）　77
ガイジシン（孩児参）　136
孩児茶（ガイジチャ）　42
カイショウシ　194
海松子（カイショウシ）　194
海人草（カイジンソウ）　338
カイソウ（海草）　67
カイソウ（海葱）属　300
海草（カイソウ）　67
海葱（カイソウ）　300
カイトウヒ　300
海桐皮（カイトウヒ）　300
海人草（カイニンソウ）　338
ガイノウコウ　137
艾納香（ガイノウコウ）　137
カイバ　226
海馬（カイバ）　226
ガイハク　68
薤白（ガイハク）　68
海螵蛸（カイヒョウショウ）　224
カイフウトウ　179
海風藤（カイフウトウ）　179
ガイヘン（艾片）　137
カイヨウ　61
槐葉（カイヨウ）　61
ガイヨウ　210
艾葉（ガイヨウ）　210
芥藍（カイラン）　92
カイリュウ　226
海竜（カイリュウ）　226
ガウクルア　68
カオウ（花王）　190
カオリン　360
カガミグサ　68
鏡草（カガミグサ）　68
カキ（牡蛎）　227
カキ（柿）　68
牡蛎（カキ）　227
柿（カキ）　68
カギカズラ　143, 325
鉤葛（カギカズラ）　143, 325
カギクルマバナルコユリ（鍵車葉鳴子百合）　62
柿渋（カキシブ）　68
カキドオシ　217
垣通し（カキドオシ）　218
籬通（カキドオシ）　218
カキネガラシ　68
垣根芥子（カキネガラシ）　68
カキノキバナ　60
蝸牛（カギュウ）　227
カギュウマツ　227
カクコウ　300
角蒿（カクコウ）　300
核酸　227
カクシツ　205
鶴虱（カクシツ）　205
カクトウシュウ（核桃楸）　105
カゲ（蘿）　118
カゲツ（花月）　60, 94
カゴソウ　300
夏枯草（カゴソウ）　300
カサンガ　226
カシ　301
訶子（カシ）　301
カシグルミ　69
菓子胡桃（カシグルミ）　69
カシス　69
カシュウ　146, 301

何首烏（カシュウ） 146, 301
カシュウイモ（何首烏芋） 63
果汁酵素 262
カシュウトウ（蝦鬚豆） 69
ガジュツ 69
莪朮（ガジュツ） 69
莪迷（ガジュツ） 69
カシュトウ 69
カショウ（花椒） 111
カスカラサグラダ 301
カズザキヨモギ（数咲き蓬） 210
カタクチイワシ 224, 229
片口鰯（カタクチイワシ） 224, 229
カタシログサ 173
片白草（カタシログサ） 173
カタツムリ 227
蝸牛（カタツムリ） 227
カタラーゼ 360
カチョウトウ（華釣藤） 143
カツアバ 70
カツオ 227
鰹（カツオ） 227
かつお節 227
鰹節（カツオブシ） 227
かつお節オリゴペプチド 227
カッコウ 301, 303
藿香（カッコウ） 301, 303
カッコウアザミ 70
勝紅薊（カッコウアザミ） 70
霍香薊（カッコウアザミ） 70
カッコン 301
葛根（カッコン） 85, 301
カッシア・アウリキュラータ 302
カッショクツリミミズ 349
カツズイシ 176
葛綉子（カツズイシ） 176
ガッタパーチャ 86
カッパリス・マサイカイ 70
カツヨウバクトウ（闊葉麦冬） 331
カテキュ 185
カテキン 248
カテキン酸 248
ガーデンアンゼリカ 47
カトウ（顆凍） 180
果糖 248
カドデタケ（門出茸） 216
カナダヒドラスチス 308
カナメノキ（要木） 156
カニ 228
蟹（カニ） 228
カニクサ 70
蟹草（カニクサ） 70
カニナバラ 153
カノコソウ 70
鹿子草（カノコソウ） 70
カバ 302, 303
カバカバ 302
カハチュウ（蚵蛂虫） 232
カバノアナタケ 71
樺穴茸（カバノアナタケ） 71
樺孔茸（カバノアナタケ） 71
カフェイン 249
ガフショクソウ 152
鵝不食草（ガフショクソウ） 152
鵞不食草（ガフショクソウ） 152
カブス（蚊無須） 137
カフン 71
花粉（カフン） 71
カホクサンショウ（華北山椒） 111
カボス（臭橙） 137
カボチャ 71
南瓜（カボチャ） 71
北瓜（カボチャ） 71
ガマ 71, 337
蒲（ガマ） 71, 337
カマキリ 233
鎌切（カマキリ） 233
螳螂（カマキリ） 233
蟷螂（カマキリ） 233
治葛（カマツ） 308
火麻仁（カマニン） 40, 339
カマラ 305
カミツレ 72
加密列（カミツレ） 72
カミヤツデ 144
紙八手（カミヤツデ） 144
カミルレ 72
カムカム 72
ガムググル 72
カメ 228
亀（カメ） 228
カメムシ 228
亀虫（カメムシ） 228
椿像（カメムシ） 228
カモウリ（甦瓜） 149, 326
カモミール 72
カヤ 174
榧（カヤ） 174
カヤツリグサ 72
蚊帳吊草（カヤツリグサ） 72
荷葉（カヨウ） 166
ガラエ 201
ガラガラヘビ 236
カラギーナン 249
β-ガラクトシダーゼ 377
カラクレナイ（韓呉藍） 186
カラグワ（唐桑） 90
カラスノエンドウ 72
烏豌豆（カラスノエンドウ） 72
カラスビシャク 332
烏柄杓（カラスビシャク） 332
カラスムギ 73
烏麦（カラスムギ） 73
カラダイオウ（唐大黄） 135
カラタチ 73
枳（カラタチ） 73
カラトウキ 150, 326
唐当帰（カラトウキ） 150, 326
ガラナ 73
カラナシ（加良奈志） 201
カラナシ（唐梨） 201
カラバル豆 302
カラフトイバラ（樺太茨） 206
カラボケ（唐木瓜） 189, 200
カラムスコン 315
カラムス根 315
カラヤマグワ 90, 195
唐山桑（カラヤマグワ） 90, 195
カリウスフォレスコリー 73
カリウム 250
カリュウコツ（花竜骨） 351
カリン 200
花梨（カリン） 201
カルケ 73
カルケージャ 73
カルケッハ 73
カルシウム 250
ガルシニアカンボジア 74
カルシフェロール 275
カルダモン 116, 177
L-カルニチン 246
カルボデナフィル 360
ガレガソウ 74
カレープラント 187
旱蓮木（カレンボク） 76
カロクジョウ（花鹿茸） 351
カロコン 302

栝楼根（カロコン） 302
カロチン 250
カロニン 74
栝楼仁（カロニン） 74
カロペプタイド 225
カロライナジャスミン 303
カワシンジュガイ（川真珠貝） 233
カワミドリ 301, 303
川緑（カワミドリ） 301, 303
カワムギ（皮麦） 64
カワヤツメ 225
カワラケツメイ 108
河原決明（カワラケツメイ） 108
カワラタケ 74, 303
瓦茸（カワラタケ） 74, 303
カワラニンジン 317
河原人参（カワラニンジン） 317
カワラヨモギ 294
河原艾（カワラヨモギ） 294
カンアオイ（寒葵） 150
カンカイ（鳫喙） 66
カンカオウトウ（甘果桜桃） 128
カンカトウ 69
カンカトウ（干花豆） 69
カンカニクジュヨウ 74
管花肉蓯容（カンカニクジュヨウ） 74
カンキョウ 116
乾姜（カンキョウ） 116
カンキョウニン 75
甘杏仁（カンキョウニン） 75
還元麦芽糖 250
カンコ（甘瓠） 207
カンコウソウ 138
ガンジツソウ 334
元日草（ガンジツソウ） 334
貫衆（カンジュウ） 299
カンショ 75
甘蔗（カンショ） 75
カンショウ（甘松） 303
カンジョウ（砍茸） 351
カンショウキョウ（幹生姜） 116
カンショウコウ 303
甘松香（カンショウコウ） 303
環状重合乳酸 251
カンジリュウ（乾地竜） 349
岩石粉 251
カンゾウ<甘草> 75
甘草（カンゾウ） 75
肝臓 228
カンチク（寒竹） 138
カンテン 148
寒天（カンテン） 148
カントウカ 304
款冬花（カントウカ） 180, 304
カントウヨウ 180
款冬葉（カントウヨウ） 180
カントリソウ（疳取草） 217
カントングワ（広東桑） 90
カントンニンジン 45
広東人参（カントンニンジン） 45
カンピョウ（干瓢） 207
ガンビール 42
カンブイ 75
カンプラ 172
カンフル 116
漢防已（カンボウイ） 314
カンボケ（寒木瓜） 189, 200
ガンマブチロラクトン 362
関木通（カンモクツウ） 295
肝油（カンユ） 228
カンヨウカンショウ（寛葉甘松） 303
寛葉香蒲（カンヨウコウホ） 71
カンヨウレンギョウ（貫葉連翹） 124
カンラン 76
橄欖（カンラン） 67, 76
カンレンソウ 138
旱蓮草（カンレンソウ） 138
カンレンボク 76

キ

キイチゴ 76
懸鉤子（キイチゴ） 76
木苺（キイチゴ） 76
キイロスズメバチ（黄色雀蜂） 235
ギカイリュウ 226
擬海竜（ギカイリュウ） 226
擬海龍（ギカイリュウ） 226
キカラスウリ 74, 302
黄烏瓜（キカラスウリ） 74, 302
キキョウ 76
桔梗（キキョウ） 76
桔梗根（キキョウコン） 76
キク（菊） 77
キク（タラの精巣） 232
キグ 76
枳椇（キグ） 76
キクイモ 77
菊芋（キクイモ） 77
キクカ 77
菊花（キクカ） 77
菊苣（キクキョ） 77
キクゴボウ（菊牛蒡） 202
キクニガナ 77
菊苦菜（キクニガナ） 77
キクバオウレン 63, 299
菊葉黄蓮（キクバオウレン） 63
菊葉黄連（キクバオウレン） 299
菊葉地縛（キクバジシバリ） 52
キクラゲ 77
木耳（キクラゲ） 77
キクワタ 232
キケン 199
奇蒿（キコウ） 213
キコク 73, 137, 155
枳殻（キコク） 73, 137, 155
枸橘（キコク） 73
ギコクタシアリ（擬黒多刺蟻） 223
キササゲ 304
木大角豆（キササゲ） 304
キサントアントラフィル 360
キシ（葵子） 150
ギシギシ 209
羊蹄（ギシギシ） 209
ギシギシダイオウ（羊蹄大黄） 209
キジツ 137, 155
枳実（キジツ） 137, 155
キジュ 76
喜樹（キジュ） 76
キシリトール 252
キセン（鬼箭） 158
キセンウ（鬼箭羽） 158
キタオットセイ（北膃肭臍） 225
キダチアロエ 77
木立蘆薈（キダチアロエ） 77
キダチキンバイ 78
木立金梅（キダチキンバイ） 78
キダチコミカンソウ 78
木立小蜜柑草（キダチコミカンソウ） 78
キダチハッカ 78
木立薄荷（キダチハッカ） 78
キダチヒャクリコウ 139
木立百里香（キダチヒャクリコウ） 139
キチン 252
キッソウコン 70

吉草根（キッソウコン） 70
キツネノタスキ（狐の襷） 118
キツネノチャブクロ 100
キトサン 252
キトサンオリゴ糖 252
キナ 304
絹 253
キヌガサタケ 78
衣笠茸（キヌガサタケ） 78
キノア 78
木灰 283
キハダ 63, 298
黄肌（キハダ） 63, 298
キバナアザミ 79
黄花薊（キバナアザミ） 79
キバナイソマツ（黄花磯松） 48
キバナオウギ 62, 151, 298
黄花黄耆（キバナオウギ） 62, 151, 298
キバナシュスラン 79, 83
黄花繻子蘭（キバナシュスラン） 79, 83
キバナノクリンザクラ（黄花の九輪桜） 125
キバナハイショウ（黄花敗醤） 66
キフゲットウ（黄斑月桃） 93
キフジ（黄藤） 61
キブシ（木附子） 160
キブネダイオウ 79
貴船大黄（キブネダイオウ） 79
キボケ（木木瓜） 201
キミガヨラン 208
君が代蘭（キミガヨラン） 208
ギムネマ 79
キムラタケ 157
金精茸（キムラタケ） 157
キャッサバ 79
キャッツクロー 80
ギャバ 251
キャラウェイ 176
キャロブ 50
キュウイン（蚯蚓） 349
牛肝（ギュウカン） 228
キュウケツソウ（吸血草） 297
九香虫（キュウコウチュウ） 228
キュウサイシ 159
韮菜子（キュウサイシ） 159
韮子（キュウシ） 159
牛髄 229
急性子（キュウセイシ） 188, 336
キュウセツチャ 80
九節茶（キュウセツチャ） 80
ギュウタン（牛胆） 350
ギュウハクトウ 80
牛白藤（ギュウハクトウ） 80
キュラソーアロエ 46
キュラソー・アロエ 293
姜黄（キョウオウ） 172
薑黄（キョウオウ） 172
キョウカ 168
姜花（キョウカ） 168
キョウカツ 56, 304
羌活（キョウカツ） 56, 304
僵蚕（キョウサン） 226
姜蚕（キョウサン） 226
ギョウジャニンニク 80
行者葫（ギョウジャニンニク） 80
キョウチクトウ 80
夾竹桃（キョウチクトウ） 81
キョウニン 304
杏仁（キョウニン） 304
キョウバク 134
蕎麦（キョウバク） 134
狭葉香蒲（キョウヨウコウホ） 71
ギョクチク 48
玉竹（ギョクチク） 48
キョクトウサソリ 230
極東蠍（キョクトウサソリ） 230
玉蓮花（ギョクレンカ） 94
キョジョウ（鋸茸） 351
魚腥草（ギョセイソウ） 115
キヨマサニンジン（清正人参） 131
魚油（ギョユ） 229
ギョリュウ 81
御柳（ギョリュウ） 81
ギョリュウモドキ 81
御柳擬き（ギョリュウモドキ） 81
キランソウ 81
金蒼小草（キランソウ） 81
金瘡小草（キランソウ） 81
キリアサ（桐麻） 49, 150
キリンケツ 81
麒麟血（キリンケツ） 81
麒麟竭（キリンケツ） 81
キリンケツヤシ 81
麒麟血椰子（キリンケツヤシ） 81
キリンソウ 82
黄輪草（キリンソウ） 82
豨薟（キレン） 199
キレンソウ 199
金 253
キンエイカ（金英花） 169
キンカイモ（金柑芋） 172
キンカン 82
金柑（キンカン） 82
錦葵花（キンキカ） 56, 130
金橘（キンキツ） 82
錦葵葉（キンキヨウ） 56, 130
キンキリバ 93
キンギンカ 82
金銀花（キンギンカ） 82
キンケリバ 93
ギンゴウカン 83
キンゴジカ 297
金午時花（キンゴジカ） 297
筋骨草（キンコツソウ） 81
金盞銀盤（キンサンギンバン） 98
ギンジ（銀茸） 118
キンシバイ 82
金糸梅（キンシバイ） 82
キンシンサイ 82
金針菜（キンシンサイ） 82
キンセンカ 150
金盞花（キンセンカ） 150
キンセンキク（金盞菊） 150
キンセンソウ 83
金銭草（キンセンソウ） 83
キンセンレン 83
金線蓮（キンセンレン） 79, 83
ギンナン 50
ギンネム 83
銀合歓（ギンネム） 83
キンバイザサ 133
金梅笹（キンバイザサ） 133
金辺土鼈 232
キンポウゲ 57
金鳳花（キンポウゲ） 57
キンマ 83
蒟醬（キンマ） 83
金精茸（キンマラタケ） 157
キンミズヒキ 83
金水引（キンミズヒキ） 83
キンモクセイ 84
金木犀（キンモクセイ） 84
キンリュウカ属 305
キンレンカ 84
金蓮花（キンレンカ） 84

ク

グアイフェネジン　361
グアガム　253
グアコ　84
グアシャトンガ　305
グアバ　84
グアヤクノキ　84
クインラン　347
クエン酸　254
クエン酸マグネシウム　254
クカ（苦茄）　122
クガイ　85
苦蓬（クガイ）　85
苦瓜子（クカシ）　157
クキ（鼓）　155
クキョウニン　304
苦杏仁（クキョウニン）　304
クキョサイ（苦苣菜）　162
苦苣苔（クキョタイ）　52
クコ　85, 314
拘杞（クコ）　314
クコシ　85
枸杞子（クコシ）　85
クコツ　173
枸骨（クコツ）　173
クコヨウ　85
枸杞葉（クコヨウ）　85
草珊瑚　133
クサスギカズラ　149, 326
草杉葛（クサスギカズラ）　326
草杉蔓（クサスギカズラ）　149
クサセンナ　170
クサダモ　154
クサノオウ　151
草の黄（クサノオウ）　151
草王（クサノオウ）　151
瘡の王（クサノオウ）　151
クサボケ　85
草木瓜（クサボケ）　85
クジチョウ　85
苦地丁（クジチョウ）　85
クジン　305
苦参（クジン）　305
クズ　85, 301
葛（クズ）　85, 301
クスノキ　86
樟（クスノキ）　86
楠（クスノキ）　86
クスノハガシワ　305
狗舌草（グゼツソウ）　64
クソウ　129
苦草（クソウ）　129
クソザクラ　58
クソニンジン　297
クチナシ　106
口無（クチナシ）　106
グッタペルカ　86
グッタペルカノキ　86
クテイチャ　109, 141, 173
苦丁茶（クテイチャ）　109, 141, 173
クヌギ　315
櫟（クヌギ）　316
グビジンソウ　175
虞美人草（グビジンソウ）　175
クマ　350
クマコケモモ　296
熊苔桃（クマコケモモ）　296
クマザサ　86
隈笹（クマザサ）　86
クマゼミ　349
熊蝉（クマゼミ）　349
クマツヅラ　86
熊葛（クマツヅラ）　86
クマノアシツメクサ　47
クマノイ（熊の胆）　350
クマヤナギ　87
熊柳（クマヤナギ）　87
クミス・クチン　87
クミスクチン　87
クミン　87
クモコ　232
クラチャイ　87
クラチャイ・ダム　183
グラビオラ　87, 306
グラミニス　112
クララ　305
クラリーセージ　66
クランベリー　88
グリシン　254
L-α-グリセリルホスホリルコリン　246
グリセリン　254
sn-グリセロ(3)ホスホコリン　246
グリフォニア・シンプリシフォリア　306
グリーンランドイソツツジ　88
クルクミン　254
グルコサミン塩酸塩　255
α-グルコシダーゼ　375
グルコマンナン　255
グルコン酸亜鉛　256
グルコン酸鉄　256
グルタチオン　361
グルタミン　256
グルタミン酸　256
グルテン　88
クルマバソウ　88
車葉草（クルマバソウ）　88
クレアチン　257
クレアチン・エチルエステル塩酸塩　257
クレノアイ（九礼乃阿井）　186
クレノアイ（呉藍）　186
クレノアイ（紅藍）　186
グレープフルーツ　88
クレン　132
苦楝（クレン）　132
クレンシ　320, 327
苦楝子（クレンシ）　320
苦楝子（クレンシ）　327
クレンピ　320, 327
苦楝皮（クレンピ）　320
苦楝皮（クレンピ）　327
クロアリ（黒蟻）　223
クロアワビ（黒鮑）　223
クロウコン（黒鬱金）　183
クロウミウマ（黒海馬）　226
黒梅擬（クロウメモドキ）　306
クロウメモドキ属　306
クロガラシ　89
黒芥子（クロガラシ）　89
クログルミ　89
黒胡桃（クログルミ）　89
黒米（クロゴメ）　90
クロショウガ（黒生姜）　183
クロスグリ　89
黒酸塊（クロスグリ）　89
クロスズメバチ（黒胡蜂）　235
クロスズメバチ（黒雀蜂）　235
クロタネソウ（黒種草）　182
クロチョウガイ（黒蝶貝）　233
クロニレ（黒楡）　159
クロバナカズラ　96
クロバナヒキオコシ　61
黒花引起（クロバナヒキオコシ）　61
クローブ　89, 143

クロフサスグリ　69, 89
黒房酸塊（クロフサスグリ）　69, 89
クロマメノキ　90
黒豆の木（クロマメノキ）　90
黒豆木（クロマメノキ）　90
クロミウムピコリネート　272
クロム（Ⅲ）　257
クロムギ（黒麦）　211
クロモジ　56
黒文字（クロモジ）　56
クロヨナ　90
九重吹（クロヨナ）　90
クロレラ　90
クロロフィル　257
クロロプレタダラフィル　362
クワ　90, 195, 322
桑（クワ）　90, 195, 322
クワガタソウ　91
鍬形草（クワガタソウ）　91
クンイソウ（薫衣草）　213
クンチ　87

ケ

ケアオダモ（毛青梻）　37
ケアリタソウ（毛有田草）　46
ケイ　91, 92
桂（ケイ）　91, 92
桂圓（ケイエン）　213
桂圓肉（ケイエンニク）　213
ケイガイ　306
荊芥（ケイガイ）　306
鶏肝（ケイカン）　228
ケイケットウ　91
鶏血藤（ケイケットウ）　91
ケイコツソウ　91
鶏骨草（ケイコツソウ）　91
荊三稜（ケイサンリョウ）　55
ケイシ　91
桂枝（ケイシ）　91
ケイジツ（茴実）　150
荊条（ケイジョウ）　160
ケイ素　258
景天三七（ケイテンサンシチ）　82
ケイトウ（鶏頭）　66, 161
ケイナイキン　235
鶏内金（ケイナイキン）　235
ケイヒ　92
桂皮（ケイヒ）　92
ケイマ　49, 150
茴麻（ケイマ）　49, 150
ケイリンサイシン　311
鶏林細辛（ケイリンサイシン）　311
ゲゲバナ（五形花）　217
ケシ　92, 306
芥子（ケシ）　92, 306
ケシアザミ（芥子薊）　162
ケツエキ　229, 347
血液（ケツエキ）　229, 347
ゲッカビジン　92
月下美人（ゲッカビジン）　92
ゲッケイジュ　92
月桂樹（ゲッケイジュ）　92
ゲッケイヨウ　92
ケツジツ　66
芡実（ケツジツ）　66
ゲットウ　93
月桃（ゲットウ）　93
ケツマ　338
蕨麻（ケツマ）　338
ケツメイシ　60
決明子（ケツメイシ）　60
ケツメイヨウ　60
決明葉（ケツメイヨウ）　60
ケナシサルトリイバラ　106, 312
ケナシ猿捕茨（ケナシサルトリイバラ）　312
ケファエリス属　307
ケープアロエ　46
ケープ・アロエ　293
ケミヤマコウゾリナ　189
毛深山顔剃菜（ケミヤマコウゾリナ）　189
毛深山髪剃菜（ケミヤマコウゾリナ）　189
ケール　92
ケルセチン　258
ケルプ　93
ゲルマニウム　258
ケン　93
莧（ケン）　93
坎気（ケンキ）　350
ゲンゲ（紫雲英）　217
ゲンゲ（翹揺）　217
ケンケレバ　93
ケンゴシ　40, 307
牽牛子（ケンゴシ）　40, 307
ケンゴロウ　237
源五郎（ゲンゴロウ）　238
ゲンサンガ　226
原蚕蛾（ゲンサンガ）　226
原蚕子（ゲンサンシ）　226
原蚕沙（ゲンサンシャ）　226
芡実（ケンジツ）　66
ゲンジン　307
玄参（ゲンジン）　307
ゲンソウ（玄草）　307
ゲンチアナ　94, 307
ゲンデナフィル　362
ゲンノショウコ　307
現之証拠（ゲンノショウコ）　307
ケンポナシ　76
玄圃梨（ケンポナシ）　76
玄米胚芽（ゲンマイハイガ）　94

コ

Commiphora属　311
コ（葫）　160
コウイカ　224
甲烏賊（コウイカ）　224
コウエン　181
香櫞（コウエン）　181
コウカ　186
紅花（コウカ）　186
ゴウカイ　225
蛤蚧（ゴウカイ）　225
コウガイモ（笄藻）　129
コウカガンショウ　94
紅花岩松（コウカガンショウ）　94
香花岩豆藤　91
コウカサイ（紅花菜）　217
紅花菜（コウカサイ）　217
コウカヒ（香加皮）　96
ゴウカンカ　161
合歓花（ゴウカンカ）　161
ゴウカンヒ　161
合歓皮（ゴウカンヒ）　161
コウキ　94
黄紀（コウキ）　94
候姜（コウキョウ）　164
紅槿（コウキン）　163
コウクジン（広狗腎）　347
コウクベン　347
広狗鞭（コウクベン）　347
コウケイテン　52
紅景天（コウケイテン）　52
コウコウ　95
降香（コウコウ）　95

コウコウダン　95
降香檀（コウコウダン）　95
コウコラン　44
紋股藍（コウコラン）　44
香荽（コウサイ）　98
コウシ　136, 155
香豉（コウシ）　136, 155
コウジコ（光慈姑）　44
ゴウシマ　229
哈士蟆（ゴウシマ）　229
コウシャジクソウ　38
紅車軸草（コウシャジクソウ）　38
コウジュ　94
香需（コウジュ）　94
香茹（コウジュ）　94
ゴウシュウアオギリ（豪州アオギリ）　37
コウジョウボク　208
交譲木（コウジョウボク）　208
コウジリュウ（広地竜）　349
コウシンコウ　95
降真香（コウシンコウ）　95
コウスイハッカ　200
コウスイボク　188
香水木（コウスイボク）　188
コウズク　156
紅豆蔻（コウズク）　156
コウズコン（広豆根）　313
孜然芹（コウゼンキン）　87
コウソウ（紅藻）　95
コウソウ（紅棗）　136
コウトウ（紅藤）　135
コウトウ（鉤藤）　143
コウトウ（香橙）　208
コウトウサン（紅豆杉）　164
コウヒモッカ（光皮木瓜）　201
コウブシ　308
香附子（コウブシ）　308
コウフン　308
鉤吻（コウフン）　308
粳米（コウベイ）　100
酵母（コウボ）　95
香茅（コウボウ）　216
広防已（コウボウイ）　295
コウボウチャ（弘法茶）　108
コウボク　308
厚朴（コウボク）　308
コウホネ　95, 319
河骨（コウホネ）　95, 319
コウホン　308
藁本（コウホン）　308
コウマ　212
紅麻（コウマ）　212
コウモウゴカ　95
紅毛五加　95
紅毛丹　213
コウモリドコロ（蝙蝠野老）　131
コウライニンジン　65
高麗人参（コウライニンジン）　65
コウリョウキョウ（高良姜）　343
コエンザイムA　259
コエンザイムQ10　259
コエンドロ　98
ゴオウ　347
牛黄（ゴオウ）　347
犀黄（ゴオウ）　347
コオウレン　96
胡黄蓮（コオウレン）　96
ゴカ　55, 96
五加（ゴカ）　55
五加参（ゴカジン）　59
ゴガツササゲ（五月豇）　53
コガネウリ（小金瓜）　153
コガネキクラゲ　97
コガネニカワタケ（黄金膠茸）　97
コガネバナ　62, 298
黄金花（コガネバナ）　62, 298
コガネヤナギ　62, 298
黄金柳（コガネヤナギ）　62, 298
五加皮（ゴカヒ）　55, 95, 96
コカマキリ（黒螵蛸）　233
コカマキリ（小刀蜋）　233
ゴガンカジュヒ　156
五眼果樹皮（ゴガンカジュヒ）　156
姑牛卵嚢　224
ゴギョウ　170
御行（ゴギョウ）　170
コクケイジュ（黒荊樹）　202
コクシンジュ（黒心樹）　138
コクダイズ　136
黒大豆（コクダイズ）　136
コクリコ（雛罌粟）　175
コクリュウ（穀粒）　100
コクワ　105
コクワヅル　105
コケイコツ（虎脛骨）　348
コケモモ　97, 309
苔桃（コケモモ）　97
コケモモヨウ　309
苔桃葉（コケモモヨウ）　309
ココツ　348
虎骨（ココツ）　348
ココナッツ　204
ココメグサ　37, 97
小米草（ココメグサ）　37, 97
ココメビユ　187
治疝草（ココメビユ）　187
ココヤシ　204
古古椰子（ココヤシ）　204
ゴサイバ（五菜葉）　39
コサン（胡蒜）　160
コシ　207
瓠子（コシ）　207
瓠子子（コシシ）　207
ゴシツ　309
牛膝（ゴシツ）　309
コシュ（虎鬚）　180
ゴシュユ　309
呉茱萸（ゴシュユ）　309
ゴショイチゴ　334
御所苺（ゴショイチゴ）　334
コショウ　97
胡椒（コショウ）　97
虎杖（コジョウ）　48
コジョウコン　309
虎杖根（コジョウコン）　309
コシロノセンダングサ　98
小白梅檀草（コシロノセンダングサ）　98
コジン　98
コズイシ　98
胡荽子（コズイシ）　98
湖水真珠（コスイシンジュ）　236
小芹葉黄蓮（コセリバオウレン）　299
コセンダングサ　98
小梅檀草（コセンダングサ）　98
五爪金龍（ゴソウキンリュウ）　201
五爪竜　201
五爪龍（ゴソウリュウ）　201
コタラヒム　104
コタラヒムブツ　104
ゴツコーラ　145
骨砕補（コツサイホ）　164
コツズイ　229, 348
骨髄（コツズイ）　229, 348
骨粉　230
梧桐子（ゴトウシ）　37

コナスビ　98
小茄子（コナスビ）　98
コナラ（小楢）　315
コニワザクラ　48
コノテガシワ　134, 330
児手柏（コノテガシワ）　134, 330
コバイケイソウ　329
小梅蕙草（コバイケイソウ）　329
ゴバイシ　160
五倍子（ゴバイシ）　160
コパイーバ・オフィシナリス　98
コパイーバ・ラングスドルフィ　99
コハク　99
コハコベ（小繁縷）　165
コバテイシ（枯葉手樹）　202
コバノシナノキ（小葉菩提樹）　190
コバノトネリコ　37
コーヒーノキ　96
コフキサルノコシカケ　99
粉吹猿腰掛（コフキサルノコシカケ）　99
コブシ　316
拳（コブシ）　316
辛夷（コブシ）　316
コブミカン　185
瘤蜜柑（コブミカン）　185
コブラ　230
虎鞭（コベン）　224
ゴボウ　99, 310
牛蒡（ゴボウ）　99, 310
ゴボウアザミ（牛蒡薊）　202
ゴボウシ　310
牛蒡子（ゴボウシ）　310
ゴホダ（五歩蛇）　236
ゴマ　100
胡麻（ゴマ）　100
ゴマ油　100
胡麻油（ゴマアブラ）　100
コマイ（氷下魚）　228
ゴマシ（胡麻子）　44
ゴマノハグサ　307
胡麻葉草（ゴマノハグサ）　307
ゴマフアザラシ　223, 347
ゴマフアザラシ（胡麻斑海豹）　223
海豹（ゴマフアザラシ）　347
コマントウ　308
胡蔓藤（コマントウ）　308
コミカンソウ　100
小蜜柑草（コミカンソウ）　100
ゴミシ　310
五味子（ゴミシ）　310
コミラ　159
古美良（コミラ）　159
コムギ　88, 100
小麦（コムギ）　100
コムソウタケ（虚無僧茸）　78
ゴムノキ　100
コメデンプン　100
米澱粉（コメデンプン）　100
コメヌカ　101
米糠（コメヌカ）　101
コモンヴィッチ　72
ゴーヤ　157
ゴーヤー　157
コヤブラン　331
小藪蘭（コヤブラン）　331
コーラ　96
ゴーラ　157
コラ　96
ゴラカ　74
コラーゲン　259
コラシ　96
コラノキ　96
コーラルサンゴ　231
コリアンダー　98
コリビ　101
狐狸尾（コリビ）　101
コリン安定化オルトケイ酸　260
コリンクチナシ（小輪梔子）　106
ゴールデンウィロー　205
ゴールデンシール　308
コルヒクム子　294
ゴレイシ　348
五霊脂（ゴレイシ）　348
コレウスフォルスコリー　73
コーレーグス（高麗薬）　113
コレン（胡蓮）　96
ゴレンシ　101
五斂子（ゴレンシ）　101
葫蘆（コロ）　177
コロシント　310
コロシントウリ　310
コロシント瓜（コロシントウリ）　310
ゴロツキアザミ　64
コロハ　101
胡芦巴（コロハ）　101
胡盧巴（コロハ）　101
コロンボ　310
コンゲンイ（混元衣）　350
コンゴウザクラ　58
コンズランゴ　310
コンドデロデンドロン属　311
コンドデンドロン属　311
コンドロイチン加水分解二糖　230
コンドロイチン硫酸　260
コンドロムコタンパク　260
コントンイ（混沌衣）　350
コンブ　101
昆布（コンブ）　101
コンフリー　102
コンブレツム　93
コンミフォラ属　311
昆明鶏血藤（コンメイケイケットウ）　91

サ

*Saccharomyces*に属する単細胞生物　95
サイカチ　102
サイカレイヨウ　351
賽加羚羊（サイカレイヨウ）　351
サイガレイヨウ　351
賽加羚羊（サイガレイヨウ）　351
サイコ　102, 311
柴胡（サイコ）　102, 311
サイシン　311
細辛（サイシン）　311
サイトウ（菜豆）　53
サイハイラン　103
采配蘭（サイハイラン）　103
サイモリバ（菜盛葉）　39
サイリウム・ハスク　184
沙苑子（サエンシ）　113
沙苑蒺藜（サエンシツリ）　113
沙苑子（サオンシ）　113
サキシマフウトウカズラ（先島風藤葛）　115
サキシマボタンヅル（先島牡丹蔓）　52
サキョウ　102, 103
沙棘（サキョウ）　102, 103
サグ　103
サクトウ（鮓荅）　350
サクナ　190
サクラシバ（桜芝）　174
サクラソウ　103
桜草（サクラソウ）　103

サクリュウカ　102, 103
醋柳果（サクリュウカ）　102, 103
ザクロ　103
石榴（ザクロ）　103
柘榴（ザクロ）　103
サケ（鮭）　232
サゴヤシ　103
サゴ椰子（サゴヤシ）　103
ササクサ　141
笹草（ササクサ）　141
サーサップ　87, 306
サージ　102, 103
沙棘（サージ）　102, 103
サジオモダカ　323
匙面高（サジオモダカ）　323
サソウ　308
沙草（サソウ）　308
サソリ　230
蝎（サソリ）　230
サッカラーゼ　358
サッサフラスノキ　104
サツマゴキブリ　232
薩摩蜚蠊（サツマゴキブリ）　232
サーディンペプチド　224
サトウキビ　75
砂糖黍（サトウキビ）　75
サトウダイコン　104
砂糖大根（サトウダイコン）　104
サトウボク（沙塘木）　95
サネブトナツメ　107
核太棗（サネブトナツメ）　107
サビナ　312
サビナビャクシン（サビナ柏槇）　312
サフラワー　186
サフラン　104
泊夫藍（サフラン）　104
サポニン　260
サボリー　78
ザボン　185
朱欒（サボン）　185
サボンソウ　104
サメ　231
鮫（サメ）　231
サメナンコツ　231
鮫軟骨（サメナンコツ）　231
サヨウ　65
鎖陽（サヨウ）　65
サラカキ　312
サラシア・オブロンガ　105
サラシア・キネンシス　105
サラシア・レティキュラータ　104
サラシナショウマ　316
晒菜升麻（サラシナショウマ）　316
サルカケミカン　312
猿掛蜜柑（サルカケミカン）　312
サルサ　109
サルサコン（サルサ根）　106
サルサパリラ　106
サルトリイバラ　106
猿捕茨（サルトリイバラ）　106
サルトリイバラ属　106, 109
サルナシ　105
猿梨（サルナシ）　105
山樝（サルナシ）　105
サルノコシカケ　74
猿の腰掛（サルノコシカケ）　74
サルビア　105
サワギキョウ　312
沢桔梗（サワギキョウ）　312
山芋（サンウ）　108
サンカクウシアブ（三角牛虻）　350
サンカクトウ　105
山核桃（サンカクトウ）　105
三角帆貝　236
酸化ケイ素　258
サンキライ　106, 312
山帰来（サンキライ）　106, 312
サンゴ　231
珊瑚（サンゴ）　231
サンコウ（山香）　115
山梗菜（サンコウサイ）　312
サンゴソウ　42
珊瑚草（サンゴソウ）　42
サンコトウ（山胡桃）　105
サンコノマツ（三鈷松）　165
サンサ（山査）　106
サンサ（山楂）　106
サンザシ　106
山査子（サンザシ）　106
山梔（サンシ）　106
サンシキスミレ　106
三色菫（サンシキスミレ）　106
サンジコ　44, 103
山慈姑（サンジコ）　44, 103
サンシシ　106
山梔子（サンシシ）　106
サンシチニンジン　107
三七人参（サンシチニンジン）　107
サンシュユ　107
山茱萸（サンシュユ）　107
参薯（サンショ）　57
サンショウ　107
山椒（サンショウ）　107
サンショウコン　337
酸漿根（サンショウコン）　337
サンショウバラ　107
山椒薔薇（サンショウバラ）　107
サンズコン　313
山豆根（サンズコン）　313
サンセイリュウシツ（三星龍虱）　237
サンセキリュウ　103
山石榴（サンセキリュウ）　103
サンソウ（酸棗）　107
サンソウニン　107, 136
酸棗仁（サンソウニン）　107, 136
サンチャ（山茶）　145
サンチャカ（山茶花）　145
サンドイモ（三度芋）　172
サントウ（酸橙）　137
サントウ（鑽凍）　180
サントウカク（山桃核）　105
サンドマメ（三度豆）　53
サントリソウ　79
サンナ　108
三奈（サンナ）　108
山奈（サンナ）　108
砂仁（サンニン）　93
サンバー　231
三白草　173
三斑海馬　226
サンペイゴボウ（三瓶牛蒡）　202
サンペンズ　108
山扁豆（サンペンズ）　108
サンヤク　108, 206
山薬（サンヤク）　108, 206
サンユニク（山萸肉）　107
三稜（サンリョウ）　55

シ

Digitalis属　313
シア　108
ジアスターゼ　356
シアノコバラミン　274
シアノバクテリア　43
シアーバターノキ　108
シイ（紫葳）　214
ジイソブ　146

爺蕎（ジイソブ） 146
爺雀斑（ジイソブ） 146
シイタケ 109
椎茸（シイタケ） 109
ジオウ 313
地黄（ジオウ） 313
シオデ属 106, 109
シオヒゲムシ 148
シオン 313
紫苑（シオン） 313
シカ 229
糸瓜花（シカカ） 186
枝核 216
糸瓜根（シカコン） 186
糸瓜子（シカシ） 186
シカジチョウ 111, 121
紫花地丁（シカジチョウ） 111, 121
シカシャ 350
紫河車（シカシャ） 350
只河車（シカシャ） 350
糸瓜藤（シカトウ） 186
糸瓜皮（シカヒ） 186
シカメガキ 227
シカラク 186
糸瓜絡（シカラク） 186
ジギタリス 313
ジギタリス属 313
シキビ（樒） 313
シキビ（櫁） 313
シキビ（梻） 313
シキミ 313
樒（シキミ） 313
ジキン（地錦） 50
ジクオウ（竺黄） 148
シクロフェニール 363
シクロペンチナフィル 363
シクンシ 109
使君子（シクンシ） 109
シケイジョテイ 109
紫茎女貞（シケイジョテイ） 109
シコウカ 109
指甲花（シコウカ） 109
匙羹藤（シコウトウ） 180
シゴカ 59, 96
刺五加（シゴカ） 59, 96
ジゴクノカマノフタ 81
地獄の釜の蓋（ジゴクノカマノフタ） 81
ジゴクノネ（地獄の根） 209
ジゴクバナ（地獄花） 318
シコクビエ 110
四国稗（シコクビエ） 110
竜爪稗（シコクビエ） 110
龍爪稗（シコクビエ） 110
ジコッピ 85, 314
地骨皮（ジコッピ） 85, 314
シコン 314
紫根（シコン） 314
紫杉（シサン） 49
梔子（シシ） 106
シシウド 110, 328
香独活（シシウド） 110, 328
猪独活（シシウド） 110, 328
紫地丁（シジチョウ） 121
シジツ 304
梓実（シジツ） 304
紫芝（シシバ） 216
ジシバリ 52
地縛（ジシバリ） 52
シジミ 231
蜆（シジミ） 231
ジジン 110
地稔（ジジン） 110
地菍（ジジン） 110
シスタチオン 261
シスチン 261
システイン 262
シセンサンショウ 111
四川山椒（シセンサンショウ） 111
シソ 110
紫蘇（シソ） 110
シソ油 110
シソウ（芝草） 216
シダレカンバ 111
枝垂樺（シダレカンバ） 111
シタン 111
紫檀（シタン） 111
シチヘンゲ（七変化） 41
ジチャ（地茶） 208
ジチョウ 111, 121
地丁（ジチョウ） 111, 121
七葉胆（シチヨウタン） 44
シッサス・クアドラングラリス 314
シツリシ 314
蒺藜子（シツリシ） 314
柿蒂（シテイ） 68
L-シトルリン 247
シトロン 181
シナガヤ（支那榧） 174
シナカラスウリ 74, 302
支那烏瓜（シナカラスウリ） 74, 302
シナカラスガイ（支那烏貝） 233
シナガワハギ 123
品川萩（シナガワハギ） 123
シナキササゲ（支那楸） 304
シナスッポン 232
支那鼈（シナスッポン） 232
シナセンニンソウ（支那仙人草） 52
シナタラノキ 112
シナナツメ（支那棗） 107
シナニッケイ 92
シナノキ 112
科の木（シナノキ） 112
級の木（シナノキ） 112
椴（シナノキ） 112
榀の木（シナノキ） 112
シナヒイラギ（支那柊） 173
シナヒキガエル 349
支那蟇（シナヒキガエル） 349
支那蟾蜍（シナヒキガエル） 349
シナボタンヅル 52, 294
支那牡丹蔓（シナボタンヅル） 294
ジネンショ（自然薯） 206
ジネンジョウ（自然生） 108, 206
シバイカ 206
ジバチ（地蜂） 235
シバムギ 112
芝麦（シバムギ） 112
ジビジビ 121
ジヒチュウ（地卑虫） 232
ジフ 112
地膚（ジフ） 112
地膚子（ジフシ） 112
ジブドウ（地葡萄） 90
ジベツ（地鼈） 232
シベット 348
シベリアジカ 351
シベリアニンジン 59
脂肪酸 262
シマカナビキソウ（島金引草） 122
シマタコノキ 113
シマツナソ（縞綱麻） 203
シマトウガラシ 113
島唐辛子（シマトウガラシ） 113
シマハスノハカズラ 314
シマボウ 202
地豆（ジマメ） 212

ジメチル-4,4'-ジメトキシ-5,6,5',6'-ジメチレンジオキシビフェニル-2,2'-ジカルボキシレート　370
紫苜蓿（シモクシュク）　46
シャウペデコウロ　113
シャエンシ　113
沙苑子（シャエンシ）　113
沙苑蒺藜（シャエンシツリ）　113
ジャガイモ（ジャガ芋）　172
シャカオ　302
ジャガタライモ（ジャガタラ芋）　172
ジャガタラカン　185
芦藤（シャカトウ）　79, 180
沙棘（シャキョク）　102, 103
ジャクゼツソウ　114
雀舌草（ジャクゼツソウ）　114
シャクナゲ　318
石南花（シャクナゲ）　318
シャクヤク　114, 315
芍薬（シャクヤク）　114, 315
芍药（シャクヤク）　114
ジャコウ　348
麝香（ジャコウ）　348
ジャコウジカ　348
麝香鹿（ジャコウジカ）　348
麝香草（ジャコウソウ）　139
ジャコウネコ　348
麝香猫（ジャコウネコ）　348
ジャショウ　315
蛇床子（ジャショウシ）　315
シャジン（沙参）　114
シャジン（砂仁）　315
沙参（シャジン）　114
砂仁（シャジン）　315
ジャスミン　114
シャゼンシ　63
車前子（シャゼンシ）　63
シャゼンソウ　63
車前草（シャゼンソウ）　63
シャゼンヨウ　63
車前葉（シャゼンヨウ）　63
シャソウ（沙草）　308
シャタバリ　114
蛇胆（ジャタン）　233
シャチュウ　232
䗪虫（シャチュウ）　232
ジャック　171
ジャックフルーツ　171
ジャドク　349
蛇毒（ジャドク）　349
ジャトバ　115
ジャトロファ　157
ジャノヒゲ　331
蛇の髭（ジャノヒゲ）　331
蛇婆　236
ジャビャクシ　115
蛇百子（ジャビャクシ）　115
蛇葡萄（ジャブドウ）　162
蛇葡萄根（ジャブドウコン）　162
蛇鞭（ジャベン）　224
ジャボン　185
シャボンソウ　104
シャミセングサ（三味線草）　154
シャミセンズル（三味線蔓）　70
シャーレーポピー　175
ジャワアナツバメ　234
ジャワザクラ（ジャワ桜）　168
ジャワナガコショウ　115
爪哇長胡椒（ジャワナガコショウ）　115
爪哇白豆蔻（ジャワビャクズク）　177
シャンピニオン　128
ジャンブル　198
ジユ（地楡）　220
シュウ（首烏）　146
茺蔚子（ジュウイシ）　216
臭化水素酸デキストロメトルファン　363
戴菜（ジュウサイ）　115
シュウソウ（臭草）　188
シュウトウ（首烏藤）　146
ジュウネン（十稔）　110
ジュウヤク　115
十薬（ジュウヤク）　115
重薬（ジュウヤク）　115
シュキン（朱槿）　182
ジュクジオウ（熟地黄）　313
シュクシャ　315
縮砂（シュクシャ）　315
シュクシャミツ　315
縮砂蜜（シュクシャミツ）　315
樹脂アルコール　284
シュショウジン　147
手掌参（シュショウジン）　147
ジュズダマ　168
数珠玉（ジュズダマ）　168
酒石酸　262
ジュゼツ　99
樹舌（ジュゼツ）　99
腫節風　133
ジュート　203
ジュルベーバ　115
ジュルベバ　115
シュロ　116
棕呂（シュロ）　116
棕梠（シュロ）　116
棕櫚（シュロ）　116
シュロソウ　329
棕櫚草（シュロソウ）　329
棕櫚皮（シュロヒ）　116
シュロヨウ　116
棕櫚葉（シュロヨウ）　116
ショウガ　116
生姜（ショウガ）　116
シヨウカ　41
紫陽花（シヨウカ）　41
松果体ホルモン　376
ショウキョウ　116
生姜（ショウキョウ）　116
生薑（ショウキョウ）　116
将軍木皮（ショウグンボクヒ）　39
小薊（ショウケイ）　161
ショウコウ（椒紅）　111
松香（ショウコウ）　99
ジョウコタケ（上戸茸）　207
常山（ジョウザン）　53
松脂（ショウシ）　194
韶子（ショウシ）　213
樟樹葉（ショウジュヨウ）　86
ショウズク　116, 177
小豆蔻（ショウズク）　116, 177
墻草（ショウソウ）　174
ショウノウ　116
樟脳（ショウノウ）　116
ショウバク（小檗）　128
ショウブ　129, 315
菖蒲（ショウブ）　129, 315
ショウブコン　315
菖蒲根（ショウブコン）　315
ショウボクヒ　194, 315
松木皮（ショウボクヒ）　194
橡木皮（ショウボクヒ）　316
ショウマ　316
升麻（ショウマ）　316
ショウマンチョウシュンカ（小蔓長春花）　177
松葉（ショウヨウ）　194

ショウヨウダイオウ（掌葉大黄） 135
ショウラン 117
松藍（ショウラン） 117
ショウリク 316
商陸（ショウリク） 316
ショウリョウバナ（精霊花） 196
ショウレンギョウ 65
小連翹（ショウレンギョウ） 65
蜀漆（ショクシツ） 53
ショクショウ（蜀椒） 111
植物性酵素 262
植物性ステロール 263
植物繊維 263
食物繊維 263
蜀羊泉（ショクヨウセン） 177
ショクヨウダイオウ 117, 135
食用ダイオウ 117, 135
食用大黄（ショクヨウダイオウ） 117, 135
食用ホオズキ 117
食用鬼灯（ショクヨウホオズキ） 117
食用酸漿（ショクヨウホオズキ） 117
ショクヨウボウフウ（食用防風） 190
女貞（ジョテイ） 159
ジョテイシ 159
女貞子（ジョテイシ） 159
ショヨ（薯蕷） 108, 206
シラカバ 117
白樺（シラカバ） 117
シラカンバ 117
白樺（シラカンバ） 117
シラクチカズラ 105
猿口葛（シラクチカズラ） 105
シラクチヅル 105
猿口蔓（シラクチヅル） 105
シラコ 232
白子（シラコ） 233
ジラシ 176
蒔蘿子（ジラシ） 176
シラネブドウ（白根葡萄） 90
シラン 117
紫蘭（シラン） 117
シリ 118
棘梨（シリ） 118
ジリュウ 349
地竜（ジリュウ） 349
地龍（ジリュウ） 349
ジリュウカン（地竜干） 349
ジリュウニク（地竜肉） 349
シルク 253
シルデナフィル 364
刺老鴉（シロウア） 140
シロカワマツ（白皮松） 165
シロキクラゲ 118
白木耳（シロキクラゲ） 118
シログワ（白桑） 90, 195
シロコヤマモモ 118
白小山桃（シロコヤマモモ） 118
シロザケ（白鮭） 232
シロダイコン（白大根） 211
白茶（シロチャ） 164
シロトウアズキ 91
シロボケ（白木瓜） 189
シロマイタケ 192
白舞茸（シロマイタケ） 192
シロマツ（白松） 165
シロミナンテン 329
白実南天（シロミナンテン） 329
シロヤマモモ（白山桃） 118
シンイ 316
辛夷（シンイ） 316
申姜（シンキョウ） 164
シンキンソウ 118
伸筋草（シンキンソウ） 118
ジンコウ 316
沈香（ジンコウ） 317, 333
シンジュ 233
真珠（シンジュ） 233
心臓 232
シントククスノキ 118
秦皮（シンピ） 37
ジンポウ（人胞） 350

ス

Smilax属 109
Streptococcus属 158
Strophanthus属 305
ズイカク 119
蕤核（ズイカク） 119
スイカズラ 82
吸葛（スイカズラ） 82
スイキシ（水亀子） 237
スイサイ 317
睡菜（スイサイ） 317
睡菜葉（スイサイヨウ） 317
スイシシ（水梔子） 106
蕤仁（ズイジン） 119
スイチョウコウ 78
水丁香（スイチョウコウ） 78
スイテツ 235
水蛭（スイテツ） 235
スイートオレンジ 67, 119
スイバ 119
酸葉（スイバ） 119
酢葉（スイバ） 119
蓚（スイバ） 119
スイベッチュウ（水鼈中） 237
スイボセツレンカ（水母雪蓮花） 130
スイボンソウ（垂盆草） 147
スイヨウバイ 136
水楊梅（スイヨウバイ） 136
水流豆（スイリュウトウ） 90
スイロク（水鹿） 231
スエツムハナ（末摘花） 186
スオウ 322
蘇芳（スオウ） 322
スカルキャップ 119, 317
スガレ 235
スカンボ 119
スカンポ（酸模） 119
スギナ 119
杉菜（スギナ） 119
スクアラミン 232
スグリ 120
酸塊（スグリ） 120
スクワレン 264
スケトウダラ（介党鱈） 228
スコッツヘザー 81
ズシ 136, 155
豆豉（ズシ） 136, 155
スズメグサ（雀草） 165
スズラン 317
鈴蘭（スズラン） 317
スターアニス 135
スターフラワー 215
スッポン 232
鼈（スッポン） 232
ステビア 120
ステビア葉 120
ストローブ 120
ストロファンツス 305
ストロファンツス子 305
ストローブマツ 120
スナジグミ（砂地茱萸） 102
スーパーオキシドディスムターゼ＜SOD＞ 263
スピルリナ 120

スペアミント　121
スペアミント油　121
スベリヒユ　165
滑莧（スベリヒユ）　165
スマ　121
スマック　121
スミイカ（墨烏賊）　224
スミノエガキ（住之江牡蠣）　227
炭焼の乾留水　264
スミレ　121
菫（スミレ）　121
スモウトリバナ　111
スリッパリーエルム　39
スリナムチェリー　139
スリムアマランス　122
ズルカマラ　122
ズルカマラ枝（茎）　122
スルフォンアミド　364
ズワイガニ（松葉蟹）　228
ズワイガニ（楚蟹）　228
ズワイガニ（津和井蟹）　228
スワンギ　185

セ

Cephaelis属　307
西河柳（セイカリュウ）　81
セイコウ　317
青蒿（セイコウ）　317
薺菜（セイサイ）　154
セイショウ　161
青葙（セイショウ）　161
青葙子（セイショウシ）　161
セイセンリュウ　122
セイソウ（茜草）　320
セイソウ（精巣）　232, 233
セイソウ（青葙）　161
茜草根（セイソウコン）　320
青葙子（セイソウシ）　161
セイタカカナビキソウ　122
セイタカミロバラン　122
セイヒ　123
青皮（セイヒ）　123
青皮竹　148
セイヨウアカネ　123
西洋茜（セイヨウアカネ）　123
セイヨウイソノキ　335
西洋磯木（セイヨウイソノキ）　335
セイヨウイラクサ　123
西洋刺草（セイヨウイラクサ）　123
西洋蕁草（セイヨウイラクサ）　123
セイヨウウスユキソウ　58
西洋薄雪草（セイヨウウスユキソウ）　58
セイヨウエビラハギ　123
西洋箙萩（セイヨウエビラハギ）　123
セイヨウオオバコ　124
西洋大葉子（セイヨウオオバコ）　124
セイヨウオトギリ（西洋弟切）　124
セイヨウオトギリソウ　124
西洋弟切草（セイヨウオトギリソウ）　124
セイヨウカノコソウ　70
セイヨウカラハナソウ（西洋唐花草）　191
セイヨウカンボク（西洋肝木）　209
セイヨウキイチゴ　124
西洋木苺（セイヨウキイチゴ）　124
セイヨウキノコ（西洋茸）　128
セイヨウキンミズヒキ　124
西洋金水引（セイヨウキンミズヒキ）　124
セイヨウグルミ　69
西洋胡桃（セイヨウグルミ）　69
セイヨウサクラソウ　125
西洋桜草（セイヨウサクラソウ）　125
セイヨウサンザシ　125
西洋山査子（セイヨウサンザシ）　125
西洋蓍草（セイヨウシソウ）　127
セイヨウシナノキ　125, 147
西洋科の木（セイヨウシナノキ）　125, 147
西洋級の木（セイヨウシナノキ）　125
西洋榀の木（セイヨウシナノキ）　125
セイヨウシロヤナギ　125
西洋白柳（セイヨウシロヤナギ）　125
セイヨウジン　45
西洋参（セイヨウジン）　45
西洋人参（セイヨウニンジン）　45
セイヨウスグリ（西洋酸塊）　120
セイヨウスノキ（西洋酢の木）　178
セイヨウスモモ　125
西洋酸桃（セイヨウスモモ）　125
セイヨウセキショウモ　129
西洋石菖藻（セイヨウセキショウモ）　129
セイヨウタンポポ　126, 189
西洋蒲公英（セイヨウタンポポ）　126, 189
西洋当帰（セイヨウトウキ）　47
セイヨウトチノキ　126, 318
西洋栃（セイヨウトチノキ）　126
西洋栃の木（セイヨウトチノキ）　318
西洋橡（セイヨウトチノキ）　126
セイヨウトネリコ　126
西洋梣（セイヨウトネリコ）　126
セイヨウナツユキソウ　126
西洋夏雪草（セイヨウナツユキソウ）　126
セイヨウニワトコ　126
西洋接骨木（セイヨウニワトコ）　126
西洋庭常（セイヨウニワトコ）　126
セイヨウニンジン　45
セイヨウニンジンボク　127
西洋人参木（セイヨウニンボク）　127
セイヨウネズ　127
西洋杜松（セイヨウネズ）　127
セイヨウノコギリソウ　127
西洋鋸草（セイヨウノコギリソウ）　127
セイヨウハシリドコロ（西洋走野老）　335
セイヨウハッカ　127
西洋薄荷（セイヨウハッカ）　127
セイヨウヒイラギ　128
西洋柊（セイヨウヒイラギ）　128
セイヨウヒメスノキ　128
西洋姫臼の木（セイヨウヒメスノキ）　128
セイヨウビャクシン　127
西洋柏槇（セイヨウビャクシン）　127
セイヨウボダイジュ　125, 147
西洋菩提樹（セイヨウボダイジュ）　125, 147
セイヨウマツタケ　128
西洋松茸（セイヨウマツタケ）　128
セイヨウミザクラ　128
西洋実桜（セイヨウミザクラ）　128
セイヨウメギ　128
西洋目木（セイヨウメギ）　128
セイヨウヤドリギ　318
西洋寄生木（セイヨウヤドリギ）　318
西洋宿木（セイヨウヤドリギ）　318
セイヨウヤブイチゴ　124
西洋藪苺（セイヨウヤブイチゴ）　124
西洋山薄荷（セイヨウヤマハッカ）　200
セイヨウリンゴ（西洋林檎）　215

セイヨウワサビ　219
西洋山葵（セイヨウワサビ）　219
セイヨヤマハッカ　200
セキイ　129
石韋（セキイ）　129
セキケツメイ　223
石決明（セキケツメイ）　223
セキコウジュ　129
石香薷（セキコウジュ）　129
セキコウジュウ（石香葇）　129
セキサン　318
石蒜（セキサン）　318
石蒜根（セキサンコン）　318
石指甲（セキシコウ）　147
セキシャク　114, 315
赤芍（セキシャク）　114, 315
セキショウ（石松）　118
セキショウ（石菖）　129, 318
セキショウコン　318
石菖根（セキショウコン）　318
セキショウズ　42
赤小豆（セキショウズ）　42
セキショウブ（石菖蒲）　129
セキショウモ　129
石菖藻（セキショウモ）　129
セキジン（赤参）　141
セキセツソウ　145, 217, 218
積雪草（セキセツソウ）　145, 217, 218
セキテッコウ　364
赤鉄鉱　364
セキナンヨウ　318
石楠葉（セキナンヨウ）　318
セキヨウ　130
赤楊（セキヨウ）　130
セキリュウ　103
石榴根皮（セキリュウコンピ）　103
石榴皮（セキリュウヒ）　103
セキレン　94
石蓮（セキレン）　94
セキレンカ（石連花）　60
石蓮子（セキレンシ）　166
セージ　105
セッカサイ（石花菜）　148
石膏　264
雪蛤（セツゴウ）　229
雪哈（セツゴウ）　229
セッコク　325
石斛（セッコク）　325
セッコツボク　80, 130
接骨木（セッコツボク）　80, 130
接骨木花（セッコツボクカ）　130
接骨木根（セッコツボクコン）　130
接骨木葉（セッコツボクヨウ）　130
雪茶（セッチャ）　208
セッテ・サングリアス　161
雪蓮（セツレン）　130
セツレンカ　130
雪蓮花（セツレンカ）　130
ゼニアオイ　56, 130
銭葵（ゼニアオイ）　56, 130
ゼニバアオイ（銭葉葵）　56, 130
セネガ　319
ゼラチン　265
セラミド　265
セリニンジン（芹人参）　159
セリン　265
セルピウムソウ　51, 131
セルリー　131
セレン　265
セロリ　131
センイ（蝉衣）　349
仙遺糧（センイリョウ）　106
センカイリュウ　226
センカイリュウ（尖海竜）　226
センカク（蝉殻）　349
センカクソウ　83
仙鶴草（センカクソウ）　83
全蝎（ゼンカツ）　230
センキュウ　131, 319
川窮（センキュウ）　131, 319
川芎（センキュウ）　131, 319
芎窮（センキュウ）　131, 319
センキョウ（鮮姜）　116
千金両（センキンリョウ）　295
ゼンコ　319
前胡（ゼンコ）　319
センコク（川穀）　168
センゴクマメ（千石豆）　188
センコツ　95, 319
川骨（センコツ）　95, 319
センザンリュウ　131
穿山竜（センザンリュウ）　131
センシソウ（染指草）　188
センショウボク（戦捷木）　155
センシンレン　131
穿心蓮（センシンレン）　131
センゼイ（蝉蛻）　349
青銭柳（センセンリュウ）　122
センソ　349
蟾酥（センソ）　349
センソウ（茜草）　320
センソウ（仙草）　132
茜草（センソウ）　320
仙草（センソウ）　132
茜草根（センソウコン）　320
センソウトウ　132
千層塔（センソウトウ）　132
センゾクダン　156
川続断（センゾクダン）　156
センタイ　349
蝉退（センタイ）　349
ゼンタイ（蝉退）　349
センタウリウムソウ　132
センダン　132, 320
栴檀（センダン）　132, 320
セントジョンズワート　124
センナ　133, 320
センナ実（センナジツ）　320
センネンフランシン（千年不爛心）　122
センプクカ　320
旋覆花（センプクカ）　320
センブリ　321
千振（センブリ）　321
センボウ　133
仙茅（センボウ）　133
センボンワケギ（千本分葱）　41
センリガンノキ（千里眼木）　198
センリコウ　133, 223
千里光（センリコウ）　133, 223
センリョウ　80, 133
千両（センリョウ）　80, 133
仙寥（センリョウ）　133
仙霊脾（センレイヒ）　295
センレン（川楝）　132
センレンシ　327
川楝子（センレンシ）　327

ソ

ソウオウ（桑黄）　198
ソウカ　321
草菓（ソウカ）　321
ソウカクシ　102
皂角刺（ソウカクシ）　102
ソウキセイ　318
桑寄生（ソウキセイ）　318
皂莢（ソウキョウ）　102

ソウキン（桑槿） 182
荘荊（ソウケイ） 160
ソウケツメイ（草決明） 60
桑根（ソウコン） 195
桑根白皮（ソウコンハクヒ） 322
ソウシ 160
葱子（ソウシ） 160
ソウシシ 321
相思子（ソウシシ） 321
ソウジシ 321
蒼耳子（ソウジシ） 321
ソウジツ 160
葱実（ソウジツ） 160
ソウジュツ 321
蒼朮（ソウジュツ） 321
ソウジュヨウ 134
草蓯蓉（ソウジュヨウ） 134
ソウジン 90
桑椹（ソウジン） 90
桑椹子（ソウジンシ） 195
ソウニン（棗仁） 107
ソウハク（葱白） 160
ソウハクヒ 90, 195, 322
桑白皮（ソウハクヒ） 90, 195, 322
ソウヒョウショウ 233
桑螵蛸（ソウヒョウショウ） 233
ソウボク 112, 140
桜木（ソウボク） 140
楤木（ソウボク） 112
ソウボクヒ（楤木皮） 112
ソウモクセイ（草木犀） 123
ソウヨウ 90, 195
桑葉（ソウヨウ） 90, 195
ゾウヨウゴカ（糙葉五加） 96
ソキクソウ 170
鼠麴草（ソキクソウ） 170
ゾクダン 156
続断（ゾクダン） 156
ソクハクヨウ 134, 330
側柏葉（ソクハクヨウ） 134, 330
素馨（ソケイ） 114
ソゴウコウ 134
蘇合香（ソゴウコウ） 134
ソテツ 322
蘇鉄（ソテツ） 322
蘇鉄子（ソテツシ） 322
蘇鉄実（ソテツジツ） 322
ソバ 134
蕎麦（ソバ） 134
ソバミツ 134
蕎麦密（ソバミツ） 134
ソボク 322
蘇木（ソボク） 322
ソヨウゴカ 96
ソリシ 306
鼠李子（ソリシ） 306
ソロバンノキ 130

タ

タイイ（胎衣） 350
ダイウイキョウ 135
大茴香（ダイウイキョウ） 135
タイウン（大雲） 157
ダイオウ 135, 322
大黄（ダイオウ） 135, 322
ダイオウウラボシ（大王裏星） 191
ダイカイバ（大海馬） 226
タイキンギク 133
堆金菊（タイキンギク） 133
タイケイ 161
大薊（タイケイ） 161
タイゲイ 98, 157
大芸（タイゲイ） 98, 157
ダイケットウ 135
大血藤（ダイケットウ） 135
ダイコン 211
大根（ダイコン） 211
ダイコンソウ 136
大根草（ダイコンソウ） 136
タイサン（大蒜） 160
ダイサン 160
大蒜（ダイサン） 160
タイシジン 136
太子参（タイシジン） 136
タイシャセキ 364
ダイショ 57
大薯（ダイショ） 57
ダイジョ（大薯） 57
ダイズ 136
大豆（ダイズ） 136
ダイズ油 136
ダイズオウケン 136
大豆黄巻（ダイズオウケン） 136
大豆サポニン 260
ダイズシ（大豆鼓） 155
大豆レシチン 286
タイセイ 117
大青（タイセイ） 117, 193
タイセイヨウ 193
大節竹 148
タイソウ（大棗） 136
タイソウ（大葱） 160
ダイダイ 137
代々（ダイダイ） 137
橙（ダイダイ） 137
大通草（ダイツウソウ） 144
タイツリオウギ（鯛釣黄耆） 62, 151
タイハクチャ（太白茶） 208
胎盤（タイバン） 233, 350
ダイフクヒ 179, 322
大腹皮（ダイフクヒ） 179, 322
ダイホウセツレンカ 130
大苞雪蓮花（ダイホウセツレンカ） 130
タイマ（大麻） 40
大麻仁（タイマニン） 40
タイム 139
タイヨウトウ（対葉豆） 169
ダイリョウキョウ（大良姜） 156
タイワンアサガオ（台湾朝顔） 201
タイワンアブラギリ 157
台湾油桐（タイワンアブラギリ） 157
タイワンアマガサ（台湾雨傘） 236
越南葛藤（タイワンクズ） 137
台湾葛（タイワンクズ） 137
タイワンシロアブ（台湾白虻） 350
タイワンスク 137
タイワンツナソ 203
台湾綱麻（タイワンツナソ） 203
タイワンテイカカズラ 137
台湾定家葛（蔓）（タイワンテイカカズラ） 137
タイワンニンジンボク 159, 160
台湾人参木（タイワンニンジンボク） 160
タイワンバナナ（台湾バナナ） 168
タイワンヤマイモ（台湾山芋） 57
タウコギ 137
田五加木（タウコギ） 137
タウリン 364
タカサゴギク 137
高砂菊（タカサゴギク） 137
タカサブロウ 138
高三郎（タカサブロウ） 138
タカノキズクスリ（鷹の傷薬） 65
タカブ 235
タガヤサン 138

鉄刀木（タガヤサン） 138
水蒿（タカヨモギ） 213
蔞蒿（タカヨモギ） 213
タクゴ（槖吾） 180
タクシャ 323
澤瀉（タクシャ） 323
タケノコ 138
竹の子（タケノコ） 138
筍（タケノコ） 138
タケ類 138
タコツ（多骨） 177
タコノアシ 138
蛸の足（タコノアシ） 138
蛸の木（タコノキ） 113
タスイカ 149
多穂柯（タスイカ） 149
タスイセキカヨウ 149
多穂石柯葉（タスイセキカヨウ） 149
タダラフィル 365
タチ 232
タチアオイ 139
立葵（タチアオイ） 139
タチキジムシロ 151
立雉莚（タチキジムシロ） 151
立雉蓆（タチキジムシロ） 151
タチジャコウソウ 139
立麝香草（タチジャコウソウ） 139
タチバナ 139
橘（タチバナ） 139
多知波奈（タチバナ） 139
タチバナアデク 139
橘アデク（タチバナアデク） 139
脱*N,N*-ジメチルシブトラミン 365
脱*N*-メチルシブトラミン 365
ダッタンソバ 139
韃靼蕎麦（ダッタンソバ） 139
タツナミソウ（立浪草） 298, 317
タツノオトシゴ 226
竜の落とし子（タツノオトシゴ） 226
ダツラ葉（ダツラヨウ） 324
タデアイ 140
蓼藍（タデアイ） 140
タテゴトアザラシ（竪琴海豹） 223
タネヒリグサ 152
タピオカ 79
タヒボ 140
タベブイア 140
ダマジカ（ダマ鹿） 231
タマツバキ 159
玉椿（タマツバキ） 159
タマリンド 74
ダミアナ 323
ターミナリア・ベリリカ 135
タムシグサ（タムシ草） 151
タムシバ 316
田虫葉（タムシバ） 316
タモ（榊） 204
タモギタケ 140
楡木茸（タモギタケ） 140
タモキノコ（タモ茸） 140
タユヤ 323
タラゴン 59
タラコンピ 112, 140
楤根皮（タラコンピ） 112, 140
タラノキ 112, 140
楤木（タラノキ） 112, 140
楤木皮（タラボクヒ） 140
タラヨウ 141
多羅葉（タラヨウ） 141
大場冬青（タラヨウ） 141
タルク 266
タングートダイオウ（唐古特大黄） 135
壇香（ダンコウ） 333
炭酸カルシウム 250
タンシ（淡豉） 155
タンジー 210
胆汁（タンジュウ） 350
タンジン 141, 323
丹参（タンジン） 141, 323
タンチク 142
淡竹（タンチク） 142
タンチクヨウ 141
淡竹葉（タンチクヨウ） 141
ダンチョウグサ（断腸草） 308
タンテイヒホウ 141
短葶飛蓬（タンテイヒホウ） 141
タントウシ（淡豆豉） 155
胆嚢（タンノウ） 233, 350
タンポポ 189

チ

チア 141
チアミン 274
チオアイルデナフィル 366
チオキナピペリフィル 366
チオクト酸 266
チオデナフィル 366
チガヤ 336
茅（チガヤ） 336
チクオウ（竹黄） 148
チクジョ 323
竹茹（チクジョ） 323
竹節草 133
チクセツニンジン 324
竹節人参（チクセツニンジン） 324
チクマハッカ 51
筑摩薄荷（チクマハッカ） 51
チクリョウ 210
竹苓（チクリョウ） 210
チクレイシ（竹鈴芝） 210
チクレキ 142
竹瀝（チクレキ） 142
チコリー 77
チシエンコン 151
チシマザサ 142
千島笹（チシマザサ） 142
チシマルリソウ 142
千島瑠璃草（チシマルリソウ） 142
チスイビル 235
チチウリ 169
乳瓜（チチウリ） 169
蜘蛛抱蛋（チチュウホウタン） 171
チドリソウ 147
千鳥草（チドリソウ） 147
チノスポラ・コルディフォリア 324
チモ 324
知母（チモ） 324
チャ 142
茶（チャ） 142
チャイロビル 235
チャーガ 71
チャデブグレ 143
チャヒキグサ（茶挽草） 73
チャービル 143
チャビン茶 60
茶葡萄 150
チャボトケイソウ 143
矮鶏時計草（チャボトケイソウ） 143
チャンチンモドキ 156
香椿擬（チャンチンモドキ） 156
チユ 220
地楡（チユ） 220
チュウゲン（丑玄） 347
チュウゴクサンショウ（中国山椒） 111
チュウソウ（虫草） 151

チュウホウ（丑宝） 347
チョウカイリュウ 226
チョウカイリュウ（刁海竜） 226
チョウコウ 89, 143
丁香（チョウコウ） 89, 143
チョウコウイクリ 48
チョウジ 89, 143
丁子（チョウジ） 89, 143
丁字（チョウジ） 89
チョウジャノキ（長者木） 198
チョウジ油 143
丁子油（チョウジユ） 143
チョウシュンボケ（長春木瓜） 189, 200
チョウショウ 56
釣樟（チョウショウ） 56
チョウセンアサガオ 324
朝鮮朝顔（チョウセンアサガオ） 324
チョウセンアサガオ属 324
チョウセンアザミ 144
朝鮮薊（チョウセンアザミ） 144
チョウセンウリ（朝鮮瓜） 149, 326
チョウセンカラスウリ（朝鮮烏瓜） 74, 302
チョウセングルミ（朝鮮胡桃） 69
チョウセンゴミシ 310
朝鮮五味子（チョウセンゴミシ） 310
チョウセンニンジン 65
朝鮮人参（チョウセンニンジン） 65
チョウトウ（釣藤） 143
チョウトウコウ 143, 325
釣藤鈎（チョウトウコウ） 325
釣藤鉤（チョウトウコウ） 143
チョウマメ 144
蝶豆（チョウマメ） 144
チョウメイギク（長命菊） 175
チョウメイソウ（長命草） 190
チョドッカツ（猪独活） 110
チョーミーグサ（沖縄：長命草） 190
チョレイ 325
猪苓（チョレイ） 325
チョレイマイタケ 325
猪苓舞茸（チョレイマイタケ） 325
チリメンジソ（皺紫蘇） 110
チロシン 266
芹菜（チンサイ） 131
チンジュ 233
珍珠（チンジュ） 233
チンネベリ・センナ 133, 320
チンピ 144
陳皮（チンピ） 144

ツ

ツウソウ 144, 341
通草（ツウソウ） 144, 341
ツウダツボク 144
通脱木（ツウダツボク） 144
ツキミグサ（月見草） 145
ツキミソウ 145, 199
月見草（ツキミソウ） 145, 199
ツキミソウ油 145
月見草油（ツキミソウユ） 145
ツクシ 119
土筆（ツクシ） 119
ツクシメナモミ 199
ツクリタケ 128
作茸（ツクリタケ） 128
ツチアケビ 145
土通草（ツチアケビ） 145
土木通（ツチアケビ） 145
角 231
ツノマタゴケ 145
角又苔（ツノマタゴケ） 145
ツバキ 145
椿（ツバキ） 145
ツバメ巣 234
ツボクサ 145
坪草（ツボクサ） 145
壺草（ツボクサ） 145
ツマキクロカメムシ（ツマキクロ亀虫） 228
ツマクレナイ（爪紅） 188
ツマクレナイノキ 109
ツマベニ（爪紅） 188
ツユクサ 146
露草（ツユクサ） 146
ツリガネダケ 146
釣鐘茸（ツリガネタケ） 146
ツリガネニンジン 114
釣鐘人参（ツリガネニンジン） 114
ツルゲンゲ 113
ツルコケモモ 88
ツルシノブ 70
蔓荵（ツルシノブ） 70
ツルドクダミ 146, 301
蔓毒痛（ツルドクダミ） 146, 301
蔓蕺（ツルドクダミ） 146, 301
ツルナ 146
蔓菜（ツルナ） 146
ツルナス（蔓茄子） 122
ツルニンジン 146
蔓人参（ツルニンジン） 146
ツルマンネングサ 147
蔓万年草（ツルマンネングサ） 147
ツルムラサキ 147
蔓紫（ツルムラサキ） 147
ツルレイシ 157
蔓茘枝（ツルレイシ） 157

テ

Dendrobium属 325
ティカナッツ 43
デイコ（梯枯） 300
デイゴ（梯梧） 300
デイジー 175, 176
テイトウ（氐冬） 180
ティートリー油 199
テイムス・セルピウム 131
ティユール 147
檉柳（テイリュウ） 81
葶藶子（テイレキシ） 50
1-デオキシノジリマイシン 367
テガタチドリ 147
手形千鳥（テガタチドリ） 147
デカルピス・ハミルトニー 148
デキストリン 267
デキストロメトルファン 367
テキラリュウゼツ 38
鉄 267
鉄クロロフィリンナトリウム 267
テツトウボク 138
鉄刀木（テツトウボク） 138
デヒドロエピアンドロステロン 367
デビルズクロー 148
テブシュカン（手仏手柑） 181
デュナリエラ 148
甜杏仁（テンキョウニン） 75
テングサ 148
天草（テングサ） 148
テンコウコクショク（天香国色） 190
デンサンシチ（田三七） 107
テンジクオウ 148
天竺黄（テンジクオウ） 148
デンシチ（田七） 107
デンシチニンジン 107
田七人参（デンシチニンジン） 107
田薯（デンショ） 57

テンダイウヤク　58, 295
天台烏薬（テンダイウヤク）　58, 295
デンチキョウ（傳致膠）　223
テンチクオウ（天竹黄）　148
テンチャ　80, 149
甜茶（テンチャ）　80, 149
デンデンムシ　227
テンドウ（天冬）　149
デンドロビウム属　325
テンナンショウ　325
天南星（テンナンショウ）　325
テンノウメ（天の梅）　204
テンバイ（天梅）　204
テンホウソウ（天蓬草）　114
テンマ　325
天麻（テンマ）　325
テンメイセイ　205
天名精（テンメイセイ）　205
テンモンドウ　149, 326
天門冬（テンモンドウ）　149, 326
テンヨウケンコウシ（甜葉懸鉤子）　149

ト

銅　268
トウアズキ　321
唐小豆（トウアズキ）　321
トウガ　326
冬瓜（トウガ）　326
トウガキ（唐柿）　49
トウカギカズラ　143, 325
唐鉤葛（トウカギカズラ）　143, 325
トウガシ　149, 326
冬瓜子（トウガシ）　149, 326
トウカニン　326
冬瓜仁（トウカニン）　326
トウガニン　149
冬瓜仁（トウガニン）　149
トウガラシ　113, 149
唐辛子（トウガラシ）　113, 149
トウカラスウリ（唐烏瓜）　74, 302
トウガン　149
冬瓜（トウガン）　149
ドウカンソウ（道灌草）　63
トウキ　150, 326
当帰（トウキ）　150, 326
トウキササゲ　304
唐楸（トウキササゲ）　304
トウキシ　150
冬葵子（トウキシ）　49, 150
トウキビ　151
唐黍（トウキビ）　151
トウキョウチクトウ（唐夾竹桃）　137
トウキンセンカ　150
唐金盞花（トウキンセンカ）　150
トウグルミ（唐胡桃）　69
トウグワ（唐桑）　90, 195
トウゲシバ（峠芝）　132
トウコツソウ（透骨草）　188, 336
トウゴマ　332
唐胡麻（トウゴマ）　332
トウサイカチ　102
唐皂莢（トウサイカチ）　102
トウササゲ（唐豇）　53
灯盞花（トウサンカ）　141
トウサンサイシン　141
灯盞細辛（トウサンサイシン）　141
トウシ（豆豉）　136
トウシ（唐柿）　153
トウシ（橙子）　208
トウシキミ（唐樒）　135
トウジシャ　181
唐萵苣（トウジシャ）　181
潼蒺藜（トウシツリ）　113
橙子皮（トウシヒ）　208
トウシャジン（唐沙参）　114
トウジン　146, 326
党参（トウジン）　146, 326
トウシンソウ　47, 327
灯心草（トウシンソウ）　327
燈芯草（トウシンソウ）　47, 327
トウスケボウフウ（藤助防風）　336
トウセンダン　327
唐栴檀（トウセンダン）　327
トウチシャ（唐萵苣）　181
トウチャ　150
藤茶（トウチャ）　150
トウチュウカソウ　151
冬虫夏草（トウチュウカソウ）　151
トウツルキンバイ　338
鵝絨委陵菜（トウツルキンバイ）　338
トウテイカカズラ（唐定家葛（蔓））　137
トウドウ（当道）　63
トウドクカツ（唐独活）　328
トウドッカツ（唐独活）　110
トウナス（唐茄子）　71
トウナベナ　156
川続断（トウナベナ）　156
トウニワトコ（接骨木）　130
トウニン　327
桃仁（トウニン）　327
トウネズミモチ　159
唐鼠黐（トウネズミモチ）　159
トウバシクルモン（紅麻）　212
トウヒ　137, 155
橙皮（トウヒ）　137, 155
トウホクオウギ　151
東北黄耆（トウホクオウギ）　151
トウムギ（唐麦）　151
トウモロコシ　151
玉蜀黍（トウモロコシ）　151
トウモロコシ油　151
トウヤク　321
当薬（トウヤク）　321
トウリョウソウ　327
冬凌草（トウリョウソウ）　327
トウリンドウ　343
唐竜胆（トウリンドウ）　343
ドオウレン　151
土黄連（ドオウレン）　151
ドカンゾウ　69
ドカンゾウ（土甘草）　69
トキワセンダン　132, 320
常盤栴檀（トキワセンダン）　320
トキンソウ　152
吐金草（トキンソウ）　152
ドクカツ　56, 328
独活（ドクカツ）　56, 328
トクサ　340
砥草（トクサ）　340
ドクダミ　115
毒痛み（ドクダミ）　115
トーグリ　157
トケイ（菟奚）　180
ドケイガイ　46
土荊芥（ドケイガイ）　46
トケイソウ　152
時計草（トケイソウ）　152
トゲナシ　118
棘梨（トゲナシ）　118
トゲバンレイシ　87, 306
刺蕃茘枝（トゲバンレイシ）　306
棘蕃茘枝（トゲバンレイシ）　87
トゲヨウジ　226
トゲヨウジ（擬海竜）　226
ドゲン（土元）　232

トケンラン　103
杜鵑蘭（トケンラン）　103
ドコサヘキサエン酸<DHA>　268
トコトリエノール　268
トコフェロール　276
トコロテン（心太）　148
トコン　307
吐根（トコン）　307
ドサイシン（土細辛）　335
土山椒　111
トシシ　328
菟絲子（トシシ）　328
トショウ　127, 152
杜松（トショウ）　127, 152
ドジョウザン　203
土常山（ドジョウザン）　203
トショウシ（杜松子）　152
トショウジツ　152
杜松実（トショウジツ）　152
ドジリュウ（土地竜）　349
ドセイ（土精）　347
トチノキ　152
栃（トチノキ）　152
橡（トチノキ）　152
トチバニンジン　324
栃葉人参（トチバニンジン）　324
トチャカ　205
トチュウ　153, 328
杜仲（トチュウ）　153, 328
ドツウソウ　145
土通草（ドツウソウ）　145
ドッカツ　110, 328
独活（ドッカツ）　110, 328
トッカリ　223
トックリイチゴ　153
徳利苺（トックリイチゴ）　153
ドッグローズ　153
トッケイ　225
トッケイヤモリ（トッケイ守宮）　225
トナカイ　231
ドナリエラ　148
ドナリエラ油　148
トネリコ　37
兎尾草（トビソウ）　101
ドブクリョウ　106, 312
土茯苓（ドブクリョウ）　106, 312
ドベツ（土鼈）(虫)　232
土別甲（ドベッコウ）　232
土鼈甲（ドベッコウ）　232
トマト　153
トーメンティル　151
ドモッコウ　328
土木香（ドモッコウ）　328
トラ　224, 348
トラガント　153
トリ　228
トリカブト　328
鳥兜（トリカブト）　329
トリカブト属　328
トリプトファン　269
ドリュウコツ（土竜骨）　351
トルラ酵母　95
トレオニン　269
トレハロース　270
ドロマイト鉱石　269
トロロ　154
トロロアオイ　154
黄蜀葵（トロロアオイ）　154
ドンカ　92
曇花（ドンカ）　92
トンカット・アリ　154
東京肉桂（トンキンニッケイ）　91, 92
トンタン（豚胆）　350
トンブリ　112
唐鰤子（トンブリ）　112
豚卵（トンラン）　224

ナ

ナイアシン　270
ナイモウオウギ　62, 298
内蒙黄耆（ナイモウオウギ）　62, 298
ナガイキグサ（長生き草）　190
ナガイモ　108
長芋（ナガイモ）　108
ナガエカサ　154
ナガコショウ（長胡椒）　115
ナカバギシギシ　209
長葉羊蹄（ナガバギシギシ）　209
ナガミツナソ（長実綱麻）　203
ナガミパンノキ（長実パンの木）　171
ナギイカダ　154
仮葉樹（ナギイカダ）　154
ナギナタコウジュ　94
薙刀香需（ナギナタコウジュ）　94
ナズナ　154
撫菜（ナズナ）　154
薺（ナズナ）　154
ナタネ　154
菜種（ナタネ）　154
ナタネ油　154
菜種油（ナタネアブラ）　154
ナツガワ（夏皮）　155
ナツカン（夏柑）　155
ナツシロギク　155
夏白菊（ナツシロギク）　155
ナツダイダイ（夏橙）　155
ナットウ　155
納豆（ナットウ）　155
ナットウ菌　155
納豆菌（ナットウキン）　155
ナツボダイジュ　190
夏菩提樹（ナツボダイジュ）　190
ナツミカン　155
夏蜜柑（ナツミカン）　155
ナツメ　136
夏芽（ナツメ）　136
棗（ナツメ）　136
ナツメグ　158
ナツメヤシ　155
棗椰子（ナツメヤシ）　155
ナトリソウ（名取草）　190
ナナカマド　156
七竈（ナナカマド）　156
ナナツボシ（七つ星）　224
ナニンジン（菜人参）　159
ナノハナ（菜の花）　154
ナベナ　156
続断（ナベナ）　156
鍋菜（ナベナ）　156
ナメタケ（滑茸）　60
ナルコユリ　62
鳴子百合（ナルコユリ）　62
ナンカ（南果）　171
南瓜子（ナンカシ）　71
南瓜子（ナンガシ）　71
ナンガニン　71
南瓜仁（ナンガニン）　71
ナンキョウ　156
南杏（ナンキョウ）　75
ナンキョウソウ　156
ナンキン（南京）　71
ナンキンマメ　212
南京豆（ナンキンマメ）　212
ナンゴカヒ　96
南五加皮（ナンゴカヒ）　96
軟骨　234
ナンサンソウ　156

南酸棗（ナンサンソウ）　156
ナンショウヤマイモ　157
ナンテン　329
南天（ナンテン）　329
ナンテンジツ　329
南天実（ナンテンジツ）　329
ナンバンガキ（南蛮柿）　49
ナンバンキカラスウリ　341
南蛮木烏瓜（ナンバンキカラスウリ）　341
ナンバンキビ　151
南蛮黍（ナンバンキビ）　151
南蠻毛（ナンバンゲ）　151
南蠻毛（ナンバンモウ）　151
ナンヨウアブラギリ　157
南洋油桐（ナンヨウアブラギリ）　157
ナンヨウギク　186
南洋菊（ナンヨウギク）　186

ニ

ニオイイガクサ　115
ニオイシタン　95
ニオイスミレ　121, 157
匂菫（ニオイスミレ）　121, 157
ニガウイ　157
ニガウリ　157
苦瓜（ニガウリ）　157
ニガカシュウ　63
苦何首烏（ニガカシュウ）　63
ニガキ　329
苦木（ニガキ）　329
ニガゴイ　157
ニガゴリ　157
荷花掌（ニカショウ）　94
ニガソバ（苦蕎麦）　139
ニガハッカ　195
苦薄荷（ニガハッカ）　195
ニガヨモギ　85
苦艾（ニガヨモギ）　85
ニクジュヨウ　98, 157
肉蓯蓉（ニクジュヨウ）　98, 157
ニクズク　158
肉豆蔻（ニクズク）　158
肉豆蔻花（ニクズクカ）　158
ニゲラ　182
ニコチン　367
ニコチン酸　270
ニシキギ　158
錦木（ニシキギ）　158
ニジョウオオムギ（二条大麦）　164
ニチニチソウ　329
日々草（ニチニチソウ）　329
ニチリンソウ　176
日輪草（ニチリンソウ）　176
ニッケイ　92
ニットボーン　102
ニッポンタチバナ（日本橘）　139
ニドイモ（二度芋）　172
ニトベギク　158
腫柄菊（ニトベギク）　158
新渡戸菊（ニトベギク）　158
N-ニトロソフェンフルラミン　359
ニトロデナフィル　368
ニホンマムシ（日本蝮）　236
ニホンヤマニンジン（日本山人参）　333
ニホンヤモリ　234
日本守宮（ニホンヤモリ）　234
ニュウコウ　337
乳香（ニュウコウ）　337
乳香樹（ニュウコウジュ）　190
乳酸桿菌（ニュウサンカンキン）　41
ニュウサンキン（乳酸菌）　41, 158
乳汁　235
乳清　270
乳糖　270
ニューカレドニアジカ　231
ニューカレドニア鹿　231
ニョテイ　159
女貞（ニョテイ）　159
女貞子（ニョテイシ）　159
ニラ　159
韮（ニラ）　159
韭（ニラ）　159
ニレ　159
楡（ニレ）　159
ニレタケ（楡茸）　140
ニワウメ　48
庭梅（ニワウメ）　48
ニワクサ（爾波久佐）　112
ニワタバコ（庭煙草）　178
ニワトコ　130
庭常（ニワトコ）　130
ニワトリ　225, 235
庭柳（ニワヤナギ）　196
扁蓄（ニワヤナギ）　196
ニンジン　159
人参（ニンジン）　65, 159
ニンジンサンシチ（人参三七）　107
ニンジンボク　159, 160
人参木（ニンジンボク）　160
ニンジン油　159
人参油（ニンジンユ）　159
ニンドウ　82
忍冬（ニンドウ）　82
忍冬藤（ニンドウ）　82
ニンニク　160
忍辱（ニンニク）　160
葫（ニンニク）　160

ヌ

ヌマスノキ（沼酢の木）　184
ヌルデ　121, 160
塩麩木（ヌルデ）　160
白膠木（ヌルデ）　121, 160

ネ

ネギ　160
葱（ネギ）　160
ネコノヒゲ　87
ネズ　152
杜松（ネズ）　152
ネズミサシ（鼠刺）　152
ネズミモチ　159
鼠黐（ネズミモチ）　159
ネットル　52
ネナシカズラ　328
根無葛（ネナシカズラ）　328
ネバリミソハギ　161
粘禊萩（ネバリミソハギ）　161
ネパールサンモ　79
ネブ（合歓）　161
ネブカ（根深）　160
ネマガリタケ　138, 142
ネマガリタケ（根曲がり竹）　138
根曲竹（ネマガリタケ）　138, 142
ネム（合歓）　161
ネムノキ　161
合歓木（ネムノキ）　161
ネムノハナ　161
ネンドウ　112

ノ

ノアザミ　161
野薊（ノアザミ）　161
ノイバラ（野茨）　296
ノウショウ（凌霄）　214

ノウゼンカズラ　214
凌霄花（ノウゼンカズラ）　214
ノウゼンハレン（凌霄葉蓮）　84
ノエンドウ（野豌豆）　218
ノグワ（野桑）　195
ノゲイトウ　161
野鶏頭（ノゲイトウ）　161
ノゲシ　162
野芥子（ノゲシ）　162
ノコギリパルメット　162
ノコギリヤシ　162
鋸椰子（ノコギリヤシ）　162
ノサンサ（野山楂）　106
ノジスミレ（野路菫）　111, 121
ノショウ（凌霄）　214
ノダケ（野竹）　319
ノダフジ（野田藤）　180
ノヂシャ（野苣）　192
ノニ　203
ノビル　68
野蒜（ノビル）　68
ノブドウ　162
野葡萄（ノブドウ）　162
ノミノフスマ　114
蚤の衾（ノミノフスマ）　114
ノルネオシルデナフィル　368
ノルホンデナフィル　368

ハ

バアソブ　162
婆蕎（バアソブ）　162
婆雀斑（バアソブ）　162
バイオレット　157
玫瑰（バイカイ）　170
バイキセイ　74, 99
梅寄生（バイキセイ）　74, 99
バイケイソウ　329
梅蕙草（バイケイソウ）　329
バイケイソウ属　329
ハイゴショウ　162
這胡椒（ハイゴショウ）　162
ハイショウ　66
敗醤（ハイショウ）　66
敗醤根（ハイショウコン）　66
ハイデソウ　81
パイナップル　163
鳳梨（パイナップル）　163
パイナップル加工品　163
ハイビスカス　163, 182
パイプマメ　144
バイモ　330
貝母（バイモ）　330
ハイラン　199, 343
佩蘭（ハイラン）　199, 343
パウダルコ　163
バエルフルーツ　187
バオバブ　163
ハカタユリ（博多百合）　209
ハカマウラボシ　164
袴裏星（ハカマウラボシ）　164
ハクエイ　177
白英（ハクエイ）　177
ハクカ　50
白果（ハクカ）　50
白瓜（ハクカ）　149
ハクガ　149
バクガ　64, 164
麦芽（バクガ）　64, 164
ハクカシ（白瓜子）　149, 326
百花蛇舌草（ハクカジャゼツソウ）　181
ハクカヒ　111
白樺皮（ハクカヒ）　111
バクキョウコウキ（膜莢黄芪）　151
ハクシジン　134, 330
柏子仁（ハクシジン）　134, 330
ハクシニン　330
柏子仁（ハクシニン）　330
ハクジュ（伯樹）　173
ハクジュ（柏樹）　173
ハクショウ（白松）　165
ハクショウトウ　165
ハクズク（白豆蔻）　177
ハクセンピ　330
白蘚皮（ハクセンピ）　330
ハクソ（白蘇）　110
バクダイ　173
莫大（バクダイ）　173
莫大海（バクダイカイ）　173
ハクチャ　164
白茶（ハクチャ）　164
ハクトウオウ　330
白頭翁（ハクトウオウ）　330
ハクトウサン　164
白豆杉（ハクトウサン）　164
白花酸藤果（ハクトウサントウカ）　61
ハクトウスギ　164, 331
白豆杉（ハクトウスギ）　164, 331
麦飯石　271
ハクヒショウ　165
白皮松（ハクヒショウ）　165
ハクヘンズ（白扁豆）　188
ハクボクジ　118
白木耳（ハクボクジ）　118
白毛夏枯草（ハクモウカゴソウ）　81
ハクモウトウ　177
白毛藤（ハクモウトウ）　177
バクモンドウ　331
麦門冬（バクモンドウ）　331
馬茎（バケイ）　224
ハゲキテン　331
巴戟天（ハゲキテン）　331
ハコシ（破故紙）　189
ハゴシ（婆固脂）　189
ハコネバラ（箱根薔薇）　107
バコパモニエラ　65
ハコベ　165
繁縷（ハコベ）　165
蘩蔞（ハコベ）　165
ハコベラ（繁縷）　165
ハゴロモカンラン　92
羽衣甘藍（ハゴロモカンラン）　92
ハゴロモグサ（羽衣草）　165
ハゴロモソウ　165
羽衣草（ハゴロモソウ）　165
バシカン　165
馬歯莧（バシケン）　165
バショウ　166
芭蕉（バショウ）　166
バジリコ　199
ハシリドコロ　331
走野老（ハシリドコロ）　331
ハシリドコロ属　331
バジル　199
ハス　166
蓮（ハス）　166
ハズ　331
巴豆（ハズ）　331
パセリ　166
旱芹菜（パセリ）　166
パセリ油　166
ハダカムギ（裸麦）　64
パタデバカ　166
バターナット　166
ハタニンジン（畑人参）　159
バーチ　111

ハチ　235
八月札（ハチガツサツ）　40
ハチク（淡竹）　138
ハチク（葉竹）　323
ハチセンカ　41
八仙花（ハチセンカ）　41
ハチノコ　235
蜂の子（ハチノコ）　235
ハチミツ　167
蜂蜜（ハチミツ）　167
パチョリ　301, 303
ハツ　232
ハッカ　167
薄荷（ハッカ）　167
ハッカクウイキョウ（八角茴香）　135
ハツカグサ（二十日草）　190
ハツカグサ（廿日草）　190
ハッカクレイシ　167
白鶴霊芝（ハッカクレイシ）　167
ハッカジャセツソウ　181
ハッカ属　197
菝葜（バッカツ）　312
白花油麻藤　91
ハッカヨウ（薄荷葉）　127
ハックツサイ　151
白屈菜（ハックツサイ）　151
ハックルベリー　167
ハッショウマメ　168
八升豆（ハッショウマメ）　168
パッションフラワー　152
パッソーラ　73
バテイソウ（馬蹄草）　217
ハトムギ　168
鳩麦（ハトムギ）　168
ハナアオイ（花葵）　139
ハナガサ（花笠）　174
ハナシバ（花柴）　313
ハナシュクシャ　168
花縮砂（ハナシュクシャ）　168
ハナスゲ　324
花菅（ハナスゲ）　324
バナナ　168
ハナノキ　313
花の木（ハナノキ）　313
バナバ　168
ハナハッカ　194
花薄荷（ハナハッカ）　194
ハナビシソウ　169
花菱草（ハナビシソウ）　169
ハナビラタケ　169
花弁茸（ハナビラタケ）　169
ハナヒリグサ　152
バニュウ　235
馬乳（バニュウ）　235
ハネセンナ　169
ハノキ　130
パパイヤ　169
パパイン　369
ハハカ　58
波波迦（ハハカ）　58
母菊（ハハギク）　72
ハハコグサ　170
母子草（ハハコグサ）　170
婆婆納（ババノウ）　50
バビンロウ　70
バ檳榔（バビンロウ）　70
ハブ　235
パフィア　121
ハブソウ　170
波布草（ハブソウ）　170
ハブ茶　170
パープルコーンフラワー　58
パープルプラム　183
バフンセキ（馬糞石）　350
バーベナ　86, 174
バベンソウ　86
馬鞭草（バベンソウ）　86
バホウ　350
馬宝（バホウ）　350
ハマウツボ　134
浜靫（ハマウツボ）　134
ハマエンドウ（浜豌豆）　218
ハマオオネ（浜大根）　336
ハマゴウ　339
浜栲（ハマゴウ）　339
ハマジシャ　146
浜千佐（ハマジシャ）　146
浜千舎（ハマジシャ）　146
ハマスガナ（波未須加奈）　170
ハマスゲ　308
浜菅（ハマスゲ）　308
ハマゼリ　170
浜芹（ハマゼリ）　170
ハマナ（浜菜）　146
ハマナシ　170
浜梨（ハマナシ）　170
ハマナス　170
浜茄子（ハマナス）　170
ハマニガナ（波未爾加奈）　170
ハマニンジン（浜人参）　170
ハマビシ　314
浜菱（ハマビシ）　314
ハマボウフウ　170
浜防風（ハマボウフウ）　171
ハママツ　42
ハマメリス　171
バラ　171
薔薇（バラ）　171
バラ科植物　171
ハラタケ（原茸）　128
ハラビロカマキリ（巨斧螳螂）　233
パラミツ　171
波羅密（パラミツ）　171
菠蘿蜜（パラミツ）　171
婆羅蜜樹（パラミツジュ）　171
ハラン（葉蘭）　171
バラン（葉蘭）　171
バラン（馬藍）　214
ハリイカ（針烏賊）　224
バリエラ　311
ハリセンボン（針千本）　207
バリン　271
ハルウコン　172
春鬱金（ハルウコン）　172
ハルオミナエシ（春女郎花）　70
ハルコガネバナ　107
春黄金花（ハルコガネバナ）　107
バルデナフィル　369
ハルニレ（春楡）　159
ハルノゲシ（春野芥子）　162
バルバドスサクラ　42
バルバドスチェリー　42
バルバロイン　356
ハルマラ　332
ハルマリン　369
パルミラヤシ　56
ハルミン　369
バレイショ　172
馬鈴薯（バレイショ）　172
バレイショデンプン　172
馬鈴薯澱粉（バレイショデンプン）　172
パレイラ根　311
パレイラ根（パレイラコン）　311
バレン　171
パロアッスル　172
バロクジョウ（馬鹿茸）　351

バンウコン　108
蕃鬱金（バンウコン）　108
バンカ（蕃果）　84
バンカ（蕃茄）　153
バンカジュ（番瓜樹）　169
バンキョウ　146
番杏（バンキョウ）　146
パンクレアチン　370
ハンゲ　332
半夏（ハンゲ）　332
ハンゲグサ（半夏草）　173
ハンゲショウ　173
半化粧（ハンゲショウ）　173
半夏生（ハンゲショウ）　173
番紅花（バンコウカ）　104
番仔藤　201
パンコムギ　100
バンザクロ　84
パンジー　106
番瀉葉（バンシャヨウ）　133, 320
バンシュウレイシ（晩秋荔枝）　157
バンショウ（蕃姜）　113
バンショウ（蕃椒）　113, 149
ハンシレン　173
半枝蓮（ハンシレン）　173
バンジロウ　84
蕃石榴（バンジロウ）　84
バンセキリュウ　84
ハンタイカイ（胖大海）　173
ハンダイカイ　173
胖大海（ハンダイカイ）　173
パントテン酸　271
パントテン酸カルシウム　271
ハンノキ　130
榛木（ハンノキ）　130
ハンビ　236
反鼻（ハンピ）　237
半辺蓮（ハンペンレン）　340
バンモッカ（番木瓜）　169
板藍（バンラン）　117
板藍根（バンランコン）　117

ヒ

Bifidobacterium属　176
ヒアルロン酸　272
ヒイラギメギ　173
柊目木（ヒイラギメギ）　173
ヒイラギモチ　128, 173
柊黐（ヒイラギモチ）　128, 173
ヒイラギモドキ（柊擬き）　173
ビオチン　272
ヒカゲノカズラ　118
日陰蔓（ヒカゲノカズラ）　118
日陰鬘（ヒカゲノカズラ）　118
ヒカゲノツルニンジン　326
日陰蔓人参（ヒカゲノツルニンジン）　326
ヒカゲミズ　174
ヒガンバナ　318
彼岸花（ヒガンバナ）　318
ヒキオコシ　61
引起（ヒキオコシ）　61
比木乎古乏（ヒキオコシ）　61
陰行草（ヒキヨモギ）　213
ヒグルマ　176
日車（ヒグルマ）　176
ピコリン酸クロム　272
瓢（ヒサゴ）　180
ヒシ　174
菱（ヒシ）　174
榧子（ヒシ）　174
ヒジツ　174
榧実（ヒジツ）　174
ヒシノミ　174
菱の実（ヒシノミ）　174
ヒシュカ　191
啤酒花（ヒシュカ）　191
ビジョザクラ　174
美女桜（ビジョザクラ）　174
ヒジリタケ（聖茸）　216
ヒスイカク　314
翡翠閣（ヒスイカク）　314
ヒスチジン　272
ビス-3-ヒドロキシ-3-メチルブチレートモノハイドレート　273
ヒゼングサ（皮癬草）　151
ヒソップ　175
ビタミンA　273
ビタミンB1　274
ビタミンB2　274
ビタミンB6　275
ビタミンB12　274
ビタミンC　275
ビタミンD　275
ビタミンE　276
ビタミンH　272
ビタミンK　276
ビタミンM　283
ヒツジ　224, 233
ビート　104
ヒトツバ　129, 171
一ツ葉（ヒトツバ）　129
ヒトモジ（一文字）　160
ヒトモジ（比止毛之）　160
ヒドラスチス根　308
ヒドロキシチオホモシルデナフィル　371
ヒドロキシトリプトファン（5-HTP）　371
4-ヒドロキシプロリン　277
ヒドロキシホモシルデナフィル　371
ヒドロキシホンデナフィル　372
ヒドロキシリシン　277
ヒナギク　175
雛菊（ヒナギク）　175
ヒナゲシ　175
雛芥子（ヒナゲシ）　175
ヒナタイノコヅチ　309
ヒナタイノコヅチ（日向猪小槌）　309
ピーナッツ　212
ヒノキ　175
桧（ヒノキ）　175
檜（ヒノキ）　175
ヒノキアスナロ（檜翌檜）　42
檜葉（ヒバ）　42
ヒハツ　54, 115
畢発（ヒハツ）　115
畢茇（ヒハツ）　54
蓽撥（ヒハツ）　54
ヒハツモドキ（畢発擬）　115
ヒバマタ　175
桧葉叉（ヒバマタ）　175
ビフィズス菌　176
鞞醯勒果（vibhitaka）　122, 135
ヒペリクムソウ　124
ピペリデナフィル　372
ヒボケ（緋木瓜）　189, 200
ヒマ　332
蓖麻（ヒマ）　332
ヒマシ油　332
蓖麻子油（ヒマシユ）　332
ヒマラヤニンジン　176
ヒマラヤハッカクレン　338
ヒマラヤ八角蓮（ヒマラヤハッカクレン）　338
ヒマワリ　176
向日葵（ヒマワリ）　176

ヒマワリ油　176
ヒメウイキョウ　176
姫茴香（ヒメウイキョウ）　176
ヒメガマ　71, 337
姫蒲（ヒメガマ）　71, 337
ヒメカモジグサ（姫髢草）　112
ヒメジョオン　176
姫女菀（ヒメジョオン）　176
ヒメシロアブ（姫白虻）　350
ヒメスイバ　119
姫酸葉（ヒメスイバ）　119
ヒメツルニチニチソウ　177
姫蔓日々草（ヒメツルニチニチソウ）　177
ヒメハブ　235
姫波布（ヒメハブ）　235
姫飯匙倩（ヒメハブ）　235
ヒメビシ（姫菱）　174
ヒメマツタケ　39
姫松茸（ヒメマツタケ）　39
ビャクゴウ　209
百合（ビャクゴウ）　209
ビャクシ　332
白芷（ビャクシ）　332
ビャクシャク　114, 315
白芍（ビャクシャク）　114, 315
ビャクジュツ　332
白朮（ビャクジュツ）　332
ビャクズク　177
白豆蔲（ビャクズク）　116, 177
白豆蔲花（ビャクズクカ）　116
白豆蔲殻（ビャクズクカク）　116, 177
ビャクダン　333
白壇（ビャクダン）　333
ビャクブ　333
百部（ビャクブ）　333
ビャクヘンズ　53, 188
白扁豆（ビャクヘンズ）　53, 188
ビャクボウコン　336
白茅根（ビャクボウコン）　336
ヒャクリコウ（百里香）　131
百里香（ヒャクリコウ）　51, 131
ビャクレン　68
白歛（ビャクレン）　68
ヒャッカオウ（百花王）　190
白花荊芥（ビャッカケイガイ）　51
百花蛇舌草（ビャッカジャゼツソウ　181
白花蛇（ビャッカダ）　236
白芨（ビャッキュウ）　117
白彊蚕（ビャッキョウサン）　226
白姜蚕（ビャッキョウサン）　226
ビャック（白蔻）　177
ヒャッポダ　236
百歩蛇（ヒャッポダ）　236
ヒユ　93
莧（ヒユ）　93
ヒュウガトウキ　333
日向当帰（ヒュウガトウキ）　333
猫髭草（ビョウシュソウ）　87
ヒョウタン　177
瓢箪（ヒョウタン）　177
ヒヨコグサ（雛草）　165
ヒヨス　333
ヒヨス属　333
ヒヨドリジョウゴ　177
蜀羊泉（ヒヨドリジョウゴ）　177
鵯上戸（ヒヨドリジョウゴ）　177
ピリドキシン　275
ヒル　235
ヒルガオ　178
昼顔（ヒルガオ）　178
ビール酵母　95
ビルベリー　128, 178
ビルマネム　178
ビルマ合歓（ビルマネム）　178
緬甸合歓（ビルマネム）　178
ヒレイケチョウガイ　236
ひれ池蝶貝（ヒレイケチョウガイ）　236
ヒレハリソウ　102
鰭玻璃草（ヒレハリソウ）　102
ビロウドマメ　168
ビロウドモウズイカ　178
天鵞絨毛蕊花（ビロウドモウズイカ）　178
ビロードアオイ　46
ヒロハ　171
ヒロハオキナグサ（広葉翁草）　330
ヒロハセネガ　319
広葉セネガ（ヒロハセネガ）　319
ピロロキノリンキノン二ナトリウム塩　273
ビワ　179
枇杷（ビワ）　179
枇杷核（ビワカク）　179
枇杷木白皮（ビワボクハクヒ）　179
枇杷葉（ビワヨウ）　179
枇杷葉露（ビワヨウロ）　179
ビンカミン　372
ヒンハンル（濱繁縷）　114
ピンピネラ　43
ビンロウ　179, 322
檳榔（ビンロウ）　179, 322
ビンロウジ　179
檳榔子（ビンロウジ）　179
檳榔皮（ビンロウヒ）　322
ビンロウヤシ（檳榔椰子）　179

フ

Physalis属　337
ファイアウィード　205
プーアルチャ　142
ファロージカ　231
ファロー鹿　231
フイ（芣苡）　63
フィクスインディカ　56
フィコシアニン　277
フィチン　245
フィトナジオン　276
フィーバーフュー　155
フイリタコノキ　113
フィリピンコブラ　230
風化造礁サンゴ　231
フウキソウ（富貴草）　190
フウセンヒルガオ（風船昼顔）　66
フウトウ（風藤）　179
フウトウカズラ　179
風藤葛（フウトウカズラ）　179
フェニルアラニン　278
プエラリア　179
プエラリア・ミリフィカ　68
プエラリアミリフィカ　179
フェリチン鉄　278
フェルラ酸　278
フェンネル　55
ブカトウ　180
武靴糖（ブカトウ）　79, 180
フカヒレ　231
鱶鰭（フカヒレ）　231
フカミグサ（深見草）　190
フキタンポポ　180, 304
蕗蒲公英（フキタンポポ）　180, 304
フキノトウ　180
蕗の薹　180
ブキュウ　131, 319
蕪芎（ブキュウ）　131, 319

フグ　236
河豚（フグ）　236
フクキツ（福橘）　123
福寿草（フクジュソウ）　334
フクジュソウ属　334
ブクシンボク　334
茯神木（ブクシンボク）　334
フクダ　236
蝮蛇（フクダ）　237
蝮蛇胆（フクダタン）　233
フグノクロヤキ　236
フクベ　180
瓢（フクベ）　180
瓠（フクベ）　180
フクボンシ　153, 212, 334
覆盆子（フクボンシ）　153, 212, 334
ブクリョウ　334
茯苓（ブクリョウ）　334
フサアカシア（房アカシア）　196
フシ（付子）　160
五倍子（フシ）　160
フジ　180, 334
藤（フジ）　180, 334
ブシ　160, 328
附子（ブシ）　160, 329
フジコブ　334
藤瘤（フジコブ）　334
フジチャ　142
普洱茶（フジチャ）　142
フシノキ（附子木）　160
フジバカマ　343
藤袴（フジバカマ）　343
フジマメ　53, 188
藤豆（フジマメ）　53, 188
ブシュ（仏手）　181
ブシュ（佛手）　181
ブシュカン　181
仏手柑（ブシュカン）　181
佛手柑（ブシュカン）　181
ブシュコウエン（仏手香櫞）　181
プソイドバルデナフィル　372
フソウゲ（扶桑花）　182
ブタ　224, 228, 229, 233, 350
フタバアオイ　335
双葉葵（フタバアオイ）　335
フタバムグサ　181
双葉葎（フタバムグラ）　181
フタモジ（二文字）　159
1,4-ブタンジオール　370
フダンソウ　181
不断草（フダンソウ）　181
フチベニベンケイ（縁紅弁慶）　60, 94
ブチュ　181
ブック　181
ブッケサ（佛袈裟）　350
ブッコ　181
フツコクカイガンショウ（仏国海岸松）　184
ブッコノキ　181
ブッシュティー　182
ブッシュマンゴー　43
フッ素　278
フッソウゲ　182
ブッソウゲ（仏桑花）　163, 182
ブッソウゲ（仏桑華）　163, 182
フーディア・ゴードニー　179
ブドウ　182
葡萄（ブドウ）　182
ブフォテニン　372
フユアオイ　150
冬葵（フユアオイ）　150
フユボダイジュ　190
冬菩提樹（フユボダイジュ）　190
フユムシナツクサタケ（冬虫夏草菌）　151
ブラジルチェリー　139
ブラジルニンジン　121
プラセンタ　233, 350
ブラッククミン　182
ブラックコホッシュ　183
ブラックジンジャー　183
ブラックプラム　183
ブラックベリー　183
ブラックルート　184
フラングラ皮　335
フラングラ皮（フラングラヒ）　335
フランスカイガンショウ　184
仏国海岸松（フランスカイガンショウ）　184
仏蘭西海岸松（フランスカイガンショウ）　184
プランタゴ・オバタ　184
フランボワーズ　212
ブリオニア　184
フリーミント　198
プルイノサ　117
β-フルクトフラノシダーゼ　358
ブルースプレー　215
プルット　185
プルプレア　58
ブルーベリー　184
フルボ酸　279
プルラン　279
プルーン　125
ブレーベリー　178
プロアントシアニジン　279
プロスタグランジン　373
プロテアーゼ　373
プロポリス　280
ブロメライン　373
プロリン　280
ブンタン　185
文旦（ブンタン）　185
ブンドウ　214
文豆（ブンドウ）　214
フンボウイ　314
粉防已（フンボウイ）　314

へ

ヘイサラバサラ　350
ベイリーフ　92
薜茘（ヘイレイ）　63
ヘキコ　234
壁虎（ヘキコ）　234
ペグアセンヤク　185
ペグ阿仙薬（ペグアセンヤク）　185
ペグノキ　185
ベスカイチゴ　59
ヘスペリジン　280
ベゾアール　350
ベータカロチン　280
ヘチマ　186
糸瓜（ヘチマ）　186
ベッコウ　232
鼈甲（ベッコウ）　232
ヘッジマスタード　68
ペドラ・ウマ・カア　75
ペドラ・ウメカ　75
ヘナ　109
ベニコウジ　186
紅麹（ベニコウジ）　186
ベニサイコ（紅柴胡）　102
ベニサンチャ（紅山茶）　145
ベニバナ　186
紅花（ベニバナ）　186
ベニバナ油　186
ベニバナセンブリ　132

紅花千振（ベニバナセンブリ） 132
ベニバナボロギク 186
紅花襤褸菊（ベニバナボロギク） 186
ベニミカン（紅蜜柑） 123
紅權（ベニムクゲ） 163
ペニーローヤルミント 198
ヘパティカ・ノビリス 335
ペパーミント 127
ヘビ 224, 236, 349
ペピーノ 186
ペピノ 186
ペプシン 374
ヘボ（地蜂（黒雀蜂）の子） 235
ヘマトコッカス藻色素 281
ヘム鉄 281
ヘラオオバコ 187
篦大葉子（ヘラオオバコ） 187
ヘラオモダカ 335
篦面高（ヘラオモダカ） 335
ベラドンナ 335
ベラドンナ根（ベラドンナコン） 335
ベラドンナ属 335
ヘラモ（篦藻） 129
ヘリクリサム・イタリカム 187
ベルコーサカンバ 111
ペルシアジョチュウギク（ペルシア除虫菊） 39
ペルシャグルミ 69
ヘルニアリアソウ 187
ベルノキ 187
ベールフルーツ 53
ベルベット 231
ベレリカミロバラン 122
ヘンカクボク（扁核木） 119
ベンガルカラタチ（ベンガル枳） 53, 187
ヘンズ 188
扁豆（ヘンズ） 188
扁蓄（ヘンチク） 196
ヘンナ 109
ペンペングサ 154
ヘンルウダ 188
ヘンルーダ 188

ホ

Boswellia属 337
Podophyllum属 338
ホアジャオ 111
ホウイ（胞衣） 350
ボウイ 336
防已（ボウイ） 336
芒果（ボウカ） 195
杧果（ボウカ） 195
ホウガジュツ（蓬莪朮） 69
ホウキギ 112
箒木（ホウキギ） 112
望江南（ボウコウナン） 170
ボウコン 336
茅根（ボウコン） 336
ホウジチャ（方児茶） 42
ボウシバナ（帽子花） 146
ボウシュウボク 188
防臭木（ボウシュウボク） 188
豊城鶏血藤（ホウジョウケイケットウ） 91
ホウセン（鳳仙） 188
ホウセンカ 188, 336
鳳仙花（ホウセンカ） 188, 336
鳳仙子（ホウセンシ） 336
ボウタン（牡丹） 190
ボウタングサ（牡丹草） 190
ボウチュウ 350
虻虫（ボウチュウ） 350
猴頭菇（ホウトウクウ） 207
ホウノキ 308
朴木（ホウノキ） 308
ホウビソウ 336
鳳尾草（ホウビソウ） 336
ボウフウ 336
防風（ボウフウ） 171, 336
ボウブラ 71
ボウマ（苘麻） 49, 150
鳳梨（ホウリ） 163
ホオウ 337
蒲黄（ホオウ） 71, 337
鬼灯（ホオズキ） 337
酸漿（ホオズキ） 337
ホオズキ属 337
母菊（ボギク） 72
ボクインキョウ 347
牝狗陰茎（ボクインキョウ） 347
ボクインケイ 347
牝狗陰茎（ボクインケイ） 347
ホークウィード 189
ボクカンレン（墨旱蓮） 138
ホクゴカヒ（北五加皮） 96
北沙参（ホクシャジン） 171
ボクソク 315
樸樕（ボクソク） 316
ボクタン（牡狗胆） 350
ホクチガラ（火口ガラ） 49
ホクチュウソウ 151
北美喬松（ホクビキョウショウ） 120
ボケ 189, 200, 201
木瓜（ボケ） 189, 200, 201
牡荊（ボケイ） 160
牡荊子（ボケイシ） 160
蒲公英（ホコウエイ） 189
ホコウエイコン 189
蒲公英根（ホコウエイコン） 189
ホコウケイテン（圃行景天） 147
ホコツシ 189
補骨脂（ホコツシ） 189
ボスウェリア・セラータ 190
ボスウェリア属 337
ホスファチジルコリン 286
ホスファチジルセリン 281
ホースミント 204
ホースラディッシュ 219
ホソバオケラ 321
細葉朮（ホソバオケラ） 321
ホソバセンナ（狭葉番瀉） 133
ホソバタイセイ 117
細葉大青（ホソバタイセイ） 117
ホソバデイコ（細葉梯沽） 67
ホソバノキリンソウ 82
ホソバメハジキ 216
細葉目弾（ホソバメハジキ） 216
細葉益母草（ホソバヤクモソウ） 216
ホソバヤマジソ（細葉山紫蘇） 129
ホソバユリ（細葉百合） 209
ボダイジュ 190
菩提樹（ボダイジュ） 190
ボダイジュミツ 190
ボタン 190, 337
牡丹（ボタン） 190, 337
ボタンピ 337
牡丹皮（ボタンピ） 337
ボタンボウフウ 190
牡丹防風（ボタンボウフウ） 190
ホッカイトウキ（北海当帰） 150
ホップ 191
忽布（ホップ） 191
ポテイトウ・ビーン 45
ポテンティラ・アンセリナ 338
ポドフィルム 338
ポドフィルム属 338

ホホバ　191
ホミカ　339
ホモシルデナフィル　374
ホモチオデナフィル　374
ボラゴソウ　215
ボラージ　215
ボリジ　215
ポリポディウム・レウコトモス　191
ボルド　191
ポルトガルプラム　183
ボルネオショウノウ（ボルネオ樟脳）　214
ボレイ　227
牡蛎（ボレイ）　227
ボレイジ　215
ホロシ（保呂之）　177
ボロホ　191
ホワイトウイロー　125
ホワイトセージ　192
ホワートルベリー　178
ホンアンズ　304
本杏（ホンアンズ）　304
ホンオニク　98, 157
塩生肉蓯蓉（ホンオニク）　157
ポンカン（凸柑）　196
ポンカン（椪柑）　196
凸柑（ポンカン）　196
椪柑（ポンカン）　196
ホンゴシュユ　309
本呉茱萸（ホンゴシュユ）　309
ポンコランチ　104, 105
ホンセッコク　325
ボンタン　185
ホンデナフィル　374
ボンバナ（盆花）　196
ホンヤシ（本椰子）　204
ホンユ（本柚）　208
ホンユズ（本柚子）　208

マ

マアザミ　192
真薊（マアザミ）　192
マイカ（真烏賊）　224
玫瑰（マイカイ）　170
マイカイカ（玫瑰花）　170
マイタケ　192
舞茸（マイタケ）　192
マイヅルテンナンショウ（異葉天南星）　325
マイヅルテンナンショウ（舞鶴天南星）　325
マイテン　192
マイワシ　224, 229
真鰯（マイワシ）　224, 229
マオウ　338
麻黄（マオウ）　338
マカ　193
マガキ　227
真牡蠣（マガキ）　227
マカマカ　193
真烏麦（マカラスムギ）　61
マキ（真木）　175
マキバクサギ　193
マキバ臭木（マキバクサギ）　193
マクキョウオウギ（膜莢黄芪）　151
マグネシウム　282
マグノフロリン　375
マクリ　338
海人草（マクリ）　338
マクリモ（万久利母）　338
マグワ　90, 195, 322
真桑（マグワ）　90, 195, 322
マゴジャクシ（孫杓子）　216
マコモ　193
菰（マコモ）　193
海帯（マコンブ）　101
マシジミ　231
真蜆（マシジミ）　231
マシニン　339
麻子仁（マシニン）　40, 339
マーシュ　192
マーシュマロウ　46
マージョラム　194
マジョラム　194
マタイセイ（真大青）　117
マダカアワビ（目高鮑）　223
マダケ　148
マダケ（真竹）　138, 323
マタタビ　200
又旅（マタタビ）　200
マダラ（真鱈）　228
マチコ　193
マチンシ　339
馬銭子（マチンシ）　339
マチン属　339
マツ　194
松（マツ）　194
マツタケ　194
松茸（マツタケ）　194
マツノミ　194
松の実（マツノミ）　194
マツバ　194
松葉（マツバ）　194
マツバゼリ（松葉芹）　131
マツホド　334
松塊（マツホド）　334
マツヤニ　194
松脂（マツヤニ）　194
マツユキソウ（待雪草）　342
マツヨイグサ　199
待宵草（マツヨイグサ）　199
マツリカ（茉莉花）　114
茉莉花（マツリカ）　114
マテ　194
マテ茶（マテチャ）　194
マニオク　79
マビンロウ　70
マ檳榔（マビンロウ）　70
マフウジュ（麻瘋樹）　157
マフグ　236
真河豚（マフグ）　236
マボケ（真木瓜）　200
マムシ　236
マメダオシ　328
豆倒し（マメダオシ）　328
マヨラナ　194
マラカスムギ　61
マリアアザミ　194
マリア薊（マリアアザミ）　194
マリーゴールド　150
マルターゼ　375
マルバキンゴジカ（丸葉金午時花）　297
マルバダイオウ　117, 135
丸葉大黄（マルバダイオウ）　117, 135
マルバタバコ　339
丸葉煙草（マルバタバコ）　339
マルバデイコ（丸葉梯沽）　67
マルバノニンジン（丸葉人参）　114
マルバハッカ　195
円葉薄荷（マルバハッカ）　43
丸葉薄荷（マルバハッカ）　195
マルベリー　195
マレイン　178
マロー　56, 130
マロウ　130
マロニエ　126, 318

マンガン　282
マンケイシ　339
蔓荊子（マンケイシ）　339
マンゴー　195
マンゴージンジャー　195
マンゴスチン　195
マンサク（万作）　334
マンシュウアカジカ　351
マンシュウウコギ　96
マンシュウジカ　351
マンジュカ（万寿果）　169
マンジュシャゲ　318
曼珠沙華（マンジュシャゲ）　318
マンジュマイ（万寿瓜）　169
曼陀羅花（マンダラゲ）　324
曼陀羅子（マンダラシ）　324
曼陀羅葉（マンダラヨウ）　324
マンダリン　144, 196
マンドラゴラ　339
マンドラゴラ属　339
マンネンタケ　216
万年茸（マンネンタケ）　216
マンネンロウ　218
万年朗（マンネンロウ）　218

ミ

ミシマサイコ　102, 311
三島柴胡（ミシマサイコ）　102, 311
ミズナラ（水楢）　315
ミズブキ　66
水蕗（ミズブキ）　66
ミスミソウ　335
三角草（ミスミソウ）　335
実千両（ミセンリョウ）　133
ミゾカクシ　312, 340
溝隠（ミゾカクシ）　312, 340
ミソハギ　196
禊萩（ミソハギ）　196
ミチヤナギ　196
道柳（ミチヤナギ）　196
路柳（ミチヤナギ）　196
ミツガシワ　317
三柏（ミツガシワ）　317
三槲（ミツガシワ）　317
密花豆　91
三白草（ミツシロソウ）　173
ミツバナ（三ツ花）　198
ミツバハナ（三葉花木）　198
ミツモウカ　340
密蒙花（ミツモウカ）　340
ミツロウ　237
蜜蝋（ミツロウ）　237
ミドリイガイ　237
緑貽貝（ミドリイガイ）　237
ミドリハッカ　121
緑薄荷（ミドリハッカ）　121
ミナミサイコ（南柴胡）　102
ミバショウ（実芭蕉）　168
ミミセンナ　302
ミモザアカシア　196
ミヤコグサ　197
都草（ミヤコグサ）　197
ミヤマコウゾウリナ　189
深山顔剃菜（ミヤマコウゾリナ）　189
深山髪剃菜（ミヤマコウゾリナ）　189
ミラ（弥良）　159
ミルナ　65
海松菜（ミルナ）　65
水松菜（ミルナ）　65
ミルラ　311
ミロバラン　301
ミント　197

ム

ムイラプアマ　197, 340
無花果（ムカカ）　49
無花果根（ムカカコン）　49
無花果葉（ムカカヨウ）　49
ムカンシ　197
無患子（ムカンシ）　197
ムギグワイ（麦慈姑）　44
無機ゲルマニウム　258
ムクロジ　197
無患子（ムクロジ）　197
無久呂之（ムクロジ）　197
無梗五加（ムコウゴカ）　96
ムコ多糖類　282
ムシゴケ　208
虫苔（ムシゴケ）　208
ムタプロデナフィル　375
ムラサキ　314
紫草（ムラサキ）　314
ムラサキウコン（紫鬱金）　69
ムラサキウマゴヤシ　46
紫馬肥（ムラサキウマゴヤシ）　46
ムラサキセンブリ　197
紫千振（ムラサキセンブリ）　197
ムラサキツメクサ　38
ムラサキナツフジ（紫夏藤）　91
ムラサキバレンギク　58
紫馬簾菊（ムラサキバレンギク）　58
ムラサキフトモモ　198
紫蒲桃（ムラサキフトモモ）　198
ムレザキフトモモ　198
ムロ（ムロノキ）（回香樹）　152
ムロ（ムロノキ）（室乃樹）　152
ムロ（ムロノキ）（天木香樹）　152
ムロ（ムロノキ）（樫）　152
ムロ（ムロノキ）（樫樫）　152
ムロウシ（無漏子）　155

メ

メイサ（榠樝）　201
迷迭香（メイテツコウ）　218
メガネヘビ（眼鏡蛇）　230
メグサハッカ　198
目草薄荷（メグサハッカ）　198
メグスリノキ　198
目薬木（メグスリノキ）　198
メシゲラック　198
メシマコブ　198
女島瘤（メシマコブ）　198
メズラ　58
メチオニン　283
メチソシルデナフィル　376
メチルサリフォニルメタン　243
メナジオン　276
メナモミ　199
雌菜揉み（メナモミ）　199
雌生揉（メナモミ）　199
メハジキ　216, 341
目弾（メハジキ）　216, 342
メビシ（雌菱）　174
メボウキ　199
目箒（メボウキ）　199
メマツヨイグサ　199
雌待宵草（メマツヨイグサ）　199
メラトニン　376
メラレウカ　199
メリッサ　200
メリロート　123
メロン　200
甜瓜（メロン）　200
メロンペア　186
メンジツ油　200
綿実油（メンジツユ）　200
メントウセツレンカ　130

綿頭雪蓮花（メントウセツレンカ）
130
メンマコン　299
綿馬根（メンマコン）　299

モ

モウオウレン　340
毛黄蓮（モウオウレン）　299, 340
檬果（モウカ）　195
毛姜（モウキョウ）　164
モウコン（毛莨）　215
毛慈姑（モウジコ）　103
モウズイカ（毛蕊花）　178
モウソウチク（孟宗竹）　138
毛龍眼　213
モウリンカ（毛輪花）　114
モエン　101
モクカ　169
木瓜（モクカ）　169
モグサ　210
野艾（モグサ）　210
艾（モグサ）　210
モクゾク　340
木賊（モクゾク）　340
モクツウ　40, 341
木通（モクツウ）　40, 341
モクテンリョウ　200
木天蓼（モクテンリョウ）　200
木天蓼子（モクテンリョウシ）　200
木乳羊（モクニュウヨウ）　323
モクベッシ　341
木鼈子（モクベッシ）　341
モクベツシ　341
木鼈子（モクベツシ）　341
モクレンシ　210
木連子（モクレンシ）　210
モケ（母計）　189
モケ（木瓜）　200
藻塩（モシオ）　101
モチグサ（餅草）　210
モチバナ（餅花）　170
モチヨモギ（餅艾）　170
モッカ　200, 201
モッカ（ボケ）　200
木瓜（モッカ）　201
モッカセイ（木花生）　157
モッコウ　341
木香（モッコウ）　341
モッショクシ　201
没食子（モッショクシ）　201
モツヤク　311
没薬（モツヤク）　311
モツヤクジュ　311
没薬樹（モツヤクジュ）　311
モミジバアサガオ（紅葉葉朝顔）　201
モミジバキセワタ　216
紅葉着せ綿（モミジバキセワタ）　216
モミジバヒルガオ（紅葉葉昼顔）　201
モミジヒルガオ　201
紅葉昼顔（モミジヒルガオ）　201
モモ　202
桃（モモ）　202
モモタマナ　202
桃玉名（モモタマナ）　202
モリアザミ　202
森薊（モリアザミ）　202
モリシマアカシア（mollissimaアカシア）　202
モリブデン　283
モロヘイヤ　203
モンケイ　119
問荊（モンケイ）　119

ヤ

ヤエナリ（八重生）　214
ヤエヤマアオキ　203
八重山青木（ヤエヤマアオキ）　203
ヤエヤマシタン（八重山紫檀）　111
ヤエンムギ　73
野燕麦（ヤエンムギ）　73
ヤオヤボウフウ（八百屋防風）　170
ヤカンゾウ　122
野甘草（ヤカンゾウ）　122
ヤクシソウ（薬師草）　65
ヤクシマアジサイ　203
屋久島紫陽花（ヤクシマアジサイ）
203
ヤクチ　341
益智（ヤクチ）　341
ヤクモソウ　216, 341
益母草（ヤクモソウ）　216, 342
ヤクヨウサルビア（薬用サルビア）
105
ヤクヨウセージ（薬用セージ）　105
ヤクヨウダイオウ　135, 322
薬用大黄（ヤクヨウダイオウ）　135,
322
ヤクヨウニンジン（薬用人参）　65
ヤグルマギク　204
矢車菊（ヤグルマギク）　204
ヤグルマソウ（矢車草）　204
ヤグルマハッカ　204
矢車薄荷（ヤグルマハッカ）　204
ヤコウトウ（夜交藤）　146
野梧桐（ヤゴドウ）　39
ヤーコン　203
ヤシ　204
椰子（ヤシ）　204
ヤシャビシャク　204
夜叉柄杓（ヤシャビシャク）　204
ヤシ油　204
椰子油（ヤシユ）　204
ヤチサンゴ　42
谷地珊瑚（ヤチサンゴ）　42
ヤチダモ　204
谷地梻（ヤチダモ）　204
ヤツメウナギ　225
八目鰻（ヤツメウナギ）　225
ヤドリギ　318
宿木（ヤドリギ）　318
ヤトロファ　157
ヤナギ　205
ヤナギハッカ　175
柳薄荷（ヤナギハッカ）　175
ヤナギラン　205
柳蘭（ヤナギラン）　205
ヤハズツノマタ　205
ヤハズ角叉（ヤハズツノマタ）　205
ヤハズニシキギ（矢筈錦木）　158
ヤバネヒイラギモチ（矢羽柊黐）　173
ヤブカンゾウ　82
藪萱草（ヤブカンゾウ）　82
ヤブタバコ　205
藪煙草（ヤブタバコ）　205
ヤブツバキ（藪椿）　145
ヤブラン　331
藪蘭（ヤブラン）　331
ヤボランジ　342
ヤマアザミ　161
ヤマイモ　206
山芋（ヤマイモ）　206
ヤマイモコン　108
ヤマウルシ　206
山漆（ヤマウルシ）　206
ヤマグワ（山桑）　195
ヤマゴボウ　202, 316
山牛蒡（ヤマゴボウ）　202, 316

ヤマザクラ 298
山桜（ヤマザクラ） 298
ヤマトシジミ 231
大和蜆（ヤマトシジミ） 231
ヤマトタチバナ（大和橘） 139
ヤマトリカブト 328
山鳥兜（ヤマトリカブト） 329
ヤマノイモ 108, 206
山芋（ヤマノイモ） 108, 206
ヤマノイモ属 206
ヤマハハコ 206
山母子（ヤマハハコ） 206
ヤマハマナス 206
山浜茄子（ヤマハマナス） 206
山浜梨（ヤマハマナス） 206
ヤマブキ 206
山吹（ヤマブキ） 206
ヤマブシタケ 207
山伏茸（ヤマブシタケ） 207
ヤマブドウ 207
山葡萄（ヤマブドウ） 207
ヤマベアオキ（ヤマベ青木） 203
ヤマモモ 207
山桃（ヤマモモ） 207
ヤラッパ 342
ヤラッパ根（ヤラッパコン） 342
ヤラッパ脂（ヤラッパシ） 342
ヤロー 127

ユ

ユウガオ 207
夕顔（ユウガオ） 207
有機ゲルマニウム 258
ユウシ（熊脂） 350
ユウシカ 111
ユウタン（熊胆） 350
ユーカリ 208
ユーカリノキ 208
ユーカリ油 208
ユカン 210
油柑（ユカン） 210
油柑枝（ユカンシ） 210
油柑木皮（ユカンボクヒ） 210
油柑葉（ユカンヨウ） 210
ユキチャ 208
雪茶（ユキチャ） 208
ユキノシタ（雪下） 60
ユキノハナ 342
雪の花（ユキノハナ） 342
ユキノハナ属 342
ユキミギク（雪見菊） 133
ユキモタセ 60
ユキワリソウ 335
雪割草（ユキワリソウ） 335
ユジツ（柚実） 208
ユズ 208
柚（ユズ） 208
柚子（ユズ） 208
ユスラ（山桜桃） 207
ユズリハ 208
譲葉（ユズリハ） 208
楪（ユズリハ） 208
ユソウボク 84
癒創木（ユソウボク） 84
ユッカ 208
ユニク（萸肉） 107
ユノス（柚子） 208
ユビキノン 259
ユリ 209
百合（ユリ） 209

ヨ

ヨイマチグサ（宵待草） 199
ヨウキセキ 376
洋金花（ヨウキンカ） 324
葉酸 283
ヨウシュオオバコ（洋種大葉子） 124
ヨウシュカンボク 209
洋種肝木（ヨウシュカンボク） 209
ヨウシュトチノキ（洋種栃の木） 318
ヨウシュトチノキ（洋種橡） 126
ヨウシュネズ（洋種杜松） 127
ヨウ素 284
ヨウテイ 209
羊蹄（ヨウテイ） 209
ヨウテイコウ（羊躑甲） 344
羊蹄根（ヨウテイコン） 209
ヨウニュウ（洋乳） 146
ヨウバイ 207
楊梅（ヨウバイ） 207
ヨウバイヒ 207
楊梅皮（ヨウバイヒ） 207
ヨウミャクアデク（葉脈アデク） 198
ヨカンシ 210
余甘子（ヨカンシ） 210
ヨクイニン 168
薏苡仁（ヨクイニン） 168
ヨグソザクラ 58
ヨクベイ 168
薏米（ヨクベイ） 168
ヨシ 41, 344
葦（ヨシ） 344
葭（ヨシ） 41
ヨシキリザメ（葦切鮫） 231
預知子（ヨチシ） 40
ヨドボケ（淀木瓜） 189, 200
ヨハンパンノキ 50
ヨヒンベ 342
ヨヒンベ皮（ヨヒンベヒ） 342
ヨモギ 210
蓬（ヨモギ） 210
ヨモギギク 210
蓬菊（ヨモギギク） 210
ヨルソケイ（夜素馨） 54
ヨロイグサ 190, 332
鎧草（ヨロイグサ） 190, 332
ヨーロッパキイチゴ 124
ヨーロッパキイチゴ（ヨーロッパ木苺） 212
ヨーロッパシラカンバ（ヨーロッパ白樺） 111
ヨーロッパスグリ（ヨーロッパ酸塊） 120
ヨーロッパスモモ 125
ヨーロッパソクズ 209
ヨーロッパ蒴藋（ヨーロッパソクズ） 209
ヨーロッパ当帰（ヨーロッパトウキ） 47
ヨーロッパブルーベリー 178

ラ

Lactobacillus属 158
Rhamnus属 306
ライ 211
ライガン 210
雷丸（ライガン） 210
ライガンキン（雷丸菌） 210
ライシ 210
雷矢（ライシ） 210
ライジツ 210
雷実（ライジツ） 210
ライチー 216
ライフクシ 211
莱菔子（ライフクシ） 211
ライムギ 211
ライ麦（ライムギ） 211

ラウオルフィア　294
ラウンド・ブック　181
ラウンドリーミント　43
ラカンカ　211
羅漢果（ラカンカ）　211
ラクキ（落葵）　147
ラークスパー　215
ラクセキ　137
絡石（ラクセキ）　137
ラクターゼ　377
ラクトフェリン　284
ラケモサ　183
ラスグラブラ　211
ラズベリー　212
ラタニア　343
ラタニア根（ラタニアコン）　343
ラッカセイ　212
落花生（ラッカセイ）　212
ラッキョウ　68
辣韮（ラッキョウ）　68
ラッショウ　113, 149
辣椒（ラッショウ）　113, 149
ラバ　223
ラパチョ　140
ラビッジ　219
ラフク（蘿菔）　211
ラフマ　212
羅布麻（ラフマ）　212
ラブラドールティー　88
ラベージ　219
ラベッジ　219
ラベンサラ　212
ラベンダー　213
ラベンダー油　213
ラムノイデス　102
羅勒（ラロク）　199
羅勒子（ラロクシ）　199
卵黄油　237
卵黄レシチン　286
卵殻　237
ランソウ　343
蘭草（ランソウ）　343
ランブータン　213
ランユ（卵油）　237

リ

リーキ　159
鯉魚胆（リギョタン）　233
リグナン　284
リコライス　75
リジン　284
鯉胆（リタン）　233
リノール酸　285
リノレン酸　285
リパーゼ　377
α-リポ酸　266
リボフラビン　274
リュウガソウ　83
竜牙草（リュウガソウ）　83
竜芽草（リュウガソウ）　83
龍牙草（リュウガソウ）　83
リュウガン　213
竜眼（リュウガン）　213
龍眼（リュウガン）　213
竜眼核（リュウガンカク）　213
竜眼殻（リュウガンカク）　213
竜眼肉（リュウガンニク）　213
リュウキ　51
竜葵（リュウキ）　51
竜葵子（リュウキシ）　51
リュウキド　213
劉寄奴（リュウキド）　213
リュウキュウアイ　214
琉球藍（リュウキュウアイ）　214
リュウキュウカワラケツメイ（琉球河原決明）　108
リュウキュウシ（留求子）　109
リュウキュウムクゲ（琉球木槿）　182
リュウコツ　351
竜骨（リュウコツ）　351
龍骨（リュウコツ）　351
リュウシツ　237
龍虱（リュウシツ）　238
リュウタン　343
竜胆（リュウタン）　343
流動パラフィン　285
リュウノウ　214
竜脳（リュウノウ）　214
リュウノウジュ（竜脳樹）　214
リュウノヒゲ　331
龍の髭（リュウノヒゲ）　331
留蘭香（リュウランコウ）　121
リョウガン（龍眼）　213
リョウキョウ　343
良姜（リョウキョウ）　343
遼藁本（リョウコウホン）　308
菱実（リョウジツ）　174
リョウショウカ　214
凌霄花（リョウショウカ）　214
リョウフンソウ　132
涼粉草（リョウフンソウ）　132
蓼藍（リョウラン）　140
リョクチャ　142
緑茶（リョクチャ）　142
リョクトウ　214
緑豆（リョクトウ）　214
リョクヨウカンラン　92
緑葉甘藍（リョクヨウカンラン）　92
藜芦根（リロコン）　329
リン　285
リンゴ　215
リンゴ酢　215
林檎酢（リンゴズ）　215
リンサンゴカ　96
リントウ　113
リンドウ　343
竜胆（リンドウ）　343

ル

ルー（Rue）　188
ルイボス　182, 215
ルサジカ（ルサ鹿）　231
ルソンシュウモウ（呂宋楸毛）　305
ルチン　286
ルテイン　286
ルバーブ　135
ルホール　219
ルリジサ（瑠璃苣）　215
ルリジシャ　215
瑠璃苣（ルリジシャ）　215
ルリハコベ　215
瑠璃繁縷（ルリハコベ）　215
ルリヒエンソウ　215
瑠璃飛燕草（ルリヒエンソウ）　215
ルンブルキナーゼ　377

レ

レイシ（霊芝）　216
レイシ（茘枝）　216
霊芝（レイシ）　216
茘枝（レイシ）　216
レイシカク　216
茘枝核（レイシカク）　216
レイシソウ（霊芝草）　216
レイシュンカ　175
麗春花（レイシュンカ）　175
レイチョウ（鱧腸）　138

レイハイカク　179
麗盃閣（レイハイカク）　179
レイビョウコウ　348
霊猫香（レイビョウコウ）　348
レイヨウカク　351
羚羊角（レイヨウカク）　351
レオヌルスソウ　216
レシチン　286
レジノール　284
E-レスベラトロール　268
trans-レスベラトロール　268
レチノール　273
レッド・クローバー　38
レッドセージ　141
レビスチクム　219
レホール　219
レモングラス　216
レモンソウ　216
レモンタイム　217
レモンバーベナ　188
レモンバーム　200
レモンマートル　217
レンカ　166
蓮花（レンカ）　166
レンギョウ　217, 344
連翹（レンギョウ）　217, 344
レンギョウウツギ（連翹空木）　217
レンゲ（蓮華）　217
レンゲソウ　217
蓮華草（レンゲソウ）　217
レンコン　166
蓮根（レンコン）　166
蓮子（レンシ）　166
蓮子心（レンシシン）　166
レンジツ　166
蓮実（レンジツ）　166
レンセンソウ　145, 217
連銭草（レンセンソウ）　145, 218
レンニク　166
蓮肉（レンニク）　166
レンヨウ　166
蓮葉（レンヨウ）　166
レンリソウ　218
連理草（レンリソウ）　218

ロ

ロイシン　287
ロウハクカ　344
老白花（ロウハクカ）　344
ロウハソウ（狼把草）　137
ロウレンシュウキュウ　203
臘蓮繍球（ロウレンシュウキュウ）　203
蘆薈（ロカイ）　46, 293
ロクインケイ（鹿陰茎）　351
ロクジュソウ（鹿寿草）　49
ロクジョウ　351
鹿茸（ロクジョウ）　351
ロクジョウオオムギ（六条大麦）　164
ロクジン　351
鹿腎（ロクジン）　351
ロクテイソウ　49
鹿蹄草（ロクテイソウ）　49
ロクベン　351
鹿鞭（ロクベン）　351
ロコン　344
芦根（ロコン）　344
ローズヒップ　153, 218
ローズマリー　218
ロゼリソウ（ロゼリ草）　163
ローゼル　163
ロゼル　163
ロッカクソウ（六角草）　60
ロッカクレイシ　216
鹿角霊芝（ロッカクレイシ）　216
ロート（莨菪）　331
露兜樹（ロトウジュ）　113
ロート根　331
莨菪根（ロートコン）　331
ロバ　223
ロヒキョウ（驢皮膠）　223
ロフク（蘆菔）　211
ロベージ　219
ロベリアソウ　344
ロベリア草（ロベリアソウ）　344
路辺青（ロヘンセイ）　193
ロヘンソウ　193
ローマカミツレ　218
ローマ加密列（ローマカミツレ）　218
ローマカミルレ　218
ローマンカモミール　218
ローヤルゼリー　238
ローレル　92

ワ

ワイルドカナダレタス　219
ワイルドチェリー　219
ワイルドブラックチェリー　219
ワイルドマンゴー　43
ワイルドレタス　219
ワキョウカツ（和羗活）　56
ワサビダイコン　219
山葵大根（ワサビダイコン）　219
ワサンキライ（和山帰来）　312
ワタゲツメクサ　47
ワダソウ　136
和田草（ワダソウ）　136
ワタフジウツギ（綿藤空木）　340
ワニナシ（鰐梨）　44
ワピチ　351
ワームウッド　85
和木瓜（ワモッカ）　85
ワレモコウ　220
吾亦紅（ワレモコウ）　220
吾木香（ワレモコウ）　220
ワレリア　70

学名索引
Scientific name index

A

Abelmoschus manihot 154
Abelmoschus manihot (L.) Medik. 154
Abrus fruticulosus Wall. ex Wighte et Arn. 91
Abrus precatorius L. 321
Abutilon avicennae Gaertn. 49, 150
Abutilon theophrasti Medik. 49, 150
Acacia catechu (L. f.) Willd. 185
Acacia dealbata Link 196
Acacia decurrens var. *dealbata* (Link) F.J. Muell. 196
Acacia decurrens var. *mollis* Lindl. 202
Acacia decurrens (Wendl. f.) Willd. var. *dealbata* (Link) F.J. Muell. 196
Acacia julibrissin (Durazz.) Willd. 161
Acacia mearnsii 202
Acacia mearnsii De Wild. 202
Acacia mollissima auct. non Willd. 202
Acacia senegal (L.) Willd. 45
Acacia verek Guill. et Perr. 45
Acanthopanax giraldii Harms 95
Acanthopanax gracilistylus W.W. Sm. 55, 96
Acanthopanax henryi (Oliv.) Harms 96
Acanthopanax pentaphyllus (Sieb. et Zucc.) Marchal 55
Acanthopanax senticosus (Rupr. et Maxim.) Harms 59, 96
Acanthopanax sessiliflorus (Rupr. et Maxim.) Seem 96
Acanthopanax sieboldianus Makino 55
Acanthopanax verticillatus G. Hoo 96
Acer maximowiczianum Miq. 198
Acer nikoense (Miq.) Maxim. 198
Achillea lanulosa Nutt. 127
Achillea millefolium L. 127
Achillea millefolium L. var. *occidentalis* DC. 127
Achyranthes bidentata Blume 309
Achyranthes fauriei H. Lév. et Vaniot 309
Aconitum L. 329
Acorus calamus L. 315
Acorus gramineus Sol. ex Aiton 129, 318
Acorus tatarinowii Schott 129, 318
Actaea racemosa (Nutt.) L. 183
Actinidia arguta (Sieb. et Zucc.) Planch. ex Miq. 105
Actinidia polygama (Sieb. et Zucc.) Planch. ex Maxim. 200
Adansonia bahobab L. 163
Adansonia baobab Gaertn. 163
Adansonia digitata L. 163
Adansonia situla Spreng. 163
Adansonia somalensis Chiov. 163
Adansonia sphaerocarpa A. Chev. 164
Adenophora hunanensis Nannfeldt 114
Adenophora stricta Miq. 114
Adenophora tetraphylla Fisch. 114
Adenophora triphylla (Thunb.) A. DC. ssp. *aperticampanulata* Kitam. 114
Adenophora triphylla (Thunb. ex Murray) A. DC. 114
Adonis amurensis Regel et Radde 334
Adonis L. 334
Aegle marmelos (L.) Correa ex Roxb. 53, 187
Aerodramus fuciphagus Thunb. 234
Aerodramus maximus Hume 234
Aesculus hippocastanum f. *memmingeri* (K. Koch) Schelle 318
Aesculus hippocastanum L. 126, 318
Aesculus turbinata Bl. 152
Agaricus bisporus (J.E. Lange) Imbach 128
Agaricus blazei Murrill 39
Agaricus fomentarius (L.) Lam. 146
Agastache rugosa (Fisch. et C.A. Mey.) Kuntze 301, 303
Agathosma betulina (P.J. Berg.) Pillans 181
Agave tequilana J.H. Weber 38
Ageratum conyzoides 70
Ageratum conyzoides L. 70
Agkistrodon halys Pallas 233
Agrimonia eupatoria L. 124
Agrimonia pilosa Ledeb. 83
Agropyron repens (L.) P. Beauv. 112
Ajuga decumbens Thunb. 81
Akebia quinata (Thunb. ex Houtt.) Decne. 40, 341
Akebia trifoliata (Thunb.) Koidz. 341
Albizia julibrissin Durazz. 161
Albizia lebbeck 178
Albizia lebbeck (L.) Benth. 178
Alcea rosea L. 139
Alchemilla vulgaris auct. non L. 165

Alchemilla xanthochlora Rothm. 165
Alisma canaliculatum A. Braun et C.D. Bouché 335
Alisma macrophyllum Kunth 113
Alisma orientale (Sam.) Juz. 323
Alisma plantago-aquatica L. var. *orientale* Sam. 323
Allium bakeri Regel 68
Allium bouddhae Debeaux 160
Allium chinense G. Don 68
Allium fistulosum 160
Allium fistulosum L. 160
Allium grayi Regel 68
Allium ledebourianum Roem. et Schult. 41
Allium macrostemon Bunge 68
Allium nipponicum Fr. et Sav. 68
Allium sativum L. 160
Allium sativum L. f. *pekinense* Makino 160
Allium sativum L. var. *japonicum* Kitam. 160
Allium sativum L. var. *pekinense* (Prokh.) F. Maek. 160
Allium schoenoprasum L. var. *foliosm* Regel 41
Allium tuberosum Rottl. ex Spreng. 159
Allium victorialis L. ssp. *platyphyllum* Hult. 80
Allium victorialis L. var. *platyphyllum* (Hult.) Makino 80
Allolobophora caliginosa Ant. Druges 349
Alnus glutinosa (L.) Gaertn. 62
Alnus japonica (Thunb.) Steud. 130
Aloe africana Mill. 47, 293
Aloe arborescens Mill. 77
Aloe barbadensis Mill. 47, 293
Aloe ferox Mill. 47, 293
Aloe spicata Baker 293
Aloe vera (L.) Burm. f. 46
Aloysia citriodora Palau 188
Aloysia triphylla (L'Hér.) Britton 188
Alpinia galanga (L.) Sw. 156
Alpinia officinarum Hance 343
Alpinia oxyphylla Miq. 341
Alpinia speciosa (J.C. Wendl.) K. Schum. 93
Alpinia zerumbet (Per.) B.L. Burtt et R.M. Sm. 93
Althaea officinalis L. 46
Althaea rosea (L.) Cav. 139
Amana edulis (Miq.) Honda 44
Amaranthus frumentaceus Buch.-Ham. 122
Amaranthus gangeticus L. 93
Amaranthus hybridus L. 122
Amaranthus hypochondriacus L. 122
Amaranthus tricolor L. ssp. *mangostanus* (L.) Aellen 93
Ambrina ambrosioides (L.) Spach 46
Amomum cardamomum L. 116, 177
Amomum compactum Sol. ex Maton 177
Amomum keplaga Sprag. et Burk. 177
Amomum kravanh Pierre ex Gagnep. 177
Amomum tsao-ko Crevost et Lemarié 321
Amomum villosum Lour. var. *xanthioides* (Wall. ex Baker) T.L. Wu et S.J. Chen 315
Amomum xanthioides Wall. ex Baker 315
Amomum zingiber L. 116
Ampelopsis brevipedunculata (Maxim.) Trautv. 162
Ampelopsis brevipedunculata (Maxim.) Trautv. var. *heterophylla* (Thunb.) Hara 162
Ampelopsis cantoniensis var. *grossedentata* 150
Ampelopsis cantoniensis var. *grossedentata* (Hook. et Aln.) Planch. 150
Ampelopsis glandulosa (Wall.) Momiyama var. *heterophylla* (Thunb.) Momiyama 162
Ampelopsis grossedentata 150
Ampelopsis grossedentata (Hand.-Mazz.) W.T. Wang 150
Ampelopsis japonica 68
Ampelopsis japonica (Thunb.) Makino 68
Ampelopsis leeoides (Maxim.) Planch. 150
Amyda japonica Temminck et Schlegel 232
Amyda sinensis Wiegmann 232
Amygdalus persica L. 202, 327
Anagallis arvensis L. 215
Anagallis arvensis L. f. *coerulea* (Schreb.) Baumg. 215
Anagallis coerulea Schreb. 215
Ananas ananas (L.) Voss 163
Ananas comosus (L.) Merr. 163
Ananas sativus Schult. f. 163
Anaphalis margaritacea (L.) Benth. et Hook. f. 206
Anavinga samyda Gaertn. f. 305
Andrographis paniculata (Burm. f.) Nees 132
Andropogon citratus DC. 217
Anemarrhena asphodeloides Bunge 324
Anemone hepatica L. 335
Anethum foeniculum L. 55
Angelica acutiloba (Sieb. et Zucc.) Kitag. 150, 326
Angelica acutiloba (Sieb. et Zucc.) Kitag. var. *sugiyamae* Hikino 150, 326
Angelica archangelica L. 47
Angelica biserrata (R.H. Shan et C.Q. Yuan) C.Q. Yuan et R.H. Shan 110
Angelica bisserata 110
Angelica dahurica (Hoffm.) Benth. et Hook. f. ex Franch. et Sav. 332
Angelica decrursiva (Miq.) Franch. et Sav. 319
Angelica furcijuga 333
Angelica furcijuga Kitag. 333
Angelica gigas Nakai 150, 326

Angelica keiskei (Miq.) Koidz. 41
Angelica laxiflora Diels 328
Angelica levisticum Baill. 219
Angelica megaphylla Diels 328
Angelica officinalis Moench 47
Angelica polymorpha Maxim. var. *sinensis* Oliv. 150
Angelica pubescens 110
Angelica pubescens Maxim. 110, 328
Angelica shishiudo Koidz. 110
Angelica sinensis (Oliv.) Diels 150, 326
Angelica tenuisecta (Makino) Makino var. *furucijuga* (Kitag.) H. Ohba 333
Angelica utilis Makino 41
Anguilla japonica Temminck et Schlegel 225
Anguilla remifera Jordan et Evermann 225
Anism officinarum Moench 43
Anisum vulgare Gaertn. 43
Annona macrocarpa auct. 306
Annona muricata L. 88, 306
Anoectochilus formosanus Hayata 79, 83
Antennaria dioica (L.) Gaertn. 59
Anthemis nobilis L. 219
Anthriscus cerefolium (L.) Hoffm. 143
Anthyllis vulneraria L. 47
Aphanizomenon A. Morren ex Bornet et Flahault 43
Aphanizomenon flos-aquae Ralfs ex Bornet et Flahault 43
Apios americana Medik. 45
Apios tuberosa Moench 45
Apis mellifera L. 235, 237, 238
Apium carvi (L.) Crantz. 176
Apium graveolens L. var. *dulce* (Mill.) Pers. 131
Apium petroselinum L. 166
Apocynum venetum L. 212
Aporrectodea trapezoides Dugès 349
Aquilaria agallocha Roxb. 317
Aquilaria crassna Pierre ex Lecomte 317
Aquilaria filaria (Oken) Merr. 317
Aquilaria malaccensis Lam. 317
Aquilaria sinensis (Lour.) Gilg. 317
Arachis hypogaea L. 212
Aralia canescens Sieb. et Zucc. 112
Aralia chinensis 112
Aralia chinensis L. 112
Aralia cordata 56, 328
Aralia cordata Thunb. 57, 328
Aralia edulis Sieb. et Zucc. 57
Aralia elata 140
Aralia elata (Miq.) Seem. 112, 140
Aralia elata var. *subinermis* Ohwi 112
Aralia mandshurica Rupr. et Maxim. 112, 140
Aralia papyrifera Hook. 144
Archangelica officinalis (Moench) Hoffm. 47
Arctium edule Beger 310
Arctium lappa L. 99, 310
Arctostaphylos uva-ursi (L.) Spreng. 296
Ardisia glabra Thunb. 133
Areca catechu L. 179, 322
Argentina anserina (L.) Rydb. 338
Arisaema amurense Maxim. 325
Arisaema erubescens (Wall.) Schott. 325
Arisaema heterophyllum Blume 325
Arisaema serratum (Thunb.) Schott. 325
Aristolochia L. 295
Armeniaca mume Sieb. 57
Armeniaca vulgaris Lam. 75, 305
Armoracia lapathifolia Gilib. ex Usteri 219
Armoracia rusticana P. Gaertn., B. Mey. et Schreb. 219
Arnica montana L. 293
Artemisia absinthium L. 85
Artemisia annua L. 297
Artemisia anomala 213
Artemisia anomala S. Moore 213
Artemisia apiacea Hance 317
Artemisia capillaris Thunb. 294
Artemisia caruifolia Buch.-Ham. ex Roxb. 317
Artemisia carvifolia var. *apiacea* (Hance) Pamp. 317
Artemisia dracunculus L. 59
Artemisia indica Willd. var. *maximowiczii* (Nakai) H. Hara 210
Artemisia montana (Nakai) Pamp. 210
Artemisia princeps Pamp. 210
Artemisia selengensis 213
Artemisia selengensis Turcz. ex Besser 213
Artemisia vulgaris L. var. *vulgatissima* Bess. 210
Arthrospira maxima Setchell et Gardener 120
Arthrospira platensis (Nordst.) Gomont 120
Artocarpus heterophyllus Lam. 171
Artocarpus integra auct. non (Thunb.) Merril 171
Artocarpus integrifolius auct. non L. f. 171
Artocarpus maxima Blanco 171
Artocarpus nanca Noranha 171
Arundinaria kurilensis Rupr. 142
Asarum caulescens Maxim. 335
Asarum heterotropoides (F. Schmidt) F. Maek. var. *mandschuricum* (Maxim.) F. Maek. 311
Asarum heterotropoides F. Schmidt var. *mandshuricum* (Maxim.) Kitag. 312

Asarum sieboldii (Miq.) F. Maek. 311
Asarum sieboldii (Miq.) var. *seoulense* Nakai 311
Aspalathus contaminatus auct. 215
Aspalathus linearis (Burm. f.) R. Dahlgren 182, 215
Asparagus cochinchinensis (Lour.) Merr. 149, 326
Asparagus lucidus Lindle. 149
Asparagus racemosus Willd. 114
Asperula odorata L. 88
Aspidistra elatior Blume 171
Aspidistra elatior Blume var. *albomaculata* Hook. 172
Aspidistra punctata Lindl. 172
Aspidium filix-mas (L.) Sw. 299
Aspongopus chinensis Dallas 228
Asterina pectinifera Müller et Troschel 226
Asteriscus pectinifera Müller et Troschel 226
Aster tataricus L. f. 313
Astilbe thunbergii (Sieb. et Zucc.) Miq. 38
Astragalus chinensis L. f. 113
Astragalus complanatus R. Br. ex Bunge 113
Astragalus gummifer Labill. 153
Astragalus lotoides Lam. 217
Astragalus membranaceus (Fisch. ex Link) Bunge 62, 298
Astragalus membranaceus (L.) (Fisch. ex Link) Bunge var. *mongholicus* (Bunge) P.K. Hsiao 62, 298
Astragalus membranaceus (Fisch.) Bunge 151
Astragalus mongholicus Bunge 62, 298
Astragalus sinicus L. 217
Atractylodes chinensis (Bunge) Koidz. 321
Atractylodes japonica Koidz. ex Kitam. 333
Atractylodes lancea (Thunb.) DC. 321
Atractylodes macrocephala Koidz. 333
Atractylodes ovata (Thunb.) DC. 332
Atropa belladonna L. 335
Atropa L. 335
Aucklandia lappa Decne. 341
Auricularia auricula (Hook.) Underw. 77
Auricularia auricula-judae (Bull. : Fr.) Wettst. 77
Avena fatua L. 73
Avena sativa L. 61
Averrhoa carambola L. 101
Azukia angularis (Willd.) Ohwi 42

B

Baccharis genistelloides (Lam.) Pers. var. *trimera* (Less.) Baker 73
Baccharis trimera (Less.) DC. 73
Bacillus natto 155
Bacillus subtilis var. *natto* 155
Backhousia citriodra F. Muell. 217
Bacopa monnieri (L.) Pennell 65
Balsamodendron mukul Hook. 72
Bambusa Schreb. 138
Bambusa spp. 324
Bambusa textilis McClure 148
Bambusa tuldoides Munro 324
Bambusa veitchii Carr. 86
Bandeiraea simplicifolia (Vahl ex DC.) Benth. 306
Baphicacanthus cusia (Nees) Bremek. 214
Barosma betulina (P.J. Berg.) Bartl. et H.L. Wendl. 181
Basella alba L. *'Rubra'* 147
Basella rubra L. 147
Bassia scoparia (L.) A.J. Scott 112
Bauhinia divaricata L. 167
Bauhinia fortificata Link 167
Bauhinia variegata L. 344
Bellis perennis L. 175
Belou marmelos W.F. Wight 187
Benincasa cerifera Savi. 149, 326
Benincasa cerifera Savi. f. *emarginata* K. Kimura et Sugiyama 149, 326
Benincasa hispida (Thunb.) Cogn. 149, 326
Benzoin strychnifolium (Sieb. et Zucc.) O. Kuntze 58
Benzoin thunbergii Sieb. et Zucc. 56
Benzoin umbellatum (Thunb.) O. Kuntze 56
Berberis aquifolium Pursh 173
Berberis vulgaris L. 128
Berchemia racemosa Sieb. et Zucc. 87
Beta cicla (L.) L. 181
Beta hortensis Mill. 181
Beta vulgaris L. 104
Beta vulgaris L. ssp *cicla* (L.) W.D.J. Koch 104
Beta vulgaris L. var. *cicla* (L.) K. Koch 181
Betula alba L. sensu Coste 111
Betula alba L. var. *japonica* Miq. 117
Betula alnus L. var. *glutinosa* L. 62
Betula glutinosa (L.) Lam. 62
Betula japonica Sieb. non Thunb. 117
Betula japonica Thunb. 130
Betula pendula Roth 111
Betula platyphylla Sukatchev var. *japonica* (Miq.) Hara 117
Betula verrucosa J.F. Ehrh. 111
Bidens acuta (Wieg.) Britt. 137
Bidens comosa (A. Gray) Wieg. 137
Bidens pilosa L. 98
Bidens tripartita L. 137
Bifidobacterium 176

Bignonia chinensis Lam. 214
Biota orientalis (L.) Endl. 134, 330
Bletilla striata (Thunb.) Rchb. f. 118
Blumea balsamifera (L.) DC. 138
Boesenbergia pandurata (Roxb.) Schult. 87
Bolboschoenus fluviatilis (Torr.) T. Koyama ssp. *yagara* (Ohwi) T. Koyama 55
Boldu boldus (Mol.) Lyons 191
Boletus applanatus Pers. 99
Boletus fomentarius L. 146
Boletus obliquus Ach. ex Pers. 71
Boletus versicolor L. 74
Bombyx mori L. 226
Borago officinalis L. 215
Borassus flabellifer L. 56
Borbonia pinifolia Marloth 215
Borojoa patinoi Cuatrec. 191
Boschniakia glabra 157
Boschniakia glabra C.A. Mey. ex Bong. 158
Boschniakia rossica 157
Boschniakia rossica (Cham. et Schltdl.) B. Fedtsch. 157
Bos taurus L. 223, 224, 228, 229, 230, 232, 233
Bos taurus L. var. *domesticus* Gmelin 347, 350
Boswellia Roxb. 337
Boswellia serrata 190
Boswellia serrata Roxb. 190
Brachyura L. 228
Bradybaena similaris Ferussac 227
Brassica alboglabra L.H. Bailey 92
Brassica campestris L. 154
Brassica campestris L. ssp. *napus* (L.) Hook. f. et Anders. var. *nippo-oleifera* Makino 154
Brassica napus L. 155
Brassica nigra (L.) W.D.J. Koch 89
Brassica oleraceae L. var. *acephala* DC. 92
Brassica rapa L. var. *rapa* 155
Bromelia ananas L. 163
Bromelia comosus L. 163
Bryonia cretica L. ssp. *dioica* (Jacq.) Tutin 184
Bryonia dioica Jacq. 184
Bryonia tayuya Vell. 323
Bubalus arnee Kerr 347
Buddleja officinalis Maxim. 340
Bufo bufo gargarizans Cantor 349
Bufo melanosticus Schneider 349
Bungarus multicinctus Blyth 236
Bupleurum falcatum L. 102, 311
Bupleurum falcatum L. var. *komarowi* Koso-Polj. 102
Bupleurum scorzonerifolium Willd. var. *stenophyllum* Nakai 102
Butea superba Roxb. 68, 179
Buthus martensii Karsch 230
Butyrospermum paradoxum (C.F. Gaertn.) Hepper ssp. *parkii* (G. Don.) Hepper 108
Butyrospermum parkii (G. Don.) Kotschy 108

C

Caesalpinia coriaria (Jacq.) Willd. 121
Caesalpinia sappan L. 322
Calendula officinalis L. 150
Callorhinus ursinus L. 225, 347
Calluna vulgaris cv. *Sunrise* 81
Calluna vulgaris (L.) Hull 81
Calystegia japonica Choisy 178
Camellia japonica L. 145
Camellia japonica L. var. *hortensis* Makino 145
Camellia sinensis (L.) O. Kuntze 142, 164
Camellia sinensis (L.) O. Kunze var. *assamica* (J.W. Mast.) Kitam. 142
Camellia thea Link 142, 164
Camphora camphora (L.) H. Karst., nom. illeg. 86, 116
Camphora officinalis Nees 86, 116
Campsis chinensis (Lam.) Voss 214
Campsis grandiflora (Thunb.) K. Schum. 214
Camptotheca acuminata Decne. 76
Canarium album 76
Canarium album (Lour.) Raeusch. 76
Candida utilis (Henneberg) Lodder et Kreger-wan Rij 95
Canis lupus familiaris L. 347
Cannabis sativa L. 40, 339
Cannabis sativa L. ssp. *sativa* 40
Capparis masaikai 70
Capparis masaikai Lévl. 70
Capsella bursa-pastoris (L.) Medik. 154
Capsicum annuum L. 149
Capsicum annuum L. var. *annuum* 113
Capsicum annuum L. var. *frutescens* (L.) Kuntze 113
Capsicum annuum L. var. *glabriusculum* (Dunal) Heiser et Pickersgill 113
Capsicum frutescens L. 113, 149
Carduus benedictus (L.) Thell. 79
Carica papaya L. 169
Carpesium abrotanoides 205
Carpesium abrotanoides L. 205
Carthamus tinctorius 186
Carthamus tinctorius L. 186
Carum carvi L. 176

Carya cathayensis Sarg.　105
Caryophyllus aromaticus L.　89, 144
Casearia parviflora L.　305
Casearia sylvestris Sw.　305
Cassia acutifolia Delile　133, 320
Cassia alata L.　169
Cassia angustifolia Vahl　133, 320
Cassia auriculata　302
Cassia auriculata L.　302
Cassia florida Vahl　138
Cassia mimosoides L. ssp. *nomame* (Sieb.) Ohashi　108
Cassia obtusifolia L.　60
Cassia occidentalis L.　170
Cassia siamea Lam.　138
Cassia tora auct. non. L.　60
Cassia torosa auct. non Cav.　170
Catalpa bungei C.A. Mey.　304
Catalpa ovata G. Don　304
Cataria vulgaris Moench　51
Catha edulis (Vahl) Forsk. ex Endl.　293
Catharanthus roseus (L.) G. Don　329
Catinbium speciosum (J.C. Wendl.) Holttum　93
Cayaponia tayuya (Vell.) Cogn.　323
Celastrus edulis Vahl　293
Celastrus maytenus Willd.　192
Celosia argentea L.　161
Celosia argentea L. var. *cristata* (L.) Kuntze　161
Centaurea benedicta (L.) L.　79
Centaurea cyanus L.　204
Centaurium erythreae Raf.　132
Centaurium minus　132
Centaurium minus auct. non Moench　132
Centaurium umbellatum Gilib.　132
Centella asiatica (L.) Urban　145
Centipeda minima (L.) A. Br. et Aschers.　152
Centipeda orbicularis Lour.　152
Cephaelis acuminata H. Karst.　307
Cephaelis ipecacuanha (Brot.) A. Rich　307
Cephaelis Sw.　307
Cerasus avium (L.) Moench　128
Cerasus japonica (Thunb.) Loisel.　48
Cerasus nigra Mill.　128
Cerasus sylvestris Lund.　128
Ceratonia siliqua L.　50
Cervus canadensis Erxleben　351
Cervus (*Cervus*) *elaphus* L. var. *xanthopygus* Milne-Edwards　351
Cervus elaphus L.　229
Cervus (*Shika*) *nippon* Temminck var. *mantchuricus* Swinhoe　351
Cetraria islandica (L.) Ach.　37
Chaenomeles cardinalis (Carriére) Nakai　189
Chaenomeles japonica (Thunb.) Lindl.　85
Chaenomeles lagenaria (Loisel.) Koidz.　189, 201
Chaenomeles maulei (T. Moore) Scheid　85
Chaenomeles sinensis (Thouin) Koehne　201
Chaenomeles speciosa (Sweet) Nakai　189, 201
Chaerofolium cerefolium (L.) Schinz.　143
Chamaecyparis obtusa (Sieb. et Zucc.) Sieb. et Zucc. ex Endl.　175
Chamaemelum nobile (L.) All.　218
Chamaenerion angustifolium (L.) Scop.　205
Chamaerops fortunei Hook.　116
Chamerion angustifolium (L.) Holub　205
Chamerion angustifolium (L.) Holub ssp. *angustifolium* 205
Chamerion angustifolium ssp. *circumvagum*　205
Chamomilla recutita (L.) Rauschert　72
Chelidonium majus L. var. *asiaticum* (Hara) Ohwi　151
Chenopodium album L. var. *centrorubrum* Makino　38
Chenopodium ambrosioides L.　46
Chenopodium anthelminticum L.　46
Chenopodium centrorubrum (Makino) Nakai　38
Chenopodium quinoa Willd.　78
Chimaphila japonica Miq.　57
Chimaphila umbellata (L.) W.C. Barton　57
Chimaphila umbellata (L.) W.C. Barton ssp. *cisatlantica* (Blake) Hultén　57
Chionoecetes opilio O. Fabricius　228
Chlamys farreri Jones et Preston　223
Chlamys farreri nipponensis Kuroda　223
Chloranthus glaber (Thunb.) Makino　80, 133
Chloranthus monander R. Br. ex Sims　80, 133
Chlorella M. Beijerinck　90
Choerospondias axillaris (Roxb.) B.L. Burtt et A.W. Hill 156
Choerospondias axillaris (Roxb.) B.L. Burtt et A.W. Hill var. *japonica* (Ohwi) Ohwi　156
Chondrodendron Ruiz et Pav. *corr.* Miers　311
Chondrodendron tomentosum Ruiz et Pav.　311
Chondrus crispus Stackh.　205
Chrysanthemum × *morifolium* Ramat.　77
Chrysanthemum arneum Bieb.　39
Chrysanthemum coccineum Willd.　39
Chrysanthemum indicum L.　77
Chrysanthemum parthenium (L.) Bernh.　155
Chrysanthemum roseum weberet Moor　39
Chrysanthemum sinense Sabine　77

Chrysanthemum vulgare (L.) Bernh. 210
Cichorium intybus L. 77
Cimicifuga cordifolia Pursh 183
Cimicifuga dahurica (Turcz.) Maxim. 316
Cimicifuga foetida L. 316
Cimicifuga heracleifolia Kom. 316
Cimicifuga racemosa (L.) Nutt. 183
Cimicifuga racemosa (L.) Nutt. var. *cordifolia* (Pursh) A. Gray 183
Cimicifuga simplex (DC.) Turcz. 316
Cinchona calisaya Wedd. 304
Cinchona ledgeriana Moens ex Trimen 304
Cinchona officinalis L. 304
Cinchona pubescens Vahl 304
Cinchona succirubra Pav. et Klotzsch 304
Cinnamomum aromaticum Nees 91, 92
Cinnamomum camphora (L.) J. Presl 86, 116
Cinnamomum cassia 91
Cinnamomum cassia Blume 91, 92
Cinnamomum cassia Presl 91, 92
Cinnamomum sintoc Bl. 119
Cirsium borealinipponense Kitam. 161
Cirsium dipsacolepis 202
Cirsium dipsacolepis (Maxim.) Matsum. 202
Cirsium japonicum 161
Cirsium japonicum Fisch. ex DC. 161
Cirsium nipponense 161
Cirsium spicatum 161
Cirsium spicatum (Maxim.) Matsum. 161
Cirsium yezoense (Maxim.) Makino 192
Cissus brevipedunculata Maxim. 162
Cissus quadrangularis L. 314
Cissus sicyoides L. 53
Cissus verticillata (L.) Nicolson et C.E. Jarvis 53
Cistanche deserticola Ma 98
Cistanche salsa 157
Cistanche salsa (C.A. Mey.) G. Beck 98, 157
Cistanche tubulosa 74
Cistanche tubulosa (Schenk) R. Wight 75
Citrullus colocynthis (L.) Schrad. 310
Citrus×aurantium L. var. *sinensis* L. 67, 119
Citrus×paradisi Macfad. 89
Citrus aurantium 137
Citrus aurantium L. 137
Citrus grandis (L.) Osbeck 185
Citrus hystrix DC. 185
Citrus junos Sieb. ex Tanaka 208
Citrus maxima (Burm.) Merr. 185
Citrus medica L. var. *sarcodactylis* (Hoola van Nooten) Swingle 181
Citrus natsudaidai 155
Citrus natsudaidai Hayata 155
Citrus papeda Miq. 185
Citrus reticulata Blanco 196
Citrus reticulata Blanco *'Satsuma'* 144
Citrus reticulata var. *unshiu* (Marcow.) Hu 123, 144
Citrus sinensis (L.) Osbeck 67, 119
Citrus tachibana 139
Citrus tachibana (Makino) T. Tanaka 139
Citrus tangerina hort. ex T. Tanaka 123
Citrus trifoliata L. 73
Citrus unshiu Marcow. 123, 144
Cladodendron frondosus (Dicks. : Fr.) Lázaro Ibiza 192 192
Clavaria crispa Wulfen 169
Clavaria erinaceus (Bull.) Paulet 207
Clematis chinensis Osbeck 52, 294
Clematis hexapetala Pall. 294
Clematis mandshurica Rupr. 294
Clematis uncinata Champ. ex Benth. 294
Clerodendranthus spicatus Wu et Li 87
Clerodendrum cyrtophyllum Turcz. 193
Clitoria ternatea 144
Clitoria ternatea L. 144
Cnicus benedictus L. 79
Cnicus dipsacolepis Maxim. 202
Cnidium japonicum Miq. 170
Cnidium monnieri (L.) Cusson 315
Cnidium officinale Makino 131, 319
Cochlearia armoracia L. 219
Cocos nucifera L. 204
Codonopsis lanceolata (Sieb. et Zucc.) Trautv. 146
Codonopsis pilosula (Franch.) Nannf. 326
Codonopsis pilosula Nannf. var. *modesta* (Nannf.) L.T. Shen 326
Codonopsis silvestris Kom. 326
Codonopsis tangshen Oliv. 326
Codonopsis ussuriensis 162
Codonopsis ussuriensis (Rupr. et Maxim.) Hemsl. 162
Coffea arabica L. 96
Coix lacryma-jobi L. 168
Coix lacryma-jobi L. var. *ma-yuen* (Roman.) Stapf 168
Coix ma-yuen Roman. 168
Cola acuminata (Brenan) Schott et Endl. 96
Cola nitida (Vent.) Schott et Endl. 96
Colchicum autumnale L. 294
Coleus barbatus (Andrews) Benth. 73
Coleus forskohlii auct. 73

Collybia shiitake J. Schroet. 109
Colocynthis vulgaris Schrad. 310
Combretum altum Perr. 93
Combretum floribundum Engle. et Diels 93
Combretum micranthum G. Don. 93
Combretum raimbautii Heck. 93
Commelina communis L. 146
Commiphora Jacq. 311
Commiphora mukul 72
Commiphora mukul (Hook. ex Stocks) Engl. 72
Conandron ramondioides Sieb. et Zucc. 52
Consolida regalis Gray 216
Convallaria majalis L. 317
Convallaria majalis L. var. *keiskei* (Miq.) Makino 317
Convallaria majalis L. var. *majalis* 317
Convallaria odorata Mill. 48
Convolvulus nil L. 40
Copaifera langsdorffii 99
Copaifera langsdorffii Desf. 99
Copaifera officinalis 98
Copaifera officinalis (Jacq.) L. 99
Coptis chinensis Franch. 63, 299, 340
Coptis deltoidea C.Y. Cheng et Hsiao 63, 299, 340
Coptis japonica (Thunb.) Makino 63, 299, 340
Coptis japonica (Thunb.) Makino var. *japonica* 63, 299, 340
Coptis japonica (Thunb.) Makino var. *major* (Miq.) Satake 63, 299, 340
Coptis teeta Wall. 63, 299, 340
Coralliidae Lamouroux 231
Corbicula japonica Prime 231
Corbicula leana Prime 231
Corchorus catharticus Blanco 203
Corchorus decemangularis Roxb. 203
Corchorus lobatus Wildem. 203
Corchorus olitorius L. 203
Corchorus quinqueloclaris Moench 203
Cordia coffeoides Warm 143
Cordia digynia Vell. 143
Cordia ecalyculata Vell. 143
Cordia salicifolia Cham. 143
Cordyceps sinensis (Berk.) Sacc. 151
Coriandrum sativum L. 98
Coridius chinensis Dallas 228
Coriolus versicolor (L.) Quél. 74, 303
Cornus officinalis Sieb. et Zucc. 107
Corydalis ambigua Cham. et Schlecht. 297
Corydalis bungeana Turcz. 85
Corydalis turtschaninovii Bess. f. *yanhusuo* Y.H. Chou et C.C. Hsu 297
Corydalis yanhusuo W.T. Wang 297
Corynanthe yohimbe K. Schum. 342
Crassocephalum crepidioides (Benth.) S. Moore 186
Crassostrea gigas Thunb. 227
Crassula argentea L. f. 60
Crassula argentea Thunb. 60
Crassula obliqua Haw. 60
Crassula ovata (Mill.) Druce 60
Crassula portulacea Lam. 61, 94
Crataegus cuneata Sieb. et Zucc. 106
Crataegus laevigata 125
Crataegus laevigata (Poir.) DC. 125
Crataegus monogyna 125
Crataegus monogyna Jacq. 125
Crataegus oxyacantha 125
Crataegus oxyacantha L. 125
Crataegus pinnatifida Bunge 106
Crataegus pinnatifida Bunge var. *major* N.E. Br. 106
Cremastra appendiculata (D. Don) Makino 103
Cremastra unguiculata Finet 103
Cremastra variabilis (Bl.) Nakai 103
Cristaria plicata Leach 234
Crocus sativus L. 104
Crotalus L. 236
Croton tiglium L. 332
Cryptotympana atrata Fabr. 349
Cucumis hispida Thunb. 207
Cucumis melo L. 200
Cucurbita hispida Thunb. 149, 326
Cucurbita lagenaria (L.) L. 177
Cucurbita maxima Duch. ex Lam. 71
Cucurbita moschata (Duch. ex Lam.) Duch. ex Poiret. 71
Cucurbita pepo L. 71
Cullen corylifolia (L.) Medik. 189
Cuminum cyminum L. 87
Cuphea balsamona Cham. et Schltdl. 161
Cuphea cartagensis (Jacq.) J.F. Macbr. 161
Cuphea carthagenensis (Jacq.) J.F. Macbr. 161
Curculigo ensifolia R. Br. 133
Curculigo orchioides Gaertn. 133
Curcuma aeruginosa Roxb. 69
Curcuma amada 195
Curcuma amada Roxb. 195
Curcuma aromatica Salisb. 172
Curcuma domestica Valet. 55
Curcuma longa L. 55
Curcuma zedoaria (Christm.) Roscoe 69
Cuscuta australis R. Br. 328

Cuscuta chinensis Lam. 328
Cuscuta epilinum Weihe 328
Cuscuta japonica Chois. 328
Cyanus segetum Hill 204
Cybister tripunctatus lateralis Fabricus 238
Cybister tripunctatus orientalis Gschwendtner 238
Cycas revoluta Thunb. 322
Cyclobalanopsis salicina (Bl.) Oerst. 58
Cyclocarya paliurus (Batal.) Iljin. 122
Cydonia japonica Loisel. non (Thunb.) Pers. 189
Cydonia japonica (Thunb.) Pers. 85
Cydonia sinensis (Dum.-Cours.) Thouin 201
Cydonia speciosa f. *eburnea* (Carriére) Hara 189
Cydonia speciosa Sweet 201
Cymbopogon citratus (DC.) Stapf 217
Cymbosepalum baroni Baker 172
Cymbosepalum baronii Baker 172
Cynara scolymus L. 144
Cynips gallae tinctoriae Olivier. 201
Cynomorium coccineum 65
Cynomorium coccineum L. 65
Cynomorium songaricum Rupr. 65
Cyperus microiria Steud. 72
Cyperus rotundus L. 308
Cyprinus carpio L. 233
Cytisus pinnatus L. 90
Cytisus scoparius (L.) Link 60, 296

D

Daemonorops draco (Willd.) Bl. 81
Dalbergia odorifera T. Chen 95
Dama dama L. 231
Daphnidium strychnifolium Seib. et Zucc. 58
Daphniphyllum himalense (Benth.) Muell. Arg. ssp. *macropodum* (Miq.) Huang 208
Daphniphyllum macropodum Miq. 208
Datura L. 324
Datura metel L. 324
Datura stramonium L. 324
Daucus carota L. ssp. *sativus* (Hoffm.) Arcang. 159
Decalepis hamiltonii Wight et Arn. 148
Deinagkistrodon acutus Günther 236
Delphinium consolida L. 216
Dendranthema grandiflorum (Ramat.) Kitam. 77
Dendrobium officinale K. Kimura et Migo 325
Dendrobium Sw. 325
Dendrocalamus spp. 324
Derris indica (Lam.) Bennett 90
Dichopsis gutta Benth. et Hook. f. 86
Dichroa febrifuga Lour. 53
Dictamnus dasycarpus Turcz. 330
Dictyophora indusiata (Vent.) Desv. 78
Digenea simplex (Wulfen) C. Agardh 338
Digitalis L. 313
Digitalis purpurea L. 313
Dimocarpus crinita Lour. 213
Dimocarpus longan Lour. 213
Dioscorea alata L. 57
Dioscorea batatas Decne. 108
Dioscorea bulbifera L. 63
Dioscorea japonica Thunb. 108
Dioscorea L. 206
Dioscorea latifolia Bent. 63
Dioscorea nipponica Makino 131
Dioscorea opposita Thunb. 108
Dioscorea oppositifolia L. 108
Diospyros kaki 68
Diospyros kaki Thunb. 68
Dipsacus asper 156
Dipsacus asper auct. 156
Dipsacus asperoides 156
Dipsacus asperoides C.Y. Cheng et T.M. Ai 156
Dipsacus asper Wall. 156
Dipsacus japonica 156
Dipsacus japonicus Miq. 156
Dolichos angularis Willd. 42
Dolichos lablab L. 53, 188
Dolichos purpureus L. 188
Dolichos soya L. 155
Draba nemorosa L. 50
Draba nemorosa L. var. *hebecarpa* Ledeb. 50
Drimia maritima (L.) Stearn 300
Drynaria fortunei (Kunze ex Mett.) J. Sm. 164
Dryobalanops aromatica 214
Dryobalanops aromatica C.F. Gaertn. 214
Dryobalanops sumatrensis (J.F. Gmel.) Kosterm. 214
Dryodon erinaceus (Bull.) P. Karst. 207
Dryopteris crassirhizoma Nakai 299
Dryopteris filix-mas (L.) Schott 299
Dunaliella bardawil Ben-Amotz et Avron 148
Dunaliella salina (Dunal) Teodor. 148

E

Echinacea angustifolia DC. 59
Echinacea pallida (Nutt.) Nutt. 59
Echinacea purpurea (L.) Moench 59
Echinodorus macrophyllus (Kunth) Micheli 113
Echinodorus macrophyllus ssp. *scaber* (Rataj) R.R. Haynes

et Holm-Niels. 113

Eclipta alba L. Hassk. 138

Eclipta erecta L. 138

Eclipta prostrata (L.) L. 138

Eisenia bicyclis (Kjellman) Setch. 46

Elasmobranchii Bonaparte 231, 232

Eleginus gracilis Tilesius 228

Elettaria cardamomum (L.) Maton var. *cardamomum* 116

Elettaria cardamomum (L.) var. *miniscula* Burkill 116

Elettaria cardamomum L. var. *minus* Watt 116

Eleusine coracana (L.) Gaertn. 110

Eleutherococcus giraldii (Harms) Nakai 95

Eleutherococcus gracilistylus (W.W. Sm.) S.Y. Hu 55, 96

Eleutherococcus henryi Oliv. 96

Eleutherococcus senticosus (Rupr. et Maxim.) Maxim. 59, 96

Eleutherococcus sessiliflorus (Rupr. et Maxim.) S.Y. Hu 96

Eleutherococcus verticillatus (G. Hoo) H. Ohashi 96

Elfvingia applanata (Pers.) P. Karst. 99

Elfvingiella fomentaria (L.) Murrill 146

Elsholtzia ciliata (Thunb.) Hyl. 94

Elymus repens (L.) Gould. 112

Elytrigia repens (L.) Desv. ex B.D. Jackson 112

Embelia ribes Burm. f. 61

Emblica officinalis Gaertn. 210

Engelhardtia chrysolepis Hance 94

Engraulis japonica Houttuyn 224

Engraulis japonicus Temminck et Schlegel 224, 229

Ephedra equisetina Bunge 338

Ephedra intermedia Schrenk et C.A. Mey. 338

Ephedra sinica Staph 338

Epilobium angustifolium L. 205

Epimedium grandiflorum C. Morr. var. *thunbergianum* Nakai 295

Epimedium koreanum Nakai 295

Epimedium sagittatum Maxim. 295

Epiphyllum oxypetalum (DC.) Haw. 92

Equisetum arvense L. 120

Equisetum hyemale L. 341

Equus asinus L. 223

Equus caballus × *Equus asinus* 223

Equus caballus L. 350

Equus caballus L. 224, 232, 235

Erica vulgaris L. 81

Erigeron annuus (L.) Pers. 177

Erigeron breviscapus (Vant.) Hand.-Mazz. 141

Eriobotrya japonica (Thunb.) Lindl. 179

Erysimum officinale L. 69

Erythraea centaurium Pers. 132

Erythrina crista-galli L. 67

Erythrina indica Lam. 300

Erythrina orientalis (L.) Merr. 300

Erythrina parcellii W. Bull 300

Erythrina pulcherrima Tod. 67

Erythrina variegata L. 300

Erythrina variegata var. *orientalis* (L.) Merr. 300

Erythroxylum catuaba A.J. Silva ex Raym.-Hamet 70

Eschscholzia californica Cham. 169

Etrumeus teres DeKay 224, 229

Eucalyptus globulus Labill. 208

Eucommia ulmoides Oliv. 153, 328

Eugenia aromatica (L.) Baill. nom. illeg. 89, 143

Eugenia caryophyllata Thunb. 89, 143

Eugenia caryophyllus (Spreng.) Bullock et S.G. Harrison 89, 144

Eugenia cumini (L.) Druce 183, 198

Eugenia jambolana Lam. 183, 198

Eugenia michelii Lam. 139

Eugenia obtusifolia Roxb. 183, 198

Eugenia uniflora L. 139

Euodia bodinieri Dode 309

Euodia officinalis Dode 309

Euodia ruticarpa (A. Juss) Hook. f. et Thomson 309

Euonymus alatus (Thunb.) Sieb. 158

Euonymus alatus (Thunb.) Sieb. f. *alatus* 158

Eupatorium fortunei Turcz. 343

Eupatorium japonicum Thunb. 343

Eupatorium rebaudianum Bertoni 120

Euphoria longana Lam. 213

Euphoria longan (Lour.) Steud. 213

Euphoria nephelium DC. 213

Euphrasia officinalis L. 37, 97

Euphrasia rostkoviana F. Hayne 37, 97

Euphrasia stricta J.P. Wolff ex J.F. Lehm. 37, 97

Eupolyphaga sinensis Walker 232

Euryale ferox Salisb. 66

Eurycoma longifolia Jack 154

Evernia prunastri (L.) Ach. 145

Evodia bodinieri Dode 309

Evodia officinalis Dode 309

Evodia rutaecarpa Benth. 309

F

Fagara mantchurica 50

Fagara schinifolium (Seib. et Zucc.) Engl. 50

Fagopyrum esculentum Moench 134

Fagopyrum esulentum 134
Fagopyrum multiflorum (Thunb.) I. Grint. 301
Fagopyrum sagittatum Gilib. 134
Fagopyrum tataricum (L.) Gaertn. 139
Fagopyrum vulgare Nees 134
Fallopia multiflora (Thunb.) Haraldson 146, 301
Fatsia papyrifera Benth. et Hook. f. 144
Felis tigris Pock 348
Ficus awkeotsang Makino 37
Ficus belgia hort. 100
Ficus carica L. 49
Ficus elastica Roxb. ex Hornem 100
Ficus pumila L. 63
Ficus religiosa 54
Ficus religiosa L. 54
Ficus repense hort. non Willd. nec Rottl. 63
Ficus rubra hort. non Roth 100
Filipendula ulmaria (L.) Maxim. 126
Firmiana plantanifolia (L. f.) Schott et Endl. 37
Firmiana simplex (L.) W.F. Wight 37
Flammulina velutipes (Curtis : Fr.) Singer 60
Foeniculum officinale All. 55
Foeniculum vulgare Mill. 55
Fomes applanatus (Pers.) Gillet 99
Fomes fomentarius (L.) J. Kickx f. 146
Fomes obliquus (Ach. ex Pers.) Cooke 71
Fordia cauliflora Hemsl. 69
Forsythia suspensa (Thunb.) Vahl 217, 344
Forsythia viridissima Lindl. 344
Fortunella japonica (Thunb.) Swingle 82
Fortunella margarita (Lour.) Swingle 82
Fortunella Swingle 82
Fragaria vesca L. 59
Frangula alnus Mill. 335
Frangula purshiana (DC.) J.G. Cooper 301
Fraxinus excelsior L. 126
Fraxinus japonica 37
Fraxinus japonica Bl. 38
Fraxinus lanuginosa 37
Fraxinus lanuginosa Koidz. 38
Fraxinus mandshurica Rupr. 204
Fraxinus mandshurica Rupr. var. *japonica* Maxim. 204
Fritillaria thunbergii Miq. 330
Fritillaria verticillata Willd. var. *thunbergii* (Miq.) Baker 330
Fucus distichus ssp. *evanescens* (C. Agardh) H.T. Powell 175
Fucus evanescens C. Agardh 175
Fucus vesiculosus L. 175
Fuscoporia obliqua (Ach. ex Pers.) Aoshima 71

G

Gadus macrocephalus Tilesius 228
Galanthus elwesii Hook. f. 342
Galanthus L. 342
Galanthus nivalis L. 342
Galega officinalis L. 74
Galeola septentrionalis Reichb. f. 145
Galium odoratum (L.) Scop. 88
Gallus gallus L. 225, 228, 235, 237
Ganoderma applanatum (Pers.) Pat. 99
Ganoderma lucidum (Curtis) P. Karst. 216
Ganoderma lucidum (Leyss. ex Fr.) Karst. 216
Ganoderma neo-japonicum Imazeki 216
Garcinia cambogia (Gaertn.) Desr. 74
Garcinia mangostana 195
Garcinia mangostana L. 196
Gardenia augusta Merr. 106
Gardenia florida L. 106
Gardenia grandiflora Lour. 106
Gardenia jasminoides f. *grandiflora* (Lour.) Makino 106
Gardenia jasminoides J. Ellis 106
Gastrochilus pandulatus (Roxb.) Ridl. 87
Gastrodia elata Blume 325
Gaylussacia Kunth 167
Gekko gecko 225
Gekko gecko L. 225
Gekko japonicus 234
Gekko japonicus Schlegel 234
Gelidium amansii (J.V. Lamouroux) J.V. Lamouroux 148
Gelidium subcostatum Okamura 148
Gelsemium elegans (Gardener et Champ.) Benth. 308
Gelsemium sempervirens (L.) J. St.-Hil. 303
Gentiana lutea L. 94, 307
Gentiana manshurica Kitag. 343
Gentiana scabra Bunge 343
Gentiana scabra Bunge var. *buergeri* (Miq.) Maxim. ex Franch. et Sav. 343
Gentiana triflora Pall. 343
Gentiana triflora Pall. var. *japonica* (Kusn.) H. Hara 343
Gentianella alborosea (Gilg) Fabris 60
Geranium nepalense var. *thunbergii* (Sieb. ex Lindl. et Paxton) Kudo 307
Geranium thunbergii Sieb. ex Lindl. et Paxton 307
Geum japonicum Thunb. 136
Ginkgo biloba L. 50
Glechoma grandis (A. Gray) Kuprian. 218
Glechoma hederacea L. ssp. *grandis* (A. Gray) H. Hara

218
Glechoma hederacea L. var. *grandis* (A. Gray) Kudo 218
Gleditsia japonica Miq. 102
Gleditsia sinensis Lam. 102
Glehnia littoralis Fr. Schm. ex Miq. 171
Gloydius blomhoffii Boie 233, 237
Gloydius halys Pallas 237
Glycine abrus L. 321
Glycine apios L. 45
Glycine gracilis Skvortsov 155
Glycine max (L.) Merr. 136, 155
Glycyrrhiza glabra L. 75
Glycyrrhiza glandulifera Waldst. et Kit. 75
Glycyrrhiza uralensis Fisch. ex DC. 75
Gnaphalium affine D. Don 170
Gnaphalium angustifolium Lam. 187
Gnaphalium luteoalbum L. ssp. *affine* (D. Don) Koster 170
Gonostemon gordonii Sweet 179
Gossypium herbaceum L. 200
Gossypium hirsutum L. 200
Gossypium L. 200
Graptopsaltria nigrofuscata Motshulsky 349
Griffonia simplicifolia (Vahl ex DC.) Baill. 306
Grifola albicans Imaz. 192
Grifola frondosa (Dicks. : Fr.) S.F. Gray 192
Grifola umbellata (Pers. : Fr.) Pilát 325
Guaiacum officinale L. 84
Gymnadenia conopsea (L.) R. Br. 147
Gymnema sylvestre (Retz.) R. Br. ex Schult. 79, 180
Gynostemma pentaphyllum (Thunb.) Makino 44

H

Haematoxylon campechianum L. 172
Haematoxylum campechianum L. 172
Haliotis discus hannai Ino 224
Haliotis discus Reeve 224
Haliotis diversicolor Reeve 224
Haliotis gigantea Gmelin 224
Haliotis madaka Habe 224
Hamamelis virginiana 171
Hamamelis virginiana L. 171
Hansenia forbessi (H. Boissieu) Pimenov et Kljuykov 304
Hansenia weberbaueriana (Fedde ex H. Wolff) Pimenov et Kljuykov 304
Harpagophytum procumbens (Burch.) DC. ex Meisn. 148
Hedychium coronarium J. König 168
Hedyotis diffusa Willd. 181
Hedyotis hedyotidea (DC.) Morr. 80
Hedysarum japonicum Basin. 217
Helianthus annuus L. 176
Helianthus tuberosus L. 77
Helichrysum angustifolium (Lam.) DC. 187
Helichrysum angustifolium ssp. *italicum* (Roth) Briq. et Cavill. 187
Helichrysum italicum (Roth) G. Don 187
Helichrysum serotinum Boiss 187
Hemerocallis fulva L. var. *kwanso* Regel 82
Hemidesmus indicus (L.) W.T. Aiton 294
Hepatica nobilis 335
Hepatica nobilis Schreb. 335
Hepatica nobilis Schreb. var. *japonica* Nakai 335
Hericium erinaceum (Bull. : Fr.) Pers. 207
Hericium erinaceus (Bull.) Pers. 207
Herniaria glabra L. 187
Herpestis monniera (L.) Kunth 65
Herpetica alata (L.) Raf. 169
Hibiscus chinensis Hort., p.p., non Roxb. 163
Hibiscus japonicus Miq. 154
Hibiscus manihot L. 154
Hibiscus rosa-sinensis L. 163, 182
Hibiscus sabdariffa L. 163
Hibiscus simplex L. 37
Hieracium japonicum Franch. et Sav. 189
Hieracium pilosella L. 189
Hierodula patellifera Serv. 233
Hippocampus coronatus Temminck et Schlegel 226
Hippocampus histrix Kaup 226
Hippocampus kelloggi Jordan et Snyder 226
Hippocampus kuda Bleeker 226
Hippocampus trimaculatus Leach 226
Hippophae rhamnoides L. 102, 103
Hirneola auricula-judae (Bull. : Fr.) Berk. 77
Hirudo nipponica Whitman 236
Holboellia cuneata Oliv. 135
Homo sapiens L. 347, 348, 350
Hoodia gordonii (Masson) Sweet ex Decne. 179
Hordeum sativum Jessen 64
Hordeum vulgare 64
Hordeum vulgare L. 64, 164
Hordeum vulgare L. var. *distichon* (L.) Hook. f. 164
Hordeum vulgare L. var. *hexastichon* Aschers. 164
Houttuynia cordata Thunb. 115
Hovenia acerba Lindl. 76
Hovenia dulcis Thunb. 76
Humulus lupulus L. 191
Huperzia serrata (Thunb.) Rothm. 132
Hydnum erinaceus Bull. 207

Hydrangea angustipetala Hayata 203
Hydrangea aspara ssp. *strigosa* 203
Hydrangea grosseserrata Engl. 203
Hydrangea hortensis Sm. 41
Hydrangea macrophylla Seringe var. *oamacha* Makino 44
Hydrangea macrophylla Seringe var. *thunbergii* Makino 44
Hydrangea macrophylla (Thunb. ex J. Murr.) Ser. f. *macrophylla* 41
Hydrangea serrata Seringe var. *thunbergii* Sugimoto 44
Hydrangea serrata (Thunb. ex Murray) Ser. var. *thumbergii* (Sieb.) H. Ohba 203
Hydrastis canadensis L. 308
Hydrocotyle asiatica L. 145
Hymenaea courbaril L. 115
Hyoscyamus L. 333
Hyoscyamus niger L. 333
Hypericum erectum Thunb. 65
Hypericum patulum Thunb. 82
Hypericum perforatum L. 124
Hyptis suaveolens (L.) Poit. 115
Hyriopsis cumingii 236
Hyriopsis cumingii Lea 236
Hyriopsis goliath Rolle 236
Hyssopus officinalis L. 175

I

Ilex aquifolium L. 128
Ilex cornuta Lindl. ex Paxt. 173
Ilex kudingcha C.J. Tseng 141
Ilex latifolia Thunb. 141
Ilex paraguariensis A. St.-Hil. 194
Illicium anisatum L. 313
Illicium japonicum Sieb. et Masam. 313
Illicium religiosum Sieb. et Zucc. 313
Illicium verum Hook. f. 135
Impatiens balsamina L. 188, 336
Imperata cylindrica (L.) P. Beauv. 336
Imperata cylindrica (L.) P. Beauv. var. *koenigii* (Retz.) Durand et Schinz 336
Imperata cylindrica (L.) P. Beauv. var. *major* (Nees) C.E. Hubb. 336
Imperatoria ostruthia L. 54
Incarvillea sinensis 300
Incarvillea sinensis Lam. 300
Indosasa crassiflora McClure 148
Inonotus linteus (Berk. et M.A. Curtis) Teixeira 198
Inonotus obliquus (Ach. ex Pers.) Pilát 71
Inula britannica L. ssp. *japonica* (Thunb.) Kitam. 320
Inula britannica var. *japonica* (Thunb.) Franch. et Sav. 320
Inula helenium L. 328
Ipomoea cairica (L.) Sweet 201
Ipomoea heptaphylla Voigt 201
Ipomoea nil (L.) Roth 40, 307
Ipomoea palmata Forssk. 201
Ipomoea pulchella Roth 201
Ipomoea purga (Wender.) Hayne 342
Ipomoea turpethum (L.) R. Br. 66
Iris florentina L. 294
Iris germanica L. var. *florentina* Dykes 294
Irvingia barteri Hook. f. 43
Irvingia gabonensis (Aubry-Lecomt ex O'Rorke) Baill. 43
Isatis canescens DC. 117
Isatis indigotica Fortune 117
Isatis littoralis Stev. 117
Isatis taurica Bieb. 117
Isatis tinctoria L. 117
Isodon japonica (Burm. f.) H. Hara 61
Isodon rubescens (Hemsl.) Hara 327
Isonandra gutta Hook. f. 86
Ixeris stolonifera A. Gray 52

J

Janipha manihot (L.) Kunth 79
Japonasarum caulescens (Maxim.) Nakai 335
Jasminum grandiflorum L. 114
Jasminum officinale f. *affine* (Royle ex Lindl.) Rehd. 114
Jasminum officinale f. *grandiflorum* (L.) Kobuski 114
Jasminum sambac (L.) Ait. 114
Jateorhiza columba Miers 310
Jatropha curcas L. 157
Jatropha manihot L. 79
Juglans cinerea L. 166
Juglans mandshurica Maxim. 105
Juglans nigra L. 89
Juglans orientis Dode 69
Juglans regia L. 69
Juglans regia var. *orientis* (Dode) Kitam. 69
Juncus decipiens (Buchenau) Nakai 47, 327
Juncus effusus 47, 327
Juncus effusus L. 47, 327
Juncus effusus L. var. *decipiens* Buchenau 47, 327
Juniperus communis L. 127
Juniperus rigida Sieb. et Zucc. 152
Juniperus sabina L. 312
Jussiaea suffruticosa auct. non L. 78

Justicia nasuta L.　167

K

Kaempferia galanga L.　108
Kaempferia pandurata Roxb.　87
Kaempferia parviflora Wall. ex Baker　183
Kaempferia parviflora　183
Kaempferia rubromarginata (S.Q. Tong) R.J. Searle　183
Katsuwonus pelamis L.　227
Kerria japonica (L.) DC.　206
Kochia scoparia (L.) Schrad.　112
Kochia scoparia (L.) Schrad. var. *littorea* (Makino) Kitam.　112
Kochia scoparia (L.) Schrad. var. *trichophylla* (Stapf) Bailey　112
Krameria lappacea (Dombey) Burdet et B.B. Simpson　343
Krameria triandra Ruiz et Pav.　343

L

Lablab niger Medik.　188
Lablab purpureus (L.) Sweet　53, 188
Laccocephalum mylittae (Cooke et Massee) Núñez et Ryvarden　210
Lachesis okinavensis Boulenger　235
Lactobacillus acidophilus　41
Lactobacillus Beijerinck　158
Lactuca virosa L.　219
Lagenaria leucantha Rusby　177
Lagenaria leucantha Rusby var. *depressa* (Ser.) Makino　180
Lagenaria leucantha Rusby var. *gourda* Makino　177
Lagenaria leucantha var. *clavata* Makino　207
Lagenaria siceraria (Molina) Standl.　207
Lagenaria siceraria (Molina) Standl. var. *gourda* (Ser.) Hara　177
Lagenaria siceraria (Molina) Standl. var. *siceraria*　177
Lagenaria siceraria (Molina) Standl. var. *depressa* (Ser.) Hara　180
Lagenaria siceraria var. *clavata* Ser.　207
Lagenaria siceraria var. *hispida* (Thunb.) Hara　207
Lagenaria vulgaris Ser.　177
Lagenaria vulgaris Ser. var. *depressa* Ser.　180
Lagerstroemia flos-reginae Retz.　168
Lagerstroemia speciosa (L.) Pers.　168
Lamium album L. var. *barbatum* (Sieb. et Zucc.) Fr. et Sav.　66
Lamium barbatum Sieb. et Zucc.　66
Languas galanga (L.) Stuntz　156
Languas speciosa (J.C. Wendl.) Small　93
Lappa edulis Sieb. ex Miq., nom. inval.　99
Lappa major Gaertn.　99, 310
Lappa officinalis All.　310
Lathyrus japonicus Willd.　218
Lathyrus quinquenervius (Miq.) Litv.　218
Laticauda colubrina Schneider　236
Laticauda semifasciata Reinwardt　236　236
Laurus camphora L.　86, 116
Laurus nobilis L.　93
Laurus persea L.　44
Laurus sassafras L.　104
Laurus sumatrensis J.F. Gmel.　214
Lavandula × intermedia Emeric ex Loisel.　213
Lavandula angustifolia Mill.　213
Lavandula dentata L.　213
Lavandula L.　213
Lavandula latifolia Medik.　213
Lavandula stoechas L.　213
Lawsonia alba Lam.　110
Lawsonia inermis L.　110
Ledebouriella seseloides auct. non (Hoffm.) H. Wolf　337
Ledum groenlandicum Oeder　88
Ledum latifolium Jacq.　88
Lentinula edodes (Berk.) Pegler　109
Lentinus edodes (Berk.) Singer　109
Leontopodium alpinum　58
Leontopodium alpinum Cass.　58
Leontopodium nivale (Ten.) Huet ex Hand.-Mazz. ssp. *alpinum* (Cass.) Greuter　58
Leonurus artemisia (Lour.) S.Y. Hu　216
Leonurus cardiaca L.　216
Leonurus heterophyllus Sweet　216
Leonurus japonicus Houtt.　216, 342
Leonurus sibiricus auct. non L.　216
Leonurus sibiricus L.　216, 342
Leo tigris Elite　348
Lepidium meyenii Walp.　193
Lepidium peruvianum G. Chacón de Popovici　193
Lepiota shiitake (J. Schroet.) Nobuj.　109
Leptandra virginica (L.) Nutt.　184
Lethenteron camtschaticum Tilesius　225
Lethenteron japonicum Martens　225
Leucaena glauca (L.) Benth.　83
Leucaena leucocephala (Lam.) De Wit　83
Levisticum officinale W.D.J. Koch　219
Ligusticum acutiloba Sieb. et Zucc.　150
Ligusticum chuanxiong Hort.　131, 319
Ligusticum ibukiense Yabe　131, 319

Ligusticum jeholense (Nakai et Kitag.) Nakai et Kitag. 308
Ligusticum sinense Oliv. 308
Ligustrum expansum Rehder 109
Ligustrum Iucidum 159
Ligustrum japonicum 159
Ligustrum japonicum Thunb. 159
Ligustrum lucidum W.T. Aiton 159
Ligustrum purpurascens Y.C. Yang. 109
Ligustrum robustum ssp. *chinense* P.S. Green 109
Ligustrum thibeticum Decne. 109
Lilium brownii F.E. Br. ex Miellez 209
Lilium brownii F.E. Br. ex Miellez var. *viridulum* Baker 209
Lilium lancifolium Thunb. 209
Lilium pumilum DC. 209
Limonium wrightii (Hance) O. Kuntze 48
Limonium wrightii (Hance) O. Kuntze f. *arbusculum* (Maxim.) Hatusima 48
Limonum wrightii (Hance) O. Kuntze var. *wrightii* 48
Lindera aggregata (Sims) Kosterm. 58, 295
Lindera hypoglauca Maxim. 56
Lindera obtusa Franch. et Sav. 56
Lindera strychnifolia (Sieb. et Zucc.) F. Vill. 58, 295
Lindera umbellata Thunb. 56
Linum usitatissimum L. 44
Lippia citriodora (Ort. ex Pers.) H.B.K. 188
Liquidambar orientalis Mill. 134
Liriope muscari Bailey 331
Liriope spicata Lour. 331
Litchi chinensis Sonn. 216
Lithocarpus polystachyus (Wall. ex A. DC.) Rehder 149
Lithospermum erythrorhizon Sieb. et Zucc. 314
Lobelia chinensis Lour. 340
Lobelia inflata L. 344
Lobelia sessilifolia Lamb. 312
Lonicera japonica Thunb. 82
Lophanthus rugosus Fisch. et C.A. Mey. 301, 303
Lophatherum gracile Brongn. 141
Lotus corniculatus L. var. *japonicus* Regel 197
Ludwigia octovalvis (Jacq.) P.H. Raven var. *sessiliflora* (Micheli) Shinners 78
Luffa aegyptiaca Mill. 186
Luffa cylindrica auct. non. M.J. Roem. 186
Luffa cylindrica (L.) M. Roem. 186
Lycium barbarum L. 85, 314
Lycium chinense Mill. 85, 314
Lycopersicon esculentum Mill. 153
Lycopersicon lycopersicum (L.) H. Karst., nom. rej. 153
Lycopodium clavatum L. 118
Lycopodium clavatum L. var. *nipponicum* Nakai 118
Lycopodium serratum Thunb. 132
Lycoris radiata (L'Hér.) Herb. 318
Lygodium japonicum 70
Lygodium japonicum (Thunb. ex Murr.) Sw. 70
Lysimachia christiniae Hance 83
Lysimachia japonica Thunb. ex Murray 98
Lythrum anceps (Koehne) Makino 196
Lythrum salicaria L. ssp. *anceps* (Kohene) H. Hara 196
Lythrum virgatum Miq. non L. 196

M

Macrocarpium officinale (Sieb. et Zucc.) Nakai 107
Macropiper excelsum 303
Macropiper excelsum (G. Forst.) Miq. 303
Magnolia biondii Pamp. 316
Magnolia denudata Desr. 316
Magnolia heptapeta (Buc'hoz) Dandy 316
Magnolia hypoleuca Sieb. et Zucc. 308
Magnolia kobus DC. 316
Magnolia obovata Thunb. 308
Magnolia officinalis Rehd. et E.H. Wils. 308
Magnolia officinalis Rehd. et E.H. Wils. var. *biloba* Rehd. et E.H. Wils. 308
Magnolia salicifolia (Sieb. et Zucc.) Maxim. 316
Magnolia sprengeri Pamp. 316
Mahonia aquifolium (Pursh) Nutt. 173
Majorana hortensis Moench 194
Mallotus japonicus (Thunb.) Müll. Arg. 39
Mallotus philippensis (Lam.) Müll. Arg. 305
Malpighia emarginata Sésse et Moç. ex DC. 42
Malpighia glabra L. 42
Malpighia punicifolia L. 42
Malus domestica Borkh. 215
Malus japonica Andr. 189
Malus pumila Mill. 215
Malus pumila Mill. var. *domestica* (Borkh.) C.K. Schneid. 215
Malva mauritiana L. 56, 130
Malva neglecta Wallr. 56, 130
Malva sylvestris L. 56, 130
Malva sylvestris L. var. *mauritiana* (L.) Boiss. 56, 130
Malva verticillata L. 49, 150
Mammalia L. 234
Mandragora L. 339
Mandragora officinarum L. 339
Mangifera indica L. 195
Mangifera mekongensis anon. 195

Manihot esculenta Crantz.　79
Manihot utilissima Pohl.　79
Manina crispa Scop.　169
Mantis religiosa L.　233
Maranta galanga L.　156
Margaritifera margaritifera L.　234
Marrubium vulgare L.　195
Marsdenia cundurango Rchb. f.　310
Masseola crispa (Wulfen) Kuntze　169
Matricaria chamomilla L.　72
Matricaria parthenium L.　155
Matricaria recutita L.　72
Matricaria suaveolens L.　72
Maytenus boaria Mol.　192
Maytenus chilensis DC.　192
Medicago sativa L.　46
Melaleuca alternifolia (Maiden et Betche) Cheel　199
Melastoma dodecandrum Lour.　110
Melia azedarach　132, 320
Melia azedarach L.　132, 320, 327
Melia azedarach var. *azedarach*　132
Melia azedarach var. *japonica* (G. Don) Makino　132
Melia dubia Cav.　132
Melia japonica G. Don　132
Melia toosendan　327
Melia toosendan Sieb. et Zucc.　132, 320, 327
Melilotus officinalis (L.) Pall.　123
Melilotus suaveolens Ledeb.　123
Melissa officinalis L.　200
Mentha×piperita L.　127
Mentha arvensis L. var. *piperascens* Malinv. ex Holmes　167
Mentha canadensis L.　167
Mentha haplocalyx Briq.　167
Mentha haplocalyx Briq. var. *piperascens* (Malinv.) Wu et Li　167
Mentha L.　197
Mentha longifolia auct. non (L.) Huds.　121
Mentha nilaca auct. non Juss. et Jacq.　121
Mentha pulegium L.　198
Mentha rotundifolia auct. non (L.) Huds.　43
Mentha roundifolia Hudson (Lamiac.)　43
Mentha spicata L.　121
Mentha suaveolens Ehrh.　43
Mentha viridis L.　121
Menyanthes trifoliata L.　317
Mertensia pterocarpa (Turcz.) Tatew. et Ohwi　142
Mesobuthus martensii Karsch　230
Mesona chinensis Benth.　132
Mesona procumbens Hemsl.　132
Mespilus japonica Thunb.　179
Metroxylon rumphii (Willd.) Mart.　103
Metroxylon sagu Rottb.　103
Mikania amara Willd.　84
Mikania guaco Humb. et Bonpl.　84
Millettia cauliflora (Hemsl.) Gagnep.　69
Millettia dielsiana Harms ex Diels　91
Millettia reticulata Benth.　91
Milobalanus embilica Burn.　210
Mimosa catechu L. f.　185
Mimosa glauca L.　83
Mimosa nemu Poir.　161
Mimosa senegal L.　45
Momordica charantia　157
Momordica charantia L.　157
Momordica charantia L. var. *pavel* Crantz.　157
Momordica cochinchinensis (Lour.) K. Spreng.　341
Momordica cylindrica L.　186
Momordica grosvenorii Swingle　211
Momordica luffa L.　186
Monarda fistulosa L.　204
Monascus albidus K. Sato　186
Monascus anka K. Sato　186
Monascus major K. Sato　186
Monascus purpureus Went.　186
Monascus rubiginosus K. Sato　186
Monascus vini Savul. et Hulea　186
Monothylaceum gordonii G. Don　179
Morella cerifera (L.) Small　118
Morella rubra Lour.　207
Morinda citrifolia L.　203
Morinda officinalis F.C. How　331
Morus alba L.　90, 195, 322
Morus alba L. var. *stylosa* Bur.　195
Morus atropurpurea Roxb.　90
Morus australis Poir.　195
Morus bombycis Koidz.　195
Morus japonica Bailey non. Sieb.　195
Moschus moschiferus L.　348
Mosla chinensis Maxim.　129
Mucuna birdwoodiana Tutcher　91
Mucuna pruriens (L.) DC. var. *utilis* (Wall ex Wight) Burk.　168
Musa acuminata Colla　168
Musa basjoo Sieb. et Zucc.　166
Myrcia multiflora (Lam.) DC.　75
Myrciaria dubia (Kunth) McVaugh　72
Myrcia sphaerocarpa DC.　75

Myrica carolinensis Mill. 118
Myrica cerifera L. 118
Myrica rubra 207
Myrica rubra Sieb. et Zucc. 207
Myristica aromatica Lam. 158
Myristica fragrans Houtt. 158
Myristica moschata Thunb. 158
Myristica officinalis L. f. 158
Myrtus cumini L. 183, 198
Mytilus viridis L. 237

N

Naja naja L. 230
Naja philippinensis Taylor 230
Nakaiomyces nipponicus Kobayashi 118
Nandina domestica Thunb. 329
Nandina domestica Thunb. f. *leucocarpa* Makino 329
Nardostachys chinensis Batalin 303
Nardostachys jatamansi (Jones ex Roxb.) DC. 303
Nasturtium armoracia (L.) Fr. 219
Nelumbium nelumbo (L.) Drucc 166
Nelumbium speciosum Willd. 166
Nelumbo nucifera Gaertn. 166
Neopicrorhiza sacrophulariiflora (Pennell) D.Y. Hong 96
Nepeta cataria L. 51
Nepeta tenuifolia Benth. 306
Nephelium lappaceum L. 213
Nephelium litchi Cambess. 216
Nephelium longana (Lam.) Camb. 213
Nephelium longan (Lour.) Hook. 213
Nerium indicum Mill. 81
Nerium odorum Sol. 81
Nerium oleander L. var. *indicum* (Mill.) Degener et Greenwell 81
Nicotiana rustica L. 339
Nigella damascena L. 182
Nigella indica Roxb. ex Flem. 182
Nigella sativa L. 182
Notopterygium forbesii H. Boissieu 304
Notopterygium incisum K.C. Ting ex H.T. Chang 304
Nuphar japonicum DC. 95, 319
Nyctanthes arbor-tristis L. 54
Nymphaea nelumbo L. 166

O

Ocimum aristatum Bl. 87
Ocimum basilicum L. 199
Ocimum basilicum var. *glabratum* Benth. 199
Ocimum basilicum var. *majus* Benth. 199
Ocimum frutescens L. 110
Ocimum spiralis (Lour.) Merr. 87
Ocimum stamineus Benth. 87
Oenothera biennis L. 199
Oenothera erythrosepala Borb. 199
Oenothera lamarckiana de Vries non Ser. 199
Oenothera odorata Jacq. 199
Oenothera stricta Ledeb. ex Link 199
Oenothera tetraptera Cav. 145
Oldenlandia diffusa (Willd.) Roxb. 181
Oldenlandia hedyotidea (DC.) Hand.-Mazz. 80
Olea europaea L. 67
Olea sativa Hoffmanns. et Link 67
Omphalia lapidescens Schroet. 210
Onagra biennis (L.) Scop. 199
Ononis campestris W.D.J. Koch et Ziz 299
Ononis spinosa L. 299
Onopordon acanthium L. 64
Operculina turpethum (L.) Silva Manso 66
Ophelia japonica (Schult.) Griseb. 321
Ophelia pseudochinensis (Hara) Toyokuni 198
Ophiopogon japonicus (L. f.) Ker Gawl. 331
Ophiopogon ohwii Okuyama 331
Opisthoplatia orientalis Burmeister 232
Opuntia ficus-indica (L.) Mill. 56
Opuntia ficus-indica (L.) Mill. var. *saboten* Makino 56
Origanum dubium Boiss. 194
Origanum majorana L. 194
Ormenis nobilis (L.) J. Gay ex Coss. et Germ. 219
Orobanche coerulescens 134
Orobanche coerulescens Steph. 134
Orthosiphon aristatus (Bl.) Miq. 87
Oryza sativa L. 51, 90, 94, 100, 101
Osmanthus fragrans Lour. var. *aurantiacus* Makino 84
Ostrea gigas Thunb. 227
Otaria ursinus Gray 347
Otoes ursinus L. 347
Ovis aries L. 224, 233
Ovophis okinavensis Boulenger 235
Oxycoccus macrocarpus (Ait.) Pers. 88

P

Pachyma hoelen Rumph. 334
Padus grayana (Maxim.) C.K. Schneid. 58
Paeonia albiflora Pall. 114, 315
Paeonia arborea Donn ex K. Koch 190
Paeonia lactiflora Pall. 114, 315
Paeonia moutan Sims 190, 337
Paeonia suffruticosa Andr. 190, 337

Paeonia veitchii Lynch 114, 315
Pagophilus groenlandicus Erxleben 223
Palaquium gutta (Hook. f.) Baill. 86
Panax bipinnatifidus Seem. 176
Panax ginseng C.A. Mey. 65
Panax japonicus (T. Nees) C.A. Mey. 324
Panax notoginseng (Burkill) F.H. Chen ex C.Y. Wu et K.M. Feng 107
Panax pseudoginseng Wall. ssp. *himalaicus* H. Hara 176
Panax pseudoginseng Wall. var. *bipinnatifidus* (Seem.) Li. 176
Panax pseudoginseng Wall. var. *japonicus* (C.A. Mey.) G. Hoo et C.J. Tseng 324
Panax pseudoginseng Wall. var. *notoginseng* (Burkill) G. Hoo et C.J. Tseng 107
Panax quinquefolium 45
Panax quinquefolius L. 45
Panax schinseng T. Nees 65
Pandanus odoratissimus L. f., nom illeg. 113
Pandanus tectorius Parkins. ex Zucc. 113
Pandanus tectorius var. *liukiuensis* Warb. 113
Pandanus veitchii hort. Veitch ex M.T. Mast. et T. Moore 113
Panthera tigris L. 224, 348
Papaver rhoeas L. 175
Papaver somniferum L. 92, 306
Papeda rumphii Hassk. 185
Paratenodera sinensis Saussure 233
Parietaria diffusa Mert. et W.D.J. Koch 174
Parietaria judaica L. 174
Parietaria micrantha Ledeb. 174
Parsonia balsamona (Cham. et Schlecht.) Arth. 161
Passiflora caerulea L. 152
Passiflora edulis Sims 152
Passiflora incarnata L. 143, 152
Passiflora trifasciata Lem. 152
Patiria pectinifera Müller et Troschel 226
Patrinia scabiosaefolia 66
Patrinia scabiosaefolia Fisch. ex Trevir. 67
Paullinia cupana Kunth 73
Pausinystalia johimbe (K. Schum.) Pierre ex Beille 342
Peganum harmala L. 332
Pelargonium reniforme Curt. 296
Pelargonium sidoides DC. 296
Pelodiscus sinensis Wiegmann 232
Penthorum chinense 138
Penthorum chinense Pursh 138
Perilla frutescens (L.) Britt. var. *acuta* Kudo 110
Perilla frutescens (L.) Britt. var. *crispa* (Thunb.) Deane 110
Perilla frutescens (L.) Britt. var. *crispa* (Thunb.) Deane f. crispa (Thunb.) Makino 110
Perilla frutescens (L.) Britt. var. *frutescens* 110
Perilla frutescens (L.) Britt. var. *japonica* Hara 110
Periploca indica L. 294
Perna viridis L. 237
Persea americana Mill. 44
Persea gratissima Gaertn. 44
Persicaria tinctoria (Lour.) H. Gross 140
Persica vulgaris 202
Petroselinum crispum (Mill.) Nym. ex A.W. Hill 166
Petroselinum hortense Hoffm. 166
Petroselinum sativum Hoffm. 166
Peucedanum decursivum (Miq.) Maxim. 319
Peucedanum japonicum 190
Peucedanum japonicum Thunb. 190
Peucedanum ostruthium (L.) W.D.J. Koch 54
Peucedanum praeruptorum Dunn 319
Peumus boldus Molina 191
Pfaffia glomerata (Spreng.) Pedersen 121
Pfaffia paniculata (Mart.) Kuntze 121
Phalacroloma annuum (L.) Dumort. 177
Phallus indusiatus Vent. 78
Pharbitis nil (L.) Choisy 40, 307
Phaseolus max L. 136, 155
Phaseolus radiatus L. 214
Phaseolus radiatus L. var. *aurea* Prain 42
Phaseolus vulgaris L. 53
Phellinus linteus (Berk. et M.A. Curtis) Teng 198
Phellinus obliquus (Ach. ex Pers.) Pat. 71
Phellodendron amurense Rupr. 63, 298
Phellodendron amurense Rupr. var. *sachalinense* F. Schmidt 298
Phellodendron chinense C.K. Schneid. 298
Phellopteris littoralis Benth. 171
Pheretima asiatica Michaelsen 349
Pheretima aspergillum E. Perrier 349
Phlebodium aureum (L.) J. Sm. 191
Phlebodium decumanum (Willd.) J. Sm. 191
Phoca groenlandica Erxleben 223
Phoca vitulina L. 223, 347
Phoenix dactylifera L. 155
Photinia serrulata Lindl. 319
Phragmites australis (Cav.) Trin. ex Steud. 41, 344
Phragmites communis Trin. 41, 344
Phyllanthus amarus Schumach. 78
Phyllanthus emblica L. 210
Phyllanthus niruri auct. non L. 78

Phyllanthus niruri L. 78
Phyllanthus niruri L. ssp. *amarus* (Schumach.) Leandri 78
Phyllanthus urinaria L. 100
Phyllostachys bambusoides Sieb. et Zucc. 148, 324
Phyllostachys henonis Bean 142
Phyllostachys heterocycla (Carr.) Mitf. 138
Phyllostachys heterocycla var. *pubescens* (Mazel) Ohwi 138
Phyllostachys nigra (Lodd.) Munro var. *henonis* (Bean) Stapf 142
Phyllostachys nigra Munro var. *henonis* Stapf ex Rendl. 324
Phyllostachys pubescens Mazel 138
Phyllostachys Sieb. et Zucc. 138
Physalis L. 337
Physalis pruinosa L. 117
Physkium natans Lour. 129
Physostigma venenosum Balf. 302
Phytolacca acinosa Roxb. 316
Phytolacca esculenta 316
Phytolacca esculenta Van Houtte 316
Phytolacca javanica Osbeck 202
Picrasma ailanthoides (Bunge) Planch. 329
Picrasma quassioides (D. Don) Benn. 329
Picrorhiza kurrooa 96
Picrorhiza kurrooa Royle ex Benth. 96
Picrorhiza scrophulariaeflora 96
Picrorhiza scrophulariiflora Pennell 96
Pilocarpus jaborandi Holmes 342
Pilocarpus microphyllus Staph ex Wardleworth 342
Pilocarpus pennatifolius Lem. 342
Pimpinella anisum L. 43
Pinctada fucata martensii Dunker 233
Pinctada margaritifera L. 234
Pinellia ternata (Thunb.) Makino ex Breitenb. 332
Pinus bungeana Zucc. ex Endl. 165
Pinus L. 99, 194
Pinus maritima Poir. 184
Pinus pinaster Ait. 184
Pinus strobus L. 120
Piper aduncum L. 193
Piper angustifolium Ruiz et Pav. 193
Piper betle L. 83
Piper celtidifolium Kunth 193
Piper elongatum Vahl 193
Piper futokadsura Sieb. 179
Piper kadsura (Choisy) Ohwi 179
Piper longum L. 54
Piper methysticum G. Forst. 302
Piper nigrum L. 97
Piper officinalm 115
Piper retrofractum Vahl 115
Piper sarmentosum Roxb. 162
Pisum maritimum L. 218
Placodes fomentarius (L.) Quél. 146
Planchonella obovata (R. Br.) Pierre 39
Plantago asiatica L. 64
Plantago ispaghula Roxb. ex Fleming 184
Plantago lanceolata L. 187
Plantago major L. 124
Plantago ovata Forssk. 184
Plantago psyllium L. 184
Platycladus orientalis (L.) Franco 134, 330
Platycodon grandiflorum (Jacq.) A. DC. 76
Plectogyne elatior hort. 171
Plectogyne variegata Link. 172
Plectranthus barbatus Andrews 73
Plectranthus trichocarpus Maxim. 61
Pleuropterus cordatus Turcz. 146, 301
Pleuropterus cuspidatus (Sieb. et Zucc.) Gross 48
Pleuropterus multiflorus (Thunb.) Turcz. ex Nakai 146
Pleurotus citrinopileatus Singer 140
Pleurotus cornucopiae citrinopileatus (Singer) O. Hilber 140
Pleurotus cornucopiae var. *citrinopileatus* (Singer) Ohira 140
Pleurotus eryngii var. *ferulae* (Lanzi) Sacc. 40
Podophyllum hexandrum Royle 338
Podophyllum L. 338
Podophyllum peltatum L. 338
Pogostemon cablin (Blanco) Benth. 301
Pogostemon patchouly Pellet. 301
Poinciana coriaria Jacq. 121
Polygala senega L. 319
Polygala senega L. var. *latifolia* Torrey et Gray 319
Polygala tenuifolia Willd. 300
Polygonatum cyrtonema Hua 62
Polygonatum falcatum A. Gray 62
Polygonatum kingianum Collett et Hemsl. 62
Polygonatum odoratum (Mill.) Druce 48
Polygonatum odoratum (Mill.) Durce var. *pluriflorum* (Miq.) Ohwi 48
Polygonatum officinale All. 48
Polygonatum sibiricum F. Delara. ex Redout. 62
Polygonum aviculare L. 196
Polygonum cuspidatum Sieb. et Zucc. 48, 309
Polygonum fagopyrum L. 134

Polygonum multiflorum Thunb. 146, 301
Polygonum tinctorium Lour. 140
Polymnia edulis Wedd. 203
Polymnia sonchifolia Poepp. et Endl. 203
Polypodium aureum L. 191
Polypodium leucatomos Poir. 191
Polypodium leucotomos 191
Polyporus applanatus (Pers.) Wall. 99
Polyporus frondosus (Dicks. : Fr.) Fr. 192
Polyporus mylittae Cooke et Massee 210
Polyporus obliquus (Ach. ex Pers.) Fr. 71
Polyporus umbellatus (Pers.) Fr. 325
Polyrhachis vicina Roger 223
Poncirus trifoliata 73
Poncirus trifoliata (L.) Rafin. 73
Pongamia glabra Vent. 90
Pongamia pinnata (L.) Pierre 90
Poria cocos (Fr.) Wolf 334
Poria versicolor (L.) Scop. 74
Portulaca oleracea L. 165
Potentilla anserina 338
Potentilla anserina L. 338
Potentilla erecta (L.) Raeusch. 151
Potentilla tormentilla Stokes 151
Poterium officinale (L.) A. Gray 220
Pouteria obovata (R. Br.) Baehni 39
Premna odorata Blanco 45
Primula officinalis Hill. 125
Primula sieboldii E. Morren 103
Primula veris L. 125
Prinsepia uniflora Batal. 119
Prionace glauca L. 231
Prunella vulgaris L. ssp. *asiatica* (Nakai) Hara 300
Prunella vulgaris L. var. *lilacina* Nakai 300
Prunus armeniaca L. 75, 305
Prunus armeniaca L. var. *ansu* Maxim. 75, 305
Prunus avium (L.) L. 128
Prunus davidiana (Carrière) Franch. 327
Prunus domestica L. 125
Prunus grayana Maxim. 58
Prunus humilis Bunge 48
Prunus jamasakura Sieb. ex Koidz. 298
Prunus japonica Thunb. 48
Prunus mume Sieb. et Zucc 57
Prunus persica (L.) Batsch. 202, 327
Prunus persica (L.) Batsch var. *davidiana* (Carrière) Maxim. 327
Prunus persica var. *persica* 202
Prunus persica var. *vulgaris* (Mill.) Maxim. 202
Prunus serotina Ehrh. 219
Prunus sibirica L. 75, 305
Prunus verecunda (Koidz.) Koehne 298
Prunus vulgaris Mill. 202, 327
Pseuderanthemum connatum Lindau 167
Pseudocydonia sinensis (Thouin) C.K. Schnied. 201
Pseudognaphalium affine (D. Don) Anderb. 170
Pseudognaphalium luteoalbum (L.) Hillard et B.L. Burtt ssp. *affine* (D. Don) Hillard et B.L. Burtt 170
Pseudomonas Migula 230
Pseudostellaria heterophylla (Miq.) Pax ex Pax et Hoffm. 136
Pseudotaxus chienii (W.C. Cheng) W.C. Cheng 164, 331
Psidium guajava L. 84
Psidium pomiferum L. 84
Psidium pyriferum L. 84
Psoralea corylifolia L. 189
Pteris multifida Poir. 336
Pterocarpus indicus 111
Pterocarpus indicus Willd. 111
Ptychopetalum olacoides Benth. 197, 340
Ptychopetalum uncinatum Anselmino 197, 340
Pueraria candollei var. *mirifica* (Airy Shaw et Suvat.) Niyomdham 68, 179
Pueraria lobata (Willd.) Ohwi 86, 302
Pueraria mirifica Airy Shaw et Suvatab. 68, 179
Pueraria montana (Lour.) Merr. 137
Pueraria montana (Lour.) Merr. var. *chinense* Maesen et S.M. Almeida 137
Pueraria montana (Lour.) Merr. var. *lobata* (Willd.) Maesen et S.M. Almeida ex Sanjappa et Predeep 86, 137, 302
Pueraria thomsonii Benth. 137
Pueraria thunbergiana (Sieb. et Zucc.) Benth. 86
Pueraria triloba (Houtt.) Makino 86
Pulsatilla chinensis (Bunge) Regel 330
Punica granatum 103
Punica granatum L. 103
Pyrethrum coccineum (Willd.) Voroch. 39
Pyrethrum parthenium Sm. 155
Pyrola asarifolia Michx. ssp. *asarifolia* 49
Pyrolaceae japonica 49
Pyrola incarnata Fisch. var. *japonica* (Klenze) Koidz. 49
Pyrola japonica Klenze 49
Pyrola rotundifolia L. 49
Pyrola rotundifolia ssp. *asarifolia* (Michx.) A. et G. Löve 49
Pyrrosia grandisimus 129
Pyrrosia hastata 129

Pyrrosia hastata (Thunb.) Ching 129
Pyrrosia lingua 129
Pyrrosia lingua (Thunb.) Farw. 129
Pyrrosia pelislosus 129
Pyrrosia tricuspis (Swartz) Tagawa 129
Pyrus japonica Thunb. 85
Pyrus pumila (Mill.) K. Koch 215

Q

Quercus acutissima Carruth. 316
Quercus infectoria Olivier 201
Quercus lusitanica Lamarck 201
Quercus mongolica Fisch. ex Ledeb. 316
Quercus salicina Bl. 58
Quercus serrata Murray 316
Quercus stenophylla Makino 58
Quercus variabilis Blume 316
Quisqualis indica L. 109

R

Rabdosia japonica (Burm. f.) H. Hara 61
Rabdosia rubescens (Hemsl.) Hara 327
Rabdosia trichocarpa (Maxim.) H. Hara 61
Radicula armoracia (L.) B.L. Rob. 219
Rajania quinata Thunb. ex Houtt. 40
Rana amurensis Boulenger 229
Rana chensinensis David 229
Rana temporaria chinensis 229
Rangifer tarandus L. 231
Rangium suspensum (Thunb.) Ohwi 217
Ranunculus japonicus Thunb. 57
Raphanus sativus L. 211
Raphanus sativus L. var. *hortensis* Backer f. *acanthiformis* Makino 211
Raphanus sativus L. var. *longipinnatus* L.H. Bailey 211
Rauvolfia L. 295
Rauvolfia serpentina (L.) Benth. ex Kurz 295
Rauvolfia vomitoria Afzel. 295
Ravensara aromatica J.F. Gmel. 212
Rehmannia glutinosa (Gaertn.) Libosch. ex Fisch. et C.A. Mey. 313
Rehmannia glutinosa Libosch. var. *purprea* Makino 313
Rehmannia glutinosa var. *huechingensis* Chao et Shih 313
Reptilia Laurenti 234
Reynoutria japonica Houtt. 48, 309
Reynoutria multiflora (Thunb.) Moldenko 301
Rhamnus frangula L. 335
Rhamnus L. 306
Rhamnus purshiana DC. 301
Rheum coreanum Nakai 322
Rheum L. 135
Rheum officinale Baill. 135, 322
Rheum palmatum L. 135, 322
Rheum palmatum L. var. *tanguticum* Maxim. ex Regel 135
Rheum rhabarbarum L. 117, 135
Rheum rhaponticum hort. non L. 117
Rheum rhaponticum L. 135
Rheum tanguticum Maxim. ex Balf. 322
Rheum undulatum L. 117
Rhinacanthus communis Nees 167
Rhinacanthus nasutus (L.) Kurz 167
Rhinoceros sinensis Owen 351
Rhodiola rosea L. 53
Rhododendron degronianum Carr. 319
Rhus chinensis Mill. 121, 160
Rhus cismontana Greene 211
Rhus coriaria L. 121
Rhus glabra L. 211
Rhus glabra var. *cismontana* (Greene) Cockerell 211
Rhus japonica L. 121, 160
Rhus javanica 160
Rhus javanica L. 121, 160
Rhus trichocarpa Miq. 206
Ribes ambiguum Maxim. 204
Ribes formosana Hayata var. *sinanense* (F. Maek.) Kitam. 120
Ribes grossularia L. 120
Ribes nigrum L. 69, 89
Ribes sinanense F. Maek. 120
Ribes uva-crispa L. 120
Ricinus communis L. 332
Rohdea japonica (Thunb.) Roth 299
Rorippa armoracia (L.) Hitchc. 219
Rosa canina L. 153, 218
Rosa davurica Pall. 206
Rosa ferox Lawrance 170
Rosa hirtula (Regel) Nakai 107
Rosa kamtschatica Vent. var. *ferox* (Lawrance) Geel 170
Rosa L. 171
Rosa lutetiana Léman 218
Rosa multiflora Thunb. ex Murray 296
Rosa roxburghii Tratt. 118
Rosa roxburghii Tratt. var. *hirtula* (Regel) Rehder et E.H. Wilson 107
Rosa rugosa Thunb. 170
Rosa rugosa var. *ferox* (Lawrance) C.A. Mey. 170
Rosa rugosa var. *thunbergiana* C.A. Mey. 170

Rosmarinus officinalis L. 218
Rosmarinus officinalis var. *prostratus* hort. 218
Rottlera tinctoria Roxb. 305
Rubia akane Nakai 320
Rubia cordifolia L. 320
Rubia tinctorum L. 123
Rubus allegheniensis T.C. Porter 183
Rubus argutus Link 183
Rubus chingii Hu 334
Rubus coreanus 153
Rubus coreanus Miq. 153
Rubus fruticosus L. 124, 183
Rubus idaeus L. 124, 212
Rubus L. 76
Rubus laciniatus Willd. 183
Rubus officinalis Koidz. 334
Rubus strigosus Michx. 124, 212
Rubus suavissimus S.K. Lee 149
Rubus tokkura Sieb. 153
Rubus ulmiformis Schott 183
Rubus ursinus Cham. et Schlecht. 183
Rudbeckia laciniata L. 64
Rumex acetosa L. 119
Rumex acetosella L. 119
Rumex crispus L. 209
Rumex crispus L. ssp. *crispus* 209
Rumex crispus L. ssp. *japonicus* (Houtt.) Kitam. 209
Rumex japonicus Houtt. 209
Rumex nepalensis Spreng. var. *andreaenus* (Makino) Kitam. 79
Rusa timorensis de Blainville 231
Rusa unicolor Kerr 231
Ruscus aculeatus L. 154
Ruta graveolens L. 188

S

Sabal serrulata (Michx.) Nutt. ex Schult. et Schult. f. 162
Saccharomyces Meyen 95
Saccharum officinarum L. 75
Saiga tatarica L. 351
Salacia chinensis L. 105
Salacia oblonga Wall. 105
Salacia prinoides (Willd.) DC. 105
Salacia reticulata Wight 104
Salicornia europaea L. 43
Salicornia herbacea L. 43
Salix alba L. 125
Salix alba L. ssp. *vitellina* (L.) Schübl. et G. Martens 205
Salix alba L. var. *vitellina* (L.) Stokes 205
Salix aurea Salisb. 125
Salix vitellina L. 205
Salsola komarovii Iljin 65
Salvia apiana Jeps. 192
Salvia hispanica L. 141
Salvia miltiorrhiza Bunge 141, 323
Salvia officinalis L. 105
Salvia sclarea 66
Salvia sclarea L. 66
Sambucus ebulus L. 209
Sambucus nigra L. 127
Sambucus racemosa L. ssp. *sieboldiana* (Miq.) Hara 130
Sambucus sieboldiana Blume ex Graebn. 130
Sambucus williamsii Hance 130
Samyda parviflora L. 305
Sanguisorba officialis 220
Sanguisorba officinalis L. 220
Sanguisorba polygama F. Nyl. 220
Santalum album L. 333
Sapindus mukorossi Gaertn. 197
Saponaria officinalis L. 104
Saposhnikovia divaricata (Turcz.) Schischk. 337
Sarcandra glabra (Thunb.) Nakai 80, 133
Sardinops melanostictus Temminck et Schlegel 224, 229
Sardinops sagax Jenyns 224, 229
Sargentodoxa cuneata (Oliv.) Rehd. et Wils. 135
Sarothamnus scoparius (L.) Wimm. ex W.D.J. Koch 60, 296
Sasa albo-marginata Makino et Shibata 86
Sasa kurilensis (Rupr.) Makino et Shibata 142
Sasa veitchii (Carr.) Rehd. 86
Sassafras albidum (Nutt.) Nees 104
Sassafras officinale T. Nees et C.H. Eberm. 104
Sassafras variifolium O. Kuntze 104
Satureja hortensis L. 78
Satureja laxiflora C. Koch 78
Satureja pachyphylla C. Koch 78
Saururus chinensis (Lour.) Baill. 173
Saussurea costus (Falc.) Lipsh. 341
Saussurea involucrata (Kar. et Kir.) Sch. Bip. 130
Saussurea laniceps Hand.-Mazz. 130
Saussurea lappa (Decne.) C.B. Clarke 341
Saussurea medusa Maxim. 130
Scandix cerefolium L. 143
Scaphium affine Pierre 173
Scaphium scaphigerum (G. Don) Guib. 173
Scaphium wallichii Schott et Endl. 173
Schisandra chinensis (Turcz.) Baill. 310
Schizonepeta tenuifolia (Benth.) Briq. 306

Schotia simplicifolia Vahl ex DC. 306
Scilla maritima L. 300
Scindalma lipsiense (Batsch) Kuntze 99
Scirpus fluviatilis auct. non (Torr.) A. Gray 55
Scirpus maritimus auct. non L. 55
Scirpus yagara Ohwi 55
Scoparia dulcis L. 122
Scoparia temata Forsk. 122
Scopolia carniolica Jacq. 331
Scopolia Jacq. 331
Scopolia japonica Maxim. 331
Scopolia parviflora (Dunn) Nakai 331
Scrophularia ningpoensis Hemsl. 307
Scutellaria baicalensis Georgi 62, 298
Scutellaria barbata D. Don 173
Scutellaria lateriflora L. 119, 317
seaweed (Gelidiaceae) 148
Secale cereale L. 211
Secale cereale L. ssp. *cereale* 211
Sedum aizoon L. 82
Sedum aizoon var. *floribundum* Nakai 82
Sedum kamtschaticum auct. non Fisch. 82
Sedum roseum (L.) Scop. 53
Sedum sarmentosum Bunge 147
Selenarctos thibetanus Cuvier 350
Selinum monnieri L. 315
Senecio aurantiacus var. *spathulatus* Miq. 64
Senecio fauriei Lev. et Vant. 64
Senecio integrifolius (L.) Clairv. ssp. *fauriei* (Lev. et Vant.) Kitam. 64
Senecio integrifolius var. *spathulatus* (Miq.) Hara 64
Senecio scandens Buch.-Ham. ex D. Don 133
Senecio wightianus DC. ex Wight 133
Senna alata (L.) Roxb. 169
Senna alexandrina Mill. 133, 320
Senna angustifolia (Vahl) Batka 133
Senna auriculata (L.) Roxb. 302
Senna obtusifolia (L.) H.S. Irwin et Barnedy 60
Senna occidentalis (L.) Link. 170
Senna siamea H.S. Irwin et Barneby 138
Sepia esculenta Hoyle 224
Serenoa repens (W. Bartram) Small 162
Serenoa serrulata (Michx.) G. Nichols 162
Serpentes L. 224, 233
Sesamum indicum L. 100
Sesamum orientale L. 100
Sida cordifolia L. 297
Sida mysorensis Wight et Arn. 297
Sida rhombifolia L. 297
Siegesbeckia orientalis 199
Siegesbeckia orientalis L. ssp. *pubescens* (Makino) Kitam ex H. Koyama 199
Siegesbeckia pubescens (Makino) Makino 199
Siesbeckia pubescens 199
Silybum marianum (L.) Gaertn. 194
Simmondsia californica Nutt. 191
Simmondsia chinensis (Link) C.K. Schneid. 191
Sinapis erysimoides Roxb. 89
Sinomenium acutum (Thunb.) Rehder et E.H. Wilson 336
Siphonostegia chinensis 213
Siphonostegia chinensis Benth. 213
Siraitia grosvenorii (Swingle) C. Jeffrey ex A.M. Lu et Zhi Y. Zhang 211
Sisymbrium officinale (L.) Scop. 69
Smallanthus sonchifolius (Poepp. et Endl.) H. Rob. 203
Smilax china L. 312
Smilax glabra 106, 312
Smilax glabra Roxb. 106, 312
Smilax L. 109
Solanum dulcamara L. 122
Solanum dulcamara var. *lyratum* (Thunb.) Sieb. et Zucc. 178
Solanum dulcamara var. *pubescens* Blume 178
Solanum incertum Dunal. 51
Solanum lycopersicum L. 153
Solanum lyratum Thunb. 178
Solanum muricatum 186
Solanum muricatum L'Hér. ex Ait. 187
Solanum nigrum L. 51
Solanum paniculatum L. 116
Solanum rubrum auct. non L. 51
Solanum tuberosum L. 172
Solegnathus hardwickii Gray 227
Solenognathus hardwickii Gray 227
Solidago japonica Kitam. 40
Solidago virgaurea L. ssp. *asiatica* Kitam. ex H. Hara 40
Solidago virgaurea var. *asiatica* Nakai 40
Sonchus oleraceus L. 162
Sophora flavescens Aiton 305
Sophora japonica L. 61, 297
Sophora subprostrata Chun et T.C. Chen 313
Sophora tonkinensis Gagnep. 313
Sorbus commixta Hedl. 156
Sorbus commixta Hedl. var. *sachalinensis* Koidz. 156
Soya max (L.) Piper 155
Sparassis crispa (Wulfen) Fr. 169
Sparassis latifolia Y.C. Dai et Zheng Wang 169

Spartium scoparium L. 60, 296
Spatholobus suberectus Dunn 91
Spiraea ulmaria L. 126
Spirulina maxima (Setchell et Gardener) Geitler 120
Spirulina P. Fischer 120
Spirulina platensis (Gomont) Geitler 120
Squalus acanthias L. 232
Stahlianthus rubromarginatus S.Q. Tong 183
Stapelia gordonii Masson 179
Statilia maculata Thunb. 233
Steccherinum quercinum Gray 207
Stegodon orientalis Owen 351
Stellaria alsine Grim. var. *undulata* (Thunb.) Ohwi 114
Stellaria media (L.) Vill. 165
Stemona japonica (Blume) Miq. 333
Stemona sessilifolia (Miq.) Franch. et Sav. 333
Stemona tuberosa Lour. 333
Stenactis annuus (L.) Cass. 177
Stephania tetranda 314
Stephania tetrandra S. Moore 314
Sterculia lychnophora Hance 173
Sterculia nitida Vent. 96
Sterculia scaphigera Wall. ex G. Don 173
Stevia rebaudiana (Bertoni) Hemsl. 120
Streptococcus Rosenback 158
Strobilanthes cusia (Nees) Kuntze 214
Strobilanthes flaccidifolia Nees 214
Strophanthus caudatus Kurz 305
Strophanthus divaricatus (Lour.) Hook. et Arn. 305
Strophanthus gratus (Wall. et Hook. ex Benth) Baill. 305
Strophanthus hispidus DC. 305
Strophanthus kombe Oliv. 305
Strychnos L. 339
Strychnos nux-vomica L. 339
Styphnolobium japonicum (L.) Schott 61
Styrax benzoin Dryand. 47
Sus scrofa domesticus Gray 350
Sus scrofa L. 224, 228, 229, 233
Swertia japonica Makino 321
Swertia japonica (Schult.) Makino 321
Swertia pseudochinensis H. Hara 198
Symphytum officinale L. 102
Syngnathoides biaculeatus Bloch 226
Syngnathus acus L. 227
Syzygium aromaticum (L.) Merr. et L.M. Perry 89, 143
Syzygium cumini 198
Syzygium cumini (L.) Skeels 183, 198
Syzygium jambolana (Lam.) DC. 183, 198

T

Tabanus amaenus Walker 350
Tabanus cordiger Meigen 350
Tabanus trigonus Coquillett 350
Tabebuia avellanedae Lorentz et Griseb. 54, 140, 163
Tabebuia heptaphylla (Vell.) Toledo 54, 140, 163
Tabebuia impetiginosa (Mart. ex DC.) Standl. 54, 140, 163
Takifugu porphyreus Temminck et Schlegel 236
Tamarix chinensis Lour. 81
Tanacetum boreale Fisch. ex DC. 210
Tanacetum parthenium (L.) Sch. Bip. 155
Tanacetum vulgare L. 210
Tanaceum coccineum (Willd) Grieson 39
Taraxacum dens-leonis Desf. 126, 189
Taraxacum japonicum Koidz. 189
Taraxacum officinale Weber ex F.H. Wigg. 126, 189
Taraxacum platycarpum Dahlst. 189
Taraxacum vulgare (Lam.) Schrank 126, 189
Taraxacum Weber 189
Taxus baccata ssp. *cuspida* (Sieb. et Zucc.) Pilg. 49
Taxus baccata var. *microcarpa* Trautv. 49
Taxus cuspidata Sieb. et Zucc. 49, 293
Taxus nucifera L. 174
Taxus sieboldii hort. 49
Taxus wallichiana Zucc. var. *wallichiana* 164, 331
Taxus yunnanensis W.C. Cheng et L.K. Fu 164, 331
Tecoma impetiginosa Mart. ex DC. 54, 140, 163
Tenodera sinensis Saussure 233
Tephroseris integrifolia (L.) Holub ssp. *kirilowii* (Turcz. ex DC.) B. Nord. 64
Terminalia bellerica (Gaertn.) Roxb. 123, 135
Terminalia bellirica 135
Terminalia bellirica (Gaertn.) Roxb. 122, 135
Terminalia catappa L. 202
Terminalia chebula Retz. 301
Testudines L. 228
Tetradapa javanorum Osbeck 300
Tetragonia expansa Thunb. ex J. Murr. 146
Tetragonia tetragonoides (Pall.) O. Kuntze 146
Tetrapanax papyrifera (Hook.) K. Koch 144
Tetrapanax papyrifer (Hook.) K. Koch 144
Tetrapanax papyriferum (Hook.) K. Koch 144
Tetrapanax papyriferus (Hook.) K. Koch 144
Thamnolia vermicularis (Sw.) Ach. ex Schaer 208
Thea sinensis L. 142, 164
Theragra chalcogramma Pallas 228
Thladiantha grosvenorii (Swingle) C. Jeffrey 211

Thuja orientalis L. 134, 330
Thujopsis dolabrata (L.f.) Sieb. et Zucc. 42
Thujopsis dolabrata (L.f.) Sieb. et Zucc. var. *hondae* Makino 42
Thymus × citriodorus (Pers.) Schreb. ex Schweigg et Körte 217
Thymus quinquecostatus Celak. 51, 131
Thymus serpyllum L. 51, 131
Thymus serpyllum L. ssp. *citriodorum* Pers. 217
Thymus serpyllum L. ssp. *quinquecostatus* (Celak.) Kitam. 51, 131
Thymus vulgaris L. 139
Tilia × europaea L. 125, 147
Tilia × intermedia DC. 147
Tilia × vulgaris Hayne 125, 147
Tilia cordata Mill. 190
Tilia grandifolia Ehrh. 190
Tilia intermedia DC. 125
Tilia japonica (Miq.) Simonk 112
Tilia miqueliana Maxim. 190
Tilia parvifolia Ehrh. 190
Tilia platyphyllos Scop. 190
Tilia ulmifolia Scop. 190
Tinospora cordifolia 324
Tinospora cordifolia (Willd.) Miers ex Hook. f. et Thoms. 324
Tinospora crispa 51
Tinospora crispa (L.) Hook. f. et Thoms. 51
Tinospora rumphii Boerl. 52
Tinospora tuberculata (Lam.) Hayne 51
Tithonia diversifolia (Hemsl.) A. Gray 158
Toddalia asiatica (L.) Lam. 312
Torilis japonica (Houtt.) DC. 315
Torilis scabra (Thunb.) DC. 315
Torreya grandis Forst. 174
Torreya nucifera (L.) Sieb. et Zucc. 174
Torula utilis Henneberg 95
Torula utilis (Henneberg) Lodder 95
Toxicodendron trichocarpum (Miq.) Kuntze 206
Trachelospermum jasminoides (Lindl.) Lem. 137
Trachomitum venetum (L.) Woodson 212
Trachycarpus excelsus (Thunb.) H. Wendl. 116
Trachycarpus excelsus var. *typicus* Makino 116
Trachycarpus fortunei (Hook.) H. Wendl. 116
Trametes versicolor (L.) Lloyd 74, 303
Trapa bispinosa Roxb. var. *iinumai* Nakano 174
Trapa incisa Sieb et Zucc. 174
Trapa japonica Flerow 174
Trapa japonica Flerow var. *rubeola* (Makino) Ohwi 174
Trapa natans L. 174
Trapa natans L. var. *rubeola* Makino 174
Tremella fuciformis Berk. 118
Tremella lutescens Pers. 97
Tremella mesenterica (Schaeff.) Retz. 97
Tremella quercina Pollini 97
Trianosperma tayuya (Vell.) Mart. 323
Tribulus terrestris L. 314
Tricholoma matsutake (S. Ito et S. Imai) Singer 194
Tricholoma shiitake (J. Schroet.) Lloyd. 109
Trichosanthes bracteata Voigt 74, 302
Trichosanthes japonica Regel. 74
Trichosanthes kirilowii Maxim. 74, 302
Trichosanthes kirilowii Maxim. var. *japonica* (Miq.) Kitam. 74, 302
Trifolium pratense L. 38
Trigonella foenum-graecum L. 101
Trimeresurus okinavensis Boulenger 235
Triticum aestivum L. 100
Triticum aestivum ssp. *vulgare* (Vill.) Mac Key 88, 100
Triticum repens L. 112
Triticum sativum L. 88
Triticum vulgare Vill. 88, 100
Trocostigma polygama Sieb. et Zucc. 200
Trogopterus xanthipes Milne-Edwards 348
Tropaeolum majus L. 84
Tulipa edulis (Miq.) Bak. 44
Turnera diffusa Willd. ex Schult. 323
Turnera microphylla Ham. 323
Tussilago farfara L. 180, 304
Typha angustata Bory et Chaub. 71, 337
Typha angustifolia L. 71, 337
Typha latifolia L. 71, 337

U

Ulmus davidiana Planch. var. *japonica* (Rehd.) Nakai 159
Ulmus fulva Michx. 39
Ulmus japonica (Rehd.) Sarg. 159
Ulmus parvifolia Jacq. 159
Ulmus rubla Muhl. 39
Uncaria gambir (W. Hunt.) Roxb. 42
Uncaria guianensis (Aubl.) J.F. Gmel. 80
Uncaria macrophylla Wall. 325
Uncaria rhynchophylla (Miq.) Jacks. 143, 325
Uncaria sinensis (Oliv.) Havil 143, 325
Uncaria tomentosa (Willd.) DC. 80
Ungulina fomentaria (L.) Pat. 146
Unio cumingii Lea 236
Uraria lagopodioides (L.) Desv. ex DC. 101

Urginea maritima (L.) Baker 300
Urginea scilla Steinh. 300
Urginea Steinh. 300
Urostachys serratus (Thunb.) Herter 132
Ursus arctos L. 350
Urtica dioica L. 123
Urtica dioica L. ssp. *dioica* 123
Urtica L. 52
Urtica thunbergiana Sieb. et Zucc. 52

V

Vaccinium angustifolium Ait. 185
Vaccinium australe Small 185
Vaccinium corymbosum L. 185
Vaccinium gaultherioides Bigelow 90
Vaccinium macrocarpon Ait. 88
Vaccinium myrtillus L. 128, 178
Vaccinium occidentale A. Gray 90
Vaccinium uliginosum L. 90
Vaccinium uliginosum L. ssp. *gaultherioides* (Bigelow) S.B. Young 90
Vaccinium uliginosum var. *alpinum* Bigelow 90
Vaccinium uliginosum var. *microphyllum* Lange 90
Vaccinium vitis-idaea L. 97, 309
Valeriana fauriei Briq. 70
Valeriana jatamansi Jones ex Roxb. 303
Valeriana officinalis L. 70
Valeriana sambucifolia var. *fauriei* (Briq.) Hara 70
Valerianella locusta (L.) Laterr. 192
Valerianella olitoria (L.) Pollich 192
Vallisneria asiatica Miki 129
Vallisneria denseserrulata Makino 129
Vallisneria gigantea Graebn. 129
Vallisneria natans (Lour.) Hara 129
Vallisneria spiralis L. 129
Varanidae Hardwicke et Gray 225
Veratrum album L. ssp. *oxysepalum* (Turcz.) Hult. 329
Veratrum L. 329
Veratrum maackii Regel var. *japonicum* (Baker) T. Shimizu 330
Veratrum stamineum Maxim. 329
Verbascum thapsus L. 178
Verbena × hortensis hort. Vilm. 174
Verbena × hybrida Voss 174
Verbena citriodora (Lam.) Cav. 188
Verbena officinalis L. 86
Verbena officinalis L. ssp. *officinalis* 86
Verbena triphylla L'Hér. 188
Veronica didyma Tenore var. *lilacina* (Hara) Yamazaki 50
Veronica miqueliana Nakai 91
Veronicastrum virginicum (L.) Farw. 184
Veronica virginica L. 184
Vespa mandarinia japonica Radoszkowski 235
Vespa simillima xanthoptera Cameron 235
Vespula flaviceps Smith 235
Viburnum macrophyllum Thunb. 41
Viburnum opulus f. *nanum* (I. David) Zabel 209
Viburnum opulus f. *xanthocarpum* (Endl.) Rehder 209
Viburnum opulus L. var. *opulus* 209
Vicia angustifolia L. 72
Vicia quinquenervia Miq. 218
Vicia sativa L. ssp. *nigra* (L.) Ehrh 72
Vigna angularis (Willd.) Ohwi et Ohashi 42
Vigna radiata (L.) R. Wilczek 214
Vinca minor L. 177
Vinca rosea L. 329
Viola × wittrockiana Hort. 106
Viola L. 121
Viola mandshurica W. Becker 111, 121
Viola odorata L. 121, 157
Viola tricolor L. 106, 121
Viola yedoensis Makino 111, 121
Viscum album L. 318
Viscum album L. var. *coloratum* (Komar.) Ohwi 318
Vitellaria paradoxa C.F. Gaertn. 108
Vitex agnus-castus L. 127
Vitex cannabifolia Sieb. et Zucc. 160
Vitex negundo L. var. *cannabifolia* (Sieb. et Zucc.) Hand.-Mazz. 160
Vitex negundo L. var. *negundo* 160 160
Vitex rotundifolia L. f. 339
Vitex trifolia L. 339
Vitis coignetiae Pulliat ex Planch. 207
Vitis L. 182
Vitis quadrangularis (L.) Wall. ex Wight et Arn. 314
Vitis vinifera L. 182
Viverra zibetha L. 348
Viverricula indica É. Geoffroy Saint-Hilaire 348

W

Wallia cinerea (L.) Alef. 166
Whitmania acranulata Whitman 236
Whitmania pigra Whitman 236
Wisteria brachybotrys Sieb. et Zucc. 334
Wisteria floribunda (Willd.) DC. 180, 334
Withania somnifera (L.) Dunal 295
Wolfiporia cocos (F.A. Wolf) Ryvarden et Gilb. 334

X

Xanthium strumarium L.　321

Y

Yucca gloriosa var. *recurvifolia* (Salisb.) Engelm.　208
Yucca gloriosa var. *tristis* Carrière　208
Yucca recurvifolia Salisb.　208

Z

Zanthoxylum americanum Mill.　45
Zanthoxylum bungeanum Maxim.　111
Zanthoxylum piperitum (L.) DC.　107
Zanthoxylum schinifolium Sieb. et Zucc.　50
Zea mays L.　151
Zingiber officinale Rosc.　116
Zizania aquatica auct. japon., non L.　193
Zizania caduciflora (Turcz.) Hand.-Mazz.　193
Zizania latifolia (Griseb.) Turcz. ex Stapf　193
Ziziphus jujuba Mill.　136
Ziziphus jujuba Mill. var. *inermis* (Bunge) Rehd.　136
Ziziphus jujuba Mill. var. *spinosa* (Bunge) Hu ex H.F. Chow　108
Ziziphus sativa Gaertn.　136
Ziziphus vulgaris Lam.　136
Ziziphus vulgaris Lam. var. *spinosa* Bunge　136
Ziziphus zizyphus (L.) H. Karst.　136

英名索引
English name index

A

Aaron's rod 40, 178
abalone 224
abata cola 96
absinthe 85
absinthe grande 85
Abyssinian tea 293
acerola 42
2-Acetamido-2-deoxy-D-glucose 246
Acetil acid 355
Acetildenafil 374
5-(5-Acetyl-2-ethoxyphenyl)-1,6-dihydro-1-methyl-3-propyl-7*H*-pyrazolo(4,3-*d*) pyrimidin-7-one 362
N-Acetyl-beta-D-glucosamine 246
N-Acetyl-D-glucosamine 246
N-Acetylglucosamine 246
N-acetyl-D-hexosaminides 252
N-Acetyl-5-methoxytryptamine 376
o-(Acetyloxy) benzoic acid 355
Acetylsalicylic acid 355
achyranthes 309
acidophilus 158
Aciglut 256
Aciletten 254
Aciport 254
aconite 329
acorus 315
Actinolite 376
Acylpyrin 355
Adam's flannel 178
adenophora 114
S-adenosyl-L-methionine 358
S-Adenosylmethionine 358
Adonitol 252
aduki bean 42
adzuki bean 42
aerial yam 63
Aeromatt 250
African baobab 164
African cucamber 157
African mango 43
African rue 332
African wild mango 43
Agalite 266
agar 148
agar-agar 148
agaricus 39
agar wood 317
Agedoite 241
ageratum 70
agnus-castus 127
agrimony 83, 124
Agstone 250
aguacate 44
aibika 154
Aildenafil 376
air potato 63
akebia 40, 341
Akoya pearl oyster 234
alagau 45
alagaw 45
alang-alang 336
(S)-Alanine 242
Alanine 242
L-(+)-Alanine 242
L-Alanine 242
L-alpha-Alanine 242
Alantin 245
Alant starch 245
Alaska pollock 229
Albolene 285
Albumin 242
alder 62, 130
alder buckthorn 335
alegria 188, 336
alehoof 218
Aleppo galls 201
Alert-pep 249
Alexandrian senna 133, 320
alfalfa 46
alga perlada 37
algaroba 50
algarroba bean 50
Ali's umbrella 154
Ali's walking stick 154
Allantoin 356
Allicin 242
alligator pear 44
dl, dl-Allo-cystathionine 261
DL-Allocystathionine 261
Alloin, Aloin 356
allo-Inositol 245
all-trans-beta-Carotene 280
all-trans-Retinol 273
all-trans-Xanthophyll 286
aloe 47
aloealoe 293
aloes wood 317
aloe vera 47, 293
Aloin A 356
Alphagloss 360
Alphalin 273
alpine cranberry 309
Alpine edelweisse 58
Alpine leek 80
Alpine strawberry 59
althaea 46
althea 46
Altheine 241
Aluminium silicate hydroxide 360
Aluminum silicate 360
Aluzime 259
Amalti syrup 250
amana 44
amaranth 122
amaranthus 122
amber 99
Ameircan agar 148
American bird cherry 219
American cranberry 88
American ginseng 45

American lovage 219
American mandrake 338
American plantain 124
American raspberry 124
American red raspberry 212
American silvertop 171
American wild cherry 219
American wormseed 46
N-Amidinosarcosine 257
Aminalon 251
Aminoacetic acid 254
((6R,12aR)-2-amino-6-(1,3-benzodioxol-5-yl)-2,3,6,7,12,12a-hexahydropyrazino(1',2':1,6)pyrido(3,4-*b*)indole-1,4-dione 355
4-Aminobutyric acid 251
gamma-Aminobutyric acid 251
N5-(Aminocarbonyl)ornithine 247
(S)-4-(2-Amino-2-carboxyethyl)imidazole 273
2-Amino-2-deoxy-D-glucosamine 255
2-Aminoethanesulfonic acid 364
Aminoethanoic acid 254
2-Aminoethylsulfonic acid 364
2-Amino-3-hydroxybutyric acid 269
2-Amino-3-hydroxypropionic acid 265
L-alpha-Aminoisocaproic acid 287
delta-Aminolevulinic acid phosphate 242
5-Aminolevulinic acid・phosphate 242
(S)-2-Amino-3-methylbutanoic acid 271
(S)-2-Amino-3-methylbutyric acid 271
2-Amino-3-methylbutyric acid 271
(S)-2-Amino-4-methylpentanoic acid 287
2-Amino-3-methylvaleric acid 244
5-Amino-4-oxopentanoic acid 242
(S)-2-Aminopropanoic acid 242
2-Aminopropionic acid 242
L-2-Aminopropionic acid 242
Amino tadalafil 355
Aminotadalafil 355
Aminutrin 284
amla 210
Amur adonis 334
Amur brown frog 229
Amur cork tree 63, 298
Amur rose 206
alpha-Amylase 356
Amylase 356
Ananas 373
Andaman redwood 111
andrographis 132
4-Androstene-3,17-dione 357
4-Androstenedione 357
Androst-4-ene-3,17-dione 357
Androstenedione 357
Androstenolone 367
Androtex 357
anemarrhena 324
Aneurin 274
angelica 41, 47
Angelica furcijuga 333
angelica tree 112, 140
angel's trumpet 324
Ang II 357
Angiotensin 357
Angiotensin II 357
angkak 186
ang-khak 186
Anhydrous citric acid 254
Anhydrous gypsum 264
anise 43
aniseed 43
anise magnolia 316
anis seed 43
annual fleabane 177
annual savory 78
annual wormwood 297
ansu apricot 305
ant 223
Anthocyanidin 243
Antiberiberi factor 274
antlers or velvet of caribou 231
antlers or velvet of fallow deer 231
antlers or velvet of reindeer 231
antlers or velvet of rusa deer 231
antlers or velvet of sambar 231
Apelagrin 270
apple 215
apple cider vinegar 215
apple mint 43
apple vinegar 215
apricot 75, 305
apricot seed (xingren) 75
apricot vine 143, 152
Arabian coffee 96
Arabian jasmine 114
Arabian tea 293
Arabino-Hexulose 249
aracaibo copaiba 99
Aragonite 250
arame 46
aramu 46
arcangel 47
archangel 66
arctic lamprey 225
arctic rose 53
areca nut 179, 322
areca nut palm 179
argaw 45
arjuna 202
arnica 293
aromatic Solomon's seal 48
aromoise 85
arrowleaf sida 297
arrow-leaf-sida 297
artichoke 144
artist's bracket 99
artist's conk 99
asatsuki 41
Ascoltin 275
Ascorbate 275
Ascorbic acid 275
L-Ascorbic acid 275
ash 126
ashwaganda 295
Asian bonnet bellflower 147
Asian clam 231
Asian flatsedge 72
Asian green mussel 237
Asian pigeon wings 144
Asian plantain 64
Asian psyllium 64
Asian trampsnail 227
Asian water plantain 323
Asian white birch 117
Asiatic cornel 107
Asiatic cornelian cherry 107
Asiatic day flower 146
Asiatic dogwood 107
Asiatic gingseng 65

Asiatic grass frog 229
Asiatic pennywort 145
Asiatic wood frog 229
Asparagic acid 241
L-Asparagic acid 241
(−)-Asparagine 241
(S)-Asparagine 241
Asparagine 241
L-Asparagine 241
Asparagine acid 241
Asparaginic acid 241
L-Asparaginic acid 241
asparagus roots 114
Asparamide 241
Aspartamic acid 241
(2S)-Aspartic acid 241
Aspartic acid 241
L-Aspartic acid 241
Aspatofort 241
Aspirin 355
H-Asp-OH 241
Assam indigo 214
Assam rubber 100
Assam tea 142
Astaxanthin 241, 281
Astaxanthine 241
Astomari 363
astragalus 298
astragarus 62
asunaro 42
aucklandia 341
Australian lemon myrtle 217
autumn crocus 294
avocado 44
awa 302
Axerophthol 273
Aztec tobacco 339

B

baby Jade 94
baby rose 296
baccharis trimera 73
bachelor's button 204
bacopa 65
bael fruit 187
bael tree 53
baheda 123, 135
bahera 123, 135
bahira 123, 135
bai bei niu wei cai 106
Baikal skullcap 62, 298
bai-zhu atractylodes 333
ba jiao hui xian 135
baker's garic 68
baker yeast 95
Balinese pepper 115
balloon flower 76
balm 200
balsam pear 157, 341
bamboo 138, 324
bamboo ginseng 324
bamboo shoot 138
banaba 168
banana 168
banda nutmeg 158
Banisterine 370
bank cress 69
bantam 225
baobab of Mahajanga 164
baphicacanthus cusia 214
barbados aloe 47, 293
Barbados cherry 42
Barbados nut 157
Barbaloin 356
barbary wolf berry 314
barbary wolfberry 85
barbat skullcap 173
barbed skullcap 173
barberry 128
barley 64, 164
barrenwort 295
barroom plant 172
basil 199
ba-sob 162
bastard cardamom 315
bastard saffron 186
Bauhinia divaricata 167
bay 93
bayberry 118, 207
bay laurel 93
bayo 53
bay tree 93
BD 370
BDD 370
bdellium tree 72
beach pea 218
beach silvertop 171
bead tree 132
bearberry 296, 301
bearded hedgehog mushroom 207
bearded tooth mushroom 207
bear's-head 207
bee balm 200
beebalm 204
beebread 215
beefsteak plant 110
Bee glue 280
beeplant 215
Bee propolis 280
beeswax 237
Beeswax acid 280
beet broomwart 122
Beflavin 274
beggar's ticks 98
begger's buttons 310
bei sha shen 171
Bejin gwenn 37
bel 53
belen 188, 336
beleric myrobalan 123, 135
belladonna 335
belleric myrobalan 123, 135
bellflower 76, 326
belliric myrobalan 123, 135
bell tree 187
belvedere 112
Belvedere broom goose foot 112
Bengal fruit 53, 187
Bengal madder 320
Bengal pepper 115
Bengal quince 53, 187
beni-koji (Japanese) 186
beni seed 100
Benjamin gum 47
Benjamin tree 47
Benzamidenafil 360
(6R,12aR)-6-(1,3-Benzodioxole-5-yl)-2,3,6,7,12,12a-hexahydro-2-methylpyrazino[1',2':1,6]pyrido[3,4-b]indole-1,4-dione 365
(6R,12aR)-6-(1,3-Benzodioxole-5-yl)-2,3,6,7,12,12a-hexahydro-2-octylpyrazino[1',2':1,6]pyrido[3,4-b]indole-1,4-dione 359
benzoin tree 47
Berubigen 274
Betaxin 274

betel 83
betel leaf pepper 83
betel nut 179
betelnut palm 179, 322
betel palm 322
betel palm nut 179
betel pepper 83
betel vine 83
Bewon 274
bezoar 350
Biamine 274
Bifendatatum 370
Bifendate 370
Bifidobacterium 176
Bifluoriden 279
bigarade 137
bigeye 229
bilberry 128, 178
bile 350
bilhitak 123, 135
bindweed 178
Bioflavonoid 286
Biotin 272
d-Biotin 272
BioZn-AAS 256
birch 111
bird cherry 128
bird's-foot-trefoil 197
Birthwort 295
Birutan 286
bis(D-Gluconato-kappaO1,kappaO2) Zinc 256
bis(3-Hydroxy-3-methylbutyrate) monohydrate(HMB) 273
bis(*p*-Acetoxyphenyl)cyclohexylidenemethane 363
bissy nut 96
bitter apple 310
bitter cardamon 341
bitter cassava 80
bitter cola 96
bitter cucumber 157, 310
bitter gourd 157, 310
bitter herb 132
bitter lettuce 219
bitter melon 157
bitter nightshade 122, 178
bitter orange 137
bitter sweet 178
bittersweet 122
black alder 62
black bamboo 142, 324
blackberry 76, 124, 183
black blood 196
black bugbane 183
black cardamom 341
black cherry 219
black choke 219
black chokecherry 219
black cohosh 183
black cumin 182
black currant 69, 89
black cutch 185
black elder 127
black fellows 98
blackfellow's bread 210
black galingale 183
blacking plant 182
black-lip oyster 234
black medicine 58, 296
black mustard 89
black myrobalan 301
black nest swiftlet 234
black nightshade 51
black pepper 97
black plum 183, 198
black rice 90
black root 184
blackroot 184
black snakeroot 183
black tang 175
black tea 142
black walnut 89
black wattle 203
bladder wrack 175
bladderwrack 93, 175
blady grass 336
blaeberry 178
blanket leaf 178
blaver 204
blessed milk thistle 194
blessed thistle 79, 194
bletilla 118
blond psyllium 184
blood of bovine 229
blood of red deer 229
blood of swine 229
bloodroot 152
bloodwoodtree 172
bloom cypress 112
blue agave 38
blue alfalfa 46
blueberry 185
bluebonnet 204
blue bottle 204
blue crown passionflower 152
blue ginseng 44
blue-green algae 43
blue gum 208
blue mallow 56, 130
blue passionflower 152
blue pimpernel 215
blue poppy 204
blue skullcap 119, 317
blushred rabdosia 327
Bodhi tree 54
bog bean 317
bog bilberry 90
bog blueberry 90
bog chickweed 114
bog Labrador tea 88
bog myrtle 317
boldo 191
Bombay black wood 138
bonavist 188
bonavista bean 188
bonavit bean 53
bon-bana 196
bone marrow of bovine 229
boneset 102
bonesetter 314
bonito 227
bookoo 181
borage 215
borecole 92
Borneo camphor 214
borojó 191
Bo-tree 54
bottle gourd 177, 180, 207
bottle tree 37
bouncing bess 104
bouncing bet 104
bourtree 127
bower actinidia 105
box holly 154
box thorn 85
boxthorn 85

bramble 124
bramble rose 296
branching larkspur 216
brank 134
Brazilian arrow root 80
Brazilian cherry 139
Brazilian copal 115
Brazilian ginseng 121
Brazilian ipecac 307
Brazilian tea 194
Brazil wood 322
bread wheat 88
brewer's yeast 95
briar bush 218
brier 171
brier bush 153
brier rose 153, 218
bright eyes 329
brindall berry 74
briony 184
British agar 37
British elecampane 320
British inula 320
broad banded blue sea snake 236
broadleaf plantain 124
Bromelain 373
Bromelains 373
brooklime 91
broom 60, 296
broomjue sida 297
broom rape 98
broomrape 158
brown cutch 42
brown mushroom 128
brown mustard 89
brown rice germ 94
Brown's lily 209
brushes 204
bryony 184
bucco 181
buchu 181
buck bean 317
buckeye 152
buckhorn 187
buckthorn 306
buckwheat 134
Buddha's hand citron 181
buddleia 340
buddleja 340
buffalo bean 168
Bufotenin 372
Bufotenine 372
bugs 228
bu gu zhi 189
buku 181
bull thistle 194
bul rush 47
bulrush 71, 327, 337
Bunge's pine 165
bupleurum 102, 311
burdock 99, 310
burijo 191
bur marygold 98
burnet bloodwort 220
burojó 191
burr rose 118
bush mango 43
bush tea 182
1,4-Butanediol 370
1,4-Butanolide 362
butcher's broom 154
butter bean 53
buttercup 57
butterfly bush 340
butterfly ginger 168
butterfly lily 168
butterfly pea 144
butter fruit 44
butternut 166
butter pear 44
butter print 150
butter-print 49
button weed 49, 150
1,4-Butylene glycol 370
4-Butyrolactone 362
gamma-Butyrolactone 362
buyo (bisaya) 83

C

cabbage palm fern 191
Caclate 361
cactus pear 56
cafe de bugre 143
cafe do mato 143
cafeillo 305
Cafeina 249
Caffeine 249
Cafipel 249
Cairo morning glory 201
calabar bean 302
calabash 177
calabash gourd 180, 207
calamus 315
Calciferol 275
Calciol 275
Calcite 250
Calcium 250
Calcium carbonate 250
Calcium magnesium salt 269
Calcium D-pantothenate 271
Calcium pantothenate 271
Calcium sulfate 264
calendula 150
California bur 321
California pilchard 229
California poppy 169
California white sage 192
call nut 160
Caloreen 267
calumba 310
camboge plant 74
campeche wood 172
camphor 86, 116
camphor tree 86, 116
camptotheca 76
camu-camu 72
Canada cocklebur 321
canary wood 203
cancharagua 122
candelabra aloe 77
candleberry 118
candle bush 169
candlestick senna 169
candlewick 178
candy leaf 120
Cang'zhu atractylodes 333
cang-zhu atractylodes 321
Canton ginger 116
cao guo 321
Cape aloe 47, 293
Cape jasmine 106
Caperase 360
capillaris 294
capillary artemisia 294
capsell 154
capsicum 149
carageen 205

carambola 101
caraway 176
5-(Carbamoylamino)hydantoin 356
N5-Carbamoyl-L-ornithine 247
Carbodenafil 360
Carbonic acid 269
3-carboxy-3-hydroxypentanedioic acid 254
6-Carboxyuracil 248
cardamom 116
cardamon 116
cardon pear 56
(-)-Carnitine 246
(-)-L-Carnitine 246
(R)-Carnitine 246
L-Carnitine 246
Carnitor 246
carob 50
Carolina jasmine 303
Carotaben 280
alpha Carotene 250
beta Carotene 280
beta-Carotene 250, 280
Carotene 250
delta-Carotene 250
gamma-Carotene 250
Carotenes 250
Carotenoid 286
caroubier 50
carqueja 73
carrageen 37, 205
carrageenan 37, 249
carrageen moss 205
carragheen moss 37
carraigín 37
carrot 159
carrot oil 159
carry-me-seed 78
cartilage of mammalia 234
cartilage of reptilia 234
cart-track plant 124
cascara 301
cascara sagrada 301
casearia 305
cassava 80
cassia 91, 92
cassia flower 84
cassia lignea 91, 92
cassia seed and leaf 60
cassis 69, 89
cast iron plant 172
castor bean 332
castor oil plant 332
Catalase 360
Catalase-peroxidase 360
Catalonian jasmine 114
cat berry 120
cat brier 106, 109
catbrier 312
(+)-Catechin 248
Catechin 248
Catechinic acid 248
catechu 179, 185, 322
Catechuic acid 248
Catergen 248
catmint 51
catnep 51
catnip 51
cat powder 200
cat's claw 80
cat's foot 59
cat's whiskers 87
cat tail 71
cat-tail 337
catuaba 70
cauliflower ears 94
cauliflower mushroom 169
cawage 168
cayenne 149
cayenne cherry 139
cayenne pepper 113, 149
Cebrogen 256
celandine 151
celera bean 214
celery 131
centaury 132
Ceramide 265
cereal rye 211
Cervonic acid 268
Ceylon spinach 147
chá de bugre 143
chaga 71
Chalk 250
chamber bitter 100
chamomile 72, 219
champignon 128
Chanca piedra 78
chapéau de couro 113
Charcoal dry distilled water 264
chard 104, 181
charga 71
charlatan ivy 133
chasteberry 127
chaste tree 127
chebulic myrobalan 301
cheesefruit 203
cheeses 56, 130
Chemfill 254
chen pi 144
chervil 143
chestnut rose 118
chia 142
chia cimarrona 115
chicken 225
chickweed 165
chickwort 165
Chicol 252
chicory 77
chikin's head 66
chili pepper 113, 149
China berry 132, 327
Chinaberry 320
China jute 49, 150
China root 312
China rose 163, 182
China squash 71
China tree 132, 320, 327
Chinese agarwood 317
Chinese allspice 58, 296
Chinese amomum 315
Chinese angelica 112, 150, 326
Chinese angelica tree 112, 140
Chinese arborvitae 134
Chinese arbutus 207
Chinese arisaema 325
Chinese asparagus 149, 326
Chinese aster 313
Chinese bamboo 329
Chinese bellflower 76
Chinese birthwort 295
Chinese bitter almond 75
Chinese black ant 223
Chinese blackberry 149
Chinese boxthorn 85, 314
Chinese brake 336
Chinese brown frog 229
Chinese cardamom 177

Chinese cardamon 177
Chinese catalpa 304
Chinese catawba 304
Chinese caterpillar fungus 151
Chinese chaste tree 160
Chinese chive 159
Chinese cimicifuga 316
Chinese cinnamon 91, 92
Chinese clematis 52, 294
Chinese colza 155
Chinese cork oak 316
Chinese cucumber 74, 302, 341
Chinese cuscuta 328
Chinese dandelion 189
Chinese date 108, 136
Chinese dodder 328
Chinese elm 159
Chinese ephedra 338
Chinese eupatorium 343
Chinese fumewort 297
Chinese galangal 343
Chinese gelsemium 308
Chinese giant hyssop 301, 303
Chinese ginger 87, 343
Chinese ginseng 65
Chinese goldthread 63, 299, 340
Chinese ground orchid 118
Chinese gutta percha 153, 328
Chinese hawthorn 106, 319
Chinese hibiscus 163, 182
Chinese hickory 105
Chinese holly 173
Chinese honey locust 102
Chinese indigo 117, 140
Chinese jointfir 338
Chinese jujube 108, 136
Chinese jute 49, 150
Chinese kale 92
Chinese key 87
Chinese knotweed 301
Chinese lantern plant 337
Chinese licorice 75
Chinese liquidambar 134
Chinese lizardtail 173
Chinese lobelia 340
Chinese lovage 308
Chinese magnolia vine 310
Chinese matrimony vine 85
Chinese mesona 132
Chinese milk vetch 217
Chinese milkvetch 113
Chinese mint 167
Chinese moccasin 236
Chinese motherwort 216, 342
Chinese mushroom 109
Chinese nardostachys 303
Chinese olive 76
Chinese onion 68
Chinese orchid 325
Chinese parasol tree 37
Chinese parsley 98
Chinese pearl barley 168
Chinese peony 114, 315
Chinese poke 316
Chinese praying mantis 233
Chinese prickly ash 111
Chinese privet 159
Chinese pulsatilla 330
Chinese quinine 53
Chinese radish 211
Chinese rhubarb 135, 322
Chinese rice paper plant 144
Chinese rubber plant 94
Chinese rubber tree 153, 328
Chinese sage 141, 323
Chinese salacia 105
Chinese salvia 141, 323
Chinese scholar tree 297
Chinese scholar-tree 61
Chinese scorpion 230
Chinese silk vine 96
Chinese skullcap 62, 298
Chinese smilax 106, 312
Chinese snake gourd 302
Chinese soapberry 197
Chinese softshell turtle 232
Chinese spikenard 303
Chinese star anise 135
Chinese strawberry tree 207
Chinese sumac 121, 160
Chinese tamarisk 81
Chinese tea 142, 164
Chinese thorough wax 102
Chinese throughwax 311
Chinese torreya 174
Chinese trumpet creeper 214
Chinese trumpet flower 214
Chinese water lily 166
Chinese white olive 76
Chinese wild ginger 312
Chinese windmill palm 116
Chinese wolfberry 85, 314
Chinese wormwood 317
Chinese yam 108
chingma 40
chinquapin rose 118
chiretta 132
D-(+)-chiro-Inositol 266
D-chiro-Inositol 266
Chisese quince 201
Chishima zasa 142
Chitin 252
Chitosamine hydrochloride 255
Chitosan 252
Chitosan oligosaccharide 252
chittam bark 301
chittem bark 301
chive 41
Chlamys farreri 223
chloranthus 133
chlorella 90
Chlorofolin 257
Chlorofyl 257
1-[1-(4-Chlorophenyl)cyclobutyl]-3-methylbutylamine 365
1-(4-Chlorophenyl)-N-methyl-α-(2-methylpropyl)-cyclobutanemethanamine Hydrochloride 365
1-(4-Chlorophenyl)-α-(2-methylpropyl)cyclobutanemethanamine 365
Chlorophyl 257
Chlorophyll 257
Chlorophyll a 257
Chlorophylls 257
Chloropretadalafil 362
chocolate vine 40, 341
Choline alfoscerate 246
Choline-stabilised orthosilicic acid 260
Chondroitin sulfate 260
Chondroitinsulfate 260
Chondromucoprotein 260
chondrus 37
ch-OSA 260
Christine loosestrife 83
Christmas-candle 169

Chromic ion 257
Chromium(3+) ions 257
Chromium (Ⅲ) 257
Chromium(Ⅲ) ion 257
Chromium(Ⅲ) picolinate 272
Chromium(Ⅲ)trispicolinate 272
Chromium ion (Cr^{3+}) 257
Chromium picolinate 272
Chromium tripicolinate 272
Chromule 257
chrysanthemum 77
chuanlong yam 131
chuan xin lian 132
church steeples 124
Chusan palm 116
Cialis® 365
cibol 160
cicada slough 349
cilantro 98
cinnamon 91, 92
cinnamon flower 84
cinnamon jasmine 168
cinnamon vine 108
Cinobufotenine 372
cinquefoil 152
Cirantin 280
Citrate 254
Citretten 254
Citric acid 254
citrin 74
Citro 254
L-Citrulline 247
clary 66
clary sage 66
clary wort 66
climbing fern 70
climbing fig 63
climbing nightshade 122, 178
clinker polypore 71
clove 89, 144
clove nutmeg 212
clove tree 144
clubmoss 118
cluster pine 184
Cluytyl alcohol 247
cnidium 315
CoA 259
Coalip 259
CoASH 259
coastal morning glory 201
Cobalamin 274
Cobavite 274
cockle bur 99
cocklebur 321
cockle burr 99
cockroach 232
cockscomb coral tree 67
cockspur coral tree 67
coconut 204
coconut palm 204
cod liver oil 228
codonopsis 326
Coenzyme A 259
Co-enzyme-A 259
Coenzyme Q_{10} 259
Coenzyme R 272
coffee 96
coffee senna 170
cogon 336
coix 168
cola 96
colchicum 294
Colecalciferol 275
colewort 92
Colfarit 355
Collagen 259
collards 92
colocynth 310
Colombian waxweed 161
colombo 310
coltsfoot 180, 304
comfrey 102
common apricot 75
common Arctic seal 223
common ash 126
common balm 200
common barberry 128
common basil 199
common bean 53
common birch 111
common bird's-foot-trefoil 197
common black currant 69, 89
common borage 215
common briar 218
common broom 60
common Californian poppy 169
common camellia 145
common cat tail 71
common cattail 337
common centaury 132
common chamomile 219
common chickweed 165
common club moss 118
common cockscomb 161
common coffee 96
common comfrey 102
common coral tree 67
common corn salad 192
common cotton thistle 64
common daisy 175
common dandelion 126
common date palm 155
common edelweisse 58
common evening primrose 199
common fig 49
common fox glove 313
common gardenia 106
common garden peony 114, 315
common garden sunflower 176
common garden verbena 174
common ginger 116
common ginger lily 168
common green minth 121
common hedge mustard 69
common holly 128
common hop 191
common horehound 195
common horse chestnut 126, 318
common horsetail 120
common hydrangea 41
common jujube 108
common juniper 127
common knotgrass 196
common lavender 213
common lime 125, 147
common linden 147
common madder 123
common mallow 56, 130
common mango 195
common marigold 150
common mint 167
common mistletoe 318
common motherwort 216
common mullein 178
common mushroom 128
common nastritium 84
common nep 51

common nettle 123
common nutmeg 158
common olive 67
common papaw 169
common peach 202
common pepper 97
common periwinkle 177
common pimpernel 215
common plantain 64, 124
common plum 125
common pomegranate 103
common purslane 165
common pyrethurum 39
common reed 41, 344
common rue 188
common rush 47
common sage 105
common sassafras 104
common sea buckthorn 102
common sida 297
common snowdrop 342
common soapwort 104
common sorrel 119
common sow thistle 162
common stinging nettle 123
common St. John's wort 124
common St. Paul's wort 199
common sunflower 176
common tansy 210
common thyme 139
common tormentil 152
common turmeric 55
common vervena 86
common vetch 72
common walnut 69
common wheat 88, 100
common willow 125
common wormwood 85
common yam 108
common yarrow 127
condor vine 311
condurango 311
cone flower 59, 64
cone head 214
confederate jasmine 137
conker tree 318
cooltankard 215
copaiba 99
Copper 268
copra 204
coptis 63, 299, 340
CoQ_{10} 259
coral 231
coral jasmine 54
coral lily 209
coral tree 76
coraltree 300
cordyceps 151
coriander 98
corn 151
corn chamomile 219
cornflower 204
corn mint 167
corn pinks 204
corn poppy 175
corn salad 192
cornsilk 151
Corydalis ambigua 297
Corydalis yanhusuo 297
Cosamin 255
Co-A-SH 259
Cossack asparagus 71, 337
costus 341
cottonseed oil 200
couch grass 112
couliflower fungus 169
country almond 202
country mallow 297
courbaril 115
cowberry 97, 309
cow clover 38
cowitch 168
cow's foot 167
cowslip 125
crab 228
crab grass 43
crab's eye 321
crack open 305
crampbark 209
cranberry 88
cranberry bush 209
crassula 61
cream tartar tree 164
creat 132
Creatin 257
Creatine 257
Creatine ethyl ester HCl(P) 257
Creatine ethyl ester hydrochloride 257
creeping fig 63
creeping ixeris 52
creeping lettuce 52
creeping lilyturf 331
creeping lobelia 340
creeping rubber plant 63
creeping thyme 51, 131
crested cockscomb 161
crested late-summer mint 94
crimson glory vine 207
Cristobalite 258
croton oil plant 332
crown wood fern 299
crue all 215
cry-baby tree 67
Crystal VI 241
Crystamine 274
Cuban jute 297
cube gambir 42
cudweed 170
culantro 98
culate mandarin 196
cultivated apple 215
culver's physic 184
culver's root 184
cumcum 72
cumin 87
Cuprein 264
cup rose 175
Cuprum 268
Curaçao aloe 47, 293
curculigo 133
curcuma 55, 254
Curcumin 254
cure leaf yucca 208
curled dock 209
curled mallow 150
curly dock 209
curly moss 37
curly parsley 166
curry plant 187
cutch tree 185
cut-leaf coneflower 64
cut-leaved coneflower 64
cuttlefish 224
Cu/Zn SOD 264
cyani 204
Cyanidanol 248

cyanobacteria 43
Cyanocobalamin 274
Cyclic polylactate (CPL) 251
Cyclobutanemethanamine 365
Cyclofenil 363
Cyclofenyl 363
(4-Cyclopentylpiperazine-1-yl) [3-(1-methyl-3-propyl-6,7-dihydro-7-oxo-1H-pyrazolo[4,3-d]pyrimidine-5-yl)-4-(ethoxy)phenyl]sulfone 363
Cyclopentynafil 363
Cycobemin 274
Cymethion 283
cynara 144
cynomorium 65
cyperus 308
DL-Cystathionine 261
L-(+)-Cystathionine 261
Cystatione 261
Cystationine 261
Cystein 262
(R)-Cysteine 262
Cysteine 262
L-(+)-Cysteine 262
L-Cysteine 262
Cysteine disulfide 261
Cystin 261
L-Cystin 261
Cystine 261
L-Cystine 261
Cystine acid 261
L-Cytrulline 247

D

Daghestan sweet clover 123
Dahlin 245
Dahurian angelica 332
Dahurian bugbane 316
daisy 177
daisy fleabane 177
Dalmatian sage 105
damiana 323
dancing mushroom 192
dancy tangerine 123
dandelion 126, 189
Danewort 209
dan shen 141, 323
dan zhu ye 141
date 155
date palm 155
date plum 68
date tree 155
day flower 146
DCI 266
Deacetylchitin 252
deadly nightshade 335
dead nettle 66
dead rat tree 164
Dehydroepiandrosterone 367
Dehydroisoandrosterone 367
dendrobium 325
dense-fruit dittany 330
Deodophyll 257
1,5-Deoxy-1,5-imino-D-mannitol 367
1-Deoxymannojirimycin 367
1-Deoxynojirimycin 367
deril-in-a-bush 182
Descarbonsildenafil 355
Des-N,N-dimethyl-sibutramine 365
desert broom rape 98
Des-N-methyl-sibutramine 365
N-(Desmethylsibutramine hydrochloride) 365
devil's backbone 314
devil's claw 148
devil's trumpet 324
devil's walking stick 112
devil's-walking-stick 140
Dextophan 363
Dextrin 267
Dextrine 267
Dextrins 267
Dextromethorphan 367
Dextromethorphan hydrobromide 363
DHA 268
DHEA 367
1,2-Diacyl-sn-glycerol 3-phospho-L-serine 281
Diallyldisulfid-S-oxid 242
Diallyl thiosulfinate 242
2,6-Diamino-5-hydroxyhexanoic acid 277
(S)-2,5-Diaminopentanoic acid 248
Diastase 356
Diatomaceous earth 258
Diatomaceous silica 258
Dicysteine 261
L-Dicysteine 261
N-Didesmethylsibutramine 365
diesel tree 99
Dietary fiber 263
Diferuloylmethane 254
difu 112
digitalis 313
Dihydro-2(3*H*)-furanone 362
3,4-Dihydroharmine 369
Dihydroharmine 369
(3R,5S)-rel-1-[[3-(4,7-Dihydro-1-methyl-3-propyl-7-thioxo-1*H*-pyrazolo[4,3-*d*]pyrimidin-5-yl)-4-ethoxyphenyl]sulfonyl]-3,5-dimethyl-piperazine 366
1-[[3-(4,7-Dihydro-1-methyl-7-oxo-3-propyl-1*H*-pyrazolo[4,3-*d*]pyrimidin-5-yl)-4-ethoxyphenyl]sulfonyl]piperidine 368
3,3'-Dihydroxy-beta-carotene-4,4'-dione 241
(10S)-1,8-Dihydroxy-3-(hydroxymethyl)-10beta-beta-D-glucopyranosyl-9,10-dihydroanthracene-9-one 356
dika 43
dikabread tree 43
dikanut 43
N-(3,4-dimethoxybenzyl)-2-((2-hydroxy-1-methylethyl)amino)-5-nitrobenzamide 360
7,7'-dimethoxy-(4,4'-bis-1,3-benzodioxole)-5,5'-dicarboxylic acid dimethyl ester 370
6,8-Dimethoxyumbelliferone 244
N-[2-Dimethylamino)ethyl]-4-ethoxy-3-(1-methyl-7-oxo-3-propyl-6,7-dihydro-1*H*-pyrazolo[4,3-*d*]pyrimidin-5-yl)benzenesulfonamide 355
Dimethyl 7,7'-dimethoxy-4,4'-bi-1,3-benzodioxole-5,5'-dicarboxylate 370
Dimethyl-4,4'-dimethoxy-5,6,5',6'-dimethylenedioxybiphenyl-2,2'-dicarboxylate 370
N,N-Dimethyl-5-hydroxytryptamine

372
N,N-Dimethylserotonin 372
Dimethyl sildenafil 376
Dimethylsildenafil 376
Dimethyl sulphone 243
di-niè 110
3,17-Dioxoandrost-4-ene 357
Dioxosilane 258
disaccharide from hydrolysed chondroitin 230
dishcloth gourd 186
dishrag gourd 186
Disodium;3-[18-(dioximethylidene)-8-ethenyl-13-ethyl-3,7,12,17-tetramethyl-20-(2-oxido-2-oxoethyl)-2,3-dihydroporphyrin-23-id-2-yl]propanoate;hydron;iron(2+) 267
beta,beta'-Dithiodialanine 261
diverse wormwood 213
divi-divi 121
DNA 227
DNJ 367
dock 209
Doconexent 268
Docosahexaenoic acid(DHA) 268
cis-4,7,10,13,16,19-Docosahexaenoic acid 268
dog 347
dogbane 212
dog brier 153
dog grass 112
dog rose 153, 218
dog tail 124
dogwood 107
doku-dami 115
dollar plant 94
Dolomite 269
domestic dog 347
dong quai 150, 326
donkey-hide gelatin 223
Donnagel 360
doorweed 196
dorset weed 37
double tawny day-lily 82
draba 50
dragon's blood 81
dragon's blood palm 81
dragon's eye 213
dried bonito 227
Drierite 264
drug eyebright 97
Drynaria 164
Duch lavender 213
dulcamara 122, 178
dumb nettle 66
dunaliella 148
durian benggala 88
Dutchman's pipe 92
Dutchman's pipe cactus 92
dwarf Cape gooseberry 117
dwarf Cavendish 168
dwarf elder 209
dwarf flowering cherry 48
dwarf Japanese quince 85
dwarf lancehead snake 235
dwarf lilyturf 331
dwarf lysimachia 98
dwarf mallow 56, 130
dwarf rubber plant 94
dwarf sedge 129
dwarf Solomon's seal 48
dyer's fucus 93
dyer's madder 123
dyer's woad 117

E

earless seal 223
ear shell 224
earth apple 203
earth nut 212
earthworm 349
eastern daisy fleabane 177
eastern white pine 120
East Indian dragon's blood 81
East-Indian galangale 108
East Indian lotus 166
East Indian rhubarb 135
East Indian sandalwood 333
East Indian sarsaparilla 294
East Indian walnut 178
ebolo 186
Echinacea 59
Echinacea angustifolia 59
Echinacea pallida 59
Echinacea purpurea 59
eclipta 138
Ecotrin 355
Ecuador sapote 39
edelweisse 58
Edemase 373
edible burdock 99, 310
edible date 155
edible nest swiftlet 234
edible stemed vine 314
eelgrass 129
Egg albumin 243
egg shell 237
Egg yolk lecithin 286
egg yolk oil 237
Eglish plantain 187
Egyptian bean 188
Egyptian lotus 166
ehytlehtivillakko 64
Eicosapentaenoic acid 244
eisenia 46
Eldrin 286
elecampane 328
eleutero 96
eleuthero 59
eleutherococcus 59
eleutherococcus gracilistylus 55
Eleutherococcus sessiliflorus 96
elm 159
elsholtzia 94
emblic 210
emblic myrobalan 210
Emitolon 259
empress candle plant 169
Endoamylase 356
English chamomile 219
English daisy 175
English gooseberry 120
English hawthorn 125
English holly 128
English knotgrass 196
English lavender 213
English twitch 112
English violet 121, 157
English walnut 69
EPA 244
epazote 46
ephedra 338
Ephedrine 359
epi-Inositol 245
Equilase 360
Erabu black banded sea krait 236

erect cinquefoil 152
erect knotgrass 196
Ergocalciferol 275
erigeron 177
erythro-L-Isoleucine 244
Escholin 375
escobilla 122
estragon 59
Ethanesulfonic acid 364
Ethiopian sour bread 164
5-[2-Ethoxy-5-[2-[4-ethylpiperazine-1-yl]acetyl]phenyl]-1-methyl-3-propyl-1*H*-pyrazolo[4,3-*d*]pyrimidine-7(6*H*)-one 374
2-[2-Ethoxy-5-(4-ethylpiperazinosulfonyl)phenyl]-5-methyl-7-propyl-3,4-dihydroimidazo[5,1-*f*][1,2,4]triazine-4-one 369
5-[2-Ethoxy-5-[2-(4-ethylpiperazin-1-yl)acetyl]phenyl]-1-methyl-3-propyl-4*H*-pyrazolo[4,3-*d*]pyrimidin-7-one 374
4-ethoxy-3-(1-methyl-7-oxo-3-propyl-6,7-dihydro-1*H*-pyrazolo[4,3-*d*]pyrimidin-5-yl)benzoic acid 355
5-(2-Ethoxy-5-nitrophenyl)-1-methyl-3-propyl-1*H*-pyrazolo[4,3-*d*]pyrimidine-7(6*H*)-one 368
5-[2-Ethoxy-5-(1-piperidinylsulfonyl)phenyl]-1,6-dihydro-1-methyl-3-propyl-7*H*-pyrazolo[4,3-*d*]pyrimidin-7-one 368
Ethyl *N*-(aminoiminomethyl)-*N*-methylglycine hydrochloride 257
Ethyl 6,7-dimethoxy-3-methyl-4-oxo-1-(3,4,5-trimethoxyphenyl)-1,2,3,4-tetrahydronaphthalene-2-carboxylate 284
3-Ethyl-8-[2-[4-(hydroxymethyl)piperidino]benzylamino]-2,3-dihydro-1*H*-imidazo[4,5-*g*]quinazoline-2-thione 366
N-Ethyl-N-nitroso-α-methyl-3-(trifluoromethyl)benzeneethanamine 359
eucalyptus 208
eucommia 153, 328
European plum 125
European alder 62
European angelica 47
European arnica 293
European ash 126
European barberry 128
European blackberry 124
European black currant 69, 89
European black elder 127
European blueberry 128, 178
European centaury 132
European corn salad 192
European cranberry bush 209
European dwarf elder 209
European elder 127
European gooseberry 120
European grape 182
European holly 128
European hop 191
European horse chestnut 126, 318
European lily of the valley 317
European lime 147
European lime tree 125
European linden 125, 147
European lowbush blueberry 178
European madder 123
European meadowsweet 126
European mistletoe 318
European pennyroyal 198
European raspberry 124
European red elder 130
European red raspberry 124, 212
European vervain 86
European water chestnut 174
European white birch 111
European wild pansy 106, 121
European willow 125
euryale 66
eurycoma 154
Eutrit 252
evening primrose 199
evening trumpet flower 303
everlasting 187
evodia 309
evodia fruit 309
ewe daisy 152
excerescence 201
eye bright 37
eyebright 37, 97
Ezo-tsunomata 37

F

fagiolo 53
fairly canndle 183
fair maids of February 342
false arborvitae 42
false daisy 138
false kamani 202
false kava 162
false myrrh 72
false saffron 186
far east Amur adonis 334
Far Eastern wood frog 229
farrer's scallop 223
fat hen 38
Fatty acid 262
feather cockscomb 161
feces of Pteromyinae spp. 348
felt fern 129
fennel 55
fennel flower 182
fenugrec 101
fenugreek 101
Ferric oxide 364
Ferritin-Fe 278
Ferroprotoporphyrin 281
Ferrous gluconate 256
Ferrous iron 267
Ferrous protoheme Ⅸ 281
Ferrum 267
Ferulate 278
(E)-Ferulic acid 278
trans-Ferulic Acid 278
Ferulic acid 278
fever bark tree 304
feverfew 155
fever flower 53
fever grass 217
fiddlewood 86
field balm 218
field corn 151
field fleawort 64
field horsetail 120
field larkspur 216
field melilot 123
field mint 167
field mustard 155

field pansy 106
field poppy 175
fig 49
fig tree 49
filé 104
fingered citoron 181
finger millet 110
fireweed 186, 205
fish oil 229
five flavor fruit 310
five leaf akebia 40, 341
five leaf morning glory 201
five leaved chaste tree 160
flacher lackporling 99
Flammulina velutipes 60
Flanders poppy 175
flannel leaf 178
flannel plant 178
flannel sida 297
flannelweed 297
flat-stem milkvetch 113
flat wrack 175
Flavin meletin 258
flax 44
fleabane 177
flea mint 198
fleeceflower 146, 301
flesh finger citron 181
Flonac C 252
Flonac N 252
Florida cranberry 163
florist's chrysanthemum 77
florist's verbena 174
florist's violet 157
floss flow 70
flowering almond 48
flowering bamboo 48
flowering plants 335
flowering quince 189
flower quince 201
Fluor 279
Fluorine 278
foetid cassia 170
Folacin 283
Folate 283
Folic acid 283
Folvite 283
food pokeberry 316
foreign henna 332
forest paper 312
forking larkspur 216
formosan sweet gum 134
forskohlii 73
forsythia 217, 344
fortune's thoroughwort 343
fossil dragon 351
fo ti 301
fo-ti 146
fourwing evening primrose 145
foxberry 97, 309
fox glove 313
fox nut 66
foxnut 66
fragrant angelica 332
fragrant olive 84
fragrant orchid 147
fragrant premna 45
fragrant rosewood 95
fragrant Solomon's seal 48
frangula 335
frankincense 190, 337
French bean 53
French lavender 213
French tarragon 59
French willow 205
fresh water clam 231
frijol 53
frijole 53
Frorentine 294
beta-Fructofuranosidase 358
D(-)-Fructose 249
D-Fructose 249
Fructose 248
fruit bromelain 373
fruit enzyme 262
fruit sugar 249
fucus 175
Fulvic acid 279
Furucton 249

G

GABA 251
Gaballon 251
gadfly 350
4-O-beta-D-Galactopyranosyl-beta-D-glucopyranose 270
beta-Galactosidase 377
galanga 156
galangale 108
galine gale 308
galla halepense 201
galla levantica 201
galla quercina 201
galla tinctoria 201
gallbladder 350
gallbladder of carp 233
gallbladder of mamushi 233
gall nut 160
galls 201
gambir 42, 143, 325
Gammalon 251
ganboge tree 74
ganges amaranth 93
ganoderma 216
garcinia 74
garden angelica 47
garden balsam 188, 336
garden basil 199
garden burnet 220
garden chamomile 219
garden chervil 143
garden daisy 175
garden heliotrope 70
gardenia 106
garden lovage 219
garden nastritium 84
garden pansy 106
garden plum 125
garden poppy 92
garden rhubarb 117, 135
garden sage 105
garden sorrel 119
garden thyme 139
garden valerian 70
garden verbena 174
garden violet 121, 157
garland flower 168
garlic 160
garlic chive 159
gastrodia 325
gastrointestinal calculous 350
gbanja kola 96
GBL 362
Ge(4+) 258
gean 128
Gelatin 265
Gelbwurz 254

gelsemium 303
Gendenafil 362
gentian 94, 307
geranium herb 307
German chamomile 72
Germanio 258
Germanium 258
Germanium element 258
German rampion 199
Germide 258
giant Cavendish 168
giant cupped oyster 227
giant knotweed 48, 309
giant oyster 227
giant Pacific oyster 227
giant reed 142
giant snowdrop 342
giant timber bamboo 148
giant vallis 129
giant white radish 211
giant whortleberry 185
gill over the ground 218
ginger 116
ginger lily 168
gingko 50
ginkgo 50
ginseng 65
glabrous greenbrier 106, 312
glasswort 43
Glavamin 256
gleditsia 102
glehnia 171
Glicoamin 254
globe artichoke 144
globe fish 236
glossy buckthorn 335
glossy privet 159
1,4-alpha-D-Glucan glucanohydrolase 356
Glucoinvertase 375
(1-6)-alpha-Glucomannan 255
Glucomannan 255
Glucomannoglycan 255
4-*O*-alpha-D-Glucopyranosyl-D-glucitol 250
alpha-D-Glucopyranosyl-alpha-D-glucopyranoside 270
(alpha-D-Glucopyranosyl-(1-4))$_n$-alpha-D-glucopyranose 356
4-*O*-alpha-D-Glucopyranosyl-D-sorbitol 250
beta-D-Glucopyranuronosyl-(1->3)-(3xi)-2-(acetylamino)-2-deoxy-beta-D-ribo-hexopyranosyl-(1->4)-beta-D-glucopyranuronosyl-(1->3)-(3xi)-2-(acetylamino)-2-deoxy-beta-D-ribo-hexopyranose 272
D-(+)-Glucosamine hydrochloride 255
Glucosamine hydrochloride 255
Glucose glycoside 247
alpha-1,4-Glucosidase 375
alpha-Glucosidase 375
alpha-D-Glucoside glucohydrolase 375
alpha-Glucoside hydrolase 375
Glucosidosucrase 375
Glumin 256
Glusate 256
Glutacid 256
L-Glutamate 256
Glutamic acid 256
L-Glutamic acid 256
Glutamic acid amide 256
Glutamicol 256
Glutamidex 256
Glutamine 256
L-(+)-Glutamine 256
L-Glutamine 256
Glutaminic acid 256
Glutaminol 256
N-[N-(L-γ-Glutamyl)-L-cysteinyl]glycine 361
Glutathione 361
Glutaton 256
gluten 88
Glycerin 254
Glycerine 254
Glyceritol 254
Glycerol 254
Glycerol guaiacolate 361
Glycero-3-phosphocholine 246
sn-Glycero-3-phosphocholine 246
L-alpha-Glycerylphosphorylcholine 246
L-alpha-Glycerylphosphorylcholine/sn-Glycero(3)phosphocholine 246
Glycine 254
Glycocoll 254
Glycogenase 356
Glycolixir 254
Glycosaminoglycans 282
Glycosthene 254
Glycyl alcohol 254
glycyrrhiza 75
Glymol 285
Glyoxaline-5-alanine 273
goat horns 305
goat nut 191
goat's rue 74
goat thorn bush 153
goat willow 125
gobo 99, 310
Gold 253
gold apple 153
goldbaldrian 67
golden apple 187
golden bell 217
goldenbells 217, 344
golden bell tree 217
golden buttons 210
golden candle 169
golden cuttlefish 224
golden eye grass 133
golden glow 64
golden gram 214
golden holly hock 139
golden needle 82
golden oyster mushroom 140
golden polypody 191
golden rod 40
golden root 53
goldenseal 308
golden serpent 191
golden tremella 97
golden willow 125, 205
gold foot fern 191
gold glow 64
goober 212
gooseberry 120
goosefoot 38
goraka 74
gorgon water lily 66
gotu kola 145
gou ju 73

graminis 112
grape 182
grapefruit 89
grape vine 182
grapple plant 148
grass-leaf calamus 129, 318
grass-leaf sweet flag 129, 318
grass nut 212
grassy-leaved sweet flag 129
graviola 88, 306
Gray's bird cherry 58
greasewood 192
great burdock 99, 310
great burnet 220
great but 99
greater burdock 310
greater celandine 151
greater galangal 156
greater plantain 124
greater snowdrop 342
greater yam 57
great lettuce 219
great morinda 203
great mullein 178
great pipefish 227
great willowherb 205
great yellow gentian 307
Grecian laurel 93
green amaranth 122
green bean 53
green brier 109
greenbrier 312
green chiretta 132
green gram 214
green-lipped mussel 237
green minth 121
green plantain 124
green purslane 165
green tangerine peel 123
green tea 142
green wattle 203
grey field-speedwell 50
griffonia 306
grifola frondosa 192
gristle moss 37
ground cherry 117
ground dragon 349
ground ivy 218
ground nut 45, 212
groundnut 45
ground pine 118
GSH 361
guaco 84
guaiac 84
Guaiacol glyceryl ether 361
guaiacum 84
Guaifenesin 361
Guaiphenesin 361
guanabana 88, 306
Guaran 253
guarana 73
guaraná 73
Guaranine 249
Guar gum 253
guassatonga 305
guava 84
guayabillo 305
guduchi 324
guelder rose 209
guggul 72
gugulipid 72
Guinea sorrel 163
guinea wheat 151
gum arabic 45
gum arabic tree 45
gum Benjamin 47
gum benzoin 47
Gum cyamopsis 253
gum guggul 72
gum Senegal 45
gum tragacanth 153
gundagai thistle 194
gurmar 79, 180
Gu-Sui-Bu 164
gutta-percha 86
Guyana arrowroot 57
gymnema 79, 180
gynostemma 44
Gypsum 264

H

Haem 281
Haematite 364
hag taper 178
hairy antler 351
hairy beggar ticks 98
hairy deer horn 351
hala screw pine 113
Haldar 254
Half cystine 262
Half-cystine 262
hand of Mary 339
han lian cao 138
Hardwicke's pipefish 227
hardy kiwi 105
hardy rubber tree 153, 328
hare foot fern 191
hare's ear 102
haricot 53
haricot bean 53
harlock 310
Harmaline 369
Harmidine 369
Harmine 369
harp seal 223
Hawaiian hibiscus 182
hawkweed 189
hawthorn 125
hawthorn (Japanese) 106
heal all 300
healing herb 102
Heartcin 259
heart leaf sida 297
heart of bovine 232
heart of horse 232
heartsease 106, 121
heather 81
heavenly bamboo 329
hedgehog mushroom 207
hedge-row thorn 125
hedyotis 181
Helichrysum 187
hellebore 330
Hematin 281
Hematite 364
Heme b 281
Heme iron 281
Hemidesmus indicus 294
Hemin 281
hemp 40, 339
hemp palm 116
hemp tree 127
henbane 333
henna 110
hen of the woods 192
henon bamboo 142, 324
hepatica 335

herb of grace 188
herb-of-grace 65
herb of snow lotus 130
hercampure 60
hercampuri 60
Hercules-club 140
Hercules-club tree 112
hermal 332
herniary breastwort 187
Hesper bitabs 280
Hesperetin-7-rhamnoglucoside 280
Hesperetin-7-rutinoside 280
Hesperidin 280
Hesperidine 280
Hesperidine-rutinoside 280
Hesperidoside 280
1,2,4/3,5,6-Hexahydroxycyclohexene 266
2,6,10,15,19,23-Hexamethyltetracosa-2,6,10,14,18,22-hexaene 264
hiba 42
hiba arbovitae 42
hibiscus 163, 182
higanbana 318
highbush blueberry 185
high bush cranberry 209
high mallow 56, 130
hill cherry 298
Himalayan mayapple 338
Himalayan panax 176
Himalayan yew 165, 331
Hindu lotus 166
hinoki 175
hinoki cypress 175
hinoki false cypress 175
Histidine 272
L-Histidine 273
Hive dross 280
HMB 273
hoarfrost juniper 312
hoelen 334
hog fennel 319
hoi 63
holly hock 139
hollyhock 139
holly-leaf barberry 173
holy herb 86, 199
holy thistle 79, 194
Homosildenafil 374
Homosildenafil thione 374
Homothiodenafil 374
honey 167
honeybee larva 235
Hongdenafil 374
hong qu 186
hoodia 179
hoodia cuctus 179
hoof fungus 146
hop 191
hops 191
horehound 195
horned holly 173
horn-of-plenty 324
horse chestnut 126, 318
horsefly 350
horse mint 204
horse radish 220
horseradish 220
horse shoe vitex 160
horsetail 120
houttuynia 115
hovenia 76
hrSOD 264
HS-CoA 259
5-HTP (5-Hydroxy-tryptophan) 371
Huang jing 62
huang qi 62
huan jing 160
huckleberry 128, 167, 178
Human angiotensin II 357
human blood 347
human bone marrow 348
human placenta 350
Hundred pace snake 236
hundred roots 114
Hungarian chamomile 72
hung-chu 186
hurtsickle 204
husk tomato 117
hyacinth bean 53, 188
hyacinth orchid 118
Hyaluronic acid 272
hydrangea 41
Hydrocerol A 254
Hydroxy acetildenafil 372
Hydroxyacetildenafil 372
beta-Hydroxyalanine 265
L-3-Hydroxy-alanine 265
3beta-Hydroxy-5-androsten-17-one 367
7-Hydroxy-6,8-dimethoxy-*2H*-1-benzopyran-2-one 244
Hydroxyhomo sildenafil 371
Hydroxyhomosildenafil 371
Hydroxyhongdenafil 372
3-Hydroxyisovaleric acid 273
beta-Hydroxyisovaleric acid 273
5-Hydroxylysine 277
Hydroxylysine 277
L-Hydroxylysine 277
4-Hydroxy-3-methoxycinnamic acid 278
3-(4-Hydroxy-3-methoxyphenyl)-2-propenoic acid 278
beta-Hydroxy-beta-methylbutylate 273
3-Hydroxy-3-methylbutyric acid (HMB) 273
8-[[2-[4-(Hydroxymethyl)piperidine-1-yl]benzyl]amino]-3-ethyl-3*H*-imidazo[4,5-*g*]quinazoline-2(1*H*)-thione 366
4-Hydroxy-L-phenylalanine 266
beta-(*p*-Hydroxyphenyl)alanine 266
4-Hydroxyproline 277
Hydroxy-L-proline 277
trans-4-Hydroxy-L-proline 277
L-4-Hydroxyproline 277
L-Hydroxyproline 277
2-hydroxy-1,2,3-propanetricarboxylic acid 254
Hydroxythiohomo sildenafil 371
Hydroxythiohomosildenafil 371
(+-)-5-Hydroxytryptophan 371
5-Hydroxy-DL-tryptophan 371
5-Hydroxy-L-tryptophan 371
DL-5-Hydroxytryptophan 371
DL-Hydroxytryptophan 371
L-5-Hydroxy-tryptophan 371
hyssop 175

I

Iceland moss 37
ice man fungus 146
Ichang lime 185
Icosa-5,8,11,14,17-Pentaenoic acid

244
Icosapentaenoic acid<EPA> 244
ikmo 83
Imidazosagatriadinone 357
immigrant oyster 227
immortelle 187
impatiens 188, 336
imperata 336
impetigo bush 169
Indian almond 202
Indian asparagus 114
Indian bael 53, 187
Indian bdellium tree 72
Indian bean 188
Indian beech 90
Indian bread 334
Indian buckwheat 139
Indian chiretta 132
Indian cobra 230
Indian coraltree 300
Indian corn mealies 151
Indian fig 56
Indian frankincense 190
Indian goldthread 63, 299, 340
Indian gooseberry 210
Indian hemp 40, 339
Indian jalap 66
Indian licorice 321
Indian lilac 320
Indian long pepper 54
Indian lotus 166
Indian madder 320
Indian mallow 49, 150
Indian mango 195
Indian mulberry 203
Indian nard 303
Indian olibanum 190
Indian pennywort 65, 145
Indian plantain 184
Indian poke 316
Indian pokeweed 316
Indian privet 160, 339
Indian psyllium 184
Indian red wood 322
Indian rubber tree 100
Indian saffron 55
Indian sarsaparilla 294
Indian scented oleander 81
Indian senna 133, 320
Indian snakeroot 295
Indian-spice 127
Indian spikenard 303
Indian spinach 147
Indian tinospora 324
Indian tobacco 339, 344
Indian wheat 139
Indian wild rice 193
Indian wormseed 46
indigo woad 117
Indole-3-alanine 269
Infusorial earth 258
Inkiapo frog 229
Inokiten 259
Inorganic germanium 258
i-Inositol 245
Inositol 245
Inulin 244
Inulin from Jerusalem artichokes 245
Invertase 358
Invertin 358
Iodine 284
iota-Carrageenan 249
ipecac 307
ipecacuanha 307
ipe roxo 54, 140, 163
ipsagol 184
Irish moss 37, 205
Irish potato 172
Iron 267
Iron(2+)bis[(2R,3S,4R,5R)-2,3,4,5,6-pentahydroxyhexanoate] 256
irris 294
isatis 117
Isinglass 246
isodon rubescens 327
Isofraxidin 244
(S)-Isoleucine 244
(S,S)-Isoleucine 244
2S,3S-Isoleucine 244
Isoleucine 244
L-Isoleucine 244
ispaghula 184

J

jaborandi 342
jaborandi pepper 54, 115
Jack 171
Jack fruit 171
Jack tree 171
Jacob's staff 178
jade plant 61, 94
jade tree 94
jalap 342
Jamaica sorrel 163
jaman 198
jambolan 183, 198
jambolang 183, 198
jambolan plum 183, 198
jambool 183, 198
jambu 198
jambul 183
Japanese abalone 224
Japanese alder 130
Japanese ampelopsis 68
Japanese anchovy 224, 229
Japanese angelica tree 140
Japanese anise tree 313
Japanese apricot 57
Japanese aralia 112, 140
Japanese arisaema 325
Japanese ash 205
Japanese asparagus 328
Japanese astilpe 38
Japanese avens 136
Japanese banana 166
Japanese bellflower 76
Japanese big-leaf magnolia 308
Japanese bindweed 178
Japanese bird cherry 58
Japanese blood grass 336
Japanese bunching onion 160
Japanese bush cherry 48
Japanese buttercup 57
Japanese catalpa 304
Japanese chestnut oak 316
Japanese climbing fern 70
Japanese cornel 107
Japanese cuscuta 328
Japanese cypress 175
Japanese dipsacus 156
Japanese dodder 328
Japanese draba 50
Japanese eel 225
Japanese elecampane 320
Japanese elm 159
Japanese false cypress 175
Japanese felt fern 129

Japanese fern palm 322
Japanese fleeceflower 48, 309
Japanese forest mushroom 109
Japanese gall 160
Japanese gentian 343
Japanese gesneria 52
Japanese ginseng 324
Japanese globeflower 206
Japanese goldenrod 40
Japanese goldthread 63, 299, 340
Japanese honey locust 102
Japanese honeysuckle 82
Japanese hornet larva 235
Japanese horse chestnut 152
Japanese hydrangea 41
Japanese kelp 101
Japanese kerria 206
Japanese knotweed 48, 309
Japanese lime 112
Japanese limonium 48
Japanese linden 112
Japanese loquat 179
Japanese male fern 299
Japanese mallotus 39
Japanese mamushi 237
Japanese medlar 179
Japanese mint 167
Japanese morning glory 40, 307
Japanese mountain ash 156
Japanese mountain cherry 298
Japanese mugwort 210
Japanese nut meg tree 174
Japanese oyster 227
Japanese pagoda 297
Japanese pagoda-tree 61
Japanese pearl oyster 234
Japanese pepper 107, 179
Japanese persimmon 68
Japanese pilchard 224, 229
Japanese plectranthus 61
Japanese plum 179
Japanese plum yew 174
Japanese prickly ash 107
Japanese privet 159
Japanese quince 189, 201
Japanese raisin-tree 76
Japanese Rohdea 299
Japanese rose 170, 206
Japanese rowan 156
Japanese rubber plant 94
Japanese rush 129
Japanese sago palm 322
Japanese sardine 224
Japanese scirpus 55
Japanese sea tangle 101
Japanese senecio 64
Japanese sophora 61, 297
Japanese speedwell 50
Japanese spikenard 328
Japanese star anise 313
Japanese stemona 333
Japanese sumac 160
Japanese summer orange 155
Japanese sweet flag 129
Japanese teasel 156
Japanese thistle 161
Japanese timber bamboo 148
Japanese torreya 174
Japanese tree peony 190
Japanese white bark magnolia 308
Japanese white birch 117
Japanese white radish 211
Japanese willow-leaf magnolia 316
Japanese willow oak 58
Japanese wisteria 180, 334
Japanese yam 108
Japanese yellow hornet larva 235
Japanese yellow loosestrife 98
Japanese yew 49, 293
Japan wood 322
jasmine 114
jatamansi 303
jatoba 115
jaundice berry 128
Java cardamom 177
Java cardamon 177
Java galanga 156
Javanese long pepper 115
Java plum 183, 198
Java tea 87
Jawa long pepper 115
jelly fig 37
jequirity 321
Jersey cudweed 170
Jerusalem artichoke 77
Jesuit's bark 304
jewel orchid 79, 83
jewelweed 188, 336
Jew's ear 77
Jew's mallow 203, 206
Jew's myrtle 154
jif 112
jimson weed 324
Job's tears 168
johimbe 342
Johnny-jump up 121
Johnny-jump-up 106
jojoba 191
Judas's ear 77
Juice bromelain 373
jujube 108, 136
jujube date 108, 136
juniper 127
jurubeba 116

K

Kacha haldi 254
kadsura pepper 179
kaempheria galanga 108
Kaffir lime 185
kaijinso 338
kail 92
kajimi 46
kakee 68
kaki 68
kale 92
kalmegh 132
kamala tree 305
kaner 81
Kangra buckwheat 139
Kaolin 360
kappa-Carrageenan 249
karavira 81
Karnitin 246
karoub 50
karum tree 90
Kashmir soapberry 197
kassod tree 138
katuka 96
kava 302
kava kava 302
kava pepper 302
kawa 303
kawakawa 303
kawaraketsumei 108
kaya 174
Kefton-2 276

keg fig 68
Keiske angelica 41
kelp 93
kendyr 212
kerosene tree 99
kerria 206
khat 293
kidney bean 53
kidney vetch 47
kidneywort 335
king's crown 53
king's fruit 196
kinkeliba 93
kinkelliba 93
kiransou 81
kirata 132
Klinit 252
knap bottle 175
knitbone 102
knotgrass 196
knotweed 196
kobus magnolia 316
Koffein 249
ko-hone 95, 319
kola 96
konara oak 316
konbu 101
kordofan pea 144
Korean black raspberry 153
Korean bramble 153
Korean cherry 48
Korean ginseng 65
Korean mint 301, 303
kothala himbutu 104
kra chai dam 183
krachai dam 183
krachaidam 183
krachaidum 183
krantz aloe 77
Kreatin 257
Krebiozon 257
ku di ding 85
ku ding cha 141
kudzu 86, 137, 302
kudzu-vine 86
kuikui pake 157
kulit lawang 119
kumis kuching 87
kumis kucin 87
kumquat 82
kunchi 87
kuromoji 56
kutki 96
kwakhur 68
kwanso 82
kwao keur 68
kwao krua 180
Kytex H 252
Kytex M 252

L

lablab bean 53, 188
Labrador tea 88
lace-bark pine 165
alpha-Lactalbumin 243
Lactase 377
Lactase-phlorizin hydrolase 377
lactic acid bacilli 158
lactic acid bacteria 158
lactic acid bacterium 158
lactic bacteria 158
Lactin 270
lactobacillus 158
lactobacillus acidophilus 41
Lactoferrin 284
Lactoflavin 274
beta-D-Lactose 270
Lactose 270
lactose galactohydrolase 377
Lactotransferrin (LTF) 284
lady bells 114
lady's delight 106
lady's finger 47
lady's mantle 165
lady's thistle 194
laitue vireuse 219
la-kwa 157
lambda Carrageenan 249
lamb minth 121
lamb's lettuce 192
lamb's quarters 38
laminaria 101
lammer 99
lamprey 225
lamp rush 327
lance-leaf plantain 187
land snail 227
lapacho 54, 140, 163
lappa 310
large cranberry 88
large flowered evening primrose 199
large Indian cress 84
large-leaf bugbane 316
large leaved linden 190
larry 189
late black wattle 203
late sweet blueberry 185
laurel 93
lavandin 213
lavender 213
lead tree 83
leaf beet 181
leaf chervil 143
lebbeck tree 178
L-alpha-Lecithin 286
Lecithin 286
ledgerbark cinchona 304
leech 236
leechee 216
leech lime 185
lemmon verbena 188
lemon balm 200
lemongrass 217
lemon ironwood 217
lemon myrtle 217
lemon scent backhousia 217
lemon scented verbena 188
lemon scent myrtle 217
lemon scent vervena 217
lemon thyme 51, 131, 217
lemon walnut 166
leopard's bane 293
lesser cat's tail 101
lesser flowering quince 189
lesser galangal 343
lesser ginger 87
lesser ginseng 136
lesser periwinkle 177
lettuce opium 219
leucaena 83
(S)-Leucine 287
Leucine 287
L-Leucine 287
Leucinum 287
Leucoharmine 370
leuconostoc 158
Levitra® 369

Levocarnitine 246
Levoglutamid 256
Levoglutamide 256
Levomethorphan 367
lichi 216
licopodium 118
licorice 75
licorice root 75
life everlasting 206
light-yellow sophora 305
Lignans 284
lignum vitae 84
lily 209
lily of China 299
lily of the valley 317
lilytree 316
Limestone 250
lime tree 190
limonium 48
linden 125, 147, 190
lindera 56, 58, 296
linen 40
lingenberry 309
lingonberry 97, 309
Linoleate 285
Linoleic acid 285
alpha-Linolenate 285
Linolenate 285
alpha-Linolenic acid 285
Linolenic acid 285
Linolic acid 285
linseed 44
linum 44
lion head mushroom 207
lion's mane mushroom 207
lion's tooth 126, 189
Lipase 377
alpha-Lipoic acid 266
Lipoic acid 266
Liquid paraffin 285
Liquimeth 283
liquorice root 75
litchi 216
lithospermum 314
liver 228
liver-leaf wintergreen 49
liver wort 335
lizard's tail 173
lobelia 344
locust bean 50
logwood 172
longan 213
longgu 351
long Jack 154
longjack 154
long net stinkhorn 78
longnosed pipefish 227
long pepper 54
long-stamen onion 68
longwood 172
loofah 186
lophatherum 141
loquat 179
lovage 219
lovage angelica 219
love apple 153
Love-in-a-mist 182
lowbush blueberry 128, 185
low-bush cranberry 88
low photinia 319
low sweet blueberry 185
lubia bean 188
lucerne 46
lucma 39
luffa 186
lumberjack's tea 115
Lumbrokinase 377
lump rush 47
lungan 213
luster-leaf holly 141
Lutein 286
trans-Lutein 286
Luteine 286
lychee 216
lycium 85, 314
lysimachia 83
L-Lysine 284
Lysine 284
Lysine acid 284

M

mabinlang 70
maca 193
macamaca 193
mace 158
mâche 192
Madagascar clove 212
Madagascar nutmeg 212
Madagascar periwinkle 329
madake 148
madder 123
maddog desert scullcap 173
mad dog scullcap 317
Madeira nut 69
Magnesium 282
Magnesium citrate 254
Magnoflorine 375
magnolia 308, 316
magnolia bark 308
magnolia vine 310
ma-huang 338
maidenhair tree 50
Maifan stone 271
maitake mashrooms 192
maize 151
makai 151
makoi 51
Makrud lime 185
makuri 338
Malabar nightshade 147
Malabar spinach 147
Malabar tamarind 74
Malayan jasmin 137
Malay camphor 214
Malay padauk 111
Malaysian ginseng 154
Malaytea scurfpea 189
Malbit 250
male fern 299
mallow 150
malt 64, 164
Maltase 375
Maltisorb 250
Maltit 250
Maltitol 250
malva 56, 130
malva nut 173
mamushi 237
mamushi pit viper 237
Manchurian ash 205
Manchurian catalpa 304
Manchurian scorpion 230
Manchurian walnut 105
Manchurian water rice 193
Manchurian wild ginger 312
Manchurian wild rice 193
Manchurian zizania 193

mandarin 196
mandarine 144
mandarine orange 144, 196
mandarin orange 196
mandrake 339
Mandrin 359
Manganese 282
mango 195
mango ginger 195
mangostan 196
mangosteen 196
mangsteen 196
manihot 80
manioc 80
manioc hibiscus 154
Manshurian gentian 343
mantids 233
mantis 233
Many banded krait 236
Maori bush basil 303
Maori kava 303
marabal almond 202
Maranhao jaborandi 342
marapuama 340
Marble 250
mare's milk 235
marigold 150
marihuana 339
marijuana 40, 339
marine turtle 228
maritime pine 184
marmalade orange 137
marronier 318
marronnier 126
marrow 71
marrow bean 53
marsh clover 317
marsh mallow 46
marshmallow 46
marsh parsely 131
marsh trefoil 317
Mary's thistle 194
masterwort 54
matara tea 302
mate 194
maté 194
Mateina 249
matico 193
matrimony vine 85, 314
mat rush 47
matsutake mushroom 194
Mauritius papeda 185
May apple 143, 152
mayapple 338
May bush 125
May flower 125
May pop 143, 152
mayten 192
mayten tree 192
May tree 125
mayweed 72
mazzard cherry 128
meadow saffron 294
meadowsweet 126
meadowsweety 126
Medicinal paraffin 285
medicinal rhubarb 135
Medicon 363
medweed 119
Melatonex® 376
Melatonin 376
Meletin 258
melia 132, 320, 327
melilot 123
melissa 200
melissa balm 200
melist 123
melon 200
melon pear 187
melon shurub 187
melon tree 169
Melovine® 376
membranaceus milk-vetch 151
membranous milkvetch 62, 298
Menadione 276
Menaquinone 4 276
Menaquinone 7 276
Menatetrenone 276
beta-Mercaptoalanine 262
meshimacobu (Japanese) 198
meso-Inositol 245
mesona 132
metel 324
L-(-)-Methionine 283
L-Methionine 283
Methionine 283
Methioninyladenylate 358
Methisosildenafil 376
d-Methorphan 367
Methoxatin disodium salt 273
5-Methoxy-N-acetyltryptamine 376
(+)-3-Methoxy-17-methylmorphinan 367
[9α,13α,14α,(+)]-3-Methoxy-17-methylmorphinan 367
(9S,13S,14S)-3-Methoxy-17-methylmorphinan monohydrobromide monohydrate 363
(+)-3-Methoxy-N-methylmorphinon 367
7-Methoxy-1-methyl-9*H*-pyrido[3,4-*b*]indole 370
[R,(-)]-α-[(S)-1-(Methylamino)ethyl]benzyl alcohol 359
(1R,2S)-2-Methylamino-1-phenylpropane-1-ol 359
(1R,2S)-2-(Methylamino)-1-phenyl-1-propanol 359
(1R,3R)-Methyl 1-(benzo[d][1,3]dioxol-5-yl)-2-(2-chloroacetyl)-2,3,4,9-tetrahydro-1*H*-pyrido[3,4-*b*]indole-3-carboxylate 362
(alpha-Methylguanido)acetic acid 257
N-Methyl-N-guanylglycine 257
O-Methylharmalol 369
methyl(3alpha,14beta,16alpha)-14-hydroxy-14,15-dihydroeburnamenine-14-carboxylate 372
1-Methyl-3-propyl-5-[2-ethoxy-5-(4-cyclopentylpiperazinosulfonyl)phenyl]-6,7-dihydro-1*H*-pyrazolo[4,3-*d*]pyrimidine-7-one 363
1-Methyl-3-propyl-5-[2-ethoxy-5-(4-methylpiperazinoacetyl)phenyl]-6,7-dihydro-1*H*-pyrazolo[4,3-*d*]pyrimidine-7-one 368
1-Methyl-3-propyl-5-[2-ethoxy-5-(4-methylpiperazinosulfonyl)phenyl]-6,7-dihydro-1*H*-pyrazolo[4,3-*d*]pyrimidine-7-thione 366
1-Methyl-3-propyl-5-[2-ethoxy-5-(4-methylpiperazinosulfonyl)phenyl]-1*H*-pyrazolo[4,3-*d*]py-

rimidine-7(6*H*)-thione 366
(S)-3-(1-methylpyrrolidin-2-yl)pyridine 368
Methyl sulfone 243
Methylsulfonylmethane 243
(1R,3R)-Methyl-1,2,3,4-tetrahydro-2-chloroacetyl-1-(3,4-methylenedioxyphenyl)-9*H*-pyrido[3,4-*b*]indole-3-carboxylate 362
Methyltheobromine 249
Mexican bamboo 48
Mexican holly 323
Mexican sunflower 158
Mexican tea 46
Mica 246
Mielogen 251
mile a minute 201
mile a minute vine 201
milfoil 127
Milk albumin 243
milk thistle 162, 194
milk vetch 217
Millettia reticulata 91
mimosa 161, 196
mimosa tree 161
Mineral oil 285
miniature pansy 106
mint 197
mirasol 176
miso-hagi 196
mistletoe 318
Mokusaku wood vinegar 264
Molybdenum 283
mond grass 331
Mongholian milkvetch 62
Mongolian milkvetch 298
Mongolian oak 316
Mongolian snake gourd 302
Mongolian snakegourd 74
monitor lizard 225
monkey bread tree 164
monkey face tree 305
monkey head mushroom 207
monkey nut 212
monkshood 329
monk's pepper tree 127
Monnier's snowparsely 315
Monosilane 258
Montanyl alcohol 247
mooli 211
moonflower gourd 207
Moranoline 367
morinda 331
morning glory 40
moron 189
mother-of-thyme 51, 131
mother's heart 154
motherwort 216
mountain black cherry 219
mountain cranberry 97, 309
mountain ebony 344
mountain grape 173
mountain peony 190, 337
mountain tabaco 293
mouse ear hawkweed 189
Moutan peony 190
muco-Inositol 245
Mucopolysaccharide 260, 282
muira puama 197, 340
mukuroji 197
mulberry 90
mullein 178
multiflora rose 296
mulukhiyah 203
mume 57
mung bean 214
muscatel sage 66
musk 348
muskmelon 200
Mussolinite 266
Mutaprodenafil 375
myo-Inositol 245
myrrh tree 311
myrtle 177
mysore cardamom 116

N

Nagi camphor tree 138
nalta jute 203
nandina 329
nangka blanda 88
nan sha shen 114
nard 303
narra 111
narrow leaf cat tail 71
narrow leaf paperbark 199
narrow-leaf plantain 187
narrow leaf tea tree 199
narrow leaf ti tree 199
native bread 210
native tobacco 339
natsudaidai 155
natsumikan 155
natto 155
Natural yellow 3 254
needle juniper 152
Neoanticid 250
Nepari hog plum 156
nettle 52, 123
Neuquinon 259
Nevulose 249
New Zealand ice plant 146
New Zealand pepper tree 303
New Zealand spinach 146
Ngai camphor plant 138
Niacin 270
Nicotine 367
Nicotinic acid 270
nigaki 329
nigella 182
Night bullet 371
night crawlers 349
night jasmine 54
nigro caffee 170
Nihon mamushi 237
Nikko maple 198
Nippon hawthorn 106
Nitrodenafil 368
Nitroprodenafil 375
N-Nitroso-bis-(2-hydroxy-propyl)amine 359
N-Nitroso-fenfluramin 359
N-Nitrosofenfluramine 359
N-nitroso-fenfluramine 359
Nitrosoprodenafil 375
niwa-ume 48
noble chamomile 219
noble sugarcane 75
noix muscade 158
nomame senna 108
noni 203
non wu jia 95
nopal 56
Norhongdenafil 368
Norneo sildenafil 368
Norneosildenafil 368
northen prickly ash 45

northern fur seal 226
northern kiwi 105
northern mountain cranberry 97, 309
northern schanzha 106
northern schisandra 310
North Indian soapnut 197
nose-bleed 127
notch-seeded buckwheat 134
notopterygium 304
nucleic acid 227
nuez moscada 158
Nujol 285
nut gall tree 121
nut grass 308
nutmeg 158
nutmeg flower 182
nut sedge 308
nux-vomica 339
nux-vomica tree 339

O

oak-leaved fern 164
oak moss 145
oakmoss 145
oat 61, 73
oat grass 73
Oceanic bonito 227
ockscomb 161
1-Octacosanol 247
n-Octacosanol 247
Octacosanol 247
Octacosyl alcohol 247
cis,cis-9,12-Octadecadienoic acid 285
9,12,15-Octadecatrienoic acid 285
octopus plant 77
(6R)-2-Octyl-6alpha-(1,3-benzodioxole-5-yl)-2,3,6,7,12,12a beta-hexahydropyrazino[1',2':1,6]pyrido[3,4-b]indole-1,4-dione 359
N-octylnortadalafil 359
ogbono 43
oilnut 166
oilseed poppy 306
Okinawa pitviper 235
old maid 329
oleander 81
Oleovitamin A 273
oligochaetes 349
Oligoglycoside 247
Oligosaccharide 247
olive 67
olive bark tree 202
Ondogyne 363
one-seed hawthorn 125
Ontosein 264
ophiopogon 331
opium 92, 306
opium lettuce 219
opium poppy 92, 306
Optidase 360
opuntia 56
orange 67, 119
orange day lily 82
orange kamala 305
orange root 308
orange tree 312
orchid tree 344
ordeal bean 302
Oregon barberry 173
Oregon grape 173
Oregongrape 173
Oregon grapeholly 173
Oregon holly 128
Organic germanium 258
Orgotein 264
oriental arborvitae 134, 330
oriental bezoar 347
oriental garlic 159
oriental lizardtail 173
oriental lotus 166
oriental senna 60
oriental sesame 100
oriental sweet gum 134
origanum 194
Ormetein 264
ornamental rhubarb 322
(S)-Ornithine 248
L-Ornithine 248
Ornithine 248
orobanche 134
Orodin 248
Oropur 248
Orotic acid 248
Orotonin 248
Oroturic 248
Orotyl 248
orris 294
gamma-Oryzanol 361
Osmoglyn 254
Ossein 259
oswego tea 204
our lady's milk thistle 194
Ovalbumin 243
Ovoester 241, 281
Oxidized L-cysteine 261
ox knee 309
oyster shell 227
gamma-OZ 361

P

Pacific cod 229
Pacific cupped oyster 227
Pacific sardine 229
paddy 51
paddy lucerne 297
Padil 254
pagoda tree 61, 132, 297, 320, 327
paigle 125
painkiller 203
painted daisy 39
pale catechu 42
pallid seahorse 227
palma christi 332
Palmitoyl ceramide 265
N-Palmitoyl 4-sphingenine 265
N-palmitoylsphingosine 265
palm-leaf raspberry 334
palmyra palm 56
palo azul 172
palo negro 172
Palosein 264
Pancreatic extracts 370
Pancreatin 370
pandan 113
pandanus palm 113
pansy 106
Pantothenate 271
D-Pantothenic acid 271
Pantothenic acid 271
Papain 369
Papaine 369
papaw 169
papaya 169
Papayotin 369
papelite 305
paprika 113, 149

Paraffin oil 285
Paraffinum liquidum 285
Paraguayan sweet herb 120
Paraguayan tea 194
Paraguay jaborandi 342
Paraguay tea 194
pareira 311
pareira brava 311
pareira root 311
parsley 166
partridge berry 309
passionflower 143
passion fruit 152
pata-de-vaca 167
patchouli plant 301
patchouly 301
patrinia 67
pau d'arco 54, 140, 163
pau da reposta 70
pawpaw 169
peach 202, 327
peanut 212
pearl oyster 234
Pearlspar 269
pearly everlasting 206
pear melon 187
peavine clover 38
pedra hume 75
pedra ume caa 75
peepal 54
peepul 54
pegu cutch 185
Pelargonium reniforme 296
Pellagrin 270
pellitory of the wall 174
pendulous yucca 208
penis or testis of bovine 224
penis or testis of deer 351
penis or testis of horse 224
penis or testis of serpent 224
penis or testis of sheep 224
penis or testis of swine 224
penis or testis of tiger 224
pennyroyal 198
peony 114, 315
pepino 187
pepino dulce 187
pepino morade 187
pepper 97
pepper bush 96
peppermint 127
pepper tree 303
Pepsin 374
Pepsin A 374
Pepsin B 374
perilla 110
Pernam buco jaborandi 342
Persian insect flower 39
Persian lilac 132, 320, 327
Persian pellitory 39
Persian silk tree 161
Persian walnut 69
persimmon 68
Peruvian bark 304
Peruvian ginseng 193
Peruvian krameria 343
Peruvian rhatany 343
Peruvian's wild grape 311
peucedanum 319
pfaffia 121
phellodendron 63, 298
3-Phenyl-L-alanine 278
beta-Phenyl-L-alanine 278
L-Phenylalanine 278
Phenylalanine 278
Philippine cobra 230
Phosphane 285
phosphate 242
3-sn-Phosphatidylcholine 286
Phosphatidylcholine 286
L-alpha-Phosphatidylcholine solution 286
3-*O*-sn-Phosphatidyl-L-serine 281
L-1-Phosphatidylserine 281
O3-Phosphatidyl-L-serine 281
Phosphatidyl-L-serine 281
Phosphatidylserine 281
Phosphine 285
Phosphorus 285
Phosphorus cation 285
Phosphorus trihydride 285
phragmites 41, 344
C-Phycocyanin 277
R-Phycocyanin 277
Phycocyanins 277
phyllanthus 78, 100
Phylloquinone 276
Phylloxanthin 286
physic nut 157
Phytin 245
Phytodolor 244
Phytonadion 276
Phytonadione 276
Phytosterol 263
pickle plant 43
picrorhiza 96
pied-de-chat 59
pie maker 150
pie-marker 49
pie plant 117
pie-plant 135
Pigment in *Haematococcus* algae 281
pignon d'inde 157
pignut 115
pig's knee 309
pigweed 38, 122
pinang 179
pindar 212
pine 194
Pineal gland hormone 376
pineapple 163
pineapple tree 163
pinellia 332
pinellia root 332
pine root of stump 334
pine tree 194
pink porcelain lily 93
pink siris 161
pink wintergreen 49
pinto bean 53
Piperadino vardenafil 372
Piperidenafil 372
Piperidic acid 251
Piperidinic acid 251
Piperidino-vardenafil 372
pipsissewa 57
piqu pichana 122
pirage 128
pitanga 139
placenta 233
plantain 64, 124
Plant enzyme 262
Plant sterol 263
platycodon 76
plum 125
plume flower 38
poet's jasmine 114

poison-nut tree 339
poisonous lettuce 219
Poliglusam 252
pollen 71
Polopiryna 355
Poly(N-acetyl-1,4-beta-D-glucopyranosamine) 252
polygala 300
polygonatum 62
polygonum indigo 140
Polyhydroxyflavan-3-ol 279
polyporus 334
polyporus mylittae 210
pomegranate 103
pomelmous 185
pomelo 185
pommelo 185
pom pom mushroom 207
pongam 90
ponkoranti 104
poonga-oil tree 90
poor man's opium 219
poor man's wealtherglass 215
poppy 92, 306
poque 158
porcelain berry 162
porcelain vine 162
porcupine orange 185
poria 334
poria cocos 334
Portugues plum 183
Potassium 250
potato 172
potato bean 45
potatoe 172
potato yam 63
pot marigold 150
powdered bones of bovine 230
powdered bones of fishes 230
praying mantis 233
precatory 321
Precipitated calcium carbonate 250
predaceous diving beetle 238
prickly ash 45
prickly custard apple 88, 306
prickly pear 56
prickly sago palm 103
prickly water-lily 66
pride-of-China 132, 327
pride-of-India 132, 168, 327
prince ginseng 136
prince's pine 57
princess vine 53
prinsepia 119
Proanthocyanidin 279
Proanthocyanidin A 279
Proanthocyanidins 279
(−)-Proline 280
L-(−)-Proline 280
L-Proline 280
Proline 280
1,2,3-Propanetriol 254
Propanetriol 254
Propolis 280
Propolis balsam 280
Propolis resin 280
Propolis wax 280
Prostaglandin 373
prostrate knotweed 196
Protease 373
Protoheme 281
Provatene 280
Provitamin A 280
prune 125
pseudoginseng 107
pseudostellaria 136
Pseudo vardenafil 372
Pseudovardenafil 372
PSF 281
psoralea 189
psyllium husk 184
Pteroylglutamic acid 283
pubescent angelica 110, 328
pudding grass 198
pu'ercha 142
Puertorican cherry 42
puke weed 344
Pullulan 279
pumelo 185
pummelo 185
pumpkin 71
puncture vine 314
puncturevine caltrop 314
purging croton 332
purging nut 157
purple beebalm 204
purple clover 38
purple cone flower 59
purple fox glove 313
purple granadilla 152
purple loosestrife 196
purple mangosteen 196
purple passion flower 143
purple passionflower 152
purple plum 183
purple puffer 236
purslane 165
Pururan 279
purut 185
pusley 165
pussy-foot 70
pyramidal yew 293
1*H*,3*H*-Pyrano(4,3-b)(1)benzopyran-9-carboxylic acid 279
pyrethrum 39
pyrethurum gardens 39
3-Pyridinecarboxylic acid 270
Pyridoxin 275
Pyridoxine 275
Pyridoxol 275
Pyroligneous acid 264
Pyroligneous vinegar 264
Pyrolysate 257
Pyrroloquinoline quinone disodium salt 273
pyrrosia 129

Q

quack grass 112
quail grass 161
Quban jute 297
queen-of-the-meadow 126
queen of the night 92
queen's crape myrtle 168
Queensland hemp 297
Quercetin 258
Quercetine 258
Quercetin 3-rutinoside 286
Quercetol 258
Quercitin 258
Quertine 258
quick-set thorn 125
quinoa 78
quinquelibas 93
quisqualis 109

R

rabbit foot fern 191
raccoon berry 338
Racemethrophan 363
radish 211
radis oriental 211
ragleaf 186
railroad creeper 201
railway creeper 201
rainbow bracket 74
rainy season bush-mango 43
rakkyo 68
ramanas rose 170
rambler rose 296
rambootta 213
rambutan 213
ram's head 192
Rangoon creeper 109
rape oil 155
rape seed 155
Raphisiderite 364
raspberry 76, 212
rat tail plantain 124
rattlesnake 236
rauwolfia 295
red algae 95
red-barried elder 130
red bryony 184
redbush tea 182
red cinchona 304
red clover 38
red cole 220
red-eye round herring 229
red eye round herrings 224
redflower 186
red fucus 93
red hawthorn 106
Red iron ore 364
red kamala 305
red kwaao khruea 180
red leaven 186
red oak 39
red peony 114
red peony root 315
red pepper 113, 149
red quinine 304
red raspberry 124, 212
red rice 186
redroot 152
red-root 314
red-root gromwell 314
red-root sage 141, 323
red spider lily 318
red sumac 211
red tangeline 196
red tangerin 144
red tea 182
reduced maltose 250
red vine spinach 147
red weed 175
red yeast 186
red yeast rice 186
reed 41
reed grass 41
reetha 197
rehmannia 313
reishi 216
reishi mushroom 216
renge 217
Resin alcohol 284
Resinols 284
restharrow 299
resurrection lily 108
Resveratrol 269
E-Resveratrol 268
trans-Resveratrol 268
Resvida 269
Retinol 273
Revatio® 364
rhapontic rhubarb 117, 135
rhatania 343
rhatany 343
rheumatism weed 183
rhodiola 53
rhubarb 117, 135
ribgrass 187
D-Ribitol 252
Ribitol 252
Riboflavin 274
ribwort plantain 187
rice 51
rice bran 101
rice leaf 51
rice paper plant 144
rice plant 51
rice polishings 101
rice starch 100
ring lichen 145
ringworm cassia 169
ringworm senna 169
Rio ipecac 307
ripplegrass 187
river bulrush 55
RNA 227
roaches 232
rock cranberry 309
Rock powder 251
rockweed 175
rock wrack 93
Roman chamomile 219
Roman coriander 182
romero 218
rooibos 182, 215
rooibos tea 215
rooirabas 296
rosary pea 321
rose 171, 206
rose balsam 188, 336
rosebay willowherb 205
rose camellia 145
rose elder 209
rose hip 153, 218
rosell 182
roselle 163
rose mallow 139
rosemary 218
rose of China 163, 182
rose of India 168
rose of sharon 163
rose-of-sharon 182
rose periwinkle 329
rose root 53
rosewood 111, 138
rose wort 53
rosy periwinkle 329
rotten cheesefruit 203
rough horsetail 341
round buchu 181
round cardamom 177
round cardamon 177
round herring 229
round herrings 224
round-leaf chaste tree 339
round leaf plantain 124
round-leaved mint 43
royal jasmine 114

royal jelly 238
rubber plant 100
Rubozine 256
rue 188
rugosa 107
rugose 107
rugose rose 170
rui ren 119
rum 214
rum cherry 219
runaway robin 218
running club moss 118
running myrtle 177
running pine 118
rupture wort 187
Russian belladonna 331
Russian chamomile 219
Russian licorice 75
Russian mulberry 195
Rutin 286
Rutin trihydrate 286
Rutoside 286
rye 211

S

sabal palm 162
Saccharase 358
sacred bamboo 329
sacred bark 301
sacred fig 54
sacred lily of China 299
sacred lotus 166
safflower 186
saffron 104
saffron cod 229
saffron crocus 104
saffron thistle 186
sagarame 46
sage 105
sage tree 127
sago cycas 322
sago palm 103
saiga tatarica horn 351
salacia 104
salad burnet 220
salad chervil 143
sallow thorn 102, 103
salsola 65
salt-wart 65
saltwort 43
SAMe 358
SAM-e 358
samphire 43
Sand 258
sandalwood 333
sand plantain 184
sanghwang (Korean) 198
sanguinary 127
sanguisorba 220
san qi 107
san sho 107
sanzashi 106
Saponin 260
sappan lignum 322
sappan wood 322
sarcandra 80
sarsaparilla 106
sassafras 104
Satsuma mandarin 123
Satsuma orange 144, 196
Satsuma tangerin 123
savin 312
savina 312
savin juniper 312
saw palmetto 162
sawtooth oak 316
Saxol 285
scabrous gentian 343
scabwort 328
scarlet pimpernel 215
scarlet sumac 211
scarlet sumach 211
scented begger ticks 98
schisandra 310
schizandra 310
schizonepeta 306
Schlegel's Japanese gecko 234
scoparium 60, 296
scopolia 331
Scotch broom 60, 296
Scotch thistle 64
scouring rush 341
screw pine 113
scrophularia 307
scrub palmetto 162
scullcap 119, 317
scurfy pea 189
scute 62, 298
scyllo-Inositol 245
sea almond 202
sea buckthorn 102, 103
Sea Cure F 252
Sea Cure Plus 252
sea-ear shell 224
seahorse 226
sea onion 300
sea pea 218
seaside pea 218
sea tangle 101
sea turtle 228
seaweed 67
seaweed (*Fucaceae, Laminariaceae, Lessoniaceae*) 93
seaweed (*Laminariaceae*) 101
seaweed pipefish 227
seaweed (*Rhodophyceae*) 95
secretion from large Indian civet 348
sedum 147
seedbox 78
segmented worm 236
seim bean 188
Selen 265
selenicereus 92
Selenium 265
Selenium atom 265
self heal 300
selfheal 300
senburi 321
seneca snakeroot 319
Senedrine 359
senega root 319
senega snakeroot 319
senkyu 319
senna 133, 320
serge 102
(S)-Serine 265
L-Serine 265
Serine 265
serpentine wood 295
sesame 100
sesame seeds 100
sessile stemona 333
sete sangrias 161
seville orange 137
shaddock 185
shan tzu ku 44
shark 231

shark liver squalamine 232
sharon fruit 68
sharp-leaf galangal 341
sha shen 114
shatavari 114
shave grass 120, 341
shavetail grass 120
shea butter 108
shea butter tree 108
sheep's head 192
sheep sorrel 79, 119
shell flower 93
shell ginger 93
shepherd's club 178
shepherd's purse 154
shield fern 299
shiitake 109
shiitake mushroom 109
shijimi clam 231
shima guwa 195
shirley poppy 175
shiso 110
shoe flower 163, 182
shop consound 102
short buchu 181
shrink 107
shrubby blackberry 124
shrubby sophora 305
shuiluosan 69
shurni 329
Siam benzoin 47
Siam cardamom 177
Siam cardamon 177
siamese cassia 138
Siamese galanga 156
siamese senna 138
Siberian apricot 305
Siberian cocklebur 321
Siberian ginseng 59, 96
Siberian motherwort 216, 342
Siberian Solomon's seal 62
Siberian tree frog 229
Siberian wood frog 229
Sichuan dang shen 326
Sichuan dipsacus 156
Sichuan lovage 308
Sichuan pepper 50, 107, 111
Sichuan peppercorn 50
Sichuan teasel 156
Sicilian sumac 121
Sickle hare's ear 311
Sickle-leaf hare's ear 311
sickle-pod senna 60
sickle sennna 60
sida retusa 297
sida weed 297
Siebold's primrose 103
Siebold's wild ginger 312
siegesbeckia 199
Silane 258
Sildenafil 364, 374
Sildenafil citrate 364
siler 337
Silica 258
Silicon 258
Silicon dust 258
Silicone 258
Silicon(Ⅳ) oxide 258
Silicon metal 258
Silicon tetrahydride 258
silk 253
silk moth 226
silk protein 253
silk tree 161
silkworm 226
silkworm mulberry 195
silky fowl 225
silver birch 111
silver ear 118
silver ear fungs 118
silver vine 200
silver wattle 196
silverweed 338
simple leaf tree 339
singer's plant 69
sintok 119
sirih 83
Siris tree 178
sirsak 88
Sitrulline 247
skipjack tuna 227
skullcap 317
skute barbata 173
skyblue bloomrape 134
slender glasswort 43
slender sweet flag 318
slim amaranth 122
slippery elm 39
smac gall nut 160
small bulrush 71
small caltrops 314
small fennel 182
small Indian civet 348
small leaf lime tree 190
small leaved European linden 190
small opium poppy 306
small reedmace 71
small spotted wintergreen 57
small tobacco 339
smooth amaranth 122
smooth loofah 186
smooth sumac 211
snake jasmine 167
snake's beard 331
snake venom 349
snow ballbush 209
snowdown rose 53
snowdrop 342
snowflake 66
soapnut tree 197
soapwort 104
SOD 263
SOD-3 264
Sodium iron chlorophyllin 267
soft rush 47, 327
soja bean 136
Solatene 280
song gen (Chinese) 198
sophora 61
Sophoretin 258
Sophorin 286
sorrel 119
sotetsu nut 322
Souchet 254
sour apple 88
sour date 136
sour dock 119, 209
sour gourd 164
sour grass 119
sour jujube 136
sour orange 137
soursop 306
sour-sop 88
South African desert cactus 179
South African red tea 182
southern bayberry 118
southern blue gum 208

southern heaven bamboo 329
southern schanzha 106
southern tsangshu 321
southern wax myrtle 118
sow thistle 162
soya bean 136
so yang 65
Soyasaponin Bb 261
Soyasaponin I 261
soybean 136
Soybean lecithin 286
Soy saponin I 261
Soy saponins 260
Spanish jasmine 114
Spanish licorice 75
Spanish needles 98
Spanish onion 160
Spanish peanut 212
Spanish saffron 104
Spanish sage 142
Spanish savin juniper 312
spatholobus 91
spearmint 121
spearminth 121
Specularite 364
speedwell 91
spider brake 336
spider fern 336
spider lily 318
spiked loosestrife 196
spiked pepper 193
spike lavender 213
spikenard 328
spinach beet 181
spiny bitter cucumber 341
spiny bitter gourd 341
spiny restharrow 299
spirulina 120
sponge gourd 186
spoon-leaf nardostachys 303
spotted seahorse 226
spotted wintergreen 57
spreading pellitory 174
Spreading sneeze weed 152
spring onion 160
spring vetch 47, 72
(E,E,E,E)-Squalene 264
Squalene 264
trans-Squalene 264
squash 71
squid 224
stalkless-flower 96
star anise 135
starfish 226
starflower 215
star fruit 101
star jasmine 137
star violet 181
starwort 165
Steatite 266
Stem bromelain 373
stemona 333
stephania 314
stevia 120
sticky weed 174
3,4',5-Stilbenetriol 269
Stimulina 256
stinging nettle 52, 123
stink bug 228
stinkhorn mushroom 78
stinking weed 170
St. John's bread 50
St. John's wort 124
St. Mary's thistle 194
stomach lining of chicken 235
stone apple 187
stone leek 160
storax 47
stramonium 324
strawberry 59
strawberry tomato 117
stringy stone crop 147
striped screw pine 113
strobe 120
strobilanthus cusia 214
strychnine tree 339
St. Thomas lidpot 66
styptic weed 170
styrax 47, 134
succory 77
Sudan gum Arabic 45
Sudismase 264
sugarcane 75
suger beet 104
Sulfoaildenafil 366
Sulfohomosildenafil 374
Sulfohydroxyhomosildenafil 371
Sulfonylbismethane 243
Sulfur 243
Sulphonamide 364
suma 121
sumac 121
Sumatra benzoin 47
Sumatra camphor 214
summer cypress 112
summer savory 78
summer squash 71
Summetrin 369
sunchoke 77
sundrops 199
sunflower 176
sunset hibiscus 154
sunset muskmallow 154
Superoxide dismutase (SOD) 263
Supraene 264
Surinam cherry 139
Surround 360
swallowroot 148
swamp blueberry 185
swamp marigold 137
swamp tickseed 137
swangi 185
Swatow orange 196
sweet Annie 297
sweet balm 200
sweet basil 199
sweet bay 93
sweet belladonna 316
sweet blue violet 121, 157
sweet broomwart 122
sweet broomweet 122
sweet bush-mango 43
sweet calamus 315
sweet chamomile 219
sweet cherry 128
sweet corn 151
sweet cumin 43
sweet false chamomile 72
sweet gourd 341
sweet hurts 185
sweet hydrangea 44
sweet leaf 120
sweet marjoram 194
sweet orange 67, 119
sweet osmanthus 84
sweet-scented bedstrow 88
sweet scented oleander 81

sweetscented squinacy 88
sweet tea 44, 149
sweet tea vine 44
sweet-tea vine 44
sweet vervena myrtle 217
sweet vervena tree 217
sweet violet 121, 157
sweet woodruff 88
sweet wormwood 297
Swiss chard 104, 181
sycamore 49
Syrian rue 332

T

taakawa 303
tabasco pepper 113, 149
tachibana mandarin 139
tachibana orange 139
Tadalafil 365
taheebo 54, 140, 163
taheebo tree 140
Taiwan engelhardtia 94
Taiwanese photinia 319
tai zi shen 136
Taka-amylase 356
Talc 266
taleflower 215
talewort 215
tall groundcover 86
tall kale 92
tall mallow 56, 130
tam 312
tamarix juniper 312
Tamil-ponkoranti 105
tamogitake 140
tangerine 144, 196
tangerine orange 196
tang kuai 150
tanner's cassia 302
tanner's sumac 121
tansy 210
tan wattle 203
tape grass 129
tapioca 80
tarajo 141
tarajo holly 141
Taraspite 269
tara vine 105
tarragon 59
Tartarian buckwheat 139
D-(-)-Tartaric acid 262
DL-Tartaric acid 262
L-(+)-Tartaric acid 262
Tartaric acid 262
tartary buckwheat 139
Tarter aster 313
Tasmanian blue gum 208
Tatar aster 313
Tatarian aster 313
tatuaba 70
L-Taurine 364
Taurine 364
tayuya 323
tea bush 115
tea tree 199
teaweed 297
teel 100
temu kunchi 87
ten-months yam 57
tequila agave 38
testis of edible fish 233
testudincs 228
(s)-5,6,6a,7-tetrahydro-1,11-dihydroxy-2,10-dimethoxy-6,6-dimethyl-4h-dibenzo[de,g]quinolinium 375
1,2,3,6-tetrahydro-2,6-dioxo-4-pyrimidinecarboxylic acid 248
Tetramethylene glycol 370
Thalictrin 375
Thalictrine 375
thatch screw pine 113
Thein 249
Thiadoxine 274
Thiamine 274
thickhead 186
thin leaf polygala 300
Thioaildenafil 366
Thioctacid 266
Thioctic acid 266
Thiodenafil 366
Thiohomo sildenafil 374
Thiohydroxyhomosildenafil 371
Thiomethisosildenafil 366
Thio-2-propene-1-sulfinic acid S-allyl ester 242
Thioquinapiperifil 366
Thioserine 262
Thiosildenafil 366
thorn apple 324
thorny acacia 45
thorny restharrow 299
thorough wax 102
thousand-seal yarrow 127
three flower gentian 343
three-lobe beggar ticks 137
L-(-)-Threonine 269
L-Threonine 269
Threonine 269
thunder ball 210
thyme 139
Tibetan goldthread 63, 299, 340
Tibetan rhubarb 322
tickseed 137
Tienchi ginseng 107
tiger bone 348
tiger lily 209
tiger's claw 300
til 100
tila 100
tilia 125, 147
timbles 204
Timnodonic acid 244
tinder conk 146
tinder fungus 146
tinder polypore 146
Tinnevelly senna 133, 320
tinospora 52
ti tree 199
toad venom 349
tocha 150
alpha-Tochopherol 276
Tocopherol 276
(2R,3'E,7'E)-alpha-Tocotrienol 268
D-alpha-Tocotrienol 268
Tocotrienol 268
todok 147
Tokay gecko 225
Tokay gekko 225
Tokyo violet 111
tomato 153
tongkat Ali 154
tongue fern 129
toothache tree 45
topped lavender 213
torches 178
torch plant 77

tormentil 152
tormentilla 152
Torula dried yeast 95
tossa jute 203
tragacanth milkvetch 153
tree mallow 56, 130
tree marigold 158
tree of sadness 54
tree peony 190, 337
alpha, alpha-Trehalose 270
alpha-D-Trehalose 270
D-Trehalose 270
Trehalose 270
tremella 118
Triacylglycerol acylhydrolase 377
Triacylglycerol lipase 377
triangle sail mussel 236
trichosanthes 74
trichosanthis semen 74
tricosanthes 302
trifoliate orange 73
1,2,3-trihydroxypropane 254
Trihydroxypropane 254
3,4',5-Trihydroxystilbene 269
Trimagnesium citrate 254
Trimagnesium dicitrate 254
Triptacin 269
triticum 112
trivrit 66
Trofan 269
tropcial almond 202
true aloe 47
true bay 93
true chamomile 72
true daikon 211
true daisy 175
true frogs 229
true ginger 116
true lavender 213
true mustard 89
true myrobalan 301
true saffron 104
true sage 105
true senna 133, 320
true tiger lily 209
true tinder polypore 146
trumpet creeper 214
trumpet flower 300
trumpet tree 54, 163
L-Tryptophan 269
Tryptophan 269
Tryptophane 269
tsao ko 321
tsaoko amomum 321
tsi 115
tuberous stemona 333
tuna 56
Turkestan rose 170
Turkey rhubarb 135, 322
Turkey tails 74, 303
Turkey wheat 151
Turkish licorice 75
turmeric 55, 254
turmeric yellow 254
turnip 155
turtle 228
twelve stamen melastoma 110
twich grass 112
two-bladed onion 160
two-lobe magnolia 308
L-Tyrosine 266
Tyrosine 266

U

ube 57
Ubidecarenone 259
Ubiquinone 259
Ubiquinone-10 259
Ubiquinone 50 259
uchiwadokoro 131
Udenafil 358
udo 57, 328
umbrella-sedge 72
Umckaloabo 296
ume 57
uña-de-gato 80
uncaria rhynchohylla 325
uncaria ryunchophylla 143
uncaria stem 143
Unshiu orange 144
upland sumach 211
Uracil-6-carboxylic acid 248
Ural licorice 75
5-Ureidoimidazolidine-2,4-dione 356
delta-Ureidonorvaline 247
urn orchid 118
Ussurian thorny 96
Ussurian thorny pepper bush 59
uva-ursi 296

V

vailed lady 78
Valencia peanut 212
valerian 70
L-Valine 271
Valine 271
Vardenafil 369
variegated thistle 194
vassourinha 122
Vegetable fiber 263
Vegitable luteol 286
veitch screw pine 113
veldt grape 314
velvet bean 168
velvet dock 328
velvet foot 60
velvet leaf 150
velvet-leaf 49
velvet plant 178
velvet weed 49
Venezuela copaiba 99
Veracruz jalap 342
Veraldon 369
verbena 188
vervain 86
vetchling 218
Viagra® 364
vibhidhaka 123, 135
vibhitaka 123, 135
Victorian blue gum 208
vidanga 61
Vietnamese sophora 313
Vincamine 372
vine 182
vinegar bush 211
vinegar tree 211
vine of Sodem 310
viola 121
violet 121
virgaurea 40
Virginia bluebells 142
Virginian skullcap 119
Vitamin A 273
Vitamin A_1 273
Vitamin B_1 274
Vitamin B_{12} 274
Vitamin B_2 274

Vitamin B_5 271
Vitamin B_6 275
Vitamin B_7 272
Vitamin B_T 246
Vitamin C 275
Vitamin D 275
Vitamin E 276
Vitamin G 274
Vitamin H 272
Vitamin K 276
Vitamin K_2(35) 276
Vitamin M 283
Vitaneuron 274
Vivanza® 369
Vivitas® 376

W

walleye pollock 229
wallwort 209
walnut 69
Warrigal greens 146
washing nut 197
wasp larva 235
water bamboo 193
water chestnut 174
water hyssop 65
water plantain 113
water yam 57
Watson pomelo 155
waxberry 118
waxflower 57
wax gourd 149, 326
wax myrtle 118, 207
waybread 124
weeping birch 111
weeping forsythia 217
weeping goldenbells 217
weeping yucca 208
weevil-wort 133
wei ling xian 52
Welsh onion 160
wermut 85
wermutkraut 85
western buckthorn 301
western pearly everlasting 206
western yarrow 127
West Indian cherry 42
West Indian lemongrass 217
West Indian locust 115
weymouth pine 120
wheat 88, 100
Whey 270
Whey factor 248
white bark pine 165
white berry yew 164, 331
white birch 111
white canary tree 76
white cutch 42
white-edge morning glory 40, 307
white flowered gourd 207
white fruit amomum 177
white fungus 118
white garland-lily 168
white gourd 149, 326
white horehound 195
white kwao keur 68, 180
white-man's foot 124
White mineral oil 285
white mulberry 90, 195, 322
white-nest swiftlet 234
white nettle 66
white peony 114
white peony root 315
white pine 120
white popinac 83
white pumpkin 149, 326
white sage 192
white sandalwood 333
white saunders 333
white thorn 125
white walnut 166
white willow 125
white wood ear 118
white worm lichen 208
whiteworm lichen 208
white yam 57
whitten tree 209
whortleberry 128, 178, 185
whtie tea 164
wild bergamot 204
wild bergamot beebalm 204
wild betel 162
wild black cherry 219
wild celery 131
wild chamomile 155
wild cherry 219
wild chrysanthemum 77
wild coffee 305
wild fennel 182
wild ghaap 179
wild gourd 310
wild grape 311
wild jalap 338
wild Korean mulberry 195
wild lemon 338
wild lettuce 219
wild mandrake 338
wild mango 43
wild mint 167
wild oat 73
wild orange tree 312
wild pansy 121
wild passionflower 143, 152
wild pepper 127, 162
wild poppy 306
wild raspberry 124
wild rue 332
wild siamese cardamom 315
wild strawberry 59
wild tamarind 83
wild thyme 51, 131
wild tobacco 339
wild turmeric 172
winberry 178
windmill palm 116
wine grape 182
wine plant 117
winged spindle tree 158
winged treebine 314
winged yam 57
winter cherry 295
wintergreen 57
winter melon 149, 326
winter mushroom 60
winter savory 78
winter squash 71
winter tares 72
witches butter 97
witch hazel 171
witch's bell 204
withania 295
woad 117
wolfbane 329
woman's tangue tree 178
wonderberry 51
Wood ash 283
woodbine 303

wood cauliflower 169
wood ear fungus 77
wood ruff 88
Wood vinegar 264
woolly grass 336
wormseed 46
wormwood 85
wounder wort 47
woundwort 40

X

Xanthaurine 258
Xanthoanthrafil 360
Xanthophyll 286
xi shu 76
xuyencoc 156
Xylite 252
D-Xylitol 252
Xylitol 252
Xyliton 252

Y

yacon 203
yacon strawberry 203
yakon 203
Yakushima rhododendron 319
yam 57, 206
yama guwa 195
yama momo 207
yama zakra 298
yangona 302
yang tao 105
yaqona 302
yarba maté 194
yarrow 127
yeast 95
yellow brain 97
yellow broom 60
yellow catalpa 304
yellow dock 209
yellow gentian 94, 307
yellow ginger 55, 172
yellow jasmine 303
yellow jessamine 303
yellow lipped sea krait 236
yellow melilot 123
yellow puccoon 308
yellow root 308
yellow sandalwood 333
yellow saunders 333
yellow sedum 82
yellow sweet clover 123
yellow zedoary 172
yin-chen wormwood 294
yohimbe 342
yomogi 210
yucca 208
yujin 172
yu lan 316
yu lan magnolia 316
yuzu 208

Z

Zea mays 151
zedoary 69
Zhejiang fritillary 330
zhi quiao zhi shi 73
zhitai (Chinese) 186
zhi zi 106
zhu ling 325
Zinc 241
Zinc bis(D-gluconate-O1,O2) 256
Zinc D-gluconate(1:2) 256
Zinc gluconate 256
Zydena 358

監修者・著者略歴
Profiles of editor and authors

■ 佐竹　元吉（さたけ　もとよし／Motoyoshi Satake, Ph.D.）学術博士

【現職】お茶の水女子大学生活環境教育研究センター研究協力員

1964～1980年　東京薬科大学卒業後、国立衛生試験所（現国立医薬品食品衛生研究所）入所（生薬部）
1980～1991年　国立衛生試験所筑波薬用植物栽培試験場育種生理研究室長を経て場長
1991～2001年　国立衛生試験所生薬部部長
2001～現在　公益財団法人日本薬剤師研修センター嘱託
2001～2002年　ペルー南大学（Peru Sur University）客員教授、日本浴用剤工業会専務理事
2001～2010年　NPO法人ミャンマー麻薬代替プロジェクト理事
2002～2006年　お茶の水女子大学生活環境研究センター（現生活環境教育研究センター）教授
2006～2013年　お茶の水女子大学生活環境研究センター客員教授
2008～2012年　富山大学和漢医薬学総合研究所客員教授

【主な所属学会・団体】

WHO（薬用植物/伝統医薬分野）コンサルタント、厚生労働科学研究費補助金評価委員会/創薬基盤推進研究事業評価委員、(財)日本薬剤師研修センター、日本生薬学会、日本薬学会、薬用植物を知ろうネットワーク（薬用植物観察会講師）、薬事審議会薬局方調査委員（第９～16改正）、厚生事業団薬事行政官研修/必須医薬品製造品質管理研修（GMP）運営委員、厚労省医薬品食品監視指導麻薬課食薬区分調査委員、内閣府食品安全衛生委員会カビ毒・自然毒等専門調査会専門委員、生薬・薬用植物国際調和会議長（FHH・WHO東南アジア）

Motoyoshi SATAKE Ph.D.

Adviser Staff, Institute of Environmental Science for Human Life, Ochanomizu University
1985-1992　Director, Tsukuba Medicinal Plant research Station, National Institute of Health Sciences, Japan
1992-2000　Director, Department of Pharmacognosy and Phytochemistry, National Institute of Health Sciences, Japan
2002-2003　Professor and Guest Professor, Ochanomizu University, Science for Human Life
2009-2012　Guest Professor, Toyama University, Institute of Natural Medicine
2001-present　Adviser, Japanese Pharmacist Education Center
2008-present　Member of the WHO Expert Advisory Panel on Traditional Medicine

■ 関田　節子（せきた　せつこ／Setsuko Sekita, Ph.D.）薬学博士

【現職】昭和薬科大学特任教授／日本薬剤師研修センター特別顧問

1966年　昭和薬科大学卒業
1966～1981年　国立衛生試験所生薬部
1981～1995年　国立衛生試験所生薬部主任研究官
1995～2001年　国立衛生試験所生薬部室長
2001～2004年　国立医薬品食品衛生研究所（1997年国立衛生試験所に改称）
筑波薬用植物栽培試験場長、和歌山薬用植物栽培試験場長（兼任）
2004～2013年　徳島文理大学香川薬学部教授

【主な所属学会・団体】

日本薬学会、日本生薬学会、日本マイコトキシン学会

【主な研究歴】

「ヤブコウジ科植物成分ardisiaquinone A、B、Cの合成研究（名取信策部長）」、「Chaetomium属の新規マイコトキシン：Chaetoglobosin等の化学的研究（同上）」、「川芎、茯苓等の新規活性成分の化学及び薬理作用に関する研究（原田正敏部長）」、「食薬区分に関連するKAWAの含有成分の定性・定量試験に関する研究（佐竹元吉部長）」、「Aristolochia 属生薬のAristolochic acidに関する研究（同上）」、「麻黄、芍薬、ハトムギ等の栽培研究」、「生薬・修治『附子』の日本薬局方規格設定に関する研究」、「抗リーシュマニア活性植物成分及びペルー、パキスタンに於ける治療に関する研究」、「麻黄のエフェドリン生合成遺伝子の研究」、「アミロイドAβ42凝集抑制作用を有する植物成分の化学及び作用機序に関する研究」

Setsuko SEKITA, Ph.D.

Professor, Showa Pharmaceutical University
1966-2001　Researcher, Senior Researcher and Head of Division of Pharmacognosy, National Institute of Health Sciences, Japan
2001-2004　Director, Tsukuba Medicinal Plant Research Station, National Institute of Health Sciences, Japan
2004-2013　Professor, Laboratory of Pharmacognosy and Natural Products Chemistry, Kagawa School of Pharmaceutical Sciences, Tokushima Bunri University

■ **大濱　宏文**（おおはま　ひろぶみ／Hirobumi Ohama, Ph.D.）医学博士、日本学術会議元連携会員

一般社団法人日本健康食品規格協会元理事長／バイオヘルスリサーチリミテッド 元代表取締役

1963～1965年　東京大学応用微生物研究所第十研究室（柳田友道教授）
1965～1973年　名古屋大学医学部第一生化学教室（八木國夫教授）
1973～1994年　東京田辺製薬株式会社研究開発本部（薬理研究室、分析・製剤研究室、安全性研究室、情報管理室、各室長）
1975～1978年　名古屋大学医学部第一生化学教室非常勤講師（生化学）
1996～1999年　厚生省「医薬品の範囲に関する研究」研究班
1999～2000年　厚生省「医薬品の範囲基準の見直しに関する検討会」委員
1998～2005年　NNFAジャパン代表、科学・法務担当ディレクター
2002～2013年　国際サプリメント業界団体連合会（IADSA）科学者会議委員（アジア地区代表）
2003～2004年　厚生労働省「健康食品に係る制度のあり方に関する検討会」委員
2006～2010年　厚生労働科学特別研究事業（主任研究者田中平三）「いわゆる健康食品」等の安全性確保方策に関する研究（分担研究者）

【主な所属学会・団体】

日本生化学会、日本生物物理学会、日本ビタミン学会、日本基礎老化学会、日本酸化ストレス学会、ゲーテ自然科学の集い、生命の起源および進化学会、（財）飯島藤十郎記念食品科学振興財団（監事）、日本臨床栄養協会（理事・情報部長）、日本臨床栄養学会（評議員）、日本健康科学学会（理事）、日本食品化学会（評議員）、日本食品安全協会（理事）、日本公衆衛生学会、日本歴史学会、日仏美術史学会

Hirobumi OHAMA, Ph.D.

Former Chairman of the Board, The Japanese Institute for Health Food Standards / Former President, Biohealth Research Ltd.

1963-1965　Researcher, Research Laboratory of Applied Microbiology, Tokyo University
1965-1973　Researcher, Department of Biochemistry, Faculty of Medicine, Nagoya University
1973-1994　Assistant Director of Research Laboratories, Tokyo Tanabe Co., Ltd.
1996-2000　Committee of the MHLW's Study Group for Deregulation of Health Foods
2002-2013　Member of Scientific Council of the International Alliance of Dietary / Food Supplement Associations (IADSA)
2006-2011　Member of the Science Council of Japan

■ **池田　秀子**（いけだ　ひでこ／Hideko Ikeda）薬剤師、臨床検査技師

【現職】一般社団法人日本健康食品規格協会理事長／バイオヘルスリサーチリミテッド取締役社長

1974年３月　北里大学薬学部薬学科卒業
1974年４月　東京田辺製薬株式会社入社（研究開発本部開発部、探索研究所）
1999～2003年　株式会社ソフィアテック東京田辺取締役
2003～現在　有限会社バイオヘルスリサーチリミテッド設立取締役
2002～2005年　NNFAジャパン科学情報担当ディレクター
2003～現在　国際サプリメント業界団体連合会（IADSA）科学者会議委員
2005～現在　一般社団法人日本健康食品規格協会（JIHFS）副理事長（現理事長）
2010～2013年　文教大学健康栄養学部非常勤講師
2006～2010年　厚生労働科学特別研究事業（主任研究者田中平三）「いわゆる健康食品」等の安全性確保方策に関する研究研究協力者
2010～2011年　厚生労働科学研究「食品の安心・安全確保推進研究事業」（主任研究員梅垣敬三）「健康食品の評価に関する研究」（分担研究員信川益明）研究協力者
2011年～現在　ISO/TC249（国際標準化機構Traditional Chinese Medicine（Provisional）専門委員会）国内委員

【主な所属学会・団体】

日本薬剤師会、公益財団法人生存科学研究所、日本臨床栄養協会（理事・情報部副部長）、日本臨床栄養学会、日本健康科学学会（評議員）、日本食品化学学会、日本公衆衛生学会、日本食品安全協会（理事）、ゲーテ自然科学の集い、日本歴史学会、日仏美術史学会

Hideko IKEDA

Chairman of the Board, The Japanese Institute for Health Food Standards / President, Biohealth Research Ltd.

1974-1993　Chief Researcher, Research Laboratories, Tokyo Tanabe Co., Ltd.
1993-1998　Director of Science and Technology, Nature's Sunshine K.K.
1999-2003　Executive Vice President, Sophiatech Tokyo Tanabe, Inc.
2003-2013　Vice President, Biohealth Research Ltd.
2003-　Member of Scientific Council of the International Alliance of Dietary / Food Supplement Associations (IADSA)

Health Food Ingredients and Scientific Names －Drug and Food Classification in Japan－
Edited by Motoyoshi Satake, Setsuko Sekita, Hirobumi Ohama, Hideko Ikeda
Published by YAKUJI NIPPO, LTD.

ISBN978-4-8408-1276-4
Cover design by Miwa Ohama
Typeset and printed in Japan by SHOWA JOHO PROCESS Co,. Ltd.

学名でひく食薬区分リスト－健康食品・医薬品に区分される成分－

2014年9月24日　第1刷発行

監　修　佐竹元吉

著　者　関田節子　大濱宏文　池田秀子

編集企画　一般財団法人医療経済研究・社会保険福祉協会
「健康食品の安全性及び品質確保のための研究会」

発　行　株式会社薬事日報社　http://www.yakuji.co.jp/
東京都千代田区神田和泉町1番地　電話03-3862-2141

表　紙　大濱美和

印　刷　昭和情報プロセス株式会社

ISBN978-4-8408-1276-4